Library of Congress Cataloging in Publication Data

Heuser, Robert L
Fertility tables for birth cohorts by color.

(DHEW publication; no. (HRA) 76-1152)
Includes bibliographical references.
1. United States–Statistics, Vital. 2. Fertility, Human. I. United States. Division of Vital Statistics. II. Title. III. Series: United States. Dept. of Health, Education, and Welfare. DHEW publication; no. (HRA) 76-1152. [DNLM: 1. Fertility–Statistics. 2. Vital statistics–United States. HB915 H595f]
HB915.H48 312'.1'73 75-619342
ISBN O-8406-0059-3

Fertility Tables for Birth Cohorts by Color:

United States, 1917-73

DHEW Publication No. (HRA) 76-1152

U.S. DEPARTMENT OF HEALTH, EDUCATION, AND WELFARE
PUBLIC HEALTH SERVICE
Health Resources Administration
National Center for Health Statistics
Rockville, Maryland
April 1976

For sale by the Superintendent of Documents, U.S. Government Printing Office
Washington, D.C. 20402 - Price $8.80

Stock Number 017-022-00490-9

CONTENTS

FERTILITY TABLES FOR BIRTH COHORTS BY COLOR

Robert L. Heuser, *Division of Vital Statistics*

INTRODUCTION

The tables in this volume present fertility data for actual groups or cohorts of women as they pass through their childbearing years of 14 through 49. The tables contain data for calendar years 1917-73. The data will be updated annually in *Vital Statistics of the United States,* Volume I, Natality, beginning with the 1974 data year. These data have been prepared as a revision and extension of the cohort fertility rates developed by Pascal K. Whelpton and Arthur A. Campbell.[1] The set of rates in this volume utilizes revised population estimates prepared by the U.S. Bureau of the Census for this purpose, and has been extended to include data for the two major color groups, white and all other,[2] as well as for all women.

This work has been done in collaboration with Arthur A. Campbell,[3] who provided invaluable assistance in developing the methods and gave advice at all stages of the project. A detailed description of the methods used in estimating the basic data, the births and populations, is included in appendixes I and II.

The cohort approach[4] refers to the study of the fertility of the same women at successive ages, the cumulative effect of this fertility at successive ages, and the completed family size of these women. A cohort consists initially of female babies born during a 12-month period centered on January 1; subsequently it consists of the survivors of these babies. A cohort is identified by the year of the date on which the births are centered. For example, women born from July 1, 1923, to June 30, 1924, centering on January 1, 1924, constitute the cohort of 1924. Since these women retain this designation throughout their childbearing years, there is a fixed relationship between the cohort identification year, the age of the member of the cohort, and the calendar year to which the fertility measure refers, and by knowing any two of these factors the third can be derived. This relationship is: cohort identification year plus age equals calendar year of the fertility measure.

Four cohort measures are shown in this volume. The central birth rates are similar to the age-specific birth rates computed annually for many geographic areas. Cumulative birth rates, the sum of central birth rates for specified cohorts, show the number of children ever born up to the indicated age. The cumulative rate at age 50, assumed to be the end of childbearing, is considered to be the completed fertility rate. The parity distribution shows a proportional distribution of all women in the cohort by parity (the number of children they have borne alive). Birth probabilities show the probability that a woman of a given age and parity will have a child in the next year. The computations of these rates are described in appendix III.

In addition to these cohort measures total fertility rates for each calendar year are shown. The total fertility rate shows the implications for completed family size of a given set of central birth rates. It states the number of births a hypothetical cohort of 1,000 women would have *if* they experienced the central birth rates of a given calendar year throughout their reproductive ages. It is the sum of the central birth rates for each single year of age in a given calendar year, and is age-adjusted in that it is based on the assumption that there are the same number of women (1,000) at each year of age.

The central birth rates have been computed using numbers of births adjusted for underregistration for all years and numbers of women adjusted for underenumeration for all censuses and for misstatement of age in all censuses except that of 1970. An additional adjustment was made so that the number of women more adequately represented the population of cohorts in calendar years as described in appendix I. These rates differ somewhat from the age-specific birth rates shown in volumes of *Vital Statistics of the United States,* for which the numbers of births have been adjusted for underregistration only through 1959 and the annual population estimates were used without the adjustments for cohorts or for underenumeration.

The data presented in this volume are intended to represent a general model of fertility trends over time and the numbers should not be taken as precise values. Small differences and fluctuations may not represent real changes because of the estimation required to obtain the births and female populations for all years and the cumulative birth rates for 1917. Comparisons of these rates with the earlier cohort rates for all women prepared by Whelpton and Campbell have been made and they appear to be reasonable. A comparison between the methods used by Whelpton and Campbell and those used for this volume is presented in appendix IV.

---

[1] National Office of Vital Statistics: Fertility tables for birth cohorts of American women, by P.K. Whelpton and A.A. Campbell. *Vital Statistics—Special Reports,* Vol. 51, No. 1. Public Health Service. Washington, D.C., Jan. 29, 1960.

[2] As used in this report, the term "all other" refers to the combined grouping of all races other than white.

[3] Deputy Director, Center for Population Research, National Institute for Child Health and Human Development, National Institutes of Health.

[4] For further discussion of the cohort approach to fertility analysis, see *Cohort Fertility,* by P.K. Whelpton, Princeton, Princeton University Press, 1954, and Chapter 13, "Cohort Fertility," in *Trends and Variations in Fertility in the United States,* by C.V. Kiser, W.H. Grabill, and A.A. Campbell, Cambridge, Harvard University Press, 1968.

LIST OF DETAILED TABLES

In each case, table A is for all women, and color is shown in separate tables designated B and C for white women and all other women, respectively.

TABLE 1A. TOTAL FERTILITY RATES FOR ALL WOMEN BY LIVE-BIRTH ORDER FOR EACH YEAR 1917-73

CALENDAR YEAR	TOTAL	LIVE-BIRTH ORDER							
		1	2	3	4	5	6	7	8 AND HIGHER
1917	3,333.3	850.4	656.1	488.9	359.6	271.1	213.2	157.5	336.5
1918	3,312.2	859.4	647.1	486.1	356.6	266.1	209.7	153.5	333.7
1919	3,067.7	699.7	626.2	463.8	344.9	257.4	199.9	149.7	326.1
1920	3,263.3	895.7	625.5	467.3	346.0	257.4	197.3	146.7	327.4
1921	3,326.2	927.7	627.5	472.7	352.3	260.7	201.7	149.3	334.3
1922	3,109.4	828.4	645.0	438.0	323.3	240.5	185.7	138.8	309.7
1923	3,101.2	809.1	652.3	446.1	320.9	240.7	185.1	138.0	309.0
1924	3,120.7	842.2	636.8	460.8	319.0	236.3	182.7	135.7	307.2
1925	3,011.6	817.9	613.3	442.7	311.9	224.2	172.7	129.4	299.5
1926	2,900.7	787.8	598.9	422.0	303.8	214.5	166.0	124.1	283.6
1927	2,824.3	776.6	579.2	407.9	293.9	210.6	160.2	119.5	276.4
1928	2,659.8	744.0	550.5	384.9	272.5	197.8	148.1	109.5	252.5
1929	2,532.0	719.8	533.5	364.8	254.3	186.8	138.0	100.8	234.0
1930	2,532.5	744.2	533.0	359.5	251.0	182.3	136.4	99.1	227.0
1931	2,401.7	706.1	512.8	341.6	237.3	169.9	128.5	93.3	212.2
1932	2,318.6	678.3	497.5	330.5	228.3	163.8	124.6	91.3	204.3
1933	2,172.0	635.2	468.9	312.3	216.4	152.8	114.4	84.1	187.9
1934	2,232.0	683.9	480.5	314.4	216.7	152.8	113.4	82.3	188.0
1935	2,188.7	710.8	468.0	299.0	204.1	143.2	105.8	78.4	179.4
1936	2,145.6	715.6	474.5	288.7	193.7	134.9	99.5	72.4	166.3
1937	2,173.3	749.7	489.9	288.7	188.6	130.9	95.3	69.6	160.6
1938	2,221.7	783.9	514.4	295.2	186.6	127.0	92.4	67.8	154.4
1939	2,171.7	770.0	518.0	292.5	180.2	120.3	86.7	62.2	141.8
1940	2,229.0	786.4	548.3	306.9	183.5	119.4	84.5	60.7	139.3
1941	2,331.5	869.6	572.1	314.5	184.7	118.1	82.0	58.3	132.2
1942	2,554.8	1,015.2	634.1	334.3	190.1	118.2	80.6	56.1	126.2
1943	2,640.2	944.4	707.0	379.7	210.7	127.8	84.6	58.2	127.8
1944	2,494.5	826.8	661.9	389.2	217.2	129.7	85.9	57.8	126.0
1945	2,421.8	794.8	640.8	378.7	213.7	128.9	83.8	57.5	123.6
1946	2,857.9	1,060.8	777.2	410.2	223.4	130.1	83.2	55.5	117.5
1947	3,181.2	1,299.0	841.2	437.5	225.1	128.8	81.4	54.3	113.9
1948	3,026.2	1,116.2	862.3	451.6	226.8	127.6	79.7	52.7	109.3
1949	3,036.2	1,034.5	899.6	481.7	243.1	131.6	81.5	53.3	110.9
1950	3,028.0	968.1	904.8	517.0	259.3	136.8	82.4	53.1	106.5
1951	3,199.1	1,027.0	926.4	562.5	288.2	148.1	86.4	54.2	106.3
1952	3,286.5	1,015.0	937.9	601.3	316.7	163.3	90.9	55.4	106.0
1953	3,349.4	1,004.5	946.3	623.7	339.2	176.4	97.2	58.1	104.0
1954	3,461.2	1,018.4	954.5	655.3	365.3	192.2	106.2	62.0	107.3
1955	3,498.3	1,002.6	950.0	671.5	382.4	204.2	113.7	65.1	108.8
1956	3,604.7	1,024.0	960.6	694.7	402.9	216.4	121.8	70.5	113.8
1957	3,682.4	1,028.0	964.2	713.6	422.7	230.2	129.8	75.1	118.8
1958	3,628.9	979.7	941.7	706.9	431.1	237.3	133.5	77.6	121.1
1959	3,638.2	952.3	927.1	712.0	445.6	248.5	142.3	82.8	127.6
1960	3,605.7	923.1	900.7	709.0	452.0	256.2	147.0	86.0	131.7
1961	3,563.9	901.5	866.3	696.5	455.4	264.4	152.8	89.6	137.4
1962	3,423.3	860.9	822.5	662.2	438.5	260.3	151.8	88.4	138.7
1963	3,297.8	841.0	786.6	625.1	418.9	252.4	147.7	88.1	138.0
1964	3,170.9	839.4	747.9	587.8	394.6	238.0	142.6	85.1	135.5
1965	2,881.6	801.9	685.6	517.7	344.3	208.8	125.9	75.2	122.2
1966	2,670.4	814.5	646.4	456.2	294.9	178.6	108.2	65.1	106.5
1967	2,525.5	793.4	637.7	425.7	266.1	157.4	94.6	57.6	93.0
1968	2,431.0	817.2	624.7	398.2	240.2	138.2	82.4	49.5	80.6
1969	2,422.9	820.3	638.7	400.7	234.1	133.5	77.4	44.9	73.3
1970	2,431.7	847.0	652.3	401.5	226.2	125.8	71.0	41.4	66.5
1971	2,245.4	793.6	620.6	364.9	200.9	110.4	62.2	35.6	57.2
1972	1,993.6	736.5	575.0	307.9	164.0	87.9	49.5	28.2	44.6
1973	1,862.5	707.5	559.8	281.3	140.6	73.1	40.2	23.2	36.8

TABLE 1B. TOTAL FERTILITY RATES FOR WHITE WOMEN BY LIVE-BIRTH ORDER FOR EACH YEAR 1917-73

CALENDAR YEAR	TOTAL	LIVE-BIRTH ORDER							
		1	2	3	4	5	6	7	8 AND HIGHER
1917	3,312.3	847.3	666.2	495.4	362.3	272.1	208.7	151.9	308.4
1918	3,288.2	855.9	659.8	488.4	359.1	268.1	204.1	149.1	303.7
1919	3,024.8	684.1	635.5	466.1	345.4	256.6	195.3	143.8	298.0
1920	3,219.0	887.1	629.7	466.5	344.7	256.4	192.8	143.0	298.8
1921	3,281.6	928.3	629.8	470.1	349.5	258.4	196.0	143.8	305.7
1922	3,071.6	832.1	649.3	435.5	320.0	237.5	180.1	133.6	283.5
1923	3,062.5	809.3	662.4	441.8	317.3	237.3	179.2	132.0	283.2
1924	3,069.3	840.3	645.7	455.2	312.2	231.0	174.9	129.2	280.8
1925	2,949.3	811.5	621.9	441.0	303.2	217.9	164.2	121.5	268.1
1926	2,838.8	784.5	605.9	421.0	295.3	207.2	156.8	115.8	252.3
1927	2,783.0	780.1	589.5	408.7	289.2	203.4	152.8	111.9	247.4
1928	2,632.4	750.7	564.1	387.2	267.9	191.5	140.6	103.3	227.1
1929	2,505.8	726.7	546.1	367.1	250.9	179.6	131.2	94.7	209.5
1930	2,505.5	751.4	545.2	362.2	247.4	175.9	129.6	92.4	201.4
1931	2,368.7	711.3	523.4	342.6	232.2	164.0	120.9	86.3	188.0
1932	2,270.7	678.4	505.1	329.1	222.9	156.9	116.6	83.3	178.4
1933	2,126.1	637.4	476.2	310.3	210.2	145.4	106.9	76.8	162.9
1934	2,181.4	687.0	488.0	312.0	209.8	144.2	104.9	75.0	160.5
1935	2,140.8	716.1	473.3	295.6	196.9	135.3	97.9	71.2	154.5
1936	2,100.9	723.4	480.5	285.7	186.1	126.0	91.3	65.4	142.5
1937	2,121.1	757.7	495.0	283.2	180.0	120.6	87.0	62.0	135.6
1938	2,174.7	794.5	521.7	289.8	176.9	118.1	83.9	60.1	129.7
1939	2,120.0	780.3	525.0	286.5	170.0	109.9	77.3	54.1	116.9
1940	2,177.0	800.3	556.9	299.9	172.0	108.5	74.8	52.0	112.6
1941	2,281.4	890.1	580.5	306.5	173.1	106.1	71.3	48.8	105.0
1942	2,525.5	1,049.4	648.1	328.1	178.0	105.9	69.5	47.3	99.2
1943	2,611.3	969.0	727.1	377.7	199.8	115.9	73.3	49.0	99.5
1944	2,451.7	842.3	679.1	387.3	205.6	117.3	73.9	48.5	97.7
1945	2,375.2	808.0	657.2	378.6	202.4	115.1	72.3	47.5	94.1
1946	2,843.1	1,098.0	800.7	410.1	212.1	116.9	71.3	45.3	88.7
1947	3,167.4	1,342.7	863.7	435.6	212.7	115.3	68.9	43.5	85.0
1948	2,968.2	1,137.3	874.7	443.8	211.8	112.7	66.6	41.8	79.5
1949	2,964.3	1,049.6	912.5	470.9	226.0	114.8	67.5	42.1	80.9
1950	2,945.4	979.0	918.8	505.2	239.6	118.2	67.0	41.4	76.2
1951	3,119.9	1,044.8	944.1	551.5	265.7	127.7	69.9	41.6	74.6
1952	3,212.6	1,034.5	959.7	595.0	294.1	140.8	73.1	41.9	73.5
1953	3,269.0	1,020.5	968.7	620.2	316.6	151.6	77.0	43.1	71.3
1954	3,372.0	1,031.0	976.6	653.2	343.4	165.6	84.4	45.8	72.0
1955	3,404.5	1,015.6	967.3	671.2	361.8	178.0	90.8	48.1	71.7
1956	3,504.3	1,036.9	976.9	694.7	382.6	190.2	97.1	51.8	74.1
1957	3,582.3	1,042.6	981.9	713.7	404.9	203.2	104.2	55.3	76.5
1958	3,532.3	994.7	959.0	707.6	414.2	212.1	109.1	58.1	77.5
1959	3,536.7	964.1	944.2	714.8	429.8	223.2	117.0	61.8	81.8
1960	3,510.2	933.9	918.0	714.1	439.0	232.7	122.3	65.4	84.8
1961	3,463.7	910.4	881.9	701.7	442.3	242.0	127.9	68.9	88.6
1962	3,320.1	866.6	834.2	666.0	427.4	238.7	128.4	68.6	90.2
1963	3,194.2	843.1	795.5	628.9	408.1	231.9	127.1	68.9	90.7
1964	3,061.3	838.8	752.6	588.8	384.1	219.7	122.0	66.9	88.4
1965	2,764.4	793.5	684.9	514.2	332.7	191.9	107.7	59.0	80.5
1966	2,562.7	804.7	644.3	451.3	283.5	163.5	92.2	52.2	71.0
1967	2,425.0	778.3	634.9	420.8	256.6	145.0	81.2	45.7	62.5
1968	2,341.1	799.0	623.1	394.0	231.5	127.3	71.4	39.9	54.9
1969	2,336.5	799.5	635.6	396.6	225.9	123.4	67.5	37.2	50.8
1970	2,337.8	824.5	645.3	394.9	216.7	115.6	61.6	33.5	45.7
1971	2,143.6	766.5	610.4	354.3	190.7	100.4	53.7	28.5	39.1
1972	1,894.3	704.2	563.5	296.9	154.1	78.9	42.3	23.0	31.4
1973	1,767.5	676.5	548.9	268.2	129.9	65.1	34.2	18.7	26.0

TABLE 1C. TOTAL FERTILITY RATES FOR ALL OTHER WOMEN BY LIVE-BIRTH ORDER FOR EACH YEAR 1917-73

CALENDAR YEAR	TOTAL	LIVE-BIRTH ORDER							
		1	2	3	4	5	6	7	8 AND HIGHER
1917------------------	3,451.1	843.8	564.1	429.0	332.2	257.0	241.3	201.4	582.3
1918------------------	3,475.0	852.0	535.4	454.3	334.0	248.2	257.2	193.2	600.7
1919------------------	3,343.5	779.6	538.3	431.5	332.0	259.6	232.7	195.7	574.1
1920------------------	3,556.3	922.4	572.2	458.1	350.9	260.2	232.3	179.2	581.0
1921------------------	3,615.0	893.0	591.0	475.2	365.0	272.3	243.9	190.7	583.9
1922------------------	3,354.3	780.2	590.5	442.0	338.8	258.1	227.2	182.7	534.8
1923------------------	3,331.9	781.3	558.2	454.9	338.1	258.2	227.1	183.8	530.3
1924------------------	3,454.4	830.6	550.8	484.7	359.1	271.7	237.8	188.4	531.3
1925------------------	3,416.6	839.0	533.3	439.5	363.4	262.1	230.7	186.5	562.1
1926------------------	3,324.0	797.8	529.9	414.1	356.6	263.4	231.4	186.3	544.5
1927------------------	3,100.7	745.9	486.5	390.8	318.3	257.9	210.5	175.4	515.4
1928------------------	2,829.4	688.3	440.2	355.9	290.9	238.3	196.2	155.0	464.6
1929------------------	2,716.2	667.0	435.5	337.3	274.6	231.2	188.4	145.6	436.6
1930------------------	2,734.4	692.5	438.1	334.4	270.9	227.5	187.0	148.5	435.5
1931------------------	2,641.3	667.6	430.0	323.8	264.9	212.2	182.4	146.2	414.2
1932------------------	2,667.6	677.3	438.4	329.5	264.9	211.5	182.5	144.2	419.3
1933------------------	2,522.9	624.9	417.1	320.6	256.6	205.6	169.9	137.7	390.5
1934------------------	2,605.3	667.7	426.8	328.1	262.2	208.4	170.4	137.2	404.5
1935------------------	2,547.7	675.2	431.1	319.9	257.5	201.1	160.6	128.1	374.2
1936------------------	2,483.0	654.1	436.5	314.3	250.0	195.4	155.8	122.5	354.4
1937------------------	2,563.0	686.8	456.1	329.4	252.3	198.7	157.4	124.8	357.5
1938------------------	2,583.8	698.7	459.3	339.9	257.2	196.9	157.9	125.8	348.1
1939------------------	2,564.0	688.9	467.4	340.1	258.2	196.1	157.1	121.5	334.7
1940------------------	2,617.7	675.7	478.6	357.2	273.1	206.0	159.7	124.9	342.5
1941------------------	2,689.8	704.2	503.8	367.9	275.1	212.0	162.4	125.6	338.8
1942------------------	2,744.0	738.0	517.5	376.8	281.4	213.2	162.7	123.3	331.1
1943------------------	2,837.1	742.5	545.3	390.4	294.7	222.1	170.2	129.0	342.9
1944------------------	2,787.4	694.8	519.5	394.6	301.8	226.9	176.6	132.1	341.1
1945------------------	2,733.3	682.1	500.2	371.6	292.9	227.9	175.5	134.3	348.8
1946------------------	2,937.2	767.1	583.7	406.7	304.9	228.0	174.3	133.8	338.7
1947------------------	3,247.4	957.3	656.9	440.9	312.7	230.7	176.5	134.8	337.6
1948------------------	3,402.3	936.4	745.1	494.0	333.8	240.7	180.1	137.2	335.0
1949------------------	3,509.3	901.3	782.1	542.0	361.8	253.6	188.4	140.2	339.9
1950------------------	3,578.9	870.0	775.8	586.2	395.5	270.4	194.9	144.1	342.0
1951------------------	3,718.4	881.6	772.9	619.0	440.1	293.2	209.7	150.4	351.5
1952------------------	3,760.3	863.7	757.9	620.6	468.8	319.3	221.8	155.3	352.9
1953------------------	3,879.7	885.7	767.3	625.7	486.0	347.9	239.6	166.6	360.9
1954------------------	4,052.6	926.0	785.5	640.4	505.7	373.0	261.4	180.5	380.1
1955------------------	4,125.9	911.8	811.6	652.1	512.1	383.2	275.6	188.5	391.0
1956------------------	4,286.2	932.5	838.3	674.3	526.3	396.6	293.1	208.6	416.5
1957------------------	4,346.5	927.0	838.3	693.4	531.1	407.6	302.6	213.7	432.8
1958------------------	4,284.6	882.2	820.7	683.9	533.8	403.9	301.4	217.0	441.7
1959------------------	4,320.5	878.3	808.6	681.8	542.3	413.2	309.2	227.9	459.2
1960------------------	4,238.0	858.9	786.3	667.5	529.0	402.6	305.3	225.9	462.5
1961------------------	4,233.8	849.5	769.8	658.2	535.5	405.0	311.7	226.3	477.8
1962------------------	4,107.8	829.4	747.7	635.1	510.1	397.1	301.7	217.1	469.6
1963------------------	4,000.1	837.0	735.7	606.5	485.9	380.9	283.1	212.4	458.6
1964------------------	3,900.0	847.2	719.3	585.1	460.2	356.3	276.2	203.7	452.0
1965------------------	3,657.2	854.0	693.0	542.0	422.0	320.9	243.1	181.7	400.5
1966------------------	3,391.1	872.9	667.3	497.0	369.3	278.4	209.4	151.4	345.4
1967------------------	3,178.4	878.4	654.3	460.4	331.8	242.0	182.3	134.0	295.2
1968------------------	2,996.0	914.9	630.6	425.9	298.6	209.4	155.6	112.0	249.0
1969------------------	2,961.0	936.3	649.1	427.2	291.1	201.7	139.6	98.8	217.2
1970------------------	2,998.4	970.2	682.5	441.4	290.1	194.6	133.1	91.3	195.2
1971------------------	2,860.1	942.5	674.0	426.5	267.8	175.7	118.6	82.5	172.5
1972------------------	2,582.6	917.1	629.3	374.7	228.2	145.0	95.3	62.4	130.6
1973------------------	2,405.5	878.1	614.2	355.4	202.9	122.4	77.9	51.3	103.3

TABLE 2A. CENTRAL BIRTH RATES FOR ALL WOMEN DURING 5-YEAR PERIODS 1920-24 TO 1965-69 BY AGE AND LIVE-BIRTH ORDER FOR SELECTED GROUPS OF COHORTS

LIVE-BIRTH ORDER AND COHORT	DIAGONAL LINE FOR CURRENT AGE	CALENDAR YEARS										COMPLETED FERTILITY RATE
		1920-24	1925-29	1930-34	1935-39	1940-44	1945-49	1950-54	1955-59	1960-64	1965-69	
TOTAL BIRTHS												
TOTAL FERTILITY RATE----------		3,184.3	2,785.4	2,331.6	2,179.9	2,450.6	2,903.9	3,265.1	3,610.1	3,412.6	2,586.0	
1871-1875----	45-49 TO 50-54	10.5										3,773.5
1876-1880----	40-44 TO 45-49	97.3	8.0									3,531.9
1881-1885----	35-39 TO 40-44	331.3	81.6	6.1								3,321.6
1886-1890----	30-34 TO 35-39	535.1	279.8	63.5	4.8							3,136.8
1891-1895----	25-29 TO 30-34	734.6	457.3	218.9	48.6	3.0						2,932.6
1896-1900----	20-24 TO 25-29	843.6	635.3	373.4	178.4	40.8	2.4					2,675.9
1901-1905----	15-19 TO 20-24	560.3	749.7	533.9	323.8	167.8	42.1	1.8				2,441.4
1906-1910----	10-14 TO 15-19	71.6	505.8	635.8	491.3	350.9	190.7	38.3	1.4			2,285.8
1911-1915----			67.9	440.9	624.1	576.9	413.6	189.0	40.3	1.6		2,354.3
1916-1920----				59.1	444.6	737.9	664.9	428.2	199.6	38.6	1.1	2,574.0
1921-1925----					64.3	505.6	869.2	743.2	456.7	187.2	29.9	...
1926-1930----						67.7	626.2	1,004.9	794.4	428.0	139.4	...
1931-1935----							94.8	753.4	1,157.3	776.3	317.8	...
1936-1940----								106.3	849.6	1,117.7	577.8	...
1941-1945----									110.8	769.4	845.1	...
1946-1950----										93.8	590.5	...
1951-1955----											84.4	...
FIRST BIRTHS												
TOTAL FERTILITY RATE----------		860.5	769.3	689.7	745.8	888.5	1,061.0	1,006.6	997.3	873.2	809.4	
1871-1875----	45-49 TO 50-54	0.2										792.8
1876-1880----	40-44 TO 45-49	2.4	0.1									783.2
1881-1885----	35-39 TO 40-44	13.7	2.2	0.1								782.6
1886-1890----	30-34 TO 35-39	41.1	12.5	1.8	0.0							789.6
1891-1895----	25-29 TO 30-34	121.1	37.2	10.8	1.5	0.1						807.3
1896-1900----	20-24 TO 25-29	283.6	105.8	34.5	10.7	1.9	0.0					805.4
1901-1905----	15-19 TO 20-24	337.4	249.9	100.0	39.2	15.5	2.9	0.1				798.1
1906-1910----	10-14 TO 15-19	61.0	303.8	222.7	115.3	57.2	21.4	3.0	0.0			784.4
1911-1915----			57.8	269.0	246.5	151.5	65.0	17.5	2.5	0.1		809.9
1916-1920----				50.8	278.1	296.5	161.1	49.4	13.4	1.7	0.0	851.0
1921-1925----					54.5	310.4	349.0	128.5	37.6	9.7	1.4	...
1926-1930----						55.4	384.9	312.5	104.8	28.0	8.0	...
1931-1935----							76.4	411.4	312.3	82.6	23.6	...
1936-1940----								84.2	440.9	277.9	79.3	...
1941-1945----									85.8	399.8	270.3	...
1946-1950----										73.4	356.4	...
1951-1955----											70.4	...
SECOND BIRTHS												
TOTAL FERTILITY RATE----------		637.5	575.0	498.6	492.8	624.7	804.2	933.9	948.7	824.9	646.6	
1871-1875----	45-49 TO 50-54	0.2										680.0
1876-1880----	40-44 TO 45-49	3.3	0.2									660.0
1881-1885----	35-39 TO 40-44	20.3	2.9	0.1								648.0
1886-1890----	30-34 TO 35-39	62.8	18.6	2.4	0.0							641.1
1891-1895----	25-29 TO 30-34	150.5	57.9	16.1	2.0	0.0						635.3
1896-1900----	20-24 TO 25-29	240.4	136.6	51.9	15.2	2.5	0.0					604.7
1901-1905----	15-19 TO 20-24	150.7	214.4	119.8	53.0	20.7	3.9	0.1				570.5
1906-1910----	10-14 TO 15-19	9.3	135.5	184.2	119.2	75.5	31.5	4.0	0.1			559.3
1911-1915----			8.9	116.8	179.5	161.7	100.6	29.8	3.9	0.1		601.3
1916-1920----				7.3	115.3	222.2	203.4	95.0	25.8	3.0	0.0	672.0
1921-1925----					8.6	131.7	279.4	221.5	78.0	18.2	2.0	...
1926-1930----						10.4	169.7	340.1	191.1	55.7	12.5	...
1931-1935----							15.7	225.0	368.0	156.0	41.3	...
1936-1940----								18.4	261.1	341.6	132.0	...
1941-1945----									20.7	233.5	282.3	...
1946-1950----										16.8	164.5	...
1951-1955----											12.0	...

TABLE 2A. CENTRAL BIRTH RATES FOR ALL WOMEN DURING 5-YEAR PERIODS 1920-24 TO 1965-69 BY AGE AND LIVE-BIRTH ORDER FOR SELECTED GROUPS OF COHORTS--CON.

LIVE-BIRTH ORDER AND COHORT	DIAGONAL LINE FOR CURRENT AGE	CALENDAR YEARS										COMPLETED FERTILITY RATE
		1920-24	1925-29	1930-34	1935-39	1940-44	1945-49	1950-54	1955-59	1960-64	1965-69	
THIRD BIRTHS												
TOTAL FERTILITY RATE----------		457.1	404.3	331.8	292.6	345.1	431.7	592.0	699.7	656.2	439.7	
1871-1875----	45-49 TO 50-54	0.3										555.8
1876-1880----	40-44 TO 45-49	4.8	0.3									528.0
1881-1885----	35-39 TO 40-44	27.9	4.1	0.2								505.5
1886-1890----	30-34 TO 35-39	74.3	25.1	3.5	0.1							487.9
1891-1895----	25-29 TO 30-34	139.6	66.3	20.8	2.8	0.1						458.1
1896-1900----	20-24 TO 25-29	157.0	120.6	55.5	18.4	3.0	0.1					409.5
1901-1905----	15-19 TO 20-24	52.0	139.6	97.6	48.9	20.8	4.4	0.1				364.3
1906-1910----	10-14 TO 15-19	1.2	47.2	113.8	84.5	58.6	30.5	4.7	0.1			340.6
1911-1915----			1.1	39.5	99.9	101.0	82.3	33.7	5.6	0.1		363.2
1916-1920----				0.9	36.9	115.1	128.8	97.1	36.5	4.9	0.1	420.3
1921-1925----					1.1	44.8	131.9	175.5	104.3	29.7	3.3	...
1926-1930----						1.7	51.3	195.8	198.3	85.2	20.1	...
1931-1935----							2.4	81.9	249.3	188.3	61.3	...
1936-1940----								3.2	101.8	251.7	140.0	...
1941-1945----									3.8	93.2	162.9	...
1946-1950----										3.1	50.2	...
1951-1955----											1.8	...
FOURTH BIRTHS												
TOTAL FERTILITY RATE----------		332.4	287.2	229.9	190.7	197.4	226.1	314.0	416.9	431.9	275.9	
1871-1875----	45-49 TO 50-54	0.6										445.8
1876-1880----	40-44 TO 45-49	6.3	0.3									414.0
1881-1885----	35-39 TO 40-44	32.7	5.4	0.3								386.2
1886-1890----	30-34 TO 35-39	74.4	28.6	4.4	0.3							358.2
1891-1895----	25-29 TO 30-34	114.6	63.3	23.0	3.6	0.1						318.8
1896-1900----	20-24 TO 25-29	88.8	95.5	50.7	19.1	3.4	0.1					272.9
1901-1905----	15-19 TO 20-24	14.9	79.8	76.0	41.5	18.4	4.1	0.2				235.0
1906-1910----	10-14 TO 15-19	0.1	14.2	63.7	61.5	41.6	23.4	4.5	0.2			209.2
1911-1915----			0.1	11.7	54.0	62.3	51.9	27.6	5.6	0.2		213.4
1916-1920----				0.1	10.6	57.6	71.3	66.3	34.0	5.7	0.1	245.7
1921-1925----					0.1	13.8	60.2	98.7	84.4	32.2	4.2	...
1926-1930----						0.2	14.8	90.5	131.9	81.9	22.9	...
1931-1935----							0.3	25.7	127.1	144.6	59.9	...
1936-1940----								0.5	33.2	135.9	98.7	...
1941-1945----									0.5	30.9	75.4	...
1946-1950----										0.5	14.5	...
1951-1955----											0.2	...
FIFTH BIRTHS												
TOTAL FERTILITY RATE----------		247.1	206.7	164.2	131.4	122.7	129.5	163.3	227.3	254.3	163.2	
1871-1875----	45-49 TO 50-54	0.6										352.2
1876-1880----	40-44 TO 45-49	7.5	0.5									321.0
1881-1885----	35-39 TO 40-44	35.7	6.2	0.4								291.2
1886-1890----	30-34 TO 35-39	70.2	29.6	5.1	0.3							258.7
1891-1895----	25-29 TO 30-34	86.1	57.1	23.4	4.1	0.2						221.0
1896-1900----	20-24 TO 25-29	43.3	70.9	45.3	18.6	3.4	0.2					185.1
1901-1905----	15-19 TO 20-24	3.7	38.8	56.7	35.3	16.2	3.8	0.1				154.6
1906-1910----	10-14 TO 15-19	*	3.6	30.5	44.5	31.3	17.8	3.8	0.2			131.7
1911-1915----			*	2.8	26.0	40.8	33.9	19.7	4.8	0.2		128.2
1916-1920----				*	2.6	27.3	42.1	40.4	25.2	5.2	0.1	142.9
1921-1925----					*	3.5	27.8	53.1	54.9	26.8	4.0	...
1926-1930----						*	3.9	39.4	75.1	60.4	20.1	...
1931-1935----							*	6.8	58.1	89.3	45.1	...
1936-1940----								*	9.0	63.8	58.1	...
1941-1945----									*	8.6	32.3	...
1946-1950----										*	3.5	...
1951-1955----											*	...

TABLE 2A. CENTRAL BIRTH RATES FOR ALL WOMEN DURING 5-YEAR PERIODS 1920-24 TO 1965-69 BY AGE AND LIVE-BIRTH ORDER FOR SELECTED GROUPS OF COHORTS--CON.

LIVE-BIRTH ORDER AND COHORT	DIAGONAL LINE FOR CURRENT AGE	CALENDAR YEARS										COMPLETED FERTILITY RATE
		1920-24	1925-29	1930-34	1935-39	1940-44	1945-49	1950-54	1955-59	1960-64	1965-69	
SIXTH BIRTHS												
TOTAL FERTILITY RATE----------		190.5	157.0	123.6	95.8	83.6	81.9	92.6	128.1	148.4	97.8	
1871-1875----	45-49 TO 50-54	0.8										277.1
1876-1880----	40-44 TO 45-49	8.9	0.5									249.0
1881-1885----	35-39 TO 40-44	37.7	7.2	0.5								219.2
1886-1890----	30-34 TO 35-39	64.4	30.3	5.8	0.4							190.7
1891-1895----	25-29 TO 30-34	58.6	52.2	23.6	4.3	0.2						159.5
1896-1900----	20-24 TO 25-29	19.0	49.0	40.8	18.1	3.5	0.2					131.6
1901-1905----	15-19 TO 20-24	1.1	16.7	39.1	30.8	14.8	3.4	0.1				106.0
1906-1910----	10-14 TO 15-19	*	1.1	13.0	30.3	25.6	14.0	3.1	0.0			87.1
1911-1915----			*	0.6	11.2	26.7	24.7	14.5	3.9	0.1		81.9
1916-1920----				*	0.7	11.8	26.1	26.4	17.8	4.2	0.1	87.1
1921-1925----					*	1.0	12.4	30.3	35.0	20.0	3.4	...
1926-1930----						*	1.1	16.4	43.2	40.9	15.6	...
1931-1935----							*	1.8	25.6	52.7	31.0	...
1936-1940----								*	2.6	28.1	33.1	...
1941-1945----									*	2.4	13.6	...
1946-1950----										*	1.0	...
1951-1955----											*	...
SEVENTH BIRTHS												
TOTAL FERTILITY RATE----------		141.8	116.7	90.0	70.1	58.3	54.5	56.7	74.1	87.5	58.4	
1871-1875----	45-49 TO 50-54	0.9										210.7
1876-1880----	40-44 TO 45-49	9.7	0.7									184.5
1881-1885----	35-39 TO 40-44	37.4	7.8	0.5								161.3
1886-1890----	30-34 TO 35-39	52.8	29.9	6.0	0.5							135.3
1891-1895----	25-29 TO 30-34	33.4	43.1	22.6	4.4	0.3						111.2
1896-1900----	20-24 TO 25-29	7.2	28.6	33.1	17.2	3.5	0.2					90.1
1901-1905----	15-19 TO 20-24	0.4	6.3	22.7	25.4	13.3	3.1	0.1				71.3
1906-1910----	10-14 TO 15-19	*	0.3	4.9	17.9	20.3	11.8	2.7	0.0			57.9
1911-1915----			*	0.2	4.4	16.0	18.4	11.2	2.8	0.1		53.1
1916-1920----				*	0.3	4.6	15.6	18.5	12.9	3.1	0.1	55.1
1921-1925----					*	0.3	5.1	17.2	22.8	14.5	2.7	...
1926-1930----						*	0.3	6.5	24.3	27.5	11.4	...
1931-1935----							*	0.5	10.6	30.0	20.5	...
1936-1940----								*	0.7	11.6	18.1	...
1941-1945----									*	0.7	5.3	...
1946-1950----										*	0.3	...
1951-1955----											*	...
EIGHTH AND HIGHER BIRTHS												
TOTAL FERTILITY RATE----------		317.4	269.2	203.8	160.7	130.3	115.0	106.0	118.0	136.2	95.0	
1871-1875----	45-49 TO 50-54	6.9										459.1
1876-1880----	40-44 TO 45-49	54.4	5.4									392.2
1881-1885----	35-39 TO 40-44	125.9	45.8	4.0								327.6
1886-1890----	30-34 TO 35-39	95.1	105.2	34.5	3.2							275.3
1891-1895----	25-29 TO 30-34	30.7	80.2	78.6	25.9	2.0						221.4
1896-1900----	20-24 TO 25-29	4.3	28.3	61.6	61.1	19.6	1.6					176.6
1901-1905----	15-19 TO 20-24	0.1	4.2	22.0	49.7	48.1	16.5	1.0				141.6
1906-1910----	10-14 TO 15-19	*	0.1	3.0	18.1	40.8	40.3	12.5	0.8			115.6
1911-1915----			*	0.1	2.6	16.9	36.8	35.0	11.2	0.7		103.3
1916-1920----				*	0.1	2.8	16.5	35.1	34.0	10.8	0.6	99.9
1921-1925----					*	0.1	3.1	18.4	39.7	36.1	8.9	...
1926-1930----						*	0.2	3.7	25.7	48.4	28.8	...
1931-1935----							*	0.3	6.3	32.8	35.1	...
1936-1940----								*	0.3	7.1	18.5	...
1941-1945----									*	0.3	3.0	...
1946-1950----										*	0.1	...
1951-1955----											*	...

TABLE 2B. CENTRAL BIRTH RATES FOR WHITE WOMEN DURING 5-YEAR PERIODS 1920-24 TO 1965-69 BY AGE AND LIVE-BIRTH ORDER FOR SELECTED GROUPS OF COHORTS

LIVE-BIRTH ORDER AND COHORT	DIAGONAL LINE FOR CURRENT AGE	CALENDAR YEARS 1920-24	1925-29	1930-34	1935-39	1940-44	1945-49	1950-54	1955-59	1960-64	1965-69	COMPLETED FERTILITY RATE
TOTAL BIRTHS												
TOTAL FERTILITY RATE----------		3,140.7	2,741.7	2,290.1	2,132.2	2,408.8	2,864.0	3,183.7	3,512.0	3,309.6	2,486.3	
1871-1875----	45-49 TO 50-54	8.3										3,663.6
1876-1880----	40-44 TO 45-49	95.1	6.7									3,444.4
1881-1885----	35-39 TO 40-44	326.5	79.5	5.2								3,253.8
1886-1890----	30-34 TO 35-39	542.3	277.2	62.2	3.7							3,092.9
1891-1895----	25-29 TO 30-34	742.9	459.9	216.1	47.4	2.4						2,890.4
1896-1900----	20-24 TO 25-29	838.0	640.4	375.0	174.9	38.8	2.4					2,631.5
1901-1905----	15-19 TO 20-24	529.0	746.4	540.7	326.2	164.2	41.2	1.5				2,399.0
1906-1910----	10-14 TO 15-19	58.6	476.4	632.8	498.7	354.9	189.5	36.5	1.5			2,248.9
1911-1915----			55.2	410.9	618.7	587.9	417.6	183.5	38.4	1.3		2,313.5
1916-1920----				47.2	412.6	737.4	675.0	424.5	192.9	36.3	0.8	2,526.7
1921-1925----					50.0	472.1	872.6	743.4	448.0	178.9	28.1	...
1926-1930----						51.1	590.3	995.7	785.3	414.7	132.1	...
1931-1935----							75.4	712.9	1,145.6	765.5	307.7	...
1936-1940----								85.7	808.2	1,105.9	570.6	...
1941-1945----									92.1	731.0	837.5	...
1946-1950----										76.0	545.7	...
1951-1955----											63.8	...
FIRST BIRTHS												
TOTAL FERTILITY RATE----------		859.3	770.9	693.0	754.3	910.3	1,087.1	1,022.0	1,010.9	878.4	795.0	
1871-1875----	45-49 TO 50-54	0.1										790.3
1876-1880----	40-44 TO 45-49	2.4	0.1									781.8
1881-1885----	35-39 TO 40-44	13.9	2.2	0.1								782.4
1886-1890----	30-34 TO 35-39	43.4	12.9	1.8	0.0							790.9
1891-1895----	25-29 TO 30-34	128.1	39.3	11.3	1.6	0.1						808.3
1896-1900----	20-24 TO 25-29	295.8	113.6	37.0	11.2	2.1	0.1					806.9
1901-1905----	15-19 TO 20-24	325.4	263.0	108.5	42.7	16.6	3.3	0.1				802.1
1906-1910----	10-14 TO 15-19	50.2	292.5	234.9	126.0	62.4	23.0	3.1	0.0			792.1
1911-1915----			47.3	258.3	261.5	165.1	69.6	18.2	2.6	0.0		822.6
1916-1920----				41.1	268.3	316.1	172.8	51.5	13.8	1.8	0.0	865.4
1921-1925----					43.0	304.5	372.2	135.9	38.9	9.9	1.4	...
1926-1930----						43.4	382.7	331.6	110.4	28.8	8.1	...
1931-1935----							63.4	411.2	330.2	86.3	24.0	...
1936-1940----								70.4	441.3	292.2	82.1	...
1941-1945----									73.7	397.8	280.8	...
1946-1950----										61.6	343.5	...
1951-1955----											55.1	...
SECOND BIRTHS												
TOTAL FERTILITY RATE----------		643.4	585.4	507.6	499.3	638.3	821.8	953.5	965.9	836.5	644.4	
1871-1875----	45-49 TO 50-54	0.1										678.2
1876-1880----	40-44 TO 45-49	3.3	0.1									659.9
1881-1885----	35-39 TO 40-44	20.9	3.0	0.1								650.2
1886-1890----	30-34 TO 35-39	66.5	19.6	2.6	0.1							646.6
1891-1895----	25-29 TO 30-34	158.4	61.9	17.1	2.0	0.1						640.8
1896-1900----	20-24 TO 25-29	244.8	146.0	56.1	16.5	2.5	0.1					614.8
1901-1905----	15-19 TO 20-24	141.9	220.3	129.2	57.9	22.4	4.2	0.1				582.6
1906-1910----	10-14 TO 15-19	7.5	127.4	189.2	129.0	82.5	34.2	4.2	0.1			574.1
1911-1915----			7.1	107.7	183.0	175.1	109.0	31.6	4.1	0.1		617.7
1916-1920----				5.6	104.5	229.5	218.6	101.3	26.9	3.1	0.0	689.5
1921-1925----					6.3	119.4	289.8	236.7	82.2	18.7	2.0	...
1926-1930----						6.8	155.2	354.3	203.5	58.0	12.6	...
1931-1935----							10.7	211.9	384.3	165.1	42.5	...
1936-1940----								13.4	248.9	356.5	138.1	...
1941-1945----									15.9	222.6	291.4	...
1946-1950----										12.4	150.0	...
1951-1955----											7.8	...

TABLE 2B. CENTRAL BIRTH RATES FOR WHITE WOMEN DURING 5-YEAR PERIODS 1920-24 TO 1965-69 BY AGE AND LIVE-BIRTH ORDER FOR SELECTED GROUPS OF COHORTS--CON.

LIVE-BIRTH ORDER AND COHORT	DIAGONAL LINE FOR CURRENT AGE	CALENDAR YEARS										COMPLETED FERTILITY RATE
		1920-24	1925-29	1930-34	1935-39	1940-44	1945-49	1950-54	1955-59	1960-64	1965-69	
THIRD BIRTHS												
TOTAL FERTILITY RATE----------		453.8	404.9	331.2	288.4	339.7	427.9	584.9	700.4	659.9	435.4	
1871-1875----	45-49 TO 50-54	0.2										550.3
1876-1880----	40-44 TO 45-49	4.9	0.2									523.8
1881-1885----	35-39 TO 40-44	28.6	4.4	0.1								502.3
1886-1890----	30-34 TO 35-39	78.0	26.3	3.7	0.1							486.3
1891-1895----	25-29 TO 30-34	143.7	70.1	21.9	3.0	0.1						456.2
1896-1900----	20-24 TO 25-29	152.0	125.3	59.2	19.7	3.1	0.1					408.9
1901-1905----	15-19 TO 20-24	45.6	136.4	102.1	52.4	22.2	4.8	0.1				364.3
1906-1910----	10-14 TO 15-19	0.8	41.5	110.2	87.9	62.6	32.9	4.9	0.1			340.9
1911-1915----			0.7	33.5	94.6	105.2	88.0	35.6	5.9	0.1		363.6
1916-1920----				0.5	30.0	109.8	134.3	102.6	38.5	5.1	0.0	420.8
1921-1925----					0.7	35.9	126.5	182.8	110.2	31.0	3.5	...
1926-1930----						0.8	40.1	189.7	208.4	89.8	20.8	...
1931-1935----							1.2	67.5	247.7	199.0	63.9	...
1936-1940----								1.7	87.3	252.3	146.3	...
1941-1945----									2.3	80.8	160.3	...
1946-1950----										1.8	39.8	...
1951-1955----											0.8	...
FOURTH BIRTHS												
TOTAL FERTILITY RATE----------		328.8	281.2	224.5	182.0	185.7	213.2	291.9	398.4	420.1	266.3	
1871-1875----	45-49 TO 50-54	0.4										437.4
1876-1880----	40-44 TO 45-49	6.5	0.3									406.9
1881-1885----	35-39 TO 40-44	33.6	5.4	0.3								379.9
1886-1890----	30-34 TO 35-39	77.4	29.8	4.6	0.2							353.9
1891-1895----	25-29 TO 30-34	115.7	65.6	24.0	3.9	0.1						314.8
1896-1900----	20-24 TO 25-29	82.9	95.2	52.9	19.9	3.5	0.2					267.5
1901-1905----	15-19 TO 20-24	12.2	73.4	76.0	43.1	19.3	4.4	0.1				228.5
1906-1910----	10-14 TO 15-19	0.1	11.4	57.8	60.4	43.0	24.6	4.6	0.2			202.1
1911-1915----			0.1	8.9	46.9	60.7	53.6	28.5	5.8	0.2		204.7
1916-1920----				0.0	7.6	49.4	69.6	67.9	35.3	5.8	0.1	235.7
1921-1925----					0.0	9.6	51.2	96.1	87.2	33.3	4.4	...
1926-1930----						0.1	9.5	76.9	131.6	85.2	23.6	...
1931-1935----							0.1	17.6	114.2	147.2	62.0	...
1936-1940----								0.2	23.9	125.3	99.2	...
1941-1945----									0.2	22.9	67.2	...
1946-1950----										0.2	9.7	...
1951-1955----											0.1	...
FIFTH BIRTHS												
TOTAL FERTILITY RATE----------		244.2	199.9	157.2	122.1	110.5	115.0	140.8	201.5	232.9	150.3	
1871-1875----	45-49 TO 50-54	0.5										341.9
1876-1880----	40-44 TO 45-49	7.6	0.5									312.1
1881-1885----	35-39 TO 40-44	36.6	6.3	0.3								283.9
1886-1890----	30-34 TO 35-39	72.4	30.5	5.2	0.2							253.7
1891-1895----	25-29 TO 30-34	85.5	58.2	24.0	4.2	0.1						216.8
1896-1900----	20-24 TO 25-29	38.8	68.4	45.9	19.0	3.5	0.2					178.5
1901-1905----	15-19 TO 20-24	2.8	33.4	54.1	35.4	16.5	3.9	0.1				146.2
1906-1910----	10-14 TO 15-19	*	2.6	25.8	41.2	30.9	17.9	3.9	0.2			122.5
1911-1915----			*	1.9	20.4	36.8	32.9	19.6	4.9	0.2		116.7
1916-1920----				*	1.7	20.6	37.5	38.8	25.3	5.2	0.1	129.2
1921-1925----					*	2.1	20.5	46.3	53.6	27.2	4.1	...
1926-1930----						*	2.1	28.3	67.6	59.9	20.3	...
1931-1935----							*	3.8	44.5	83.9	44.9	...
1936-1940----								*	5.4	51.1	54.0	...
1941-1945----									*	5.4	24.9	...
1946-1950----										*	2.0	...
1951-1955----											*	...

TABLE 2B. CENTRAL BIRTH RATES FOR WHITE WOMEN DURING 5-YEAR PERIODS 1920-24 TO 1965-69 BY AGE AND LIVE-BIRTH ORDER FOR SELECTED GROUPS OF COHORTS--CON.

LIVE-BIRTH ORDER AND COHORT	DIAGONAL LINE FOR CURRENT AGE	CALENDAR YEARS										COMPLETED FERTILITY RATE
		1920-24	1925-29	1930-34	1935-39	1940-44	1945-49	1950-54	1955-59	1960-64	1965-69	
SIXTH BIRTHS												
TOTAL FERTILITY RATE----------		184.5	149.2	115.6	87.6	72.5	69.4	74.4	103.5	125.5	84.0	
1871-1875----	45-49 TO 50-54	0.6										264.7
1876-1880----	40-44 TO 45-49	9.0	0.5									238.1
1881-1885----	35-39 TO 40-44	37.9	7.2	0.4								209.7
1886-1890----	30-34 TO 35-39	65.0	30.6	5.8	0.3							183.4
1891-1895----	25-29 TO 30-34	55.8	51.8	23.7	4.4	0.2						152.6
1896-1900----	20-24 TO 25-29	15.5	45.3	40.0	18.1	3.5	0.2					123.3
1901-1905----	15-19 TO 20-24	0.7	13.1	35.3	29.8	14.4	3.4	0.1				96.8
1906-1910----	10-14 TO 15-19	*	0.7	9.9	26.5	23.9	13.7	3.0	0.1			77.8
1911-1915----			*	0.5	8.1	22.1	22.4	13.8	3.6	0.1		70.6
1916-1920----				*	0.4	7.9	21.1	23.4	17.0	4.0	0.1	73.9
1921-1925----					*	0.5	8.0	23.4	31.5	19.2	3.3	...
1926-1930----						*	0.6	9.9	33.8	38.1	15.0	...
1931-1935----							*	0.8	16.3	44.0	29.0	...
1936-1940----								*	1.2	18.9	27.4	...
1941-1945----									*	1.2	8.7	...
1946-1950----										*	0.5	...
1951-1955----											*	...
SEVENTH BIRTHS												
TOTAL FERTILITY RATE----------		136.4	109.3	82.8	62.5	49.1	44.0	42.6	55.1	67.8	46.9	
1871-1875----	45-49 TO 50-54	0.7										198.0
1876-1880----	40-44 TO 45-49	9.8	0.5									173.9
1881-1885----	35-39 TO 40-44	37.4	7.7	0.5								151.9
1886-1890----	30-34 TO 35-39	52.4	29.7	6.0	0.3							128.6
1891-1895----	25-29 TO 30-34	30.4	41.8	22.4	4.5	0.2						104.8
1896-1900----	20-24 TO 25-29	5.4	25.0	31.3	16.7	3.4	0.2					82.2
1901-1905----	15-19 TO 20-24	0.3	4.4	19.2	23.5	12.6	3.1	0.0				63.1
1906-1910----	10-14 TO 15-19	*	0.2	3.3	14.7	18.0	11.0	2.5	0.1			49.8
1911-1915----			*	0.1	2.7	12.1	15.6	9.9	2.7	0.1		43.2
1916-1920----				*	0.1	2.7	11.1	15.1	11.5	3.0	0.1	43.6
1921-1925----					*	0.1	2.9	11.7	18.6	13.2	2.6	...
1926-1930----						*	0.1	3.3	16.3	23.1	10.5	...
1931-1935----							*	0.1	5.7	21.7	17.6	...
1936-1940----								*	0.2	6.5	13.1	...
1941-1945----									*	0.2	2.9	...
1946-1950----										*	0.1	...
1951-1955----											*	...
EIGHTH AND HIGHER BIRTHS												
TOTAL FERTILITY RATE----------		290.3	240.9	178.2	136.0	102.7	85.6	73.6	76.3	88.5	64.0	
1871-1875----	45-49 TO 50-54	5.7										402.8
1876-1880----	40-44 TO 45-49	51.6	4.5									347.9
1881-1885----	35-39 TO 40-44	117.6	43.3	3.4								293.5
1886-1890----	30-34 TO 35-39	87.2	97.8	32.5	2.5							249.5
1891-1895----	25-29 TO 30-34	25.3	71.2	71.7	23.8	1.5						196.1
1896-1900----	20-24 TO 25-29	2.8	21.6	52.6	53.8	17.2	1.3					149.4
1901-1905----	15-19 TO 20-24	0.1	2.4	16.3	41.4	40.2	14.1	0.9				115.4
1906-1910----	10-14 TO 15-19	*	0.1	1.7	13.0	31.6	32.2	10.3	0.7			89.6
1911-1915----			*	0.0	1.5	10.8	26.5	26.3	8.8	0.5		74.4
1916-1920----				*	0.0	1.4	10.0	23.9	24.6	8.3	0.4	68.6
1921-1925----					*	0.0	1.5	10.5	25.8	26.4	6.8	...
1926-1930----						*	0.0	1.7	13.7	31.8	21.2	...
1931-1935----							*	0.0	2.7	18.3	23.8	...
1936-1940----								*	0.0	3.1	10.4	...
1941-1945----									*	0.1	1.3	...
1946-1950----										*	0.1	...
1951-1955----											*	...

TABLE 2C. CENTRAL BIRTH RATES FOR ALL OTHER WOMEN DURING 5-YEAR PERIODS 1920-24 TO 1965-69 BY AGE AND LIVE-BIRTH ORDER FOR SELECTED GROUPS OF COHORTS

LIVE-BIRTH ORDER AND COHORT	DIAGONAL LINE FOR CURRENT AGE	CALENDAR YEARS										COMPLETED FERTILITY RATE
		1920-24	1925-29	1930-34	1935-39	1940-44	1945-49	1950-54	1955-59	1960-64	1965-69	
TOTAL BIRTHS												
TOTAL FERTILITY RATE----------		3,462.5	3,077.3	2,634.6	2,548.0	2,735.2	3,166.0	3,797.9	4,272.7	4,095.5	3,236.9	
1871-1875----	45-49 TO 50-54	27.5										4,770.8
1876-1880----	40-44 TO 45-49	117.1	19.7									4,254.7
1881-1885----	35-39 TO 40-44	376.3	102.7	16.0								3,865.0
1886-1890----	30-34 TO 35-39	480.6	298.0	74.6	12.4							3,451.4
1891-1895----	25-29 TO 30-34	667.1	435.7	241.7	62.7	8.2						3,212.5
1896-1900----	20-24 TO 25-29	881.6	593.6	361.2	208.0	54.9	6.8					2,967.7
1901-1905----	15-19 TO 20-24	758.0	768.2	483.6	309.0	193.9	52.0	4.2				2,706.7
1906-1910----	10-14 TO 15-19	154.3	703.7	656.4	437.9	319.3	204.3	49.6	3.6			2,529.1
1911-1915----			155.7	655.3	664.5	493.4	381.9	231.7	55.5	3.2		2,641.2
1916-1920----				145.8	684.5	739.5	585.2	455.1	256.4	55.1	2.6	2,924.2
1921-1925----					169.0	743.0	843.2	740.4	524.5	248.3	45.7	...
1926-1930----						183.0	872.8	1,069.5	857.5	514.6	190.8	...
1931-1935----							219.8	1,010.5	1,229.4	845.2	384.5	...
1936-1940----								236.9	1,112.7	1,194.0	626.3	...
1941-1945----									233.1	1,021.5	896.4	...
1946-1950----										213.6	882.0	...
1951-1955----											208.6	...
FIRST BIRTHS												
TOTAL FERTILITY RATE----------		841.4	747.6	666.1	680.7	711.2	848.8	885.3	906.4	844.3	891.4	
1871-1875----	45-49 TO 50-54	0.7										814.3
1876-1880----	40-44 TO 45-49	2.6	0.6									792.3
1881-1885----	35-39 TO 40-44	11.7	2.1	0.4								776.9
1886-1890----	30-34 TO 35-39	23.8	8.7	1.4	0.3							768.1
1891-1895----	25-29 TO 30-34	65.9	18.6	6.1	1.2	0.2						777.7
1896-1900----	20-24 TO 25-29	195.9	48.5	14.9	5.3	1.0	0.2					772.6
1901-1905----	15-19 TO 20-24	410.9	160.1	39.3	13.4	6.3	1.5	0.1				749.6
1906-1910----	10-14 TO 15-19	129.9	378.8	136.1	37.5	18.5	9.8	1.9	0.0			712.5
1911-1915----			130.2	345.9	135.4	49.2	28.9	12.2	2.0	0.1		703.9
1916-1920----				122.0	349.8	147.5	69.2	32.6	11.0	1.6	0.1	733.8
1921-1925----					137.8	349.7	182.2	74.5	28.5	8.3	1.2	...
1926-1930----						138.8	397.0	180.9	65.7	22.2	7.1	...
1931-1935----							160.0	411.4	196.5	59.3	20.5	...
1936-1940----								171.7	437.1	186.3	61.8	...
1941-1945----									165.6	413.6	201.0	...
1946-1950----										152.9	437.2	...
1951-1955----											162.5	...
SECOND BIRTHS												
TOTAL FERTILITY RATE----------		572.5	485.1	430.3	449.9	513.1	653.6	771.8	823.6	751.7	658.9	
1871-1875----	45-49 TO 50-54	0.6										696.1
1876-1880----	40-44 TO 45-49	3.1	0.6									658.3
1881-1885----	35-39 TO 40-44	15.1	2.2	0.3								625.4
1886-1890----	30-34 TO 35-39	32.8	9.4	1.3	0.3							592.2
1891-1895----	25-29 TO 30-34	87.3	24.8	7.1	1.1	0.1						571.0
1896-1900----	20-24 TO 25-29	207.1	65.3	18.9	6.4	1.2	0.1					517.6
1901-1905----	15-19 TO 20-24	206.0	171.8	51.5	17.8	7.9	1.7	0.1				473.7
1906-1910----	10-14 TO 15-19	20.5	189.5	149.4	49.4	23.0	11.7	2.3	0.1			445.9
1911-1915----			21.5	181.8	153.0	60.8	36.0	15.7	2.7	0.0		471.5
1916-1920----				20.0	195.9	165.8	85.2	46.1	16.6	2.1	0.1	531.8
1921-1925----					26.0	218.7	202.1	109.1	47.0	13.9	2.0	...
1926-1930----						35.6	268.7	240.0	105.2	39.5	11.2	...
1931-1935----							48.1	307.8	261.7	97.6	34.6	...
1936-1940----								50.7	338.3	246.2	92.5	...
1941-1945----									52.0	305.6	222.5	...
1946-1950----										46.8	258.4	...
1951-1955----											37.6	...

TABLE 2C. CENTRAL BIRTH RATES FOR ALL OTHER WOMEN DURING 5-YEAR PERIODS 1920-24 TO 1965-69 BY AGE AND LIVE-BIRTH ORDER FOR SELECTED GROUPS OF COHORTS--CON.

LIVE-BIRTH ORDER AND COHORT	DIAGONAL LINE FOR CURRENT AGE	CALENDAR YEARS										COMPLETED FERTILITY RATE
		1920-24	1925-29	1930-34	1935-39	1940-44	1945-49	1950-54	1955-59	1960-64	1965-69	
THIRD BIRTHS												
TOTAL FERTILITY RATE----------		463.0	387.4	327.3	328.7	377.4	450.9	618.5	677.0	630.4	470.5	
1871-1875----	45-49 TO 50-54	0.9										602.5
1876-1880----	40-44 TO 45-49	4.1	0.7									558.8
1881-1885----	35-39 TO 40-44	21.1	3.1	0.4								525.6
1886-1890----	30-34 TO 35-39	43.4	14.3	1.9	0.3							486.3
1891-1895----	25-29 TO 30-34	106.4	35.5	10.0	1.5	0.2						458.6
1896-1900----	20-24 TO 25-29	190.6	84.4	25.9	9.2	1.4	0.3					403.5
1901-1905----	15-19 TO 20-24	93.1	160.1	64.9	23.5	9.6	2.0	0.1				355.9
1906-1910----	10-14 TO 15-19	3.4	85.8	138.7	60.0	27.1	13.5	2.7	0.2			331.4
1911-1915----			3.5	82.2	140.4	68.4	38.5	18.9	3.2	0.1		355.2
1916-1920----				3.3	89.3	154.5	86.0	53.4	21.1	3.2	0.1	410.9
1921-1925----					4.5	108.8	170.0	120.9	60.0	19.9	2.9	...
1926-1930----						7.4	130.5	236.2	126.8	52.9	15.8	...
1931-1935----							10.1	174.1	257.0	120.7	44.2	...
1936-1940----								12.2	195.7	247.2	99.5	...
1941-1945----									13.0	174.7	181.5	...
1946-1950----										11.7	119.2	...
1951-1955----											7.3	...
FOURTH BIRTHS												
TOTAL FERTILITY RATE----------		350.4	320.7	264.0	255.1	285.0	321.4	459.0	529.1	504.1	342.6	
1871-1875----	45-49 TO 50-54	1.1										520.5
1876-1880----	40-44 TO 45-49	5.1	0.8									471.4
1881-1885----	35-39 TO 40-44	25.3	4.5	0.6								429.1
1886-1890----	30-34 TO 35-39	49.5	18.5	2.9	0.5							389.7
1891-1895----	25-29 TO 30-34	105.7	43.8	14.1	2.2	0.3						344.1
1896-1900----	20-24 TO 25-29	130.5	96.6	33.2	12.0	2.1	0.3					306.0
1901-1905----	15-19 TO 20-24	32.7	122.8	75.3	29.2	11.9	2.6	0.1				274.9
1906-1910----	10-14 TO 15-19	0.5	33.2	105.9	69.3	31.0	15.1	3.0	0.2			258.2
1911-1915----			0.5	31.5	107.3	73.8	39.7	20.2	3.8	0.1		276.9
1916-1920----				0.5	33.9	119.8	84.2	53.4	23.8	4.0	0.1	319.7
1921-1925----					0.7	44.9	125.7	116.8	63.6	23.6	3.5	...
1926-1930----						1.2	52.2	184.6	133.0	59.1	17.9	...
1931-1935----							1.6	78.6	209.4	128.1	46.7	...
1936-1940----								2.3	92.8	203.9	95.5	...
1941-1945----									2.5	83.1	130.3	...
1946-1950----										2.2	47.4	...
1951-1955----											1.2	...
FIFTH BIRTHS												
TOTAL FERTILITY RATE----------		264.0	250.7	212.9	197.5	216.2	236.2	320.7	400.9	388.3	250.4	
1871-1875----	45-49 TO 50-54	1.3										444.1
1876-1880----	40-44 TO 45-49	6.1	0.9									391.5
1881-1885----	35-39 TO 40-44	28.0	5.2	0.8								343.8
1886-1890----	30-34 TO 35-39	52.8	22.0	3.8	0.6							296.4
1891-1895----	25-29 TO 30-34	90.1	48.6	18.2	2.9	0.4						251.5
1896-1900----	20-24 TO 25-29	76.0	88.2	40.8	15.1	2.8	0.3					231.7
1901-1905----	15-19 TO 20-24	9.7	75.3	75.1	34.7	14.7	2.9	0.2				212.6
1906-1910----	10-14 TO 15-19	*	10.5	64.9	67.8	35.3	16.3	3.1	0.2			198.1
1911-1915----			*	9.3	66.1	71.7	40.9	20.3	4.2	0.3		212.8
1916-1920----				*	10.3	77.1	78.3	51.7	25.2	4.4	0.2	247.2
1921-1925----					*	14.2	81.1	101.5	64.8	24.3	3.8	...
1926-1930----						*	16.4	117.5	127.4	61.3	18.9	...
1931-1935----							*	26.4	146.3	123.4	46.8	...
1936-1940----								*	32.8	145.1	84.8	...
1941-1945----									*	29.5	82.0	...
1946-1950----										*	13.9	...
1951-1955----											*	...

TABLE 2C. CENTRAL BIRTH RATES FOR ALL OTHER WOMEN DURING 5-YEAR PERIODS 1920-24 TO 1965-69 BY AGE AND LIVE-BIRTH ORDER FOR SELECTED GROUPS OF COHORTS--CON.

LIVE-BIRTH ORDER AND COHORT	DIAGONAL LINE FOR CURRENT AGE	CALENDAR YEARS										COMPLETED FERTILITY RATE
		1920-24	1925-29	1930-34	1935-39	1940-44	1945-49	1950-54	1955-59	1960-64	1965-69	
SIXTH BIRTHS												
TOTAL FERTILITY RATE----------		233.7	211.4	178.4	157.7	166.2	179.0	225.7	296.3	295.5	185.9	
1871-1875----	45-49 TO 50-54	1.4										388.0
1876-1880----	40-44 TO 45-49	7.8	1.2									336.8
1881-1885----	35-39 TO 40-44	35.6	6.9	1.0								302.3
1886-1890----	30-34 TO 35-39	60.3	27.1	4.9	0.8							244.0
1891-1895----	25-29 TO 30-34	80.4	54.7	22.8	3.6	0.4						211.1
1896-1900----	20-24 TO 25-29	44.5	76.1	47.1	18.4	3.3	0.5					192.9
1901-1905----	15-19 TO 20-24	3.7	41.6	65.3	38.6	16.7	3.4	0.3				169.6
1906-1910----	10-14 TO 15-19	*	3.8	34.2	57.8	37.5	17.5	3.5	0.3			154.6
1911-1915----			*	3.1	35.0	62.1	41.5	20.4	4.4	0.2		166.7
1916-1920----				*	3.5	41.5	65.8	49.2	24.7	4.6	0.1	189.4
1921-1925----					*	4.7	44.9	81.3	61.4	24.7	4.0	...
1926-1930----						*	5.4	62.4	108.7	60.0	19.2	...
1931-1935----							*	8.6	85.5	107.9	43.5	...
1936-1940----								*	11.3	87.6	70.0	...
1941-1945----									*	10.5	44.9	...
1946-1950----										*	4.2	...
1951-1955----											*	...
SEVENTH BIRTHS												
TOTAL FERTILITY RATE----------		185.2	169.6	142.9	124.5	126.9	136.1	159.3	211.2	217.2	135.6	
1871-1875----	45-49 TO 50-54	2.0										322.7
1876-1880----	40-44 TO 45-49	9.0	1.4									272.0
1881-1885----	35-39 TO 40-44	38.0	7.5	1.1								238.2
1886-1890----	30-34 TO 35-39	56.8	30.4	5.9	0.9							186.0
1891-1895----	25-29 TO 30-34	57.2	53.7	24.6	4.6	0.6						162.7
1896-1900----	20-24 TO 25-29	21.0	55.6	47.1	21.2	3.8	0.5					150.3
1901-1905----	15-19 TO 20-24	1.2	19.7	47.9	39.1	18.6	3.7	0.3				130.5
1906-1910----	10-14 TO 15-19	*	1.3	15.4	41.6	37.9	18.8	3.7	0.3			119.0
1911-1915----			*	0.9	15.9	45.4	40.6	20.5	4.2	0.3		127.8
1916-1920----				*	1.2	19.2	49.3	45.1	24.9	4.7	0.1	144.5
1921-1925----					*	1.4	21.5	58.4	55.1	24.3	4.0	...
1926-1930----						*	1.7	28.8	80.6	56.7	18.7	...
1931-1935----							*	2.5	42.8	83.0	39.6	...
1936-1940----								*	3.3	45.0	51.2	...
1941-1945----									*	3.2	20.8	...
1946-1950----										*	1.2	...
1951-1955----											*	...
EIGHTH AND HIGHER BIRTHS												
TOTAL FERTILITY RATE----------		552.3	504.8	412.7	353.9	339.2	340.0	357.6	428.2	464.0	301.6	
1871-1875----	45-49 TO 50-54	19.5										982.6
1876-1880----	40-44 TO 45-49	79.3	13.5									773.6
1881-1885----	35-39 TO 40-44	201.5	71.2	11.4								623.7
1886-1890----	30-34 TO 35-39	161.2	167.6	52.5	8.7							488.7
1891-1895----	25-29 TO 30-34	74.1	156.0	138.8	45.6	6.0						435.8
1896-1900----	20-24 TO 25-29	16.0	78.9	133.3	120.4	39.3	4.6					393.1
1901-1905----	15-19 TO 20-24	0.7	16.8	64.3	112.7	108.2	34.2	3.0				339.9
1906-1910----	10-14 TO 15-19	*	0.8	11.8	54.5	109.0	101.6	29.4	2.3			309.4
1911-1915----			*	0.6	11.4	62.0	115.8	103.5	31.0	2.1		326.4
1916-1920----				*	0.6	14.1	67.2	123.6	109.1	30.5	1.8	346.9
1921-1925----					*	0.6	15.7	77.9	144.1	109.3	24.3	...
1926-1930----						*	0.9	19.1	110.1	162.9	82.0	...
1931-1935----							*	1.1	30.2	125.2	108.6	...
1936-1940----								*	1.4	32.7	71.0	...
1941-1945----									*	1.3	13.4	...
1946-1950----										*	0.5	...
1951-1955----											*	...

TABLE 3A. CENTRAL BIRTH RATES FOR ALL WOMEN DURING EACH YEAR 1917-73 BY AGE AND LIVE-BIRTH ORDER FOR GROUPS OF COHORTS FROM 1868-72 TO 1954-58

(RATES ARE SIMPLE AVERAGES OF THE RATES FOR SINGLE COHORTS IN TABLE 4A)

CURRENT AGE AND COHORT	CALENDAR YEAR	TOTAL	LIVE-BIRTH ORDER							
			1	2	3	4	5	6	7	8 AND HIGHER
15-19 YEARS										
1898-1902----------	1917	60.3	45.7	12.1	2.2	0.3	*	*	*	*
1899-1903----------	1918	59.1	44.7	11.8	2.3	0.3	*	*	*	*
1900-1904----------	1919	51.7	38.1	11.2	2.1	0.3	*	*	*	*
1901-1905----------	1920	62.6	49.0	11.2	2.1	0.3	*	*	*	*
1902-1906----------	1921	67.1	52.2	12.3	2.3	0.3	*	*	*	*
1903-1907----------	1922	61.5	46.1	12.9	2.1	0.4	*	*	*	*
1904-1908----------	1923	61.7	45.7	13.2	2.4	0.4	*	*	*	*
1905-1909----------	1924	64.0	48.6	12.6	2.4	0.4	*	*	*	*
1906-1910----------	1925	62.5	47.5	12.3	2.3	0.4	*	*	*	*
1907-1911----------	1926	61.2	46.0	12.5	2.3	0.4	*	*	*	*
1908-1912----------	1927	60.5	45.4	12.4	2.3	0.4	*	*	*	*
1909-1913----------	1928	57.6	43.2	11.7	2.3	0.4	*	*	*	*
1910-1914----------	1929	55.4	41.6	11.3	2.1	0.4	*	*	*	*
1911-1915----------	1930	56.7	43.0	11.2	2.1	0.4	*	*	*	*
1912-1916----------	1931	53.2	40.2	10.7	2.0	0.3	*	*	*	*
1913-1917----------	1932	51.4	38.8	10.4	1.9	0.3	*	*	*	*
1914-1918----------	1933	47.7	36.0	9.6	1.8	0.3	*	*	*	*
1915-1919----------	1934	50.1	38.5	9.5	1.8	0.3	*	*	*	*
1916-1920----------	1935	50.8	39.4	9.4	1.7	0.3	*	*	*	*
1917-1921----------	1936	50.1	38.3	9.8	1.7	0.3	*	*	*	*
1918-1922----------	1937	52.3	40.0	10.2	1.8	0.3	*	*	*	*
1919-1923----------	1938	54.1	41.4	10.5	1.9	0.3	*	*	*	*
1920-1924----------	1939	52.3	39.3	10.7	2.0	0.3	*	*	*	*
1921-1925----------	1940	53.4	38.8	11.7	2.5	0.4	*	*	*	*
1922-1926----------	1941	56.0	41.3	11.8	2.5	0.4	*	*	*	*
1923-1927----------	1942	60.2	45.1	12.0	2.6	0.5	*	*	*	*
1924-1928----------	1943	60.4	44.5	12.7	2.7	0.5	*	*	*	*
1925-1929----------	1944	53.7	39.1	11.4	2.7	0.5	*	*	*	*
1926-1930----------	1945	50.5	37.4	10.3	2.3	0.5	*	*	*	*
1927-1931----------	1946	58.5	44.0	11.6	2.4	0.5	*	*	*	*
1928-1932----------	1947	77.2	60.7	13.4	2.6	0.5	*	*	*	*
1929-1933----------	1948	79.4	59.3	16.5	3.1	0.5	*	*	*	*
1930-1934----------	1949	80.3	57.0	18.8	3.8	0.7	*	*	*	*
1931-1935----------	1950	79.4	55.3	19.2	4.2	0.7	*	*	*	*
1932-1936----------	1951	85.4	60.0	19.9	4.6	0.9	*	*	*	*
1933-1937----------	1952	85.1	59.0	20.3	4.9	0.9	*	*	*	*
1934-1938----------	1953	87.8	60.8	21.0	5.0	1.0	*	*	*	*
1935-1939----------	1954	90.0	62.4	21.3	5.2	1.1	*	*	*	*
1936-1940----------	1955	90.4	61.8	22.2	5.3	1.1	*	*	*	*
1937-1941----------	1956	95.0	65.0	23.3	5.6	1.1	*	*	*	*
1938-1942----------	1957	97.3	66.4	23.8	5.9	1.2	*	*	*	*
1939-1943----------	1958	95.0	63.7	24.2	5.9	1.2	*	*	*	*
1940-1944----------	1959	94.1	62.4	24.2	6.3	1.2	*	*	*	*
1941-1945----------	1960	91.0	60.2	23.4	6.1	1.3	*	*	*	*
1942-1946----------	1961	88.7	59.3	22.3	5.9	1.2	*	*	*	*
1943-1947----------	1962	85.2	56.8	21.6	5.6	1.2	*	*	*	*
1944-1948----------	1963	82.2	55.6	20.3	5.2	1.1	*	*	*	*
1945-1949----------	1964	78.4	53.9	18.7	4.8	1.0	*	*	*	*
1946-1950----------	1965	73.3	51.8	16.5	4.1	0.9	*	*	*	*
1947-1951----------	1966	70.9	51.8	15.0	3.4	0.7	*	*	*	*
1948-1952----------	1967	68.5	50.3	14.5	3.1	0.6	*	*	*	*
1949-1953----------	1968	67.0	50.5	13.3	2.7	0.5	*	*	*	*
1950-1954----------	1969	67.3	51.0	13.2	2.6	0.5	*	*	*	*
1951-1955----------	1970	69.7	53.5	13.3	2.5	0.4	*	*	*	*
1952-1956----------	1971	66.1	50.7	12.7	2.3	0.4	*	*	*	*
1953-1957----------	1972	63.0	49.1	11.6	2.0	0.3	*	*	*	*
1954-1958----------	1973	60.4	47.2	11.1	1.8	0.3	*	*	*	*

TABLE 3A. CENTRAL BIRTH RATES FOR ALL WOMEN DURING EACH YEAR 1917-73 BY AGE AND LIVE-BIRTH ORDER FOR GROUPS OF COHORTS FROM 1868-72 TO 1954-58--CON.

(RATES ARE SIMPLE AVERAGES OF THE RATES FOR SINGLE COHORTS IN TABLE 4A)

CURRENT AGE AND COHORT	CALENDAR YEAR	TOTAL	LIVE-BIRTH ORDER							
			1	2	3	4	5	6	7	8 AND HIGHER
20-24 YEARS										
1893-1897----------	1917	171.9	73.4	53.4	28.2	11.3	3.8	1.2	0.4	0.2
1894-1898----------	1918	171.2	73.9	52.3	28.2	11.4	3.6	1.2	0.4	0.2
1895-1899----------	1919	150.8	57.5	50.1	26.8	11.1	3.6	1.1	0.4	0.2
1896-1900----------	1920	168.7	76.0	49.3	26.7	11.2	3.7	1.2	0.4	0.2
1897-1901----------	1921	171.3	77.7	48.9	27.1	11.7	4.0	1.3	0.4	0.2
1898-1902----------	1922	160.6	68.4	51.2	24.7	10.8	3.7	1.2	0.4	0.2
1899-1903----------	1923	161.2	66.6	52.0	25.9	10.9	3.9	1.3	0.4	0.2
1900-1904----------	1924	164.7	69.8	50.6	27.5	11.0	3.9	1.3	0.4	0.2
1901-1905----------	1925	158.6	67.2	48.2	26.5	11.1	3.7	1.3	0.4	0.2
1902-1906----------	1926	154.4	64.9	47.3	25.1	11.2	3.9	1.3	0.4	0.3
1903-1907----------	1927	150.0	63.5	45.6	24.4	10.9	3.8	1.2	0.4	0.2
1904-1908----------	1928	142.3	60.7	43.1	23.1	10.0	3.6	1.2	0.4	0.2
1905-1909----------	1929	136.4	58.4	41.7	21.8	9.4	3.5	1.1	0.3	0.2
1906-1910----------	1930	136.8	60.1	41.2	21.4	9.3	3.3	1.0	0.3	0.2
1907-1911----------	1931	130.0	56.9	39.7	20.3	8.7	3.0	1.0	0.3	0.1
1908-1912----------	1932	125.8	54.7	38.7	19.7	8.4	2.9	0.9	0.3	0.2
1909-1913----------	1933	118.2	51.4	36.4	18.7	7.9	2.7	0.8	0.2	0.1
1910-1914----------	1934	123.3	55.7	36.9	18.7	8.0	2.8	0.8	0.3	0.1
1911-1915----------	1935	123.1	58.0	35.6	17.8	7.7	2.7	0.9	0.3	0.1
1912-1916----------	1936	122.9	58.3	36.3	17.1	7.4	2.6	0.8	0.3	0.1
1913-1917----------	1937	126.4	60.4	37.5	17.4	7.3	2.6	0.8	0.3	0.1
1914-1918----------	1938	129.9	62.2	38.8	17.9	7.2	2.6	0.8	0.3	0.1
1915-1919----------	1939	126.7	60.2	38.2	17.5	7.1	2.5	0.8	0.3	0.1
1916-1920----------	1940	131.1	61.2	39.4	18.5	7.8	2.8	0.9	0.3	0.2
1917-1921----------	1941	140.0	68.7	40.6	18.8	7.8	2.8	0.9	0.3	0.1
1918-1922----------	1942	157.7	82.2	44.0	19.3	8.0	2.9	0.9	0.3	0.1
1919-1923----------	1943	156.4	74.6	47.7	21.0	8.6	3.1	1.0	0.3	0.1
1920-1924----------	1944	143.9	66.7	43.0	20.7	8.8	3.2	1.1	0.3	0.1
1921-1925----------	1945	131.9	63.7	37.9	17.9	7.9	3.1	1.0	0.3	0.1
1922-1926----------	1946	172.7	88.7	51.6	19.7	8.2	3.0	1.0	0.3	0.2
1923-1927----------	1947	200.1	109.2	57.1	21.3	8.0	3.0	1.0	0.3	0.2
1924-1928----------	1948	191.1	91.9	62.4	23.7	8.5	3.1	1.0	0.3	0.2
1925-1929----------	1949	192.2	84.5	66.5	26.5	9.6	3.4	1.1	0.4	0.2
1926-1930----------	1950	190.0	78.3	66.6	29.3	10.5	3.6	1.1	0.4	0.2
1927-1931----------	1951	203.6	84.6	68.8	32.2	12.1	4.1	1.2	0.4	0.2
1928-1932----------	1952	208.8	84.7	70.3	33.7	13.4	4.7	1.4	0.4	0.2
1929-1933----------	1953	215.3	84.3	73.6	35.4	14.4	5.3	1.6	0.5	0.2
1930-1934----------	1954	225.4	87.1	76.1	38.1	15.5	5.8	1.9	0.6	0.3
1931-1935----------	1955	231.3	87.4	78.3	40.0	16.4	6.2	2.1	0.6	0.3
1932-1936----------	1956	241.8	90.1	81.5	42.7	17.6	6.6	2.3	0.7	0.3
1933-1937----------	1957	248.0	90.4	83.7	44.8	18.6	7.1	2.4	0.7	0.3
1934-1938----------	1958	245.8	86.8	83.4	45.5	19.2	7.3	2.5	0.8	0.3
1935-1939----------	1959	247.1	85.0	84.0	46.8	20.0	7.5	2.6	0.9	0.3
1936-1940----------	1960	246.1	83.4	82.7	47.7	20.5	7.8	2.7	0.9	0.4
1937-1941----------	1961	242.3	82.0	80.3	47.1	20.9	7.9	2.8	0.9	0.4
1938-1942----------	1962	233.2	78.7	76.8	45.5	20.2	8.0	2.7	0.9	0.4
1939-1943----------	1963	222.9	77.1	73.6	42.3	18.7	7.4	2.6	0.8	0.4
1940-1944----------	1964	211.4	76.6	69.4	38.5	16.8	6.7	2.3	0.7	0.4
1941-1945----------	1965	190.0	72.6	62.9	32.4	13.9	5.4	1.9	0.6	0.3
1942-1946----------	1966	178.9	74.6	58.9	27.6	11.2	4.3	1.6	0.5	0.2
1943-1947----------	1967	170.2	72.4	57.8	25.0	9.7	3.6	1.2	0.4	0.1
1944-1948----------	1968	163.6	73.1	55.3	22.6	8.3	2.9	1.0	0.3	0.1
1945-1949----------	1969	162.8	73.6	55.4	22.0	7.8	2.6	0.9	0.3	0.2
1946-1950----------	1970	163.1	74.9	55.8	21.6	7.2	2.4	0.7	0.3	0.2
1947-1951----------	1971	149.1	68.2	52.2	19.6	6.3	2.0	0.6	0.1	0.1
1948-1952----------	1972	128.8	59.7	46.1	16.0	5.0	1.5	0.4	0.1	0.0
1949-1953----------	1973	119.4	55.5	43.6	14.3	4.3	1.3	0.3	0.1	0.0

TABLE 3A. CENTRAL BIRTH RATES FOR ALL WOMEN DURING EACH YEAR 1917-73 BY AGE AND LIVE-BIRTH ORDER FOR GROUPS OF COHORTS FROM 1868-72 TO 1954-58--CON.

(RATES ARE SIMPLE AVERAGES OF THE RATES FOR SINGLE COHORTS IN TABLE 4A)

CURRENT AGE AND COHORT	CALENDAR YEAR	TOTAL	LIVE-BIRTH ORDER							
			1	2	3	4	5	6	7	8 AND HIGHER
25-29 YEARS										
1888-1892----------	1917	172.6	34.0	40.4	36.1	27.1	17.7	9.9	4.4	3.0
1889-1893----------	1918	171.2	35.2	40.1	35.7	26.9	17.1	9.4	4.1	2.7
1890-1894----------	1919	158.7	28.0	38.8	33.6	25.8	16.7	9.1	4.1	2.6
1891-1895----------	1920	167.2	35.9	38.9	33.9	26.0	16.7	9.1	4.0	2.7
1892-1896----------	1921	169.9	37.0	38.3	34.2	26.1	17.2	9.7	4.4	3.0
1893-1897----------	1922	159.0	33.4	39.1	31.3	23.9	15.6	8.8	4.1	2.8
1894-1898----------	1923	158.6	32.3	39.6	31.4	23.4	15.8	9.0	4.2	2.9
1895-1899----------	1924	158.2	32.7	38.6	32.2	23.1	15.4	9.0	4.2	3.0
1896-1900----------	1925	152.4	31.6	37.3	30.9	22.4	14.6	8.4	4.1	3.1
1897-1901----------	1926	146.7	30.4	35.8	29.2	21.9	14.0	8.4	4.0	3.0
1898-1902----------	1927	142.8	30.0	34.4	28.1	21.4	14.1	8.0	3.9	2.9
1899-1903----------	1928	135.0	29.2	32.8	26.3	19.7	13.2	7.5	3.6	2.7
1900-1904----------	1929	129.1	28.6	31.8	24.8	18.3	12.6	7.1	3.3	2.6
1901-1905----------	1930	128.6	29.7	32.0	24.4	17.9	12.1	6.9	3.2	2.4
1902-1906----------	1931	122.9	28.8	30.8	23.1	17.0	11.3	6.5	3.1	2.3
1903-1907----------	1932	118.2	27.4	29.7	22.5	16.4	10.8	6.3	3.0	2.1
1904-1908----------	1933	111.2	25.9	28.3	21.2	15.5	10.0	5.7	2.7	1.9
1905-1909----------	1934	114.5	27.9	29.2	21.5	15.5	10.1	5.7	2.6	2.0
1906-1910----------	1935	111.6	29.3	28.3	20.1	14.4	9.5	5.4	2.6	2.0
1907-1911----------	1936	110.3	30.4	28.4	19.4	13.7	9.0	5.2	2.4	1.8
1908-1912----------	1937	112.3	32.4	29.3	19.2	13.3	8.8	5.1	2.4	1.8
1909-1913----------	1938	116.1	34.6	31.1	19.7	13.2	8.5	4.9	2.4	1.7
1910-1914----------	1939	114.9	34.9	31.4	19.3	12.6	8.0	4.7	2.3	1.7
1911-1915----------	1940	119.7	36.7	33.3	20.1	12.7	8.0	4.7	2.4	1.8
1912-1916----------	1941	126.6	41.2	35.2	20.7	12.8	8.0	4.6	2.3	1.8
1913-1917----------	1942	140.7	49.1	40.3	22.1	13.0	7.8	4.5	2.2	1.7
1914-1918----------	1943	146.4	43.6	45.8	25.3	14.4	8.5	4.7	2.3	1.8
1915-1919----------	1944	136.0	36.1	42.4	25.6	14.5	8.5	4.8	2.3	1.8
1916-1920----------	1945	131.2	34.4	41.5	24.6	13.9	8.2	4.6	2.3	1.7
1917-1921----------	1946	159.1	49.8	50.4	26.9	14.8	8.4	4.7	2.3	1.8
1918-1922----------	1947	173.0	56.7	55.2	29.3	14.8	8.3	4.6	2.3	1.8
1919-1923----------	1948	161.9	45.1	54.1	30.3	15.0	8.4	4.7	2.4	1.9
1920-1924----------	1949	163.1	40.8	55.9	32.4	16.1	8.6	4.8	2.5	2.0
1921-1925----------	1950	164.4	37.3	56.5	34.9	17.4	8.9	4.9	2.5	2.0
1922-1926----------	1951	172.8	38.4	57.5	38.1	19.4	9.7	5.2	2.5	2.0
1923-1927----------	1952	178.9	37.5	57.8	41.2	21.3	10.8	5.5	2.7	2.1
1924-1928----------	1953	180.5	35.4	56.9	42.5	22.9	11.7	6.0	2.9	2.2
1925-1929----------	1954	184.9	34.3	56.2	44.6	24.8	12.9	6.6	3.2	2.3
1926-1930----------	1955	186.4	33.0	54.6	45.9	26.1	13.6	7.1	3.5	2.6
1927-1931----------	1956	190.9	32.3	54.0	47.6	27.9	14.6	7.8	3.8	2.9
1928-1932----------	1957	195.7	31.8	53.8	49.2	29.6	15.7	8.3	4.1	3.2
1929-1933----------	1958	194.3	29.8	51.6	49.0	30.7	16.5	8.7	4.4	3.6
1930-1934----------	1959	196.2	28.2	50.2	49.9	32.5	17.5	9.3	4.8	3.8
1931-1935----------	1960	196.0	27.0	48.6	50.1	33.3	18.2	9.8	5.0	4.0
1932-1936----------	1961	194.2	25.9	46.5	49.4	33.8	19.1	10.2	5.1	4.2
1933-1937----------	1962	187.2	24.6	43.9	47.2	33.0	18.9	10.2	5.1	4.3
1934-1938----------	1963	180.5	24.0	42.5	45.1	31.6	18.2	9.8	5.1	4.2
1935-1939----------	1964	174.3	24.9	41.5	43.1	29.9	17.1	9.2	4.7	3.9
1936-1940----------	1965	157.3	24.2	39.1	38.5	25.8	14.5	7.9	4.0	3.3
1937-1941----------	1966	143.9	25.2	38.0	34.5	21.8	12.1	6.4	3.3	2.6
1938-1942----------	1967	137.4	25.6	38.5	32.8	19.6	10.4	5.5	2.8	2.2
1939-1943----------	1968	134.9	28.3	39.6	31.6	17.9	8.9	4.6	2.2	1.8
1940-1944----------	1969	137.2	28.6	42.1	32.7	17.7	8.6	4.1	1.9	1.5
1941-1945----------	1970	138.9	29.9	43.9	33.3	17.2	8.0	3.7	1.6	1.3
1942-1946----------	1971	129.3	29.3	42.2	30.2	15.2	7.0	3.1	1.3	1.0
1943-1947----------	1972	114.6	28.0	40.3	25.0	12.0	5.3	2.3	1.0	0.7
1944-1948----------	1973	108.2	28.2	40.2	22.6	10.0	4.2	1.8	0.7	0.5

TABLE 3A. CENTRAL BIRTH RATES FOR ALL WOMEN DURING EACH YEAR 1917-73 BY AGE AND LIVE-BIRTH ORDER FOR GROUPS OF COHORTS FROM 1868-72 TO 1954-58--CON.

(RATES ARE SIMPLE AVERAGES OF THE RATES FOR SINGLE COHORTS IN TABLE 4A)

CURRENT AGE AND COHORT	CALENDAR YEAR	TOTAL	LIVE-BIRTH ORDER							
			1	2	3	4	5	6	7	8 AND HIGHER
30-34 YEARS										
1883-1887----------	1917	127.5	11.3	17.5	20.3	20.0	18.2	15.6	11.2	13.4
1884-1888----------	1918	126.6	12.0	17.4	19.9	19.6	18.0	15.5	11.0	13.2
1885-1889----------	1919	121.6	10.6	17.2	19.4	18.9	17.1	14.7	10.6	13.1
1886-1890----------	1920	122.9	12.2	17.7	19.7	18.8	17.0	14.2	10.3	13.0
1887-1891----------	1921	125.6	12.3	17.9	20.0	19.4	16.9	14.6	10.7	13.8
1888-1892----------	1922	118.1	11.8	17.9	19.0	17.6	15.7	13.5	9.8	12.8
1889-1893----------	1923	117.5	11.4	17.8	19.0	17.5	15.6	13.4	9.8	13.0
1890-1894----------	1924	116.9	11.5	17.7	19.4	17.3	15.3	13.2	9.7	12.8
1891-1895----------	1925	112.6	11.3	17.2	18.6	16.7	14.5	12.4	9.2	12.7
1892-1896----------	1926	107.6	10.7	16.8	17.9	16.1	13.6	11.7	8.8	12.0
1893-1897----------	1927	104.8	10.7	16.3	17.2	15.5	13.3	11.4	8.6	11.8
1894-1898----------	1928	98.1	10.3	15.7	16.2	14.4	12.4	10.5	7.8	10.8
1895-1899----------	1929	93.5	10.2	15.3	15.6	13.5	11.7	9.8	7.2	10.2
1896-1900----------	1930	93.3	10.8	15.5	15.4	13.3	11.5	9.7	7.1	10.0
1897-1901----------	1931	88.8	10.4	15.0	14.8	12.6	10.8	9.1	6.7	9.4
1898-1902----------	1932	86.0	10.0	14.5	14.1	12.1	10.5	9.0	6.6	9.2
1899-1903----------	1933	80.7	9.4	13.8	13.4	11.5	9.8	8.3	6.1	8.4
1900-1904----------	1934	82.1	10.2	14.6	13.5	11.5	9.7	8.1	6.0	8.5
1901-1905----------	1935	79.0	10.7	14.5	12.9	10.8	8.9	7.5	5.6	8.1
1902-1906----------	1936	76.5	11.3	14.5	12.5	10.1	8.4	6.9	5.2	7.6
1903-1907----------	1937	76.4	12.1	15.0	12.4	9.8	8.1	6.7	5.0	7.3
1904-1908----------	1938	77.3	13.2	16.1	12.5	9.5	7.8	6.4	4.8	7.0
1905-1909----------	1939	76.7	13.9	16.7	12.6	9.3	7.3	5.9	4.4	6.6
1906-1910----------	1940	78.6	14.6	18.1	13.0	9.3	7.0	5.7	4.3	6.6
1907-1911----------	1941	81.1	16.1	19.2	13.5	9.4	7.0	5.5	4.1	6.3
1908-1912----------	1942	87.9	19.0	22.0	14.7	9.7	7.0	5.4	4.0	6.1
1909-1913----------	1943	95.2	18.1	25.1	17.4	11.0	7.6	5.7	4.1	6.2
1910-1914----------	1944	94.2	15.6	24.8	18.5	11.4	7.7	5.8	4.1	6.3
1911-1915----------	1945	96.8	15.3	26.6	19.6	11.7	7.8	5.6	4.1	6.1
1912-1916----------	1946	105.8	20.1	29.1	21.1	12.3	7.8	5.6	3.9	5.9
1913-1917----------	1947	109.3	22.5	29.6	22.0	12.6	7.7	5.3	3.8	5.8
1914-1918----------	1948	101.4	17.7	27.4	21.5	12.5	7.6	5.3	3.7	5.7
1915-1919----------	1949	101.0	16.0	27.1	21.9	13.2	7.8	5.4	3.7	5.9
1916-1920----------	1950	101.7	14.4	27.2	23.1	13.9	8.2	5.4	3.7	5.8
1917-1921----------	1951	106.2	14.4	27.5	24.9	15.2	8.8	5.6	3.9	5.9
1918-1922----------	1952	110.7	14.0	27.5	26.9	16.9	9.6	5.9	3.9	6.0
1919-1923----------	1953	111.8	12.9	26.5	27.9	18.0	10.3	6.2	4.0	6.0
1920-1924----------	1954	115.1	12.5	26.0	28.6	19.4	11.1	6.8	4.3	6.4
1921-1925----------	1955	114.6	11.5	24.2	28.6	20.2	11.9	7.2	4.5	6.5
1922-1926----------	1956	115.7	10.9	23.0	28.6	21.1	12.7	7.7	4.8	6.9
1923-1927----------	1957	117.2	10.6	21.8	28.6	21.8	13.5	8.3	5.2	7.4
1924-1928----------	1958	114.4	9.8	20.0	27.3	22.0	13.7	8.5	5.4	7.7
1925-1929----------	1959	114.2	9.3	18.7	26.4	22.2	14.4	9.1	5.7	8.4
1926-1930----------	1960	113.5	8.7	17.8	25.5	22.3	14.9	9.5	6.0	8.8
1927-1931----------	1961	113.0	8.2	16.7	24.9	22.4	15.3	9.9	6.3	9.3
1928-1932----------	1962	108.5	7.6	15.5	23.2	21.3	15.2	9.9	6.3	9.5
1929-1933----------	1963	105.8	7.2	14.7	22.2	20.9	15.0	9.9	6.4	9.5
1930-1934----------	1964	103.1	7.8	14.1	21.4	20.2	14.4	9.7	6.2	9.3
1931-1935----------	1965	94.1	7.3	13.3	19.6	18.2	13.1	8.7	5.6	8.3
1932-1936----------	1966	84.2	7.1	12.4	17.7	16.1	11.4	7.6	4.7	7.2
1933-1937----------	1967	77.7	6.5	12.1	16.7	14.9	10.4	6.7	4.3	6.1
1934-1938----------	1968	73.0	7.2	12.3	16.0	13.7	9.2	5.8	3.6	5.2
1935-1939----------	1969	72.7	7.0	12.7	16.5	13.7	9.1	5.7	3.4	4.6
1936-1940----------	1970	72.0	7.2	13.2	16.8	13.5	8.8	5.3	3.1	4.1
1937-1941----------	1971	66.6	7.0	13.1	15.5	12.3	7.9	4.7	2.7	3.4
1938-1942----------	1972	58.9	6.9	13.3	13.7	10.3	6.3	3.8	2.1	2.5
1939-1943----------	1973	54.6	7.1	13.5	13.0	9.0	5.3	3.0	1.7	2.0

TABLE 3A. CENTRAL BIRTH RATES FOR ALL WOMEN DURING EACH YEAR 1917-73 BY AGE AND LIVE-BIRTH ORDER FOR GROUPS OF COHORTS FROM 1868-72 TO 1954-58--CON.

(RATES ARE SIMPLE AVERAGES OF THE RATES FOR SINGLE COHORTS IN TABLE 4A)

CURRENT AGE AND COHORT	CALENDAR YEAR	TOTAL	LIVE-BIRTH ORDER							
			1	2	3	4	5	6	7	8 AND HIGHER
35-39 YEARS										
1878-1882----------	1917	93.1	4.0	6.4	8.9	10.4	11.3	11.8	11.3	29.0
1879-1883----------	1918	92.2	4.2	6.5	8.9	10.4	11.1	11.8	11.0	28.3
1880-1884----------	1919	90.9	4.1	6.5	8.7	10.1	10.9	11.3	10.9	28.4
1881-1885----------	1920	90.5	4.3	6.5	8.9	10.1	10.8	11.1	10.6	28.2
1882-1886----------	1921	90.9	4.5	6.7	9.0	10.2	10.7	10.9	10.4	28.5
1883-1887----------	1922	84.9	4.2	6.4	8.5	9.5	10.0	10.2	9.7	26.4
1884-1888----------	1923	83.9	4.1	6.5	8.6	9.4	9.8	9.9	9.4	26.2
1885-1889----------	1924	83.2	4.2	6.4	8.6	9.4	9.6	9.7	9.3	26.0
1886-1890----------	1925	80.3	4.1	6.3	8.3	9.2	9.2	9.2	8.8	25.2
1887-1891----------	1926	76.7	3.8	6.1	8.1	8.9	8.8	8.7	8.4	23.9
1888-1892----------	1927	74.5	4.0	6.0	7.8	8.4	8.4	8.5	8.0	23.4
1889-1893----------	1928	68.9	3.8	5.7	7.4	7.9	7.9	7.8	7.3	21.1
1890-1894----------	1929	64.0	3.5	5.5	7.0	7.3	7.3	7.2	6.7	19.5
1891-1895----------	1930	63.3	3.7	5.6	6.9	7.3	7.3	7.1	6.6	18.8
1892-1896----------	1931	59.5	3.6	5.3	6.6	7.0	6.8	6.6	6.1	17.5
1893-1897----------	1932	57.0	3.3	5.1	6.4	6.6	6.4	6.4	6.0	16.8
1894-1898----------	1933	53.0	3.1	4.8	6.0	6.3	6.0	5.9	5.5	15.4
1895-1899----------	1934	53.2	3.2	5.0	6.1	6.3	6.0	5.9	5.4	15.3
1896-1900----------	1935	51.4	3.4	5.0	5.9	6.0	5.7	5.5	5.1	14.8
1897-1901----------	1936	48.9	3.5	5.0	5.8	5.7	5.3	5.1	4.7	13.8
1898-1902----------	1937	47.8	3.6	5.1	5.7	5.5	5.1	4.8	4.5	13.5
1899-1903----------	1938	47.4	3.9	5.4	5.7	5.5	5.0	4.7	4.3	12.9
1900-1904----------	1939	45.8	4.2	5.7	5.8	5.3	4.7	4.4	3.9	11.8
1901-1905----------	1940	45.1	4.4	6.1	5.9	5.1	4.5	4.1	3.7	11.3
1902-1906----------	1941	45.3	4.8	6.5	6.1	5.2	4.4	4.0	3.6	10.7
1903-1907----------	1942	47.2	5.9	7.4	6.7	5.4	4.4	3.9	3.4	10.1
1904-1908----------	1943	51.5	6.2	8.7	7.9	6.1	4.8	4.1	3.5	10.2
1905-1909----------	1944	52.8	6.0	9.3	8.6	6.5	4.9	4.1	3.4	10.0
1906-1910----------	1945	54.7	6.1	10.1	9.4	6.8	5.1	4.0	3.4	9.8
1907-1911----------	1946	56.7	7.3	10.9	10.0	7.0	5.1	3.9	3.2	9.3
1908-1912----------	1947	57.4	8.0	10.9	10.2	7.3	5.1	3.9	3.1	8.9
1909-1913----------	1948	53.9	6.7	10.2	9.7	7.1	4.9	3.7	3.0	8.6
1910-1914----------	1949	53.2	6.2	9.8	9.7	7.2	5.0	3.7	3.0	8.6
1911-1915----------	1950	53.1	5.7	9.7	10.0	7.5	5.2	3.8	2.9	8.3
1912-1916----------	1951	54.6	5.6	9.8	10.6	8.1	5.4	4.0	2.9	8.2
1913-1917----------	1952	56.1	5.4	9.8	11.3	8.7	5.8	4.0	3.0	8.1
1914-1918----------	1953	56.7	5.1	9.4	11.5	9.4	6.2	4.2	3.1	7.8
1915-1919----------	1954	58.4	4.9	9.3	12.0	9.9	6.7	4.5	3.2	7.9
1916-1920----------	1955	58.4	4.5	8.9	11.9	10.2	7.0	4.7	3.3	7.9
1917-1921----------	1956	58.9	4.2	8.5	11.9	10.4	7.3	4.9	3.5	8.2
1918-1922----------	1957	59.6	4.1	8.1	11.7	10.8	7.7	5.3	3.6	8.3
1919-1923----------	1958	58.1	3.8	7.4	11.2	10.6	7.8	5.4	3.7	8.2
1920-1924----------	1959	57.9	3.5	6.8	10.7	10.6	8.1	5.6	3.9	8.7
1921-1925----------	1960	56.9	3.3	6.4	10.1	10.5	8.1	5.7	4.0	8.8
1922-1926----------	1961	56.5	3.1	6.0	9.8	10.2	8.2	5.9	4.2	9.1
1923-1927----------	1962	53.6	2.8	5.4	8.9	9.6	7.9	5.7	4.1	9.2
1924-1928----------	1963	51.7	2.6	5.1	8.3	9.1	7.7	5.7	4.0	9.2
1925-1929----------	1964	50.7	2.9	4.8	8.0	8.8	7.4	5.5	4.1	9.2
1926-1930----------	1965	46.7	2.8	4.4	7.2	8.1	6.9	5.1	3.6	8.6
1927-1931----------	1966	42.1	2.6	4.0	6.5	7.2	6.2	4.6	3.4	7.6
1928-1932----------	1967	38.6	2.2	3.8	6.1	6.7	5.6	4.3	3.1	6.8
1929-1933----------	1968	35.8	2.5	3.7	5.6	6.1	5.2	3.9	2.7	6.1
1930-1934----------	1969	33.7	2.1	3.6	5.3	5.8	5.0	3.7	2.6	5.6
1931-1935----------	1970	32.0	2.1	3.5	5.1	5.5	4.7	3.4	2.5	5.2
1932-1936----------	1971	29.0	1.9	3.2	4.6	5.0	4.3	3.2	2.2	4.6
1933-1937----------	1972	25.1	1.8	3.1	4.1	4.3	3.6	2.7	1.8	3.7
1934-1938----------	1973	22.2	1.7	3.1	3.8	3.7	3.1	2.2	1.6	3.0

TABLE 3A. CENTRAL BIRTH RATES FOR ALL WOMEN DURING EACH YEAR 1917-73 BY AGE AND LIVE-BIRTH ORDER FOR GROUPS OF COHORTS FROM 1868-72 TO 1954-58--CON.

(RATES ARE SIMPLE AVERAGES OF THE RATES FOR SINGLE COHORTS IN TABLE 4A)

CURRENT AGE AND COHORT	CALENDAR YEAR	TOTAL	LIVE-BIRTH ORDER							
			1	2	3	4	5	6	7	8 AND HIGHER
40-44 YEARS										
1873-1877----------	1917	35.0	0.8	1.3	1.9	2.5	2.9	3.6	3.7	18.3
1874-1878----------	1918	35.2	0.9	1.3	2.0	2.5	3.0	3.5	3.8	18.2
1875-1879----------	1919	34.1	0.9	1.4	1.9	2.5	2.9	3.4	3.6	17.5
1876-1880----------	1920	34.5	1.0	1.4	1.9	2.5	2.9	3.4	3.6	17.8
1877-1881----------	1921	34.8	1.0	1.4	1.9	2.5	3.0	3.4	3.6	18.0
1878-1882----------	1922	32.5	0.9	1.3	1.9	2.4	2.8	3.1	3.4	16.7
1879-1883----------	1923	31.9	0.9	1.3	1.9	2.3	2.7	3.1	3.3	16.4
1880-1884----------	1924	31.8	0.9	1.3	1.9	2.3	2.7	3.0	3.2	16.5
1881-1885----------	1925	30.6	0.9	1.3	1.8	2.3	2.5	2.8	3.1	15.9
1882-1886----------	1926	28.8	0.9	1.2	1.7	2.1	2.4	2.7	2.9	14.9
1883-1887----------	1927	27.8	0.8	1.2	1.7	2.0	2.3	2.6	2.7	14.5
1884-1888----------	1928	25.9	0.8	1.2	1.6	1.9	2.2	2.4	2.5	13.3
1885-1889----------	1929	24.1	0.8	1.1	1.5	1.8	2.1	2.2	2.4	12.2
1886-1890----------	1930	24.0	0.8	1.1	1.6	1.9	2.1	2.3	2.3	11.9
1887-1891----------	1931	22.4	0.8	1.0	1.4	1.7	1.9	2.2	2.2	11.2
1888-1892----------	1932	21.7	0.7	1.0	1.4	1.7	1.9	2.1	2.2	10.7
1889-1893----------	1933	20.3	0.7	1.0	1.3	1.6	1.8	1.9	2.0	10.0
1890-1894----------	1934	20.0	0.7	0.9	1.3	1.6	1.8	1.9	1.9	9.9
1891-1895----------	1935	18.7	0.6	0.9	1.3	1.5	1.7	1.7	1.8	9.2
1892-1896----------	1936	17.5	0.7	0.9	1.2	1.4	1.6	1.6	1.7	8.4
1893-1897----------	1937	16.6	0.7	0.9	1.1	1.4	1.5	1.5	1.5	8.0
1894-1898----------	1938	16.4	0.7	1.0	1.2	1.4	1.4	1.5	1.5	7.7
1895-1899----------	1939	15.4	0.7	0.9	1.2	1.4	1.4	1.4	1.4	7.0
1896-1900----------	1940	15.0	0.7	1.0	1.2	1.3	1.4	1.3	1.3	6.8
1897-1901----------	1941	14.8	0.8	1.0	1.3	1.3	1.3	1.3	1.3	6.5
1898-1902----------	1942	14.7	0.9	1.1	1.3	1.4	1.3	1.3	1.2	6.2
1899-1903----------	1943	15.7	1.0	1.3	1.5	1.5	1.4	1.4	1.3	6.3
1900-1904----------	1944	16.3	1.2	1.5	1.7	1.6	1.5	1.4	1.3	6.1
1901-1905----------	1945	16.6	1.2	1.6	1.9	1.7	1.5	1.4	1.3	6.0
1902-1906----------	1946	16.4	1.4	1.8	1.9	1.7	1.5	1.3	1.2	5.6
1903-1907----------	1947	16.5	1.5	1.9	2.0	1.8	1.5	1.3	1.2	5.3
1904-1908----------	1948	15.3	1.3	1.8	2.0	1.7	1.4	1.2	1.1	4.8
1905-1909----------	1949	15.1	1.3	1.8	1.9	1.7	1.4	1.2	1.0	4.8
1906-1910----------	1950	14.9	1.3	1.8	1.9	1.7	1.5	1.2	1.0	4.5
1907-1911----------	1951	15.2	1.2	1.8	2.1	1.9	1.5	1.2	1.0	4.5
1908-1912----------	1952	15.5	1.2	1.8	2.2	2.0	1.6	1.3	1.1	4.3
1909-1913----------	1953	15.8	1.2	1.8	2.3	2.1	1.7	1.4	1.1	4.2
1910-1914----------	1954	16.1	1.1	1.8	2.4	2.3	1.9	1.4	1.1	4.1
1911-1915----------	1955	16.2	1.1	1.8	2.4	2.3	2.0	1.5	1.1	4.0
1912-1916----------	1956	16.3	1.0	1.7	2.4	2.4	2.0	1.5	1.2	4.1
1913-1917----------	1957	16.3	1.0	1.6	2.4	2.5	2.0	1.6	1.2	4.0
1914-1918----------	1958	15.8	0.9	1.5	2.3	2.4	2.1	1.5	1.2	3.9
1915-1919----------	1959	15.8	0.8	1.4	2.3	2.5	2.1	1.6	1.2	3.9
1916-1920----------	1960	15.7	0.8	1.3	2.2	2.4	2.1	1.7	1.2	4.0
1917-1921----------	1961	15.8	0.7	1.3	2.1	2.5	2.2	1.7	1.3	4.0
1918-1922----------	1962	15.2	0.7	1.2	1.9	2.3	2.1	1.7	1.3	4.0
1919-1923----------	1963	14.5	0.6	1.1	1.8	2.2	2.0	1.6	1.3	3.9
1920-1924----------	1964	14.1	0.7	1.0	1.7	2.1	1.9	1.6	1.2	3.9
1921-1925----------	1965	13.3	0.7	1.0	1.6	1.9	1.8	1.5	1.2	3.6
1922-1926----------	1966	12.0	0.6	0.8	1.4	1.8	1.6	1.4	1.1	3.3
1923-1927----------	1967	11.1	0.5	0.8	1.3	1.7	1.5	1.2	1.0	3.1
1924-1928----------	1968	9.9	0.6	0.8	1.1	1.4	1.3	1.1	0.9	2.7
1925-1929----------	1969	9.1	0.4	0.7	1.1	1.3	1.3	1.0	0.8	2.5
1926-1930----------	1970	8.7	0.4	0.7	1.0	1.2	1.2	1.0	0.8	2.4
1927-1931----------	1971	7.4	0.4	0.6	0.8	1.0	1.0	0.8	0.7	2.1
1928-1932----------	1972	6.5	0.4	0.6	0.7	0.9	0.8	0.7	0.6	1.8
1929-1933----------	1973	6.1	0.4	0.5	0.7	0.8	0.8	0.7	0.5	1.7

TABLE 3A. CENTRAL BIRTH RATES FOR ALL WOMEN DURING EACH YEAR 1917-73 BY AGE AND LIVE-BIRTH ORDER FOR GROUPS OF COHORTS FROM 1868-72 TO 1954-58--CON.

(RATES ARE SIMPLE AVERAGES OF THE RATES FOR SINGLE COHORTS IN TABLE 4A)

CURRENT AGE AND COHORT	CALENDAR YEAR	TOTAL	LIVE-BIRTH ORDER							
			1	2	3	4	5	6	7	8 AND HIGHER
45-49 YEARS										
1868-1872----------	1917	5.3	0.1	0.1	0.1	0.3	0.3	0.4	0.5	3.5
1869-1873----------	1918	6.2	0.1	0.1	0.2	0.3	0.4	0.5	0.5	4.1
1870-1874----------	1919	5.0	0.1	0.1	0.1	0.2	0.3	0.4	0.4	3.4
1871-1875----------	1920	5.7	0.1	0.2	0.2	0.3	0.4	0.4	0.5	3.6
1872-1876----------	1921	5.0	0.1	0.1	0.1	0.3	0.3	0.3	0.4	3.4
1873-1877----------	1922	4.6	0.1	0.1	0.1	0.2	0.3	0.3	0.4	3.1
1874-1878----------	1923	4.6	0.1	0.1	0.1	0.2	0.3	0.4	0.4	3.0
1875-1879----------	1924	4.5	0.1	0.1	0.1	0.2	0.3	0.3	0.4	3.0
1876-1880----------	1925	4.4	0.1	0.1	0.2	0.2	0.3	0.3	0.3	2.9
1877-1881----------	1926	4.1	0.1	0.1	0.1	0.2	0.2	0.3	0.4	2.7
1878-1882----------	1927	3.8	0.1	0.1	0.1	0.2	0.2	0.3	0.3	2.5
1879-1883----------	1928	3.7	0.1	0.1	0.1	0.2	0.2	0.3	0.3	2.4
1880-1884----------	1929	3.4	0.1	0.1	0.1	0.1	0.2	0.3	0.3	2.2
1881-1885----------	1930	3.2	0.1	0.1	0.1	0.1	0.2	0.2	0.3	2.1
1882-1886----------	1931	3.0	0.1	0.1	0.1	0.1	0.2	0.2	0.2	2.0
1883-1887----------	1932	2.9	0.0	0.1	0.1	0.1	0.2	0.2	0.3	1.9
1884-1888----------	1933	2.7	0.0	0.1	0.1	0.1	0.2	0.2	0.2	1.8
1885-1889----------	1934	2.5	0.0	0.0	0.1	0.1	0.2	0.2	0.2	1.7
1886-1890----------	1935	2.5	0.1	0.0	0.1	0.1	0.2	0.2	0.2	1.6
1887-1891----------	1936	2.2	0.0	0.0	0.1	0.1	0.1	0.2	0.2	1.5
1888-1892----------	1937	2.1	0.0	0.0	0.1	0.1	0.1	0.2	0.2	1.4
1889-1893----------	1938	2.0	0.0	0.0	0.1	0.1	0.1	0.2	0.2	1.3
1890-1894----------	1939	1.8	0.0	0.0	0.1	0.1	0.1	0.1	0.2	1.2
1891-1895----------	1940	1.6	0.0	0.0	0.1	0.1	0.1	0.1	0.1	1.1
1892-1896----------	1941	1.6	0.0	0.1	0.1	0.1	0.1	0.1	0.1	1.0
1893-1897----------	1942	1.6	0.0	0.1	0.1	0.1	0.1	0.1	0.1	1.0
1894-1898----------	1943	1.6	0.1	0.1	0.1	0.1	0.1	0.1	0.1	0.9
1895-1899----------	1944	1.6	0.1	0.1	0.1	0.1	0.1	0.1	0.1	0.9
1896-1900----------	1945	1.6	0.1	0.1	0.1	0.1	0.1	0.1	0.1	0.9
1897-1901----------	1946	1.5	0.1	0.1	0.1	0.1	0.1	0.1	0.1	0.8
1898-1902----------	1947	1.5	0.1	0.1	0.1	0.1	0.1	0.1	0.1	0.8
1899-1903----------	1948	1.4	0.1	0.1	0.1	0.1	0.1	0.1	0.1	0.7
1900-1904----------	1949	1.4	0.1	0.1	0.1	0.1	0.1	0.1	0.1	0.7
1901-1905----------	1950	1.3	0.1	0.1	0.1	0.1	0.1	0.1	0.1	0.6
1902-1906----------	1951	1.2	0.1	0.1	0.1	0.1	0.1	0.1	0.1	0.5
1903-1907----------	1952	1.2	0.1	0.1	0.1	0.1	0.1	0.1	0.1	0.5
1904-1908----------	1953	1.2	0.1	0.1	0.1	0.1	0.1	0.1	0.1	0.5
1905-1909----------	1954	1.2	0.1	0.1	0.1	0.1	0.1	0.1	0.1	0.5
1906-1910----------	1955	1.1	0.1	0.1	0.1	0.1	0.1	0.1	0.1	0.4
1907-1911----------	1956	1.2	0.1	0.1	0.1	0.1	0.1	0.1	0.1	0.5
1908-1912----------	1957	1.2	0.1	0.1	0.1	0.1	0.1	0.1	0.1	0.5
1909-1913----------	1958	1.1	0.0	0.1	0.1	0.1	0.1	0.1	0.1	0.5
1910-1914----------	1959	1.1	0.1	0.1	0.1	0.1	0.1	0.1	0.1	0.4
1911-1915----------	1960	1.0	0.0	0.1	0.1	0.1	0.1	0.1	0.1	0.4
1912-1916----------	1961	1.0	0.0	0.1	0.1	0.1	0.1	0.1	0.1	0.4
1913-1917----------	1962	1.0	0.0	0.1	0.1	0.1	0.1	0.1	0.1	0.4
1914-1918----------	1963	1.0	0.0	0.1	0.1	0.1	0.1	0.1	0.1	0.4
1915-1919----------	1964	0.8	0.0	0.0	0.1	0.1	0.1	0.1	0.1	0.3
1916-1920----------	1965	0.8	0.0	0.0	0.1	0.1	0.1	0.1	0.1	0.3
1917-1921----------	1966	0.8	0.0	0.0	0.1	0.1	0.1	0.1	0.1	0.3
1918-1922----------	1967	0.8	0.0	0.0	0.1	0.1	0.1	0.1	0.1	0.3
1919-1923----------	1968	0.8	0.0	0.0	0.1	0.1	0.1	0.1	0.1	0.3
1920-1924----------	1969	0.7	0.0	0.0	0.0	0.1	0.1	0.1	0.1	0.3
1921-1925----------	1970	0.6	0.0	0.0	0.0	0.1	0.1	0.1	0.1	0.2
1922-1926----------	1971	0.4	0.0	0.0	0.0	0.1	0.0	0.1	0.0	0.2
1923-1927----------	1972	0.2	0.0	0.0	0.0	0.0	0.0	0.0	0.0	0.2
1924-1928----------	1973	0.1	0.0	0.0	0.0	0.0	0.0	0.0	0.0	0.1

TABLE 3B. CENTRAL BIRTH RATES FOR WHITE WOMEN DURING EACH YEAR 1917-73 BY AGE AND LIVE-BIRTH ORDER FOR GROUPS OF COHORTS FROM 1868-72 TO 1954-58

(RATES ARE SIMPLE AVERAGES OF THE RATES FOR SINGLE COHORTS IN TABLE 4B)

CURRENT AGE AND COHORT	CALENDAR YEAR	TOTAL	LIVE-BIRTH ORDER							
			1	2	3	4	5	6	7	8 AND HIGHER
15-19 YEARS										
1898-1902----------	1917	53.7	40.9	10.7	1.9	0.2	*	*	*	*
1899-1903----------	1918	52.7	40.1	10.5	1.9	0.2	*	*	*	*
1900-1904----------	1919	45.0	33.2	9.9	1.7	0.2	*	*	*	*
1901-1905----------	1920	55.6	43.9	9.8	1.7	0.2	*	*	*	*
1902-1906----------	1921	60.0	47.5	10.5	1.8	0.2	*	*	*	*
1903-1907----------	1922	55.5	42.1	11.4	1.7	0.3	*	*	*	*
1904-1908----------	1923	54.9	41.1	11.7	1.8	0.3	*	*	*	*
1905-1909----------	1924	56.8	43.7	10.9	1.9	0.3	*	*	*	*
1906-1910----------	1925	55.0	42.3	10.7	1.8	0.2	*	*	*	*
1907-1911----------	1926	53.8	40.9	10.8	1.8	0.3	*	*	*	*
1908-1912----------	1927	53.8	40.9	10.7	1.9	0.3	*	*	*	*
1909-1913----------	1928	51.2	39.1	10.1	1.7	0.3	*	*	*	*
1910-1914----------	1929	49.4	37.7	9.8	1.6	0.3	*	*	*	*
1911-1915----------	1930	50.6	39.0	9.7	1.6	0.3	*	*	*	*
1912-1916----------	1931	47.1	36.2	9.2	1.5	0.2	*	*	*	*
1913-1917----------	1932	44.9	34.5	8.8	1.4	0.2	*	*	*	*
1914-1918----------	1933	41.6	32.1	8.0	1.3	0.2	*	*	*	*
1915-1919----------	1934	43.8	34.4	7.9	1.3	0.2	*	*	*	*
1916-1920----------	1935	44.1	35.1	7.6	1.2	0.2	*	*	*	*
1917-1921----------	1936	43.5	34.1	8.0	1.2	0.2	*	*	*	*
1918-1922----------	1937	45.0	35.4	8.2	1.2	0.2	*	*	*	*
1919-1923----------	1938	46.5	36.6	8.5	1.3	0.1	*	*	*	*
1920-1924----------	1939	44.6	34.6	8.5	1.3	0.2	*	*	*	*
1921-1925----------	1940	45.6	34.3	9.4	1.7	0.2	*	*	*	*
1922-1926----------	1941	47.8	36.8	9.2	1.6	0.2	*	*	*	*
1923-1927----------	1942	51.9	40.8	9.3	1.6	0.2	*	*	*	*
1924-1928----------	1943	52.0	40.1	9.9	1.7	0.3	*	*	*	*
1925-1929----------	1944	45.6	34.8	8.8	1.7	0.3	*	*	*	*
1926-1930----------	1945	42.2	33.1	7.5	1.4	0.2	*	*	*	*
1927-1931----------	1946	50.6	40.2	8.8	1.4	0.2	*	*	*	*
1928-1932----------	1947	68.8	56.8	10.3	1.5	0.2	*	*	*	*
1929-1933----------	1948	69.7	54.8	12.9	1.8	0.2	*	*	*	*
1930-1934----------	1949	70.2	52.6	15.0	2.3	0.3	*	*	*	*
1931-1935----------	1950	69.3	50.9	15.4	2.7	0.3	*	*	*	*
1932-1936----------	1951	75.3	55.9	16.1	2.9	0.4	*	*	*	*
1933-1937----------	1952	75.5	55.2	16.7	3.1	0.5	*	*	*	*
1934-1938----------	1953	78.2	56.9	17.5	3.3	0.5	*	*	*	*
1935-1939----------	1954	80.1	58.2	17.9	3.5	0.5	*	*	*	*
1936-1940----------	1955	80.4	57.7	18.6	3.6	0.5	*	*	*	*
1937-1941----------	1956	85.3	61.1	19.7	3.9	0.6	*	*	*	*
1938-1942----------	1957	87.9	62.9	20.3	4.1	0.6	*	*	*	*
1939-1943----------	1958	86.4	60.6	20.9	4.2	0.7	*	*	*	*
1940-1944----------	1959	85.5	59.2	21.0	4.6	0.7	*	*	*	*
1941-1945----------	1960	82.5	57.0	20.3	4.5	0.7	*	*	*	*
1942-1946----------	1961	80.4	56.0	19.4	4.3	0.7	*	*	*	*
1943-1947----------	1962	76.9	53.5	18.6	4.1	0.7	*	*	*	*
1944-1948----------	1963	73.7	52.0	17.3	3.8	0.6	*	*	*	*
1945-1949----------	1964	69.3	49.9	15.5	3.3	0.6	*	*	*	*
1946-1950----------	1965	63.8	47.4	13.3	2.7	0.4	*	*	*	*
1947-1951----------	1966	61.1	46.9	11.8	2.1	0.3	*	*	*	*
1948-1952----------	1967	58.3	44.8	11.3	1.9	0.3	*	*	*	*
1949-1953----------	1968	56.8	44.7	10.2	1.6	0.3	*	*	*	*
1950-1954----------	1969	56.8	44.9	10.1	1.6	0.2	*	*	*	*
1951-1955----------	1970	59.0	47.1	10.2	1.5	0.2	*	*	*	*
1952-1956----------	1971	55.2	44.1	9.7	1.3	0.1	*	*	*	*
1953-1957----------	1972	52.3	42.3	8.7	1.2	0.1	*	*	*	*
1954-1958----------	1973	50.3	40.7	8.4	1.1	0.1	*	*	*	*

TABLE 3B. CENTRAL BIRTH RATES FOR WHITE WOMEN DURING EACH YEAR 1917-73 BY AGE AND LIVE-BIRTH ORDER FOR GROUPS OF COHORTS FROM 1868-72 TO 1954-58--CON.

(RATES ARE SIMPLE AVERAGES OF THE RATES FOR SINGLE COHORTS IN TABLE 4B)

CURRENT AGE AND COHORT	CALENDAR YEAR	TOTAL	LIVE-BIRTH ORDER							
			1	2	3	4	5	6	7	8 AND HIGHER
20-24 YEARS										
1893-1897----------	1917	170.3	75.2	53.2	27.1	10.2	3.3	0.9	0.3	0.1
1894-1898----------	1918	169.6	75.7	52.5	26.8	10.3	3.1	0.8	0.3	0.1
1895-1899----------	1919	147.3	57.6	50.0	25.5	10.1	3.0	0.8	0.2	0.1
1896-1900----------	1920	165.5	77.3	48.6	25.2	10.1	3.1	0.9	0.2	0.1
1897-1901----------	1921	168.0	79.8	48.1	25.2	10.4	3.3	0.9	0.2	0.1
1898-1902----------	1922	157.7	70.5	50.5	22.9	9.5	3.0	0.9	0.3	0.1
1899-1903----------	1923	158.4	68.6	51.9	23.9	9.5	3.2	0.9	0.3	0.1
1900-1904----------	1924	161.2	71.6	50.3	25.4	9.5	3.1	0.9	0.3	0.1
1901-1905----------	1925	155.1	68.8	47.9	24.8	9.5	3.0	0.8	0.2	0.1
1902-1906----------	1926	150.9	66.6	46.9	23.5	9.6	3.1	0.9	0.2	0.1
1903-1907----------	1927	147.8	65.8	45.5	22.8	9.5	3.0	0.8	0.3	0.1
1904-1908----------	1928	140.7	63.1	43.2	21.7	8.7	2.9	0.8	0.2	0.1
1905-1909----------	1929	134.8	60.6	41.8	20.5	8.2	2.7	0.7	0.2	0.1
1906-1910----------	1930	135.0	62.3	41.1	20.0	8.0	2.6	0.7	0.2	0.1
1907-1911----------	1931	127.8	58.7	39.4	18.8	7.5	2.4	0.7	0.2	0.1
1908-1912----------	1932	122.3	56.1	38.1	18.0	7.1	2.2	0.6	0.1	0.1
1909-1913----------	1933	115.0	52.8	35.8	17.0	6.6	2.0	0.6	0.1	0.1
1910-1914----------	1934	119.9	57.3	36.2	16.9	6.6	2.0	0.6	0.2	0.1
1911-1915----------	1935	119.7	59.9	34.7	16.0	6.3	2.0	0.6	0.1	0.1
1912-1916----------	1936	119.9	60.5	35.5	15.3	6.0	1.9	0.5	0.1	0.1
1913-1917----------	1937	122.8	62.6	36.6	15.3	5.8	1.8	0.5	0.1	0.1
1914-1918----------	1938	126.8	64.8	38.1	15.8	5.7	1.8	0.5	0.1	0.0
1915-1919----------	1939	123.1	62.5	37.4	15.4	5.5	1.7	0.5	0.1	0.0
1916-1920----------	1940	127.5	63.7	38.7	16.4	6.0	1.9	0.6	0.1	0.1
1917-1921----------	1941	137.0	72.0	39.9	16.5	6.0	1.9	0.5	0.1	0.1
1918-1922----------	1942	156.6	86.9	43.8	17.2	6.1	1.9	0.5	0.1	0.1
1919-1923----------	1943	154.8	78.5	47.8	18.9	6.7	2.1	0.6	0.1	0.1
1920-1924----------	1944	141.2	70.0	42.9	18.6	6.8	2.1	0.6	0.1	0.1
1921-1925----------	1945	128.9	66.8	37.4	15.8	6.1	2.0	0.6	0.1	0.1
1922-1926----------	1946	172.5	94.0	51.8	17.5	6.3	2.0	0.6	0.2	0.1
1923-1927----------	1947	200.0	115.4	57.2	18.9	6.0	1.9	0.5	0.1	0.0
1924-1928----------	1948	188.0	96.3	62.0	20.8	6.3	1.9	0.6	0.1	0.0
1925-1929----------	1949	188.2	88.4	66.4	23.3	7.1	2.1	0.6	0.2	0.1
1926-1930----------	1950	185.3	82.0	66.7	25.9	7.7	2.2	0.6	0.1	0.1
1927-1931----------	1951	200.0	89.3	69.5	28.8	9.0	2.5	0.6	0.2	0.1
1928-1932----------	1952	205.8	89.6	71.7	30.6	10.1	2.9	0.7	0.1	0.1
1929-1933----------	1953	212.2	88.9	75.3	32.6	11.1	3.2	0.8	0.2	0.1
1930-1934----------	1954	222.0	91.7	77.9	35.4	12.2	3.6	0.9	0.2	0.1
1931-1935----------	1955	227.5	91.8	79.8	37.4	13.1	4.0	1.1	0.2	0.1
1932-1936----------	1956	237.6	94.6	82.9	40.0	14.2	4.3	1.2	0.3	0.1
1933-1937----------	1957	243.7	94.9	85.4	42.1	15.1	4.6	1.2	0.3	0.1
1934-1938----------	1958	241.6	91.1	85.2	42.9	15.8	4.9	1.3	0.3	0.1
1935-1939----------	1959	243.1	89.1	86.0	44.5	16.5	5.1	1.4	0.4	0.1
1936-1940----------	1960	242.6	87.4	84.9	45.6	17.3	5.4	1.5	0.4	0.1
1937-1941----------	1961	238.8	85.9	82.3	45.3	17.7	5.6	1.5	0.4	0.1
1938-1942----------	1962	229.4	82.1	78.6	43.6	17.3	5.7	1.6	0.4	0.1
1939-1943----------	1963	218.8	80.1	75.1	40.5	15.9	5.2	1.5	0.4	0.1
1940-1944----------	1964	206.8	79.3	70.4	36.6	14.1	4.7	1.3	0.3	0.1
1941-1945----------	1965	184.6	74.6	63.3	30.2	11.4	3.7	1.1	0.2	0.1
1942-1946----------	1966	174.1	76.7	59.1	25.4	9.0	2.8	0.8	0.2	0.1
1943-1947----------	1967	166.1	74.0	58.0	23.0	7.8	2.4	0.6	0.2	0.1
1944-1948----------	1968	160.0	74.6	55.5	20.7	6.6	1.9	0.6	0.1	0.0
1945-1949----------	1969	159.0	74.9	55.3	20.1	6.2	1.8	0.5	0.1	0.1
1946-1950----------	1970	158.6	76.1	55.3	19.5	5.6	1.6	0.4	0.1	0.0
1947-1951----------	1971	143.9	68.8	51.2	17.4	4.8	1.3	0.3	0.1	0.0
1948-1952----------	1972	123.7	59.9	45.0	13.9	3.8	0.9	0.2	0.0	0.0
1949-1953----------	1973	114.3	55.6	42.3	12.3	3.1	0.8	0.2	0.0	0.0

TABLE 3B. CENTRAL BIRTH RATES FOR WHITE WOMEN DURING EACH YEAR 1917-73 BY AGE AND LIVE-BIRTH ORDER FOR GROUPS OF COHORTS FROM 1868-72 TO 1954-58--CON.

(RATES ARE SIMPLE AVERAGES OF THE RATES FOR SINGLE COHORTS IN TABLE 4B)

CURRENT AGE AND COHORT	CALENDAR YEAR	TOTAL	LIVE-BIRTH ORDER							
			1	2	3	4	5	6	7	8 AND HIGHER
25-29 YEARS										
1888-1892----------	1917	176.1	36.0	42.7	37.3	27.5	17.4	9.2	3.8	2.2
1889-1893----------	1918	174.9	37.2	42.4	36.7	27.2	16.9	8.8	3.6	2.1
1890-1894----------	1919	160.4	29.3	40.8	34.4	25.9	16.3	8.3	3.5	1.9
1891-1895----------	1920	168.6	37.6	40.6	34.5	25.8	16.3	8.3	3.5	2.0
1892-1896----------	1921	170.7	39.2	40.0	34.6	25.8	16.6	8.8	3.6	2.1
1893-1897----------	1922	160.1	35.5	40.9	31.7	23.6	15.0	8.0	3.4	2.0
1894-1898----------	1923	160.2	34.5	41.8	31.9	23.1	15.2	8.1	3.5	2.1
1895-1899----------	1924	158.7	34.9	40.9	32.4	22.5	14.6	7.9	3.4	2.1
1896-1900----------	1925	152.5	33.7	39.4	31.4	21.6	13.7	7.4	3.2	2.1
1897-1901----------	1926	146.7	32.6	37.8	29.8	21.1	13.0	7.2	3.2	2.0
1898-1902----------	1927	143.7	32.3	36.6	28.8	21.0	13.0	7.0	3.1	1.9
1899-1903----------	1928	136.8	31.6	35.2	27.1	19.3	12.3	6.6	2.9	1.8
1900-1904----------	1929	130.7	31.0	34.1	25.6	18.0	11.6	6.1	2.6	1.7
1901-1905----------	1930	130.5	32.2	34.2	25.2	17.5	11.2	6.0	2.6	1.6
1902-1906----------	1931	124.4	31.2	33.0	23.8	16.5	10.4	5.6	2.4	1.5
1903-1907----------	1932	119.4	29.6	31.8	23.1	15.9	9.9	5.4	2.3	1.4
1904-1908----------	1933	112.2	28.0	30.3	21.7	15.0	9.1	4.7	2.1	1.3
1905-1909----------	1934	115.3	30.2	31.3	21.9	14.9	9.1	4.7	2.0	1.2
1906-1910----------	1935	112.7	31.8	30.3	20.5	13.8	8.5	4.5	2.0	1.3
1907-1911----------	1936	111.5	33.0	30.3	19.8	13.1	7.9	4.3	1.9	1.2
1908-1912----------	1937	113.3	35.3	31.3	19.4	12.6	7.7	4.1	1.8	1.1
1909-1913----------	1938	117.5	37.7	33.2	19.9	12.5	7.4	3.9	1.8	1.1
1910-1914----------	1939	115.9	38.0	33.5	19.5	11.8	6.9	3.6	1.6	1.0
1911-1915----------	1940	121.0	40.0	35.7	20.4	11.8	6.8	3.6	1.7	1.0
1912-1916----------	1941	128.2	44.9	37.7	20.9	12.0	6.7	3.5	1.5	1.0
1913-1917----------	1942	143.9	53.6	43.3	22.5	12.2	6.6	3.3	1.5	0.9
1914-1918----------	1943	149.6	47.3	49.3	26.1	13.6	7.2	3.6	1.5	1.0
1915-1919----------	1944	137.5	38.8	45.4	26.2	13.7	7.3	3.6	1.6	0.9
1916-1920----------	1945	132.6	36.9	44.5	25.2	13.2	6.9	3.5	1.5	0.9
1917-1921----------	1946	162.5	53.8	54.1	27.6	14.0	7.1	3.5	1.5	0.9
1918-1922----------	1947	177.1	61.2	59.2	30.0	13.9	7.0	3.4	1.5	0.9
1919-1923----------	1948	163.4	48.2	57.6	30.9	13.9	6.9	3.4	1.5	1.0
1920-1924----------	1949	164.3	43.5	59.5	33.0	15.0	7.1	3.5	1.6	1.1
1921-1925----------	1950	164.6	39.7	60.2	35.5	16.0	7.2	3.4	1.6	1.0
1922-1926----------	1951	173.4	40.9	61.5	38.9	18.0	7.9	3.6	1.6	1.0
1923-1927----------	1952	178.9	39.8	61.8	42.3	19.9	8.7	3.8	1.6	1.0
1924-1928----------	1953	180.0	37.6	60.8	43.8	21.5	9.4	4.1	1.7	1.1
1925-1929----------	1954	184.1	36.3	60.1	46.2	23.4	10.5	4.6	1.9	1.1
1926-1930----------	1955	185.4	35.0	58.2	47.7	25.0	11.3	5.0	2.0	1.2
1927-1931----------	1956	189.3	34.2	57.6	49.4	26.8	12.2	5.5	2.2	1.4
1928-1932----------	1957	194.6	33.8	57.4	51.3	28.9	13.3	5.9	2.5	1.5
1929-1933----------	1958	193.3	31.6	55.2	51.3	30.1	14.3	6.4	2.7	1.7
1930-1934----------	1959	194.5	29.8	53.5	52.3	32.0	15.3	6.9	2.9	1.8
1931-1935----------	1960	194.6	28.4	51.8	52.6	33.1	16.1	7.4	3.2	2.0
1932-1936----------	1961	192.2	27.1	49.4	51.9	33.6	17.1	7.7	3.3	2.1
1933-1937----------	1962	184.7	25.8	46.5	49.4	32.8	16.9	7.9	3.3	2.1
1934-1938----------	1963	178.1	25.1	44.9	47.2	31.5	16.3	7.7	3.3	2.1
1935-1939----------	1964	172.3	26.2	43.9	45.1	29.7	15.4	7.1	3.0	1.9
1936-1940----------	1965	155.0	25.2	41.2	40.1	25.4	12.9	6.0	2.6	1.6
1937-1941----------	1966	142.6	26.4	40.0	35.8	21.4	10.7	4.9	2.1	1.3
1938-1942----------	1967	136.7	26.8	40.5	34.0	19.2	9.2	4.1	1.8	1.1
1939-1943----------	1968	135.5	29.5	41.8	32.9	17.5	7.9	3.5	1.5	0.9
1940-1944----------	1969	138.4	29.8	44.3	34.0	17.4	7.6	3.2	1.3	0.8
1941-1945----------	1970	139.7	31.1	46.0	34.3	16.7	7.0	2.8	1.1	0.7
1942-1946----------	1971	129.5	30.4	44.0	30.8	14.6	6.0	2.3	0.9	0.5
1943-1947----------	1972	114.5	28.8	41.9	25.4	11.3	4.5	1.7	0.6	0.3
1944-1948----------	1973	108.5	29.1	41.9	22.6	9.3	3.5	1.3	0.5	0.3

TABLE 3B. CENTRAL BIRTH RATES FOR WHITE WOMEN DURING EACH YEAR 1917-73 BY AGE AND LIVE-BIRTH ORDER FOR GROUPS OF COHORTS FROM 1868-72 TO 1954-58--CON.

(RATES ARE SIMPLE AVERAGES OF THE RATES FOR SINGLE COHORTS IN TABLE 4B)

CURRENT AGE AND COHORT	CALENDAR YEAR	TOTAL	LIVE-BIRTH ORDER							
			1	2	3	4	5	6	7	8 AND HIGHER
30-34 YEARS										
1883-1887----------	1917	130.1	11.9	18.6	21.5	20.9	18.8	15.6	10.9	11.9
1884-1888----------	1918	129.4	12.6	18.4	21.0	20.5	18.6	15.5	10.8	12.0
1885-1889----------	1919	124.1	11.1	18.3	20.5	19.7	17.6	14.8	10.3	11.8
1886-1890----------	1920	125.7	12.8	18.7	20.7	19.6	17.5	14.4	10.2	11.8
1887-1891----------	1921	128.1	13.0	19.0	21.0	20.2	17.4	14.6	10.5	12.4
1888-1892----------	1922	120.4	12.6	19.0	20.0	18.2	16.1	13.5	9.6	11.4
1889-1893----------	1923	119.6	12.1	18.9	19.9	18.1	16.0	13.4	9.5	11.7
1890-1894----------	1924	118.5	12.2	18.9	20.3	17.9	15.6	13.0	9.3	11.3
1891-1895----------	1925	113.7	12.0	18.4	19.5	17.2	14.7	12.2	8.8	10.9
1892-1896----------	1926	108.5	11.4	17.9	18.9	16.5	13.7	11.5	8.4	10.2
1893-1897----------	1927	105.9	11.4	17.5	18.2	16.0	13.4	11.2	8.1	10.1
1894-1898----------	1928	99.8	11.1	17.0	17.3	14.9	12.5	10.3	7.4	9.3
1895-1899----------	1929	95.1	11.0	16.6	16.6	14.0	11.8	9.6	6.8	8.7
1896-1900----------	1930	94.9	11.6	16.8	16.5	13.9	11.6	9.5	6.6	8.4
1897-1901----------	1931	90.1	11.2	16.2	15.8	13.1	10.9	8.9	6.2	7.8
1898-1902----------	1932	86.7	10.7	15.7	15.1	12.6	10.5	8.6	6.0	7.5
1899-1903----------	1933	81.3	10.2	14.9	14.3	11.9	9.7	7.9	5.6	6.8
1900-1904----------	1934	82.6	11.0	15.9	14.4	11.9	9.6	7.7	5.4	6.7
1901-1905----------	1935	80.0	11.7	15.7	13.8	11.1	8.9	7.1	5.1	6.6
1902-1906----------	1936	77.7	12.3	15.9	13.4	10.4	8.3	6.6	4.7	6.1
1903-1907----------	1937	77.7	13.3	16.5	13.2	10.1	7.9	6.3	4.5	5.9
1904-1908----------	1938	78.7	14.4	17.6	13.4	9.8	7.6	6.0	4.3	5.6
1905-1909----------	1939	78.0	15.2	18.3	13.4	9.5	7.1	5.5	3.9	5.1
1906-1910----------	1940	80.1	16.0	19.8	13.9	9.5	6.8	5.3	3.7	5.1
1907-1911----------	1941	82.5	17.7	21.0	14.4	9.5	6.7	5.0	3.5	4.7
1908-1912----------	1942	89.8	20.8	24.0	15.7	9.9	6.8	4.8	3.4	4.4
1909-1913----------	1943	97.4	19.6	27.5	18.7	11.2	7.4	5.1	3.4	4.5
1910-1914----------	1944	95.7	16.7	27.0	19.8	11.7	7.4	5.2	3.5	4.4
1911-1915----------	1945	98.4	16.4	29.1	21.0	11.9	7.4	5.0	3.3	4.3
1912-1916----------	1946	108.4	21.7	31.6	22.7	12.6	7.5	5.0	3.2	4.1
1913-1917----------	1947	111.7	24.2	32.1	23.5	12.9	7.4	4.7	3.0	3.9
1914-1918----------	1948	102.2	18.8	29.4	22.8	12.7	7.2	4.6	2.9	3.8
1915-1919----------	1949	101.4	16.8	29.1	23.1	13.4	7.4	4.6	3.0	4.0
1916-1920----------	1950	101.8	15.2	29.2	24.3	14.1	7.6	4.7	2.9	3.8
1917-1921----------	1951	105.9	15.1	29.4	26.3	15.3	8.2	4.8	3.0	3.8
1918-1922----------	1952	110.5	14.7	29.4	28.4	17.1	9.0	5.1	3.0	3.8
1919-1923----------	1953	111.5	13.5	28.2	29.6	18.3	9.7	5.3	3.1	3.8
1920-1924----------	1954	114.2	13.0	27.7	30.3	19.8	10.4	5.8	3.2	4.0
1921-1925----------	1955	113.7	12.0	25.7	30.3	20.7	11.3	6.2	3.5	4.0
1922-1926----------	1956	114.0	11.3	24.3	30.2	21.6	12.1	6.6	3.7	4.2
1923-1927----------	1957	115.3	11.0	23.1	30.3	22.5	12.9	7.1	4.0	4.4
1924-1928----------	1958	112.3	10.2	21.1	29.0	22.6	13.3	7.4	4.1	4.6
1925-1929----------	1959	111.7	9.6	19.7	28.0	23.0	14.0	8.0	4.4	5.0
1926-1930----------	1960	110.6	9.0	18.6	27.0	23.1	14.5	8.4	4.7	5.3
1927-1931----------	1961	110.4	8.5	17.6	26.3	23.3	15.1	8.9	5.0	5.7
1928-1932----------	1962	105.8	7.8	16.2	24.6	22.2	15.0	9.0	5.1	5.9
1929-1933----------	1963	103.4	7.5	15.3	23.5	21.8	14.9	9.1	5.3	6.0
1930-1934----------	1964	100.6	8.0	14.7	22.6	21.1	14.3	8.9	5.1	5.9
1931-1935----------	1965	91.4	7.5	13.7	20.6	18.9	12.9	8.0	4.6	5.2
1932-1936----------	1966	82.1	7.3	12.8	18.6	16.6	11.3	6.9	4.0	4.6
1933-1937----------	1967	75.8	6.7	12.5	17.5	15.4	10.2	6.1	3.5	3.9
1934-1938----------	1968	71.6	7.4	12.6	16.7	14.1	9.1	5.3	3.0	3.4
1935-1939----------	1969	71.1	7.0	13.0	17.2	14.0	8.9	5.2	2.8	3.0
1936-1940----------	1970	70.6	7.3	13.5	17.4	13.8	8.6	4.8	2.5	2.7
1937-1941----------	1971	64.9	7.0	13.3	15.9	12.5	7.6	4.2	2.2	2.2
1938-1942----------	1972	57.7	6.9	13.5	14.1	10.4	6.1	3.3	1.7	1.7
1939-1943----------	1973	53.5	7.1	13.7	13.3	9.0	5.0	2.7	1.4	1.3

TABLE 3B. CENTRAL BIRTH RATES FOR WHITE WOMEN DURING EACH YEAR 1917-73 BY AGE AND LIVE-BIRTH ORDER FOR GROUPS OF COHORTS FROM 1868-72 TO 1954-58--CON.

(RATES ARE SIMPLE AVERAGES OF THE RATES FOR SINGLE COHORTS IN TABLE 4B)

CURRENT AGE AND COHORT	CALENDAR YEAR	TOTAL	LIVE-BIRTH ORDER							
			1	2	3	4	5	6	7	8 AND HIGHER
35-39 YEARS										
1878-1882----------	1917	92.3	4.1	6.6	9.2	10.8	11.6	12.0	11.2	26.8
1879-1883----------	1918	91.3	4.2	6.7	9.1	10.8	11.5	11.7	10.9	26.4
1880-1884----------	1919	89.4	4.2	6.7	9.0	10.4	11.1	11.3	10.7	26.0
1881-1885----------	1920	88.9	4.4	6.7	9.1	10.3	11.0	11.1	10.5	25.8
1882-1886----------	1921	90.2	4.7	7.0	9.3	10.5	11.0	11.0	10.4	26.3
1883-1887----------	1922	84.0	4.3	6.7	8.8	9.8	10.2	10.2	9.6	24.4
1884-1888----------	1923	83.6	4.2	6.8	8.9	9.8	10.1	10.0	9.4	24.4
1885-1889----------	1924	82.8	4.3	6.8	9.0	9.7	9.9	9.8	9.2	24.1
1886-1890----------	1925	79.4	4.2	6.6	8.7	9.6	9.4	9.3	8.6	23.0
1887-1891----------	1926	75.6	4.0	6.4	8.4	9.2	9.0	8.7	8.2	21.7
1888-1892----------	1927	73.8	4.1	6.3	8.2	8.8	8.6	8.6	7.9	21.3
1889-1893----------	1928	68.6	3.9	6.1	7.8	8.2	8.1	7.8	7.3	19.4
1890-1894----------	1929	63.8	3.7	5.8	7.4	7.7	7.5	7.2	6.7	17.8
1891-1895----------	1930	63.0	3.9	6.0	7.4	7.7	7.4	7.1	6.5	17.0
1892-1896----------	1931	59.0	3.7	5.6	7.0	7.3	7.0	6.6	6.0	15.8
1893-1897----------	1932	56.2	3.5	5.4	6.7	6.9	6.6	6.3	5.8	15.0
1894-1898----------	1933	52.3	3.2	5.1	6.3	6.6	6.2	5.9	5.4	13.6
1895-1899----------	1934	52.3	3.4	5.4	6.4	6.6	6.2	5.8	5.2	13.3
1896-1900----------	1935	50.5	3.5	5.4	6.3	6.2	5.8	5.4	4.9	13.0
1897-1901----------	1936	48.2	3.7	5.4	6.2	5.9	5.4	5.1	4.5	12.0
1898-1902----------	1937	47.1	3.9	5.5	6.1	5.8	5.1	4.8	4.3	11.6
1899-1903----------	1938	46.7	4.2	5.9	6.1	5.7	5.1	4.6	4.1	11.0
1900-1904----------	1939	45.0	4.5	6.2	6.2	5.5	4.7	4.3	3.7	9.9
1901-1905----------	1940	44.5	4.8	6.6	6.3	5.3	4.6	4.0	3.5	9.4
1902-1906----------	1941	44.4	5.2	7.1	6.5	5.4	4.4	3.8	3.3	8.7
1903-1907----------	1942	46.7	6.3	8.0	7.2	5.6	4.5	3.8	3.1	8.2
1904-1908----------	1943	51.4	6.7	9.4	8.5	6.4	4.9	3.9	3.3	8.3
1905-1909----------	1944	52.7	6.5	10.1	9.2	6.8	5.0	4.0	3.1	8.0
1906-1910----------	1945	54.8	6.6	11.0	10.2	7.2	5.1	3.9	3.1	7.7
1907-1911----------	1946	56.9	7.9	11.8	10.7	7.4	5.1	3.8	2.9	7.3
1908-1912----------	1947	57.6	8.7	11.9	10.9	7.6	5.1	3.7	2.8	6.9
1909-1913----------	1948	53.3	7.2	10.9	10.4	7.4	4.9	3.5	2.6	6.4
1910-1914----------	1949	52.2	6.5	10.5	10.3	7.4	4.9	3.5	2.6	6.5
1911-1915----------	1950	52.1	6.0	10.4	10.6	7.8	5.1	3.5	2.6	6.1
1912-1916----------	1951	53.1	5.7	10.4	11.2	8.3	5.3	3.7	2.5	6.0
1913-1917----------	1952	55.1	5.6	10.4	12.0	9.0	5.8	3.8	2.6	5.9
1914-1918----------	1953	55.4	5.3	9.9	12.2	9.7	6.2	3.9	2.6	5.6
1915-1919----------	1954	56.9	5.0	9.8	12.7	10.3	6.6	4.1	2.8	5.6
1916-1920----------	1955	56.9	4.7	9.3	12.6	10.6	6.9	4.4	2.8	5.6
1917-1921----------	1956	57.2	4.3	8.9	12.6	10.8	7.3	4.6	3.0	5.7
1918-1922----------	1957	57.7	4.2	8.4	12.3	11.2	7.7	4.9	3.1	5.9
1919-1923----------	1958	56.1	3.8	7.7	11.7	11.0	7.8	5.1	3.3	5.7
1920-1924----------	1959	55.8	3.6	7.1	11.2	11.0	8.1	5.3	3.4	6.1
1921-1925----------	1960	54.7	3.3	6.6	10.6	10.9	8.2	5.4	3.5	6.2
1922-1926----------	1961	54.1	3.1	6.2	10.2	10.5	8.3	5.7	3.7	6.4
1923-1927----------	1962	51.2	2.8	5.6	9.3	9.9	8.0	5.5	3.6	6.5
1924-1928----------	1963	49.6	2.7	5.2	8.8	9.5	7.7	5.5	3.6	6.6
1925-1929----------	1964	48.5	3.0	5.0	8.3	9.2	7.5	5.3	3.7	6.5
1926-1930----------	1965	44.7	2.8	4.5	7.5	8.4	7.0	5.0	3.3	6.2
1927-1931----------	1966	40.1	2.6	4.1	6.8	7.5	6.2	4.4	3.1	5.4
1928-1932----------	1967	36.8	2.3	3.9	6.3	6.9	5.7	4.1	2.7	4.9
1929-1933----------	1968	34.1	2.5	3.7	5.7	6.3	5.2	3.8	2.5	4.4
1930-1934----------	1969	32.1	2.1	3.6	5.4	6.0	5.0	3.5	2.4	4.1
1931-1935----------	1970	30.4	2.1	3.5	5.2	5.6	4.7	3.3	2.2	3.8
1932-1936----------	1971	27.2	1.9	3.2	4.6	5.1	4.2	3.0	1.9	3.3
1933-1937----------	1972	23.5	1.8	3.0	4.1	4.3	3.5	2.5	1.6	2.7
1934-1938----------	1973	20.8	1.7	3.0	3.7	3.7	3.0	2.1	1.4	2.2

TABLE 3B. CENTRAL BIRTH RATES FOR WHITE WOMEN DURING EACH YEAR 1917-73 BY AGE AND LIVE-BIRTH ORDER FOR GROUPS OF COHORTS FROM 1868-72 TO 1954-58--CON.

(RATES ARE SIMPLE AVERAGES OF THE RATES FOR SINGLE COHORTS IN TABLE 4B)

CURRENT AGE AND COHORT	CALENDAR YEAR	TOTAL	LIVE-BIRTH ORDER							
			1	2	3	4	5	6	7	8 AND HIGHER
40-44 YEARS										
1873-1877----------	1917	35.0	0.9	1.4	1.9	2.6	3.1	3.7	3.8	17.6
1874-1878----------	1918	34.7	0.9	1.4	2.0	2.6	3.2	3.6	3.8	17.2
1875-1879----------	1919	34.1	1.0	1.3	2.0	2.6	3.1	3.5	3.7	16.9
1876-1880----------	1920	34.3	1.0	1.4	2.0	2.6	3.0	3.5	3.7	17.1
1877-1881----------	1921	34.6	1.0	1.4	2.0	2.6	3.1	3.5	3.7	17.3
1878-1882----------	1922	32.1	0.9	1.3	1.9	2.5	2.8	3.2	3.5	16.0
1879-1883----------	1923	31.5	0.9	1.3	1.8	2.4	2.8	3.2	3.4	15.7
1880-1884----------	1924	31.5	0.9	1.3	1.9	2.4	2.8	3.1	3.3	15.8
1881-1885----------	1925	30.1	0.9	1.3	1.9	2.3	2.6	2.9	3.1	15.1
1882-1886----------	1926	28.3	0.9	1.3	1.7	2.2	2.5	2.7	2.9	14.1
1883-1887----------	1927	27.8	0.9	1.2	1.8	2.1	2.4	2.7	2.8	13.9
1884-1888----------	1928	25.9	0.9	1.2	1.6	2.0	2.3	2.5	2.6	12.8
1885-1889----------	1929	23.9	0.8	1.1	1.6	1.9	2.1	2.3	2.4	11.7
1886-1890----------	1930	23.8	0.8	1.1	1.6	2.0	2.2	2.4	2.3	11.4
1887-1891----------	1931	22.3	0.8	1.1	1.5	1.8	2.0	2.2	2.2	10.7
1888-1892----------	1932	21.5	0.8	1.1	1.4	1.8	2.0	2.1	2.2	10.1
1889-1893----------	1933	20.0	0.7	1.0	1.4	1.7	1.9	2.0	2.0	9.3
1890-1894----------	1934	19.6	0.7	0.9	1.4	1.7	1.8	1.9	2.0	9.2
1891-1895----------	1935	18.4	0.7	0.9	1.3	1.6	1.7	1.8	1.8	8.6
1892-1896----------	1936	17.2	0.7	0.9	1.3	1.5	1.6	1.7	1.7	7.8
1893-1897----------	1937	16.3	0.7	0.9	1.3	1.5	1.5	1.6	1.5	7.3
1894-1898----------	1938	16.1	0.7	1.0	1.3	1.5	1.5	1.6	1.5	7.0
1895-1899----------	1939	15.4	0.8	1.0	1.3	1.5	1.5	1.5	1.4	6.4
1896-1900----------	1940	14.7	0.8	1.0	1.3	1.4	1.4	1.4	1.3	6.1
1897-1901----------	1941	14.2	0.9	1.1	1.3	1.4	1.4	1.3	1.2	5.6
1898-1902----------	1942	14.3	1.0	1.2	1.4	1.4	1.4	1.3	1.2	5.4
1899-1903----------	1943	15.3	1.1	1.4	1.6	1.6	1.5	1.4	1.3	5.4
1900-1904----------	1944	16.0	1.2	1.6	1.8	1.7	1.6	1.4	1.3	5.4
1901-1905----------	1945	16.3	1.3	1.8	2.0	1.8	1.5	1.4	1.3	5.2
1902-1906----------	1946	16.2	1.5	2.0	2.1	1.8	1.6	1.3	1.2	4.7
1903-1907----------	1947	16.4	1.6	2.1	2.2	1.9	1.6	1.3	1.1	4.6
1904-1908----------	1948	15.1	1.4	2.0	2.1	1.8	1.5	1.2	1.0	4.1
1905-1909----------	1949	14.5	1.4	1.9	2.0	1.8	1.4	1.1	0.9	4.0
1906-1910----------	1950	14.5	1.3	1.9	2.1	1.8	1.5	1.2	1.0	3.7
1907-1911----------	1951	14.7	1.3	1.9	2.2	2.0	1.5	1.2	1.0	3.6
1908-1912----------	1952	15.0	1.3	1.9	2.4	2.1	1.7	1.2	1.0	3.4
1909-1913----------	1953	15.2	1.2	2.0	2.4	2.3	1.7	1.3	1.0	3.3
1910-1914----------	1954	15.6	1.2	1.9	2.6	2.3	1.9	1.4	1.0	3.3
1911-1915----------	1955	15.5	1.1	1.9	2.6	2.4	2.0	1.4	1.0	3.1
1912-1916----------	1956	15.4	1.0	1.8	2.6	2.4	2.0	1.4	1.1	3.1
1913-1917----------	1957	15.7	1.0	1.7	2.5	2.6	2.1	1.6	1.1	3.1
1914-1918----------	1958	15.1	0.9	1.6	2.4	2.5	2.1	1.5	1.1	3.0
1915-1919----------	1959	15.2	0.9	1.5	2.3	2.6	2.1	1.6	1.2	3.0
1916-1920----------	1960	15.1	0.8	1.4	2.3	2.5	2.2	1.7	1.2	3.0
1917-1921----------	1961	15.2	0.8	1.4	2.2	2.6	2.2	1.6	1.3	3.1
1918-1922----------	1962	14.5	0.7	1.3	2.1	2.4	2.1	1.6	1.2	3.1
1919-1923----------	1963	14.0	0.7	1.2	1.9	2.2	2.1	1.6	1.2	3.1
1920-1924----------	1964	13.4	0.7	1.0	1.8	2.1	2.0	1.6	1.2	3.0
1921-1925----------	1965	12.7	0.7	1.0	1.7	2.0	1.9	1.5	1.1	2.8
1922-1926----------	1966	11.4	0.6	0.9	1.5	1.8	1.7	1.3	1.0	2.6
1923-1927----------	1967	10.2	0.5	0.8	1.3	1.7	1.5	1.2	0.9	2.3
1924-1928----------	1968	9.3	0.6	0.7	1.2	1.4	1.3	1.1	0.9	2.1
1925-1929----------	1969	8.6	0.4	0.7	1.1	1.3	1.3	1.0	0.8	2.0
1926-1930----------	1970	7.9	0.4	0.7	1.0	1.2	1.2	0.9	0.7	1.8
1927-1931----------	1971	6.8	0.4	0.6	0.8	1.0	1.0	0.8	0.6	1.6
1928-1932----------	1972	6.0	0.4	0.5	0.7	0.9	0.8	0.7	0.6	1.4
1929-1933----------	1973	5.2	0.3	0.5	0.6	0.7	0.7	0.6	0.5	1.3

TABLE 3B. CENTRAL BIRTH RATES FOR WHITE WOMEN DURING EACH YEAR 1917-73 BY AGE AND LIVE-BIRTH ORDER FOR GROUPS OF COHORTS FROM 1868-72 TO 1954-58--CON.

(RATES ARE SIMPLE AVERAGES OF THE RATES FOR SINGLE COHORTS IN TABLE 4B)

CURRENT AGE AND COHORT	CALENDAR YEAR	TOTAL	LIVE-BIRTH ORDER							
			1	2	3	4	5	6	7	8 AND HIGHER
45-49 YEARS										
1868-1872----------	1917	4.6	0.1	0.1	0.1	0.3	0.3	0.3	0.4	3.0
1869-1873----------	1918	4.7	0.1	0.1	0.1	0.3	0.3	0.4	0.4	3.0
1870-1874----------	1919	4.3	0.1	0.1	0.1	0.2	0.3	0.3	0.3	2.9
1871-1875----------	1920	4.7	0.1	0.1	0.1	0.3	0.3	0.4	0.4	3.0
1872-1876----------	1921	4.4	0.1	0.1	0.1	0.2	0.3	0.3	0.3	3.0
1873-1877----------	1922	4.0	0.1	0.1	0.1	0.2	0.2	0.3	0.3	2.7
1874-1878----------	1923	3.9	0.1	0.1	0.1	0.2	0.2	0.3	0.3	2.6
1875-1879----------	1924	3.9	0.1	0.1	0.1	0.2	0.2	0.3	0.3	2.6
1876-1880----------	1925	3.8	0.1	0.1	0.1	0.2	0.2	0.3	0.3	2.5
1877-1881----------	1926	3.6	0.1	0.1	0.1	0.2	0.2	0.3	0.3	2.3
1878-1882----------	1927	3.5	0.1	0.1	0.1	0.2	0.2	0.3	0.3	2.2
1879-1883----------	1928	3.1	0.1	0.1	0.1	0.1	0.2	0.2	0.3	2.0
1880-1884----------	1929	2.9	0.1	0.1	0.1	0.1	0.2	0.2	0.2	1.9
1881-1885----------	1930	2.8	0.1	0.1	0.1	0.1	0.2	0.2	0.2	1.8
1882-1886----------	1931	2.5	0.0	0.1	0.1	0.1	0.1	0.2	0.2	1.7
1883-1887----------	1932	2.5	0.0	0.1	0.1	0.1	0.2	0.2	0.2	1.6
1884-1888----------	1933	2.4	0.0	0.1	0.1	0.1	0.2	0.2	0.2	1.5
1885-1889----------	1934	2.2	0.0	0.0	0.1	0.1	0.2	0.1	0.2	1.5
1886-1890----------	1935	2.0	0.0	0.0	0.1	0.1	0.1	0.1	0.2	1.4
1887-1891----------	1936	1.9	0.0	0.0	0.1	0.1	0.1	0.1	0.2	1.3
1888-1892----------	1937	1.8	0.0	0.0	0.1	0.1	0.1	0.1	0.2	1.2
1889-1893----------	1938	1.6	0.0	0.0	0.1	0.1	0.1	0.1	0.1	1.1
1890-1894----------	1939	1.6	0.0	0.0	0.1	0.1	0.1	0.1	0.2	1.0
1891-1895----------	1940	1.4	0.0	0.0	0.1	0.1	0.1	0.1	0.1	0.9
1892-1896----------	1941	1.4	0.0	0.1	0.1	0.1	0.1	0.1	0.1	0.8
1893-1897----------	1942	1.4	0.0	0.1	0.1	0.1	0.1	0.1	0.1	0.8
1894-1898----------	1943	1.5	0.1	0.1	0.1	0.1	0.1	0.1	0.1	0.8
1895-1899----------	1944	1.4	0.1	0.1	0.1	0.1	0.1	0.1	0.1	0.7
1896-1900----------	1945	1.4	0.1	0.1	0.1	0.1	0.1	0.1	0.1	0.7
1897-1901----------	1946	1.4	0.1	0.1	0.1	0.1	0.1	0.1	0.1	0.7
1898-1902----------	1947	1.4	0.1	0.1	0.1	0.1	0.1	0.1	0.1	0.7
1899-1903----------	1948	1.3	0.1	0.1	0.1	0.1	0.1	0.1	0.1	0.6
1900-1904----------	1949	1.3	0.1	0.1	0.1	0.1	0.1	0.1	0.1	0.6
1901-1905----------	1950	1.2	0.1	0.1	0.1	0.1	0.1	0.1	0.1	0.5
1902-1906----------	1951	1.2	0.1	0.1	0.1	0.1	0.1	0.1	0.1	0.5
1903-1907----------	1952	1.1	0.1	0.1	0.1	0.1	0.1	0.1	0.1	0.4
1904-1908----------	1953	1.1	0.1	0.1	0.1	0.1	0.1	0.1	0.1	0.4
1905-1909----------	1954	1.1	0.1	0.1	0.1	0.1	0.1	0.1	0.1	0.4
1906-1910----------	1955	1.1	0.1	0.1	0.1	0.1	0.1	0.1	0.1	0.4
1907-1911----------	1956	1.1	0.1	0.1	0.1	0.1	0.1	0.1	0.1	0.4
1908-1912----------	1957	1.1	0.1	0.1	0.1	0.1	0.1	0.1	0.1	0.4
1909-1913----------	1958	1.0	0.1	0.1	0.1	0.1	0.1	0.1	0.1	0.3
1910-1914----------	1959	1.0	0.1	0.1	0.1	0.1	0.1	0.1	0.1	0.3
1911-1915----------	1960	0.9	0.0	0.1	0.1	0.1	0.1	0.1	0.1	0.3
1912-1916----------	1961	0.9	0.0	0.1	0.1	0.1	0.1	0.1	0.1	0.3
1913-1917----------	1962	0.9	0.0	0.1	0.1	0.1	0.1	0.1	0.1	0.3
1914-1918----------	1963	0.9	0.0	0.1	0.1	0.1	0.1	0.1	0.1	0.3
1915-1919----------	1964	0.8	0.0	0.0	0.1	0.1	0.1	0.1	0.1	0.3
1916-1920----------	1965	0.7	0.0	0.0	0.1	0.1	0.1	0.1	0.1	0.2
1917-1921----------	1966	0.8	0.0	0.0	0.1	0.1	0.1	0.1	0.1	0.3
1918-1922----------	1967	0.7	0.0	0.0	0.1	0.1	0.1	0.1	0.1	0.2
1919-1923----------	1968	0.7	0.0	0.0	0.1	0.1	0.1	0.1	0.1	0.2
1920-1924----------	1969	0.5	0.0	0.0	0.0	0.1	0.1	0.1	0.0	0.2
1921-1925----------	1970	0.4	0.0	0.0	0.0	0.1	0.1	0.1	0.0	0.1
1922-1926----------	1971	0.2	0.0	0.0	0.0	0.0	0.0	0.1	0.0	0.1
1923-1927----------	1972	0.1	0.0	0.0	0.0	0.0	0.0	0.0	0.0	0.1
1924-1928----------	1973	0.1	0.0	0.0	0.0	0.0	0.0	0.0	0.0	0.1

TABLE 3C. CENTRAL BIRTH RATES FOR ALL OTHER WOMEN DURING EACH YEAR 1917-73 BY AGE AND LIVE-BIRTH ORDER FOR GROUPS OF COHORTS FROM 1868-72 TO 1954-58

(RATES ARE SIMPLE AVERAGES OF THE RATES FOR SINGLE COHORTS IN TABLE 4C)

CURRENT AGE AND COHORT	CALENDAR YEAR	TOTAL	LIVE-BIRTH ORDER							
			1	2	3	4	5	6	7	8 AND HIGHER
15-19 YEARS										
1898-1902----------	1917	103.2	76.3	21.3	4.7	0.9	*	*	*	*
1899-1903----------	1918	99.6	73.9	20.0	4.9	0.8	*	*	*	*
1900-1904----------	1919	93.2	68.6	19.1	4.6	0.9	*	*	*	*
1901-1905----------	1920	106.1	80.9	19.7	4.7	0.8	*	*	*	*
1902-1906----------	1921	111.3	81.7	23.4	5.2	1.0	*	*	*	*
1903-1907----------	1922	100.4	71.5	22.9	5.0	1.0	*	*	*	*
1904-1908----------	1923	104.5	75.1	22.5	5.7	1.2	*	*	*	*
1905-1909----------	1924	110.6	80.2	23.2	5.9	1.3	*	*	*	*
1906-1910----------	1925	112.0	82.0	22.9	5.7	1.4	*	*	*	*
1907-1911----------	1926	111.1	79.6	24.1	6.0	1.4	*	*	*	*
1908-1912----------	1927	106.4	75.6	23.5	6.0	1.3	*	*	*	*
1909-1913----------	1928	100.8	71.6	21.9	5.9	1.4	*	*	*	*
1910-1914----------	1929	97.9	69.1	22.0	5.6	1.2	*	*	*	*
1911-1915----------	1930	99.9	71.4	21.9	5.4	1.2	*	*	*	*
1912-1916----------	1931	96.8	68.8	21.4	5.4	1.2	*	*	*	*
1913-1917----------	1932	98.3	69.8	21.8	5.5	1.2	*	*	*	*
1914-1918----------	1933	92.1	64.9	20.8	5.2	1.2	*	*	*	*
1915-1919----------	1934	96.9	69.0	21.3	5.5	1.1	*	*	*	*
1916-1920----------	1935	100.6	71.2	22.6	5.6	1.2	*	*	*	*
1917-1921----------	1936	99.5	69.2	23.2	5.9	1.2	*	*	*	*
1918-1922----------	1937	106.1	73.9	24.7	6.2	1.3	*	*	*	*
1919-1923----------	1938	108.7	75.7	25.1	6.5	1.4	*	*	*	*
1920-1924----------	1939	108.1	73.3	26.4	7.0	1.4	*	*	*	*
1921-1925----------	1940	109.5	70.6	28.4	8.5	2.0	*	*	*	*
1922-1926----------	1941	113.6	72.9	29.9	8.8	2.0	*	*	*	*
1923-1927----------	1942	117.3	75.0	30.8	9.4	2.1	*	*	*	*
1924-1928----------	1943	119.7	75.3	32.4	9.7	2.3	*	*	*	*
1925-1929----------	1944	110.4	68.3	30.1	9.6	2.4	*	*	*	*
1926-1930----------	1945	107.3	67.0	29.2	8.8	2.3	*	*	*	*
1927-1931----------	1946	111.7	69.8	30.4	9.3	2.2	*	*	*	*
1928-1932----------	1947	133.5	86.1	34.6	10.3	2.5	*	*	*	*
1929-1933----------	1948	141.9	87.6	40.1	11.5	2.7	*	*	*	*
1930-1934----------	1949	144.4	84.6	43.5	13.4	2.9	*	*	*	*
1931-1935----------	1950	145.0	83.2	43.9	14.5	3.4	*	*	*	*
1932-1936----------	1951	148.2	85.7	43.6	15.2	3.7	*	*	*	*
1933-1937----------	1952	145.7	83.4	42.7	15.5	4.1	*	*	*	*
1934-1938----------	1953	148.3	85.6	43.1	15.4	4.2	*	*	*	*
1935-1939----------	1954	153.0	89.3	43.5	15.9	4.3	*	*	*	*
1936-1940----------	1955	152.5	87.1	45.0	16.0	4.4	*	*	*	*
1937-1941----------	1956	156.9	89.3	46.5	16.6	4.5	*	*	*	*
1938-1942----------	1957	156.7	89.2	46.0	16.9	4.6	*	*	*	*
1939-1943----------	1958	151.9	84.4	45.6	17.1	4.8	*	*	*	*
1940-1944----------	1959	150.9	84.3	44.8	17.0	4.8	*	*	*	*
1941-1945----------	1960	146.6	81.8	43.5	16.5	4.8	*	*	*	*
1942-1946----------	1961	143.8	80.9	41.9	16.3	4.7	*	*	*	*
1943-1947----------	1962	140.1	79.0	40.9	15.7	4.5	*	*	*	*
1944-1948----------	1963	139.3	79.6	40.3	15.0	4.4	*	*	*	*
1945-1949----------	1964	139.7	81.1	39.8	14.7	4.1	*	*	*	*
1946-1950----------	1965	136.4	81.1	37.8	13.6	3.9	*	*	*	*
1947-1951----------	1966	134.4	83.1	36.1	12.0	3.2	*	*	*	*
1948-1952----------	1967	132.5	84.2	34.6	10.9	2.8	*	*	*	*
1949-1953----------	1968	130.2	86.0	32.4	9.5	2.3	*	*	*	*
1950-1954----------	1969	129.9	87.5	31.5	8.9	2.0	*	*	*	*
1951-1955----------	1970	133.4	90.8	32.2	8.6	1.8	*	*	*	*
1952-1956----------	1971	129.1	88.9	30.8	7.8	1.6	*	*	*	*
1953-1957----------	1972	124.7	88.3	28.3	6.8	1.3	*	*	*	*
1954-1958----------	1973	118.4	84.3	26.6	6.3	1.2	*	*	*	*

TABLE 3C. CENTRAL BIRTH RATES FOR ALL OTHER WOMEN DURING EACH YEAR 1917-73 BY AGE AND LIVE-BIRTH ORDER FOR GROUPS OF COHORTS FROM 1868-72 TO 1954-58--CON.

(RATES ARE SIMPLE AVERAGES OF THE RATES FOR SINGLE COHORTS IN TABLE 4C)

CURRENT AGE AND COHORT	CALENDAR YEAR	TOTAL	LIVE-BIRTH ORDER							
			1	2	3	4	5	6	7	8 AND HIGHER
20-24 YEARS										
1893-1897----------	1917	183.3	60.2	53.9	36.4	19.0	8.0	3.6	1.4	0.8
1894-1898----------	1918	182.5	61.1	50.6	38.4	19.3	7.6	3.5	1.1	0.9
1895-1899----------	1919	174.0	56.0	50.4	35.8	18.4	7.9	3.3	1.4	0.8
1896-1900----------	1920	188.0	66.6	53.2	36.5	18.7	7.8	3.4	1.1	0.7
1897-1901----------	1921	191.5	62.8	54.0	39.5	20.6	8.6	3.8	1.3	0.9
1898-1902----------	1922	180.3	54.4	55.0	36.8	19.6	8.5	3.8	1.3	0.9
1899-1903----------	1923	179.3	52.8	52.3	39.0	20.0	8.9	3.9	1.5	0.9
1900-1904----------	1924	188.9	57.2	52.6	41.8	21.2	9.4	4.3	1.5	0.9
1901-1905----------	1925	182.3	56.5	50.2	37.5	22.1	9.1	4.2	1.7	1.0
1902-1906----------	1926	176.6	53.3	49.7	35.5	21.6	9.4	4.3	1.6	1.2
1903-1907----------	1927	164.4	48.1	45.7	34.9	19.9	9.4	3.8	1.5	1.1
1904-1908----------	1928	152.6	44.1	41.7	32.6	18.8	9.0	3.8	1.5	1.1
1905-1909----------	1929	147.3	43.4	41.1	31.0	17.8	8.6	3.4	1.2	0.8
1906-1910----------	1930	149.4	45.0	41.6	31.1	17.9	8.4	3.3	1.2	0.9
1907-1911----------	1931	145.4	43.8	41.3	30.1	17.3	7.8	3.3	1.1	0.7
1908-1912----------	1932	148.9	44.8	43.1	31.2	17.5	7.7	2.9	1.0	0.7
1909-1913----------	1933	141.6	41.0	40.7	30.4	17.3	7.6	3.0	1.0	0.6
1910-1914----------	1934	148.6	44.4	41.9	31.6	18.0	7.9	3.0	1.1	0.7
1911-1915----------	1935	148.4	44.0	41.8	31.0	18.4	8.2	3.2	1.1	0.7
1912-1916----------	1936	145.5	42.0	42.3	30.5	17.8	8.0	3.1	1.1	0.7
1913-1917----------	1937	151.9	43.6	44.0	32.4	18.4	8.3	3.3	1.2	0.7
1914-1918----------	1938	152.7	43.2	43.8	33.3	18.7	8.4	3.4	1.2	0.7
1915-1919----------	1939	153.0	42.8	44.2	33.1	18.8	8.8	3.4	1.2	0.7
1916-1920----------	1940	158.4	42.4	44.0	34.9	21.1	9.8	3.9	1.5	0.8
1917-1921----------	1941	163.2	44.1	45.6	35.5	21.2	10.4	4.1	1.4	0.9
1918-1922----------	1942	166.3	46.5	45.5	35.7	21.7	10.6	4.1	1.4	0.8
1919-1923----------	1943	168.6	45.4	46.9	36.2	22.3	10.9	4.5	1.6	0.8
1920-1924----------	1944	162.3	42.5	43.4	35.7	22.7	11.2	4.5	1.5	0.8
1921-1925----------	1945	153.3	41.2	40.8	32.6	21.1	10.8	4.4	1.6	0.8
1922-1926----------	1946	175.0	50.6	50.0	35.2	21.5	10.8	4.4	1.6	0.9
1923-1927----------	1947	199.8	65.2	56.3	38.1	21.9	11.0	4.6	1.7	1.0
1924-1928----------	1948	212.8	60.8	64.8	44.0	24.2	11.5	4.7	1.8	1.0
1925-1929----------	1949	219.2	56.5	66.7	48.4	27.0	12.7	5.1	1.8	1.0
1926-1930----------	1950	221.9	52.6	65.1	52.9	29.4	13.7	5.3	1.9	1.0
1927-1931----------	1951	227.6	51.9	63.6	55.0	33.4	15.3	5.7	1.8	0.9
1928-1932----------	1952	228.2	51.3	60.5	54.2	35.7	16.9	6.5	2.1	1.0
1929-1933----------	1953	234.3	53.7	61.4	53.2	36.5	18.8	7.2	2.4	1.1
1930-1934----------	1954	246.4	57.6	64.3	55.3	36.9	19.9	8.3	2.9	1.2
1931-1935----------	1955	255.5	58.8	68.1	56.8	37.9	20.7	8.7	3.1	1.4
1932-1936----------	1956	268.9	61.2	72.5	59.9	39.9	21.3	9.2	3.4	1.5
1933-1937----------	1957	275.1	61.6	72.9	62.4	40.7	22.6	9.8	3.4	1.7
1934-1938----------	1958	273.3	58.8	71.8	62.6	41.8	23.2	10.0	3.4	1.7
1935-1939----------	1959	273.2	58.1	70.9	61.8	42.8	23.5	10.4	3.9	1.8
1936-1940----------	1960	267.6	57.8	68.4	60.8	41.2	23.1	10.5	4.0	1.8
1937-1941----------	1961	264.8	57.4	67.6	59.0	41.3	23.1	10.6	4.0	1.8
1938-1942----------	1962	257.0	56.8	65.2	57.2	39.2	22.7	10.4	3.8	1.7
1939-1943----------	1963	249.7	57.6	64.5	54.1	37.1	21.4	9.6	3.7	1.7
1940-1944----------	1964	242.2	58.9	63.3	51.5	34.6	19.6	9.1	3.4	1.8
1941-1945----------	1965	226.2	59.2	60.6	46.9	30.8	17.1	7.5	2.9	1.2
1942-1946----------	1966	211.9	60.9	58.1	42.6	26.4	14.3	6.4	2.2	1.0
1943-1947----------	1967	198.6	61.2	56.7	38.3	22.6	12.0	5.1	1.9	0.8
1944-1948----------	1968	188.4	63.3	54.1	35.4	19.9	9.8	3.9	1.4	0.6
1945-1949----------	1969	187.6	64.9	55.8	34.5	18.5	8.7	3.4	1.2	0.6
1946-1950----------	1970	189.9	66.6	58.6	35.1	17.6	7.6	2.9	1.0	0.5
1947-1951----------	1971	179.7	63.4	57.7	33.1	15.6	6.5	2.3	0.7	0.4
1948-1952----------	1972	159.8	58.7	52.0	28.5	13.1	5.1	1.6	0.5	0.3
1949-1953----------	1973	149.2	54.7	50.5	26.7	11.3	4.1	1.3	0.4	0.2

TABLE 3C. CENTRAL BIRTH RATES FOR ALL OTHER WOMEN DURING EACH YEAR 1917-73 BY AGE AND LIVE-BIRTH ORDER FOR GROUPS OF COHORTS FROM 1868-72 TO 1954-58--CON.

(RATES ARE SIMPLE AVERAGES OF THE RATES FOR SINGLE COHORTS IN TABLE 4C)

CURRENT AGE AND COHORT	CALENDAR YEAR	TOTAL	LIVE-BIRTH ORDER							
			1	2	3	4	5	6	7	8 AND HIGHER
25-29 YEARS										
1888-1892----------	1917	145.4	19.1	23.2	26.9	24.8	19.1	15.0	8.9	8.4
1889-1893----------	1918	141.3	20.2	21.7	27.6	24.2	18.0	14.4	7.9	7.3
1890-1894----------	1919	145.4	18.3	23.5	27.3	24.9	19.8	14.5	8.9	8.2
1891-1895----------	1920	156.6	22.2	25.9	29.5	27.3	20.2	15.2	8.4	7.9
1892-1896----------	1921	162.6	20.0	25.4	30.8	28.3	21.6	16.4	10.4	9.7
1893-1897----------	1922	149.5	17.2	25.2	27.7	26.0	20.0	15.5	9.2	8.7
1894-1898----------	1923	147.1	16.1	23.2	28.0	25.7	20.3	15.2	9.4	9.2
1895-1899----------	1924	153.9	16.3	21.7	29.9	27.6	21.8	16.9	10.2	9.5
1896-1900----------	1925	151.0	16.5	21.5	27.0	28.3	20.9	16.0	10.0	10.8
1897-1901----------	1926	146.6	14.9	20.8	24.9	27.4	21.2	16.7	9.8	10.9
1898-1902----------	1927	136.4	13.8	18.2	22.9	24.5	21.6	15.4	9.8	10.2
1899-1903----------	1928	122.9	12.0	15.9	20.6	22.2	19.5	14.2	8.8	9.7
1900-1904----------	1929	116.8	11.6	15.3	19.2	20.7	19.3	13.8	8.1	8.8
1901-1905----------	1930	114.3	12.1	15.6	18.9	20.2	18.0	13.2	8.1	8.2
1902-1906----------	1931	110.7	11.5	15.1	18.4	20.0	17.2	13.0	7.8	7.7
1903-1907----------	1932	109.7	11.6	15.0	18.3	20.1	17.3	12.5	7.6	7.3
1904-1908----------	1933	105.0	10.4	14.3	18.0	19.2	17.0	12.2	7.2	6.7
1905-1909----------	1934	107.3	11.3	14.5	18.0	19.8	17.2	12.3	7.1	7.1
1906-1910----------	1935	103.1	11.0	14.3	17.3	18.9	16.5	11.6	6.8	6.7
1907-1911----------	1936	101.8	11.0	14.6	16.8	18.6	16.3	11.6	6.6	6.3
1908-1912----------	1937	104.6	11.1	15.0	17.5	18.7	16.7	11.9	7.1	6.6
1909-1913----------	1938	106.8	11.6	15.4	18.3	19.1	16.7	12.1	7.1	6.5
1910-1914----------	1939	107.4	12.1	15.2	18.1	19.2	16.7	12.2	7.2	6.7
1911-1915----------	1940	109.8	12.3	15.4	18.1	19.5	16.9	12.6	7.6	7.4
1912-1916----------	1941	113.2	13.2	16.4	18.7	19.5	17.4	12.8	7.7	7.5
1913-1917----------	1942	115.3	14.6	17.3	19.0	19.4	17.3	12.7	7.6	7.4
1914-1918----------	1943	121.6	15.3	18.9	19.9	20.5	18.1	13.1	8.0	7.8
1915-1919----------	1944	123.4	15.2	18.8	20.5	20.6	18.4	13.7	8.2	8.0
1916-1920----------	1945	120.4	14.9	18.1	19.3	20.0	18.2	13.6	8.4	7.9
1917-1921----------	1946	132.7	18.5	22.4	21.9	21.1	18.6	13.6	8.4	8.2
1918-1922----------	1947	142.1	22.8	25.1	23.6	21.7	18.4	13.6	8.6	8.3
1919-1923----------	1948	149.6	21.8	27.6	26.1	22.9	19.4	14.1	8.9	8.8
1920-1924----------	1949	154.9	21.0	28.8	27.9	24.4	20.0	14.7	9.1	9.0
1921-1925----------	1950	160.8	20.2	28.9	30.1	26.7	21.3	15.3	9.3	9.0
1922-1926----------	1951	169.1	20.2	28.8	32.3	29.5	22.9	16.5	9.7	9.2
1923-1927----------	1952	176.3	20.3	29.0	32.5	31.5	25.3	17.5	10.6	9.6
1924-1928----------	1953	183.9	19.9	29.3	33.1	32.9	27.6	19.2	11.6	10.3
1925-1929----------	1954	192.0	20.3	29.2	33.1	34.4	29.8	21.0	12.7	11.5
1926-1930----------	1955	194.3	19.1	29.1	33.4	34.1	30.4	22.3	13.5	12.4
1927-1931----------	1956	200.8	19.1	29.1	33.8	34.7	31.1	23.9	15.1	14.0
1928-1932----------	1957	202.8	18.6	29.3	34.5	34.2	31.3	24.4	15.4	15.1
1929-1933----------	1958	202.0	17.9	28.3	33.5	34.3	31.0	24.6	16.1	16.3
1930-1934----------	1959	206.0	18.0	28.7	34.1	35.3	31.7	24.7	16.7	16.8
1931-1935----------	1960	203.4	17.9	28.1	33.5	34.3	31.2	24.8	16.7	16.9
1932-1936----------	1961	206.5	17.7	27.9	33.5	35.0	31.9	25.7	16.8	18.0
1933-1937----------	1962	201.4	17.1	27.3	32.5	34.0	31.2	24.7	16.6	18.0
1934-1938----------	1963	195.6	17.3	26.6	31.4	32.3	30.2	23.5	16.5	17.8
1935-1939----------	1964	186.8	16.7	26.1	30.4	30.6	28.1	22.7	15.3	16.9
1936-1940----------	1965	172.0	17.6	25.5	28.5	28.2	24.8	19.6	13.4	14.4
1937-1941----------	1966	153.7	17.9	25.2	26.2	24.5	21.2	16.2	11.0	11.5
1938-1942----------	1967	140.6	18.0	25.4	25.0	22.2	18.1	13.8	9.0	9.1
1939-1943----------	1968	130.4	20.2	25.3	23.3	20.4	15.4	11.5	7.1	7.2
1940-1944----------	1969	129.5	20.9	27.5	24.4	20.1	14.9	10.2	5.8	5.7
1941-1945----------	1970	133.6	22.4	30.1	26.3	20.5	14.7	9.4	5.4	4.8
1942-1946----------	1971	127.4	22.2	30.2	26.3	19.3	13.3	7.9	4.4	3.8
1943-1947----------	1972	113.4	22.2	29.2	23.0	16.4	10.5	6.3	3.2	2.6
1944-1948----------	1973	106.1	22.3	29.4	22.1	14.5	8.6	4.9	2.4	1.9

TABLE 3C. CENTRAL BIRTH RATES FOR ALL OTHER WOMEN DURING EACH YEAR 1917-73 BY AGE AND LIVE-BIRTH ORDER FOR GROUPS OF COHORTS FROM 1868-72 TO 1954-58--CON.

(RATES ARE SIMPLE AVERAGES OF THE RATES FOR SINGLE COHORTS IN TABLE 4C)

CURRENT AGE AND COHORT	CALENDAR YEAR	TOTAL	LIVE-BIRTH ORDER							
			1	2	3	4	5	6	7	8 AND HIGHER
30-34 YEARS										
1883-1887----------	1917	106.8	6.5	8.7	10.7	12.3	13.2	15.3	13.8	26.3
1884-1888----------	1918	103.3	7.1	8.7	11.1	12.1	12.9	15.2	12.9	23.3
1885-1889----------	1919	101.8	6.4	8.8	11.0	12.4	13.0	13.8	12.4	24.0
1886-1890----------	1920	100.7	7.2	9.0	11.8	12.7	12.3	13.2	11.4	23.1
1887-1891----------	1921	105.6	6.6	9.4	11.6	12.9	13.4	14.5	12.3	24.9
1888-1892----------	1922	100.6	6.1	9.3	11.2	12.3	12.8	13.5	11.9	23.5
1889-1893----------	1923	100.0	5.8	8.4	11.0	12.4	12.8	13.9	12.1	23.6
1890-1894----------	1924	103.8	5.7	8.2	12.0	12.9	13.0	14.5	12.4	25.1
1891-1895----------	1925	104.4	5.9	7.7	10.9	12.6	13.0	14.2	12.5	27.6
1892-1896----------	1926	101.1	4.9	7.5	10.1	12.6	12.9	13.6	12.8	26.7
1893-1897----------	1927	93.2	4.7	6.2	9.0	11.0	12.1	12.6	12.2	25.4
1894-1898----------	1928	83.9	4.2	5.4	7.7	9.7	11.3	11.8	10.5	23.3
1895-1899----------	1929	80.4	3.9	5.4	7.4	9.3	10.9	11.4	10.1	22.0
1896-1900----------	1930	81.9	4.4	5.6	7.3	9.1	11.1	11.7	10.4	22.3
1897-1901----------	1931	80.1	4.2	5.3	7.0	9.0	10.2	11.5	10.8	22.1
1898-1902----------	1932	80.0	4.1	5.2	7.0	9.0	10.6	11.7	10.6	21.8
1899-1903----------	1933	76.6	3.8	5.1	6.9	8.6	10.1	11.0	10.4	20.7
1900-1904----------	1934	76.9	3.9	5.2	6.9	8.5	10.1	10.8	10.1	21.4
1901-1905----------	1935	70.4	3.6	5.0	6.5	8.2	9.3	9.9	9.0	18.9
1902-1906----------	1936	66.6	3.5	4.7	6.1	7.5	8.8	9.4	8.5	18.1
1903-1907----------	1937	66.7	3.5	4.8	6.2	7.4	8.9	9.3	8.7	17.9
1904-1908----------	1938	67.1	3.8	4.9	6.4	7.6	8.8	9.3	8.9	17.4
1905-1909----------	1939	66.8	4.0	5.1	6.4	7.8	8.5	9.2	8.5	17.3
1906-1910----------	1940	68.6	4.2	5.4	6.5	7.6	8.9	9.1	8.7	18.2
1907-1911----------	1941	71.1	4.7	5.9	7.0	8.0	8.9	9.3	8.8	18.5
1908-1912----------	1942	73.5	5.2	6.7	7.5	8.3	9.1	9.4	8.8	18.5
1909-1913----------	1943	78.8	6.0	7.4	8.2	9.0	9.7	10.0	9.1	19.4
1910-1914----------	1944	82.4	6.4	8.0	8.7	9.5	9.9	10.5	9.4	20.0
1911-1915----------	1945	83.6	6.5	8.1	8.9	9.6	10.3	10.2	9.6	20.4
1912-1916----------	1946	86.6	7.4	9.4	9.9	10.3	10.1	10.1	9.4	20.0
1913-1917----------	1947	90.9	9.1	10.5	10.5	10.5	10.4	10.2	9.6	20.1
1914-1918----------	1948	93.3	8.5	11.3	11.4	10.9	10.7	10.5	9.7	20.3
1915-1919----------	1949	97.3	9.0	11.7	12.4	11.6	11.2	10.8	9.8	20.8
1916-1920----------	1950	101.2	8.7	11.8	13.2	12.6	12.1	11.2	10.1	21.5
1917-1921----------	1951	107.4	9.0	12.6	14.0	13.9	12.9	12.2	10.9	21.9
1918-1922----------	1952	111.6	8.7	13.2	14.8	14.8	14.0	12.7	10.8	22.6
1919-1923----------	1953	115.5	8.7	13.2	15.6	15.4	14.8	13.2	11.3	23.3
1920-1924----------	1954	121.6	8.8	13.4	15.7	16.5	16.0	14.3	12.2	24.7
1921-1925----------	1955	124.1	8.3	13.3	16.0	16.9	16.4	14.9	12.4	25.9
1922-1926----------	1956	128.7	8.0	13.1	16.4	17.2	17.3	15.9	13.6	27.2
1923-1927----------	1957	132.1	7.4	13.1	16.5	17.4	17.7	16.5	14.5	29.0
1924-1928----------	1958	130.1	7.1	12.2	15.6	16.9	16.9	16.5	14.6	30.3
1925-1929----------	1959	132.6	7.0	11.8	15.3	16.6	17.6	16.7	15.3	32.3
1926-1930----------	1960	130.0	6.6	11.7	14.9	16.3	16.8	16.0	14.9	32.8
1927-1931----------	1961	130.7	6.3	11.1	14.9	16.7	16.5	16.3	14.9	34.0
1928-1932----------	1962	126.2	6.0	10.7	14.1	15.6	16.2	15.9	14.1	33.6
1929-1933----------	1963	122.2	5.9	10.7	13.8	15.3	15.6	14.8	13.5	32.6
1930-1934----------	1964	118.9	5.8	10.0	13.5	14.6	15.0	14.8	13.4	31.8
1931-1935----------	1965	110.6	5.9	10.2	12.9	14.0	14.0	13.2	12.1	28.3
1932-1936----------	1966	99.7	6.0	9.8	12.4	12.8	12.7	11.9	10.0	24.1
1933-1937----------	1967	91.4	5.6	9.8	11.8	12.2	11.7	10.6	9.2	20.5
1934-1938----------	1968	83.6	6.4	10.1	11.5	11.1	10.3	9.3	7.7	17.2
1935-1939----------	1969	81.8	6.7	10.7	12.1	11.4	10.4	8.7	7.2	14.6
1936-1940----------	1970	81.2	6.8	11.5	12.7	11.7	10.5	8.6	6.6	12.8
1937-1941----------	1971	77.9	6.8	12.0	12.8	11.2	9.7	8.0	6.2	11.2
1938-1942----------	1972	67.7	7.1	12.0	11.6	9.6	8.3	6.5	4.6	8.0
1939-1943----------	1973	62.2	7.0	12.3	11.2	9.0	7.2	5.4	3.9	6.2

TABLE 3C. CENTRAL BIRTH RATES FOR ALL OTHER WOMEN DURING EACH YEAR 1917-73 BY AGE AND LIVE-BIRTH ORDER FOR GROUPS OF COHORTS FROM 1868-72 TO 1954-58--CON.

(RATES ARE SIMPLE AVERAGES OF THE RATES FOR SINGLE COHORTS IN TABLE 4C)

CURRENT AGE AND COHORT	CALENDAR YEAR	TOTAL	LIVE-BIRTH ORDER							
			1	2	3	4	5	6	7	8 AND HIGHER
35-39 YEARS										
1878-1882----------	1917	99.8	3.1	4.4	5.7	7.2	8.5	10.9	12.3	47.7
1879-1883----------	1918	101.6	4.0	4.8	6.6	7.5	8.3	12.6	11.8	46.0
1880-1884----------	1919	105.1	3.5	4.6	6.2	7.8	8.7	11.7	12.4	50.2
1881-1885----------	1920	106.2	3.9	5.0	7.2	8.3	8.8	11.2	11.1	50.7
1882-1886----------	1921	100.3	3.6	4.5	6.2	7.7	8.5	10.8	10.3	48.7
1883-1887----------	1922	92.8	3.3	4.5	6.0	6.9	8.0	9.6	10.4	44.1
1884-1888----------	1923	87.3	2.8	4.0	5.6	6.5	7.1	9.3	9.9	42.1
1885-1889----------	1924	86.3	2.8	3.5	5.6	6.5	7.5	8.7	9.9	41.8
1886-1890----------	1925	87.2	2.9	3.2	5.2	6.3	7.1	8.8	9.8	43.9
1887-1891----------	1926	83.7	2.5	3.1	4.8	6.3	7.0	8.8	9.6	41.6
1888-1892----------	1927	78.8	2.8	2.8	4.2	5.4	6.5	7.8	8.8	40.5
1889-1893----------	1928	69.2	2.1	2.3	3.6	4.8	6.0	7.2	7.6	35.6
1890-1894----------	1929	66.1	1.9	2.6	3.5	4.6	5.8	6.8	7.3	33.6
1891-1895----------	1930	66.4	2.1	2.3	3.3	4.4	6.1	7.0	7.3	33.9
1892-1896----------	1931	62.6	1.9	2.3	3.1	4.3	5.4	6.6	7.1	31.9
1893-1897----------	1932	62.8	1.8	2.0	3.0	4.0	5.1	7.1	7.3	32.5
1894-1898----------	1933	58.5	1.6	2.1	2.8	3.9	4.9	6.0	6.7	30.5
1895-1899----------	1934	60.3	1.7	2.0	2.9	3.9	5.0	6.1	7.0	31.7
1896-1900----------	1935	56.9	1.6	2.0	2.9	3.7	4.8	5.7	6.7	29.5
1897-1901----------	1936	54.8	1.7	2.0	2.9	3.8	4.6	5.5	6.3	28.0
1898-1902----------	1937	55.3	1.6	2.1	3.0	3.6	4.6	5.4	6.2	28.8
1899-1903----------	1938	54.5	1.7	2.2	2.9	3.8	4.5	5.4	6.1	27.9
1900-1904----------	1939	52.0	1.8	2.2	2.8	3.6	4.1	5.2	5.8	26.5
1901-1905----------	1940	50.7	1.8	2.2	2.7	3.5	4.4	4.9	5.4	25.8
1902-1906----------	1941	51.0	1.9	2.4	2.9	3.4	4.5	4.9	5.6	25.4
1903-1907----------	1942	50.3	2.1	2.6	3.0	3.7	4.4	4.8	5.2	24.5
1904-1908----------	1943	52.7	2.3	2.9	3.4	3.9	4.6	5.0	5.4	25.2
1905-1909----------	1944	53.8	2.5	3.1	3.7	4.1	4.6	5.2	5.7	24.9
1906-1910----------	1945	55.8	2.7	3.2	3.9	4.4	4.9	5.3	5.5	25.9
1907-1911----------	1946	56.1	3.1	3.8	4.3	4.6	4.9	5.2	5.6	24.6
1908-1912----------	1947	58.1	3.5	4.2	4.6	4.8	5.1	5.4	5.6	24.9
1909-1913----------	1948	58.9	3.5	4.4	4.9	5.0	5.4	5.4	5.6	24.7
1910-1914----------	1949	60.7	3.8	4.7	5.1	5.2	5.4	5.7	5.8	25.0
1911-1915----------	1950	61.9	3.8	4.6	5.5	5.7	5.6	5.7	5.9	25.1
1912-1916----------	1951	64.9	3.9	4.9	6.0	6.1	6.1	6.0	6.0	25.9
1913-1917----------	1952	64.5	3.7	5.1	5.9	6.3	6.2	6.1	5.9	25.3
1914-1918----------	1953	66.8	3.9	5.2	6.4	6.6	6.7	6.5	6.4	25.1
1915-1919----------	1954	70.1	3.7	5.5	6.6	7.2	7.2	7.0	6.6	26.3
1916-1920----------	1955	71.4	3.7	5.5	6.7	7.3	7.4	7.3	7.0	26.5
1917-1921----------	1956	73.9	3.5	5.3	6.8	7.3	7.7	7.6	7.6	28.1
1918-1922----------	1957	74.1	3.2	5.2	6.8	7.7	7.9	7.8	7.6	27.9
1919-1923----------	1958	72.4	3.1	5.1	6.7	7.3	7.9	7.4	7.4	27.5
1920-1924----------	1959	73.6	3.0	4.5	6.6	7.2	7.9	8.1	7.7	28.6
1921-1925----------	1960	72.2	2.8	4.5	6.4	7.4	7.4	7.7	7.4	28.6
1922-1926----------	1961	73.0	2.6	4.5	6.4	7.5	7.7	7.6	7.5	29.2
1923-1927----------	1962	70.2	2.4	4.4	6.2	7.0	7.4	7.4	7.0	28.4
1924-1928----------	1963	67.0	2.4	4.1	5.6	6.4	7.1	6.9	6.8	27.7
1925-1929----------	1964	66.3	2.3	3.8	5.6	6.4	6.7	6.8	6.7	28.0
1926-1930----------	1965	61.4	2.2	3.8	5.2	5.9	6.4	6.4	6.1	25.4
1927-1931----------	1966	55.4	2.2	3.4	5.0	5.4	5.9	5.7	5.5	22.3
1928-1932----------	1967	50.5	2.0	3.5	4.8	5.2	5.3	5.3	5.1	19.3
1929-1933----------	1968	46.1	2.3	3.4	4.5	4.7	5.0	5.0	4.5	16.7
1930-1934----------	1969	43.9	2.2	3.5	4.5	4.9	5.0	4.3	4.3	15.2
1931-1935----------	1970	42.7	2.2	3.5	4.6	5.0	4.8	4.4	4.1	14.1
1932-1936----------	1971	39.8	2.1	3.4	4.4	4.6	4.5	4.3	4.0	12.5
1933-1937----------	1972	34.9	2.0	3.6	4.2	4.2	4.0	3.6	3.2	10.1
1934-1938----------	1973	30.7	2.0	3.3	4.0	3.8	3.6	3.1	2.8	8.1

TABLE 3C. CENTRAL BIRTH RATES FOR ALL OTHER WOMEN DURING EACH YEAR 1917-73 BY AGE AND LIVE-BIRTH ORDER FOR GROUPS OF COHORTS FROM 1868-72 TO 1954-58--CON.

(RATES ARE SIMPLE AVERAGES OF THE RATES FOR SINGLE COHORTS IN TABLE 4C)

CURRENT AGE AND COHORT	CALENDAR YEAR	TOTAL	LIVE-BIRTH ORDER							
			1	2	3	4	5	6	7	8 AND HIGHER
40-44 YEARS										
1873-1877----------	1917	36.2	0.6	0.9	1.0	1.7	2.0	2.8	2.8	24.4
1874-1878----------	1918	41.5	1.1	1.1	1.5	1.7	2.1	3.6	3.3	27.1
1875-1879----------	1919	35.1	0.6	1.1	1.0	1.6	2.0	2.6	3.0	23.2
1876-1880----------	1920	37.0	0.9	1.2	1.5	1.9	2.2	2.7	2.8	23.8
1877-1881----------	1921	38.2	0.8	1.2	1.5	2.0	2.0	2.8	3.2	24.7
1878-1882----------	1922	35.2	0.8	1.1	1.4	1.5	1.9	2.6	3.0	22.9
1879-1883----------	1923	35.2	0.9	1.0	1.4	1.6	1.9	2.5	3.0	22.9
1880-1884----------	1924	34.5	0.7	0.8	1.3	1.9	2.1	2.5	2.9	22.3
1881-1885----------	1925	34.5	0.7	0.8	1.3	1.7	1.9	2.5	2.6	23.0
1882-1886----------	1926	32.8	0.7	0.7	1.1	1.5	1.7	2.3	2.6	22.2
1883-1887----------	1927	29.6	0.7	0.6	1.0	1.3	1.6	1.9	2.4	20.1
1884-1888----------	1928	25.5	0.6	0.6	0.7	1.1	1.5	1.7	1.9	17.4
1885-1889----------	1929	24.4	0.5	0.5	0.8	1.0	1.3	1.7	1.9	16.7
1886-1890----------	1930	24.7	0.5	0.5	0.7	1.1	1.5	1.7	2.2	16.5
1887-1891----------	1931	23.2	0.5	0.4	0.6	1.0	1.3	1.7	2.0	15.7
1888-1892----------	1932	24.4	0.5	0.5	0.7	1.0	1.3	1.8	1.9	16.7
1889-1893----------	1933	22.6	0.4	0.4	0.7	1.0	1.2	1.5	1.9	15.5
1890-1894----------	1934	22.8	0.4	0.4	0.6	1.0	1.2	1.5	1.8	15.9
1891-1895----------	1935	21.7	0.4	0.4	0.6	0.9	1.2	1.4	1.7	15.1
1892-1896----------	1936	20.3	0.4	0.4	0.6	0.8	1.1	1.3	1.6	14.1
1893-1897----------	1937	19.7	0.3	0.4	0.5	0.8	0.9	1.3	1.5	14.0
1894-1898----------	1938	19.2	0.3	0.4	0.5	0.7	0.9	1.2	1.5	13.7
1895-1899----------	1939	17.9	0.3	0.4	0.5	0.7	0.9	1.2	1.3	12.6
1896-1900----------	1940	19.0	0.4	0.4	0.5	0.8	1.0	1.2	1.5	13.2
1897-1901----------	1941	18.7	0.4	0.4	0.6	0.8	1.0	1.2	1.4	12.9
1898-1902----------	1942	18.3	0.4	0.5	0.6	0.8	1.0	1.1	1.3	12.6
1899-1903----------	1943	18.9	0.4	0.5	0.6	0.9	1.0	1.2	1.4	12.9
1900-1904----------	1944	19.1	0.5	0.6	0.7	1.0	1.1	1.3	1.4	12.5
1901-1905----------	1945	19.4	0.6	0.6	0.8	1.0	1.2	1.3	1.5	12.4
1902-1906----------	1946	18.8	0.6	0.7	0.7	1.0	1.1	1.3	1.5	11.9
1903-1907----------	1947	18.4	0.6	0.7	0.9	1.1	1.1	1.3	1.4	11.3
1904-1908----------	1948	17.3	0.6	0.7	0.9	1.1	1.1	1.1	1.3	10.5
1905-1909----------	1949	18.4	0.8	0.9	0.9	1.1	1.2	1.3	1.4	10.8
1906-1910----------	1950	18.2	0.7	0.9	1.0	1.1	1.2	1.4	1.5	10.4
1907-1911----------	1951	19.7	0.8	1.1	1.2	1.3	1.4	1.4	1.5	11.0
1908-1912----------	1952	19.5	0.8	1.1	1.2	1.4	1.3	1.5	1.5	10.7
1909-1913----------	1953	20.5	0.8	1.1	1.3	1.4	1.6	1.6	1.6	11.1
1910-1914----------	1954	21.0	0.8	1.1	1.4	1.7	1.6	1.6	1.7	11.1
1911-1915----------	1955	20.8	0.8	1.2	1.4	1.6	1.6	1.7	1.6	10.9
1912-1916----------	1956	21.8	0.8	1.1	1.4	1.5	1.8	1.9	1.8	11.5
1913-1917----------	1957	21.7	0.8	1.1	1.4	1.6	1.8	1.8	1.7	11.5
1914-1918----------	1958	21.2	0.7	1.1	1.2	1.6	1.7	1.7	1.8	11.4
1915-1919----------	1959	21.4	0.7	1.0	1.4	1.6	1.9	1.7	1.9	11.2
1916-1920----------	1960	21.8	0.7	0.9	1.4	1.7	1.9	1.9	2.0	11.3
1917-1921----------	1961	21.8	0.6	0.9	1.5	1.7	1.7	2.0	1.9	11.5
1918-1922----------	1962	21.1	0.6	0.9	1.3	1.6	1.8	1.8	1.9	11.2
1919-1923----------	1963	20.4	0.5	0.9	1.2	1.7	1.8	1.7	1.8	10.8
1920-1924----------	1964	20.5	0.6	0.9	1.3	1.5	1.7	1.8	1.8	10.9
1921-1925----------	1965	19.2	0.6	0.8	1.2	1.6	1.7	1.8	1.7	9.8
1922-1926----------	1966	18.0	0.5	0.8	1.2	1.4	1.6	1.7	1.5	9.3
1923-1927----------	1967	16.5	0.5	0.8	1.2	1.2	1.3	1.5	1.5	8.5
1924-1928----------	1968	14.7	0.5	0.7	1.0	1.2	1.2	1.3	1.5	7.3
1925-1929----------	1969	14.1	0.5	0.8	1.0	1.3	1.3	1.3	1.3	6.6
1926-1930----------	1970	13.0	0.4	0.7	0.9	1.2	1.3	1.2	1.1	6.2
1927-1931----------	1971	12.1	0.4	0.7	0.8	1.1	1.0	1.1	1.1	5.9
1928-1932----------	1972	10.3	0.3	0.7	0.8	0.9	1.0	1.0	1.0	4.6
1929-1933----------	1973	9.0	0.4	0.6	0.7	0.8	0.9	0.9	0.8	3.9

TABLE 3C. CENTRAL BIRTH RATES FOR ALL OTHER WOMEN DURING EACH YEAR 1917-73 BY AGE AND LIVE-BIRTH ORDER FOR GROUPS OF COHORTS FROM 1868-72 TO 1954-58--CON.

(RATES ARE SIMPLE AVERAGES OF THE RATES FOR SINGLE COHORTS IN TABLE 4C)

CURRENT AGE AND COHORT	CALENDAR YEAR	TOTAL	LIVE-BIRTH ORDER							
			1	2	3	4	5	6	7	8 AND HIGHER
45-49 YEARS										
1868-1872----------	1917	12.8	0.4	0.4	0.4	0.5	0.6	0.7	1.0	8.8
1869-1873----------	1918	22.8	0.6	0.2	0.8	1.2	0.7	2.1	1.7	15.5
1870-1874----------	1919	11.6	0.2	0.2	0.3	0.4	0.5	0.6	1.0	8.4
1871-1875----------	1920	14.1	0.3	0.4	0.5	0.5	0.6	0.8	1.0	10.0
1872-1876----------	1921	10.3	0.3	0.1	0.3	0.5	0.4	0.4	0.6	7.7
1873-1877----------	1922	9.5	0.3	0.1	0.3	0.3	0.4	0.5	0.8	6.8
1874-1878----------	1923	10.4	0.2	0.2	0.3	0.3	0.6	0.6	0.9	7.3
1875-1879----------	1924	9.9	0.3	0.2	0.4	0.4	0.6	0.6	0.7	6.7
1876-1880----------	1925	8.7	0.2	0.3	0.3	0.3	0.4	0.5	0.6	6.1
1877-1881----------	1926	9.5	0.3	0.2	0.4	0.5	0.4	0.6	0.8	6.3
1878-1882----------	1927	8.1	0.3	0.2	0.2	0.3	0.4	0.5	0.5	5.7
1879-1883----------	1928	8.2	0.2	0.2	0.2	0.3	0.4	0.5	0.6	5.8
1880-1884----------	1929	7.8	0.1	0.2	0.2	0.3	0.4	0.6	0.5	5.5
1881-1885----------	1930	7.4	0.1	0.1	0.2	0.3	0.4	0.4	0.5	5.4
1882-1886----------	1931	6.7	0.2	0.1	0.2	0.2	0.4	0.4	0.5	4.7
1883-1887----------	1932	6.8	0.1	0.1	0.2	0.3	0.3	0.5	0.5	4.8
1884-1888----------	1933	5.6	0.1	0.1	0.1	0.3	0.2	0.3	0.4	4.1
1885-1889----------	1934	5.7	0.1	0.1	0.2	0.2	0.2	0.4	0.4	4.1
1886-1890----------	1935	5.3	0.1	0.1	0.1	0.2	0.3	0.3	0.3	3.9
1887-1891----------	1936	5.2	0.1	0.1	0.1	0.2	0.2	0.3	0.4	3.8
1888-1892----------	1937	4.9	0.2	0.1	0.1	0.1	0.2	0.3	0.3	3.6
1889-1893----------	1938	4.6	0.1	0.1	0.1	0.1	0.1	0.2	0.4	3.5
1890-1894----------	1939	4.2	0.1	0.1	0.1	0.1	0.2	0.2	0.3	3.1
1891-1895----------	1940	4.1	0.1	0.0	0.1	0.1	0.2	0.2	0.3	3.1
1892-1896----------	1941	3.5	0.1	0.1	0.1	0.1	0.2	0.1	0.2	2.6
1893-1897----------	1942	3.5	0.1	0.1	0.1	0.2	0.2	0.2	0.2	2.4
1894-1898----------	1943	3.3	0.0	0.1	0.1	0.1	0.1	0.2	0.2	2.5
1895-1899----------	1944	2.9	0.0	0.0	0.1	0.1	0.2	0.2	0.2	2.1
1896-1900----------	1945	3.3	0.0	0.0	0.1	0.2	0.2	0.2	0.2	2.4
1897-1901----------	1946	3.1	0.1	0.1	0.1	0.2	0.2	0.2	0.2	2.0
1898-1902----------	1947	2.8	0.1	0.0	0.1	0.1	0.1	0.2	0.2	2.0
1899-1903----------	1948	2.4	0.1	0.1	0.1	0.1	0.1	0.1	0.2	1.6
1900-1904----------	1949	2.3	0.0	0.1	0.1	0.1	0.1	0.2	0.2	1.5
1901-1905----------	1950	2.2	0.1	0.1	0.1	0.1	0.1	0.1	0.1	1.5
1902-1906----------	1951	2.0	0.0	0.1	0.1	0.1	0.1	0.1	0.1	1.4
1903-1907----------	1952	2.0	0.1	0.0	0.1	0.1	0.1	0.1	0.2	1.3
1904-1908----------	1953	2.0	0.1	0.1	0.1	0.1	0.1	0.1	0.1	1.3
1905-1909----------	1954	1.9	0.1	0.1	0.0	0.2	0.1	0.1	0.1	1.2
1906-1910----------	1955	1.8	0.0	0.0	0.1	0.1	0.2	0.1	0.2	1.1
1907-1911----------	1956	1.8	0.0	0.1	0.1	0.1	0.1	0.1	0.1	1.2
1908-1912----------	1957	2.0	0.0	0.1	0.1	0.1	0.1	0.1	0.1	1.4
1909-1913----------	1958	2.0	0.1	0.1	0.1	0.1	0.1	0.2	0.1	1.2
1910-1914----------	1959	2.0	0.1	0.0	0.1	0.1	0.1	0.2	0.2	1.2
1911-1915----------	1960	1.9	0.1	0.0	0.1	0.1	0.2	0.1	0.2	1.1
1912-1916----------	1961	1.7	0.0	0.0	0.1	0.1	0.1	0.2	0.1	1.1
1913-1917----------	1962	1.6	0.0	0.0	0.1	0.1	0.1	0.1	0.1	1.1
1914-1918----------	1963	1.8	0.1	0.1	0.1	0.1	0.1	0.1	0.2	1.0
1915-1919----------	1964	1.6	0.0	0.0	0.1	0.1	0.1	0.1	0.1	1.1
1916-1920----------	1965	1.5	0.0	0.0	0.1	0.1	0.1	0.1	0.1	1.0
1917-1921----------	1966	1.5	0.0	0.0	0.1	0.1	0.1	0.1	0.1	1.0
1918-1922----------	1967	1.3	0.0	0.0	0.1	0.1	0.1	0.1	0.1	0.8
1919-1923----------	1968	1.2	0.0	0.0	0.1	0.1	0.1	0.1	0.1	0.7
1920-1924----------	1969	1.2	0.1	0.0	0.1	0.1	0.1	0.1	0.1	0.6
1921-1925----------	1970	1.2	0.0	0.0	0.1	0.1	0.1	0.1	0.1	0.7
1922-1926----------	1971	1.1	0.0	0.0	0.1	0.1	0.1	0.1	0.1	0.6
1923-1927----------	1972	0.9	0.0	0.0	0.0	0.1	0.1	0.1	0.1	0.5
1924-1928----------	1973	0.5	0.0	0.0	0.0	0.0	0.1	0.0	0.0	0.4

TABLE 4A. CENTRAL BIRTH RATES FOR ALL WOMEN DURING EACH YEAR 1917-73 BY AGE AND LIVE-BIRTH ORDER FOR EACH COHORT FROM 1868 TO 1959

LIVE-BIRTH ORDER AND COHORT	DIAGONAL LINE FOR CALENDAR YEAR	CURRENT AGE											
		14	15	16	17	18	19	20	21	22	23	24	25
TOTAL BIRTHS													
1892-------													180.8
1893-------												183.2	178.7
1894-------											185.5	181.6	163.2
1895-------										175.3	184.2	163.9	175.7
1896-------									167.3	174.5	163.3	178.2	179.5
1897-------								148.5	167.1	153.0	179.4	181.7	169.7
1898-------							122.6	148.2	145.4	172.2	183.4	173.2	171.9
1899-------						86.2	121.1	128.1	164.8	173.2	171.7	173.2	171.2
1900-------					54.2	84.0	105.2	148.2	165.4	161.7	173.2	175.1	164.2
1901-------				27.0	52.4	73.7	123.8	151.9	153.3	161.4	176.1	168.7	158.0
1902-------			11.5	26.5	46.7	90.5	131.9	143.1	154.6	167.5	169.3	162.5	153.5
1903-------	1917	3.5	11.4	23.6	57.8	98.7	122.9	143.6	158.5	162.7	164.8	158.7	146.2
1904-------	1918	3.6	9.8	29.0	61.8	90.6	122.6	146.3	153.0	158.9	159.6	150.8	140.5
1905-------	1919	3.0	12.0	30.5	55.6	91.1	125.8	140.1	148.5	153.4	150.8	143.8	139.8
1906-------	1920	3.6	12.7	27.2	55.9	94.7	120.8	136.3	144.9	144.9	144.1	143.3	132.8
1907-------	1921	3.8	11.2	27.3	58.5	92.1	118.0	133.6	137.9	139.4	144.1	136.3	128.2
1908-------	1922	3.4	11.4	28.9	58.2	90.0	115.6	127.1	132.7	139.6	136.3	131.0	119.9
1909-------	1923	3.5	12.1	29.5	57.1	87.9	110.2	121.8	133.7	133.1	131.9	123.4	124.5
1910-------	1924	3.7	12.4	28.7	56.5	83.8	105.3	123.1	126.6	128.3	124.0	127.6	121.4
1911-------	1925	3.9	12.5	29.5	54.0	80.5	107.6	117.4	123.6	121.6	129.5	126.5	122.0
1912-------	1926	3.9	12.9	27.7	52.4	82.3	101.4	114.0	115.8	126.4	128.2	126.3	124.6
1913-------	1927	4.1	12.0	27.2	53.7	77.4	98.5	106.3	121.3	126.5	128.0	129.9	129.0
1914-------	1928	3.7	11.7	27.8	49.9	74.8	91.4	111.9	121.8	126.8	132.4	134.5	127.6
1915-------	1929	3.7	12.0	26.1	48.3	69.3	96.2	112.6	121.7	130.9	136.7	132.5	133.0
1916-------	1930	3.8	11.2	25.0	44.4	72.5	96.6	111.9	124.6	133.9	133.3	136.7	140.9
1917-------	1931	3.5	10.8	23.0	46.6	73.2	95.1	114.0	127.6	130.2	137.1	145.4	159.1
1918-------	1932	3.3	9.9	24.2	47.4	71.8	97.7	116.9	123.0	133.4	145.2	166.3	162.5
1919-------	1933	3.2	10.4	25.2	47.1	75.3	101.5	114.4	128.9	144.2	169.9	167.9	149.3
1920-------	1934	3.4	11.3	25.0	49.8	78.1	98.8	119.5	137.9	163.7	168.8	153.6	139.4
1921-------	1935	3.7	11.3	26.9	51.8	76.4	102.8	127.6	152.1	160.4	154.5	142.2	179.2
1922-------	1936	3.5	11.7	27.2	49.1	76.8	107.0	137.3	149.2	148.0	140.1	184.5	196.4
1923-------	1937	3.7	11.9	25.8	49.3	80.2	116.1	136.1	138.3	135.1	184.9	205.0	184.4
1924-------	1938	3.8	11.4	26.2	52.1	87.0	116.1	124.6	126.9	180.2	209.5	194.3	186.8
1925-------	1939	3.7	11.9	28.0	55.0	87.4	104.1	115.5	166.8	207.7	198.7	196.3	187.0
1926-------	1940	3.8	12.7	29.2	55.6	77.0	96.6	147.0	197.9	197.3	200.0	195.3	197.7
1927-------	1941	4.1	13.3	29.7	49.2	72.3	117.8	180.5	189.8	198.0	197.5	206.3	202.8
1928-------	1942	4.1	13.4	26.1	46.4	84.0	150.6	175.4	190.0	195.4	210.0	211.0	205.1
1929-------	1943	4.2	12.0	25.2	51.8	111.6	149.6	176.6	187.9	209.9	216.6	216.6	212.3
1930-------	1944	3.8	11.8	26.6	70.3	113.8	150.2	173.6	202.6	216.0	221.5	225.0	216.3
1931-------	1945	3.9	12.2	37.2	74.5	115.5	148.4	189.0	208.9	223.2	233.3	231.0	225.4
1932-------	1946	3.8	16.3	40.2	75.3	113.7	160.7	192.4	215.2	234.2	239.6	241.0	231.6
1933-------	1947	5.2	18.3	41.3	75.0	123.2	162.3	199.6	226.3	241.5	250.4	247.9	230.5
1934-------	1948	5.8	18.8	41.4	80.2	122.6	168.6	208.3	232.5	252.6	257.7	246.8	232.4
1935-------	1949	5.7	18.8	43.4	79.0	126.5	173.2	212.0	243.1	258.9	255.7	247.5	231.8
1936-------	1950	5.8	19.4	42.5	81.5	129.6	174.8	222.0	248.7	256.1	255.5	246.8	228.8
1937-------	1951	6.0	18.9	43.5	82.7	129.8	183.7	227.2	246.0	256.5	255.8	243.9	220.6
1938-------	1952	5.7	19.1	44.6	82.3	136.5	187.8	224.6	248.0	256.4	252.0	234.3	211.7
1939-------	1953	5.8	20.1	44.7	87.2	140.5	186.3	228.0	247.0	253.3	242.9	225.6	203.3
1940-------	1954	6.3	19.9	46.8	89.3	138.1	187.6	224.2	243.2	244.5	232.9	215.3	183.5
1941-------	1955	6.1	20.9	47.9	86.3	136.1	181.9	219.1	234.2	232.9	221.4	193.7	170.7
1942-------	1956	6.2	20.8	45.4	83.7	131.2	176.4	210.0	222.5	220.3	198.5	181.3	164.6
1943-------	1957	6.1	19.5	43.8	80.2	127.1	169.1	200.5	209.8	197.1	186.2	174.1	161.2
1944-------	1958	5.8	19.3	42.6	79.1	122.6	163.3	190.3	188.9	185.6	178.2	168.7	162.5
1945-------	1959	6.0	19.2	42.3	76.3	119.0	155.3	172.0	177.9	175.9	170.5	168.0	163.0
1946-------	1960	6.0	18.8	40.3	73.4	113.4	142.4	163.5	168.3	168.8	171.2	170.1	151.2
1947-------	1961	5.5	17.4	38.6	70.1	105.4	136.1	154.3	161.5	167.8	171.2	156.8	133.2
1948-------	1962	5.1	16.7	37.0	66.4	101.8	129.5	148.9	160.1	167.4	157.1	136.4	125.1
1949-------	1963	5.1	16.7	36.0	64.8	97.5	125.2	146.7	159.2	153.0	135.3	126.6	
1950-------	1964	5.2	16.5	35.5	63.2	95.7	124.5	147.1	144.5	130.9	125.1		
1951-------	1965	5.2	16.4	35.3	62.6	95.7	126.0	133.9	124.6	120.8			
1952-------	1966	5.3	16.5	35.2	63.1	98.3	116.1	117.2	115.0				
1953-------	1967	5.3	16.7	35.8	66.6	92.4	105.0	108.8					
1954-------	1968	5.7	17.4	38.8	64.2	87.1	98.5						
1955-------	1969	6.0	19.2	38.3	63.5	83.1							
1956-------	1970	6.6	19.2	39.3	61.5								
1957-------	1971	6.7	20.1	38.8									
1958-------	1972	7.1	20.2										
1959-------	1973	7.4											

TABLE 4A. CENTRAL BIRTH RATES FOR ALL WOMEN DURING EACH YEAR 1917-73 BY AGE AND LIVE-BIRTH ORDER FOR EACH COHORT FROM 1868 TO 1959--CON.

LIVE-BIRTH ORDER AND COHORT	DIAGONAL LINE FOR CALENDAR YEAR	CURRENT AGE											
		26	27	28	29	30	31	32	33	34	35	36	37
TOTAL BIRTHS--CON.													
1880-------													95.3
1881-------												101.3	94.2
1882-------											109.6	100.1	93.2
1883-------										114.7	108.2	98.6	92.6
1884-------									121.0	113.1	105.5	98.2	92.7
1885-------								122.3	119.7	109.2	105.2	98.7	86.2
1886-------							134.5	121.9	115.1	109.6	106.9	92.3	85.3
1887-------						144.9	134.6	117.3	115.9	112.1	100.3	91.7	84.8
1888-------					166.2	144.1	129.1	118.2	118.5	105.3	99.6	90.8	81.6
1889-------				170.7	164.1	136.8	130.5	120.7	111.6	104.6	98.8	88.0	78.4
1890-------			174.6	168.9	155.2	140.0	133.4	114.2	111.7	104.5	95.0	83.8	76.1
1891-------	1917	171.1	173.6	157.9	160.3	142.6	126.4	114.0	111.4	101.1	91.0	81.9	70.5
1892-------	1918	170.2	160.9	164.3	162.0	133.2	125.2	113.2	106.9	95.6	87.5	74.6	64.6
1893-------	1919	156.8	168.6	165.5	150.4	131.5	124.6	109.0	100.8	92.5	80.8	69.6	63.6
1894-------	1920	167.1	171.4	153.7	148.9	131.0	120.0	104.2	98.5	85.9	76.0	68.7	60.4
1895-------	1921	170.7	160.4	152.8	148.2	126.7	115.5	101.9	92.4	81.4	75.6	65.3	57.9
1896-------	1922	160.7	159.5	151.4	142.6	122.3	112.2	95.2	87.0	80.5	70.8	62.4	53.5
1897-------	1923	160.0	158.8	145.5	137.1	118.0	105.6	90.1	86.1	75.4	68.5	57.9	53.3
1898-------	1924	161.1	152.6	139.8	132.0	111.3	100.9	90.2	81.5	72.9	63.8	58.1	51.0
1899-------	1925	156.8	148.2	136.9	126.5	108.0	101.8	87.1	81.5	70.2	66.0	57.3	49.7
1900-------	1926	150.2	144.1	128.9	120.6	108.0	96.9	84.9	76.5	71.6	64.1	55.2	49.0
1901-------	1927	147.3	135.4	122.6	119.5	102.9	93.6	79.2	77.3	68.5	60.8	53.5	48.0
1902-------	1928	138.1	128.5	121.8	113.3	97.5	86.1	79.4	73.1	64.6	58.7	52.4	45.8
1903-------	1929	132.9	128.5	117.1	108.7	91.3	87.9	76.1	70.4	63.5	58.5	50.6	45.0
1904-------	1930	133.0	123.5	113.1	102.8	94.4	85.6	74.6	70.3	63.9	57.4	50.9	45.5
1905-------	1931	127.4	118.9	106.3	105.6	91.6	83.2	74.6	70.7	62.7	57.4	51.3	47.2
1906-------	1932	122.3	111.9	108.9	102.5	89.4	83.4	75.3	69.8	63.7	58.0	52.6	51.5
1907-------	1933	115.3	115.2	106.3	100.0	90.3	85.0	75.0	71.1	64.9	61.8	57.8	53.0
1908-------	1934	118.1	111.7	103.6	100.3	91.8	84.0	76.7	72.3	70.2	67.6	59.9	54.6
1909-------	1935	116.0	110.4	105.7	103.6	91.7	87.0	79.5	80.0	76.7	69.0	62.9	56.6
1910-------	1936	115.0	112.4	109.3	102.4	95.2	89.9	86.1	87.0	77.5	72.0	65.5	57.4
1911-------	1937	118.3	117.3	108.4	106.7	99.2	95.5	93.8	86.4	80.5	75.9	66.9	54.1
1912-------	1938	122.0	115.1	112.6	110.9	107.5	104.1	93.0	88.8	85.0	76.7	62.2	52.9
1913-------	1939	120.8	119.9	118.6	121.3	115.1	102.6	95.6	95.3	86.7	71.6	61.1	52.6
1914-------	1940	126.6	127.7	132.0	128.7	111.6	105.5	104.7	97.9	81.0	70.9	61.2	54.3
1915-------	1941	134.6	141.9	138.4	122.7	113.4	117.0	108.0	91.2	80.2	71.2	63.3	56.2
1916-------	1942	149.3	147.7	129.2	122.4	127.0	120.8	99.6	89.8	80.2	73.0	64.9	56.4
1917-------	1943	154.0	136.8	127.3	140.0	133.3	112.2	99.0	90.3	82.6	74.9	65.8	58.1
1918-------	1944	141.8	131.5	147.6	147.6	122.6	111.2	99.1	92.8	85.0	75.6	67.1	57.4
1919-------	1945	135.9	159.9	160.6	138.4	124.6	113.2	104.8	98.2	87.5	79.1	68.2	59.1
1920-------	1946	168.9	174.4	150.1	139.8	126.0	118.6	109.7	99.6	90.2	78.9	68.6	59.5
1921-------	1947	186.2	163.3	151.8	141.5	132.1	124.2	110.8	102.7	90.5	79.7	69.6	58.1
1922-------	1948	172.7	163.1	152.1	146.5	136.7	124.1	112.9	101.6	90.2	80.0	67.0	57.1
1923-------	1949	174.3	164.4	159.5	152.2	137.2	127.3	112.7	102.5	91.7	77.9	66.8	56.2
1924-------	1950	176.3	174.2	166.0	153.8	141.8	127.6	114.3	104.5	89.4	77.9	66.2	56.0
1925-------	1951	186.2	180.3	167.4	157.9	141.3	129.1	115.8	101.6	88.9	77.2	65.9	53.2
1926-------	1952	192.0	181.5	171.7	158.0	142.7	130.0	112.7	100.6	87.8	76.0	62.3	51.2
1927-------	1953	194.2	184.9	171.4	159.7	144.2	127.2	112.0	99.4	86.9	72.5	60.3	50.0
1928-------	1954	198.0	185.8	172.9	161.1	141.5	127.1	110.8	98.3	82.4	69.7	58.6	45.8
1929-------	1955	200.9	190.1	177.7	159.6	143.0	126.8	111.7	95.0	80.7	68.8	54.2	41.8
1930-------	1956	206.3	194.7	175.6	161.0	142.3	126.4	107.0	92.8	79.2	63.1	49.0	38.3
1931-------	1957	213.7	194.0	177.6	160.7	142.4	121.8	104.7	90.9	72.5	57.1	45.2	35.3
1932-------	1958	212.2	195.9	177.3	159.7	136.3	118.7	101.6	83.0	65.1	52.1	41.8	32.9
1933-------	1959	213.9	195.5	176.6	153.0	132.3	115.1	92.8	74.0	60.0	48.8	39.5	31.3
1934-------	1960	213.7	194.1	169.9	148.7	128.8	105.1	83.1	68.1	55.5	46.7	37.7	28.6
1935-------	1961	211.4	187.2	164.3	145.0	116.5	94.0	76.5	63.3	53.8	44.5	34.3	24.9
1936-------	1962	204.7	180.7	159.8	130.6	105.1	86.5	71.2	61.8	51.8	40.5	29.6	21.8
1937-------	1963	196.9	174.5	143.7	118.3	97.9	82.2	70.8	60.2	47.2	34.8	26.2	
1938-------	1964	189.1	157.2	130.0	110.3	93.0	81.9	70.0	54.9	41.1	31.1		
1939-------	1965	171.3	143.7	123.5	107.1	94.6	82.6	65.0	48.8	37.5			
1940-------	1966	157.4	137.1	121.1	109.4	96.0	76.5	57.4	44.6				
1941-------	1967	151.1	135.3	123.7	111.3	89.6	67.9	53.2					
1942-------	1968	149.6	139.1	126.4	104.0	79.6	63.5						
1943-------	1969	151.7	140.6	117.8	92.1	74.6							
1944-------	1970	153.2	130.9	104.7	87.3								
1945-------	1971	142.1	116.1	99.2									
1946-------	1972	126.2	110.8										
1947-------	1973	119.3											

TABLE 4A. CENTRAL BIRTH RATES FOR ALL WOMEN DURING EACH YEAR 1917-73 BY AGE AND LIVE-BIRTH ORDER FOR EACH COHORT FROM 1868 TO 1959--CON.

LIVE-BIRTH ORDER AND COHORT	DIAGONAL LINE FOR CALENDAR YEAR	CURRENT AGE											
		38	39	40	41	42	43	44	45	46	47	48	49
TOTAL BIRTHS--CON.													
1868-------													1.1
1869-------												2.3	1.4
1870-------											4.1	2.8	1.1
1871-------										7.5	5.1	2.1	1.3
1872-------									11.7	9.1	3.9	2.4	1.0
1873-------								17.8	12.8	7.3	4.4	2.0	0.9
1874-------							25.4	18.4	11.2	7.9	3.9	1.9	0.9
1875-------						32.2	25.1	16.9	11.9	7.1	3.5	1.9	0.9
1876-------					44.2	32.1	24.4	17.3	11.1	6.6	3.6	1.8	0.7
1877-------				55.8	44.6	31.0	24.6	17.0	10.3	6.6	3.4	1.7	0.7
1878-------			75.1	56.0	43.2	31.3	25.1	16.1	10.4	6.4	3.0	1.7	0.6
1879-------	1917	84.3	75.2	54.9	44.1	31.9	23.4	16.0	10.3	6.2	3.0	1.4	0.5
1880-------	1918	83.6	74.3	55.5	44.3	29.8	23.2	15.9	9.9	6.0	2.8	1.5	0.7
1881-------	1919	82.9	74.4	55.9	41.3	29.6	23.2	15.1	9.2	5.4	2.6	1.3	0.6
1882-------	1920	82.5	74.6	51.8	40.6	29.5	22.2	14.2	8.7	5.2	2.7	1.2	0.4
1883-------	1921	82.6	69.0	50.9	40.3	28.2	21.0	13.4	8.2	4.8	2.5	1.1	0.4
1884-------	1922	76.5	67.8	50.3	38.8	26.9	19.9	12.6	7.6	4.5	2.2	1.2	0.5
1885-------	1923	75.2	66.9	48.5	36.7	25.8	18.6	11.5	7.4	4.3	2.0	1.2	0.5
1886-------	1924	74.8	64.1	45.4	35.3	23.9	16.9	11.4	7.0	4.2	1.9	1.1	0.7
1887-------	1925	72.5	61.2	44.9	33.0	22.3	17.0	10.7	6.6	3.8	1.8	1.0	0.6
1888-------	1926	68.6	59.3	41.4	30.4	22.0	15.8	10.2	6.1	3.5	1.7	1.0	0.5
1889-------	1927	67.7	55.6	39.0	30.5	21.0	15.6	9.8	5.9	3.6	1.6	0.9	0.4
1890-------	1928	62.4	51.6	38.8	28.6	20.2	14.8	9.5	5.7	3.3	1.5	1.0	0.4
1891-------	1929	57.9	51.2	36.1	27.5	19.1	14.6	8.8	5.2	2.9	1.4	0.9	0.2
1892-------	1930	57.3	47.3	34.4	25.7	18.7	13.4	8.2	4.9	2.9	1.2	0.7	0.2
1893-------	1931	53.6	45.3	32.3	25.2	17.3	12.4	7.5	4.7	2.6	1.1	0.4	0.2
1894-------	1932	51.1	42.0	31.9	23.8	16.1	11.5	7.6	4.3	2.4	1.1	0.3	0.2
1895-------	1933	47.8	41.7	30.2	22.3	15.4	11.3	6.9	4.0	2.3	0.9	0.3	0.1
1896-------	1934	47.3	39.4	28.2	21.2	15.2	10.4	6.4	3.8	2.2	0.7	0.3	0.2
1897-------	1935	44.9	36.9	27.3	20.9	14.1	10.1	6.1	3.9	2.0	0.8	0.3	0.1
1898-------	1936	42.4	35.8	27.1	19.9	13.9	9.7	6.9	4.2	2.1	1.1	0.3	0.2
1899-------	1937	42.4	36.2	26.3	19.6	13.7	10.0	6.8	3.9	2.3	1.0	0.3	0.2
1900-------	1938	42.3	34.6	25.9	19.5	13.5	10.5	6.9	4.0	2.2	1.0	0.3	0.1
1901-------	1939	40.2	33.3	25.2	18.4	14.2	10.8	6.8	3.8	2.1	0.8	0.3	0.1
1902-------	1940	39.2	33.0	25.3	20.2	15.0	10.9	6.6	3.6	1.7	0.7	0.2	0.1
1903-------	1941	38.8	33.9	27.0	20.8	15.4	10.7	6.5	3.3	1.7	0.6	0.2	0.1
1904-------	1942	40.8	36.4	27.7	21.7	14.9	10.6	5.8	3.2	1.6	0.5	0.2	0.1
1905-------	1943	44.0	37.1	28.7	21.4	15.1	9.8	5.9	3.0	1.4	0.5	0.2	0.1
1906-------	1944	45.0	38.2	28.7	21.4	14.0	9.5	5.4	3.0	1.4	0.5	0.2	0.1
1907-------	1945	46.4	38.9	29.2	20.3	13.7	9.3	5.5	3.0	1.4	0.5	0.1	0.1
1908-------	1946	47.1	38.6	27.1	19.7	13.1	9.1	5.5	2.9	1.6	0.5	0.1	0.1
1909-------	1947	47.9	36.6	27.0	19.5	13.6	9.5	5.7	2.9	1.5	0.5	0.2	0.1
1910-------	1948	45.2	36.5	27.0	20.0	14.0	9.6	5.7	2.8	1.5	0.5	0.2	0.1
1911-------	1949	44.7	36.1	27.6	20.5	14.2	9.8	5.8	3.0	1.5	0.6	0.1	0.1
1912-------	1950	44.2	36.7	28.1	20.7	14.8	9.8	5.7	3.0	1.4	0.6	0.1	0.1
1913-------	1951	45.1	37.7	28.4	21.3	14.6	9.9	5.6	2.8	1.5	0.6	0.1	0.1
1914-------	1952	47.0	38.2	29.3	21.2	14.9	9.9	5.6	3.0	1.5	0.5	0.1	0.1
1915-------	1953	47.4	39.2	29.4	21.7	14.9	9.5	5.7	2.8	1.4	0.6	0.1	0.0
1916-------	1954	48.2	39.2	28.9	21.6	14.2	9.6	5.5	3.0	1.5	0.3	0.1	0.0
1917-------	1955	48.5	39.3	29.6	21.0	14.4	9.3	5.6	2.8	1.2	0.4	0.1	0.0
1918-------	1956	48.1	39.2	28.5	20.8	14.1	9.4	5.2	2.5	1.2	0.2	0.1	0.0
1919-------	1957	49.4	38.9	29.1	20.9	14.5	9.2	5.3	2.5	1.0	0.2	0.1	0.0
1920-------	1958	48.2	39.0	28.8	21.2	14.0	8.8	5.0	2.4	1.0	0.2	0.1	0.0
1921-------	1959	48.1	38.1	28.9	20.2	13.6	8.7	4.7	2.3	0.9	0.2	0.1	0.0
1922-------	1960	46.9	37.7	27.1	19.3	12.8	7.8	4.4	2.2	0.8	0.2	0.0	0.0
1923-------	1961	46.6	35.7	26.0	18.8	12.1	7.2	4.1	1.9	0.7	0.1	0.0	0.0
1924-------	1962	44.2	34.6	25.8	17.5	11.0	6.7	3.7	1.8	0.8	0.1	0.0	0.0
1925-------	1963	42.8	34.1	24.0	16.0	10.0	6.1	3.3	1.7	0.7	0.1	0.0	
1926-------	1964	42.0	31.7	21.6	14.6	9.3	5.6	3.1	1.4	0.5	0.1		
1927-------	1965	38.7	28.3	19.7	13.2	8.4	5.0	2.4	1.1	0.4			
1928-------	1966	34.6	25.6	17.8	12.0	7.8	4.4	2.1	1.0				
1929-------	1967	32.1	23.7	16.8	11.4	6.7	4.0	2.0					
1930-------	1968	29.3	22.0	15.8	9.8	5.9	3.4						
1931-------	1969	27.3	21.0	13.7	8.7	5.4							
1932-------	1970	25.9	18.4	12.0	7.7								
1933-------	1971	23.0	15.9	10.6									
1934-------	1972	20.4	14.1										
1935-------	1973	17.8											

TABLE 4A. CENTRAL BIRTH RATES FOR ALL WOMEN DURING EACH YEAR 1917-73 BY AGE AND LIVE-BIRTH ORDER FOR EACH COHORT FROM 1868 TO 1959--CON.

LIVE-BIRTH ORDER AND COHORT	DIAGONAL LINE FOR CALENDAR YEAR	CURRENT AGE 14	15	16	17	18	19	20	21	22	23	24	25
FIRST BIRTHS													
1892-------													47.8
1893-------												56.9	48.6
1894-------											67.3	57.5	38.1
1895-------										74.6	67.6	44.5	49.8
1896-------									83.0	75.1	51.7	58.8	51.5
1897-------								85.4	83.8	57.7	68.9	60.5	46.3
1898-------							81.8	85.7	65.1	77.2	70.8	54.2	45.2
1899-------						65.7	80.7	68.4	85.6	78.2	61.9	52.3	46.0
1900-------					45.6	63.9	66.7	89.3	86.5	68.3	60.1	54.0	44.1
1901-------				24.4	44.1	54.9	86.3	92.4	75.7	66.4	63.0	52.3	42.6
1902-------			10.9	24.0	38.6	71.3	91.7	82.0	74.0	70.1	60.9	50.3	42.0
1903-------	1917	3.5	10.9	21.1	49.6	76.9	81.3	80.4	77.4	67.9	58.9	49.8	40.9
1904-------	1918	3.6	9.3	26.5	52.6	67.9	79.8	84.3	74.6	65.9	57.6	48.1	39.6
1905-------	1919	3.0	11.5	27.8	46.2	67.4	84.3	80.5	71.7	64.0	55.2	46.0	40.9
1906-------	1920	3.6	12.1	24.4	46.1	72.0	80.9	77.5	70.3	61.0	52.8	47.4	39.1
1907-------	1921	3.8	10.6	24.4	49.1	69.8	78.0	75.9	66.9	59.0	54.5	45.3	37.4
1908-------	1922	3.4	10.8	26.1	48.7	67.4	76.1	72.2	64.8	60.6	51.4	43.2	35.1
1909-------	1923	3.5	11.5	26.5	47.2	65.6	72.7	69.2	66.7	57.3	49.4	40.5	37.7
1910-------	1924	3.7	11.8	25.6	46.6	62.9	69.3	71.3	62.8	54.9	46.0	43.5	39.3
1911-------	1925	3.9	11.8	26.3	44.6	60.2	71.8	67.5	60.8	51.8	50.0	45.7	40.9
1912-------	1926	3.9	12.2	24.7	43.3	62.3	67.3	65.2	57.1	56.2	52.3	47.1	43.2
1913-------	1927	4.1	11.3	24.3	44.7	58.1	65.3	61.4	62.3	58.8	53.2	49.6	45.6
1914-------	1928	3.7	11.1	25.0	41.4	56.2	60.9	66.6	64.7	59.4	55.9	52.0	45.5
1915-------	1929	3.7	11.4	23.4	40.1	52.2	65.8	68.5	64.4	61.6	58.0	51.1	47.2
1916-------	1930	3.8	10.6	22.4	36.9	55.7	66.9	67.3	66.0	63.3	56.1	51.9	52.9
1917-------	1931	3.5	10.2	20.6	39.2	56.5	64.8	68.7	67.7	61.1	56.4	58.6	64.6
1918-------	1932	3.3	9.4	21.8	40.0	54.6	66.6	70.2	64.7	61.5	63.4	72.3	57.5
1919-------	1933	3.2	9.9	22.7	39.1	57.3	69.2	67.9	67.2	70.3	79.6	64.7	48.6
1920-------	1934	3.4	10.7	22.3	41.4	59.3	66.2	69.1	75.2	85.0	71.2	56.0	46.0
1921-------	1935	3.7	10.6	23.9	43.0	56.7	66.4	76.2	87.5	76.0	63.3	53.4	67.7
1922-------	1936	3.5	11.0	24.2	40.2	54.6	70.8	86.7	79.4	68.6	59.9	77.4	77.6
1923-------	1937	3.7	11.2	22.8	39.2	57.9	80.0	81.5	72.3	65.4	85.9	90.1	62.4
1924-------	1938	3.8	10.7	22.7	41.8	64.6	77.4	73.2	69.2	92.7	102.3	73.4	57.0
1925-------	1939	3.7	10.9	24.4	44.1	64.1	68.3	70.5	95.1	113.1	84.2	67.0	52.1
1926-------	1940	3.8	11.7	25.0	44.1	55.8	65.3	92.6	119.8	94.1	77.0	61.5	54.3
1927-------	1941	4.1	11.9	25.1	38.6	53.2	81.9	120.8	101.8	86.0	70.7	64.4	53.3
1928-------	1942	4.1	12.0	22.0	36.7	63.3	110.2	106.0	93.5	79.5	75.0	63.7	50.8
1929-------	1943	4.2	10.7	21.3	41.6	87.9	101.2	98.8	87.3	85.9	75.2	61.6	50.6
1930-------	1944	3.8	10.5	22.6	58.5	84.8	95.1	92.7	95.2	86.3	73.1	62.4	49.5
1931-------	1945	3.9	10.8	32.3	59.8	81.2	90.6	102.4	95.9	85.2	75.4	62.1	49.4
1932-------	1946	3.8	14.7	34.2	57.9	78.2	99.9	102.2	96.7	88.6	75.8	62.4	48.7
1933-------	1947	5.2	16.3	34.1	57.0	85.8	98.8	104.7	100.4	89.4	76.9	61.8	45.5
1934-------	1948	5.8	16.5	34.1	61.2	84.2	102.3	108.7	100.9	92.0	76.7	58.3	43.5
1935-------	1949	5.7	16.6	35.9	60.0	86.8	105.2	108.6	105.4	92.2	73.0	56.1	42.0
1936-------	1950	5.8	17.2	35.2	61.8	89.1	104.3	113.9	106.0	88.3	70.4	54.6	41.0
1937-------	1951	6.0	16.8	36.2	62.9	88.1	109.8	115.5	102.3	86.1	69.4	53.5	39.0
1938-------	1952	5.7	17.1	37.0	62.0	92.5	112.0	112.0	100.7	84.9	68.0	50.7	38.4
1939-------	1953	5.8	17.9	36.8	65.5	95.2	108.9	111.5	99.2	83.4	64.7	50.0	38.9
1940-------	1954	6.3	17.6	38.5	67.1	91.9	107.9	109.0	98.0	80.1	63.4	50.5	38.0
1941-------	1955	6.1	18.5	39.4	63.8	89.8	104.3	107.2	94.6	78.1	64.0	49.0	40.8
1942-------	1956	6.2	18.5	36.9	61.7	86.4	102.5	103.6	92.3	78.4	61.7	52.7	41.7
1943-------	1957	6.1	17.2	35.7	59.0	84.6	98.9	101.5	91.0	74.0	64.6	52.4	44.7
1944-------	1958	5.8	17.1	34.6	58.4	81.6	97.3	99.2	85.5	76.0	63.0	54.0	45.1
1945-------	1959	6.0	16.9	34.3	55.9	80.2	94.2	92.6	86.0	73.2	63.4	54.4	46.5
1946-------	1960	6.0	16.5	32.4	54.5	77.6	89.3	93.6	83.4	74.2	65.3	57.2	45.2
1947-------	1961	5.5	15.2	31.4	52.7	74.1	89.5	89.8	83.9	75.3	67.1	54.0	42.1
1948-------	1962	5.1	14.7	30.5	51.2	74.2	86.0	90.2	84.1	76.4	61.9	48.7	40.9
1949-------	1963	5.1	14.7	29.9	50.7	71.2	85.6	89.1	84.0	68.8	54.0	45.8	
1950-------	1964	5.2	14.6	29.9	49.8	71.5	85.4	89.8	75.3	59.4	50.4		
1951-------	1965	5.2	14.7	29.7	50.2	71.9	87.0	80.9	65.3	54.9			
1952-------	1966	5.3	14.8	30.2	51.1	74.7	79.7	71.3	60.2				
1953-------	1967	5.3	15.2	30.9	54.4	70.1	72.7	66.0					
1954-------	1968	5.7	15.9	33.7	52.5	66.8	68.0						
1955-------	1969	6.0	17.6	33.4	52.7	63.7							
1956-------	1970	6.6	17.6	34.7	51.2								
1957-------	1971	6.7	18.6	34.4									
1958-------	1972	7.1	18.8										
1959-------	1973	7.4											

TABLE 4A. CENTRAL BIRTH RATES FOR ALL WOMEN DURING EACH YEAR 1917-73 BY AGE AND LIVE-BIRTH ORDER FOR EACH COHORT FROM 1868 TO 1959--CON.

LIVE-BIRTH ORDER AND COHORT	DIAGONAL LINE FOR CALENDAR YEAR	CURRENT AGE											
		26	27	28	29	30	31	32	33	34	35	36	37
FIRST BIRTHS--CON.													
1880-------													3.9
1881-------												4.8	4.1
1882-------											6.1	5.0	4.0
1883-------										7.2	6.3	4.9	4.2
1884-------									8.7	7.5	6.0	5.1	4.4
1885-------								10.1	9.3	6.9	6.4	5.4	4.1
1886-------							13.2	10.9	8.3	7.7	6.7	5.0	3.9
1887-------						17.1	14.2	9.7	9.4	7.8	6.3	4.9	4.0
1888-------					22.9	18.1	12.7	11.0	9.4	7.5	6.1	5.0	4.0
1889-------				27.8	24.0	15.4	14.4	11.0	9.2	7.3	6.2	5.0	3.7
1890-------			33.3	29.0	19.8	18.4	14.4	10.8	8.9	7.4	6.1	4.6	3.9
1891-------	1917	38.3	34.7	23.1	24.5	18.7	14.1	10.5	9.0	7.4	5.7	4.8	3.7
1892-------	1918	39.8	27.5	29.4	24.8	17.4	13.6	10.5	8.8	6.8	5.8	4.5	3.4
1893-------	1919	31.6	35.0	30.2	22.6	16.7	13.6	10.4	8.2	6.8	5.5	4.2	3.5
1894-------	1920	40.6	36.3	27.1	21.7	16.8	13.4	9.9	8.4	6.5	5.2	4.3	3.4
1895-------	1921	42.3	32.8	26.0	21.9	16.5	12.9	9.9	8.0	6.4	5.5	4.3	3.2
1896-------	1922	38.4	31.6	26.2	21.3	15.9	12.8	9.5	7.9	6.7	5.3	4.0	3.0
1897-------	1923	37.0	31.9	25.3	20.4	15.6	12.4	9.4	8.3	6.4	5.0	3.7	3.0
1898-------	1924	37.6	30.7	24.2	19.9	15.1	12.3	9.9	7.8	5.9	4.6	3.8	3.1
1899-------	1925	36.6	29.8	24.1	19.7	15.2	13.0	9.6	7.7	5.9	5.0	4.2	3.4
1900-------	1926	35.1	29.2	23.3	19.3	15.9	12.5	9.3	7.3	6.2	5.3	4.3	3.5
1901-------	1927	35.0	28.4	22.9	20.1	15.5	12.2	8.8	7.8	6.5	5.5	4.5	3.7
1902-------	1928	33.6	27.8	23.8	19.6	14.8	11.2	9.4	8.1	6.7	5.7	4.8	3.9
1903-------	1929	33.2	29.0	23.5	18.7	13.8	12.2	9.9	8.5	7.1	6.2	5.2	4.1
1904-------	1930	34.5	28.3	22.3	17.7	15.2	13.1	10.6	9.1	7.9	6.7	5.5	4.5
1905-------	1931	33.3	26.8	21.0	19.3	16.1	13.7	11.3	9.9	8.4	7.0	6.1	5.6
1906-------	1932	31.7	25.5	22.9	20.3	16.9	14.6	12.3	10.5	8.8	7.7	6.9	5.9
1907-------	1933	30.0	27.5	24.2	21.2	18.3	16.0	13.1	11.0	9.7	9.5	7.4	5.8
1908-------	1934	32.0	28.9	24.9	22.6	19.7	16.8	13.7	12.0	12.1	9.6	7.3	6.0
1909-------	1935	33.7	29.8	26.9	24.6	20.7	17.8	15.2	15.4	11.9	9.0	7.4	7.1
1910-------	1936	35.0	31.9	28.9	25.2	21.9	19.6	18.0	14.8	10.7	9.1	8.9	7.8
1911-------	1937	37.3	34.4	29.4	26.7	24.2	21.9	17.4	12.7	10.8	11.1	9.9	6.5
1912-------	1938	39.6	34.5	31.0	29.6	27.4	21.0	14.9	12.7	13.3	12.1	8.1	6.0
1913-------	1939	39.9	36.5	34.8	34.0	25.3	18.1	14.8	16.0	14.7	9.9	7.4	5.6
1914-------	1940	42.3	41.2	41.0	30.7	21.4	17.6	19.2	17.9	11.9	9.1	6.9	5.4
1915-------	1941	47.5	48.9	36.3	25.6	20.7	23.6	21.7	14.2	10.8	8.4	6.7	5.3
1916-------	1942	57.0	43.2	29.7	24.5	28.3	26.4	16.9	12.8	9.8	8.1	6.5	5.0
1917-------	1943	50.3	35.3	28.6	34.4	31.9	20.8	15.2	11.5	9.6	7.9	6.1	4.8
1918-------	1944	41.2	33.4	40.4	38.4	24.8	18.5	13.6	11.4	9.3	7.2	5.7	4.4
1919-------	1945	39.3	48.7	46.0	30.4	22.5	16.9	13.7	11.2	8.7	7.0	5.4	4.2
1920-------	1946	57.7	55.5	36.3	27.5	20.4	16.9	13.4	10.3	8.3	6.5	5.1	4.0
1921-------	1947	66.1	44.0	32.8	24.9	20.4	16.4	12.3	10.0	7.7	6.1	4.8	3.7
1922-------	1948	52.3	39.5	29.8	25.0	19.7	15.0	11.9	9.1	7.2	5.8	4.5	3.4
1923-------	1949	47.3	36.2	30.2	24.2	18.4	14.7	10.9	8.7	7.0	5.4	4.2	3.2
1924-------	1950	43.6	37.3	29.5	22.5	17.7	13.4	10.4	8.4	6.4	5.1	3.9	3.0
1925-------	1951	45.2	36.3	27.6	21.6	16.4	12.8	10.0	7.8	6.1	4.8	3.7	2.7
1926-------	1952	44.0	34.0	26.3	20.3	15.5	12.3	9.3	7.3	5.7	4.4	3.3	2.5
1927-------	1953	41.9	32.6	24.9	19.3	15.1	11.5	8.8	6.8	5.3	4.1	3.1	2.8
1928-------	1954	40.5	31.1	23.8	18.9	14.1	10.9	8.2	6.4	4.9	3.8	3.4	2.7
1929-------	1955	39.2	30.3	23.6	17.7	13.3	10.3	7.8	5.9	4.6	4.2	3.3	2.5
1930-------	1956	38.6	29.8	22.1	16.6	12.6	9.7	7.2	5.6	5.1	4.0	3.1	2.2
1931-------	1957	38.2	28.0	20.7	15.8	11.9	8.9	6.8	6.1	4.7	3.7	2.7	2.4
1932-------	1958	35.6	26.4	19.7	14.8	10.9	8.6	7.3	5.7	4.4	3.3	3.0	2.0
1933-------	1959	33.7	25.1	18.6	13.6	10.6	9.0	6.9	5.4	4.0	3.6	2.6	2.0
1934-------	1960	32.2	23.8	17.5	13.4	11.3	8.6	6.6	4.9	4.4	3.2	2.5	1.8
1935-------	1961	31.1	22.8	17.0	14.3	10.6	8.4	6.0	5.4	3.9	3.1	2.3	1.7
1936-------	1962	30.0	22.1	18.2	13.5	10.5	7.7	6.7	4.9	4.0	2.9	2.2	1.6
1937-------	1963	29.2	23.1	17.5	13.7	10.1	8.6	6.4	5.1	3.7	2.8	2.1	
1938-------	1964	30.0	22.6	17.6	13.4	11.1	8.4	6.6	4.7	3.7	2.7		
1939-------	1965	29.4	23.2	17.6	14.9	11.2	8.8	6.4	4.8	3.6			
1940-------	1966	30.9	23.7	19.9	14.9	11.7	8.5	6.2	4.7				
1941-------	1967	31.8	26.7	20.1	16.0	11.6	8.4	6.4					
1942-------	1968	35.3	27.3	21.5	15.7	11.4	8.8						
1943-------	1969	35.8	28.5	21.3	15.3	11.9							
1944-------	1970	37.1	28.1	20.6	16.1								
1945-------	1971	36.1	27.1	21.3									
1946-------	1972	34.8	28.0										
1947-------	1973	34.7											

TABLE 4A. CENTRAL BIRTH RATES FOR ALL WOMEN DURING EACH YEAR 1917-73 BY AGE AND LIVE-BIRTH ORDER FOR EACH COHORT FROM 1868 TO 1959--CON.

LIVE-BIRTH ORDER AND COHORT	DIAGONAL LINE FOR CALENDAR YEAR	CURRENT AGE											
		38	39	40	41	42	43	44	45	46	47	48	49
FIRST BIRTHS--CON.													
1868-------													0.0
1869-------												0.1	0.0
1870-------											0.1	0.1	0.0
1871-------										0.1	0.1	0.0	0.0
1872-------									0.2	0.2	0.1	0.0	0.0
1873-------								0.3	0.2	0.1	0.1	0.0	0.0
1874-------							0.5	0.4	0.2	0.1	0.1	0.1	0.0
1875-------						0.7	0.5	0.3	0.2	0.1	0.1	0.0	0.0
1876-------					1.1	0.8	0.6	0.3	0.2	0.1	0.1	0.0	0.0
1877-------				1.6	1.2	0.8	0.6	0.3	0.2	0.1	0.1	0.1	0.0
1878-------			2.4	1.7	1.2	0.8	0.6	0.3	0.2	0.1	0.1	0.0	0.0
1879-------	1917	3.0	2.6	1.7	1.3	0.8	0.6	0.3	0.2	0.1	0.0	0.0	0.0
1880-------	1918	3.2	2.6	1.8	1.3	0.8	0.6	0.3	0.2	0.1	0.0	0.0	0.0
1881-------	1919	3.1	2.7	1.9	1.2	0.8	0.6	0.3	0.2	0.1	0.0	0.1	0.0
1882-------	1920	3.3	2.8	1.7	1.2	0.8	0.5	0.3	0.2	0.1	0.1	0.0	0.0
1883-------	1921	3.4	2.6	1.7	1.2	0.7	0.5	0.3	0.2	0.1	0.1	0.0	0.0
1884-------	1922	3.2	2.5	1.7	1.2	0.8	0.5	0.3	0.2	0.1	0.0	0.0	0.0
1885-------	1923	3.0	2.5	1.7	1.1	0.7	0.5	0.3	0.2	0.1	0.0	0.0	0.0
1886-------	1924	3.1	2.5	1.6	1.1	0.7	0.4	0.3	0.2	0.1	0.0	0.0	0.0
1887-------	1925	3.1	2.3	1.6	1.1	0.7	0.4	0.3	0.1	0.1	0.0	0.0	0.0
1888-------	1926	2.9	2.4	1.5	1.0	0.7	0.4	0.2	0.1	0.0	0.0	0.0	0.0
1889-------	1927	3.0	2.3	1.5	1.0	0.7	0.4	0.2	0.1	0.1	0.0	0.0	0.0
1890-------	1928	2.9	2.2	1.5	1.0	0.6	0.4	0.2	0.2	0.1	0.0	0.0	0.0
1891-------	1929	2.7	2.2	1.4	1.0	0.6	0.4	0.2	0.1	0.0	0.0	0.0	0.0
1892-------	1930	2.8	2.1	1.4	0.9	0.6	0.4	0.2	0.1	0.1	0.0	0.0	0.0
1893-------	1931	2.7	2.0	1.2	0.9	0.5	0.4	0.2	0.1	0.1	0.0	0.0	0.0
1894-------	1932	2.5	1.8	1.2	0.8	0.5	0.4	0.2	0.1	0.1	0.0	0.0	0.0
1895-------	1933	2.3	1.8	1.2	0.9	0.6	0.4	0.2	0.1	0.1	0.0	0.0	0.0
1896-------	1934	2.3	1.8	1.3	0.9	0.6	0.4	0.2	0.1	0.1	0.0	0.0	0.0
1897-------	1935	2.4	1.9	1.3	0.9	0.6	0.4	0.2	0.1	0.1	0.0	0.0	0.0
1898-------	1936	2.5	1.9	1.3	0.9	0.6	0.4	0.2	0.2	0.1	0.0	0.0	0.0
1899-------	1937	2.6	2.0	1.5	1.0	0.7	0.4	0.3	0.2	0.1	0.0	0.0	0.0
1900-------	1938	2.8	2.2	1.5	1.1	0.7	0.5	0.3	0.2	0.1	0.0	0.0	0.0
1901-------	1939	3.0	2.2	1.7	1.2	0.8	0.6	0.4	0.2	0.1	0.0	0.0	0.0
1902-------	1940	3.1	2.5	2.0	1.4	1.0	0.7	0.4	0.2	0.1	0.0	0.0	0.0
1903-------	1941	3.4	3.1	2.2	1.6	1.0	0.7	0.4	0.2	0.1	0.0	0.0	0.0
1904-------	1942	4.3	3.3	2.3	1.6	1.1	0.7	0.3	0.2	0.1	0.0	0.0	0.0
1905-------	1943	4.6	3.3	2.4	1.8	1.2	0.7	0.4	0.2	0.1	0.0	0.0	0.0
1906-------	1944	4.5	3.5	2.8	2.0	1.1	0.7	0.4	0.2	0.1	0.0	0.0	0.0
1907-------	1945	4.7	4.1	3.1	1.8	1.1	0.7	0.4	0.2	0.1	0.0	0.0	0.0
1908-------	1946	5.5	4.4	2.8	1.8	1.0	0.6	0.4	0.2	0.1	0.0	0.0	0.0
1909-------	1947	6.0	3.9	2.6	1.7	1.0	0.7	0.4	0.2	0.1	0.0	0.0	0.0
1910-------	1948	5.2	3.7	2.5	1.6	1.1	0.7	0.4	0.2	0.1	0.0	0.0	0.0
1911-------	1949	4.7	3.4	2.4	1.6	1.1	0.6	0.4	0.2	0.1	0.0	0.0	0.0
1912-------	1950	4.4	3.3	2.4	1.6	1.0	0.6	0.3	0.2	0.0	0.0	0.0	0.0
1913-------	1951	4.3	3.3	2.2	1.5	1.0	0.6	0.3	0.1	0.1	0.0	0.0	0.0
1914-------	1952	4.2	3.1	2.2	1.4	0.9	0.6	0.3	0.2	0.1	0.0	0.0	0.0
1915-------	1953	4.0	3.0	2.0	1.3	0.9	0.5	0.3	0.1	0.1	0.0	0.0	0.0
1916-------	1954	3.8	2.8	1.8	1.3	0.8	0.5	0.2	0.1	0.0	0.0	0.0	0.0
1917-------	1955	3.6	2.5	1.8	1.2	0.7	0.4	0.2	0.1	0.0	0.0	0.0	0.0
1918-------	1956	3.3	2.5	1.6	1.1	0.7	0.4	0.2	0.1	0.0	0.0	0.0	0.0
1919-------	1957	3.2	2.3	1.6	1.0	0.6	0.4	0.2	0.1	0.0	0.0	0.0	0.0
1920-------	1958	2.9	2.1	1.5	1.0	0.6	0.3	0.2	0.1	0.0	0.0	0.0	0.0
1921-------	1959	2.7	2.0	1.4	0.9	0.6	0.4	0.2	0.1	0.0	0.0	0.0	0.0
1922-------	1960	2.5	1.9	1.2	0.8	0.6	0.4	0.2	0.1	0.0	0.0	0.0	0.0
1923-------	1961	2.4	1.7	1.2	1.0	0.6	0.3	0.2	0.1	0.0	0.0	0.0	0.0
1924-------	1962	2.2	1.6	1.3	0.9	0.5	0.3	0.2	0.1	0.0	0.0	0.0	0.0
1925-------	1963	2.0	1.8	1.2	0.8	0.4	0.3	0.1	0.1	0.0	0.0	0.0	
1926-------	1964	2.3	1.7	1.1	0.7	0.5	0.2	0.1	0.1	0.0	0.0		
1927-------	1965	2.2	1.5	1.0	0.8	0.4	0.2	0.1	0.0	0.0			
1928-------	1966	2.0	1.3	1.1	0.6	0.4	0.2	0.1	0.0				
1929-------	1967	1.7	1.5	0.9	0.6	0.3	0.2	0.1					
1930-------	1968	1.9	1.2	0.9	0.5	0.3	0.2						
1931-------	1969	1.6	1.2	0.8	0.5	0.3							
1932-------	1970	1.6	1.0	0.7	0.5								
1933-------	1971	1.4	1.0	0.7									
1934-------	1972	1.3	0.9										
1935-------	1973	1.2											

TABLE 4A. CENTRAL BIRTH RATES FOR ALL WOMEN DURING EACH YEAR 1917-73 BY AGE AND LIVE-BIRTH ORDER FOR EACH COHORT FROM 1868 TO 1959--CON.

LIVE-BIRTH ORDER AND COHORT	DIAGONAL LINE FOR CALENDAR YEAR	CURRENT AGE 14	15	16	17	18	19	20	21	22	23	24	25
SECOND BIRTHS													
1892-------													49.6
1893-------												54.1	48.6
1894-------											58.1	52.9	46.9
1895-------										56.5	56.7	50.8	46.9
1896-------									53.6	55.2	54.1	50.3	46.4
1897-------								44.7	52.5	52.9	53.1	49.8	48.1
1898-------							32.1	44.0	50.6	52.3	52.9	52.5	49.4
1899-------						17.5	31.5	42.0	49.5	51.3	55.1	53.0	47.6
1900-------					7.7	17.1	30.0	41.3	48.6	53.4	55.9	51.5	45.0
1901-------				2.4	7.4	16.0	29.4	41.7	50.5	54.1	54.5	48.9	43.3
1902-------			0.6	2.3	7.2	16.3	31.5	44.3	51.7	53.4	51.4	47.2	41.4
1903-------	1917	*	0.5	2.3	7.3	18.6	33.4	45.2	50.4	51.3	50.3	45.3	39.7
1904-------	1918	*	0.5	2.3	8.2	19.6	33.8	43.4	48.2	50.3	48.0	43.1	38.5
1905-------	1919	*	0.5	2.5	8.5	20.0	32.3	41.4	47.4	48.2	45.2	41.6	38.3
1906-------	1920	*	0.6	2.6	8.7	19.0	31.0	41.1	46.1	45.3	43.8	41.1	36.9
1907-------	1921	*	0.6	2.7	8.3	18.7	31.2	40.3	43.6	44.0	43.3	39.8	35.9
1908-------	1922	*	0.6	2.6	8.5	19.0	30.7	38.1	42.2	43.4	41.6	38.4	33.8
1909-------	1923	*	0.6	2.8	8.8	18.8	29.0	36.8	41.7	42.0	40.5	36.4	34.7
1910-------	1924	*	0.6	2.9	8.8	17.5	28.0	36.3	39.9	40.8	38.2	37.0	33.2
1911-------	1925	*	0.7	3.0	8.3	17.1	27.9	35.0	39.4	38.6	39.1	35.7	33.6
1912-------	1926	*	0.7	2.8	8.1	16.9	26.6	34.5	36.8	39.2	37.4	36.2	34.7
1913-------	1927	*	0.7	2.7	8.0	16.3	26.0	31.8	37.3	37.7	38.1	37.5	36.7
1914-------	1928	*	0.6	2.6	7.6	15.8	23.9	32.0	35.9	38.5	39.6	39.4	36.8
1915-------	1929	*	0.6	2.5	7.3	14.5	23.8	31.1	36.8	40.0	41.2	39.2	38.5
1916-------	1930	*	0.6	2.4	6.7	14.2	23.2	31.9	37.8	41.1	40.5	40.2	40.3
1917-------	1931	*	0.6	2.2	6.6	14.1	24.0	32.5	38.9	40.2	41.1	41.8	45.8
1918-------	1932	*	0.5	2.2	6.6	14.6	24.5	33.4	37.8	40.9	42.1	48.1	51.3
1919-------	1933	*	0.5	2.3	7.1	15.3	25.4	33.3	39.4	42.5	49.3	53.0	46.8
1920-------	1934	*	0.6	2.5	7.5	15.8	25.6	35.3	40.3	46.2	53.2	47.6	43.1
1921-------	1935	*	0.7	2.8	7.8	16.4	27.9	36.2	41.2	49.7	47.3	43.0	57.3
1922-------	1936	*	0.7	2.8	7.8	17.9	27.8	35.2	44.7	44.7	41.5	58.5	63.1
1923-------	1937	*	0.7	2.8	8.6	18.0	27.4	38.1	40.6	39.1	57.8	64.7	63.7
1924-------	1938	*	0.7	3.2	8.8	18.1	29.4	34.6	35.5	54.8	64.1	67.1	66.8
1925-------	1939	*	0.9	3.3	9.3	18.9	26.5	30.4	48.0	60.4	67.9	70.5	67.4
1926-------	1940	*	0.9	3.8	9.8	16.9	23.4	38.8	53.1	65.9	71.5	70.7	69.2
1927-------	1941	*	1.3	4.1	8.9	15.3	27.6	43.3	60.3	69.9	71.3	72.5	69.2
1928-------	1942	*	1.3	3.7	8.2	16.8	31.4	51.0	64.6	69.7	73.3	72.8	69.7
1929-------	1943	*	1.2	3.5	8.7	19.5	38.2	55.8	64.9	72.1	74.6	75.0	70.2
1930-------	1944	*	1.2	3.6	10.1	24.2	42.6	56.2	67.3	74.0	77.3	76.3	69.7
1931-------	1945	*	1.3	4.4	12.7	27.9	43.6	58.8	69.8	78.1	80.3	76.9	71.1
1932-------	1946	*	1.5	5.4	14.8	28.6	45.1	60.5	73.4	81.3	81.9	79.6	72.2
1933-------	1947	*	1.8	6.4	15.3	29.7	46.7	64.0	76.7	83.9	85.3	81.5	70.7
1934-------	1948	*	2.1	6.5	15.9	30.3	49.0	66.1	79.9	87.7	87.8	80.5	69.7
1935-------	1949	*	2.0	6.6	16.0	31.4	49.6	68.8	83.1	90.3	87.4	79.6	68.0
1936-------	1950	*	2.0	6.4	16.5	31.8	51.8	71.7	85.3	89.8	87.0	78.3	65.5
1937-------	1951	*	1.9	6.4	16.6	33.0	54.3	73.5	85.5	90.3	85.9	75.7	62.3
1938-------	1952	*	1.8	6.7	17.1	34.7	55.2	74.0	87.2	89.2	83.5	72.1	60.4
1939-------	1953	*	2.0	7.0	18.2	35.6	56.4	76.0	85.8	87.3	79.8	70.0	58.7
1940-------	1954	*	2.1	7.3	18.6	36.3	57.5	74.1	83.6	83.9	77.3	67.5	54.9
1941-------	1955	*	2.2	7.5	18.9	35.9	55.4	71.4	80.2	80.4	73.7	62.7	53.5
1942-------	1956	*	2.1	7.5	18.3	34.7	52.6	68.2	76.2	75.6	67.7	60.5	54.5
1943-------	1957	*	2.1	7.1	17.7	32.8	50.3	64.2	70.8	68.4	64.3	61.0	55.0
1944-------	1958	*	2.0	7.0	17.1	31.8	47.6	59.6	63.1	64.0	64.1	60.4	57.1
1945-------	1959	*	2.1	7.0	16.8	30.0	44.1	52.7	58.2	62.2	61.6	60.8	57.8
1946-------	1960	*	2.1	6.9	15.7	27.6	38.6	47.7	55.9	59.5	62.4	62.1	54.8
1947-------	1961	*	2.0	6.3	14.3	24.3	34.7	45.6	52.6	59.5	62.9	58.3	50.7
1948-------	1962	*	1.8	5.7	12.6	21.9	33.2	42.6	52.4	59.6	58.8	52.7	49.4
1949-------	1963	*	1.8	5.3	11.8	21.1	30.6	41.9	52.3	55.6	51.9	50.2	
1950-------	1964	*	1.7	5.0	11.4	19.6	30.4	42.1	48.8	48.5	49.1		
1951-------	1965	*	1.6	5.0	10.5	19.4	30.7	39.5	42.6	45.7			
1952-------	1966	*	1.6	4.5	10.3	19.4	28.9	34.8	40.0				
1953-------	1967	*	1.4	4.4	10.5	18.6	25.9	32.8					
1954-------	1968	*	1.4	4.6	10.2	17.1	24.6						
1955-------	1969	*	1.5	4.5	9.5	16.4							
1956-------	1970	*	1.5	4.2	9.1								
1957-------	1971	*	1.4	4.1									
1958-------	1972	*	1.3										
1959-------	1973	*											

TABLE 4A. CENTRAL BIRTH RATES FOR ALL WOMEN DURING EACH YEAR 1917-73 BY AGE AND LIVE-BIRTH ORDER FOR EACH COHORT FROM 1868 TO 1959--CON.

LIVE-BIRTH ORDER AND COHORT	DIAGONAL LINE FOR CALENDAR YEAR	CURRENT AGE											
		26	27	28	29	30	31	32	33	34	35	36	37
SECOND BIRTHS--CON.													
1880-------													6.2
1881-------												7.8	6.3
1882-------											9.6	7.9	6.3
1883-------										11.5	9.6	7.8	6.3
1884-------									14.0	11.4	9.5	7.9	6.5
1885-------								16.4	13.8	11.3	9.7	8.2	6.2
1886-------							20.3	16.3	13.8	11.6	10.0	7.8	6.3
1887-------						25.2	20.3	16.2	14.2	11.9	9.7	7.9	6.2
1888-------					31.9	25.0	20.1	16.7	14.4	11.8	9.8	7.8	6.0
1889-------				36.7	31.7	24.6	20.7	16.9	14.5	11.7	9.7	7.6	5.8
1890-------			40.8	36.6	31.0	25.1	21.1	17.1	14.4	11.7	9.6	7.4	5.8
1891-------	1917	43.1	40.7	35.5	31.3	25.1	21.2	16.9	14.4	11.6	9.2	7.3	5.5
1892-------	1918	42.8	39.3	35.4	30.8	25.1	20.9	16.9	14.1	11.0	8.9	6.8	5.2
1893-------	1919	41.4	39.3	34.4	30.9	24.9	20.9	16.3	13.4	10.7	8.5	6.6	5.4
1894-------	1920	41.8	38.6	34.9	30.9	24.6	20.2	15.9	13.2	10.4	8.2	6.8	5.1
1895-------	1921	41.3	39.4	35.2	30.3	24.0	20.0	15.6	12.9	10.1	8.5	6.5	4.9
1896-------	1922	42.3	39.8	34.2	29.5	23.5	19.3	15.1	12.4	10.3	8.0	6.2	4.6
1897-------	1923	42.9	38.8	33.4	28.8	22.6	18.6	14.6	12.5	9.8	7.8	5.8	4.7
1898-------	1924	42.1	37.4	31.9	27.2	21.5	18.1	14.7	11.9	9.4	7.3	6.0	4.7
1899-------	1925	41.0	36.2	30.9	26.3	21.4	18.5	14.5	12.0	9.2	7.8	6.2	4.8
1900-------	1926	38.9	34.6	29.2	25.6	21.6	17.8	14.1	11.3	9.7	7.9	6.2	4.9
1901-------	1927	37.7	32.9	28.5	25.9	20.9	17.3	13.3	11.9	9.7	7.9	6.4	5.1
1902-------	1928	35.7	31.7	28.6	24.7	19.8	16.1	14.0	11.8	9.7	8.0	6.7	5.4
1903-------	1929	34.7	32.1	27.7	23.8	18.9	17.2	13.9	11.9	10.0	8.6	7.0	5.7
1904-------	1930	34.9	31.0	26.6	22.8	20.2	17.1	14.1	12.3	10.7	9.1	7.7	6.2
1905-------	1931	33.8	29.8	25.4	23.8	19.8	17.1	14.6	13.2	11.2	9.7	8.2	7.0
1906-------	1932	32.4	28.4	26.4	23.4	19.9	17.7	15.7	13.8	12.1	10.3	8.9	8.3
1907-------	1933	31.0	29.4	25.8	23.5	20.6	19.0	16.4	14.9	12.9	11.9	10.6	9.0
1908-------	1934	31.7	28.4	25.8	24.0	21.7	19.6	17.7	15.7	15.0	13.8	11.5	9.7
1909-------	1935	30.7	28.4	26.5	25.5	22.6	21.4	19.0	18.6	17.3	14.4	12.5	10.5
1910-------	1936	30.6	29.3	28.2	26.0	24.4	22.7	21.5	21.3	17.6	15.6	13.4	10.6
1911-------	1937	31.9	31.3	28.7	27.9	25.9	25.1	24.6	21.1	18.9	16.8	13.4	9.9
1912-------	1938	33.7	31.4	30.5	29.4	29.6	28.8	24.3	22.6	20.4	16.8	12.5	9.4
1913-------	1939	34.0	33.4	32.3	34.2	33.7	28.4	26.3	24.5	20.4	15.5	12.0	9.3
1914-------	1940	36.3	35.6	38.0	39.0	32.5	30.7	28.8	24.7	18.8	15.0	11.8	9.4
1915-------	1941	38.5	40.9	43.4	36.9	34.7	33.6	29.0	22.6	18.3	14.8	11.9	9.5
1916-------	1942	42.6	46.6	40.1	38.4	38.2	34.2	26.5	22.0	18.1	14.8	11.9	9.0
1917-------	1943	48.5	43.1	40.9	43.1	39.7	31.9	26.3	22.0	18.2	14.8	11.4	9.0
1918-------	1944	44.9	42.3	46.6	45.5	37.0	31.5	26.2	21.9	18.0	14.1	11.1	8.5
1919-------	1945	43.0	51.0	51.1	43.4	37.5	31.8	26.8	22.1	17.5	14.1	10.8	8.3
1920-------	1946	54.1	56.2	49.1	44.2	37.8	32.3	26.7	21.4	17.3	13.3	10.3	7.8
1921-------	1947	60.2	54.9	50.5	44.7	38.3	32.4	25.7	21.1	16.2	12.7	9.7	7.3
1922-------	1948	59.4	56.3	50.7	44.7	38.4	31.0	25.0	19.6	15.4	12.0	8.9	6.5
1923-------	1949	61.7	56.9	51.4	45.0	36.7	30.3	23.4	18.7	14.6	10.9	8.1	6.1
1924-------	1950	62.7	58.2	51.8	43.4	36.2	28.4	22.2	17.6	13.2	10.1	7.7	5.8
1925-------	1951	64.1	58.4	50.1	42.5	33.6	26.8	20.9	16.0	12.3	9.6	7.3	5.3
1926-------	1952	64.4	57.3	49.2	40.1	31.9	25.4	19.2	14.9	11.6	8.9	6.5	4.9
1927-------	1953	64.1	56.0	46.8	38.5	30.6	23.4	17.7	14.0	10.8	8.0	6.2	4.6
1928-------	1954	63.3	54.1	45.2	37.0	28.3	21.8	16.8	13.0	9.8	7.6	5.8	4.2
1929-------	1955	62.1	53.3	44.5	34.6	26.9	20.8	15.9	12.2	9.3	7.3	5.3	3.9
1930-------	1956	61.9	52.8	41.8	33.2	25.7	19.7	14.8	11.5	9.0	6.6	4.9	3.7
1931-------	1957	62.5	50.6	40.3	31.8	24.3	18.2	14.0	11.0	8.1	6.2	4.7	3.5
1932-------	1958	60.4	49.2	38.8	30.1	22.5	17.3	13.4	10.2	7.6	5.8	4.4	3.4
1933-------	1959	58.8	47.1	36.8	27.7	21.3	16.6	12.5	9.4	7.3	5.7	4.3	3.3
1934-------	1960	57.1	45.2	34.6	26.8	20.6	15.9	11.7	9.1	7.0	5.6	4.3	3.0
1935-------	1961	54.8	42.7	33.3	26.0	19.6	14.7	11.3	9.0	7.1	5.6	4.0	3.0
1936-------	1962	52.4	41.3	32.7	24.8	18.7	14.4	11.4	9.2	7.1	5.2	3.9	2.8
1937-------	1963	50.6	40.6	30.9	23.9	18.6	14.9	11.7	9.3	6.8	5.1	3.8	
1938-------	1964	49.5	38.2	30.1	23.8	19.0	15.4	12.1	9.0	6.7	5.1		
1939-------	1965	46.5	37.3	30.4	24.6	20.2	16.2	12.1	9.0	6.9			
1940-------	1966	45.3	37.8	31.4	26.7	21.5	16.2	12.2	9.2				
1941-------	1967	46.1	39.1	34.0	28.5	21.6	16.5	12.4					
1942-------	1968	47.7	42.6	36.6	28.4	22.1	16.8						
1943-------	1969	50.2	44.6	35.6	28.3	22.3							
1944-------	1970	51.9	43.0	34.8	28.6								
1945-------	1971	49.3	40.9	35.2									
1946-------	1972	46.6	41.6										
1947-------	1973	46.3											

TABLE 4A. CENTRAL BIRTH RATES FOR ALL WOMEN DURING EACH YEAR 1917-73 BY AGE AND LIVE-BIRTH ORDER FOR EACH COHORT FROM 1868 TO 1959--CON.

LIVE-BIRTH ORDER AND COHORT	DIAGONAL LINE FOR CALENDAR YEAR	CURRENT AGE											
		38	39	40	41	42	43	44	45	46	47	48	49
SECOND BIRTHS--CON.													
1868-------													0.0
1869-------												0.1	0.0
1870-------											0.1	0.0	0.0
1871-------										0.2	0.1	0.0	0.1
1872-------									0.3	0.2	0.1	0.1	0.0
1873-------								0.5	0.3	0.2	0.1	0.0	0.0
1874-------							0.7	0.5	0.3	0.2	0.0	0.0	0.0
1875-------						1.1	0.8	0.5	0.3	0.1	0.1	0.0	0.0
1876-------					1.7	1.1	0.8	0.5	0.2	0.1	0.1	0.0	0.0
1877-------				2.5	1.8	1.1	0.8	0.4	0.2	0.2	0.1	0.0	0.0
1878-------			3.7	2.5	1.8	1.1	0.8	0.4	0.3	0.2	0.0	0.1	0.0
1879-------	1917	4.8	3.8	2.6	1.8	1.2	0.8	0.5	0.3	0.1	0.1	0.0	0.0
1880-------	1918	4.9	3.8	2.6	1.8	1.1	0.7	0.5	0.2	0.2	0.1	0.0	0.0
1881-------	1919	4.9	3.8	2.7	1.8	1.1	0.7	0.4	0.2	0.1	0.1	0.0	0.0
1882-------	1920	4.9	3.9	2.5	1.7	1.1	0.8	0.4	0.2	0.1	0.1	0.0	0.0
1883-------	1921	5.1	3.7	2.5	1.7	1.1	0.7	0.4	0.2	0.1	0.1	0.0	0.0
1884-------	1922	4.8	3.7	2.5	1.7	1.0	0.6	0.4	0.2	0.1	0.0	0.0	0.0
1885-------	1923	4.8	3.7	2.4	1.7	1.0	0.7	0.3	0.2	0.1	0.0	0.0	0.0
1886-------	1924	4.8	3.5	2.4	1.5	1.0	0.6	0.3	0.2	0.1	0.0	0.0	0.0
1887-------	1925	4.6	3.5	2.3	1.5	0.9	0.6	0.3	0.2	0.1	0.0	0.0	0.0
1888-------	1926	4.4	3.4	2.2	1.4	0.9	0.5	0.3	0.2	0.1	0.0	0.0	0.0
1889-------	1927	4.5	3.3	2.1	1.4	0.9	0.6	0.3	0.1	0.1	0.0	0.0	0.0
1890-------	1928	4.3	3.2	2.1	1.4	0.8	0.5	0.2	0.1	0.1	0.0	0.0	0.0
1891-------	1929	4.1	3.2	2.0	1.3	0.8	0.5	0.2	0.1	0.0	0.0	0.0	0.0
1892-------	1930	4.2	3.0	1.9	1.3	0.7	0.5	0.2	0.1	0.1	0.0	0.0	0.0
1893-------	1931	3.9	2.9	1.9	1.2	0.7	0.5	0.2	0.1	0.0	0.0	0.0	0.0
1894-------	1932	3.7	2.7	1.8	1.2	0.7	0.4	0.3	0.1	0.0	0.0	0.0	0.0
1895-------	1933	3.6	2.8	1.8	1.2	0.7	0.5	0.2	0.1	0.1	0.0	0.0	0.0
1896-------	1934	3.7	2.6	1.7	1.2	0.8	0.4	0.2	0.2	0.1	0.0	0.0	0.0
1897-------	1935	3.6	2.6	1.8	1.3	0.7	0.5	0.3	0.2	0.1	0.0	0.0	0.0
1898-------	1936	3.5	2.7	1.9	1.2	0.8	0.5	0.3	0.2	0.1	0.0	0.0	0.0
1899-------	1937	3.7	2.9	2.0	1.4	0.8	0.5	0.3	0.2	0.1	0.0	0.0	0.0
1900-------	1938	3.9	3.0	2.2	1.4	0.9	0.6	0.4	0.2	0.1	0.0	0.0	0.0
1901-------	1939	4.1	3.2	2.2	1.5	1.0	0.7	0.4	0.2	0.1	0.1	0.0	0.0
1902-------	1940	4.3	3.3	2.5	1.8	1.2	0.7	0.5	0.2	0.1	0.0	0.0	0.0
1903-------	1941	4.6	3.8	2.9	2.0	1.3	0.9	0.5	0.2	0.1	0.0	0.0	0.0
1904-------	1942	5.3	4.5	3.2	2.3	1.4	0.9	0.5	0.2	0.1	0.0	0.0	0.0
1905-------	1943	6.2	4.8	3.5	2.4	1.6	0.9	0.5	0.2	0.1	0.0	0.0	0.0
1906-------	1944	6.7	5.2	3.8	2.6	1.5	0.9	0.5	0.2	0.1	0.0	0.0	0.0
1907-------	1945	7.3	5.8	4.0	2.5	1.5	0.9	0.4	0.2	0.1	0.0	0.0	0.0
1908-------	1946	7.9	5.9	3.7	2.4	1.4	0.8	0.5	0.2	0.1	0.0	0.0	0.0
1909-------	1947	8.0	5.5	3.7	2.4	1.4	0.9	0.5	0.2	0.1	0.0	0.0	0.0
1910-------	1948	7.6	5.4	3.7	2.5	1.6	0.9	0.5	0.2	0.1	0.0	0.0	0.0
1911-------	1949	7.3	5.4	3.8	2.5	1.5	0.9	0.5	0.2	0.1	0.0	0.0	0.0
1912-------	1950	7.2	5.5	3.7	2.5	1.6	0.9	0.5	0.2	0.1	0.0	0.0	0.0
1913-------	1951	7.2	5.4	3.8	2.5	1.5	0.9	0.4	0.2	0.1	0.0	0.0	0.0
1914-------	1952	7.4	5.4	3.7	2.4	1.5	0.8	0.4	0.2	0.1	0.0	0.0	0.0
1915-------	1953	7.1	5.3	3.6	2.4	1.4	0.8	0.4	0.2	0.1	0.0	0.0	0.0
1916-------	1954	7.0	5.1	3.4	2.2	1.3	0.8	0.4	0.2	0.1	0.0	0.0	0.0
1917-------	1955	6.7	4.9	3.3	2.1	1.3	0.7	0.4	0.2	0.1	0.0	0.0	0.0
1918-------	1956	6.3	4.7	3.0	1.9	1.2	0.7	0.4	0.2	0.0	0.0	0.0	0.0
1919-------	1957	6.1	4.4	2.8	1.8	1.1	0.6	0.4	0.1	0.0	0.0	0.0	0.0
1920-------	1958	5.7	4.0	2.6	1.8	1.1	0.6	0.3	0.1	0.0	0.0	0.0	0.0
1921-------	1959	5.2	3.6	2.6	1.6	1.0	0.5	0.3	0.1	0.0	0.0	0.0	0.0
1922-------	1960	4.8	3.6	2.3	1.5	0.8	0.5	0.2	0.1	0.0	0.0	0.0	0.0
1923-------	1961	4.6	3.1	2.1	1.3	0.8	0.5	0.2	0.1	0.0	0.0	0.0	0.0
1924-------	1962	4.1	2.9	2.0	1.3	0.7	0.4	0.2	0.1	0.0	0.0	0.0	0.0
1925-------	1963	3.8	2.8	1.9	1.2	0.7	0.4	0.2	0.1	0.0	0.0	0.0	
1926-------	1964	3.6	2.6	1.6	1.1	0.7	0.4	0.2	0.1	0.0	0.0		
1927-------	1965	3.3	2.3	1.6	1.0	0.6	0.3	0.1	0.1	0.0			
1928-------	1966	2.9	2.1	1.5	1.0	0.6	0.3	0.2	0.1				
1929-------	1967	2.9	2.1	1.4	0.9	0.5	0.3	0.1					
1930-------	1968	2.7	2.0	1.3	0.8	0.5	0.2						
1931-------	1969	2.6	1.9	1.2	0.7	0.4							
1932-------	1970	2.5	1.7	1.1	0.7								
1933-------	1971	2.2	1.5	1.0									
1934-------	1972	2.2	1.5										
1935-------	1973	2.1											

TABLE 4A. CENTRAL BIRTH RATES FOR ALL WOMEN DURING EACH YEAR 1917-73 BY AGE AND LIVE-BIRTH ORDER FOR EACH COHORT FROM 1868 TO 1959--CON.

LIVE-BIRTH ORDER AND COHORT	DIAGONAL LINE FOR CALENDAR YEAR	CURRENT AGE											
		14	15	16	17	18	19	20	21	22	23	24	25
THIRD BIRTHS													
1892-------													38.8
1893-------												38.2	38.2
1894-------											36.0	37.9	36.1
1895-------										29.8	36.0	35.9	36.4
1896-------									22.7	29.9	34.1	35.9	37.0
1897-------								14.5	22.8	28.4	33.8	36.5	34.0
1898-------							7.5	14.6	21.8	28.4	34.6	33.8	35.1
1899-------						2.7	7.6	13.9	21.6	28.6	31.3	34.7	36.0
1900-------					0.8	2.7	7.2	13.7	21.8	26.0	32.9	36.4	34.4
1901-------				0.2	0.8	2.5	6.9	13.8	19.5	26.9	34.8	35.1	32.2
1902-------			0.0	0.2	0.8	2.6	7.4	12.9	20.9	29.3	33.4	32.8	31.1
1903-------	1917	*	0.0	0.2	0.8	2.9	6.9	13.9	22.4	28.5	31.6	31.9	29.4
1904-------	1918	*	0.0	0.2	0.9	2.7	7.6	14.5	21.5	27.1	30.5	30.0	27.7
1905-------	1919	*	0.0	0.2	0.8	3.2	7.8	13.9	20.5	26.2	28.6	28.3	27.3
1906-------	1920	*	0.0	0.2	1.0	3.2	7.5	13.4	20.0	24.7	27.1	27.8	25.6
1907-------	1921	*	0.0	0.2	1.0	3.1	7.4	13.3	19.3	23.5	26.5	26.1	25.0
1908-------	1922	*	0.0	0.2	0.9	3.1	7.4	12.8	18.2	22.9	24.9	25.3	23.5
1909-------	1923	*	0.0	0.2	1.0	3.1	7.2	12.1	17.9	21.9	24.3	24.1	23.8
1910-------	1924	*	0.0	0.2	1.0	3.0	6.7	11.8	17.0	21.2	23.2	24.2	22.2
1911-------	1925	*	0.0	0.2	1.0	2.8	6.6	11.4	16.6	20.3	23.4	22.9	21.6
1912-------	1926	*	0.0	0.2	0.9	2.7	6.3	11.0	15.6	20.1	22.0	22.0	21.4
1913-------	1927	*	0.0	0.2	0.9	2.6	6.1	10.2	15.5	19.2	21.0	22.1	22.1
1914-------	1928	*	0.0	0.2	0.8	2.5	5.6	10.2	14.9	18.5	21.3	22.7	21.6
1915-------	1929	*	0.0	0.2	0.8	2.3	5.6	9.9	14.4	18.9	22.0	22.3	22.5
1916-------	1930	*	0.0	0.2	0.7	2.3	5.5	9.6	14.7	19.3	21.5	23.2	23.0
1917-------	1931	*	0.0	0.2	0.7	2.3	5.3	9.9	15.1	18.9	22.5	23.6	23.8
1918-------	1932	*	0.0	0.2	0.7	2.3	5.6	10.3	14.7	19.8	22.7	24.5	26.8
1919-------	1933	*	0.0	0.2	0.8	2.4	5.9	10.2	15.7	20.1	24.0	27.1	26.7
1920-------	1934	*	0.0	0.2	0.8	2.6	6.0	11.5	15.8	20.7	26.0	26.6	24.4
1921-------	1935	*	0.0	0.2	0.9	2.9	7.2	11.6	16.1	22.2	25.3	23.8	27.2
1922-------	1936	*	0.0	0.2	1.0	3.7	7.1	11.4	17.3	21.9	21.8	26.1	29.4
1923-------	1937	*	0.0	0.2	1.3	3.7	7.2	12.3	17.3	18.8	24.0	28.3	31.6
1924-------	1938	*	0.0	0.3	1.3	3.7	7.7	12.3	14.8	20.7	26.0	31.1	34.2
1925-------	1939	*	0.1	0.3	1.4	3.8	7.6	10.4	16.2	22.4	28.8	33.8	37.0
1926-------	1940	*	0.1	0.4	1.5	3.7	6.4	11.4	17.5	24.9	31.6	36.7	40.5
1927-------	1941	*	0.1	0.5	1.5	3.2	6.8	12.2	19.6	27.9	34.6	40.0	43.1
1928-------	1942	*	0.1	0.4	1.3	3.3	7.4	13.9	22.5	30.9	37.8	42.1	44.6
1929-------	1943	*	0.1	0.4	1.3	3.6	8.5	16.5	25.4	34.1	39.8	44.3	47.4
1930-------	1944	*	0.1	0.4	1.5	4.2	10.4	18.7	28.1	35.6	41.7	47.3	49.8
1931-------	1945	*	0.1	0.5	1.8	5.5	11.8	20.8	29.4	37.6	45.3	50.0	53.0
1932-------	1946	*	0.1	0.6	2.3	6.0	12.9	21.7	30.6	40.6	47.6	53.5	55.4
1933-------	1947	*	0.2	0.7	2.4	6.6	13.7	22.6	33.2	42.7	51.3	56.0	56.3
1934-------	1948	*	0.2	0.7	2.7	6.9	14.1	24.3	34.9	45.8	53.8	57.3	58.0
1935-------	1949	*	0.2	0.8	2.7	7.1	14.9	25.0	36.8	47.9	54.8	59.0	58.5
1936-------	1950	*	0.2	0.8	2.8	7.4	15.2	26.3	38.8	48.6	55.9	59.5	58.0
1937-------	1951	*	0.2	0.8	2.8	7.4	16.0	27.7	39.0	49.6	57.0	59.2	55.7
1938-------	1952	*	0.2	0.8	2.8	7.9	16.8	27.8	40.1	50.9	56.6	57.0	53.0
1939-------	1953	*	0.2	0.8	3.1	8.2	17.0	29.3	41.5	50.5	54.9	54.1	49.9
1940-------	1954	*	0.2	0.9	3.2	8.4	18.0	29.7	40.5	49.2	51.6	50.2	43.8
1941-------	1955	*	0.2	0.9	3.2	8.9	17.9	28.8	39.1	45.4	47.1	43.1	38.4
1942-------	1956	*	0.2	0.9	3.3	8.5	17.1	27.1	35.6	40.8	39.6	37.1	36.2
1943-------	1957	*	0.2	0.9	3.1	8.2	16.0	24.8	31.8	33.9	33.7	34.5	34.0
1944-------	1958	*	0.2	0.9	3.2	7.8	14.8	22.5	26.7	28.8	31.0	32.0	34.4
1945-------	1959	*	0.2	0.9	3.2	7.4	13.7	18.9	22.5	26.0	28.2	31.7	34.3
1946-------	1960	*	0.2	0.9	2.8	6.9	11.6	15.8	19.8	23.1	27.5	31.5	30.7
1947-------	1961	*	0.2	0.8	2.7	5.8	9.5	13.8	17.5	22.3	27.0	28.2	25.0
1948-------	1962	*	0.2	0.7	2.3	4.8	8.4	12.0	16.7	21.8	24.3	22.8	22.1
1949-------	1963	*	0.2	0.7	2.0	4.4	7.4	11.6	16.4	20.0	19.8	20.2	
1950-------	1964	*	0.2	0.6	1.8	3.9	7.2	11.4	15.0	16.2	17.7		
1951-------	1965	*	0.1	0.6	1.7	3.8	6.9	10.4	12.3	14.6			
1952-------	1966	*	0.1	0.5	1.5	3.6	6.3	8.7	11.2				
1953-------	1967	*	0.1	0.5	1.5	3.2	5.4	7.9					
1954-------	1968	*	0.1	0.5	1.4	2.8	5.0						
1955-------	1969	*	0.1	0.4	1.2	2.6							
1956-------	1970	*	0.1	0.4	1.1								
1957-------	1971	*	0.1	0.3									
1958-------	1972	*	0.1										
1959-------	1973	*											

TABLE 4A. CENTRAL BIRTH RATES FOR ALL WOMEN DURING EACH YEAR 1917-73 BY AGE AND LIVE-BIRTH ORDER FOR EACH COHORT FROM 1868 TO 1959--CON.

LIVE-BIRTH ORDER AND COHORT	DIAGONAL LINE FOR CALENDAR YEAR	CURRENT AGE											
		26	27	28	29	30	31	32	33	34	35	36	37
THIRD BIRTHS--CON.													
1880-------													8.7
1881-------												10.6	8.8
1882-------											12.8	10.6	8.6
1883-------										15.0	12.7	10.4	8.8
1884-------									17.6	14.7	12.4	10.6	8.9
1885-------								19.3	17.2	14.3	12.6	10.7	8.4
1886-------							22.9	18.9	16.8	14.6	12.8	10.2	8.4
1887-------						26.8	22.5	18.6	17.1	14.9	12.3	10.3	8.5
1888-------					32.5	26.4	22.0	18.8	17.3	14.2	12.3	10.3	8.1
1889-------				35.3	32.0	25.4	22.3	19.1	16.6	14.2	12.5	9.9	8.0
1890-------			37.0	35.0	30.5	25.7	22.6	18.3	16.7	14.6	11.9	9.7	7.7
1891-------	1917	37.0	36.6	32.9	30.8	25.9	21.7	18.4	17.2	14.0	11.6	9.3	7.3
1892-------	1918	36.5	34.4	33.0	30.8	24.1	21.6	18.8	16.4	13.5	11.0	8.8	6.8
1893-------	1919	34.3	34.6	32.9	28.2	23.9	22.1	18.0	15.6	12.9	10.4	8.3	6.7
1894-------	1920	34.8	34.8	29.9	28.0	24.5	21.2	17.4	15.0	12.3	9.9	8.3	6.5
1895-------	1921	35.3	31.8	29.8	28.6	23.5	20.3	16.8	14.3	11.7	10.0	7.9	6.3
1896-------	1922	32.4	31.8	30.2	27.4	22.6	19.6	15.8	13.7	11.7	9.5	7.7	5.9
1897-------	1923	32.5	32.4	29.0	26.2	21.6	18.4	15.1	13.5	11.1	9.2	7.2	5.9
1898-------	1924	33.6	31.1	27.6	24.8	20.3	17.7	15.0	12.8	10.7	8.6	7.3	5.7
1899-------	1925	32.6	29.6	26.5	23.6	19.6	17.6	14.6	12.7	10.2	9.0	7.3	5.7
1900-------	1926	30.4	28.5	24.7	22.4	19.3	16.8	13.9	11.9	10.5	8.7	7.0	5.7
1901-------	1927	29.7	26.4	23.3	21.9	18.5	16.0	13.2	12.1	10.1	8.4	6.9	5.6
1902-------	1928	27.5	24.8	22.8	20.6	17.4	15.1	13.2	11.4	9.6	8.2	6.8	5.6
1903-------	1929	26.0	24.5	21.8	19.9	16.5	15.1	12.6	11.1	9.6	8.2	6.9	5.7
1904-------	1930	25.7	23.3	21.2	18.9	16.8	14.5	12.3	11.1	9.6	8.4	7.1	6.0
1905-------	1931	24.4	22.8	19.9	19.1	15.9	14.0	12.2	11.1	9.7	8.6	7.4	6.6
1906-------	1932	23.7	21.4	20.2	18.0	15.4	13.9	12.3	11.2	10.0	8.9	8.0	7.8
1907-------	1933	22.4	21.7	19.0	17.4	15.3	14.1	12.4	11.6	10.4	9.8	9.5	8.5
1908-------	1934	22.5	20.1	18.2	17.0	15.4	14.0	12.8	12.0	11.4	11.6	10.4	9.2
1909-------	1935	21.1	19.4	18.1	17.4	15.5	14.6	13.4	13.2	13.6	12.5	11.4	9.8
1910-------	1936	20.3	19.2	18.5	17.2	16.1	15.2	14.6	15.7	14.6	13.7	12.1	10.1
1911-------	1937	20.4	19.9	18.2	17.9	16.6	16.3	17.3	16.8	15.8	14.6	12.4	9.6
1912-------	1938	20.8	19.3	18.9	18.3	18.2	19.3	18.5	17.9	16.8	14.8	11.8	9.5
1913-------	1939	20.3	20.1	19.4	20.3	21.3	20.5	19.6	19.2	17.3	14.3	11.8	9.7
1914-------	1940	21.2	20.8	21.6	23.5	22.3	21.7	21.3	19.9	16.8	14.2	12.1	10.3
1915-------	1941	21.8	22.4	24.8	24.2	23.0	23.6	22.1	19.4	16.8	14.8	12.9	11.1
1916-------	1942	22.6	25.7	25.1	24.3	24.8	24.4	21.5	19.3	17.4	15.6	13.7	11.2
1917-------	1943	25.8	25.9	24.7	26.4	26.3	24.0	21.8	20.3	18.5	16.7	14.0	11.8
1918-------	1944	26.1	24.7	26.5	27.9	25.7	24.5	22.7	21.4	19.7	17.1	14.6	11.5
1919-------	1945	24.8	27.3	29.1	28.2	27.1	26.1	24.8	23.4	20.5	17.8	14.4	11.7
1920-------	1946	27.1	29.9	29.6	29.7	28.9	28.2	26.7	24.3	21.1	17.6	14.4	11.4
1921-------	1947	30.1	30.9	31.5	32.0	31.5	30.7	27.9	24.8	21.1	17.5	14.2	10.9
1922-------	1948	31.2	32.9	33.7	34.4	34.0	31.8	28.3	24.7	20.8	17.2	13.4	10.3
1923-------	1949	33.7	35.2	36.7	37.5	35.2	32.4	28.3	24.5	20.7	16.4	12.8	9.8
1924-------	1950	36.4	38.9	40.0	38.9	36.4	32.6	28.3	24.6	19.7	15.7	12.2	9.5
1925-------	1951	40.0	42.1	41.5	40.2	36.5	32.8	28.3	23.2	18.6	14.9	11.8	8.7
1926-------	1952	43.1	43.3	43.3	40.7	36.6	32.6	26.8	22.1	17.8	14.3	10.7	8.1
1927-------	1953	44.4	45.4	44.0	41.3	36.9	31.3	25.8	21.1	17.1	13.1	10.0	7.7
1928-------	1954	46.6	46.5	44.5	41.6	35.7	30.4	24.7	20.3	15.6	12.3	9.5	6.9
1929-------	1955	48.6	48.3	45.9	40.7	35.3	29.4	24.2	18.8	15.0	11.8	8.7	6.3
1930-------	1956	50.7	49.8	45.1	40.7	34.4	28.8	22.5	18.1	14.3	10.7	7.9	5.9
1931-------	1957	53.1	49.6	45.7	40.1	34.0	27.0	21.6	17.4	13.2	9.7	7.4	5.3
1932-------	1958	53.5	50.4	45.6	39.6	32.0	25.8	20.7	15.9	11.9	9.1	6.8	5.0
1933-------	1959	54.8	50.8	44.9	37.3	30.4	25.0	19.0	14.4	11.1	8.5	6.4	4.8
1934-------	1960	55.4	50.1	42.6	35.6	29.5	22.9	17.2	13.4	10.5	8.3	6.3	4.4
1935-------	1961	54.4	47.8	40.8	34.7	26.9	20.7	16.2	12.8	10.3	8.0	5.7	3.9
1936-------	1962	52.5	45.8	39.4	31.5	24.5	19.6	15.3	12.9	10.2	7.3	5.1	3.6
1937-------	1963	50.2	43.9	35.6	28.7	23.4	18.8	15.9	12.8	9.3	6.5	4.7	
1938-------	1964	47.5	39.4	32.3	27.2	22.5	19.6	16.1	11.8	8.3	6.1		
1939-------	1965	42.4	35.5	30.9	26.7	23.7	20.2	14.9	10.6	7.9			
1940-------	1966	37.6	33.9	30.2	27.9	24.6	18.6	13.3	10.1				
1941-------	1967	35.8	32.8	31.6	29.0	22.7	16.5	12.7					
1942-------	1968	34.3	34.3	32.6	26.7	19.9	15.8						
1943-------	1969	35.3	34.9	29.8	22.9	18.7							
1944-------	1970	35.5	31.6	25.0	21.2								
1945-------	1971	32.0	26.1	22.8									
1946-------	1972	26.1	23.6										
1947-------	1973	23.3											

TABLE 4A. CENTRAL BIRTH RATES FOR ALL WOMEN DURING EACH YEAR 1917-73 BY AGE AND LIVE-BIRTH ORDER FOR EACH COHORT FROM 1868 TO 1959--CON.

LIVE-BIRTH ORDER AND COHORT	DIAGONAL LINE FOR CALENDAR YEAR	CURRENT AGE											
		38	39	40	41	42	43	44	45	46	47	48	49
THIRD BIRTHS--CON.													
1868-------													0.0
1869-------												0.0	0.0
1870-------											0.1	0.1	0.0
1871-------										0.2	0.2	0.0	0.0
1872-------									0.4	0.4	0.1	0.1	0.0
1873-------								0.7	0.5	0.2	0.2	0.0	0.0
1874-------							1.1	0.7	0.4	0.3	0.1	0.0	0.0
1875-------						1.6	1.1	0.7	0.5	0.2	0.1	0.0	0.0
1876-------					2.4	1.7	1.1	0.7	0.4	0.2	0.1	0.0	0.0
1877-------				3.5	2.7	1.6	1.1	0.7	0.4	0.2	0.1	0.0	0.0
1878-------			5.3	3.7	2.5	1.6	1.1	0.7	0.4	0.2	0.1	0.1	0.0
1879-------	1917	6.9	5.5	3.5	2.6	1.6	1.1	0.7	0.4	0.3	0.1	0.0	0.0
1880-------	1918	6.9	5.4	3.7	2.6	1.6	1.1	0.7	0.4	0.2	0.1	0.1	0.0
1881-------	1919	6.8	5.5	3.7	2.4	1.6	1.1	0.6	0.3	0.2	0.1	0.0	0.0
1882-------	1920	7.0	5.6	3.5	2.4	1.6	1.0	0.6	0.3	0.2	0.1	0.0	0.0
1883-------	1921	7.0	5.2	3.5	2.4	1.5	1.0	0.5	0.3	0.2	0.0	0.1	0.0
1884-------	1922	6.6	5.2	3.5	2.4	1.4	0.9	0.5	0.3	0.1	0.1	0.0	0.0
1885-------	1923	6.6	5.2	3.4	2.2	1.4	0.9	0.5	0.3	0.2	0.1	0.0	0.0
1886-------	1924	6.7	5.0	3.2	2.3	1.4	0.8	0.5	0.3	0.1	0.1	0.0	0.0
1887-------	1925	6.4	4.9	3.2	2.1	1.3	0.8	0.5	0.3	0.1	0.0	0.0	0.0
1888-------	1926	6.2	4.8	3.0	2.0	1.3	0.8	0.4	0.2	0.1	0.1	0.0	0.0
1889-------	1927	6.1	4.5	3.0	2.1	1.3	0.8	0.4	0.2	0.1	0.0	0.0	0.0
1890-------	1928	5.8	4.3	3.1	1.9	1.2	0.8	0.4	0.2	0.1	0.0	0.0	0.0
1891-------	1929	5.5	4.3	2.7	1.8	1.1	0.8	0.4	0.2	0.1	0.0	0.0	0.0
1892-------	1930	5.4	4.0	2.6	1.8	1.1	0.7	0.4	0.2	0.1	0.0	0.0	0.0
1893-------	1931	5.1	3.8	2.5	1.7	1.1	0.6	0.3	0.2	0.1	0.0	0.0	0.0
1894-------	1932	4.9	3.7	2.5	1.7	1.0	0.6	0.4	0.2	0.1	0.0	0.0	0.0
1895-------	1933	4.7	3.6	2.5	1.6	0.9	0.6	0.4	0.2	0.1	0.0	0.0	0.0
1896-------	1934	4.6	3.5	2.4	1.5	1.0	0.6	0.4	0.2	0.1	0.0	0.0	0.0
1897-------	1935	4.5	3.5	2.3	1.6	1.0	0.6	0.4	0.2	0.1	0.0	0.0	0.0
1898-------	1936	4.4	3.4	2.4	1.6	1.0	0.6	0.4	0.2	0.1	0.0	0.0	0.0
1899-------	1937	4.5	3.5	2.5	1.6	1.1	0.7	0.4	0.2	0.1	0.0	0.0	0.0
1900-------	1938	4.6	3.5	2.5	1.7	1.1	0.8	0.5	0.3	0.1	0.1	0.0	0.0
1901-------	1939	4.6	3.5	2.6	1.7	1.2	0.9	0.5	0.3	0.1	0.0	0.0	0.0
1902-------	1940	4.6	3.6	2.7	2.0	1.4	1.0	0.5	0.2	0.1	0.0	0.0	0.0
1903-------	1941	4.7	3.9	3.1	2.3	1.6	1.0	0.5	0.3	0.1	0.0	0.0	0.0
1904-------	1942	5.2	4.6	3.4	2.5	1.6	1.1	0.6	0.3	0.1	0.0	0.0	0.0
1905-------	1943	6.1	5.0	3.8	2.6	1.7	1.1	0.6	0.2	0.1	0.0	0.0	0.0
1906-------	1944	6.6	5.4	3.8	2.7	1.7	1.0	0.5	0.3	0.1	0.0	0.0	0.0
1907-------	1945	7.3	5.7	4.1	2.7	1.6	1.0	0.6	0.3	0.1	0.0	0.0	0.0
1908-------	1946	7.6	5.9	3.9	2.6	1.6	1.1	0.6	0.3	0.1	0.0	0.0	0.0
1909-------	1947	7.9	5.6	3.9	2.6	1.7	1.1	0.6	0.3	0.1	0.0	0.0	0.0
1910-------	1948	7.4	5.7	4.0	2.8	1.9	1.2	0.7	0.3	0.1	0.1	0.0	0.0
1911-------	1949	7.5	5.7	4.2	3.0	1.9	1.3	0.7	0.3	0.2	0.1	0.0	0.0
1912-------	1950	7.6	6.0	4.5	3.1	2.1	1.2	0.7	0.3	0.2	0.0	0.0	0.0
1913-------	1951	8.0	6.4	4.6	3.3	2.1	1.3	0.7	0.3	0.1	0.0	0.0	0.0
1914-------	1952	8.7	6.6	4.8	3.3	2.1	1.3	0.7	0.3	0.1	0.0	0.0	0.0
1915-------	1953	8.8	6.8	4.9	3.4	2.1	1.2	0.7	0.3	0.1	0.1	0.0	0.0
1916-------	1954	9.0	6.9	4.7	3.3	1.9	1.2	0.7	0.3	0.2	0.0	0.0	0.0
1917-------	1955	9.1	6.9	4.8	3.1	1.9	1.2	0.6	0.3	0.1	0.0	0.0	0.0
1918-------	1956	9.0	6.6	4.5	3.0	1.8	1.1	0.6	0.3	0.1	0.0	0.0	0.0
1919-------	1957	9.0	6.5	4.5	2.9	1.9	1.0	0.6	0.3	0.1	0.0	0.0	0.0
1920-------	1958	8.6	6.3	4.3	2.9	1.7	1.0	0.5	0.2	0.1	0.0	0.0	0.0
1921-------	1959	8.2	6.0	4.2	2.6	1.6	0.9	0.5	0.2	0.1	0.0	0.0	0.0
1922-------	1960	7.8	5.7	3.8	2.5	1.5	0.9	0.4	0.2	0.1	0.0	0.0	0.0
1923-------	1961	7.5	5.3	3.5	2.4	1.4	0.8	0.4	0.2	0.0	0.0	0.0	0.0
1924-------	1962	6.9	4.9	3.4	2.1	1.2	0.7	0.4	0.1	0.1	0.0	0.0	0.0
1925-------	1963	6.4	4.7	3.0	1.9	1.1	0.6	0.3	0.1	0.1	0.0	0.0	
1926-------	1964	6.1	4.3	2.8	1.8	1.0	0.6	0.3	0.1	0.1	0.0		
1927-------	1965	5.5	3.8	2.6	1.5	1.0	0.5	0.2	0.1	0.0			
1928-------	1966	5.0	3.6	2.2	1.4	0.8	0.4	0.2	0.1				
1929-------	1967	4.7	3.1	2.1	1.3	0.7	0.4	0.2					
1930-------	1968	4.2	2.9	1.9	1.2	0.6	0.3						
1931-------	1969	3.8	2.8	1.7	1.0	0.6							
1932-------	1970	3.7	2.4	1.5	0.9								
1933-------	1971	3.3	2.1	1.3									
1934-------	1972	3.0	1.9										
1935-------	1973	2.7											

TABLE 4A. CENTRAL BIRTH RATES FOR ALL WOMEN DURING EACH YEAR 1917-73 BY AGE AND LIVE-BIRTH ORDER FOR EACH COHORT FROM 1868 TO 1959--CON.

LIVE-BIRTH ORDER AND COHORT	DIAGONAL LINE FOR CALENDAR YEAR	CURRENT AGE											
		14	15	16	17	18	19	20	21	22	23	24	25
FOURTH BIRTHS													
1892-------													24.6
1893-------												20.7	24.4
1894-------											16.1	20.7	23.6
1895-------										10.4	16.3	20.2	23.9
1896-------									6.1	10.5	15.9	20.4	24.4
1897-------								3.0	6.2	10.3	15.9	21.1	22.6
1898-------							1.2	3.1	6.1	10.4	16.8	19.7	22.7
1899-------						0.3	1.3	3.0	6.2	10.9	15.4	19.7	22.3
1900-------					0.1	0.3	1.3	3.0	6.5	10.0	15.7	19.7	21.9
1901-------				0.0	0.1	0.3	1.2	3.1	5.7	9.9	15.6	19.5	21.4
1902-------			0.0	0.0	0.1	0.3	1.3	3.0	6.0	10.4	15.6	19.3	21.0
1903-------	1917	*	0.0	0.0	0.1	0.3	1.3	3.1	6.2	10.8	15.8	19.0	19.5
1904-------	1918	*	0.0	0.0	0.1	0.4	1.4	3.1	6.5	11.0	15.4	17.5	18.4
1905-------	1919	*	0.0	0.0	0.1	0.5	1.4	3.3	6.6	10.6	14.1	16.5	17.8
1906-------	1920	*	0.0	0.0	0.1	0.5	1.4	3.3	6.3	9.6	13.2	16.1	16.7
1907-------	1921	*	0.0	0.0	0.1	0.5	1.4	3.1	5.8	9.1	13.0	15.0	16.2
1908-------	1922	*	0.0	0.0	0.1	0.5	1.4	3.0	5.5	9.1	12.1	14.5	15.1
1909-------	1923	*	0.0	0.0	0.1	0.4	1.3	2.8	5.5	8.5	11.8	13.6	15.5
1910-------	1924	*	0.0	0.0	0.1	0.4	1.3	2.8	5.1	8.2	11.1	13.9	14.4
1911-------	1925	*	0.0	0.0	0.1	0.4	1.3	2.6	5.0	7.8	11.3	13.2	13.9
1912-------	1926	*	0.0	0.0	0.1	0.4	1.2	2.5	4.7	7.8	10.8	12.6	13.5
1913-------	1927	*	0.0	0.0	0.1	0.4	1.1	2.3	4.7	7.6	10.3	12.4	13.3
1914-------	1928	*	0.0	0.0	0.1	0.3	1.0	2.4	4.7	7.3	10.2	12.2	12.8
1915-------	1929	*	0.0	0.0	0.1	0.3	1.0	2.4	4.5	7.3	10.1	11.9	13.3
1916-------	1930	*	0.0	0.0	0.1	0.3	1.0	2.4	4.5	7.2	9.9	12.7	13.2
1917-------	1931	*	0.0	0.0	0.1	0.3	1.0	2.3	4.4	7.0	10.9	12.6	13.2
1918-------	1932	*	0.0	0.0	0.1	0.3	1.0	2.3	4.3	7.8	10.9	12.5	14.5
1919-------	1933	*	0.0	0.0	0.1	0.3	1.0	2.3	4.8	7.9	10.9	13.5	14.6
1920-------	1934	*	0.0	0.0	0.1	0.4	1.0	2.7	4.8	8.2	11.7	13.7	13.7
1921-------	1935	*	0.0	0.0	0.1	0.4	1.3	2.7	5.3	8.7	11.9	12.7	14.6
1922-------	1936	*	0.0	0.0	0.1	0.6	1.3	3.0	5.7	8.9	10.6	13.2	14.1
1923-------	1937	*	0.0	0.0	0.2	0.6	1.5	3.2	5.9	8.0	11.0	12.7	14.4
1924-------	1938	*	0.0	0.0	0.2	0.6	1.6	3.4	5.3	8.2	10.7	13.3	15.8
1925-------	1939	*	0.0	0.0	0.2	0.6	1.7	3.1	5.3	8.0	11.3	14.8	17.1
1926-------	1940	*	0.0	0.0	0.2	0.6	1.5	3.1	5.3	8.6	12.7	16.0	19.1
1927-------	1941	*	0.0	0.0	0.2	0.6	1.5	3.1	5.8	9.8	13.7	18.0	21.1
1928-------	1942	*	0.0	0.0	0.2	0.6	1.6	3.4	6.7	10.7	15.8	19.7	22.4
1929-------	1943	*	0.0	0.0	0.2	0.6	1.7	4.1	7.5	12.6	17.5	21.4	24.4
1930-------	1944	*	0.0	0.0	0.2	0.6	2.1	4.6	8.9	13.9	18.7	23.0	25.9
1931-------	1945	*	0.0	0.0	0.2	0.9	2.4	5.4	10.0	15.1	20.3	24.5	28.2
1932-------	1946	*	0.0	0.0	0.3	0.9	2.8	6.1	10.4	16.0	21.4	26.5	30.1
1933-------	1947	*	0.0	0.1	0.3	1.1	3.1	6.5	11.3	17.1	23.1	28.3	31.3
1934-------	1948	*	0.0	0.1	0.4	1.2	3.2	6.9	11.9	18.3	24.5	29.3	33.2
1935-------	1949	*	0.0	0.1	0.3	1.2	3.5	7.2	12.6	19.0	25.2	30.6	34.1
1936-------	1950	*	0.0	0.1	0.4	1.3	3.5	7.6	13.1	19.8	26.3	31.5	34.4
1937-------	1951	*	0.0	0.1	0.4	1.3	3.6	7.9	13.7	20.4	27.0	32.0	33.8
1938-------	1952	*	0.0	0.1	0.4	1.4	3.8	8.2	14.2	21.0	27.4	31.2	31.8
1939-------	1953	*	0.0	0.1	0.4	1.5	4.0	8.5	14.5	21.5	26.8	29.4	29.6
1940-------	1954	*	0.0	0.1	0.4	1.5	4.2	8.7	14.9	20.7	24.9	26.8	25.0
1941-------	1955	*	0.0	0.1	0.4	1.5	4.3	8.9	14.1	19.1	22.3	22.4	20.5
1942-------	1956	*	0.0	0.1	0.4	1.6	4.2	8.2	12.8	16.8	18.2	17.9	17.8
1943-------	1957	*	0.0	0.1	0.4	1.5	3.9	7.5	11.3	13.8	14.6	15.5	15.9
1944-------	1958	*	0.0	0.1	0.4	1.4	3.6	6.7	9.4	11.2	12.7	13.7	15.4
1945-------	1959	*	0.0	0.1	0.4	1.4	3.3	5.8	7.8	9.7	11.2	13.1	14.7
1946-------	1960	*	0.0	0.1	0.4	1.3	2.9	4.7	6.5	8.2	10.4	12.2	12.7
1947-------	1961	*	0.0	0.1	0.4	1.2	2.4	3.9	5.4	7.4	9.5	10.6	9.8
1948-------	1962	*	0.0	0.1	0.3	0.9	1.9	3.2	4.9	6.8	8.3	8.2	8.2
1949-------	1963	*	0.0	0.1	0.3	0.8	1.6	3.0	4.7	6.1	6.7	7.0	
1950-------	1964	*	0.0	0.0	0.2	0.7	1.5	2.8	4.0	5.0	5.6		
1951-------	1965	*	0.0	0.0	0.2	0.6	1.4	2.4	3.4	4.2			
1952-------	1966	*	0.0	0.0	0.2	0.6	1.2	1.9	2.8				
1953-------	1967	*	0.0	0.0	0.2	0.5	1.0	1.7					
1954-------	1968	*	0.0	0.0	0.1	0.4	0.9						
1955-------	1969	*	0.0	0.0	0.1	0.4							
1956-------	1970	*	0.0	0.0	0.1								
1957-------	1971	*	0.0	0.0									
1958-------	1972	*	0.0										
1959-------	1973	*											

TABLE 4A. CENTRAL BIRTH RATES FOR ALL WOMEN DURING EACH YEAR 1917-73 BY AGE AND LIVE-BIRTH ORDER FOR EACH COHORT FROM 1868 TO 1959--CON.

LIVE-BIRTH ORDER AND COHORT	DIAGONAL LINE FOR CALENDAR YEAR	CURRENT AGE											
		26	27	28	29	30	31	32	33	34	35	36	37
FOURTH BIRTHS--CON.													
1880-------													10.4
1881-------												12.2	10.4
1882-------											14.4	12.2	10.1
1883-------										16.3	14.2	11.8	10.0
1884-------									18.3	15.9	13.8	11.7	10.1
1885-------								19.2	17.8	15.4	13.7	11.9	9.4
1886-------							21.8	18.8	17.2	15.3	14.0	11.1	9.4
1887-------						24.2	21.4	18.2	17.2	15.8	12.9	11.1	9.4
1888-------					28.0	23.9	20.7	18.1	17.7	14.4	12.9	11.0	9.3
1889-------				28.6	27.6	22.9	20.6	18.7	16.1	14.4	12.8	10.8	8.9
1890-------			28.3	28.3	26.6	22.9	21.3	17.0	16.1	14.4	12.3	10.4	8.5
1891-------	1917	26.2	28.1	27.2	26.6	23.3	19.3	17.0	16.0	13.8	12.0	9.9	8.0
1892-------	1918	25.9	26.9	27.3	26.7	21.1	19.2	16.8	15.4	13.4	11.4	9.2	7.3
1893-------	1919	24.8	27.0	27.0	24.1	20.7	19.1	16.3	14.8	12.8	10.6	8.5	7.3
1894-------	1920	25.1	27.0	24.6	23.5	20.4	18.4	15.7	14.3	11.9	9.9	8.5	7.0
1895-------	1921	25.4	24.8	23.9	23.2	19.6	17.7	15.1	13.3	11.1	9.8	8.1	6.6
1896-------	1922	23.4	24.1	23.4	22.2	18.9	17.0	14.0	12.3	10.9	9.3	7.7	6.3
1897-------	1923	22.9	23.7	22.4	21.4	18.1	15.8	13.1	12.1	10.3	8.9	7.3	6.3
1898-------	1924	22.9	23.1	21.8	20.6	16.8	14.8	13.0	11.5	9.8	8.4	7.3	5.9
1899-------	1925	22.5	22.7	21.3	19.3	16.0	14.8	12.5	11.3	9.6	8.6	7.0	5.7
1900-------	1926	22.0	22.2	19.7	17.9	15.8	14.0	12.1	10.8	9.7	8.2	6.7	5.5
1901-------	1927	21.7	20.3	18.1	17.5	14.9	13.4	11.4	10.7	9.0	7.7	6.4	5.6
1902-------	1928	19.9	18.7	17.7	16.5	14.1	12.5	11.2	10.0	8.5	7.3	6.4	5.3
1903-------	1929	18.5	18.2	16.9	15.7	13.4	12.5	10.5	9.3	8.1	7.3	6.2	5.1
1904-------	1930	18.1	17.5	16.4	15.2	13.4	11.8	9.8	9.0	8.0	7.1	6.0	5.2
1905-------	1931	17.2	16.9	15.7	15.1	12.6	11.0	9.6	8.8	7.7	6.9	6.1	5.4
1906-------	1932	16.7	16.0	15.3	14.0	11.8	10.7	9.3	8.6	7.7	7.0	6.2	6.2
1907-------	1933	15.6	15.9	14.3	13.1	11.5	10.4	9.1	8.5	7.8	7.2	7.0	6.5
1908-------	1934	15.6	14.7	13.4	12.6	11.2	10.1	9.1	8.6	8.1	8.2	7.5	6.8
1909-------	1935	14.7	14.1	13.1	12.6	10.8	10.1	9.2	9.1	9.2	8.6	8.0	7.1
1910-------	1936	14.0	13.6	13.1	12.0	10.9	10.2	9.6	10.3	9.7	9.1	8.2	7.3
1911-------	1937	13.7	13.7	12.5	12.1	11.0	10.4	10.9	10.7	10.1	9.5	8.6	7.1
1912-------	1938	13.5	12.9	12.5	12.1	11.4	11.8	11.4	11.0	10.5	9.8	8.3	7.1
1913-------	1939	12.9	12.9	12.6	12.4	12.7	12.3	11.6	11.7	10.9	9.6	8.4	7.4
1914-------	1940	12.9	13.1	13.0	13.8	13.1	12.6	12.4	11.9	10.8	9.8	8.9	8.0
1915-------	1941	13.0	13.3	14.4	14.1	13.2	13.3	12.6	11.9	11.2	10.5	9.6	8.7
1916-------	1942	13.3	14.7	14.5	13.8	13.8	13.5	12.5	12.3	11.8	11.2	10.3	9.3
1917-------	1943	14.6	14.8	14.0	14.7	14.1	13.4	13.2	13.0	12.6	12.0	11.2	9.9
1918-------	1944	14.7	14.1	14.7	14.8	13.9	14.2	13.7	13.9	13.6	12.9	11.6	10.0
1919-------	1945	14.1	15.2	15.1	15.0	15.1	15.0	15.2	15.5	14.8	13.8	12.2	10.4
1920-------	1946	15.0	15.2	15.2	16.1	16.0	16.6	17.0	16.6	15.8	14.2	12.3	10.7
1921-------	1947	14.8	15.4	16.4	17.2	17.8	18.6	18.1	17.9	16.5	14.6	13.0	10.5
1922-------	1948	14.8	16.3	17.4	18.8	19.6	19.6	19.3	18.4	16.8	15.1	12.5	10.4
1923-------	1949	16.1	17.6	19.5	20.7	20.7	21.1	20.2	19.1	17.5	14.9	12.5	10.3
1924-------	1950	17.5	19.8	21.3	22.3	22.7	22.2	21.2	19.9	17.4	14.9	12.5	10.0
1925-------	1951	19.6	21.7	23.0	24.3	23.8	23.3	21.9	19.9	17.3	14.8	12.1	9.4
1926-------	1952	21.5	23.4	25.1	25.6	25.1	24.0	21.9	19.7	17.2	14.4	11.4	8.9
1927-------	1953	23.2	25.3	26.2	26.9	25.9	24.3	22.0	19.6	16.8	13.5	10.9	8.6
1928-------	1954	25.0	26.6	27.7	27.9	26.3	24.7	22.0	19.4	15.7	13.0	10.4	7.8
1929-------	1955	26.4	28.3	29.3	28.7	27.4	24.9	22.3	18.5	15.4	12.7	9.6	7.1
1930-------	1956	28.3	30.1	30.2	30.1	27.6	25.3	21.1	18.1	15.0	11.6	8.6	6.5
1931-------	1957	30.5	31.5	31.9	30.5	28.3	24.2	20.9	17.6	13.6	10.3	8.1	6.0
1932-------	1958	31.9	33.4	32.6	31.0	27.1	23.8	20.0	16.0	12.1	9.6	7.3	5.6
1933-------	1959	33.8	34.4	33.3	30.1	26.5	22.8	18.1	14.1	11.4	8.9	7.0	5.3
1934-------	1960	34.8	34.8	32.4	29.2	25.6	20.6	16.1	13.2	10.4	8.5	6.7	4.9
1935-------	1961	35.3	34.1	31.4	28.2	22.6	18.2	15.1	12.0	10.2	8.2	6.1	4.2
1936-------	1962	34.5	32.8	30.0	24.8	20.0	16.7	13.6	11.9	9.9	7.4	5.2	3.6
1937-------	1963	33.0	30.9	26.1	21.6	18.3	15.4	13.7	11.6	8.9	6.3	4.6	
1938-------	1964	30.8	26.6	22.3	19.7	17.0	15.5	13.5	10.5	7.6	5.6		
1939-------	1965	26.5	22.7	20.6	18.3	17.1	15.5	12.4	9.1	6.8			
1940-------	1966	22.1	20.4	19.0	18.5	17.2	14.1	10.4	8.0				
1941-------	1967	19.5	18.7	19.0	18.3	15.6	11.7	9.2					
1942-------	1968	17.6	18.6	18.6	16.5	12.6	10.2						
1943-------	1969	17.2	17.9	16.5	13.3	10.9							
1944-------	1970	16.6	15.8	13.2	11.3								
1945-------	1971	14.5	12.5	11.1									
1946-------	1972	11.2	10.3										
1947-------	1973	9.3											

TABLE 4A. CENTRAL BIRTH RATES FOR ALL WOMEN DURING EACH YEAR 1917-73 BY AGE AND LIVE-BIRTH ORDER FOR EACH COHORT FROM 1868 TO 1959--CON.

LIVE-BIRTH ORDER AND COHORT	DIAGONAL LINE FOR CALENDAR YEAR	CURRENT AGE											
		38	39	40	41	42	43	44	45	46	47	48	49
FOURTH BIRTHS--CON.													
1868-------													0.1
1869-------												0.1	0.1
1870-------											0.2	0.2	0.1
1871-------										0.3	0.2	0.1	0.1
1872-------									0.6	0.4	0.1	0.1	0.1
1873-------								1.0	0.6	0.3	0.2	0.1	0.1
1874-------							1.5	1.0	0.5	0.4	0.2	0.1	0.1
1875-------						2.2	1.4	0.9	0.6	0.3	0.1	0.1	0.1
1876-------					3.3	2.1	1.5	1.0	0.6	0.3	0.1	0.1	0.0
1877-------				4.7	3.2	2.1	1.5	0.9	0.5	0.3	0.1	0.1	0.0
1878-------			6.8	4.7	3.3	2.1	1.5	0.9	0.5	0.3	0.1	0.1	0.0
1879-------	1917	8.4	6.8	4.6	3.4	2.1	1.4	0.9	0.5	0.3	0.1	0.1	0.0
1880-------	1918	8.5	6.7	4.7	3.3	2.0	1.4	0.9	0.5	0.3	0.2	0.1	0.0
1881-------	1919	8.3	6.8	4.7	3.1	2.0	1.4	0.8	0.5	0.3	0.1	0.0	0.0
1882-------	1920	8.2	6.8	4.4	3.1	2.0	1.3	0.8	0.5	0.3	0.1	0.0	0.0
1883-------	1921	8.3	6.3	4.3	3.1	2.0	1.3	0.7	0.4	0.2	0.1	0.0	0.0
1884-------	1922	7.7	6.2	4.3	3.1	1.9	1.2	0.7	0.4	0.2	0.1	0.1	0.0
1885-------	1923	7.6	6.2	4.3	2.8	1.8	1.1	0.7	0.4	0.2	0.1	0.1	0.0
1886-------	1924	7.6	6.1	3.9	2.7	1.7	1.1	0.7	0.4	0.2	0.1	0.0	0.0
1887-------	1925	7.6	5.8	3.8	2.6	1.6	1.1	0.6	0.3	0.2	0.1	0.0	0.0
1888-------	1926	7.2	5.5	3.6	2.4	1.6	1.0	0.6	0.3	0.2	0.1	0.1	0.0
1889-------	1927	6.9	5.3	3.4	2.5	1.5	1.0	0.6	0.3	0.2	0.1	0.0	0.0
1890-------	1928	6.5	4.9	3.5	2.3	1.5	1.0	0.6	0.3	0.2	0.1	0.1	0.0
1891-------	1929	6.0	5.0	3.3	2.3	1.4	1.0	0.5	0.3	0.2	0.1	0.0	0.0
1892-------	1930	6.1	4.7	3.1	2.1	1.4	0.9	0.5	0.3	0.2	0.0	0.0	0.0
1893-------	1931	5.8	4.4	3.0	2.1	1.3	0.8	0.5	0.3	0.1	0.0	0.0	0.0
1894-------	1932	5.4	4.2	3.0	2.0	1.2	0.8	0.5	0.3	0.1	0.0	0.0	0.0
1895-------	1933	5.2	4.2	2.8	1.9	1.3	0.8	0.5	0.2	0.1	0.0	0.0	0.0
1896-------	1934	5.2	3.9	2.7	1.9	1.2	0.8	0.4	0.2	0.1	0.0	0.0	0.0
1897-------	1935	4.9	3.8	2.7	1.8	1.2	0.8	0.4	0.2	0.1	0.1	0.0	0.0
1898-------	1936	4.6	3.6	2.5	1.9	1.2	0.8	0.5	0.3	0.2	0.1	0.0	0.0
1899-------	1937	4.5	3.6	2.6	1.8	1.2	0.8	0.5	0.3	0.2	0.1	0.0	0.0
1900-------	1938	4.6	3.5	2.5	1.8	1.2	0.9	0.6	0.3	0.2	0.0	0.0	0.0
1901-------	1939	4.4	3.3	2.5	1.8	1.3	1.0	0.6	0.3	0.1	0.0	0.0	0.0
1902-------	1940	4.2	3.4	2.6	2.0	1.4	1.0	0.6	0.3	0.1	0.0	0.0	0.0
1903-------	1941	4.2	3.6	2.9	2.1	1.5	1.0	0.6	0.3	0.1	0.1	0.0	0.0
1904-------	1942	4.5	4.1	3.0	2.3	1.5	1.0	0.5	0.3	0.2	0.0	0.0	0.0
1905-------	1943	5.1	4.3	3.3	2.3	1.6	1.0	0.6	0.3	0.1	0.1	0.0	0.0
1906-------	1944	5.4	4.6	3.3	2.4	1.5	1.0	0.5	0.3	0.1	0.1	0.0	0.0
1907-------	1945	5.7	4.6	3.5	2.4	1.5	1.0	0.6	0.3	0.2	0.1	0.0	0.0
1908-------	1946	5.7	4.7	3.3	2.3	1.5	1.0	0.6	0.3	0.2	0.1	0.0	0.0
1909-------	1947	6.0	4.6	3.3	2.3	1.7	1.1	0.7	0.3	0.2	0.1	0.0	0.0
1910-------	1948	5.9	4.6	3.4	2.5	1.7	1.2	0.6	0.3	0.2	0.0	0.0	0.0
1911-------	1949	5.9	4.7	3.7	2.7	1.8	1.2	0.7	0.3	0.1	0.1	0.0	0.0
1912-------	1950	6.0	5.0	4.0	2.8	2.0	1.3	0.7	0.4	0.2	0.1	0.0	0.0
1913-------	1951	6.5	5.5	4.2	3.1	2.0	1.3	0.7	0.3	0.2	0.1	0.0	0.0
1914-------	1952	7.1	5.8	4.5	3.1	2.1	1.3	0.7	0.4	0.2	0.0	0.0	0.0
1915-------	1953	7.6	6.3	4.6	3.2	2.2	1.3	0.8	0.4	0.1	0.1	0.0	0.0
1916-------	1954	8.0	6.3	4.5	3.4	2.1	1.4	0.7	0.4	0.2	0.0	0.0	0.0
1917-------	1955	8.2	6.5	4.9	3.3	2.2	1.3	0.8	0.4	0.1	0.0	0.0	0.0
1918-------	1956	8.2	6.6	4.7	3.3	2.1	1.3	0.7	0.3	0.1	0.0	0.0	0.0
1919-------	1957	8.6	6.5	4.7	3.3	2.2	1.3	0.7	0.3	0.1	0.0	0.0	0.0
1920-------	1958	8.4	6.6	4.7	3.3	2.1	1.2	0.7	0.3	0.1	0.0	0.0	0.0
1921-------	1959	8.4	6.5	4.7	3.2	1.9	1.2	0.6	0.3	0.1	0.0	0.0	0.0
1922-------	1960	8.3	6.3	4.4	2.9	1.8	1.0	0.6	0.3	0.1	0.0	0.0	0.0
1923-------	1961	8.0	5.9	4.1	2.8	1.7	1.0	0.6	0.2	0.1	0.0	0.0	0.0
1924-------	1962	7.6	5.6	4.0	2.6	1.6	1.0	0.5	0.2	0.1	0.0	0.0	0.0
1925-------	1963	7.2	5.5	3.7	2.3	1.5	0.8	0.4	0.2	0.1	0.0	0.0	
1926-------	1964	7.0	5.0	3.3	2.2	1.2	0.7	0.4	0.2	0.0	0.0		
1927-------	1965	6.3	4.5	3.0	1.9	1.1	0.7	0.3	0.1	0.0			
1928-------	1966	5.7	4.1	2.7	1.7	1.1	0.5	0.2	0.1				
1929-------	1967	5.2	3.7	2.6	1.6	0.9	0.5	0.2					
1930-------	1968	4.8	3.5	2.4	1.3	0.8	0.4						
1931-------	1969	4.5	3.3	2.0	1.2	0.7							
1932-------	1970	4.2	2.8	1.7	1.0								
1933-------	1971	3.7	2.4	1.5									
1934-------	1972	3.3	2.1										
1935-------	1973	2.8											

TABLE 4A. CENTRAL BIRTH RATES FOR ALL WOMEN DURING EACH YEAR 1917-73 BY AGE AND LIVE-BIRTH ORDER FOR EACH COHORT FROM 1868 TO 1959--CON.

LIVE-BIRTH ORDER AND COHORT	DIAGONAL LINE FOR CALENDAR YEAR	CURRENT AGE											
		14	15	16	17	18	19	20	21	22	23	24	25
FIFTH BIRTHS													
1892-------													12.4
1893-------												8.7	11.8
1894-------											5.5	8.3	11.6
1895-------										2.8	5.2	8.3	11.8
1896-------									1.4	2.7	5.2	8.5	12.4
1897-------								0.6	1.3	2.7	5.3	9.0	11.5
1898-------							*	0.5	1.3	2.8	5.7	8.4	11.9
1899-------						*	*	0.5	1.4	3.0	5.4	8.8	11.6
1900-------					*	*	*	0.6	1.5	2.8	5.8	8.6	11.1
1901-------				*	*	*	*	0.6	1.4	2.9	5.6	8.2	10.9
1902-------			*	*	*	*	*	0.6	1.5	3.0	5.3	8.2	10.8
1903-------	1917	*	*	*	*	*	*	0.7	1.6	2.9	5.5	8.2	10.2
1904-------	1918	*	*	*	*	*	*	0.7	1.6	3.2	5.5	7.8	10.0
1905-------	1919	*	*	*	*	*	*	0.7	1.7	3.1	5.2	7.5	9.4
1906-------	1920	*	*	*	*	*	*	0.7	1.6	2.9	5.0	7.1	8.8
1907-------	1921	*	*	*	*	*	*	0.7	1.6	2.7	4.7	6.5	8.4
1908-------	1922	*	*	*	*	*	*	0.7	1.5	2.6	4.3	6.3	7.7
1909-------	1923	*	*	*	*	*	*	0.6	1.4	2.4	4.1	5.8	7.9
1910-------	1924	*	*	*	*	*	*	0.6	1.3	2.3	3.8	6.0	7.5
1911-------	1925	*	*	*	*	*	*	0.6	1.3	2.2	4.0	5.8	7.2
1912-------	1926	*	*	*	*	*	*	0.6	1.2	2.2	3.9	5.4	7.1
1913-------	1927	*	*	*	*	*	*	0.5	1.1	2.3	3.7	5.4	6.9
1914-------	1928	*	*	*	*	*	*	0.5	1.2	2.2	3.7	5.4	6.6
1915-------	1929	*	*	*	*	*	*	0.5	1.2	2.2	3.7	5.2	6.9
1916-------	1930	*	*	*	*	*	*	0.5	1.2	2.1	3.6	5.6	6.9
1917-------	1931	*	*	*	*	*	*	0.5	1.1	2.1	4.2	5.7	6.9
1918-------	1932	*	*	*	*	*	*	0.5	1.1	2.4	4.2	5.7	7.4
1919-------	1933	*	*	*	*	*	*	0.5	1.3	2.4	4.2	6.1	7.5
1920-------	1934	*	*	*	*	*	*	0.6	1.3	2.6	4.5	6.2	7.1
1921-------	1935	*	*	*	*	*	*	0.6	1.5	2.7	4.6	5.9	7.3
1922-------	1936	*	*	*	*	*	*	0.7	1.6	2.8	4.3	5.8	7.1
1923-------	1937	*	*	*	*	*	*	0.7	1.7	2.7	4.2	5.7	7.2
1924-------	1938	*	*	*	*	*	*	0.8	1.6	2.7	4.2	5.9	7.5
1925-------	1939	*	*	*	*	*	*	0.8	1.6	2.7	4.3	6.3	7.8
1926-------	1940	*	*	*	*	*	*	0.8	1.6	2.7	4.8	6.6	8.8
1927-------	1941	*	*	*	*	*	*	0.8	1.7	3.1	4.9	7.4	9.7
1928-------	1942	*	*	*	*	*	*	0.8	2.0	3.3	5.6	8.2	10.5
1929-------	1943	*	*	*	*	*	*	1.0	2.1	3.8	6.5	9.3	11.8
1930-------	1944	*	*	*	*	*	*	1.0	2.4	4.5	7.4	10.2	12.5
1931-------	1945	*	*	*	*	*	*	1.2	2.9	5.2	8.1	11.0	13.7
1932-------	1946	*	*	*	*	*	*	1.4	3.1	5.5	8.6	11.7	14.5
1933-------	1947	*	*	*	*	*	*	1.4	3.5	5.9	9.1	12.6	15.4
1934-------	1948	*	*	*	*	*	*	1.7	3.7	6.2	9.8	13.2	16.0
1935-------	1949	*	*	*	*	*	*	1.8	3.9	6.7	10.2	13.6	16.6
1936-------	1950	*	*	*	*	*	*	1.9	4.2	6.8	10.4	14.1	17.2
1937-------	1951	*	*	*	*	*	*	2.0	4.2	7.1	10.9	14.5	17.0
1938-------	1952	*	*	*	*	*	*	2.0	4.3	7.3	10.9	14.3	15.9
1939-------	1953	*	*	*	*	*	*	2.1	4.5	7.5	11.1	13.5	14.9
1940-------	1954	*	*	*	*	*	*	2.1	4.6	7.5	10.3	12.4	12.4
1941-------	1955	*	*	*	*	*	*	2.2	4.7	7.0	9.3	10.1	10.0
1942-------	1956	*	*	*	*	*	*	2.2	4.2	6.1	7.4	8.0	8.2
1943-------	1957	*	*	*	*	*	*	1.9	3.7	4.9	5.8	6.6	6.8
1944-------	1958	*	*	*	*	*	*	1.8	3.1	3.9	4.9	5.5	6.4
1945-------	1959	*	*	*	*	*	*	1.5	2.5	3.4	4.1	5.1	6.0
1946-------	1960	*	*	*	*	*	*	1.3	2.1	2.7	3.7	4.6	5.0
1947-------	1961	*	*	*	*	*	*	1.0	1.6	2.3	3.2	3.8	3.7
1948-------	1962	*	*	*	*	*	*	0.7	1.4	2.0	2.7	2.8	3.0
1949-------	1963	*	*	*	*	*	*	0.7	1.3	1.8	2.1	2.4	
1950-------	1964	*	*	*	*	*	*	0.7	1.1	1.4	1.8		
1951-------	1965	*	*	*	*	*	*	0.6	0.8	1.1			
1952-------	1966	*	*	*	*	*	*	0.4	0.7				
1953-------	1967	*	*	*	*	*	*	0.3					
1954-------	1968	*	*	*	*	*	*						
1955-------	1969	*	*	*	*	*							
1956-------	1970	*	*	*	*								
1957-------	1971	*	*	*									
1958-------	1972	*	*										
1959-------	1973	*											

TABLE 4A. CENTRAL BIRTH RATES FOR ALL WOMEN DURING EACH YEAR 1917-73 BY AGE AND LIVE-BIRTH ORDER FOR EACH COHORT FROM 1868 TO 1959--CON.

LIVE-BIRTH ORDER AND COHORT	DIAGONAL LINE FOR CALENDAR YEAR	CURRENT AGE											
		26	27	28	29	30	31	32	33	34	35	36	37
FIFTH BIRTHS--CON.													
1880-------													11.4
1881-------												12.8	11.2
1882-------											14.8	12.6	11.0
1883-------										16.1	14.5	12.4	10.9
1884-------									17.6	15.9	14.0	12.3	10.8
1885-------								17.8	17.4	15.1	13.9	12.2	10.0
1886-------							19.4	17.7	16.4	15.0	13.9	11.4	9.9
1887-------						20.1	19.4	16.7	16.3	15.0	12.9	11.2	9.7
1888-------					21.8	19.8	18.3	16.6	16.2	14.0	12.7	11.0	9.3
1889-------				20.4	21.2	18.8	18.1	16.5	15.1	13.8	12.5	10.6	9.0
1890-------			18.5	19.7	20.5	18.8	18.1	15.4	15.1	13.7	11.8	10.1	8.5
1891-------	1917	15.2	17.9	19.3	20.5	18.9	16.9	15.4	14.8	13.0	11.2	9.6	8.0
1892-------	1918	14.7	17.5	19.3	20.8	17.3	16.7	15.0	13.9	12.1	10.6	8.9	7.4
1893-------	1919	14.4	17.5	19.7	18.8	17.1	16.3	14.3	12.9	11.7	9.9	8.3	7.3
1894-------	1920	14.5	18.1	17.7	18.7	16.8	15.5	13.4	12.6	10.9	9.5	8.3	6.9
1895-------	1921	15.1	16.4	17.8	18.3	16.0	14.6	13.1	11.9	10.3	9.3	7.8	6.5
1896-------	1922	13.8	16.5	17.3	17.2	15.1	14.3	12.2	11.0	10.0	8.6	7.4	6.1
1897-------	1923	13.9	16.2	16.2	16.0	14.7	13.3	11.4	10.8	9.3	8.4	6.9	6.1
1898-------	1924	13.8	15.2	15.3	16.0	13.9	12.6	11.2	10.1	9.1	7.7	6.8	5.6
1899-------	1925	13.2	14.7	15.6	15.3	13.3	12.5	10.7	10.1	8.6	7.9	6.5	5.4
1900-------	1926	13.0	14.9	14.7	14.4	13.0	11.7	10.5	9.5	8.6	7.4	6.2	5.2
1901-------	1927	13.0	13.8	13.8	13.9	12.1	11.3	9.7	9.4	8.0	6.9	5.8	5.1
1902-------	1928	12.0	13.1	13.3	12.9	11.5	10.4	9.5	8.5	7.3	6.5	5.6	4.7
1903-------	1929	11.6	12.6	12.4	12.3	10.7	10.3	8.7	8.0	7.0	6.3	5.2	4.6
1904-------	1930	11.1	11.8	12.1	11.6	10.7	9.5	8.2	7.7	6.8	5.9	5.1	4.5
1905-------	1931	10.4	11.4	11.2	11.6	9.9	9.0	8.0	7.5	6.4	5.7	5.0	4.5
1906-------	1932	10.0	10.5	11.1	10.8	9.3	8.7	7.6	7.0	6.2	5.6	5.0	4.9
1907-------	1933	9.2	10.6	10.4	10.1	9.0	8.3	7.2	6.7	6.1	5.6	5.4	5.0
1908-------	1934	9.3	9.9	9.7	9.7	8.6	7.7	6.9	6.6	6.2	6.1	5.5	5.1
1909-------	1935	8.8	9.4	9.6	9.4	8.1	7.5	6.9	6.7	6.7	6.2	5.8	5.2
1910-------	1936	8.4	9.2	9.3	8.8	7.9	7.4	7.0	7.3	6.8	6.5	5.8	5.1
1911-------	1937	8.3	9.0	8.8	8.7	7.9	7.4	7.6	7.4	7.1	6.5	5.8	5.0
1912-------	1938	8.0	8.4	8.6	8.6	7.8	8.1	7.7	7.5	7.0	6.4	5.6	5.0
1913-------	1939	7.5	8.3	8.6	8.3	8.5	8.2	7.7	7.5	6.9	6.3	5.6	5.2
1914-------	1940	7.5	8.3	8.3	9.1	8.5	8.1	7.7	7.5	6.9	6.4	5.9	5.5
1915-------	1941	7.5	8.1	9.0	9.1	8.4	8.2	7.8	7.4	7.0	6.7	6.3	5.9
1916-------	1942	7.5	8.8	9.1	8.9	8.6	8.1	7.6	7.5	7.2	7.1	6.7	6.4
1917-------	1943	8.1	8.9	8.8	9.0	8.4	8.0	7.7	7.8	7.7	7.5	7.2	6.7
1918-------	1944	8.1	8.4	8.9	8.8	8.3	8.1	8.0	8.2	8.2	7.9	7.7	6.9
1919-------	1945	7.9	8.8	8.9	8.9	8.7	8.7	8.8	9.2	8.9	8.8	8.1	7.3
1920-------	1946	8.1	8.7	9.0	9.2	9.1	9.3	9.8	9.8	9.7	9.2	8.5	7.8
1921-------	1947	8.1	8.8	9.2	9.5	9.8	10.4	10.4	10.6	10.3	9.8	9.1	7.9
1922-------	1948	8.0	8.8	9.3	10.2	10.6	11.0	11.0	11.2	10.8	10.2	9.0	8.1
1923-------	1949	8.2	9.2	10.1	11.1	11.4	11.8	11.9	11.9	11.4	10.3	9.4	8.1
1924-------	1950	8.7	10.1	11.3	12.2	12.5	12.8	12.7	12.6	11.7	10.8	9.5	8.2
1925-------	1951	9.5	11.3	12.2	13.3	13.4	13.7	13.6	12.9	12.1	11.0	9.7	7.9
1926-------	1952	10.6	12.1	13.4	14.1	14.3	14.6	13.8	13.3	12.3	11.0	9.3	7.6
1927-------	1953	11.5	13.2	14.2	15.0	15.2	14.7	14.4	13.7	12.5	10.7	9.1	7.3
1928-------	1954	12.6	14.0	14.9	15.9	15.6	15.6	14.8	13.9	12.1	10.4	8.7	6.7
1929-------	1955	13.4	15.0	16.2	16.7	16.7	16.3	15.4	13.8	12.0	10.1	8.1	6.2
1930-------	1956	14.5	16.2	17.0	17.7	17.4	16.8	15.2	13.6	11.6	9.4	7.3	5.6
1931-------	1957	15.7	17.0	18.1	18.5	18.0	16.8	15.1	13.1	10.8	8.4	6.6	5.2
1932-------	1958	16.5	18.1	18.9	19.3	17.9	16.7	14.5	12.2	9.5	7.6	6.1	4.9
1933-------	1959	17.4	18.8	19.9	19.2	17.8	15.9	13.3	10.6	8.7	7.1	5.9	4.6
1934-------	1960	18.1	19.9	19.7	18.8	17.0	14.3	11.6	9.7	7.9	6.9	5.6	4.3
1935-------	1961	19.1	19.7	19.3	18.0	14.9	12.5	10.5	8.7	7.8	6.5	5.1	3.6
1936-------	1962	18.7	19.1	18.2	15.5	13.0	11.3	9.3	8.5	7.4	5.9	4.2	3.1
1937-------	1963	18.0	17.8	15.5	13.3	11.7	10.0	9.2	8.2	6.6	4.9	3.6	
1938-------	1964	16.6	15.0	13.0	11.8	10.2	9.8	9.0	7.3	5.5	4.1		
1939-------	1965	14.0	12.5	11.4	10.4	10.2	9.6	8.0	6.1	4.7			
1940-------	1966	11.5	10.8	10.1	10.3	9.9	8.6	6.6	5.1				
1941-------	1967	9.7	9.3	9.8	9.8	8.8	6.8	5.5					
1942-------	1968	8.1	8.9	9.1	8.6	6.7	5.6						
1943-------	1969	7.6	8.2	8.0	6.5	5.5							
1944-------	1970	7.1	7.1	6.1	5.4								
1945-------	1971	6.1	5.5	4.9									
1946-------	1972	4.6	4.3										
1947-------	1973	3.5											

TABLE 4A. CENTRAL BIRTH RATES FOR ALL WOMEN DURING EACH YEAR 1917-73 BY AGE AND LIVE-BIRTH ORDER FOR EACH COHORT FROM 1868 TO 1959--CON.

LIVE-BIRTH ORDER AND COHORT	DIAGONAL LINE FOR CALENDAR YEAR	CURRENT AGE 38	39	40	41	42	43	44	45	46	47	48	49
FIFTH BIRTHS--CON.													
1868-------													0.1
1869-------												0.1	0.1
1870-------											0.2	0.1	0.1
1871-------										0.5	0.3	0.1	0.1
1872-------									0.7	0.5	0.2	0.1	0.0
1873-------								1.2	0.8	0.5	0.3	0.1	0.0
1874-------							1.8	1.2	0.7	0.5	0.2	0.1	0.0
1875-------						2.5	1.9	1.2	0.8	0.4	0.2	0.1	0.0
1876-------					3.8	2.6	1.8	1.2	0.7	0.4	0.2	0.1	0.1
1877-------				5.4	4.0	2.5	1.8	1.2	0.6	0.4	0.2	0.1	0.0
1878-------			7.9	5.5	3.8	2.5	1.9	1.1	0.7	0.4	0.2	0.1	0.0
1879-------	1917	9.6	7.9	5.4	3.8	2.6	1.7	1.1	0.7	0.4	0.2	0.1	0.0
1880-------	1918	9.4	7.8	5.3	3.9	2.4	1.7	1.1	0.6	0.3	0.2	0.1	0.0
1881-------	1919	9.3	7.7	5.4	3.7	2.4	1.7	1.0	0.5	0.3	0.1	0.1	0.0
1882-------	1920	9.2	7.7	5.0	3.6	2.4	1.6	0.9	0.5	0.3	0.1	0.1	0.0
1883-------	1921	9.1	7.1	4.9	3.5	2.2	1.5	0.9	0.5	0.3	0.2	0.0	0.0
1884-------	1922	8.4	7.0	4.8	3.3	2.2	1.5	0.9	0.5	0.3	0.1	0.1	0.0
1885-------	1923	8.2	6.8	4.5	3.2	2.1	1.4	0.8	0.5	0.3	0.1	0.1	0.0
1886-------	1924	8.1	6.4	4.3	3.0	1.9	1.3	0.8	0.4	0.3	0.1	0.1	0.1
1887-------	1925	7.8	6.2	4.2	2.9	1.8	1.3	0.7	0.4	0.2	0.1	0.1	0.0
1888-------	1926	7.5	6.0	4.0	2.7	1.8	1.2	0.7	0.4	0.2	0.1	0.0	0.0
1889-------	1927	7.3	5.7	3.7	2.8	1.7	1.2	0.7	0.4	0.2	0.1	0.1	0.0
1890-------	1928	6.8	5.3	3.8	2.6	1.7	1.2	0.7	0.4	0.2	0.1	0.1	0.0
1891-------	1929	6.2	5.3	3.5	2.5	1.7	1.1	0.6	0.4	0.2	0.1	0.1	0.0
1892-------	1930	6.3	4.9	3.3	2.4	1.6	1.0	0.6	0.3	0.2	0.1	0.1	0.0
1893-------	1931	5.9	4.5	3.2	2.4	1.5	1.0	0.5	0.3	0.2	0.1	0.0	0.0
1894-------	1932	5.4	4.3	3.2	2.2	1.4	0.9	0.5	0.3	0.2	0.1	0.0	0.0
1895-------	1933	5.2	4.3	3.0	2.1	1.3	0.9	0.5	0.3	0.1	0.0	0.0	0.0
1896-------	1934	5.1	4.0	2.8	2.0	1.3	0.9	0.5	0.2	0.1	0.0	0.0	0.0
1897-------	1935	4.8	3.7	2.7	1.9	1.3	0.8	0.4	0.3	0.1	0.0	0.0	0.0
1898-------	1936	4.5	3.6	2.6	1.9	1.2	0.8	0.6	0.3	0.1	0.1	0.0	0.0
1899-------	1937	4.4	3.6	2.6	1.8	1.2	0.8	0.6	0.3	0.2	0.1	0.0	0.0
1900-------	1938	4.3	3.5	2.5	1.8	1.2	0.9	0.6	0.3	0.2	0.1	0.0	0.0
1901-------	1939	4.1	3.3	2.4	1.7	1.3	0.9	0.6	0.3	0.2	0.0	0.0	0.0
1902-------	1940	3.9	3.2	2.4	1.9	1.4	0.9	0.6	0.3	0.1	0.1	0.0	0.0
1903-------	1941	3.8	3.2	2.5	1.9	1.4	1.0	0.5	0.3	0.2	0.0	0.0	0.0
1904-------	1942	3.9	3.4	2.6	2.0	1.4	0.9	0.5	0.3	0.1	0.1	0.0	0.0
1905-------	1943	4.2	3.5	2.7	2.0	1.4	0.8	0.5	0.3	0.1	0.0	0.0	0.0
1906-------	1944	4.3	3.7	2.7	2.0	1.3	0.8	0.5	0.3	0.1	0.0	0.0	0.0
1907-------	1945	4.4	3.7	2.8	1.9	1.3	0.9	0.5	0.3	0.1	0.1	0.0	0.0
1908-------	1946	4.4	3.6	2.6	1.9	1.3	0.9	0.5	0.3	0.2	0.1	0.0	0.0
1909-------	1947	4.4	3.5	2.6	2.0	1.3	0.9	0.6	0.3	0.2	0.1	0.0	0.0
1910-------	1948	4.2	3.5	2.7	2.0	1.4	1.0	0.6	0.3	0.2	0.1	0.0	0.0
1911-------	1949	4.3	3.6	2.8	2.2	1.5	1.1	0.7	0.3	0.2	0.0	0.0	0.0
1912-------	1950	4.4	3.7	3.0	2.2	1.7	1.2	0.6	0.3	0.1	0.1	0.0	0.0
1913-------	1951	4.6	4.1	3.1	2.5	1.8	1.1	0.6	0.3	0.2	0.1	0.0	0.0
1914-------	1952	5.0	4.3	3.4	2.6	1.8	1.1	0.7	0.4	0.2	0.1	0.0	0.0
1915-------	1953	5.4	4.6	3.6	2.7	1.8	1.2	0.7	0.3	0.2	0.1	0.0	0.0
1916-------	1954	5.6	4.8	3.7	2.7	1.8	1.2	0.7	0.4	0.2	0.1	0.0	0.0
1917-------	1955	5.9	4.9	3.7	2.8	1.9	1.2	0.7	0.3	0.2	0.1	0.0	0.0
1918-------	1956	6.1	5.0	3.8	2.8	1.9	1.3	0.6	0.3	0.2	0.0	0.0	0.0
1919-------	1957	6.4	5.2	3.9	2.9	2.0	1.2	0.7	0.3	0.1	0.0	0.0	0.0
1920-------	1958	6.5	5.3	4.0	2.9	1.9	1.2	0.6	0.3	0.1	0.0	0.0	0.0
1921-------	1959	6.8	5.3	4.0	2.8	1.9	1.1	0.6	0.3	0.1	0.0	0.0	0.0
1922-------	1960	6.7	5.4	3.8	2.7	1.7	1.0	0.6	0.3	0.1	0.0	0.0	0.0
1923-------	1961	6.8	5.1	3.7	2.6	1.7	0.9	0.5	0.2	0.1	0.0	0.0	0.0
1924-------	1962	6.5	5.0	3.6	2.5	1.5	0.8	0.4	0.2	0.1	0.0	0.0	0.0
1925-------	1963	6.3	4.8	3.4	2.2	1.3	0.8	0.5	0.2	0.0	0.0	0.0	
1926-------	1964	6.0	4.5	3.0	2.0	1.2	0.8	0.4	0.1	0.1	0.0		
1927-------	1965	5.6	4.0	2.7	1.8	1.2	0.6	0.3	0.1	0.1			
1928-------	1966	5.1	3.5	2.4	1.7	1.0	0.6	0.2	0.1				
1929-------	1967	4.6	3.3	2.4	1.6	0.9	0.5	0.2					
1930-------	1968	4.2	3.2	2.3	1.3	0.7	0.4						
1931-------	1969	4.0	3.0	1.8	1.2	0.7							
1932-------	1970	3.8	2.6	1.6	1.0								
1933-------	1971	3.4	2.3	1.5									
1934-------	1972	2.9	2.0										
1935-------	1973	2.5											

TABLE 4A. CENTRAL BIRTH RATES FOR ALL WOMEN DURING EACH YEAR 1917-73 BY AGE AND LIVE-BIRTH ORDER FOR EACH COHORT FROM 1868 TO 1959--CON.

LIVE-BIRTH ORDER AND COHORT	DIAGONAL LINE FOR CALENDAR YEAR	CURRENT AGE 14	15	16	17	18	19	20	21	22	23	24	25
SIXTH BIRTHS													
1892-------													5.0
1893-------												3.0	4.7
1894-------											1.7	2.8	4.5
1895-------										0.8	1.6	2.8	4.6
1896-------									0.4	0.8	1.5	2.9	5.1
1897-------								0.2	0.4	0.7	1.6	3.2	4.7
1898-------							*	0.2	0.4	0.8	1.8	3.0	4.9
1899-------						*	*	0.2	0.4	0.9	1.8	3.1	5.0
1900-------					*	*	*	0.2	0.4	0.8	1.9	3.2	4.8
1901-------				*	*	*	*	0.2	0.4	0.8	1.8	3.1	4.8
1902-------			*	*	*	*	*	0.2	0.4	0.9	1.8	3.0	4.5
1903-------	1917	*	*	*	*	*	*	0.2	0.4	0.9	1.8	2.9	4.1
1904-------	1918	*	*	*	*	*	*	0.2	0.5	0.9	1.7	2.8	4.1
1905-------	1919	*	*	*	*	*	*	0.2	0.5	0.9	1.7	2.6	3.9
1906-------	1920	*	*	*	*	*	*	0.2	0.5	0.9	1.5	2.5	3.7
1907-------	1921	*	*	*	*	*	*	0.2	0.5	0.8	1.4	2.4	3.4
1908-------	1922	*	*	*	*	*	*	0.2	0.4	0.7	1.4	2.2	3.1
1909-------	1923	*	*	*	*	*	*	0.2	0.4	0.7	1.2	2.0	3.2
1910-------	1924	*	*	*	*	*	*	0.2	0.4	0.6	1.2	2.0	3.1
1911-------	1925	*	*	*	*	*	*	0.2	0.3	0.6	1.2	2.1	3.1
1912-------	1926	*	*	*	*	*	*	0.2	0.3	0.6	1.2	2.0	3.0
1913-------	1927	*	*	*	*	*	*	0.1	0.3	0.6	1.2	1.9	2.9
1914-------	1928	*	*	*	*	*	*	0.1	0.3	0.6	1.1	1.9	2.8
1915-------	1929	*	*	*	*	*	*	0.1	0.3	0.6	1.1	1.9	2.9
1916-------	1930	*	*	*	*	*	*	0.1	0.3	0.6	1.1	2.0	2.9
1917-------	1931	*	*	*	*	*	*	0.1	0.3	0.6	1.3	2.0	3.1
1918-------	1932	*	*	*	*	*	*	0.1	0.3	0.7	1.3	2.1	3.2
1919-------	1933	*	*	*	*	*	*	0.1	0.4	0.7	1.3	2.3	3.3
1920-------	1934	*	*	*	*	*	*	0.2	0.4	0.7	1.5	2.4	3.2
1921-------	1935	*	*	*	*	*	*	0.2	0.4	0.8	1.5	2.2	3.3
1922-------	1936	*	*	*	*	*	*	0.2	0.4	0.8	1.4	2.3	3.2
1923-------	1937	*	*	*	*	*	*	0.2	0.4	0.8	1.4	2.3	3.2
1924-------	1938	*	*	*	*	*	*	0.2	0.4	0.8	1.5	2.3	3.4
1925-------	1939	*	*	*	*	*	*	0.2	0.4	0.8	1.5	2.5	3.5
1926-------	1940	*	*	*	*	*	*	0.2	0.4	0.8	1.6	2.5	3.7
1927-------	1941	*	*	*	*	*	*	0.2	0.4	0.9	1.6	2.7	4.1
1928-------	1942	*	*	*	*	*	*	0.2	0.5	0.9	1.8	3.0	4.5
1929-------	1943	*	*	*	*	*	*	0.2	0.5	1.0	2.1	3.4	5.1
1930-------	1944	*	*	*	*	*	*	0.2	0.5	1.2	2.3	3.9	5.6
1931-------	1945	*	*	*	*	*	*	0.2	0.6	1.4	2.8	4.4	6.3
1932-------	1946	*	*	*	*	*	*	0.3	0.7	1.6	3.0	4.9	6.6
1933-------	1947	*	*	*	*	*	*	0.3	0.9	1.8	3.3	5.1	6.9
1934-------	1948	*	*	*	*	*	*	0.4	0.9	1.9	3.5	5.4	7.3
1935-------	1949	*	*	*	*	*	*	0.4	1.0	2.1	3.6	5.6	7.7
1936-------	1950	*	*	*	*	*	*	0.4	1.0	2.1	3.8	5.8	7.8
1937-------	1951	*	*	*	*	*	*	0.4	1.0	2.2	3.9	5.9	7.9
1938-------	1952	*	*	*	*	*	*	0.4	1.1	2.3	3.9	5.9	7.4
1939-------	1953	*	*	*	*	*	*	0.5	1.1	2.3	3.9	5.6	6.8
1940-------	1954	*	*	*	*	*	*	0.4	1.2	2.3	3.7	5.2	5.8
1941-------	1955	*	*	*	*	*	*	0.5	1.1	2.1	3.4	4.2	4.6
1942-------	1956	*	*	*	*	*	*	0.5	1.0	1.9	2.7	3.4	3.8
1943-------	1957	*	*	*	*	*	*	0.4	0.9	1.5	2.2	2.7	3.0
1944-------	1958	*	*	*	*	*	*	0.3	0.8	1.3	1.8	2.1	2.6
1945-------	1959	*	*	*	*	*	*	0.3	0.7	1.0	1.4	2.0	2.3
1946-------	1960	*	*	*	*	*	*	0.3	0.5	0.8	1.3	1.6	1.8
1947-------	1961	*	*	*	*	*	*	0.2	0.4	0.7	1.0	1.3	1.3
1948-------	1962	*	*	*	*	*	*	0.1	0.4	0.5	0.8	0.9	1.0
1949-------	1963	*	*	*	*	*	*	0.2	0.3	0.5	0.6	0.7	
1950-------	1964	*	*	*	*	*	*	0.1	0.2	0.3	0.4		
1951-------	1965	*	*	*	*	*	*	0.1	0.2	0.2			
1952-------	1966	*	*	*	*	*	*	0.1	0.1				
1953-------	1967	*	*	*	*	*	*	0.1					
1954-------	1968	*	*	*	*	*	*						
1955-------	1969	*	*	*	*	*							
1956-------	1970	*	*	*	*								
1957-------	1971	*	*	*									
1958-------	1972	*	*										
1959-------	1973	*											

TABLE 4A. CENTRAL BIRTH RATES FOR ALL WOMEN DURING EACH YEAR 1917-73 BY AGE AND LIVE-BIRTH ORDER FOR EACH COHORT FROM 1868 TO 1959--CON.

LIVE-BIRTH ORDER AND COHORT	DIAGONAL LINE FOR CALENDAR YEAR	CURRENT AGE 26	27	28	29	30	31	32	33	34	35	36	37
SIXTH BIRTHS--CON.													
1880-------													12.2
1881-------												13.3	12.1
1882-------											14.6	13.2	11.7
1883-------										15.4	14.5	12.7	11.5
1884-------									16.0	15.2	13.8	12.5	11.2
1885-------								15.6	15.8	14.4	13.5	12.2	10.4
1886-------							16.0	15.6	15.0	14.0	13.4	11.4	10.1
1887-------						15.1	16.0	14.8	14.5	14.2	12.6	11.1	10.0
1888-------					15.0	14.9	15.1	14.3	14.9	13.2	12.3	10.9	9.4
1889-------				12.4	14.4	14.1	14.6	14.6	13.7	13.0	12.0	10.4	9.0
1890-------			10.1	11.7	13.8	13.8	15.1	13.5	13.7	12.8	11.4	9.9	8.7
1891-------	1917	7.2	9.6	11.3	13.7	14.4	13.9	13.5	13.5	12.1	10.9	9.7	8.0
1892-------	1918	6.8	9.2	11.3	14.3	13.1	13.8	13.2	12.6	11.4	10.4	8.7	7.3
1893-------	1919	6.5	9.2	12.0	13.0	13.0	13.5	12.3	11.8	11.0	9.6	8.1	7.2
1894-------	1920	6.6	9.9	10.8	13.0	12.8	12.8	11.6	11.5	10.0	8.9	7.8	6.8
1895-------	1921	7.1	9.0	11.0	12.9	12.3	12.1	11.5	10.6	9.4	8.6	7.5	6.5
1896-------	1922	6.5	9.2	11.0	12.2	11.8	11.7	10.4	9.7	9.1	8.0	7.1	6.0
1897-------	1923	6.7	9.3	10.2	11.8	11.2	10.9	9.5	9.6	8.4	7.8	6.6	5.9
1898-------	1924	6.8	8.5	10.1	11.3	10.5	10.2	9.7	9.0	8.4	7.4	6.6	5.6
1899-------	1925	6.5	8.7	9.8	10.7	10.0	10.3	9.2	9.2	8.0	7.4	6.1	5.2
1900-------	1926	6.5	8.4	9.2	10.2	10.0	9.8	9.1	8.5	7.9	6.8	5.9	5.0
1901-------	1927	6.2	7.8	8.5	9.9	9.3	9.4	8.3	8.3	7.2	6.4	5.4	4.8
1902-------	1928	5.7	7.1	8.4	9.2	8.9	8.5	8.0	7.5	6.6	5.9	5.1	4.5
1903-------	1929	5.5	7.0	7.9	9.0	8.1	8.3	7.3	6.9	6.2	5.6	4.8	4.2
1904-------	1930	5.3	6.7	7.9	8.1	8.1	7.8	6.9	6.7	6.0	5.3	4.6	4.1
1905-------	1931	5.1	6.5	7.0	8.1	7.6	7.2	6.7	6.4	5.5	5.0	4.4	4.0
1906-------	1932	4.8	5.9	7.0	7.6	7.0	7.0	6.4	5.9	5.3	4.8	4.3	4.1
1907-------	1933	4.4	5.9	6.6	7.1	6.9	6.8	5.9	5.7	5.1	4.8	4.4	4.2
1908-------	1934	4.4	5.5	6.2	6.9	6.6	6.2	5.7	5.4	5.1	5.0	4.5	4.1
1909-------	1935	4.3	5.3	6.1	6.7	6.1	6.0	5.5	5.4	5.4	5.1	4.5	4.0
1910-------	1936	4.1	5.2	5.9	6.2	6.0	5.7	5.3	5.7	5.5	4.9	4.4	4.0
1911-------	1937	4.1	5.1	5.6	6.2	5.8	5.5	5.7	5.8	5.2	4.8	4.4	3.8
1912-------	1938	3.9	4.9	5.6	6.0	5.5	5.9	5.8	5.5	5.2	4.8	4.2	3.8
1913-------	1939	3.8	4.8	5.5	5.6	5.8	5.9	5.5	5.5	5.1	4.5	4.2	3.8
1914-------	1940	3.8	4.8	5.2	5.9	6.0	5.8	5.6	5.3	4.8	4.7	4.2	4.1
1915-------	1941	3.7	4.6	5.4	6.0	5.8	5.8	5.3	5.2	5.0	4.7	4.5	4.1
1916-------	1942	3.8	4.8	5.5	5.8	5.7	5.5	5.3	5.3	5.0	4.9	4.5	4.3
1917-------	1943	4.0	4.9	5.3	5.7	5.5	5.5	5.3	5.3	5.1	4.9	4.7	4.5
1918-------	1944	4.1	4.8	5.3	5.6	5.5	5.5	5.4	5.4	5.3	5.1	4.9	4.7
1919-------	1945	4.1	4.9	5.2	5.7	5.7	5.7	5.6	5.8	5.7	5.6	5.4	5.0
1920-------	1946	4.1	4.8	5.4	5.9	5.8	6.0	6.0	6.1	6.2	6.0	5.7	5.4
1921-------	1947	4.0	5.0	5.6	6.0	6.1	6.3	6.2	6.7	6.6	6.3	6.1	5.5
1922-------	1948	4.1	5.0	5.5	6.2	6.3	6.4	6.8	6.9	6.8	6.7	6.1	5.7
1923-------	1949	4.2	5.0	5.9	6.4	6.6	7.0	7.1	7.3	7.3	6.9	6.4	5.7
1924-------	1950	4.3	5.5	6.1	6.9	7.2	7.6	7.7	8.0	7.5	7.2	6.6	6.0
1925-------	1951	4.6	5.8	6.7	7.6	7.9	8.3	8.4	8.1	7.9	7.4	6.8	5.7
1926-------	1952	5.0	6.3	7.4	8.2	8.6	8.8	8.5	8.6	8.1	7.6	6.7	5.7
1927-------	1953	5.5	6.9	7.9	8.9	9.0	9.0	9.1	8.9	8.4	7.6	6.6	5.5
1928-------	1954	6.0	7.4	8.5	9.2	9.3	9.8	9.4	9.2	8.4	7.4	6.4	5.1
1929-------	1955	6.6	8.1	9.1	9.7	10.2	10.2	10.0	9.3	8.3	7.4	5.9	4.6
1930-------	1956	7.2	8.7	9.6	10.5	10.7	10.6	10.0	9.3	8.3	6.7	5.3	4.3
1931-------	1957	7.9	9.2	10.3	11.1	11.2	10.8	10.0	9.3	7.5	6.1	5.0	4.0
1932-------	1958	8.2	9.7	10.8	11.5	11.2	10.7	9.8	8.3	6.7	5.5	4.6	3.6
1933-------	1959	8.7	10.2	11.3	11.5	11.0	10.4	8.8	7.3	6.1	5.1	4.3	3.4
1934-------	1960	9.1	10.7	11.3	11.3	10.6	9.3	7.7	6.5	5.4	4.9	4.0	3.2
1935-------	1961	9.5	10.6	10.9	10.9	9.5	8.0	6.8	5.7	5.4	4.5	3.7	2.7
1936-------	1962	9.5	10.2	10.5	9.4	8.1	7.0	5.9	5.6	4.9	4.2	3.1	2.3
1937-------	1963	9.0	9.6	8.9	8.0	7.0	6.1	5.7	5.3	4.5	3.4	2.5	
1938-------	1964	8.3	8.1	7.3	6.8	6.0	5.8	5.4	4.7	3.7	2.8		
1939-------	1965	7.1	6.6	6.3	5.9	5.8	5.6	4.9	3.9	3.1			
1940-------	1966	5.7	5.7	5.4	5.6	5.4	4.9	3.9	3.2				
1941-------	1967	4.7	4.7	4.9	5.0	4.6	3.8	3.2					
1942-------	1968	3.8	4.2	4.4	4.2	3.5	3.0						
1943-------	1969	3.4	3.7	3.7	3.1	2.7							
1944-------	1970	3.0	3.1	2.8	2.5								
1945-------	1971	2.5	2.4	2.2									
1946-------	1972	1.8	1.9										
1947-------	1973	1.4											

TABLE 4A. CENTRAL BIRTH RATES FOR ALL WOMEN DURING EACH YEAR 1917-73 BY AGE AND LIVE-BIRTH ORDER FOR EACH COHORT FROM 1868 TO 1959--CON.

LIVE-BIRTH ORDER AND COHORT	DIAGONAL LINE FOR CALENDAR YEAR	CURRENT AGE											
		38	39	40	41	42	43	44	45	46	47	48	49
SIXTH BIRTHS--CON.													
1868-------													0.1
1869-------												0.2	0.1
1870-------											0.3	0.2	0.1
1871-------										0.6	0.4	0.2	0.1
1872-------									0.9	0.8	0.3	0.2	0.1
1873-------								1.5	1.1	0.6	0.3	0.1	0.0
1874-------							2.3	1.6	0.9	0.6	0.2	0.1	0.1
1875-------						3.2	2.2	1.4	0.9	0.5	0.2	0.2	0.1
1876-------					4.7	3.1	2.1	1.4	0.8	0.5	0.3	0.2	0.0
1877-------				6.3	4.6	3.0	2.1	1.4	0.8	0.5	0.2	0.1	0.1
1878-------			8.8	6.2	4.4	3.0	2.2	1.3	0.8	0.5	0.2	0.1	0.0
1879-------	1917	10.3	8.8	6.0	4.5	3.1	2.0	1.3	0.7	0.4	0.2	0.1	0.0
1880-------	1918	10.3	8.5	6.0	4.5	2.8	2.0	1.3	0.8	0.5	0.2	0.1	0.1
1881-------	1919	9.9	8.4	6.0	4.1	2.8	2.0	1.2	0.7	0.4	0.2	0.1	0.1
1882-------	1920	9.8	8.3	5.5	4.1	2.7	1.9	1.2	0.7	0.4	0.2	0.1	0.0
1883-------	1921	9.6	7.6	5.4	4.0	2.5	1.8	1.0	0.6	0.4	0.2	0.1	0.0
1884-------	1922	8.8	7.4	5.2	3.7	2.5	1.7	1.0	0.6	0.3	0.2	0.1	0.0
1885-------	1923	8.5	7.2	4.9	3.6	2.3	1.5	0.9	0.5	0.3	0.1	0.1	0.0
1886-------	1924	8.4	6.9	4.6	3.4	2.1	1.4	0.9	0.5	0.3	0.1	0.1	0.1
1887-------	1925	8.1	6.4	4.6	3.1	2.0	1.5	0.9	0.5	0.3	0.1	0.1	0.1
1888-------	1926	7.5	6.3	4.2	2.9	2.0	1.4	0.9	0.5	0.3	0.1	0.1	0.1
1889-------	1927	7.4	5.8	3.9	3.0	2.0	1.4	0.8	0.5	0.3	0.2	0.1	0.0
1890-------	1928	6.8	5.3	4.0	2.8	1.9	1.3	0.8	0.4	0.3	0.1	0.1	0.0
1891-------	1929	6.2	5.5	3.7	2.7	1.7	1.3	0.7	0.4	0.2	0.1	0.1	0.0
1892-------	1930	6.3	5.0	3.6	2.5	1.7	1.1	0.7	0.4	0.2	0.1	0.0	0.0
1893-------	1931	5.9	4.9	3.3	2.4	1.6	1.1	0.6	0.4	0.2	0.1	0.0	0.0
1894-------	1932	5.7	4.5	3.3	2.3	1.5	1.0	0.6	0.3	0.2	0.1	0.0	0.0
1895-------	1933	5.2	4.4	3.0	2.1	1.4	1.0	0.6	0.3	0.2	0.1	0.0	0.0
1896-------	1934	5.2	4.1	2.8	1.9	1.4	0.9	0.5	0.3	0.2	0.0	0.0	0.0
1897-------	1935	4.7	3.7	2.6	2.0	1.3	0.8	0.5	0.3	0.1	0.0	0.0	0.0
1898-------	1936	4.4	3.5	2.6	1.9	1.2	0.8	0.6	0.3	0.1	0.1	0.0	0.0
1899-------	1937	4.3	3.6	2.5	1.8	1.2	0.9	0.6	0.3	0.2	0.1	0.0	0.0
1900-------	1938	4.2	3.4	2.4	1.8	1.2	0.9	0.5	0.3	0.2	0.1	0.0	0.0
1901-------	1939	3.9	3.1	2.3	1.6	1.3	0.9	0.5	0.3	0.2	0.1	0.0	0.0
1902-------	1940	3.7	3.0	2.2	1.8	1.3	0.9	0.5	0.3	0.1	0.1	0.0	0.0
1903-------	1941	3.5	3.0	2.3	1.8	1.3	0.9	0.6	0.2	0.1	0.1	0.0	0.0
1904-------	1942	3.6	3.1	2.3	1.9	1.2	0.9	0.4	0.2	0.1	0.0	0.0	0.0
1905-------	1943	3.7	3.1	2.4	1.8	1.2	0.8	0.4	0.2	0.1	0.0	0.0	0.0
1906-------	1944	3.7	3.1	2.3	1.6	1.1	0.7	0.4	0.2	0.1	0.1	0.0	0.0
1907-------	1945	3.6	3.0	2.2	1.6	1.1	0.8	0.4	0.2	0.1	0.0	0.0	0.0
1908-------	1946	3.5	2.9	2.0	1.5	1.1	0.7	0.4	0.2	0.1	0.0	0.0	0.0
1909-------	1947	3.5	2.7	2.1	1.6	1.1	0.8	0.5	0.2	0.1	0.0	0.0	0.0
1910-------	1948	3.3	2.7	2.1	1.6	1.1	0.8	0.5	0.2	0.1	0.0	0.0	0.0
1911-------	1949	3.3	2.8	2.2	1.7	1.3	0.8	0.5	0.3	0.1	0.1	0.0	0.0
1912-------	1950	3.3	2.9	2.3	1.8	1.3	0.9	0.5	0.3	0.1	0.1	0.0	0.0
1913-------	1951	3.4	3.0	2.4	1.9	1.3	0.9	0.6	0.3	0.2	0.0	0.0	0.0
1914-------	1952	3.5	3.1	2.6	2.0	1.4	1.0	0.5	0.3	0.1	0.1	0.0	0.0
1915-------	1953	3.8	3.4	2.7	2.0	1.5	0.9	0.6	0.3	0.2	0.1	0.0	0.0
1916-------	1954	3.9	3.5	2.7	2.1	1.4	1.0	0.6	0.3	0.2	0.0	0.0	0.0
1917-------	1955	4.1	3.5	2.8	2.0	1.5	1.0	0.6	0.3	0.1	0.1	0.0	0.0
1918-------	1956	4.2	3.6	2.8	2.1	1.5	1.0	0.6	0.2	0.2	0.0	0.0	0.0
1919-------	1957	4.5	3.8	3.0	2.2	1.6	1.0	0.5	0.3	0.1	0.0	0.0	0.0
1920-------	1958	4.6	4.0	3.0	2.3	1.5	0.9	0.6	0.3	0.1	0.0	0.0	0.0
1921-------	1959	4.9	4.0	3.1	2.2	1.5	1.0	0.5	0.2	0.1	0.0	0.0	0.0
1922-------	1960	4.9	4.1	3.0	2.2	1.5	0.9	0.5	0.2	0.1	0.0	0.0	0.0
1923-------	1961	5.1	3.9	3.0	2.1	1.4	0.8	0.4	0.2	0.1	0.0	0.0	0.0
1924-------	1962	4.8	3.9	2.9	2.0	1.3	0.7	0.4	0.2	0.1	0.0	0.0	0.0
1925-------	1963	4.8	3.8	2.8	1.9	1.1	0.7	0.4	0.2	0.1	0.0	0.0	
1926-------	1964	4.6	3.6	2.5	1.6	1.1	0.6	0.4	0.2	0.1	0.0		
1927-------	1965	4.4	3.2	2.2	1.5	0.9	0.6	0.3	0.1	0.0			
1928-------	1966	3.8	2.9	2.0	1.4	0.9	0.5	0.2	0.1				
1929-------	1967	3.7	2.7	1.9	1.3	0.7	0.4	0.2					
1930-------	1968	3.3	2.5	1.8	1.1	0.7	0.4						
1931-------	1969	3.0	2.4	1.6	1.0	0.6							
1932-------	1970	2.9	2.2	1.4	0.9								
1933-------	1971	2.6	1.8	1.2									
1934-------	1972	2.3	1.6										
1935-------	1973	1.9											

TABLE 4A. CENTRAL BIRTH RATES FOR ALL WOMEN DURING EACH YEAR 1917-73 BY AGE AND LIVE-BIRTH ORDER FOR EACH COHORT FROM 1868 TO 1959--CON.

LIVE-BIRTH ORDER AND COHORT	DIAGONAL LINE FOR CALENDAR YEAR	CURRENT AGE											
		14	15	16	17	18	19	20	21	22	23	24	25
SEVENTH BIRTHS													
1892-------													1.7
1893-------												1.0	1.5
1894-------											0.5	0.9	1.6
1895-------										0.3	0.5	0.9	1.5
1896-------									0.1	0.2	0.5	0.9	1.7
1897-------								0.1	0.1	0.2	0.5	1.0	1.6
1898-------							*	0.1	0.1	0.2	0.5	1.0	1.7
1899-------						*	*	0.1	0.1	0.2	0.5	1.0	1.7
1900-------					*	*	*	0.1	0.1	0.3	0.6	1.0	1.8
1901-------				*	*	*	*	0.1	0.1	0.3	0.5	1.0	1.7
1902-------			*	*	*	*	*	0.1	0.1	0.3	0.6	1.0	1.6
1903-------	1917	*	*	*	*	*	*	0.1	0.1	0.3	0.5	0.9	1.5
1904-------	1918	*	*	*	*	*	*	0.1	0.1	0.3	0.5	0.9	1.4
1905-------	1919	*	*	*	*	*	*	0.1	0.1	0.3	0.5	0.8	1.4
1906-------	1920	*	*	*	*	*	*	0.1	0.1	0.3	0.4	0.8	1.3
1907-------	1921	*	*	*	*	*	*	0.1	0.1	0.2	0.4	0.8	1.2
1908-------	1922	*	*	*	*	*	*	0.1	0.1	0.2	0.4	0.7	1.0
1909-------	1923	*	*	*	*	*	*	0.1	0.1	0.2	0.4	0.6	1.1
1910-------	1924	*	*	*	*	*	*	0.1	0.1	0.2	0.3	0.6	1.1
1911-------	1925	*	*	*	*	*	*	0.1	0.1	0.2	0.3	0.7	1.1
1912-------	1926	*	*	*	*	*	*	0.0	0.1	0.2	0.4	0.6	1.1
1913-------	1927	*	*	*	*	*	*	0.0	0.1	0.2	0.3	0.6	1.0
1914-------	1928	*	*	*	*	*	*	0.1	0.1	0.2	0.4	0.6	1.0
1915-------	1929	*	*	*	*	*	*	0.1	0.1	0.2	0.4	0.6	1.1
1916-------	1930	*	*	*	*	*	*	0.1	0.1	0.2	0.4	0.7	1.1
1917-------	1931	*	*	*	*	*	*	0.0	0.1	0.2	0.4	0.7	1.1
1918-------	1932	*	*	*	*	*	*	0.1	0.1	0.2	0.4	0.7	1.2
1919-------	1933	*	*	*	*	*	*	0.1	0.1	0.2	0.4	0.8	1.2
1920-------	1934	*	*	*	*	*	*	0.1	0.1	0.2	0.5	0.7	1.2
1921-------	1935	*	*	*	*	*	*	0.1	0.1	0.2	0.4	0.8	1.2
1922-------	1936	*	*	*	*	*	*	0.1	0.1	0.2	0.4	0.8	1.2
1923-------	1937	*	*	*	*	*	*	0.1	0.1	0.2	0.4	0.8	1.3
1924-------	1938	*	*	*	*	*	*	0.1	0.1	0.2	0.5	0.8	1.3
1925-------	1939	*	*	*	*	*	*	0.1	0.1	0.2	0.5	0.9	1.4
1926-------	1940	*	*	*	*	*	*	0.1	0.1	0.2	0.5	0.9	1.4
1927-------	1941	*	*	*	*	*	*	0.1	0.1	0.3	0.5	0.9	1.5
1928-------	1942	*	*	*	*	*	*	0.1	0.1	0.3	0.5	1.0	1.7
1929-------	1943	*	*	*	*	*	*	0.1	0.1	0.3	0.6	1.1	1.9
1930-------	1944	*	*	*	*	*	*	0.1	0.1	0.3	0.7	1.3	2.2
1931-------	1945	*	*	*	*	*	*	0.1	0.2	0.4	0.8	1.5	2.5
1932-------	1946	*	*	*	*	*	*	0.1	0.2	0.4	0.9	1.7	2.7
1933-------	1947	*	*	*	*	*	*	0.1	0.2	0.5	1.0	1.8	2.8
1934-------	1948	*	*	*	*	*	*	0.1	0.2	0.5	1.1	1.9	3.1
1935-------	1949	*	*	*	*	*	*	0.1	0.2	0.5	1.1	2.1	3.2
1936-------	1950	*	*	*	*	*	*	0.1	0.2	0.5	1.2	2.1	3.2
1937-------	1951	*	*	*	*	*	*	0.1	0.2	0.6	1.2	2.1	3.2
1938-------	1952	*	*	*	*	*	*	0.1	0.3	0.6	1.2	2.1	3.1
1939-------	1953	*	*	*	*	*	*	0.1	0.3	0.6	1.2	2.0	2.9
1940-------	1954	*	*	*	*	*	*	0.1	0.3	0.6	1.2	1.8	2.4
1941-------	1955	*	*	*	*	*	*	0.1	0.3	0.6	1.1	1.5	1.9
1942-------	1956	*	*	*	*	*	*	0.1	0.3	0.5	0.9	1.2	1.6
1943-------	1957	*	*	*	*	*	*	0.1	0.2	0.4	0.7	1.0	1.2
1944-------	1958	*	*	*	*	*	*	0.1	0.2	0.3	0.5	0.7	1.0
1945-------	1959	*	*	*	*	*	*	0.1	0.2	0.3	0.4	0.6	0.9
1946-------	1960	*	*	*	*	*	*	0.1	0.1	0.2	0.4	0.6	0.6
1947-------	1961	*	*	*	*	*	*	0.0	0.1	0.2	0.3	0.4	0.4
1948-------	1962	*	*	*	*	*	*	0.1	0.1	0.2	0.2	0.2	0.3
1949-------	1963	*	*	*	*	*	*	0.1	0.1	0.1	0.1	0.2	
1950-------	1964	*	*	*	*	*	*	0.1	0.0	0.1	0.1		
1951-------	1965	*	*	*	*	*	*	0.0	0.0	0.1			
1952-------	1966	*	*	*	*	*	*	0.0	0.0				
1953-------	1967	*	*	*	*	*	*	0.0					
1954-------	1968	*	*	*	*	*	*						
1955-------	1969	*	*	*	*	*							
1956-------	1970	*	*	*	*								
1957-------	1971	*	*	*									
1958-------	1972	*	*										
1959-------	1973	*											

TABLE 4A. CENTRAL BIRTH RATES FOR ALL WOMEN DURING EACH YEAR 1917-73 BY AGE AND LIVE-BIRTH ORDER FOR EACH COHORT FROM 1868 TO 1959--CON.

LIVE-BIRTH ORDER AND COHORT	DIAGONAL LINE FOR CALENDAR YEAR	CURRENT AGE											
		26	27	28	29	30	31	32	33	34	35	36	37
SEVENTH BIRTHS--CON.													
1880-------													11.9
1881-------												12.4	11.5
1882-------											12.8	12.0	11.5
1883-------										12.7	12.5	11.9	11.2
1884-------									12.5	12.4	12.2	11.6	10.9
1885-------								11.3	12.3	11.9	11.8	11.4	10.1
1886-------							10.7	11.2	11.7	11.6	11.9	10.6	9.8
1887-------						8.9	10.6	10.7	11.4	11.9	11.0	10.4	9.7
1888-------					8.0	8.7	10.1	10.4	11.8	11.0	10.9	10.2	9.1
1889-------				5.7	7.5	8.4	9.8	10.8	10.8	10.9	10.7	9.7	8.7
1890-------			4.1	5.2	7.4	8.1	10.2	9.9	10.9	10.8	10.1	9.2	8.3
1891-------	1917	2.6	3.8	5.3	7.2	8.6	9.4	9.9	10.8	10.3	9.8	8.9	7.7
1892-------	1918	2.4	3.9	5.2	7.7	7.9	9.4	9.8	10.2	9.8	9.3	8.0	6.9
1893-------	1919	2.5	3.8	5.6	7.1	7.9	9.2	9.3	9.6	9.5	8.4	7.3	6.7
1894-------	1920	2.4	4.2	5.2	7.2	7.8	8.7	8.9	9.4	8.5	7.7	7.1	6.4
1895-------	1921	2.7	3.9	5.4	7.1	7.5	8.5	8.7	8.4	7.9	7.6	6.7	6.2
1896-------	1922	2.5	4.0	5.3	6.8	7.4	8.2	7.8	7.8	7.6	7.1	6.5	5.6
1897-------	1923	2.6	4.0	5.2	6.7	7.1	7.5	7.2	7.5	7.1	6.8	6.0	5.5
1898-------	1924	2.7	3.9	5.0	6.5	6.6	7.0	7.1	7.2	6.9	6.5	5.9	5.2
1899-------	1925	2.7	3.8	5.0	6.1	6.2	7.0	6.8	7.2	6.7	6.5	5.7	4.9
1900-------	1926	2.6	3.8	4.6	5.6	6.2	6.6	6.8	6.8	6.7	6.2	5.3	4.7
1901-------	1927	2.4	3.5	4.2	5.5	5.9	6.5	6.3	6.6	6.2	5.6	4.9	4.5
1902-------	1928	2.3	3.1	4.1	5.2	5.6	5.8	6.0	6.1	5.6	5.2	4.7	4.0
1903-------	1929	2.1	3.1	4.0	5.1	5.1	5.7	5.6	5.6	5.3	5.0	4.2	3.8
1904-------	1930	2.1	3.0	3.9	4.6	5.0	5.4	5.3	5.5	5.1	4.5	4.1	3.7
1905-------	1931	2.0	2.9	3.6	4.5	4.8	5.1	5.1	5.2	4.7	4.3	3.9	3.5
1906-------	1932	1.9	2.6	3.4	4.4	4.5	4.9	4.9	4.8	4.5	4.1	3.7	3.6
1907-------	1933	1.7	2.5	3.4	4.0	4.3	4.7	4.5	4.6	4.3	4.0	3.8	3.5
1908-------	1934	1.6	2.5	3.1	4.0	4.3	4.3	4.3	4.3	4.1	4.1	3.7	3.5
1909-------	1935	1.7	2.4	3.1	4.0	3.9	4.2	4.1	4.3	4.3	4.1	3.7	3.3
1910-------	1936	1.6	2.4	3.1	3.7	3.9	4.0	4.1	4.4	4.3	4.0	3.6	3.2
1911-------	1937	1.6	2.4	2.9	3.8	3.8	3.9	4.2	4.4	4.2	3.8	3.5	3.1
1912-------	1938	1.6	2.2	3.1	3.6	3.6	4.0	4.2	4.3	4.0	3.6	3.3	3.1
1913-------	1939	1.5	2.3	3.0	3.3	3.7	4.0	4.1	4.0	3.8	3.5	3.3	3.0
1914-------	1940	1.6	2.3	2.7	3.4	3.7	4.0	3.9	3.9	3.7	3.6	3.2	3.0
1915-------	1941	1.6	2.2	2.8	3.5	3.7	3.9	3.8	3.8	3.7	3.5	3.2	3.1
1916-------	1942	1.6	2.3	2.9	3.5	3.6	3.8	3.7	3.8	3.7	3.5	3.3	3.2
1917-------	1943	1.7	2.3	2.8	3.4	3.6	3.7	3.7	3.8	3.7	3.5	3.4	3.3
1918-------	1944	1.7	2.3	2.9	3.4	3.5	3.8	3.7	3.9	3.7	3.7	3.6	3.3
1919-------	1945	1.7	2.4	2.9	3.4	3.7	3.8	4.0	4.0	3.9	4.0	3.7	3.6
1920-------	1946	1.8	2.4	3.0	3.6	3.7	4.0	4.0	4.1	4.1	4.0	3.9	3.7
1921-------	1947	1.8	2.5	3.1	3.6	3.8	4.0	4.1	4.3	4.3	4.3	4.1	3.8
1922-------	1948	1.8	2.5	3.1	3.6	3.8	4.1	4.3	4.4	4.5	4.5	4.1	3.9
1923-------	1949	1.9	2.5	3.1	3.7	3.9	4.3	4.4	4.7	4.8	4.5	4.4	4.0
1924-------	1950	1.9	2.6	3.3	3.9	4.3	4.6	4.9	5.2	4.9	4.9	4.5	4.2
1925-------	1951	2.0	2.7	3.5	4.3	4.6	5.0	5.3	5.3	5.3	5.0	4.7	4.1
1926-------	1952	2.1	3.0	3.9	4.6	5.1	5.4	5.4	5.6	5.5	5.3	4.6	4.1
1927-------	1953	2.3	3.3	4.1	5.0	5.5	5.7	5.7	5.8	5.8	5.2	4.6	4.1
1928-------	1954	2.6	3.6	4.5	5.3	5.7	6.0	6.0	6.1	5.6	5.1	4.6	3.6
1929-------	1955	2.9	4.0	4.9	5.7	6.1	6.4	6.5	6.1	5.7	5.2	4.1	3.4
1930-------	1956	3.2	4.2	5.2	6.0	6.4	6.6	6.4	6.2	5.7	4.6	3.8	3.1
1931-------	1957	3.6	4.6	5.6	6.4	6.7	6.8	6.5	6.2	5.1	4.3	3.4	2.7
1932-------	1958	3.7	5.0	5.9	6.5	6.7	6.7	6.4	5.5	4.6	3.8	3.1	2.6
1933-------	1959	4.1	5.2	6.2	6.6	6.7	6.5	5.7	4.8	4.1	3.4	3.0	2.5
1934-------	1960	4.3	5.4	6.1	6.6	6.4	5.8	4.8	4.4	3.6	3.3	2.8	2.2
1935-------	1961	4.4	5.3	6.1	6.2	5.7	4.8	4.4	3.8	3.4	3.1	2.5	1.9
1936-------	1962	4.3	5.3	5.6	5.4	4.7	4.3	3.7	3.5	3.2	2.8	2.1	1.6
1937-------	1963	4.2	4.9	4.8	4.5	4.1	3.7	3.5	3.2	2.9	2.2	1.8	
1938-------	1964	3.9	4.1	4.0	3.8	3.4	3.4	3.2	2.9	2.3	1.9		
1939-------	1965	3.3	3.4	3.4	3.2	3.1	3.1	2.8	2.3	1.9			
1940-------	1966	2.7	2.8	2.8	2.8	2.8	2.7	2.2	1.9				
1941-------	1967	2.2	2.3	2.3	2.4	2.4	2.0	1.8					
1942-------	1968	1.7	1.9	2.0	2.1	1.8	1.6						
1943-------	1969	1.4	1.6	1.7	1.5	1.4							
1944-------	1970	1.2	1.3	1.3	1.2								
1945-------	1971	1.0	1.0	1.0									
1946-------	1972	0.7	0.7										
1947-------	1973	0.5											

TABLE 4A. CENTRAL BIRTH RATES FOR ALL WOMEN DURING EACH YEAR 1917-73 BY AGE AND LIVE-BIRTH ORDER FOR EACH COHORT FROM 1868 TO 1959--CON.

LIVE-BIRTH ORDER AND COHORT	DIAGONAL LINE FOR CALENDAR YEAR	CURRENT AGE											
		38	39	40	41	42	43	44	45	46	47	48	49
SEVENTH BIRTHS--CON.													
1868-------													0.1
1869-------												0.2	0.1
1870-------											0.3	0.2	0.1
1871-------										0.7	0.4	0.2	0.1
1872-------									1.1	0.7	0.3	0.2	0.1
1873-------								1.7	1.1	0.6	0.3	0.2	0.1
1874-------							2.6	1.7	1.0	0.7	0.3	0.2	0.1
1875-------						3.4	2.6	1.6	1.1	0.6	0.3	0.2	0.1
1876-------					4.7	3.4	2.4	1.6	0.9	0.6	0.3	0.2	0.0
1877-------				6.2	4.8	3.2	2.5	1.5	0.9	0.6	0.3	0.1	0.1
1878-------			8.8	6.3	4.6	3.3	2.5	1.5	0.9	0.5	0.2	0.2	0.1
1879-------	1917	10.4	8.7	6.1	4.7	3.3	2.3	1.5	0.9	0.5	0.3	0.1	0.0
1880-------	1918	10.1	8.6	6.1	4.7	3.1	2.3	1.4	0.9	0.5	0.2	0.1	0.1
1881-------	1919	10.1	8.5	6.0	4.4	3.1	2.2	1.4	0.8	0.5	0.2	0.1	0.1
1882-------	1920	9.8	8.3	5.7	4.3	3.0	2.1	1.2	0.7	0.4	0.2	0.1	0.0
1883-------	1921	9.6	7.8	5.5	4.2	2.8	2.0	1.1	0.7	0.4	0.2	0.1	0.0
1884-------	1922	8.9	7.5	5.3	4.0	2.6	1.8	1.1	0.6	0.4	0.2	0.1	0.1
1885-------	1923	8.6	7.3	5.1	3.8	2.4	1.8	1.0	0.6	0.3	0.2	0.1	0.1
1886-------	1924	8.5	6.9	4.8	3.6	2.3	1.6	1.0	0.6	0.4	0.2	0.1	0.1
1887-------	1925	8.0	6.6	4.7	3.3	2.2	1.6	0.9	0.6	0.3	0.2	0.1	0.1
1888-------	1926	7.5	6.3	4.2	3.0	2.1	1.5	0.9	0.5	0.3	0.1	0.1	0.1
1889-------	1927	7.4	5.9	4.0	3.0	2.0	1.5	0.9	0.5	0.3	0.1	0.1	0.1
1890-------	1928	6.7	5.4	4.0	2.8	2.0	1.4	0.8	0.5	0.2	0.1	0.1	0.1
1891-------	1929	6.2	5.3	3.6	2.8	1.9	1.3	0.8	0.4	0.2	0.1	0.1	0.0
1892-------	1930	6.1	4.8	3.6	2.6	1.8	1.2	0.7	0.4	0.2	0.1	0.1	0.0
1893-------	1931	5.6	4.8	3.3	2.5	1.6	1.1	0.7	0.4	0.2	0.1	0.0	0.0
1894-------	1932	5.5	4.3	3.2	2.3	1.6	1.0	0.7	0.4	0.2	0.1	0.0	0.0
1895-------	1933	5.0	4.3	3.0	2.2	1.4	1.0	0.6	0.3	0.2	0.1	0.0	0.0
1896-------	1934	4.9	4.0	2.7	2.0	1.4	0.9	0.5	0.3	0.2	0.1	0.0	0.0
1897-------	1935	4.6	3.6	2.6	1.9	1.3	0.9	0.5	0.3	0.2	0.1	0.0	0.0
1898-------	1936	4.2	3.5	2.6	1.8	1.2	0.8	0.6	0.3	0.2	0.1	0.0	0.0
1899-------	1937	4.1	3.4	2.4	1.7	1.2	0.9	0.6	0.3	0.2	0.1	0.0	0.0
1900-------	1938	4.0	3.1	2.3	1.7	1.1	0.9	0.6	0.3	0.2	0.1	0.0	0.0
1901-------	1939	3.6	2.9	2.1	1.5	1.2	0.9	0.5	0.3	0.2	0.1	0.0	0.0
1902-------	1940	3.4	2.8	2.0	1.6	1.2	0.9	0.5	0.3	0.1	0.0	0.0	0.0
1903-------	1941	3.3	2.7	2.1	1.6	1.3	0.8	0.5	0.2	0.1	0.0	0.0	0.0
1904-------	1942	3.1	2.8	2.1	1.7	1.1	0.8	0.4	0.2	0.1	0.0	0.0	0.0
1905-------	1943	3.2	2.7	2.1	1.6	1.1	0.7	0.4	0.2	0.1	0.0	0.0	0.0
1906-------	1944	3.1	2.7	2.0	1.5	1.0	0.7	0.4	0.2	0.1	0.0	0.0	0.0
1907-------	1945	3.1	2.6	1.9	1.4	0.9	0.6	0.4	0.2	0.1	0.0	0.0	0.0
1908-------	1946	2.9	2.4	1.8	1.3	0.9	0.6	0.4	0.2	0.1	0.0	0.0	0.0
1909-------	1947	2.9	2.3	1.7	1.3	1.0	0.7	0.4	0.2	0.1	0.0	0.0	0.0
1910-------	1948	2.7	2.3	1.8	1.4	1.0	0.7	0.4	0.2	0.1	0.0	0.0	0.0
1911-------	1949	2.7	2.3	1.8	1.4	1.0	0.7	0.4	0.2	0.1	0.0	0.0	0.0
1912-------	1950	2.7	2.3	1.8	1.4	1.0	0.7	0.4	0.2	0.1	0.0	0.0	0.0
1913-------	1951	2.7	2.2	1.8	1.4	1.0	0.7	0.4	0.2	0.1	0.1	0.0	0.0
1914-------	1952	2.7	2.4	1.9	1.4	1.1	0.8	0.4	0.2	0.1	0.0	0.0	0.0
1915-------	1953	2.8	2.4	1.9	1.6	1.1	0.8	0.4	0.2	0.1	0.0	0.0	0.0
1916-------	1954	2.9	2.5	2.0	1.6	1.1	0.8	0.4	0.3	0.1	0.0	0.0	0.0
1917-------	1955	3.0	2.7	2.1	1.6	1.2	0.7	0.5	0.2	0.1	0.0	0.0	0.0
1918-------	1956	3.0	2.7	2.1	1.6	1.1	0.8	0.4	0.2	0.1	0.0	0.0	0.0
1919-------	1957	3.2	2.8	2.2	1.7	1.2	0.8	0.4	0.2	0.1	0.0	0.0	0.0
1920-------	1958	3.3	2.9	2.3	1.8	1.2	0.8	0.4	0.2	0.1	0.0	0.0	0.0
1921-------	1959	3.4	3.0	2.4	1.7	1.2	0.8	0.4	0.2	0.1	0.0	0.0	0.0
1922-------	1960	3.5	3.0	2.3	1.7	1.1	0.7	0.4	0.2	0.1	0.0	0.0	0.0
1923-------	1961	3.6	2.9	2.2	1.6	1.1	0.6	0.4	0.2	0.1	0.0	0.0	0.0
1924-------	1962	3.5	2.9	2.2	1.5	1.0	0.6	0.4	0.2	0.1	0.0	0.0	0.0
1925-------	1963	3.5	2.9	2.1	1.4	0.9	0.6	0.3	0.2	0.1	0.0	0.0	
1926-------	1964	3.5	2.7	1.9	1.3	0.9	0.5	0.3	0.1	0.0	0.0		
1927-------	1965	3.2	2.4	1.8	1.2	0.7	0.5	0.2	0.1	0.1			
1928-------	1966	2.9	2.3	1.6	1.0	0.7	0.4	0.2	0.1				
1929-------	1967	2.7	2.0	1.4	1.0	0.6	0.4	0.2					
1930-------	1968	2.4	1.8	1.4	0.9	0.5	0.3						
1931-------	1969	2.3	1.8	1.2	0.8	0.4							
1932-------	1970	2.1	1.6	1.1	0.6								
1933-------	1971	1.9	1.4	0.9									
1934-------	1972	1.6	1.2										
1935-------	1973	1.4											

TABLE 4A. CENTRAL BIRTH RATES FOR ALL WOMEN DURING EACH YEAR 1917-73 BY AGE AND LIVE-BIRTH ORDER FOR EACH COHORT FROM 1868 TO 1959--CON.

LIVE-BIRTH ORDER AND COHORT	DIAGONAL LINE FOR CALENDAR YEAR	CURRENT AGE											
		14	15	16	17	18	19	20	21	22	23	24	25
EIGHTH AND HIGHER BIRTHS													
1892-------													0.9
1893-------												0.6	0.9
1894-------											0.3	0.6	0.8
1895-------										0.1	0.3	0.5	0.8
1896-------									0.0	0.1	0.3	0.5	1.0
1897-------								0.0	0.0	0.1	0.3	0.6	0.9
1898-------							*	0.0	0.0	0.1	0.3	0.6	1.0
1899-------						*	*	0.0	0.0	0.1	0.3	0.6	1.0
1900-------					*	*	*	0.0	0.0	0.1	0.3	0.7	1.1
1901-------				*	*	*	*	0.0	0.0	0.1	0.3	0.6	1.1
1902-------			*	*	*	*	*	0.0	0.0	0.1	0.3	0.7	1.1
1903-------	1917	*	*	*	*	*	*	0.0	0.0	0.1	0.4	0.7	0.9
1904-------	1918	*	*	*	*	*	*	0.0	0.0	0.2	0.4	0.6	0.8
1905-------	1919	*	*	*	*	*	*	0.0	0.0	0.1	0.3	0.5	0.8
1906-------	1920	*	*	*	*	*	*	0.0	0.0	0.2	0.3	0.5	0.7
1907-------	1921	*	*	*	*	*	*	0.0	0.1	0.1	0.3	0.4	0.7
1908-------	1922	*	*	*	*	*	*	0.0	0.0	0.1	0.2	0.4	0.6
1909-------	1923	*	*	*	*	*	*	0.0	0.0	0.1	0.2	0.4	0.6
1910-------	1924	*	*	*	*	*	*	0.0	0.0	0.1	0.2	0.4	0.6
1911-------	1925	*	*	*	*	*	*	0.0	0.1	0.1	0.2	0.4	0.6
1912-------	1926	*	*	*	*	*	*	0.0	0.0	0.1	0.2	0.4	0.6
1913-------	1927	*	*	*	*	*	*	0.0	0.0	0.1	0.2	0.4	0.5
1914-------	1928	*	*	*	*	*	*	0.0	0.0	0.1	0.2	0.3	0.5
1915-------	1929	*	*	*	*	*	*	0.0	0.0	0.1	0.2	0.3	0.6
1916-------	1930	*	*	*	*	*	*	0.0	0.0	0.1	0.2	0.4	0.6
1917-------	1931	*	*	*	*	*	*	0.0	0.0	0.1	0.3	0.4	0.6
1918-------	1932	*	*	*	*	*	*	0.0	0.0	0.1	0.2	0.4	0.6
1919-------	1933	*	*	*	*	*	*	0.0	0.0	0.1	0.2	0.4	0.6
1920-------	1934	*	*	*	*	*	*	0.0	0.0	0.1	0.2	0.4	0.7
1921-------	1935	*	*	*	*	*	*	0.0	0.0	0.1	0.2	0.4	0.6
1922-------	1936	*	*	*	*	*	*	0.0	0.0	0.1	0.2	0.4	0.7
1923-------	1937	*	*	*	*	*	*	0.0	0.0	0.1	0.2	0.4	0.6
1924-------	1938	*	*	*	*	*	*	0.0	0.0	0.1	0.2	0.4	0.8
1925-------	1939	*	*	*	*	*	*	0.0	0.1	0.1	0.2	0.5	0.7
1926-------	1940	*	*	*	*	*	*	0.0	0.1	0.1	0.3	0.4	0.7
1927-------	1941	*	*	*	*	*	*	0.0	0.1	0.1	0.2	0.4	0.8
1928-------	1942	*	*	*	*	*	*	0.0	0.1	0.1	0.2	0.5	0.9
1929-------	1943	*	*	*	*	*	*	0.1	0.1	0.1	0.3	0.5	0.9
1930-------	1944	*	*	*	*	*	*	0.1	0.1	0.2	0.3	0.6	1.1
1931-------	1945	*	*	*	*	*	*	0.1	0.1	0.2	0.3	0.6	1.2
1932-------	1946	*	*	*	*	*	*	0.1	0.1	0.2	0.4	0.7	1.4
1933-------	1947	*	*	*	*	*	*	0.0	0.1	0.2	0.4	0.8	1.6
1934-------	1948	*	*	*	*	*	*	0.1	0.1	0.2	0.5	0.9	1.6
1935-------	1949	*	*	*	*	*	*	0.1	0.1	0.2	0.4	0.9	1.7
1936-------	1950	*	*	*	*	*	*	0.1	0.1	0.2	0.5	0.9	1.7
1937-------	1951	*	*	*	*	*	*	0.1	0.1	0.2	0.5	1.0	1.7
1938-------	1952	*	*	*	*	*	*	0.1	0.1	0.2	0.5	1.0	1.7
1939-------	1953	*	*	*	*	*	*	0.0	0.1	0.2	0.5	1.0	1.6
1940-------	1954	*	*	*	*	*	*	0.1	0.1	0.2	0.5	0.9	1.2
1941-------	1955	*	*	*	*	*	*	0.0	0.1	0.2	0.5	0.7	1.0
1942-------	1956	*	*	*	*	*	*	0.1	0.1	0.2	0.3	0.5	0.8
1943-------	1957	*	*	*	*	*	*	0.1	0.1	0.2	0.3	0.4	0.6
1944-------	1958	*	*	*	*	*	*	0.1	0.1	0.1	0.2	0.3	0.5
1945-------	1959	*	*	*	*	*	*	0.1	0.0	0.1	0.2	0.3	0.5
1946-------	1960	*	*	*	*	*	*	0.0	0.0	0.1	0.2	0.3	0.4
1947-------	1961	*	*	*	*	*	*	0.0	0.0	0.1	0.2	0.2	0.2
1948-------	1962	*	*	*	*	*	*	0.0	0.1	0.1	0.1	0.1	0.2
1949-------	1963	*	*	*	*	*	*	0.1	0.1	0.1	0.1	0.1	
1950-------	1964	*	*	*	*	*	*	0.1	0.1	0.0	0.0		
1951-------	1965	*	*	*	*	*	*	0.0	0.0	0.0			
1952-------	1966	*	*	*	*	*	*	0.0	0.0				
1953-------	1967	*	*	*	*	*	*	0.0					
1954-------	1968	*	*	*	*	*	*						
1955-------	1969	*	*	*	*	*							
1956-------	1970	*	*	*	*								
1957-------	1971	*	*	*									
1958-------	1972	*	*										
1959-------	1973	*											

TABLE 4A. CENTRAL BIRTH RATES FOR ALL WOMEN DURING EACH YEAR 1917-73 BY AGE AND LIVE-BIRTH ORDER FOR EACH COHORT FROM 1868 TO 1959--CON.

LIVE-BIRTH ORDER AND COHORT	DIAGONAL LINE FOR CALENDAR YEAR	CURRENT AGE											
		26	27	28	29	30	31	32	33	34	35	36	37
EIGHTH AND HIGHER BIRTHS--CON.													
1880-------													30.6
1881-------												27.4	29.8
1882-------											24.5	26.6	30.0
1883-------										20.5	23.9	26.7	29.7
1884-------									16.3	20.1	23.8	26.5	29.9
1885-------								12.6	16.1	19.9	23.6	26.7	27.6
1886-------							10.2	12.5	15.9	19.8	24.2	24.8	27.5
1887-------						7.5	10.2	12.4	15.8	20.6	22.6	24.8	27.3
1888-------					6.1	7.3	10.1	12.3	16.8	19.2	22.6	24.6	26.4
1889-------				3.8	5.7	7.2	10.0	13.1	15.6	19.3	22.4	24.0	25.3
1890-------			2.5	3.4	5.6	7.2	10.6	12.2	15.9	19.1	21.8	22.5	24.7
1891-------	1917	1.5	2.2	3.3	5.7	7.7	9.9	12.4	15.7	18.9	20.6	22.4	22.3
1892-------	1918	1.3	2.2	3.4	6.1	7.2	10.0	12.2	15.5	17.6	20.1	19.7	20.3
1893-------	1919	1.3	2.2	3.7	5.7	7.3	9.9	12.1	14.5	17.1	17.9	18.3	19.5
1894-------	1920	1.3	2.5	3.5	5.9	7.3	9.8	11.4	14.1	15.4	16.7	17.6	18.3
1895-------	1921	1.5	2.3	3.7	5.9	7.3	9.4	11.2	13.0	14.5	16.3	16.5	17.7
1896-------	1922	1.4	2.5	3.8	6.0	7.1	9.3	10.4	12.2	14.2	15.0	15.8	16.0
1897-------	1923	1.5	2.5	3.8	5.8	7.1	8.7	9.8	11.8	13.0	14.6	14.4	15.9
1898-------	1924	1.6	2.7	3.9	5.7	6.6	8.2	9.6	11.2	12.7	13.3	14.4	15.2
1899-------	1925	1.7	2.7	3.7	5.5	6.3	8.1	9.2	11.3	12.0	13.8	14.3	14.6
1900-------	1926	1.7	2.5	3.5	5.2	6.2	7.7	9.1	10.4	12.3	13.6	13.6	14.5
1901-------	1927	1.6	2.3	3.3	4.8	5.8	7.5	8.2	10.5	11.8	12.4	13.2	13.6
1902-------	1928	1.4	2.2	3.1	4.6	5.4	6.5	8.1	9.7	10.6	11.9	12.3	12.4
1903-------	1929	1.3	2.0	2.9	4.2	4.8	6.6	7.6	9.1	10.2	11.3	11.1	11.8
1904-------	1930	1.3	1.9	2.7	3.9	5.0	6.4	7.4	8.9	9.8	10.4	10.8	11.3
1905-------	1931	1.2	1.8	2.5	4.1	4.9	6.1	7.1	8.6	9.1	10.2	10.2	10.6
1906-------	1932	1.1	1.6	2.6	4.0	4.6	5.9	6.8	8.0	9.1	9.6	9.6	10.7
1907-------	1933	1.0	1.7	2.6	3.6	4.4	5.7	6.4	8.1	8.6	9.0	9.7	10.5
1908-------	1934	1.0	1.7	2.3	3.5	4.3	5.3	6.5	7.7	8.2	9.2	9.5	10.2
1909-------	1935	1.0	1.6	2.3	3.4	4.0	5.4	6.2	7.3	8.3	9.1	9.6	9.6
1910-------	1936	1.0	1.6	2.3	3.3	4.1	5.1	6.0	7.5	8.3	9.1	9.1	9.3
1911-------	1937	1.0	1.5	2.3	3.4	4.0	5.0	6.1	7.5	8.4	8.8	8.9	9.1
1912-------	1938	0.9	1.5	2.4	3.3	4.0	5.2	6.2	7.3	7.8	8.4	8.4	9.0
1913-------	1939	0.9	1.6	2.4	3.2	4.1	5.2	6.0	6.9	7.6	8.0	8.4	8.6
1914-------	1940	1.0	1.6	2.2	3.3	4.1	5.0	5.8	6.8	7.3	8.1	8.2	8.6
1915-------	1941	1.0	1.5	2.3	3.3	3.9	5.0	5.7	6.7	7.4	7.8	8.2	8.5
1916-------	1942	0.9	1.6	2.3	3.2	4.0	4.9	5.6	6.8	7.2	7.8	8.0	8.0
1917-------	1943	1.0	1.6	2.2	3.3	3.8	4.9	5.8	6.6	7.2	7.6	7.8	8.1
1918-------	1944	1.0	1.5	2.3	3.2	3.9	5.1	5.8	6.7	7.2	7.6	7.9	8.1
1919-------	1945	1.0	1.6	2.3	3.4	4.3	5.2	5.9	7.0	7.5	8.0	8.2	8.6
1920-------	1946	1.0	1.7	2.5	3.6	4.3	5.3	6.1	7.0	7.7	8.1	8.4	8.7
1921-------	1947	1.1	1.8	2.7	3.6	4.4	5.4	6.1	7.3	7.8	8.4	8.6	8.5
1922-------	1948	1.1	1.8	2.6	3.6	4.3	5.2	6.3	7.3	7.9	8.5	8.5	8.8
1923-------	1949	1.2	1.8	2.6	3.6	4.3	5.7	6.5	7.6	8.4	8.6	9.0	9.0
1924-------	1950	1.2	1.8	2.7	3.7	4.8	6.0	6.9	8.2	8.6	9.2	9.3	9.3
1925-------	1951	1.2	2.0	2.8	4.1	5.1	6.4	7.4	8.4	9.3	9.7	9.8	9.4
1926-------	1952	1.3	2.1	3.1	4.4	5.6	6.9	7.8	9.1	9.6	10.1	9.8	9.4
1927-------	1953	1.3	2.2	3.3	4.8	6.0	7.3	8.5	9.5	10.2	10.3	9.8	9.4
1928-------	1954	1.4	2.5	3.8	5.3	6.5	7.9	8.9	10.0	10.3	10.1	9.8	8.8
1929-------	1955	1.7	2.8	4.2	5.8	7.1	8.5	9.6	10.4	10.4	10.1	9.2	7.8
1930-------	1956	1.9	3.1	4.6	6.2	7.5	8.9	9.8	10.4	10.2	9.5	8.1	7.0
1931-------	1957	2.2	3.5	5.0	6.5	8.0	9.1	9.8	10.2	9.5	8.4	7.3	6.2
1932-------	1958	2.4	3.7	5.0	6.9	8.0	9.1	9.5	9.2	8.3	7.4	6.5	5.8
1933-------	1959	2.6	3.9	5.6	7.0	8.0	8.9	8.5	8.0	7.3	6.5	6.0	5.4
1934-------	1960	2.7	4.2	5.7	7.0	7.8	7.7	7.4	6.9	6.3	6.0	5.5	4.8
1935-------	1961	2.8	4.2	5.5	6.7	6.7	6.7	6.2	5.9	5.7	5.5	4.9	3.9
1936-------	1962	2.8	4.1	5.2	5.7	5.6	5.5	5.3	5.3	5.1	4.8	3.8	3.2
1937-------	1963	2.7	3.7	4.4	4.6	4.7	4.7	4.7	4.7	4.5	3.6	3.1	
1938-------	1964	2.5	3.2	3.4	3.8	3.8	4.0	4.1	4.0	3.3	2.8		
1939-------	1965	2.1	2.5	2.9	3.1	3.3	3.6	3.5	3.0	2.6			
1940-------	1966	1.6	2.0	2.3	2.7	2.9	2.9	2.6	2.4				
1941-------	1967	1.3	1.7	2.0	2.3	2.3	2.2	2.0					
1942-------	1968	1.1	1.3	1.6	1.8	1.6	1.7						
1943-------	1969	0.8	1.2	1.2	1.2	1.2							
1944-------	1970	0.8	0.9	0.9	1.0								
1945-------	1971	0.6	0.6	0.7									
1946-------	1972	0.4	0.4										
1947-------	1973	0.3											

TABLE 4A. CENTRAL BIRTH RATES FOR ALL WOMEN DURING EACH YEAR 1917-73 BY AGE AND LIVE-BIRTH ORDER FOR EACH COHORT FROM 1868 TO 1959--CON.

LIVE-BIRTH ORDER AND COHORT	DIAGONAL LINE FOR CALENDAR YEAR	CURRENT AGE											
		38	39	40	41	42	43	44	45	46	47	48	49
EIGHTH AND HIGHER BIRTHS--CON.													
1868-------													0.7
1869-------												1.5	1.0
1870-------											2.8	1.9	0.7
1871-------										4.9	3.4	1.5	0.8
1872-------									7.5	5.9	2.7	1.6	0.7
1873-------								10.9	8.2	4.8	2.9	1.5	0.7
1874-------							14.9	11.3	7.2	5.1	2.8	1.3	0.6
1875-------						17.5	14.6	10.3	7.5	4.9	2.4	1.3	0.6
1876-------					22.5	17.3	14.1	10.6	7.3	4.4	2.4	1.2	0.6
1877-------				25.6	22.3	16.7	14.2	10.6	6.7	4.3	2.3	1.2	0.5
1878-------			31.4	25.4	21.6	16.9	14.5	9.9	6.6	4.2	2.1	1.0	0.5
1879-------	1917	30.9	31.1	25.0	22.0	17.2	13.5	9.7	6.6	4.1	2.0	1.0	0.5
1880-------	1918	30.3	30.9	25.3	22.2	16.0	13.4	9.7	6.3	3.9	1.8	1.0	0.5
1881-------	1919	30.5	31.0	25.5	20.6	15.8	13.5	9.4	6.0	3.5	1.8	0.9	0.4
1882-------	1920	30.3	31.2	23.5	20.2	15.9	13.0	8.8	5.6	3.4	1.8	0.9	0.4
1883-------	1921	30.5	28.7	23.1	20.2	15.4	12.2	8.5	5.3	3.1	1.6	0.8	0.4
1884-------	1922	28.1	28.3	23.0	19.4	14.5	11.7	7.7	4.8	3.0	1.5	0.8	0.4
1885-------	1923	27.9	28.0	22.2	18.3	14.1	10.7	7.0	4.7	2.8	1.4	0.8	0.4
1886-------	1924	27.6	26.8	20.6	17.7	12.8	9.7	6.9	4.4	2.7	1.3	0.8	0.4
1887-------	1925	26.9	25.5	20.5	16.4	11.8	9.7	6.5	4.2	2.5	1.3	0.7	0.4
1888-------	1926	25.4	24.6	18.7	15.0	11.6	9.0	6.2	3.9	2.3	1.2	0.7	0.3
1889-------	1927	25.1	22.8	17.4	14.7	10.9	8.7	5.9	3.8	2.3	1.1	0.6	0.3
1890-------	1928	22.6	21.0	16.8	13.8	10.5	8.2	5.8	3.6	2.1	1.1	0.6	0.3
1891-------	1929	21.0	20.4	15.9	13.1	9.9	8.2	5.4	3.3	2.0	1.0	0.6	0.2
1892-------	1930	20.1	18.8	14.9	12.1	9.8	7.6	4.9	3.1	1.8	0.9	0.5	0.2
1893-------	1931	18.7	18.0	13.9	12.0	9.0	6.9	4.5	2.9	1.7	0.8	0.4	0.2
1894-------	1932	18.0	16.5	13.7	11.3	8.2	6.4	4.4	2.6	1.5	0.8	0.3	0.2
1895-------	1933	16.6	16.3	12.9	10.3	7.8	6.1	3.9	2.5	1.4	0.7	0.3	0.1
1896-------	1934	16.3	15.5	11.8	9.8	7.5	5.5	3.7	2.3	1.3	0.6	0.3	0.2
1897-------	1935	15.4	14.1	11.3	9.5	6.7	5.3	3.4	2.3	1.2	0.6	0.3	0.1
1898-------	1936	14.3	13.6	11.2	8.7	6.7	5.0	3.7	2.4	1.2	0.7	0.3	0.2
1899-------	1937	14.3	13.6	10.2	8.5	6.3	5.0	3.5	2.1	1.2	0.6	0.3	0.2
1900-------	1938	13.9	12.4	10.0	8.2	6.1	5.0	3.4	2.1	1.1	0.6	0.3	0.1
1901-------	1939	12.5	11.8	9.4	7.4	6.1	4.9	3.3	1.9	1.1	0.5	0.3	0.1
1902-------	1940	12.0	11.2	8.9	7.7	6.1	4.8	3.0	1.8	1.0	0.5	0.2	0.1
1903-------	1941	11.3	10.6	9.0	7.5	6.0	4.4	2.9	1.6	0.9	0.4	0.2	0.1
1904-------	1942	10.9	10.6	8.8	7.4	5.6	4.3	2.6	1.5	0.8	0.4	0.2	0.1
1905-------	1943	10.9	10.4	8.5	6.9	5.3	3.8	2.5	1.4	0.7	0.4	0.2	0.1
1906-------	1944	10.7	10.0	8.0	6.6	4.8	3.7	2.2	1.3	0.7	0.3	0.2	0.1
1907-------	1945	10.3	9.4	7.6	6.0	4.7	3.4	2.2	1.3	0.6	0.3	0.1	0.1
1908-------	1946	9.6	8.8	7.0	5.9	4.3	3.4	2.1	1.2	0.7	0.3	0.1	0.1
1909-------	1947	9.2	8.5	7.1	5.6	4.4	3.3	2.0	1.2	0.6	0.3	0.2	0.1
1910-------	1948	8.9	8.6	6.8	5.6	4.2	3.1	2.0	1.1	0.6	0.3	0.2	0.1
1911-------	1949	9.0	8.2	6.7	5.4	4.1	3.2	1.9	1.2	0.6	0.3	0.1	0.1
1912-------	1950	8.6	8.0	6.4	5.3	4.1	3.0	2.0	1.1	0.6	0.3	0.1	0.1
1913-------	1951	8.4	7.8	6.3	5.1	3.9	3.1	1.9	1.1	0.5	0.3	0.1	0.1
1914-------	1952	8.4	7.5	6.2	5.0	4.0	3.0	1.9	1.0	0.6	0.3	0.1	0.1
1915-------	1953	7.9	7.4	6.1	5.1	3.9	2.8	1.8	1.0	0.5	0.2	0.1	0.0
1916-------	1954	8.0	7.3	6.1	5.0	3.8	2.7	1.8	1.0	0.5	0.2	0.1	0.0
1917-------	1955	7.9	7.4	6.2	4.9	3.7	2.8	1.8	1.0	0.5	0.2	0.1	0.0
1918-------	1956	8.0	7.5	6.0	5.0	3.8	2.8	1.7	0.9	0.5	0.2	0.1	0.0
1919-------	1957	8.4	7.4	6.4	5.1	3.9	2.9	1.8	0.9	0.5	0.2	0.1	0.0
1920-------	1958	8.2	7.8	6.4	5.2	3.9	2.8	1.7	0.9	0.5	0.2	0.1	0.0
1921-------	1959	8.5	7.7	6.5	5.2	3.9	2.8	1.6	0.9	0.4	0.2	0.1	0.0
1922-------	1960	8.4	7.7	6.3	5.0	3.8	2.4	1.5	0.8	0.3	0.2	0.0	0.0
1923-------	1961	8.6	7.8	6.2	5.0	3.4	2.3	1.4	0.7	0.3	0.1	0.0	0.0
1924-------	1962	8.6	7.8	6.4	4.6	3.2	2.2	1.2	0.7	0.3	0.1	0.0	0.0
1925-------	1963	8.8	7.8	5.9	4.3	3.0	1.9	1.1	0.6	0.3	0.1	0.0	
1926-------	1964	8.9	7.3	5.4	3.9	2.7	1.8	1.0	0.5	0.2	0.1		
1927-------	1965	8.2	6.6	4.8	3.5	2.5	1.6	0.9	0.5	0.2			
1928-------	1966	7.2	5.8	4.3	3.2	2.3	1.5	0.8	0.4				
1929-------	1967	6.6	5.3	4.1	3.1	2.1	1.3	0.8					
1930-------	1968	5.8	4.9	3.8	2.7	1.8	1.2						
1931-------	1969	5.5	4.6	3.4	2.3	1.7							
1932-------	1970	5.1	4.1	2.9	2.1								
1933-------	1971	4.5	3.4	2.5									
1934-------	1972	3.8	2.9										
1935-------	1973	3.2											

TABLE 4B. CENTRAL BIRTH RATES FOR WHITE WOMEN DURING EACH YEAR 1917-73 BY AGE AND LIVE-BIRTH ORDER FOR EACH COHORT FROM 1868 TO 1959

LIVE-BIRTH ORDER AND COHORT	DIAGONAL LINE FOR CALENDAR YEAR	CURRENT AGE											
		14	15	16	17	18	19	20	21	22	23	24	25
TOTAL BIRTHS													
1892-------													182.1
1893-------												183.5	180.2
1894-------											185.1	181.8	162.9
1895-------										174.4	183.4	162.6	175.4
1896-------									164.7	173.7	161.0	177.2	179.0
1897-------								143.8	164.6	150.3	177.8	180.6	169.7
1898-------							115.0	143.8	140.6	170.0	181.5	172.1	172.1
1899-------						77.9	113.7	122.1	160.4	171.1	169.8	172.4	170.5
1900-------					46.2	76.1	96.8	142.3	161.2	159.3	171.1	173.4	163.0
1901-------				21.3	44.7	65.6	115.5	146.0	149.2	159.4	173.4	167.0	156.9
1902-------			7.8	21.0	38.8	81.9	123.4	137.8	150.9	164.7	166.9	161.2	154.4
1903-------	1917	2.0	7.9	18.1	49.3	90.0	115.5	138.3	153.9	159.8	163.0	158.9	148.0
1904-------	1918	2.1	6.4	23.0	53.4	83.2	114.6	140.3	148.2	156.2	158.7	151.7	142.2
1905-------	1919	1.6	8.2	24.6	48.4	82.6	116.9	134.0	143.9	151.6	150.5	144.7	141.9
1906-------	1920	2.0	8.8	22.0	47.8	85.7	112.0	130.0	141.4	143.8	144.0	144.1	134.0
1907-------	1921	2.2	7.9	21.6	50.1	82.8	109.4	128.7	134.9	138.5	144.0	136.8	128.8
1908-------	1922	2.0	7.8	23.0	49.1	81.0	108.3	122.6	129.7	138.5	135.5	130.5	120.3
1909-------	1923	2.0	8.3	23.0	48.2	80.0	103.4	117.1	130.4	131.2	130.1	122.4	124.5
1910-------	1924	2.1	8.3	22.3	48.4	76.2	98.2	118.2	123.0	125.5	121.8	126.3	121.5
1911-------	1925	2.1	8.1	23.4	46.2	73.1	100.4	112.1	118.4	118.7	126.9	125.4	122.5
1912-------	1926	2.1	8.9	21.9	45.2	75.0	94.2	107.7	111.5	123.2	126.0	125.6	124.7
1913-------	1927	2.4	8.1	21.9	46.5	69.8	90.5	100.8	116.8	123.4	126.1	129.1	130.0
1914-------	1928	2.1	8.3	22.5	42.6	66.8	84.0	106.0	117.1	123.9	130.1	134.2	127.9
1915-------	1929	2.2	8.6	20.8	40.7	61.8	88.4	106.7	117.3	127.6	135.0	131.6	133.4
1916-------	1930	2.3	7.9	19.5	37.4	64.6	88.8	106.4	119.7	131.3	131.0	135.8	141.8
1917-------	1931	2.0	7.3	17.9	39.2	64.9	87.6	108.0	123.2	126.9	134.2	144.7	161.6
1918-------	1932	1.8	6.7	18.9	39.5	63.9	89.5	110.9	118.2	130.3	143.0	167.9	164.8
1919-------	1933	1.8	7.2	19.4	38.9	66.5	93.2	108.1	124.5	141.9	170.3	169.0	150.3
1920-------	1934	1.9	7.5	19.1	41.1	68.8	90.0	112.7	134.1	163.1	168.7	153.6	139.6
1921-------	1935	2.1	7.4	20.4	42.9	66.6	93.8	121.2	149.5	159.3	153.3	141.5	182.6
1922-------	1936	1.9	7.6	20.6	40.2	66.8	97.8	132.3	146.1	146.1	138.7	187.3	200.7
1923-------	1937	2.0	7.5	19.3	40.4	69.8	108.1	130.6	134.4	132.7	186.8	208.8	186.4
1924-------	1938	2.0	7.3	19.6	42.6	77.1	107.7	118.6	122.4	180.6	211.7	194.8	187.8
1925-------	1939	1.9	7.4	21.0	45.0	77.1	95.3	109.2	164.9	208.3	197.6	195.7	186.7
1926-------	1940	1.9	8.0	21.5	45.2	67.0	87.8	142.0	195.9	194.7	198.0	193.8	197.9
1927-------	1941	2.1	8.2	21.8	39.4	62.2	110.0	176.0	184.9	194.6	194.7	205.3	202.6
1928-------	1942	2.1	8.3	18.8	36.4	74.7	142.8	168.4	184.3	191.2	207.9	210.3	204.6
1929-------	1943	2.1	7.2	17.6	42.2	101.7	139.9	168.6	181.4	207.0	214.7	215.6	211.8
1930-------	1944	1.9	6.8	19.3	60.1	102.7	140.0	165.3	197.7	213.5	219.9	224.1	215.7
1931-------	1945	1.9	7.2	28.8	63.1	103.7	137.9	182.1	204.6	220.7	231.6	230.2	224.5
1932-------	1946	1.9	10.6	31.0	63.4	101.6	151.0	186.1	211.4	231.8	237.8	239.8	231.1
1933-------	1947	2.8	12.0	31.8	62.9	111.6	153.5	193.4	221.5	238.1	248.1	246.7	229.6
1934-------	1948	3.2	12.3	31.6	68.1	111.4	159.6	201.0	227.0	248.9	255.2	245.0	230.7
1935-------	1949	3.0	12.3	33.5	67.2	115.1	163.3	203.9	237.1	255.1	252.8	244.9	230.3
1936-------	1950	3.1	12.7	33.0	69.7	117.9	164.8	214.0	243.0	252.1	252.2	244.8	227.2
1937-------	1951	3.2	12.5	34.1	70.9	118.1	173.8	219.2	240.5	252.9	253.9	242.3	218.7
1938-------	1952	3.1	12.8	35.0	70.8	124.9	178.5	217.6	243.4	254.0	250.3	232.5	210.1
1939-------	1953	3.2	13.6	35.2	75.5	129.6	177.6	221.6	242.8	250.6	240.9	223.6	201.8
1940-------	1954	3.5	13.6	37.5	78.1	127.6	179.2	217.8	238.4	241.5	230.6	213.4	181.7
1941-------	1955	3.5	14.6	38.8	75.8	125.7	173.5	212.6	229.2	229.5	218.7	191.5	169.7
1942-------	1956	3.6	14.8	36.9	73.3	121.2	168.5	203.0	217.1	216.3	195.3	180.1	164.4
1943-------	1957	3.6	14.0	35.3	70.2	117.5	161.0	193.0	203.6	192.1	183.9	173.9	162.6
1944-------	1958	3.5	13.7	34.4	69.0	112.6	154.5	181.9	181.2	181.3	176.8	169.6	164.1
1945-------	1959	3.6	13.6	34.1	66.3	108.6	145.3	162.4	170.9	172.0	169.3	168.7	163.8
1946-------	1960	3.6	13.4	32.2	63.4	102.3	131.8	154.4	162.1	165.4	170.2	170.1	151.8
1947-------	1961	3.2	12.1	30.5	59.5	93.9	125.5	145.3	155.3	164.7	169.9	156.1	133.3
1948-------	1962	3.0	11.5	28.8	55.6	90.0	118.7	140.1	154.1	163.6	154.7	135.6	125.1
1949-------	1963	2.9	11.0	27.2	53.3	85.1	114.1	137.3	152.2	148.1	132.7	125.5	
1950-------	1964	2.8	10.5	26.4	51.4	83.0	112.8	137.0	137.4	126.0	122.5		
1951-------	1965	2.7	10.5	25.8	50.7	82.8	114.0	123.7	117.2	116.1			
1952-------	1966	2.8	10.1	25.7	51.2	85.2	103.9	107.2	107.9				
1953-------	1967	2.7	10.5	26.5	54.3	79.5	93.2	99.1					
1954-------	1968	2.9	11.1	29.0	51.8	74.4	87.1						
1955-------	1969	3.2	12.6	28.6	51.2	70.9							
1956-------	1970	3.6	12.4	29.5	50.0								
1957-------	1971	3.7	13.2	29.5									
1958-------	1972	4.1	13.6										
1959-------	1973	4.3											

TABLE 4B. CENTRAL BIRTH RATES FOR WHITE WOMEN DURING EACH YEAR 1917-73 BY AGE AND LIVE-BIRTH ORDER FOR EACH COHORT FROM 1868 TO 1959--CON.

LIVE-BIRTH ORDER AND COHORT	DIAGONAL LINE FOR CALENDAR YEAR	CURRENT AGE											
		26	27	28	29	30	31	32	33	34	35	36	37
TOTAL BIRTHS--CON.													
1880-------													94.6
1881-------												100.1	93.4
1882-------											108.9	98.5	91.3
1883-------										114.8	107.4	96.7	90.8
1884-------									123.2	113.6	104.4	96.3	91.7
1885-------								125.4	122.4	109.6	104.5	97.7	85.3
1886-------							137.4	125.7	117.6	110.5	106.9	91.5	84.9
1887-------						149.2	137.9	120.8	119.2	113.4	100.5	91.5	84.5
1888-------					170.3	148.4	131.8	122.2	121.6	106.5	100.2	90.5	80.6
1889-------				175.8	168.6	140.0	133.4	124.1	114.3	106.0	99.2	87.2	77.5
1890-------			178.8	174.4	157.8	143.4	135.9	117.4	114.3	105.3	94.6	82.6	75.4
1891-------	1917	173.9	178.0	161.2	162.5	145.2	128.4	116.9	113.2	101.2	90.5	81.1	70.3
1892-------	1918	173.2	163.1	167.1	163.5	135.4	127.2	115.5	107.8	95.4	87.4	74.6	64.5
1893-------	1919	157.6	170.1	167.6	151.5	133.4	126.0	110.6	101.8	92.7	80.9	69.3	63.2
1894-------	1920	167.6	172.2	155.8	150.5	132.5	120.8	105.6	99.6	86.8	76.2	68.6	60.0
1895-------	1921	171.1	161.8	155.4	149.1	127.8	116.6	103.6	94.0	82.0	76.0	65.4	57.2
1896-------	1922	161.8	161.6	152.8	142.9	123.5	113.6	97.5	88.6	81.3	71.1	62.0	52.8
1897-------	1923	161.4	159.6	146.5	137.6	119.6	107.3	92.5	87.8	76.0	68.3	57.7	52.4
1898-------	1924	161.3	152.9	140.8	133.1	113.5	102.6	92.4	82.6	73.0	63.6	57.5	50.5
1899-------	1925	156.5	148.3	138.2	127.8	109.7	103.2	88.8	81.9	69.9	65.1	56.6	48.9
1900-------	1926	149.5	144.8	130.7	121.5	109.5	98.1	86.0	76.5	70.9	63.4	54.3	47.7
1901-------	1927	148.1	137.0	124.4	120.6	104.4	94.3	80.0	77.4	68.3	60.4	52.6	47.0
1902-------	1928	140.0	130.5	124.0	114.4	98.8	87.3	80.4	73.9	65.2	58.6	52.1	44.8
1903-------	1929	135.1	131.0	119.1	109.7	92.8	89.1	77.8	71.8	63.8	58.5	50.3	44.1
1904-------	1930	135.5	125.6	114.8	103.4	95.8	87.3	76.4	71.1	64.5	57.4	50.6	44.6
1905-------	1931	129.2	120.5	107.5	106.3	93.3	84.7	76.1	71.6	63.3	57.7	50.9	46.7
1906-------	1932	123.3	113.0	110.3	103.6	90.9	84.9	77.2	70.7	64.2	58.2	52.6	51.3
1907-------	1933	116.4	116.6	108.1	101.4	92.1	86.7	76.6	72.1	65.3	62.2	58.4	52.9
1908-------	1934	119.2	113.5	105.5	101.5	93.8	85.7	78.4	73.2	71.2	68.2	60.4	54.5
1909-------	1935	117.2	111.9	107.3	104.9	93.5	88.8	81.1	81.3	77.7	69.4	63.2	56.5
1910-------	1936	116.1	113.5	110.9	103.6	97.3	91.7	88.1	88.6	78.1	72.3	66.0	57.3
1911-------	1937	119.4	118.7	109.9	108.1	101.7	97.9	96.4	87.7	81.2	76.6	67.0	53.3
1912-------	1938	123.6	116.3	114.2	112.5	110.3	106.5	94.8	90.1	86.5	77.5	61.7	52.0
1913-------	1939	121.8	121.6	120.6	124.1	118.3	104.3	97.6	97.2	87.9	71.4	60.4	51.3
1914-------	1940	128.1	129.5	135.2	131.7	113.4	107.5	107.4	99.7	81.2	70.5	60.5	52.7
1915-------	1941	136.8	145.6	142.2	124.3	115.6	119.9	110.7	91.5	80.2	70.6	62.2	55.0
1916-------	1942	152.9	151.6	131.2	124.1	130.4	123.9	100.7	90.0	79.7	72.1	64.2	55.0
1917-------	1943	157.4	138.7	129.4	143.2	136.8	113.6	99.8	90.1	82.1	74.4	64.8	56.5
1918-------	1944	143.3	133.2	150.9	150.9	124.2	111.8	99.3	92.3	84.4	74.6	65.8	55.7
1919-------	1945	137.0	163.2	164.5	139.4	125.3	113.5	104.6	97.5	86.3	77.5	66.5	57.2
1920-------	1946	172.6	178.3	151.4	140.2	126.4	118.3	109.5	98.7	88.7	77.4	66.9	57.1
1921-------	1947	190.8	164.8	152.8	141.7	132.2	124.2	110.3	101.4	89.0	77.9	67.6	56.1
1922-------	1948	175.1	164.9	153.0	146.9	137.1	124.0	112.3	100.5	88.7	78.2	65.0	55.1
1923-------	1949	176.1	165.1	160.4	152.7	137.6	126.8	111.9	100.9	89.7	76.1	64.9	54.1
1924-------	1950	176.8	175.3	166.9	153.3	141.3	126.4	113.2	102.5	87.5	75.3	64.0	53.7
1925-------	1951	186.8	180.6	167.0	156.7	140.2	127.2	113.9	99.3	86.2	74.6	63.3	50.8
1926-------	1952	192.2	180.8	170.4	156.1	140.7	127.7	110.5	97.5	85.0	73.4	59.7	49.1
1927-------	1953	194.0	184.0	170.1	157.3	142.1	124.9	109.5	96.6	84.1	69.5	57.8	47.6
1928-------	1954	197.6	184.5	171.2	158.6	139.6	124.4	108.4	95.2	79.5	67.4	56.5	43.7
1929-------	1955	200.1	188.6	176.2	157.6	140.8	124.1	108.9	91.8	78.3	66.1	52.0	39.6
1930-------	1956	205.6	193.7	174.5	158.9	140.1	123.7	104.5	90.2	76.6	60.8	46.8	36.6
1931-------	1957	213.1	193.1	176.0	158.9	140.4	119.4	102.3	88.5	70.2	54.7	43.2	33.7
1932-------	1958	211.9	194.6	176.4	157.5	134.1	116.2	99.4	80.4	63.2	50.4	40.0	31.3
1933-------	1959	212.7	194.6	174.5	150.7	130.0	112.5	90.2	71.8	58.1	46.9	37.8	29.8
1934-------	1960	212.7	191.9	167.3	146.0	126.4	102.2	80.6	65.9	53.6	44.8	35.8	26.8
1935-------	1961	209.7	184.7	161.5	142.0	113.9	91.4	74.3	61.4	52.0	42.6	32.3	23.2
1936-------	1962	202.6	178.1	157.4	127.6	102.9	84.4	69.5	59.9	49.8	38.4	27.9	20.3
1937-------	1963	194.9	172.6	141.2	116.1	96.2	80.5	69.3	58.4	45.1	33.3	24.6	
1938-------	1964	187.6	155.1	128.6	109.0	92.2	81.0	68.3	53.1	39.4	29.7		
1939-------	1965	169.4	142.5	122.5	106.4	93.8	81.2	63.0	47.1	36.0			
1940-------	1966	156.4	136.6	121.0	109.1	95.5	74.9	55.8	43.3				
1941-------	1967	151.1	136.2	124.5	111.6	88.4	66.6	51.9					
1942-------	1968	151.1	140.7	127.3	103.4	78.8	62.4						
1943-------	1969	153.8	141.7	117.8	91.8	73.9							
1944-------	1970	154.4	131.5	104.4	86.6								
1945-------	1971	142.9	116.3	99.4									
1946-------	1972	126.8	111.3										
1947-------	1973	120.0											

TABLE 4B. CENTRAL BIRTH RATES FOR WHITE WOMEN DURING EACH YEAR 1917-73 BY AGE AND LIVE-BIRTH ORDER FOR EACH COHORT FROM 1868 TO 1959--CON.

LIVE-BIRTH ORDER AND COHORT	DIAGONAL LINE FOR CALENDAR YEAR	CURRENT AGE											
		38	39	40	41	42	43	44	45	46	47	48	49
TOTAL BIRTHS--CON.													
1868-------													0.7
1869-------												1.6	0.7
1870-------											3.4	1.6	0.6
1871-------										6.5	3.6	1.5	0.7
1872-------									10.9	6.7	3.1	1.7	0.6
1873-------								17.1	10.9	6.2	3.4	1.6	0.6
1874-------							25.4	16.8	10.3	6.7	3.1	1.5	0.5
1875-------						32.3	25.1	16.2	10.7	6.3	3.1	1.4	0.5
1876-------					44.3	31.9	24.4	16.7	10.5	5.7	2.8	1.4	0.4
1877-------				55.7	43.9	31.2	24.9	16.5	9.7	5.5	2.8	1.3	0.3
1878-------			74.4	55.6	43.3	31.9	25.1	15.6	9.5	5.5	2.6	1.1	0.4
1879-------	1917	83.8	73.9	54.8	43.7	32.1	23.6	15.3	9.4	5.4	2.4	1.2	0.3
1880-------	1918	83.0	73.0	54.8	44.0	30.0	23.3	15.4	9.1	5.1	2.4	1.0	0.3
1881-------	1919	81.5	72.5	55.0	40.9	29.4	23.2	14.6	8.5	4.8	2.2	0.9	0.3
1882-------	1920	80.7	72.8	51.0	40.0	29.3	22.0	13.5	8.0	4.5	2.2	0.8	0.3
1883-------	1921	81.3	67.4	49.9	39.9	28.2	20.5	13.0	7.6	4.2	2.0	0.9	0.3
1884-------	1922	75.4	66.4	49.8	38.1	26.5	19.8	12.2	7.1	3.9	2.0	0.8	0.3
1885-------	1923	74.6	66.0	47.6	36.1	26.1	18.7	11.2	6.9	3.8	1.7	0.9	0.3
1886-------	1924	74.3	62.8	45.0	35.2	24.1	16.9	11.0	6.4	3.6	1.6	0.8	0.2
1887-------	1925	71.6	60.2	44.7	33.3	22.4	17.1	10.5	6.1	3.4	1.5	0.6	0.2
1888-------	1926	67.6	58.3	41.4	30.7	22.2	15.8	9.7	5.7	3.1	1.4	0.6	0.2
1889-------	1927	66.8	55.1	39.0	30.4	21.0	15.5	9.4	5.5	3.1	1.3	0.6	0.2
1890-------	1928	62.2	51.2	38.4	28.4	20.3	14.6	9.3	5.1	2.6	1.2	0.6	0.2
1891-------	1929	57.7	50.3	35.8	27.3	19.1	14.3	8.7	4.9	2.4	1.2	0.6	0.1
1892-------	1930	56.7	46.4	33.9	25.3	18.7	13.4	8.0	4.5	2.5	1.0	0.3	0.1
1893-------	1931	52.8	44.0	31.8	24.7	17.2	12.2	7.3	4.4	2.3	0.9	0.3	0.1
1894-------	1932	50.1	41.1	31.3	23.3	16.0	11.2	7.3	4.0	2.1	0.9	0.2	0.1
1895-------	1933	46.9	40.6	29.6	21.7	15.3	11.3	6.6	3.8	2.1	0.6	0.2	0.1
1896-------	1934	46.4	38.3	27.6	20.8	15.0	10.5	6.1	3.4	1.9	0.7	0.2	0.1
1897-------	1935	44.1	35.9	26.7	20.5	14.2	9.7	5.8	3.6	1.8	0.7	0.2	0.1
1898-------	1936	41.8	34.6	26.6	19.6	13.8	9.3	6.5	3.8	1.9	0.9	0.2	0.1
1899-------	1937	41.4	34.9	25.7	19.0	13.5	9.7	6.4	3.7	2.0	0.9	0.2	0.1
1900-------	1938	41.1	33.5	25.0	18.7	13.0	10.1	6.6	3.7	2.0	0.8	0.2	0.1
1901-------	1939	38.9	32.1	24.2	18.0	14.0	10.4	6.5	3.5	1.8	0.5	0.2	0.1
1902-------	1940	38.1	31.4	24.6	19.8	14.8	10.5	6.3	3.4	1.5	0.5	0.2	0.1
1903-------	1941	37.6	32.8	26.5	20.7	15.2	10.3	6.3	3.1	1.5	0.4	0.1	0.1
1904-------	1942	39.7	35.6	27.3	21.4	14.8	10.5	5.7	3.0	1.5	0.3	0.1	0.1
1905-------	1943	43.3	36.4	28.4	21.0	14.9	9.4	5.5	2.9	1.3	0.3	0.1	0.1
1906-------	1944	44.5	37.7	28.7	21.4	13.9	8.9	5.2	2.9	1.3	0.6	0.1	0.1
1907-------	1945	46.1	38.4	28.8	20.0	13.2	8.9	5.4	2.8	1.4	0.5	0.1	0.0
1908-------	1946	47.0	38.3	26.7	19.1	13.0	8.7	5.3	2.7	1.4	0.3	0.1	0.1
1909-------	1947	47.4	35.9	26.2	19.0	13.1	9.2	5.4	2.7	1.3	0.5	0.1	0.0
1910-------	1948	44.2	35.4	26.0	19.1	13.6	9.1	5.4	2.6	1.5	0.3	0.1	0.1
1911-------	1949	43.5	34.8	26.4	19.6	13.6	9.3	5.5	3.0	1.3	0.4	0.1	0.1
1912-------	1950	42.9	35.1	27.0	19.9	14.1	9.2	5.4	2.8	1.3	0.5	0.1	0.1
1913-------	1951	43.5	36.4	27.2	20.7	14.0	9.4	5.4	2.8	1.4	0.4	0.1	0.0
1914-------	1952	45.7	36.7	28.4	20.7	14.1	9.3	5.3	2.8	1.3	0.3	0.1	0.0
1915-------	1953	45.7	37.7	28.5	20.8	14.3	8.9	5.3	2.6	1.3	0.5	0.1	0.0
1916-------	1954	46.6	37.9	27.6	20.8	13.7	9.0	5.2	2.8	1.3	0.3	0.1	0.0
1917-------	1955	47.2	37.8	28.6	20.2	13.9	8.7	5.2	2.6	1.1	0.3	0.0	0.0
1918-------	1956	46.4	37.6	27.2	19.9	13.7	8.8	4.8	2.3	0.8	0.2	0.1	0.0
1919-------	1957	47.6	37.1	28.0	20.0	13.8	8.8	4.9	2.3	0.9	0.2	0.0	0.0
1920-------	1958	46.2	37.1	27.5	20.2	13.2	8.2	4.6	2.1	0.8	0.1	0.0	0.0
1921-------	1959	46.2	36.3	27.4	19.2	12.8	8.0	4.3	2.1	0.8	0.1	0.0	0.0
1922-------	1960	44.7	35.9	26.0	18.6	12.1	7.4	4.1	2.0	0.8	0.1	0.0	0.0
1923-------	1961	44.4	33.9	25.0	17.9	11.5	6.8	3.8	1.7	0.6	0.1	0.0	0.0
1924-------	1962	42.1	33.0	24.5	16.7	10.4	6.3	3.5	1.5	0.7	0.1	0.0	0.0
1925-------	1963	40.8	32.3	22.6	14.9	9.4	5.7	3.1	1.4	0.5	0.1	0.0	
1926-------	1964	39.8	29.7	20.4	13.5	8.5	5.2	2.7	1.2	0.4	0.1		
1927-------	1965	36.4	26.7	18.2	12.4	7.8	4.5	2.2	1.0	0.3			
1928-------	1966	32.8	24.0	16.9	11.3	7.3	4.0	1.8	0.9				
1929-------	1967	30.3	22.2	15.7	10.6	6.2	3.6	1.8					
1930-------	1968	27.6	20.6	14.7	8.9	5.5	3.1						
1931-------	1969	25.9	19.6	12.7	8.1	4.7							
1932-------	1970	24.5	17.0	11.1	6.8								
1933-------	1971	21.5	14.7	9.5									
1934-------	1972	19.0	12.9										
1935-------	1973	16.4											

TABLE 4B. CENTRAL BIRTH RATES FOR WHITE WOMEN DURING EACH YEAR 1917-73 BY AGE AND LIVE-BIRTH ORDER FOR EACH COHORT FROM 1868 TO 1959--CON.

LIVE-BIRTH ORDER AND COHORT	DIAGONAL LINE FOR CALENDAR YEAR	CURRENT AGE											
		14	15	16	17	18	19	20	21	22	23	24	25
FIRST BIRTHS													
1892-------													50.3
1893-------												59.7	51.1
1894-------											70.2	60.2	39.6
1895-------										77.1	70.4	46.0	52.1
1896-------									84.3	77.6	52.9	61.3	54.5
1897-------								84.7	85.0	58.5	71.4	63.8	49.2
1898-------							78.1	85.1	64.4	79.4	74.1	57.3	48.2
1899-------						60.2	77.1	66.3	86.2	81.1	65.0	55.4	48.9
1900-------					39.3	58.6	62.1	88.0	87.9	71.0	63.1	57.1	46.8
1901-------				19.4	38.0	49.3	82.1	91.9	77.1	69.1	66.0	55.1	45.4
1902-------			7.4	19.1	32.4	65.5	88.3	81.9	75.5	72.7	63.6	53.4	45.2
1903-------	1917	2.0	7.5	16.3	42.9	71.8	78.6	80.0	78.5	70.2	61.9	53.2	44.3
1904-------	1918	2.1	6.1	21.2	46.3	63.6	76.4	83.6	75.5	68.2	60.9	51.8	42.9
1905-------	1919	1.6	7.9	22.7	40.8	62.1	80.5	79.5	72.7	67.0	58.6	49.4	44.2
1906-------	1920	2.0	8.5	20.0	39.9	66.5	76.9	76.7	72.0	64.0	56.0	50.8	42.2
1907-------	1921	2.2	7.5	19.5	42.7	63.9	74.4	75.9	68.6	61.8	57.7	48.6	40.3
1908-------	1922	2.0	7.4	21.0	41.7	62.0	73.4	72.5	66.4	63.4	54.3	46.0	37.8
1909-------	1923	2.0	7.9	20.9	40.5	61.0	70.3	69.2	68.2	59.6	51.8	43.1	40.5
1910-------	1924	2.1	7.9	20.1	40.7	58.6	66.7	71.2	63.9	56.8	48.4	46.2	42.4
1911-------	1925	2.1	7.7	21.1	38.9	56.0	69.1	67.2	61.6	53.8	52.6	48.8	44.3
1912-------	1926	2.1	8.5	19.8	38.0	58.0	64.6	64.5	58.1	58.3	55.3	50.5	46.8
1913-------	1927	2.4	7.7	19.8	39.3	53.7	62.2	60.8	63.4	61.3	56.3	53.2	49.4
1914-------	1928	2.1	7.9	20.5	36.1	51.4	58.1	66.0	66.1	62.1	59.1	55.8	49.1
1915-------	1929	2.2	8.2	18.9	34.5	47.8	62.8	68.2	66.0	64.4	61.7	54.8	51.0
1916-------	1930	2.3	7.5	17.7	31.8	51.0	64.2	67.5	67.5	66.5	59.5	55.7	57.3
1917-------	1931	2.0	6.9	16.3	33.8	51.8	62.5	68.6	69.5	63.9	59.8	63.0	70.1
1918-------	1932	1.8	6.4	17.3	34.3	50.3	63.8	70.3	66.4	64.5	67.6	78.0	62.1
1919-------	1933	1.8	6.9	17.8	33.3	52.4	66.4	67.9	69.2	74.2	85.2	69.5	52.2
1920-------	1934	1.9	7.2	17.3	35.1	54.3	63.4	69.3	78.0	90.5	76.0	60.0	49.4
1921-------	1935	2.1	7.0	18.5	36.6	51.6	63.9	77.1	91.9	80.5	67.4	57.1	73.2
1922-------	1936	1.9	7.2	18.7	33.9	49.9	68.6	89.1	83.0	72.5	63.9	83.5	83.8
1923-------	1937	2.0	7.2	17.4	33.3	53.3	79.0	83.3	75.3	69.2	92.3	97.0	66.9
1924-------	1938	2.0	6.9	17.4	35.7	60.4	76.1	74.6	72.1	98.9	109.5	78.3	61.0
1925-------	1939	1.9	7.0	18.8	37.9	59.7	66.7	71.7	100.1	120.1	89.3	71.4	55.5
1926-------	1940	1.9	7.6	19.2	37.7	51.5	63.7	95.3	125.7	99.2	81.7	65.4	58.1
1927-------	1941	2.1	7.7	19.3	32.7	49.0	81.2	124.6	106.1	90.6	74.9	68.9	57.0
1928-------	1942	2.1	7.7	16.6	30.7	59.7	110.5	108.5	97.4	83.8	80.0	68.2	54.3
1929-------	1943	2.1	6.7	15.7	36.0	84.5	100.6	101.1	91.0	91.3	80.5	65.9	54.0
1930-------	1944	1.9	6.4	17.3	52.7	81.0	94.7	95.1	100.3	92.0	78.0	66.7	52.8
1931-------	1945	1.9	6.8	26.3	53.5	77.7	90.3	106.2	101.2	90.5	80.3	66.4	52.7
1932-------	1946	1.9	10.1	27.8	51.7	74.6	100.5	106.2	101.7	94.0	80.8	66.5	51.9
1933-------	1947	2.8	11.3	27.7	50.8	82.8	99.8	108.4	105.3	94.6	81.8	65.8	48.5
1934-------	1948	3.2	11.2	27.5	55.2	81.4	103.1	112.1	105.6	97.3	81.4	62.0	46.1
1935-------	1949	3.0	11.3	29.3	54.1	83.9	105.4	111.7	110.2	97.3	77.4	59.4	44.4
1936-------	1950	3.1	11.8	28.8	55.9	85.8	104.5	117.4	110.8	93.1	74.4	57.8	43.2
1937-------	1951	3.2	11.7	29.8	56.9	84.9	110.3	119.1	107.1	90.8	73.5	56.7	41.2
1938-------	1952	3.1	12.0	30.5	56.2	89.6	112.9	115.8	105.5	89.6	72.1	53.7	40.4
1939-------	1953	3.2	12.6	30.5	59.8	92.9	110.1	115.3	103.8	87.9	68.4	52.7	41.1
1940-------	1954	3.5	12.6	32.4	61.7	89.7	109.0	112.5	102.3	84.1	66.8	53.2	39.9
1941-------	1955	3.5	13.4	33.4	58.9	87.6	105.2	110.6	98.4	81.8	67.2	51.4	42.9
1942-------	1956	3.6	13.6	31.5	56.7	84.1	103.4	106.1	95.6	81.7	64.5	55.4	43.8
1943-------	1957	3.6	12.8	30.1	54.1	82.3	99.2	103.5	93.8	76.6	67.6	55.0	46.9
1944-------	1958	3.5	12.5	29.2	53.4	79.0	97.0	100.6	87.3	78.7	65.7	56.7	47.3
1945-------	1959	3.6	12.4	28.9	51.1	77.2	93.2	93.1	87.8	75.5	66.0	57.1	48.6
1946-------	1960	3.6	12.1	27.2	49.4	74.0	87.8	93.9	84.7	76.2	67.9	59.6	47.2
1947-------	1961	3.2	11.0	26.0	47.2	70.1	87.4	89.3	84.7	77.2	69.6	56.1	43.6
1948-------	1962	3.0	10.5	25.0	45.4	69.5	83.1	89.2	84.7	78.3	63.9	50.2	42.5
1949-------	1963	2.9	10.2	23.8	44.2	65.8	82.1	87.7	84.7	70.0	55.4	47.4	
1950-------	1964	2.8	9.8	23.4	42.8	65.5	81.4	88.3	75.4	60.1	51.8		
1951-------	1965	2.7	9.8	22.9	42.8	65.6	83.0	78.8	64.8	55.6			
1952-------	1966	2.8	9.5	23.1	43.4	68.2	75.2	68.8	59.6				
1953-------	1967	2.7	9.9	23.8	46.5	63.3	67.9	63.4					
1954-------	1968	2.9	10.5	26.2	44.4	59.8	63.3						
1955-------	1969	3.2	11.8	25.8	44.3	57.0							
1956-------	1970	3.6	11.7	26.9	43.2								
1957-------	1971	3.7	12.6	26.9									
1958-------	1972	4.1	12.9										
1959-------	1973	4.3											

TABLE 4B. CENTRAL BIRTH RATES FOR WHITE WOMEN DURING EACH YEAR 1917-73 BY AGE AND LIVE-BIRTH ORDER FOR EACH COHORT FROM 1868 TO 1959--CON.

LIVE-BIRTH ORDER AND COHORT	DIAGONAL LINE FOR CALENDAR YEAR	CURRENT AGE											
		26	27	28	29	30	31	32	33	34	35	36	37
FIRST BIRTHS--CON.													
1880-------													4.0
1881-------												4.9	4.1
1882-------											6.2	5.0	4.0
1883-------										7.4	6.4	5.0	4.2
1884-------									9.1	7.8	6.1	5.2	4.5
1885-------								10.7	9.7	7.2	6.6	5.6	4.1
1886-------							14.0	11.5	8.7	8.0	6.9	5.2	4.0
1887-------						18.2	15.0	10.3	9.9	8.2	6.6	5.1	4.1
1888-------					24.3	19.2	13.3	11.7	10.0	8.0	6.5	5.2	4.1
1889-------				29.6	25.4	16.2	15.1	11.7	9.8	7.7	6.5	5.1	3.9
1890-------			35.3	30.8	20.7	19.4	15.3	11.6	9.5	7.8	6.3	4.8	4.0
1891-------	1917	40.5	36.7	24.3	25.6	19.7	15.0	11.2	9.6	7.7	6.0	4.9	3.8
1892-------	1918	41.9	28.9	30.9	26.2	18.5	14.4	11.2	9.3	7.2	6.0	4.7	3.5
1893-------	1919	33.0	36.8	32.0	23.9	17.7	14.4	11.0	8.7	7.1	5.7	4.4	3.7
1894-------	1920	42.6	38.5	28.8	23.0	17.8	14.2	10.5	8.9	6.9	5.5	4.6	3.6
1895-------	1921	44.9	34.9	27.8	23.2	17.6	13.8	10.6	8.6	6.8	5.9	4.5	3.3
1896-------	1922	40.9	33.7	28.0	22.7	17.0	13.7	10.3	8.5	7.2	5.6	4.2	3.1
1897-------	1923	39.6	34.1	27.1	21.9	16.8	13.4	10.2	8.9	6.8	5.3	3.9	3.2
1898-------	1924	40.2	32.8	26.0	21.4	16.4	13.3	10.7	8.4	6.3	4.9	4.1	3.3
1899-------	1925	39.0	32.0	25.9	21.2	16.4	14.0	10.5	8.2	6.3	5.3	4.4	3.5
1900-------	1926	37.5	31.5	25.2	20.9	17.2	13.6	10.0	7.9	6.7	5.6	4.6	3.7
1901-------	1927	37.7	30.7	24.9	21.8	16.8	13.2	9.5	8.4	6.9	5.8	4.8	4.0
1902-------	1928	36.5	30.2	25.9	21.3	16.0	12.2	10.2	8.8	7.2	6.2	5.2	4.1
1903-------	1929	36.1	31.5	25.5	20.3	15.1	13.2	10.9	9.3	7.8	6.7	5.6	4.4
1904-------	1930	37.5	30.8	24.2	19.3	16.6	14.4	11.6	10.0	8.5	7.2	6.0	4.9
1905-------	1931	36.2	29.1	22.9	21.0	17.6	15.1	12.4	10.8	9.1	7.7	6.6	6.0
1906-------	1932	34.2	27.7	25.0	22.2	18.5	16.1	13.5	11.5	9.6	8.4	7.5	6.4
1907-------	1933	32.5	30.0	26.4	23.1	20.1	17.6	14.4	12.1	10.6	10.3	8.1	6.3
1908-------	1934	34.7	31.5	27.2	24.7	21.7	18.5	15.0	13.2	13.2	10.5	7.9	6.4
1909-------	1935	36.6	32.5	29.5	26.9	22.7	19.5	16.7	16.8	12.9	9.7	8.0	7.6
1910-------	1936	38.0	34.8	31.7	27.6	24.0	21.4	19.8	16.0	11.5	9.7	9.6	8.4
1911-------	1937	40.7	37.6	32.2	29.2	26.6	24.0	18.9	13.7	11.5	11.9	10.7	7.0
1912-------	1938	43.1	37.7	34.0	32.3	30.0	22.8	16.1	13.6	14.3	13.0	8.6	6.3
1913-------	1939	43.4	39.9	38.2	37.2	27.6	19.4	15.8	17.3	15.8	10.5	7.8	5.8
1914-------	1940	46.1	45.0	44.8	33.4	23.0	18.9	20.9	19.2	12.6	9.6	7.2	5.6
1915-------	1941	51.8	53.4	39.5	27.5	22.3	25.5	23.3	15.1	11.3	8.8	6.9	5.5
1916-------	1942	62.3	46.9	32.0	26.3	30.6	28.5	18.0	13.4	10.2	8.4	6.7	5.2
1917-------	1943	54.5	38.0	30.7	37.1	34.4	22.1	16.0	12.1	10.0	8.2	6.3	4.9
1918-------	1944	44.3	35.9	43.7	41.4	26.4	19.5	14.3	11.9	9.7	7.5	5.9	4.5
1919-------	1945	42.2	52.6	49.6	32.4	23.8	17.8	14.3	11.7	9.0	7.2	5.6	4.3
1920-------	1946	62.4	59.8	38.7	29.1	21.5	17.7	14.1	10.7	8.5	6.7	5.2	4.1
1921-------	1947	71.4	47.0	34.8	26.3	21.5	17.2	12.8	10.4	8.0	6.3	4.9	3.8
1922-------	1948	56.1	42.1	31.6	26.5	20.7	15.7	12.3	9.5	7.4	6.0	4.6	3.4
1923-------	1949	50.6	38.5	32.1	25.5	19.4	15.3	11.3	9.0	7.2	5.5	4.2	3.2
1924-------	1950	46.5	39.7	31.3	23.8	18.4	14.0	10.8	8.7	6.6	5.2	4.0	3.0
1925-------	1951	48.2	38.6	29.1	22.6	17.2	13.3	10.4	8.0	6.2	4.9	3.7	2.7
1926-------	1952	46.8	36.0	27.6	21.2	16.2	12.8	9.6	7.5	5.8	4.5	3.4	2.6
1927-------	1953	44.6	34.4	26.3	20.2	15.8	11.9	9.1	7.1	5.4	4.2	3.1	2.9
1928-------	1954	43.1	33.0	25.1	19.8	14.7	11.2	8.5	6.5	5.0	3.9	3.6	2.7
1929-------	1955	41.7	32.0	25.0	18.6	13.8	10.7	8.0	6.1	4.7	4.4	3.4	2.5
1930-------	1956	41.0	31.6	23.4	17.4	13.1	10.0	7.4	5.8	5.3	4.1	3.1	2.2
1931-------	1957	40.7	29.7	21.8	16.6	12.4	9.2	7.1	6.3	4.9	3.7	2.7	2.4
1932-------	1958	37.9	27.9	20.7	15.5	11.2	8.9	7.5	5.8	4.5	3.4	3.0	2.0
1933-------	1959	35.7	26.4	19.4	14.1	11.0	9.3	7.0	5.5	4.1	3.7	2.6	2.0
1934-------	1960	34.0	24.9	18.2	13.8	11.8	8.8	6.8	5.0	4.4	3.2	2.5	1.7
1935-------	1961	32.7	23.8	17.6	14.8	10.9	8.6	6.0	5.5	3.9	3.2	2.3	1.7
1936-------	1962	31.5	23.1	19.0	13.9	10.9	7.9	6.8	4.9	4.0	2.9	2.2	1.6
1937-------	1963	30.6	24.3	18.1	14.1	10.4	8.8	6.4	5.1	3.7	2.8	2.1	
1938-------	1964	31.6	23.5	18.3	13.9	11.4	8.5	6.6	4.7	3.6	2.7		
1939-------	1965	30.7	24.3	18.3	15.3	11.3	8.9	6.4	4.7	3.6			
1940-------	1966	32.4	24.7	20.5	15.2	11.9	8.6	6.2	4.7				
1941-------	1967	33.3	27.8	20.7	16.4	11.7	8.4	6.4					
1942-------	1968	37.0	28.4	22.2	16.0	11.4	8.8						
1943-------	1969	37.5	29.6	21.8	15.5	12.0							
1944-------	1970	38.6	29.1	21.1	16.3								
1945-------	1971	37.7	27.9	21.8									
1946-------	1972	36.1	28.9										
1947-------	1973	36.0											

TABLE 4B. CENTRAL BIRTH RATES FOR WHITE WOMEN DURING EACH YEAR 1917-73 BY AGE AND LIVE-BIRTH ORDER FOR EACH COHORT FROM 1868 TO 1959--CON.

LIVE-BIRTH ORDER AND COHORT	DIAGONAL LINE FOR CALENDAR YEAR	CURRENT AGE											
		38	39	40	41	42	43	44	45	46	47	48	49
FIRST BIRTHS--CON.													
1868-------													0.0
1869-------												0.0	0.0
1870-------											0.0	0.0	0.0
1871-------										0.1	0.1	0.0	0.0
1872-------									0.2	0.1	0.0	0.0	0.0
1873-------								0.3	0.2	0.1	0.0	0.0	0.0
1874-------							0.5	0.3	0.2	0.1	0.0	0.0	0.0
1875-------						0.8	0.5	0.3	0.2	0.1	0.1	0.0	0.0
1876-------					1.2	0.8	0.6	0.3	0.2	0.1	0.0	0.0	0.0
1877-------				1.7	1.2	0.8	0.6	0.3	0.2	0.1	0.0	0.0	0.0
1878-------			2.5	1.7	1.3	0.8	0.6	0.3	0.2	0.1	0.1	0.0	0.0
1879-------	1917	3.1	2.5	1.8	1.3	0.9	0.6	0.3	0.2	0.1	0.0	0.0	0.0
1880-------	1918	3.2	2.6	1.8	1.4	0.8	0.6	0.3	0.2	0.1	0.0	0.0	0.0
1881-------	1919	3.2	2.7	1.9	1.2	0.8	0.6	0.3	0.2	0.1	0.0	0.0	0.0
1882-------	1920	3.3	2.8	1.7	1.2	0.8	0.5	0.3	0.2	0.1	0.1	0.0	0.0
1883-------	1921	3.5	2.6	1.7	1.2	0.7	0.5	0.3	0.2	0.1	0.1	0.0	0.0
1884-------	1922	3.2	2.5	1.7	1.2	0.8	0.5	0.3	0.2	0.1	0.0	0.0	0.0
1885-------	1923	3.1	2.6	1.7	1.2	0.8	0.5	0.3	0.2	0.1	0.0	0.0	0.0
1886-------	1924	3.2	2.5	1.6	1.2	0.8	0.4	0.3	0.1	0.1	0.0	0.0	0.0
1887-------	1925	3.2	2.4	1.7	1.2	0.7	0.4	0.2	0.1	0.1	0.0	0.0	0.0
1888-------	1926	3.0	2.4	1.6	1.1	0.7	0.4	0.2	0.1	0.0	0.0	0.0	0.0
1889-------	1927	3.1	2.4	1.6	1.1	0.7	0.5	0.2	0.1	0.1	0.0	0.0	0.0
1890-------	1928	3.0	2.3	1.5	1.1	0.7	0.4	0.2	0.1	0.0	0.0	0.0	0.0
1891-------	1929	2.9	2.3	1.5	1.0	0.6	0.4	0.3	0.1	0.0	0.0	0.0	0.0
1892-------	1930	2.9	2.2	1.4	0.9	0.6	0.4	0.2	0.1	0.0	0.0	0.0	0.0
1893-------	1931	2.8	2.0	1.3	0.9	0.6	0.4	0.2	0.1	0.1	0.0	0.0	0.0
1894-------	1932	2.6	1.9	1.3	0.9	0.6	0.4	0.2	0.1	0.1	0.0	0.0	0.0
1895-------	1933	2.4	1.9	1.3	0.9	0.6	0.4	0.2	0.1	0.1	0.0	0.0	0.0
1896-------	1934	2.5	1.8	1.3	0.9	0.6	0.4	0.2	0.1	0.1	0.0	0.0	0.0
1897-------	1935	2.5	1.9	1.3	0.9	0.7	0.4	0.3	0.1	0.1	0.0	0.0	0.0
1898-------	1936	2.6	2.0	1.4	1.0	0.7	0.5	0.3	0.2	0.1	0.0	0.0	0.0
1899-------	1937	2.8	2.2	1.6	1.1	0.8	0.5	0.3	0.2	0.1	0.0	0.0	0.0
1900-------	1938	3.0	2.3	1.6	1.2	0.8	0.6	0.3	0.2	0.1	0.0	0.0	0.0
1901-------	1939	3.2	2.4	1.8	1.2	0.9	0.6	0.4	0.2	0.1	0.0	0.0	0.0
1902-------	1940	3.3	2.6	2.1	1.5	1.0	0.7	0.4	0.2	0.1	0.0	0.0	0.0
1903-------	1941	3.7	3.3	2.4	1.7	1.1	0.8	0.4	0.2	0.1	0.0	0.0	0.0
1904-------	1942	4.6	3.6	2.5	1.8	1.3	0.8	0.4	0.2	0.1	0.0	0.0	0.0
1905-------	1943	4.9	3.6	2.7	2.0	1.3	0.7	0.4	0.2	0.1	0.0	0.0	0.0
1906-------	1944	4.8	3.8	3.1	2.2	1.2	0.7	0.4	0.2	0.1	0.0	0.0	0.0
1907-------	1945	5.1	4.5	3.3	1.9	1.2	0.7	0.4	0.2	0.1	0.0	0.0	0.0
1908-------	1946	5.9	4.8	2.9	1.9	1.1	0.6	0.4	0.2	0.1	0.0	0.0	0.0
1909-------	1947	6.5	4.2	2.7	1.8	1.1	0.7	0.4	0.2	0.1	0.0	0.0	0.0
1910-------	1948	5.5	3.9	2.6	1.7	1.1	0.7	0.4	0.2	0.1	0.0	0.0	0.0
1911-------	1949	5.0	3.6	2.5	1.7	1.1	0.6	0.4	0.2	0.1	0.0	0.0	0.0
1912-------	1950	4.6	3.4	2.5	1.6	1.0	0.6	0.3	0.2	0.1	0.0	0.0	0.0
1913-------	1951	4.4	3.4	2.3	1.6	1.0	0.6	0.3	0.2	0.1	0.0	0.0	0.0
1914-------	1952	4.4	3.2	2.3	1.5	0.9	0.6	0.3	0.2	0.1	0.0	0.0	0.0
1915-------	1953	4.1	3.1	2.1	1.3	0.9	0.5	0.3	0.1	0.1	0.0	0.0	0.0
1916-------	1954	4.0	2.9	1.8	1.4	0.8	0.5	0.2	0.1	0.0	0.0	0.0	0.0
1917-------	1955	3.7	2.6	1.9	1.2	0.8	0.4	0.2	0.1	0.0	0.0	0.0	0.0
1918-------	1956	3.3	2.5	1.6	1.1	0.7	0.4	0.2	0.1	0.0	0.0	0.0	0.0
1919-------	1957	3.3	2.3	1.7	1.1	0.7	0.4	0.2	0.1	0.0	0.0	0.0	0.0
1920-------	1958	3.0	2.2	1.5	1.1	0.6	0.4	0.2	0.1	0.0	0.0	0.0	0.0
1921-------	1959	2.8	2.0	1.4	0.9	0.6	0.4	0.2	0.1	0.0	0.0	0.0	0.0
1922-------	1960	2.6	1.9	1.3	0.9	0.7	0.4	0.2	0.1	0.0	0.0	0.0	0.0
1923-------	1961	2.4	1.7	1.2	1.0	0.6	0.3	0.2	0.1	0.0	0.0	0.0	0.0
1924-------	1962	2.2	1.6	1.4	0.9	0.5	0.3	0.2	0.1	0.0	0.0	0.0	0.0
1925-------	1963	2.1	1.9	1.2	0.8	0.4	0.3	0.1	0.1	0.0	0.0	0.0	
1926-------	1964	2.3	1.7	1.1	0.7	0.5	0.2	0.1	0.1	0.0	0.0		
1927-------	1965	2.2	1.6	0.9	0.8	0.4	0.2	0.1	0.0	0.0			
1928-------	1966	2.0	1.3	1.1	0.6	0.4	0.2	0.1	0.0				
1929-------	1967	1.7	1.5	0.9	0.6	0.3	0.2	0.1					
1930-------	1968	1.9	1.2	0.9	0.5	0.3	0.2						
1931-------	1969	1.6	1.2	0.8	0.5	0.3							
1932-------	1970	1.6	1.0	0.7	0.4								
1933-------	1971	1.4	1.0	0.6									
1934-------	1972	1.3	0.9										
1935-------	1973	1.2											

TABLE 4B. CENTRAL BIRTH RATES FOR WHITE WOMEN DURING EACH YEAR 1917-73 BY AGE AND LIVE-BIRTH ORDER FOR EACH COHORT FROM 1868 TO 1959--CON.

LIVE-BIRTH ORDER AND COHORT	DIAGONAL LINE FOR CALENDAR YEAR	CURRENT AGE 14	15	16	17	18	19	20	21	22	23	24	25
SECOND BIRTHS													
1892-------													51.6
1893-------												55.5	50.8
1894-------											58.9	54.6	48.7
1895-------										56.5	57.8	52.2	48.3
1896-------									52.5	55.6	54.9	51.2	47.9
1897-------								42.7	51.9	52.9	53.3	50.8	49.8
1898-------							29.5	42.4	49.6	51.7	53.1	53.6	51.6
1899-------						15.3	29.2	40.3	47.8	50.7	55.5	54.7	49.8
1900-------					6.3	15.1	27.7	39.0	46.8	52.9	56.8	53.0	46.9
1901-------				1.8	6.1	14.1	26.7	39.0	48.7	54.1	55.1	50.4	45.0
1902-------			0.4	1.8	5.9	14.2	28.1	41.8	50.5	53.2	52.1	48.6	43.7
1903-------	1917	*	0.4	1.7	5.9	15.8	30.4	43.2	49.1	51.1	51.0	47.1	42.1
1904-------	1918	*	0.3	1.7	6.5	17.2	31.1	41.1	46.8	50.1	49.0	45.0	40.9
1905-------	1919	*	0.3	1.8	7.0	17.8	29.2	39.2	45.9	48.2	46.3	43.4	40.6
1906-------	1920	*	0.3	1.9	7.2	16.5	28.1	38.7	44.9	45.6	44.9	42.8	38.9
1907-------	1921	*	0.4	2.0	6.7	16.2	28.1	38.3	42.8	44.3	44.3	41.3	37.7
1908-------	1922	*	0.4	1.9	6.8	16.4	27.9	36.3	41.3	43.6	42.3	39.7	35.7
1909-------	1923	*	0.4	2.0	7.0	16.3	26.4	34.9	40.6	41.8	40.9	37.6	36.5
1910-------	1924	*	0.4	2.1	6.9	15.1	25.2	34.2	38.7	40.3	38.6	38.1	34.7
1911-------	1925	*	0.4	2.1	6.6	14.7	25.1	32.9	37.7	38.1	39.3	36.7	35.2
1912-------	1926	*	0.4	2.0	6.5	14.6	23.9	31.9	35.2	38.6	37.5	37.2	36.4
1913-------	1927	*	0.4	2.0	6.5	14.0	23.0	29.4	35.5	37.0	38.3	38.6	38.6
1914-------	1928	*	0.4	1.9	6.0	13.4	21.0	29.5	34.0	37.8	39.7	40.7	38.6
1915-------	1929	*	0.4	1.8	5.7	12.1	20.8	28.4	35.0	39.3	41.6	40.4	40.6
1916-------	1930	*	0.4	1.7	5.2	11.8	20.0	29.2	35.9	40.6	40.7	41.6	42.4
1917-------	1931	*	0.4	1.5	5.0	11.4	20.7	29.7	37.1	39.5	41.5	43.2	48.4
1918-------	1932	*	0.3	1.5	4.8	11.9	21.1	30.6	35.9	40.5	42.5	50.2	54.4
1919-------	1933	*	0.3	1.5	5.2	12.3	21.9	30.3	37.8	42.1	50.5	55.5	49.6
1920-------	1934	*	0.3	1.7	5.5	12.7	21.8	32.3	38.7	46.2	54.8	49.8	45.5
1921-------	1935	*	0.4	1.8	5.7	13.0	24.0	33.0	39.6	50.0	48.5	44.7	60.7
1922-------	1936	*	0.4	1.8	5.7	14.2	23.6	32.3	43.4	44.9	42.3	61.3	67.0
1923-------	1937	*	0.3	1.8	6.3	13.9	23.4	35.2	39.3	39.0	59.6	68.0	67.3
1924-------	1938	*	0.4	2.0	6.1	14.2	25.3	31.8	33.8	55.3	66.0	69.8	70.6
1925-------	1939	*	0.4	2.0	6.3	14.8	22.5	27.4	46.8	60.7	69.3	73.5	71.2
1926-------	1940	*	0.4	2.1	6.7	13.0	19.2	35.8	51.5	65.7	73.3	73.9	73.4
1927-------	1941	*	0.5	2.3	5.9	11.2	23.5	40.0	58.2	70.1	73.3	76.1	73.6
1928-------	1942	*	0.6	2.0	5.1	12.9	26.8	47.2	62.9	70.2	75.9	76.8	74.3
1929-------	1943	*	0.5	1.7	5.6	15.0	33.0	52.0	63.4	73.3	77.7	79.3	74.9
1930-------	1944	*	0.4	1.8	6.7	19.1	37.2	52.7	66.4	75.9	81.0	80.8	74.3
1931-------	1945	*	0.4	2.3	8.7	22.4	38.3	55.7	69.8	80.4	84.1	81.4	75.8
1932-------	1946	*	0.5	3.0	10.5	23.0	40.1	58.2	73.8	83.8	85.5	84.2	76.9
1933-------	1947	*	0.7	3.8	10.8	24.3	42.2	61.9	77.0	86.1	89.0	86.2	75.4
1934-------	1948	*	1.0	3.8	11.5	25.1	44.5	63.8	79.8	89.7	91.7	85.1	74.1
1935-------	1949	*	0.9	3.9	11.7	26.2	45.1	66.1	82.7	92.7	91.2	84.0	72.4
1936-------	1950	*	0.9	3.9	12.2	26.7	47.0	68.9	85.5	92.1	90.9	82.8	69.6
1937-------	1951	*	0.8	4.0	12.4	27.7	49.4	71.1	85.8	93.1	90.1	80.0	66.0
1938-------	1952	*	0.8	4.2	12.9	29.4	50.6	72.0	88.0	92.3	87.5	76.1	63.9
1939-------	1953	*	1.0	4.4	13.9	30.5	52.3	74.2	86.8	90.1	83.4	73.7	62.2
1940-------	1954	*	1.0	4.7	14.4	31.4	53.5	72.4	84.3	86.4	80.6	71.0	58.0
1941-------	1955	*	1.1	5.0	14.8	31.1	51.5	69.7	80.8	82.6	76.6	65.7	56.5
1942-------	1956	*	1.1	5.0	14.4	30.2	49.0	66.5	76.4	77.1	69.9	63.3	57.4
1943-------	1957	*	1.1	4.8	14.0	28.6	46.8	62.2	70.3	69.2	66.4	63.8	58.2
1944-------	1958	*	1.1	4.8	13.5	27.5	43.7	57.0	62.0	64.5	66.2	63.4	60.0
1945-------	1959	*	1.1	4.8	13.1	25.6	39.8	49.6	56.9	62.7	63.6	63.4	60.4
1946-------	1960	*	1.2	4.6	12.1	23.0	34.1	44.6	54.6	60.0	64.1	64.3	57.0
1947-------	1961	*	1.0	4.1	10.6	19.7	30.3	42.5	51.2	59.7	64.2	59.9	52.5
1948-------	1962	*	0.9	3.5	9.0	17.3	28.9	39.4	50.8	59.3	59.4	54.1	51.1
1949-------	1963	*	0.8	3.1	8.0	16.5	26.2	38.5	50.2	54.8	52.4	51.4	
1950-------	1964	*	0.7	2.8	7.6	15.0	25.8	38.3	46.4	47.7	49.3		
1951-------	1965	*	0.7	2.7	7.0	14.8	25.8	35.6	40.1	44.6			
1952-------	1966	*	0.6	2.4	7.0	14.8	24.1	30.9	37.4				
1953-------	1967	*	0.6	2.5	7.0	14.2	21.4	29.0					
1954-------	1968	*	0.6	2.6	6.8	12.8	20.3						
1955-------	1969	*	0.7	2.6	6.3	12.3							
1956-------	1970	*	0.7	2.4	6.2								
1957-------	1971	*	0.6	2.4									
1958-------	1972	*	0.7										
1959-------	1973	*											

TABLE 4B. CENTRAL BIRTH RATES FOR WHITE WOMEN DURING EACH YEAR 1917-73 BY AGE AND LIVE-BIRTH ORDER FOR EACH COHORT FROM 1868 TO 1959--CON.

LIVE-BIRTH ORDER AND COHORT	DIAGONAL LINE FOR CALENDAR YEAR	CURRENT AGE											
		26	27	28	29	30	31	32	33	34	35	36	37
SECOND BIRTHS--CON.													
1880-------													6.4
1881-------												8.1	6.5
1882-------											10.0	8.1	6.4
1883-------										12.1	9.9	8.1	6.5
1884-------									14.8	11.9	9.9	8.1	6.7
1885-------								17.4	14.6	11.9	10.1	8.5	6.4
1886-------							21.6	17.3	14.6	12.2	10.5	8.1	6.5
1887-------						26.9	21.5	17.3	15.1	12.6	10.2	8.3	6.5
1888-------					34.0	26.7	21.4	17.8	15.3	12.5	10.3	8.2	6.3
1889-------				39.1	33.8	26.2	22.0	18.0	15.4	12.5	10.3	8.1	6.2
1890-------			43.3	39.1	32.9	26.6	22.4	18.2	15.4	12.5	10.2	7.8	6.1
1891-------	1917	45.4	43.3	37.6	33.0	26.6	22.4	18.1	15.4	12.4	9.8	7.7	5.9
1892-------	1918	45.2	41.5	37.2	32.3	26.5	22.3	18.0	15.0	11.7	9.4	7.3	5.5
1893-------	1919	43.4	41.1	36.2	32.4	26.4	22.2	17.4	14.3	11.4	9.1	7.0	5.8
1894-------	1920	43.4	40.4	36.7	32.7	26.2	21.5	17.0	14.1	11.2	8.8	7.3	5.4
1895-------	1921	43.0	41.3	37.4	32.2	25.6	21.4	16.8	13.9	10.8	9.1	7.0	5.2
1896-------	1922	44.2	42.2	36.4	31.4	25.2	20.8	16.4	13.3	11.1	8.6	6.7	4.9
1897-------	1923	45.2	41.3	35.6	30.7	24.4	20.1	15.9	13.6	10.5	8.4	6.3	5.1
1898-------	1924	44.6	39.7	34.1	29.3	23.4	19.6	16.0	12.9	10.2	7.8	6.5	5.1
1899-------	1925	43.2	38.4	33.1	28.5	23.2	20.0	15.8	13.0	9.9	8.5	6.7	5.2
1900-------	1926	40.9	36.9	31.6	27.7	23.4	19.3	15.3	12.2	10.5	8.4	6.7	5.3
1901-------	1927	40.0	35.4	30.7	27.9	22.7	18.7	14.5	12.9	10.4	8.6	6.8	5.6
1902-------	1928	38.3	34.2	30.8	26.7	21.5	17.5	15.2	12.8	10.6	8.7	7.3	5.8
1903-------	1929	37.2	34.5	30.0	25.7	20.6	18.7	15.2	13.1	10.9	9.3	7.7	6.2
1904-------	1930	37.4	33.4	28.8	24.6	22.0	18.7	15.5	13.5	11.7	9.9	8.3	6.7
1905-------	1931	36.1	32.0	27.4	25.8	21.6	18.7	16.0	14.4	12.3	10.6	8.9	7.6
1906-------	1932	34.6	30.5	28.5	25.4	21.7	19.4	17.2	15.1	13.2	11.3	9.7	9.0
1907-------	1933	33.1	31.7	28.0	25.5	22.5	20.8	18.0	16.3	14.1	13.0	11.5	9.8
1908-------	1934	33.9	30.6	27.9	26.0	23.8	21.5	19.5	17.2	16.4	15.1	12.5	10.6
1909-------	1935	32.7	30.5	28.6	27.7	24.7	23.5	20.8	20.3	18.9	15.7	13.7	11.4
1910-------	1936	32.5	31.4	30.4	28.2	26.7	24.8	23.5	23.3	19.1	17.0	14.6	11.5
1911-------	1937	33.9	33.5	31.0	30.4	28.3	27.5	27.0	23.0	20.7	18.3	14.5	10.6
1912-------	1938	35.9	33.7	33.0	31.9	32.3	31.5	26.5	24.7	22.2	18.2	13.4	10.1
1913-------	1939	36.2	35.9	34.8	37.1	36.9	30.9	28.8	26.6	22.1	16.6	12.9	9.9
1914-------	1940	38.7	38.2	41.1	42.4	35.3	33.5	31.3	26.7	20.2	16.1	12.7	10.0
1915-------	1941	41.1	44.1	47.1	39.9	37.7	36.5	31.5	24.2	19.7	15.9	12.7	10.1
1916-------	1942	45.6	50.4	43.4	41.6	41.4	37.1	28.6	23.6	19.4	15.8	12.6	9.5
1917-------	1943	52.0	46.3	44.2	46.6	43.0	34.3	28.3	23.6	19.4	15.7	12.1	9.4
1918-------	1944	47.9	45.5	50.3	49.1	39.7	33.8	28.1	23.4	19.1	14.9	11.7	8.9
1919-------	1945	45.9	54.8	55.0	46.5	40.2	34.2	28.6	23.6	18.6	14.9	11.3	8.7
1920-------	1946	57.9	60.4	52.6	47.2	40.6	34.5	28.5	22.7	18.3	14.0	10.8	8.1
1921-------	1947	64.4	58.6	53.9	47.9	41.0	34.6	27.3	22.4	17.0	13.4	10.1	7.6
1922-------	1948	63.2	60.2	54.4	47.9	41.1	33.1	26.7	20.7	16.2	12.6	9.2	6.8
1923-------	1949	65.8	60.8	55.2	48.3	39.3	32.4	24.8	19.7	15.3	11.4	8.5	6.3
1924-------	1950	66.8	62.4	55.6	46.4	38.7	30.1	23.5	18.6	13.8	10.5	8.0	6.0
1925-------	1951	68.5	62.5	53.5	45.4	35.7	28.4	22.1	16.8	12.8	9.9	7.5	5.4
1926-------	1952	68.8	61.2	52.5	42.7	33.9	26.8	20.2	15.5	12.0	9.3	6.7	5.0
1927-------	1953	68.5	60.0	49.9	41.0	32.5	24.7	18.6	14.6	11.3	8.3	6.4	4.7
1928-------	1954	67.7	57.8	48.2	39.3	30.1	23.0	17.6	13.6	10.1	7.9	6.0	4.2
1929-------	1955	66.3	56.9	47.5	36.9	28.5	21.9	16.7	12.6	9.7	7.5	5.4	4.0
1930-------	1956	66.2	56.4	44.8	35.3	27.1	20.7	15.5	11.9	9.3	6.8	5.0	3.8
1931-------	1957	66.8	54.1	43.0	33.7	25.7	19.1	14.5	11.5	8.3	6.4	4.7	3.6
1932-------	1958	64.7	52.5	41.4	31.9	23.7	18.1	14.0	10.4	7.9	5.9	4.5	3.4
1933-------	1959	62.8	50.3	39.1	29.3	22.4	17.3	13.0	9.7	7.5	5.8	4.4	3.3
1934-------	1960	61.0	48.0	36.5	28.2	21.5	16.5	12.0	9.3	7.1	5.6	4.3	3.0
1935-------	1961	58.3	45.2	35.2	27.2	20.5	15.1	11.7	9.2	7.2	5.5	4.0	2.8
1936-------	1962	55.6	43.7	34.5	25.9	19.4	14.9	11.6	9.3	7.1	5.2	3.8	2.7
1937-------	1963	53.7	43.0	32.4	24.9	19.3	15.3	11.9	9.3	6.8	5.0	3.7	
1938-------	1964	52.5	40.3	31.6	24.8	19.8	15.9	12.3	9.0	6.6	5.1		
1939-------	1965	49.2	39.3	31.9	25.7	20.8	16.5	12.2	9.0	6.9			
1940-------	1966	47.9	39.8	33.0	27.8	22.2	16.5	12.3	9.3				
1941-------	1967	48.7	41.3	35.7	29.7	22.1	16.8	12.5					
1942-------	1968	50.6	45.0	38.4	29.5	22.7	17.1						
1943-------	1969	53.0	46.9	37.2	29.3	22.9							
1944-------	1970	54.5	45.0	36.2	29.6								
1945-------	1971	51.5	42.8	36.8									
1946-------	1972	48.6	43.5										
1947-------	1973	48.3											

TABLE 4B. CENTRAL BIRTH RATES FOR WHITE WOMEN DURING EACH YEAR 1917-73 BY AGE AND LIVE-BIRTH ORDER FOR EACH COHORT FROM 1868 TO 1959--CON.

LIVE-BIRTH ORDER AND COHORT	DIAGONAL LINE FOR CALENDAR YEAR	CURRENT AGE											
		38	39	40	41	42	43	44	45	46	47	48	49
SECOND BIRTHS--CON.													
1868-------													0.0
1869-------												0.0	0.0
1870-------											0.1	0.0	0.0
1871-------										0.2	0.1	0.0	0.0
1872-------									0.3	0.2	0.1	0.0	0.0
1873-------								0.5	0.3	0.1	0.1	0.0	0.0
1874-------							0.8	0.5	0.2	0.2	0.0	0.0	0.0
1875-------						1.1	0.8	0.4	0.3	0.1	0.1	0.0	0.0
1876-------					1.8	1.1	0.8	0.5	0.2	0.1	0.1	0.0	0.0
1877-------				2.6	1.8	1.1	0.8	0.4	0.2	0.1	0.1	0.0	0.0
1878-------			3.8	2.6	1.8	1.2	0.8	0.4	0.2	0.1	0.0	0.0	0.0
1879-------	1917	4.9	3.8	2.6	1.8	1.2	0.8	0.4	0.2	0.1	0.0	0.0	0.0
1880-------	1918	5.0	3.9	2.7	1.9	1.1	0.8	0.4	0.2	0.1	0.0	0.0	0.0
1881-------	1919	5.0	3.9	2.7	1.8	1.1	0.8	0.4	0.3	0.1	0.0	0.0	0.0
1882-------	1920	5.0	4.0	2.6	1.7	1.1	0.8	0.4	0.2	0.1	0.0	0.0	0.0
1883-------	1921	5.2	3.8	2.5	1.8	1.2	0.7	0.4	0.2	0.1	0.0	0.0	0.0
1884-------	1922	4.9	3.8	2.6	1.7	1.0	0.7	0.4	0.2	0.1	0.0	0.0	0.0
1885-------	1923	5.0	3.8	2.5	1.7	1.1	0.7	0.3	0.2	0.1	0.0	0.0	0.0
1886-------	1924	5.0	3.7	2.5	1.6	1.0	0.6	0.3	0.2	0.1	0.0	0.0	0.0
1887-------	1925	4.9	3.7	2.4	1.6	0.9	0.6	0.4	0.2	0.1	0.0	0.0	0.0
1888-------	1926	4.7	3.5	2.3	1.5	0.9	0.6	0.3	0.2	0.1	0.0	0.0	0.0
1889-------	1927	4.7	3.5	2.3	1.5	0.9	0.6	0.3	0.1	0.1	0.0	0.0	0.0
1890-------	1928	4.6	3.4	2.2	1.5	0.9	0.6	0.3	0.1	0.1	0.0	0.0	0.0
1891-------	1929	4.4	3.4	2.1	1.5	0.9	0.5	0.2	0.1	0.0	0.0	0.0	0.0
1892-------	1930	4.5	3.1	2.1	1.4	0.8	0.5	0.2	0.1	0.0	0.0	0.0	0.0
1893-------	1931	4.1	3.0	2.0	1.2	0.7	0.5	0.2	0.1	0.0	0.0	0.0	0.0
1894-------	1932	3.9	2.9	1.9	1.2	0.8	0.4	0.3	0.1	0.0	0.0	0.0	0.0
1895-------	1933	3.8	3.0	1.9	1.2	0.7	0.5	0.2	0.1	0.1	0.0	0.0	0.0
1896-------	1934	3.9	2.8	1.9	1.2	0.8	0.5	0.2	0.2	0.1	0.0	0.0	0.0
1897-------	1935	3.9	2.8	1.9	1.4	0.8	0.5	0.3	0.2	0.1	0.0	0.0	0.0
1898-------	1936	3.8	2.8	2.1	1.3	0.8	0.5	0.3	0.2	0.1	0.0	0.0	0.0
1899-------	1937	4.0	3.1	2.2	1.4	0.9	0.6	0.4	0.2	0.1	0.0	0.0	0.0
1900-------	1938	4.2	3.3	2.3	1.5	0.9	0.7	0.4	0.2	0.1	0.0	0.0	0.0
1901-------	1939	4.4	3.4	2.4	1.6	1.1	0.7	0.4	0.2	0.1	0.0	0.0	0.0
1902-------	1940	4.7	3.6	2.7	1.9	1.3	0.8	0.5	0.2	0.1	0.0	0.0	0.0
1903-------	1941	5.0	4.1	3.1	2.2	1.5	0.9	0.5	0.2	0.1	0.0	0.0	0.0
1904-------	1942	5.7	4.8	3.5	2.5	1.6	1.0	0.5	0.2	0.1	0.0	0.0	0.0
1905-------	1943	6.7	5.3	3.8	2.7	1.7	0.9	0.5	0.2	0.1	0.0	0.0	0.0
1906-------	1944	7.3	5.7	4.2	2.8	1.6	0.9	0.5	0.2	0.1	0.0	0.0	0.0
1907-------	1945	8.0	6.3	4.3	2.7	1.5	0.9	0.5	0.2	0.1	0.0	0.0	0.0
1908-------	1946	8.6	6.4	4.1	2.6	1.5	0.9	0.5	0.2	0.1	0.0	0.0	0.0
1909-------	1947	8.7	6.0	4.0	2.5	1.5	1.0	0.5	0.2	0.1	0.0	0.0	0.0
1910-------	1948	8.1	5.8	3.9	2.6	1.7	1.0	0.5	0.2	0.1	0.0	0.0	0.0
1911-------	1949	7.8	5.7	4.0	2.6	1.6	1.0	0.5	0.3	0.1	0.0	0.0	0.0
1912-------	1950	7.7	5.8	3.9	2.7	1.6	0.9	0.5	0.2	0.1	0.0	0.0	0.0
1913-------	1951	7.6	5.7	4.0	2.6	1.6	1.0	0.5	0.2	0.1	0.0	0.0	0.0
1914-------	1952	7.8	5.7	3.9	2.5	1.6	0.9	0.4	0.2	0.1	0.0	0.0	0.0
1915-------	1953	7.4	5.5	3.8	2.5	1.5	0.8	0.4	0.2	0.1	0.0	0.0	0.0
1916-------	1954	7.3	5.3	3.5	2.3	1.3	0.8	0.4	0.2	0.1	0.0	0.0	0.0
1917-------	1955	7.0	5.1	3.4	2.2	1.3	0.7	0.4	0.2	0.1	0.0	0.0	0.0
1918-------	1956	6.6	4.8	3.1	2.0	1.2	0.7	0.4	0.2	0.0	0.0	0.0	0.0
1919-------	1957	6.4	4.5	2.9	1.9	1.2	0.7	0.4	0.1	0.0	0.0	0.0	0.0
1920-------	1958	5.9	4.1	2.7	1.8	1.1	0.6	0.3	0.1	0.0	0.0	0.0	0.0
1921-------	1959	5.4	3.7	2.7	1.7	1.0	0.5	0.3	0.1	0.0	0.0	0.0	0.0
1922-------	1960	4.9	3.7	2.4	1.6	0.8	0.5	0.2	0.1	0.0	0.0	0.0	0.0
1923-------	1961	4.7	3.2	2.2	1.4	0.9	0.5	0.2	0.1	0.0	0.0	0.0	0.0
1924-------	1962	4.2	3.0	2.0	1.4	0.8	0.4	0.2	0.1	0.0	0.0	0.0	0.0
1925-------	1963	3.9	2.9	1.9	1.2	0.7	0.4	0.2	0.1	0.0	0.0	0.0	
1926-------	1964	3.7	2.6	1.7	1.1	0.6	0.4	0.2	0.1	0.0	0.0		
1927-------	1965	3.3	2.3	1.5	1.0	0.6	0.3	0.1	0.1	0.0			
1928-------	1966	3.0	2.2	1.5	1.0	0.6	0.3	0.1	0.1				
1929-------	1967	2.9	2.1	1.5	0.9	0.5	0.3	0.1					
1930-------	1968	2.7	2.0	1.3	0.8	0.5	0.2						
1931-------	1969	2.6	1.8	1.2	0.7	0.4							
1932-------	1970	2.5	1.7	1.1	0.6								
1933-------	1971	2.2	1.5	1.0									
1934-------	1972	2.1	1.4										
1935-------	1973	2.0											

TABLE 4B. CENTRAL BIRTH RATES FOR WHITE WOMEN DURING EACH YEAR 1917-73 BY AGE AND LIVE-BIRTH ORDER FOR EACH COHORT FROM 1868 TO 1959--CON.

LIVE-BIRTH ORDER AND COHORT	DIAGONAL LINE FOR CALENDAR YEAR	CURRENT AGE											
		14	15	16	17	18	19	20	21	22	23	24	25
THIRD BIRTHS													
1892-------													39.0
1893-------												37.8	38.2
1894-------											35.0	37.1	36.0
1895-------										28.5	34.5	35.2	36.1
1896-------									21.2	28.2	32.8	35.1	36.4
1897-------								13.2	21.0	26.9	32.4	35.3	33.5
1898-------							6.4	13.1	20.1	26.7	32.6	32.6	34.6
1899-------						2.2	6.4	12.5	19.7	26.5	29.5	33.4	35.3
1900-------					0.6	2.2	6.1	12.2	19.6	23.9	30.8	35.0	34.1
1901-------				0.1	0.6	2.0	5.8	12.0	17.4	24.7	32.6	34.2	32.1
1902-------			0.0	0.1	0.5	2.0	6.1	11.2	18.5	26.9	31.8	32.0	31.2
1903-------	1917	*	0.0	0.1	0.5	2.2	5.6	12.0	19.9	26.6	30.2	31.3	29.5
1904-------	1918	*	0.0	0.1	0.6	2.1	6.1	12.5	19.4	25.3	29.1	29.5	27.8
1905-------	1919	*	0.0	0.1	0.5	2.4	6.3	12.1	18.4	24.3	27.4	27.9	27.5
1906-------	1920	*	0.0	0.1	0.6	2.4	6.1	11.5	17.9	23.1	26.0	27.3	25.6
1907-------	1921	*	0.0	0.1	0.6	2.4	5.9	11.4	17.4	22.0	25.4	25.5	24.8
1908-------	1922	*	0.0	0.1	0.6	2.3	6.0	11.1	16.4	21.3	23.7	24.5	23.2
1909-------	1923	*	0.0	0.1	0.6	2.4	5.8	10.4	15.9	20.2	22.8	23.2	23.5
1910-------	1924	*	0.0	0.1	0.7	2.2	5.4	10.1	15.1	19.3	21.5	23.1	21.8
1911-------	1925	*	0.0	0.2	0.6	2.1	5.3	9.6	14.3	18.3	21.6	21.8	21.2
1912-------	1926	*	0.0	0.1	0.6	2.1	4.9	9.1	13.6	18.1	20.3	21.0	20.8
1913-------	1927	*	0.0	0.1	0.6	1.9	4.6	8.5	13.4	17.1	19.3	20.8	21.6
1914-------	1928	*	0.0	0.1	0.5	1.8	4.3	8.4	12.7	16.4	19.4	21.5	21.1
1915-------	1929	*	0.0	0.1	0.5	1.7	4.2	8.0	12.1	16.5	20.0	21.0	22.0
1916-------	1930	*	0.0	0.1	0.4	1.6	4.0	7.7	12.2	16.9	19.5	21.9	22.4
1917-------	1931	*	0.0	0.1	0.4	1.5	3.8	7.8	12.6	16.5	20.4	22.2	23.4
1918-------	1932	*	0.0	0.1	0.4	1.5	4.0	8.1	12.2	17.3	20.5	23.4	26.6
1919-------	1933	*	0.0	0.1	0.4	1.6	4.3	8.0	13.2	17.6	22.1	26.1	26.5
1920-------	1934	*	0.0	0.1	0.5	1.7	4.2	9.0	13.2	18.3	24.3	25.7	24.1
1921-------	1935	*	0.0	0.1	0.6	1.8	5.2	9.0	13.3	20.0	23.6	22.8	26.9
1922-------	1936	*	0.0	0.1	0.6	2.4	4.9	8.7	14.6	19.6	20.1	25.1	29.2
1923-------	1937	*	0.0	0.1	0.7	2.3	4.9	9.6	14.6	16.5	22.2	27.3	31.2
1924-------	1938	*	0.0	0.2	0.7	2.2	5.4	9.6	12.0	18.2	24.1	29.7	33.8
1925-------	1939	*	0.0	0.2	0.7	2.3	5.2	7.8	13.3	19.7	26.4	32.3	36.4
1926-------	1940	*	0.0	0.2	0.7	2.2	4.2	8.5	14.3	21.6	29.0	35.0	40.1
1927-------	1941	*	0.0	0.2	0.7	1.8	4.5	9.1	15.9	24.4	31.8	38.5	43.1
1928-------	1942	*	0.0	0.2	0.6	1.9	4.8	10.3	18.4	27.2	35.1	41.1	44.8
1929-------	1943	*	0.0	0.2	0.6	2.0	5.5	12.4	21.0	30.5	37.4	43.6	48.1
1930-------	1944	*	0.0	0.2	0.7	2.3	7.0	14.3	23.6	32.2	39.9	46.9	50.8
1931-------	1945	*	0.0	0.2	0.8	3.2	8.1	16.3	25.1	34.6	43.6	49.9	54.1
1932-------	1946	*	0.0	0.2	1.1	3.6	9.0	17.3	26.7	37.6	46.1	53.5	56.8
1933-------	1947	*	0.0	0.3	1.2	4.0	9.8	18.3	29.1	39.7	49.8	56.2	57.8
1934-------	1948	*	0.1	0.3	1.3	4.3	10.3	19.8	30.7	42.7	52.4	57.5	59.6
1935-------	1949	*	0.1	0.3	1.3	4.5	10.9	20.5	32.5	44.7	53.2	59.3	60.4
1936-------	1950	*	0.0	0.3	1.5	4.8	11.3	21.7	34.4	45.6	54.7	60.1	59.8
1937-------	1951	*	0.0	0.3	1.5	4.9	12.0	22.9	34.8	46.9	56.1	60.0	57.6
1938-------	1952	*	0.0	0.3	1.6	5.3	12.8	23.2	36.4	48.6	56.0	57.8	54.8
1939-------	1953	*	0.0	0.3	1.7	5.5	12.9	25.1	37.9	48.4	54.3	54.8	51.4
1940-------	1954	*	0.0	0.4	1.8	5.7	14.2	25.5	37.1	47.0	51.0	50.7	44.8
1941-------	1955	*	0.1	0.4	1.9	6.2	14.2	24.8	35.7	43.3	46.2	43.1	39.0
1942-------	1956	*	0.1	0.4	2.0	6.1	13.5	23.3	32.4	38.6	38.3	36.9	36.8
1943-------	1957	*	0.1	0.4	1.9	5.8	12.6	21.1	28.6	31.4	32.3	34.2	34.7
1944-------	1958	*	0.1	0.4	1.9	5.4	11.6	18.8	23.2	26.3	29.7	31.7	35.0
1945-------	1959	*	0.1	0.4	1.9	5.1	10.3	15.2	19.2	23.6	26.8	31.3	34.5
1946-------	1960	*	0.1	0.4	1.7	4.6	8.3	12.3	16.9	20.9	26.1	30.8	30.5
1947-------	1961	*	0.1	0.4	1.5	3.6	6.6	10.6	14.7	20.1	25.4	27.2	24.6
1948-------	1962	*	0.1	0.3	1.1	2.9	5.7	9.2	14.1	19.4	22.5	21.7	21.4
1949-------	1963	*	0.0	0.3	1.0	2.5	4.9	8.8	13.4	17.5	18.0	18.9	
1950-------	1964	*	0.0	0.2	0.9	2.2	4.8	8.4	12.3	13.8	15.8		
1951-------	1965	*	0.0	0.2	0.8	2.1	4.5	7.7	9.7	12.3			
1952-------	1966	*	0.0	0.2	0.7	2.0	4.1	6.2	8.7				
1953-------	1967	*	0.0	0.2	0.7	1.8	3.4	5.6					
1954-------	1968	*	0.0	0.2	0.6	1.6	3.1						
1955-------	1969	*	0.1	0.2	0.6	1.5							
1956-------	1970	*	0.0	0.2	0.6								
1957-------	1971	*	0.0	0.2									
1958-------	1972	*	0.0										
1959-------	1973	*											

TABLE 4B. CENTRAL BIRTH RATES FOR WHITE WOMEN DURING EACH YEAR 1917-73 BY AGE AND LIVE-BIRTH ORDER FOR EACH COHORT FROM 1868 TO 1959--CON.

LIVE-BIRTH ORDER AND COHORT	DIAGONAL LINE FOR CALENDAR YEAR	CURRENT AGE											
		26	27	28	29	30	31	32	33	34	35	36	37
THIRD BIRTHS--CON.													
1880-------													9.0
1881-------												10.9	9.0
1882-------											13.4	10.8	8.8
1883-------										15.8	13.1	10.6	8.9
1884-------									18.7	15.4	12.9	10.8	9.1
1885-------								20.5	18.2	15.1	13.0	11.1	8.6
1886-------							24.1	20.1	17.8	15.3	13.4	10.5	8.7
1887-------						28.4	23.7	19.7	18.1	15.7	12.8	10.7	8.8
1888-------					34.2	27.8	23.1	19.9	18.4	15.0	12.9	10.7	8.5
1889-------				37.1	33.5	26.6	23.3	20.2	17.6	15.0	13.1	10.4	8.3
1890-------			38.4	36.6	31.8	26.9	23.7	19.4	17.7	15.4	12.5	10.2	8.1
1891-------	1917	37.8	37.9	34.3	31.9	27.1	22.7	19.4	18.1	14.7	12.2	9.8	7.8
1892-------	1918	37.2	35.4	34.2	31.8	25.2	22.6	19.8	17.3	14.2	11.7	9.3	7.2
1893-------	1919	34.7	35.2	33.9	29.1	24.9	23.0	19.0	16.5	13.6	11.1	8.7	7.1
1894-------	1920	34.9	35.3	30.8	29.0	25.4	22.2	18.4	15.9	13.1	10.5	8.8	6.9
1895-------	1921	35.4	32.4	30.7	29.5	24.5	21.4	17.8	15.3	12.5	10.7	8.5	6.6
1896-------	1922	32.6	32.4	31.0	28.3	23.8	20.8	17.0	14.6	12.5	10.2	8.1	6.2
1897-------	1923	32.6	32.8	29.9	27.3	22.8	19.6	16.2	14.5	11.9	9.8	7.6	6.3
1898-------	1924	33.5	31.7	28.5	26.0	21.6	18.9	16.2	13.7	11.5	9.2	7.7	6.1
1899-------	1925	32.8	30.3	27.5	24.8	20.8	18.8	15.6	13.6	10.9	9.5	7.7	6.1
1900-------	1926	30.7	29.2	25.9	23.5	20.5	17.9	14.9	12.7	11.2	9.3	7.5	6.0
1901-------	1927	30.1	27.3	24.4	23.0	19.7	17.0	14.1	12.9	10.8	9.0	7.3	6.0
1902-------	1928	28.0	25.7	23.9	21.7	18.5	16.1	14.1	12.2	10.4	8.8	7.3	6.0
1903-------	1929	26.6	25.5	22.8	20.9	17.5	16.2	13.5	12.0	10.2	8.8	7.4	6.1
1904-------	1930	26.3	24.0	22.2	19.8	17.8	15.5	13.2	11.9	10.4	9.0	7.6	6.4
1905-------	1931	24.8	23.5	20.7	20.0	16.9	14.9	13.1	12.0	10.4	9.2	7.9	7.0
1906-------	1932	24.0	22.0	21.1	18.8	16.3	14.8	13.2	12.0	10.7	9.5	8.6	8.4
1907-------	1933	22.7	22.3	19.8	18.3	16.2	15.0	13.3	12.4	11.1	10.5	10.3	9.1
1908-------	1934	22.7	20.7	19.0	17.8	16.3	14.9	13.7	12.8	12.3	12.4	11.2	10.0
1909-------	1935	21.2	19.9	18.7	18.1	16.3	15.5	14.3	14.2	14.6	13.4	12.3	10.5
1910-------	1936	20.5	19.5	19.0	17.9	17.0	16.1	15.6	16.9	15.7	14.8	13.1	10.8
1911-------	1937	20.4	20.2	18.8	18.7	17.6	17.3	18.6	18.0	17.1	15.7	13.3	10.2
1912-------	1938	20.8	19.6	19.5	19.1	19.3	20.6	19.8	19.3	18.2	15.9	12.6	10.1
1913-------	1939	20.3	20.5	20.0	21.2	22.7	21.9	21.1	20.7	18.5	15.3	12.5	10.3
1914-------	1940	21.2	21.1	22.3	24.8	23.6	23.1	22.8	21.3	17.9	15.1	12.9	10.9
1915-------	1941	21.8	22.9	26.0	25.4	24.5	25.2	23.7	20.6	17.8	15.7	13.6	11.8
1916-------	1942	22.7	26.6	26.1	25.6	26.4	26.0	22.8	20.5	18.4	16.5	14.6	11.9
1917-------	1943	26.3	26.7	25.8	27.8	27.8	25.4	23.1	21.4	19.5	17.7	14.9	12.4
1918-------	1944	26.5	25.5	27.6	29.3	27.1	25.8	24.0	22.6	20.9	18.1	15.4	12.1
1919-------	1945	25.1	28.1	30.3	29.4	28.4	27.5	26.3	24.7	21.7	18.8	15.3	12.4
1920-------	1946	27.4	30.7	30.6	30.9	30.3	29.8	28.2	25.7	22.3	18.6	15.3	12.0
1921-------	1947	30.5	31.6	32.5	33.3	33.1	32.5	29.5	26.2	22.3	18.5	15.0	11.4
1922-------	1948	31.5	33.7	34.9	36.0	35.9	33.6	30.0	26.2	22.0	18.1	14.1	10.8
1923-------	1949	34.0	36.1	38.1	39.4	37.3	34.3	30.0	25.9	21.9	17.3	13.5	10.3
1924-------	1950	36.7	40.0	41.8	40.8	38.5	34.5	30.0	26.1	20.8	16.5	12.8	9.9
1925-------	1951	40.4	43.5	43.4	42.3	38.6	34.6	30.0	24.5	19.7	15.7	12.3	9.1
1926-------	1952	43.9	44.8	45.3	42.8	38.7	34.4	28.4	23.3	18.7	15.1	11.2	8.5
1927-------	1953	45.4	47.2	46.1	43.4	39.0	33.2	27.3	22.3	18.0	13.7	10.5	8.0
1928-------	1954	48.0	48.4	46.8	43.8	38.0	32.2	26.2	21.4	16.4	13.0	9.9	7.2
1929-------	1955	50.2	50.4	48.4	43.1	37.5	31.2	25.6	19.8	15.8	12.3	9.0	6.5
1930-------	1956	52.5	52.2	47.7	43.2	36.6	30.5	23.9	19.1	15.0	11.2	8.2	6.1
1931-------	1957	55.2	52.2	48.4	42.6	36.2	28.7	22.9	18.4	13.8	10.1	7.6	5.4
1932-------	1958	55.9	53.1	48.5	42.1	34.0	27.4	21.9	16.8	12.4	9.5	6.9	5.1
1933-------	1959	57.1	53.7	47.7	39.5	32.2	26.5	20.0	15.1	11.5	8.7	6.6	4.9
1934-------	1960	58.0	52.9	45.0	37.7	31.3	24.1	18.0	14.0	10.8	8.4	6.4	4.4
1935-------	1961	57.0	50.3	43.0	36.7	28.4	21.7	17.0	13.3	10.6	8.2	5.7	3.9
1936-------	1962	54.8	48.2	41.6	33.1	25.8	20.5	16.0	13.3	10.4	7.3	5.1	3.5
1937-------	1963	52.4	46.1	37.4	30.2	24.6	19.6	16.6	13.2	9.4	6.6	4.6	
1938-------	1964	49.6	41.2	33.9	28.6	23.6	20.5	16.7	12.0	8.5	6.0		
1939-------	1965	44.0	37.0	32.4	28.1	24.8	21.1	15.2	10.8	7.9			
1940-------	1966	38.9	35.4	31.8	29.3	25.7	19.2	13.5	10.3				
1941-------	1967	37.0	34.5	33.2	30.4	23.5	16.9	13.0					
1942-------	1968	35.5	35.9	34.1	27.6	20.6	16.2						
1943-------	1969	36.6	36.2	30.8	23.7	19.2							
1944-------	1970	36.4	32.5	25.7	21.7								
1945-------	1971	32.4	26.6	23.2									
1946-------	1972	26.2	23.8										
1947-------	1973	23.1											

TABLE 4B. CENTRAL BIRTH RATES FOR WHITE WOMEN DURING EACH YEAR 1917-73 BY AGE AND LIVE-BIRTH ORDER FOR EACH COHORT FROM 1868 TO 1959--CON.

LIVE-BIRTH ORDER AND COHORT	DIAGONAL LINE FOR CALENDAR YEAR	CURRENT AGE											
		38	39	40	41	42	43	44	45	46	47	48	49
THIRD BIRTHS--CON.													
1868-------													0.0
1869-------												0.0	0.0
1870-------											0.1	0.0	0.0
1871-------										0.2	0.1	0.0	0.0
1872-------									0.4	0.2	0.1	0.0	0.0
1873-------								0.7	0.4	0.2	0.1	0.0	0.0
1874-------							1.1	0.7	0.4	0.2	0.1	0.0	0.0
1875-------						1.6	1.2	0.7	0.4	0.2	0.1	0.0	0.0
1876-------					2.6	1.7	1.1	0.7	0.4	0.2	0.1	0.0	0.0
1877-------				3.7	2.7	1.7	1.2	0.7	0.4	0.2	0.1	0.0	0.0
1878-------			5.6	3.9	2.6	1.7	1.2	0.7	0.4	0.2	0.1	0.0	0.0
1879-------	1917	7.1	5.7	3.7	2.7	1.7	1.1	0.6	0.4	0.2	0.1	0.0	0.0
1880-------	1918	7.1	5.6	3.8	2.6	1.6	1.1	0.7	0.3	0.2	0.1	0.0	0.0
1881-------	1919	7.0	5.6	3.8	2.5	1.6	1.1	0.6	0.3	0.2	0.1	0.0	0.0
1882-------	1920	7.1	5.7	3.6	2.4	1.6	1.1	0.6	0.3	0.2	0.1	0.0	0.0
1883-------	1921	7.2	5.4	3.5	2.5	1.6	1.0	0.6	0.3	0.2	0.0	0.0	0.0
1884-------	1922	6.8	5.3	3.6	2.5	1.4	1.0	0.5	0.3	0.1	0.1	0.0	0.0
1885-------	1923	6.8	5.4	3.5	2.3	1.5	1.0	0.5	0.3	0.2	0.1	0.0	0.0
1886-------	1924	6.9	5.2	3.4	2.4	1.4	0.8	0.5	0.3	0.1	0.1	0.0	0.0
1887-------	1925	6.7	5.1	3.4	2.2	1.3	0.9	0.5	0.3	0.1	0.0	0.0	0.0
1888-------	1926	6.4	5.0	3.1	2.1	1.4	0.9	0.4	0.2	0.1	0.0	0.0	0.0
1889-------	1927	6.4	4.7	3.1	2.2	1.3	0.8	0.4	0.2	0.1	0.0	0.0	0.0
1890-------	1928	6.2	4.6	3.2	2.0	1.3	0.8	0.4	0.2	0.1	0.0	0.0	0.0
1891-------	1929	5.8	4.5	2.9	1.9	1.2	0.8	0.4	0.2	0.1	0.0	0.0	0.0
1892-------	1930	5.7	4.2	2.7	1.8	1.2	0.7	0.4	0.2	0.1	0.0	0.0	0.0
1893-------	1931	5.4	3.9	2.7	1.8	1.1	0.7	0.4	0.2	0.1	0.0	0.0	0.0
1894-------	1932	5.2	3.8	2.6	1.8	1.1	0.7	0.4	0.2	0.1	0.0	0.0	0.0
1895-------	1933	4.9	3.8	2.6	1.7	1.1	0.7	0.4	0.2	0.1	0.0	0.0	0.0
1896-------	1934	4.9	3.7	2.5	1.7	1.1	0.7	0.4	0.2	0.1	0.0	0.0	0.0
1897-------	1935	4.8	3.7	2.4	1.7	1.1	0.7	0.4	0.2	0.1	0.0	0.0	0.0
1898-------	1936	4.7	3.5	2.6	1.7	1.1	0.7	0.4	0.2	0.1	0.0	0.0	0.0
1899-------	1937	4.7	3.7	2.7	1.7	1.1	0.7	0.4	0.3	0.1	0.0	0.0	0.0
1900-------	1938	4.8	3.8	2.7	1.8	1.1	0.8	0.5	0.3	0.1	0.1	0.0	0.0
1901-------	1939	4.9	3.7	2.7	1.9	1.3	1.0	0.6	0.3	0.2	0.0	0.0	0.0
1902-------	1940	4.9	3.8	2.9	2.2	1.5	1.0	0.6	0.3	0.1	0.0	0.0	0.0
1903-------	1941	5.0	4.2	3.3	2.5	1.7	1.1	0.6	0.3	0.1	0.0	0.0	0.0
1904-------	1942	5.5	4.9	3.7	2.7	1.8	1.2	0.6	0.3	0.1	0.0	0.0	0.0
1905-------	1943	6.5	5.3	4.1	2.8	1.8	1.1	0.6	0.3	0.1	0.0	0.0	0.0
1906-------	1944	7.1	5.9	4.2	2.9	1.8	1.1	0.5	0.3	0.1	0.0	0.0	0.0
1907-------	1945	7.9	6.1	4.3	2.9	1.7	1.1	0.6	0.3	0.1	0.0	0.0	0.0
1908-------	1946	8.2	6.3	4.2	2.7	1.7	1.1	0.6	0.3	0.1	0.0	0.0	0.0
1909-------	1947	8.4	6.0	4.1	2.8	1.8	1.2	0.7	0.3	0.1	0.0	0.0	0.0
1910-------	1948	7.9	6.0	4.2	2.9	2.0	1.2	0.7	0.3	0.2	0.0	0.0	0.0
1911-------	1949	7.9	6.0	4.4	3.2	2.0	1.3	0.7	0.4	0.1	0.0	0.0	0.0
1912-------	1950	8.0	6.3	4.8	3.2	2.2	1.3	0.8	0.3	0.1	0.0	0.0	0.0
1913-------	1951	8.5	6.8	4.8	3.5	2.2	1.4	0.7	0.3	0.1	0.0	0.0	0.0
1914-------	1952	9.2	7.0	5.1	3.5	2.3	1.3	0.7	0.3	0.1	0.0	0.0	0.0
1915-------	1953	9.3	7.2	5.2	3.6	2.2	1.2	0.7	0.3	0.1	0.1	0.0	0.0
1916-------	1954	9.5	7.3	5.0	3.4	2.0	1.2	0.7	0.3	0.2	0.0	0.0	0.0
1917-------	1955	9.7	7.2	5.1	3.2	2.0	1.2	0.6	0.3	0.1	0.0	0.0	0.0
1918-------	1956	9.5	7.0	4.7	3.1	2.0	1.2	0.6	0.3	0.1	0.0	0.0	0.0
1919-------	1957	9.5	6.8	4.7	3.0	1.9	1.1	0.6	0.3	0.1	0.0	0.0	0.0
1920-------	1958	8.9	6.6	4.5	3.0	1.8	1.0	0.5	0.2	0.1	0.0	0.0	0.0
1921-------	1959	8.6	6.3	4.3	2.8	1.7	0.9	0.5	0.2	0.1	0.0	0.0	0.0
1922-------	1960	8.1	6.0	4.0	2.6	1.5	0.9	0.4	0.2	0.1	0.0	0.0	0.0
1923-------	1961	7.8	5.5	3.7	2.5	1.5	0.8	0.4	0.2	0.0	0.0	0.0	0.0
1924-------	1962	7.1	5.2	3.5	2.2	1.3	0.7	0.4	0.1	0.1	0.0	0.0	0.0
1925-------	1963	6.7	4.9	3.2	2.0	1.1	0.6	0.3	0.1	0.0	0.0	0.0	
1926-------	1964	6.3	4.4	2.9	1.8	1.0	0.6	0.3	0.1	0.1	0.0		
1927-------	1965	5.7	4.0	2.7	1.6	1.0	0.5	0.2	0.1	0.0			
1928-------	1966	5.1	3.7	2.3	1.5	0.9	0.4	0.2	0.1				
1929-------	1967	4.8	3.2	2.1	1.4	0.7	0.4	0.2					
1930-------	1968	4.3	3.0	2.0	1.1	0.6	0.3						
1931-------	1969	3.9	2.8	1.7	1.0	0.5							
1932-------	1970	3.7	2.4	1.5	0.8								
1933-------	1971	3.3	2.1	1.2									
1934-------	1972	3.0	1.9										
1935-------	1973	2.6											

TABLE 4B. CENTRAL BIRTH RATES FOR WHITE WOMEN DURING EACH YEAR 1917-73 BY AGE AND LIVE-BIRTH ORDER FOR EACH COHORT FROM 1868 TO 1959--CON.

LIVE-BIRTH ORDER AND COHORT	DIAGONAL LINE FOR CALENDAR YEAR	CURRENT AGE											
		14	15	16	17	18	19	20	21	22	23	24	25
FOURTH BIRTHS													
1892-------													23.9
1893-------												19.5	23.7
1894-------											14.6	19.5	22.7
1895-------										9.2	14.8	19.0	22.8
1896-------									5.2	9.3	14.5	19.1	23.2
1897-------								2.5	5.3	9.1	14.5	19.6	21.4
1898-------							1.0	2.6	5.2	9.2	15.1	18.1	21.4
1899-------						0.2	1.0	2.5	5.2	9.5	13.7	18.0	20.7
1900-------					0.0	0.2	0.9	2.5	5.4	8.5	13.9	17.7	20.2
1901-------				0.0	0.0	0.2	0.9	2.5	4.7	8.5	13.6	17.4	19.8
1902-------			0.0	0.0	0.0	0.2	0.9	2.3	4.9	8.7	13.5	17.3	20.0
1903-------	1917	*	0.0	0.0	0.0	0.2	0.9	2.4	4.9	9.0	13.8	17.5	18.5
1904-------	1918	*	0.0	0.0	0.0	0.3	1.0	2.4	5.1	9.3	13.7	16.1	17.4
1905-------	1919	*	0.0	0.0	0.1	0.3	0.9	2.5	5.3	9.0	12.5	15.1	16.8
1906-------	1920	*	0.0	0.0	0.1	0.3	0.9	2.5	5.1	8.1	11.7	14.7	15.6
1907-------	1921	*	0.0	0.0	0.1	0.3	1.0	2.4	4.6	7.7	11.4	13.6	15.0
1908-------	1922	*	0.0	0.0	0.0	0.3	1.0	2.2	4.4	7.6	10.6	13.0	13.8
1909-------	1923	*	0.0	0.0	0.1	0.3	0.9	2.1	4.4	7.1	10.2	11.9	14.1
1910-------	1924	*	0.0	0.0	0.1	0.3	0.9	2.1	4.1	6.8	9.3	12.2	13.1
1911-------	1925	*	0.0	0.0	0.1	0.3	0.9	1.9	3.8	6.3	9.4	11.5	12.6
1912-------	1926	*	0.0	0.0	0.1	0.3	0.8	1.8	3.6	6.2	8.9	10.9	12.1
1913-------	1927	*	0.0	0.0	0.1	0.2	0.7	1.7	3.5	6.0	8.5	10.6	11.9
1914-------	1928	*	0.0	0.0	0.0	0.2	0.6	1.7	3.4	5.7	8.3	10.4	11.3
1915-------	1929	*	0.0	0.0	0.0	0.2	0.6	1.7	3.3	5.5	8.1	10.0	11.6
1916-------	1930	*	0.0	0.0	0.0	0.2	0.6	1.6	3.2	5.5	7.9	10.6	11.7
1917-------	1931	*	0.0	0.0	0.0	0.2	0.6	1.5	3.1	5.3	8.6	10.6	11.6
1918-------	1932	*	0.0	0.0	0.0	0.2	0.6	1.5	3.0	5.9	8.6	10.4	12.9
1919-------	1933	*	0.0	0.0	0.0	0.2	0.6	1.5	3.4	5.9	8.7	11.5	13.0
1920-------	1934	*	0.0	0.0	0.0	0.1	0.6	1.7	3.3	6.1	9.5	11.6	12.1
1921-------	1935	*	0.0	0.0	0.0	0.2	0.7	1.7	3.7	6.6	9.6	10.7	13.0
1922-------	1936	*	0.0	0.0	0.0	0.3	0.7	1.8	4.0	6.8	8.5	11.2	12.4
1923-------	1937	*	0.0	0.0	0.1	0.3	0.8	2.0	4.1	5.9	8.8	10.7	12.6
1924-------	1938	*	0.0	0.0	0.1	0.3	0.9	2.1	3.5	6.1	8.4	11.0	13.7
1925-------	1939	*	0.0	0.0	0.1	0.3	0.9	1.8	3.6	5.8	8.7	12.2	14.8
1926-------	1940	*	0.0	0.0	0.1	0.3	0.7	1.9	3.4	6.1	9.8	13.1	16.6
1927-------	1941	*	0.0	0.0	0.1	0.2	0.8	1.8	3.7	7.0	10.5	14.7	18.4
1928-------	1942	*	0.0	0.0	0.0	0.2	0.7	1.9	4.3	7.6	12.2	16.4	19.8
1929-------	1943	*	0.0	0.0	0.0	0.2	0.8	2.4	4.8	9.1	13.7	18.0	21.8
1930-------	1944	*	0.0	0.0	0.0	0.3	1.1	2.7	5.9	10.2	14.9	19.7	23.5
1931-------	1945	*	0.0	0.0	0.1	0.4	1.2	3.3	6.7	11.3	16.6	21.4	25.8
1932-------	1946	*	0.0	0.0	0.1	0.4	1.4	3.7	7.2	12.3	17.7	23.3	28.1
1933-------	1947	*	0.0	0.0	0.1	0.5	1.7	4.0	8.0	13.2	19.2	25.3	29.3
1934-------	1948	*	0.0	0.0	0.1	0.6	1.7	4.4	8.5	14.2	20.7	26.3	31.2
1935-------	1949	*	0.0	0.0	0.1	0.5	1.9	4.7	9.1	15.0	21.4	27.5	32.3
1936-------	1950	*	0.0	0.0	0.1	0.6	2.0	5.0	9.5	15.7	22.4	28.6	32.8
1937-------	1951	*	0.0	0.0	0.1	0.6	2.1	5.1	10.0	16.3	23.5	29.3	32.3
1938-------	1952	*	0.0	0.0	0.1	0.6	2.2	5.4	10.5	17.2	24.1	28.8	30.5
1939-------	1953	*	0.0	0.0	0.1	0.7	2.3	5.7	11.1	17.7	23.7	27.1	28.1
1940-------	1954	*	0.0	0.0	0.2	0.8	2.5	6.0	11.4	17.3	21.9	24.5	23.5
1941-------	1955	*	0.0	0.0	0.2	0.8	2.6	6.1	10.9	15.7	19.4	20.1	19.0
1942-------	1956	*	0.0	0.0	0.2	0.8	2.6	5.7	9.7	13.6	15.5	15.9	16.4
1943-------	1957	*	0.0	0.0	0.2	0.8	2.4	5.1	8.4	10.9	12.2	13.8	14.7
1944-------	1958	*	0.0	0.0	0.2	0.7	2.2	4.5	6.7	8.7	10.7	12.1	14.2
1945-------	1959	*	0.0	0.0	0.2	0.7	2.0	3.6	5.4	7.5	9.2	11.5	13.4
1946-------	1960	*	0.0	0.0	0.2	0.7	1.6	2.9	4.6	6.2	8.6	10.6	11.4
1947-------	1961	*	0.0	0.0	0.2	0.5	1.2	2.3	3.7	5.7	7.7	9.0	8.6
1948-------	1962	*	0.0	0.0	0.1	0.3	1.0	1.9	3.4	5.1	6.6	6.9	7.0
1949-------	1963	*	0.0	0.0	0.1	0.3	0.9	1.8	3.1	4.5	5.2	5.7	
1950-------	1964	*	0.0	0.0	0.1	0.3	0.8	1.6	2.6	3.5	4.2		
1951-------	1965	*	0.0	0.0	0.1	0.3	0.7	1.3	2.1	2.8			
1952-------	1966	*	0.0	0.0	0.1	0.2	0.5	1.1	1.7				
1953-------	1967	*	0.0	0.0	0.1	0.2	0.5	0.9					
1954-------	1968	*	0.0	0.0	0.0	0.2	0.4						
1955-------	1969	*	0.0	0.0	0.0	0.1							
1956-------	1970	*	0.0	0.0	0.0								
1957-------	1971	*	0.0	0.0									
1958-------	1972	*	0.0										
1959-------	1973	*											

TABLE 4B. CENTRAL BIRTH RATES FOR WHITE WOMEN DURING EACH YEAR 1917-73 BY AGE AND LIVE-BIRTH ORDER FOR EACH COHORT FROM 1868 TO 1959--CON.

LIVE-BIRTH ORDER AND COHORT	DIAGONAL LINE FOR CALENDAR YEAR	CURRENT AGE											
		26	27	28	29	30	31	32	33	34	35	36	37
FOURTH BIRTHS--CON.													
1880-------													10.8
1881-------												12.5	10.8
1882-------											14.9	12.5	10.4
1883-------										16.9	14.7	12.1	10.3
1884-------									19.2	16.6	14.1	12.0	10.5
1885-------								20.2	18.7	15.9	14.0	12.2	9.7
1886-------							22.8	19.9	18.0	15.9	14.5	11.4	9.8
1887-------						25.3	22.4	19.2	18.0	16.5	13.4	11.5	9.7
1888-------					29.0	24.9	21.5	19.1	18.6	15.0	13.4	11.4	9.6
1889-------				29.5	28.5	23.8	21.3	19.6	16.8	15.0	13.3	11.2	9.2
1890-------			28.8	29.2	27.3	23.7	22.1	17.8	16.8	14.9	12.8	10.7	8.9
1891-------	1917	26.2	28.6	27.9	27.1	24.0	19.9	17.8	16.7	14.4	12.5	10.3	8.3
1892-------	1918	25.9	27.1	27.7	27.1	21.6	19.8	17.5	16.0	13.8	11.9	9.6	7.7
1893-------	1919	24.6	26.9	27.2	24.4	21.1	19.6	16.9	15.3	13.3	11.0	8.9	7.6
1894-------	1920	24.6	26.7	24.8	23.8	20.8	18.8	16.2	14.9	12.4	10.3	8.9	7.3
1895-------	1921	24.7	24.6	24.1	23.3	19.9	18.1	15.7	13.9	11.6	10.3	8.5	7.0
1896-------	1922	22.8	24.0	23.3	22.1	19.2	17.5	14.6	12.9	11.5	9.7	8.1	6.6
1897-------	1923	22.3	23.2	22.1	21.3	18.5	16.3	13.8	12.8	10.8	9.3	7.7	6.6
1898-------	1924	21.9	22.3	21.6	20.7	17.3	15.3	13.7	12.0	10.3	8.8	7.6	6.2
1899-------	1925	21.3	21.9	21.3	19.4	16.4	15.3	13.0	11.8	10.0	9.0	7.3	6.0
1900-------	1926	20.8	21.8	19.6	18.0	16.1	14.4	12.6	11.2	10.0	8.5	6.9	5.8
1901-------	1927	21.0	19.9	18.1	17.6	15.2	13.7	11.9	11.2	9.4	8.0	6.7	5.8
1902-------	1928	19.2	18.4	17.7	16.6	14.4	12.9	11.7	10.4	8.8	7.7	6.7	5.5
1903-------	1929	17.9	17.9	16.8	15.8	13.7	12.9	10.9	9.7	8.5	7.6	6.4	5.3
1904-------	1930	17.5	17.1	16.3	15.2	13.7	12.1	10.3	9.4	8.3	7.4	6.3	5.5
1905-------	1931	16.4	16.5	15.6	15.0	12.8	11.3	10.0	9.1	8.1	7.2	6.4	5.7
1906-------	1932	15.8	15.6	15.1	14.0	12.0	10.9	9.7	8.9	8.0	7.3	6.4	6.5
1907-------	1933	14.8	15.4	14.1	13.1	11.6	10.6	9.4	8.9	8.1	7.5	7.4	6.9
1908-------	1934	14.8	14.2	13.2	12.4	11.2	10.2	9.4	8.8	8.4	8.5	7.8	7.2
1909-------	1935	13.8	13.5	12.7	12.4	10.8	10.3	9.5	9.3	9.5	9.0	8.4	7.4
1910-------	1936	13.1	12.9	12.6	11.7	10.9	10.3	9.8	10.6	10.0	9.5	8.5	7.6
1911-------	1937	12.7	12.9	12.0	11.8	11.0	10.6	11.2	11.1	10.5	9.9	9.0	7.4
1912-------	1938	12.5	12.1	11.9	11.8	11.4	12.0	11.7	11.3	10.9	10.2	8.6	7.4
1913-------	1939	11.7	12.1	12.1	12.2	12.8	12.5	12.0	12.0	11.3	9.9	8.7	7.7
1914-------	1940	11.8	12.3	12.6	13.6	13.1	12.7	12.7	12.3	11.1	10.2	9.2	8.2
1915-------	1941	11.9	12.6	14.0	13.9	13.2	13.5	13.0	12.2	11.6	10.8	10.0	9.0
1916-------	1942	12.1	14.1	14.1	13.6	13.9	13.8	12.8	12.7	12.1	11.6	10.7	9.6
1917-------	1943	13.5	14.1	13.7	14.5	14.1	13.6	13.5	13.3	13.0	12.5	11.6	10.3
1918-------	1944	13.6	13.4	14.3	14.5	13.8	14.2	13.9	14.1	14.0	13.3	12.1	10.4
1919-------	1945	13.0	14.4	14.5	14.5	15.0	15.1	15.4	15.9	15.2	14.3	12.6	10.8
1920-------	1946	13.8	14.3	14.4	15.6	15.9	16.6	17.3	17.0	16.3	14.7	12.8	11.0
1921-------	1947	13.6	14.3	15.8	16.8	17.6	18.8	18.4	18.4	17.0	15.1	13.4	10.9
1922-------	1948	13.5	15.3	16.6	18.4	19.6	19.9	19.9	19.0	17.4	15.7	13.1	10.9
1923-------	1949	14.6	16.3	18.7	20.4	20.8	21.5	20.7	19.7	18.2	15.6	13.1	10.7
1924-------	1950	15.7	18.6	20.6	21.9	22.8	22.6	21.9	20.6	18.1	15.5	13.0	10.3
1925-------	1951	17.7	20.4	22.2	23.9	24.0	23.7	22.6	20.6	18.0	15.4	12.5	9.7
1926-------	1952	19.6	22.1	24.3	25.3	25.4	24.6	22.6	20.5	18.0	14.9	11.8	9.3
1927-------	1953	21.3	24.0	25.7	26.8	26.4	24.9	22.9	20.4	17.4	14.0	11.3	8.9
1928-------	1954	23.1	25.5	27.3	28.1	26.9	25.6	22.9	20.1	16.4	13.6	10.9	8.2
1929-------	1955	24.8	27.4	29.2	29.1	28.2	25.8	23.2	19.2	16.1	13.2	10.0	7.3
1930-------	1956	26.9	29.6	30.4	30.6	28.6	26.3	22.0	18.9	15.7	12.0	8.9	6.7
1931-------	1957	29.3	31.1	32.2	31.4	29.3	25.3	21.8	18.4	14.2	10.7	8.4	6.2
1932-------	1958	30.8	33.2	33.3	31.8	28.2	24.7	21.0	16.7	12.6	10.0	7.6	5.7
1933-------	1959	32.9	34.5	33.8	31.0	27.5	23.8	18.8	14.6	11.9	9.2	7.2	5.4
1934-------	1960	34.1	34.8	32.9	30.0	26.5	21.3	16.6	13.6	10.8	8.8	6.8	5.0
1935-------	1961	34.6	34.1	31.9	28.8	23.3	18.7	15.4	12.4	10.5	8.4	6.2	4.2
1936-------	1962	33.9	32.8	30.4	25.3	20.5	17.1	14.0	12.2	10.1	7.5	5.2	3.6
1937-------	1963	32.4	30.9	26.3	21.9	18.8	15.8	14.1	12.0	9.0	6.4	4.6	
1938-------	1964	30.2	26.4	22.5	20.1	17.4	15.9	13.8	10.8	7.7	5.6		
1939-------	1965	25.7	22.4	20.6	18.6	17.5	15.8	12.6	9.3	6.8			
1940-------	1966	21.3	20.1	19.0	18.8	17.5	14.3	10.6	8.0				
1941-------	1967	18.7	18.4	19.1	18.5	15.7	11.9	9.2					
1942-------	1968	16.9	18.3	18.5	16.5	12.6	10.2						
1943-------	1969	16.5	17.5	16.3	13.1	10.8							
1944-------	1970	15.8	15.3	12.7	11.0								
1945-------	1971	13.6	11.8	10.6									
1946-------	1972	10.3	9.6										
1947-------	1973	8.4											

TABLE 4B. CENTRAL BIRTH RATES FOR WHITE WOMEN DURING EACH YEAR 1917-73 BY AGE AND LIVE-BIRTH ORDER FOR EACH COHORT FROM 1868 TO 1959--CON.

LIVE-BIRTH ORDER AND COHORT	DIAGONAL LINE FOR CALENDAR YEAR	CURRENT AGE											
		38	39	40	41	42	43	44	45	46	47	48	49
FOURTH BIRTHS--CON.													
1868-------													0.1
1869-------												0.1	0.1
1870-------											0.2	0.1	0.1
1871-------										0.3	0.2	0.1	0.1
1872-------									0.6	0.3	0.1	0.1	0.1
1873-------								0.9	0.6	0.3	0.2	0.1	0.1
1874-------							1.6	0.9	0.5	0.3	0.1	0.1	0.0
1875-------						2.2	1.6	0.9	0.6	0.3	0.1	0.1	0.0
1876-------					3.4	2.2	1.6	1.0	0.5	0.3	0.1	0.1	0.0
1877-------				4.9	3.4	2.2	1.6	0.9	0.5	0.3	0.1	0.1	0.0
1878-------			7.0	4.8	3.4	2.3	1.6	0.9	0.5	0.3	0.1	0.0	0.0
1879-------	1917	8.8	7.0	4.8	3.5	2.2	1.5	0.9	0.5	0.3	0.1	0.1	0.0
1880-------	1918	8.8	6.9	4.8	3.4	2.2	1.5	0.9	0.5	0.3	0.1	0.0	0.0
1881-------	1919	8.5	6.8	4.8	3.3	2.1	1.5	0.8	0.4	0.2	0.1	0.0	0.0
1882-------	1920	8.4	6.9	4.5	3.2	2.1	1.4	0.8	0.4	0.2	0.1	0.0	0.0
1883-------	1921	8.5	6.4	4.4	3.2	2.0	1.3	0.7	0.4	0.2	0.1	0.0	0.0
1884-------	1922	7.9	6.4	4.4	3.1	2.0	1.2	0.7	0.4	0.2	0.1	0.0	0.0
1885-------	1923	7.9	6.3	4.4	2.9	1.8	1.2	0.7	0.4	0.2	0.1	0.0	0.0
1886-------	1924	7.9	6.3	4.1	2.8	1.7	1.1	0.7	0.3	0.2	0.1	0.0	0.0
1887-------	1925	7.9	6.0	4.0	2.7	1.7	1.2	0.6	0.4	0.2	0.1	0.0	0.0
1888-------	1926	7.4	5.8	3.8	2.6	1.7	1.1	0.6	0.3	0.2	0.1	0.0	0.0
1889-------	1927	7.2	5.5	3.6	2.6	1.6	1.1	0.6	0.3	0.2	0.1	0.0	0.0
1890-------	1928	6.8	5.2	3.7	2.4	1.6	1.0	0.6	0.3	0.1	0.1	0.0	0.0
1891-------	1929	6.3	5.2	3.4	2.4	1.5	1.0	0.6	0.3	0.2	0.1	0.0	0.0
1892-------	1930	6.4	4.8	3.2	2.2	1.5	1.0	0.5	0.3	0.2	0.0	0.0	0.0
1893-------	1931	6.0	4.6	3.1	2.2	1.4	0.9	0.5	0.3	0.1	0.0	0.0	0.0
1894-------	1932	5.6	4.4	3.2	2.1	1.3	0.9	0.5	0.3	0.1	0.0	0.0	0.0
1895-------	1933	5.4	4.4	2.9	2.0	1.3	0.9	0.5	0.3	0.1	0.0	0.0	0.0
1896-------	1934	5.4	4.1	2.8	2.0	1.3	0.9	0.5	0.2	0.1	0.1	0.0	0.0
1897-------	1935	5.1	3.9	2.8	1.9	1.3	0.8	0.4	0.2	0.1	0.1	0.0	0.0
1898-------	1936	4.9	3.8	2.7	2.0	1.3	0.8	0.5	0.3	0.2	0.1	0.0	0.0
1899-------	1937	4.8	3.7	2.7	1.9	1.3	0.8	0.5	0.3	0.1	0.1	0.0	0.0
1900-------	1938	4.7	3.7	2.6	1.9	1.2	0.9	0.6	0.3	0.2	0.0	0.0	0.0
1901-------	1939	4.5	3.4	2.6	1.9	1.4	1.0	0.6	0.3	0.1	0.0	0.0	0.0
1902-------	1940	4.3	3.5	2.7	2.2	1.5	1.1	0.6	0.3	0.1	0.0	0.0	0.0
1903-------	1941	4.4	3.8	3.1	2.2	1.6	1.0	0.6	0.3	0.1	0.1	0.0	0.0
1904-------	1942	4.7	4.3	3.2	2.5	1.6	1.0	0.6	0.3	0.2	0.0	0.0	0.0
1905-------	1943	5.4	4.5	3.4	2.4	1.7	1.0	0.6	0.3	0.1	0.0	0.0	0.0
1906-------	1944	5.7	4.8	3.5	2.6	1.6	1.0	0.6	0.3	0.1	0.1	0.0	0.0
1907-------	1945	6.0	4.9	3.7	2.5	1.6	1.0	0.6	0.3	0.2	0.1	0.0	0.0
1908-------	1946	6.1	4.9	3.5	2.4	1.6	1.1	0.6	0.3	0.2	0.0	0.0	0.0
1909-------	1947	6.2	4.8	3.5	2.5	1.7	1.1	0.7	0.3	0.1	0.1	0.0	0.0
1910-------	1948	6.1	4.8	3.5	2.6	1.8	1.3	0.6	0.3	0.2	0.0	0.0	0.0
1911-------	1949	6.1	4.9	3.8	2.8	2.0	1.2	0.7	0.3	0.1	0.1	0.0	0.0
1912-------	1950	6.3	5.1	4.1	3.0	2.0	1.3	0.7	0.4	0.2	0.1	0.0	0.0
1913-------	1951	6.7	5.7	4.4	3.2	2.1	1.3	0.8	0.4	0.2	0.1	0.0	0.0
1914-------	1952	7.3	6.0	4.7	3.3	2.1	1.4	0.8	0.4	0.2	0.0	0.0	0.0
1915-------	1953	7.8	6.5	4.8	3.4	2.3	1.4	0.8	0.4	0.2	0.1	0.0	0.0
1916-------	1954	8.3	6.6	4.7	3.5	2.2	1.4	0.8	0.4	0.2	0.0	0.0	0.0
1917-------	1955	8.6	6.7	5.1	3.4	2.3	1.3	0.8	0.4	0.1	0.0	0.0	0.0
1918-------	1956	8.5	6.9	4.8	3.4	2.2	1.4	0.7	0.3	0.1	0.0	0.0	0.0
1919-------	1957	8.9	6.7	4.9	3.4	2.3	1.4	0.7	0.3	0.1	0.0	0.0	0.0
1920-------	1958	8.7	6.8	4.9	3.5	2.2	1.2	0.7	0.3	0.1	0.0	0.0	0.0
1921-------	1959	8.8	6.8	4.9	3.3	2.0	1.2	0.6	0.3	0.1	0.0	0.0	0.0
1922-------	1960	8.5	6.5	4.6	3.0	1.8	1.1	0.6	0.3	0.1	0.0	0.0	0.0
1923-------	1961	8.3	6.1	4.2	2.8	1.8	1.0	0.6	0.2	0.1	0.0	0.0	0.0
1924-------	1962	7.9	5.8	4.1	2.7	1.6	1.0	0.5	0.2	0.1	0.0	0.0	0.0
1925-------	1963	7.4	5.7	3.8	2.3	1.5	0.8	0.4	0.2	0.1	0.0	0.0	
1926-------	1964	7.3	5.1	3.4	2.3	1.3	0.7	0.4	0.1	0.0	0.0		
1927-------	1965	6.5	4.6	3.1	1.9	1.1	0.7	0.3	0.1	0.0			
1928-------	1966	5.9	4.2	2.7	1.7	1.1	0.5	0.2	0.1				
1929-------	1967	5.4	3.7	2.6	1.6	0.9	0.5	0.2					
1930-------	1968	4.9	3.5	2.4	1.3	0.8	0.4						
1931-------	1969	4.6	3.3	2.0	1.2	0.6							
1932-------	1970	4.3	2.8	1.7	1.0								
1933-------	1971	3.8	2.4	1.5									
1934-------	1972	3.3	2.1										
1935-------	1973	2.8											

TABLE 4B. CENTRAL BIRTH RATES FOR WHITE WOMEN DURING EACH YEAR 1917-73 BY AGE AND LIVE-BIRTH ORDER FOR EACH COHORT FROM 1868 TO 1959--CON.

LIVE-BIRTH ORDER AND COHORT	DIAGONAL LINE FOR CALENDAR YEAR	CURRENT AGE											
		14	15	16	17	18	19	20	21	22	23	24	25
FIFTH BIRTHS													
1892-------													11.4
1893-------												7.7	11.0
1894-------											4.7	7.4	10.6
1895-------										2.3	4.4	7.2	10.8
1896-------									1.1	2.2	4.3	7.4	11.2
1897-------								0.5	1.0	2.1	4.5	7.8	10.3
1898-------							*	0.4	1.0	2.2	4.8	7.2	10.6
1899-------						*	*	0.4	1.1	2.4	4.4	7.5	10.2
1900-------					*	*	*	0.5	1.1	2.2	4.7	7.2	9.7
1901-------				*	*	*	*	0.5	1.0	2.2	4.4	6.8	9.4
1902-------			*	*	*	*	*	0.4	1.1	2.3	4.2	6.8	9.3
1903-------	1917	*	*	*	*	*	*	0.5	1.1	2.2	4.4	6.8	8.9
1904-------	1918	*	*	*	*	*	*	0.5	1.1	2.4	4.3	6.5	8.6
1905-------	1919	*	*	*	*	*	*	0.5	1.2	2.3	4.1	6.2	8.2
1906-------	1920	*	*	*	*	*	*	0.5	1.1	2.2	3.9	5.9	7.6
1907-------	1921	*	*	*	*	*	*	0.5	1.1	2.0	3.7	5.4	7.1
1908-------	1922	*	*	*	*	*	*	0.4	1.0	1.9	3.4	5.1	6.5
1909-------	1923	*	*	*	*	*	*	0.4	1.0	1.8	3.2	4.6	6.6
1910-------	1924	*	*	*	*	*	*	0.4	0.9	1.7	2.9	4.7	6.2
1911-------	1925	*	*	*	*	*	*	0.4	0.8	1.6	2.9	4.6	5.8
1912-------	1926	*	*	*	*	*	*	0.3	0.8	1.5	2.9	4.2	5.6
1913-------	1927	*	*	*	*	*	*	0.3	0.7	1.5	2.7	4.0	5.5
1914-------	1928	*	*	*	*	*	*	0.3	0.7	1.4	2.6	4.1	5.1
1915-------	1929	*	*	*	*	*	*	0.3	0.7	1.4	2.6	3.8	5.3
1916-------	1930	*	*	*	*	*	*	0.3	0.7	1.4	2.5	4.1	5.2
1917-------	1931	*	*	*	*	*	*	0.3	0.7	1.3	2.8	4.0	5.2
1918-------	1932	*	*	*	*	*	*	0.3	0.6	1.5	2.8	4.0	5.7
1919-------	1933	*	*	*	*	*	*	0.3	0.7	1.5	2.8	4.4	5.8
1920-------	1934	*	*	*	*	*	*	0.3	0.7	1.6	3.0	4.5	5.5
1921-------	1935	*	*	*	*	*	*	0.3	0.8	1.7	3.1	4.3	5.6
1922-------	1936	*	*	*	*	*	*	0.3	0.9	1.8	2.8	4.2	5.4
1923-------	1937	*	*	*	*	*	*	0.4	0.9	1.6	2.8	4.0	5.4
1924-------	1938	*	*	*	*	*	*	0.4	0.8	1.6	2.7	4.1	5.5
1925-------	1939	*	*	*	*	*	*	0.4	0.8	1.5	2.8	4.3	5.7
1926-------	1940	*	*	*	*	*	*	0.4	0.8	1.6	3.0	4.4	6.4
1927-------	1941	*	*	*	*	*	*	0.4	0.8	1.8	3.1	5.0	7.1
1928-------	1942	*	*	*	*	*	*	0.4	1.0	1.9	3.5	5.6	7.6
1929-------	1943	*	*	*	*	*	*	0.5	1.0	2.2	4.1	6.3	8.6
1930-------	1944	*	*	*	*	*	*	0.4	1.2	2.6	4.6	7.1	9.4
1931-------	1945	*	*	*	*	*	*	0.5	1.5	3.0	5.2	7.7	10.5
1932-------	1946	*	*	*	*	*	*	0.6	1.6	3.3	5.7	8.5	11.3
1933-------	1947	*	*	*	*	*	*	0.7	1.8	3.6	6.1	9.1	12.2
1934-------	1948	*	*	*	*	*	*	0.8	2.0	3.8	6.5	9.8	12.7
1935-------	1949	*	*	*	*	*	*	0.8	2.1	4.1	7.0	10.1	13.4
1936-------	1950	*	*	*	*	*	*	0.9	2.3	4.3	7.2	10.7	14.2
1937-------	1951	*	*	*	*	*	*	0.9	2.3	4.5	7.8	11.3	13.9
1938-------	1952	*	*	*	*	*	*	1.0	2.4	4.8	7.8	11.1	13.1
1939-------	1953	*	*	*	*	*	*	1.1	2.6	4.9	8.1	10.4	12.3
1940-------	1954	*	*	*	*	*	*	1.1	2.7	5.1	7.4	9.6	9.9
1941-------	1955	*	*	*	*	*	*	1.2	2.8	4.7	6.7	7.6	7.9
1942-------	1956	*	*	*	*	*	*	1.2	2.5	4.0	5.1	5.8	6.5
1943-------	1957	*	*	*	*	*	*	1.0	2.1	3.1	3.9	4.9	5.4
1944-------	1958	*	*	*	*	*	*	0.9	1.7	2.4	3.3	4.0	5.1
1945-------	1959	*	*	*	*	*	*	0.8	1.3	2.1	2.7	3.8	4.7
1946-------	1960	*	*	*	*	*	*	0.6	1.1	1.6	2.5	3.4	3.9
1947-------	1961	*	*	*	*	*	*	0.5	0.8	1.4	2.2	2.8	2.8
1948-------	1962	*	*	*	*	*	*	0.3	0.8	1.2	1.8	2.0	2.2
1949-------	1963	*	*	*	*	*	*	0.3	0.7	1.1	1.3	1.6	
1950-------	1964	*	*	*	*	*	*	0.3	0.6	0.7	1.1		
1951-------	1965	*	*	*	*	*	*	0.3	0.4	0.7			
1952-------	1966	*	*	*	*	*	*	0.2	0.4				
1953-------	1967	*	*	*	*	*	*	0.2					
1954-------	1968	*	*	*	*	*	*						
1955-------	1969	*	*	*	*	*							
1956-------	1970	*	*	*	*								
1957-------	1971	*	*	*									
1958-------	1972	*	*										
1959-------	1973	*											

TABLE 4B. CENTRAL BIRTH RATES FOR WHITE WOMEN DURING EACH YEAR 1917-73 BY AGE AND LIVE-BIRTH ORDER FOR EACH COHORT FROM 1868 TO 1959--CON.

LIVE-BIRTH ORDER AND COHORT	DIAGONAL LINE FOR CALENDAR YEAR	CURRENT AGE											
		26	27	28	29	30	31	32	33	34	35	36	37
FIFTH BIRTHS--CON.													
1880-------													11.8
1881-------												13.1	11.6
1882-------											15.1	12.9	11.3
1883-------										16.5	14.9	12.6	11.2
1884-------									18.2	16.3	14.3	12.4	11.1
1885-------								18.4	18.0	15.4	14.2	12.4	10.3
1886-------							20.0	18.4	17.0	15.4	14.2	11.6	10.2
1887-------						20.7	20.0	17.3	17.0	15.4	13.3	11.5	10.1
1888-------					22.2	20.4	18.8	17.3	16.8	14.4	13.1	11.3	9.5
1889-------				20.6	21.7	19.3	18.6	17.1	15.7	14.2	12.9	10.9	9.2
1890-------			18.3	20.0	20.7	19.2	18.5	15.9	15.6	14.0	12.1	10.2	8.7
1891-------	1917	14.6	17.8	19.3	20.7	19.2	17.2	15.8	15.2	13.3	11.4	9.8	8.3
1892-------	1918	14.2	17.1	19.3	20.8	17.5	16.9	15.4	14.1	12.3	10.9	9.2	7.6
1893-------	1919	13.6	17.1	19.5	18.7	17.3	16.5	14.5	13.2	11.9	10.1	8.5	7.5
1894-------	1920	13.7	17.5	17.5	18.6	16.8	15.6	13.6	12.9	11.1	9.7	8.4	7.1
1895-------	1921	14.1	15.8	17.6	18.0	16.0	14.6	13.3	12.1	10.5	9.5	8.0	6.7
1896-------	1922	12.9	16.0	16.8	16.8	14.9	14.3	12.4	11.3	10.2	8.8	7.6	6.3
1897-------	1923	13.0	15.3	15.6	15.6	14.5	13.3	11.6	11.0	9.5	8.6	7.0	6.2
1898-------	1924	12.6	14.3	14.7	15.5	13.7	12.6	11.4	10.3	9.2	7.9	7.0	5.8
1899-------	1925	12.0	13.6	14.9	14.8	13.0	12.4	10.9	10.2	8.7	8.0	6.6	5.5
1900-------	1926	11.6	13.8	14.0	13.7	12.8	11.7	10.6	9.5	8.6	7.5	6.2	5.2
1901-------	1927	11.6	12.9	13.0	13.4	11.9	11.2	9.7	9.4	8.1	6.9	5.9	5.1
1902-------	1928	10.9	12.1	12.7	12.4	11.2	10.2	9.5	8.6	7.4	6.5	5.7	4.8
1903-------	1929	10.5	11.8	11.8	11.7	10.4	10.1	8.7	8.1	7.0	6.4	5.3	4.7
1904-------	1930	10.1	11.0	11.4	10.9	10.3	9.4	8.3	7.6	6.8	6.0	5.2	4.5
1905-------	1931	9.4	10.5	10.4	10.9	9.6	8.8	7.9	7.4	6.4	5.8	5.0	4.6
1906-------	1932	8.9	9.5	10.3	10.1	8.9	8.4	7.6	6.9	6.2	5.6	5.0	5.0
1907-------	1933	8.1	9.5	9.7	9.4	8.6	8.1	7.0	6.6	6.0	5.6	5.5	5.1
1908-------	1934	8.1	9.0	8.9	9.0	8.2	7.4	6.8	6.5	6.1	6.1	5.6	5.1
1909-------	1935	7.7	8.3	8.7	8.7	7.6	7.2	6.7	6.6	6.7	6.2	5.8	5.2
1910-------	1936	7.1	8.1	8.4	8.1	7.4	7.1	6.8	7.2	6.7	6.4	5.8	5.2
1911-------	1937	6.9	7.9	7.8	7.9	7.4	7.1	7.5	7.3	6.9	6.4	5.7	5.0
1912-------	1938	6.7	7.2	7.7	7.8	7.2	7.7	7.5	7.2	6.9	6.3	5.5	5.0
1913-------	1939	6.1	7.1	7.6	7.5	7.9	7.7	7.3	7.3	6.8	6.2	5.5	5.1
1914-------	1940	6.1	7.0	7.2	8.2	7.9	7.7	7.5	7.3	6.7	6.2	5.8	5.4
1915-------	1941	6.1	6.9	8.0	8.2	7.8	7.8	7.5	7.1	6.8	6.5	6.2	5.9
1916-------	1942	6.1	7.6	8.0	8.0	8.0	7.7	7.3	7.2	7.0	6.9	6.7	6.3
1917-------	1943	6.7	7.6	7.6	8.2	7.8	7.5	7.4	7.4	7.5	7.4	7.1	6.6
1918-------	1944	6.7	7.1	7.8	7.9	7.6	7.6	7.6	7.9	7.9	7.8	7.6	6.9
1919-------	1945	6.4	7.4	7.8	7.8	7.9	8.0	8.3	8.7	8.6	8.5	8.0	7.3
1920-------	1946	6.6	7.3	7.7	8.1	8.2	8.6	9.2	9.4	9.3	9.1	8.5	7.7
1921-------	1947	6.5	7.3	7.9	8.3	8.8	9.6	9.8	10.0	10.0	9.6	9.1	7.9
1922-------	1948	6.4	7.3	7.9	8.9	9.6	10.2	10.4	10.8	10.7	10.1	9.0	8.1
1923-------	1949	6.5	7.4	8.6	9.7	10.3	11.0	11.4	11.6	11.2	10.2	9.5	8.2
1924-------	1950	6.7	8.3	9.6	10.7	11.4	12.0	12.3	12.2	11.6	10.7	9.6	8.3
1925-------	1951	7.4	9.1	10.4	11.8	12.3	12.9	13.1	12.6	11.9	11.0	9.8	8.0
1926-------	1952	8.2	9.7	11.4	12.5	13.1	13.8	13.4	13.0	12.2	11.0	9.3	7.7
1927-------	1953	8.8	10.8	12.2	13.4	14.1	14.1	14.0	13.5	12.5	10.7	9.1	7.4
1928-------	1954	9.8	11.6	13.0	14.4	14.7	15.0	14.5	13.8	12.1	10.4	8.8	6.8
1929-------	1955	10.6	12.6	14.3	15.4	15.9	15.8	15.2	13.7	12.0	10.2	8.2	6.2
1930-------	1956	11.7	13.8	15.3	16.5	16.7	16.4	15.1	13.6	11.7	9.5	7.4	5.7
1931-------	1957	12.9	14.9	16.5	17.4	17.5	16.6	15.1	13.2	10.9	8.4	6.7	5.2
1932-------	1958	13.8	16.0	17.4	18.3	17.5	16.5	14.5	12.2	9.6	7.7	6.1	4.9
1933-------	1959	14.7	16.8	18.5	18.4	17.3	15.7	13.2	10.6	8.7	7.0	5.9	4.7
1934-------	1960	15.5	17.9	18.4	17.9	16.6	14.0	11.4	9.7	7.9	6.9	5.6	4.2
1935-------	1961	16.5	17.7	17.9	17.2	14.4	12.2	10.4	8.6	7.7	6.4	5.0	3.5
1936-------	1962	16.2	17.2	17.0	14.6	12.5	11.0	9.2	8.4	7.2	5.8	4.1	3.0
1937-------	1963	15.6	16.1	14.4	12.6	11.2	9.7	9.0	8.0	6.5	4.8	3.5	
1938-------	1964	14.4	13.4	12.0	11.1	9.9	9.6	8.8	7.2	5.4	4.0		
1939-------	1965	12.0	11.2	10.5	9.8	9.8	9.3	7.8	5.9	4.5			
1940-------	1966	9.7	9.6	9.3	9.7	9.5	8.2	6.3	4.9				
1941-------	1967	8.2	8.3	9.0	9.2	8.2	6.4	5.2					
1942-------	1968	6.9	7.9	8.3	7.9	6.3	5.3						
1943-------	1969	6.5	7.1	7.1	5.9	5.1							
1944-------	1970	5.9	6.1	5.3	4.8								
1945-------	1971	5.0	4.6	4.2									
1946-------	1972	3.7	3.5										
1947-------	1973	2.8											

TABLE 4B. CENTRAL BIRTH RATES FOR WHITE WOMEN DURING EACH YEAR 1917-73 BY AGE AND LIVE-BIRTH ORDER FOR EACH COHORT FROM 1868 TO 1959--CON.

LIVE-BIRTH ORDER AND COHORT	DIAGONAL LINE FOR CALENDAR YEAR	CURRENT AGE											
		38	39	40	41	42	43	44	45	46	47	48	49
FIFTH BIRTHS--CON.													
1868-------													0.0
1869-------												0.1	0.0
1870-------											0.2	0.1	0.0
1871-------										0.4	0.3	0.1	0.0
1872-------									0.7	0.5	0.2	0.1	0.0
1873-------								1.2	0.8	0.5	0.2	0.1	0.0
1874-------							1.9	1.3	0.7	0.5	0.2	0.1	0.0
1875-------						2.7	2.0	1.2	0.7	0.4	0.2	0.1	0.0
1876-------					4.0	2.7	1.9	1.2	0.7	0.3	0.2	0.1	0.0
1877-------				5.6	4.1	2.6	1.9	1.2	0.6	0.3	0.2	0.1	0.0
1878-------			8.2	5.7	4.0	2.6	1.9	1.1	0.6	0.3	0.1	0.1	0.0
1879-------	1917	9.9	8.2	5.6	3.9	2.7	1.8	1.1	0.6	0.3	0.2	0.1	0.0
1880-------	1918	9.8	8.0	5.4	4.1	2.5	1.8	1.1	0.6	0.3	0.2	0.1	0.0
1881-------	1919	9.5	7.9	5.5	3.7	2.5	1.8	1.0	0.5	0.3	0.1	0.0	0.0
1882-------	1920	9.4	7.9	5.1	3.7	2.4	1.6	0.9	0.5	0.3	0.1	0.0	0.0
1883-------	1921	9.3	7.2	5.0	3.6	2.3	1.5	0.9	0.5	0.3	0.1	0.0	0.0
1884-------	1922	8.6	7.1	4.9	3.5	2.2	1.5	0.9	0.5	0.3	0.1	0.0	0.0
1885-------	1923	8.5	7.0	4.6	3.3	2.2	1.4	0.8	0.5	0.2	0.1	0.1	0.0
1886-------	1924	8.4	6.6	4.5	3.2	2.0	1.3	0.8	0.4	0.3	0.1	0.1	0.0
1887-------	1925	8.0	6.4	4.4	3.1	1.9	1.4	0.8	0.4	0.2	0.1	0.0	0.0
1888-------	1926	7.7	6.2	4.2	2.8	1.9	1.2	0.7	0.4	0.2	0.1	0.0	0.0
1889-------	1927	7.5	5.9	3.9	2.9	1.8	1.2	0.7	0.4	0.2	0.1	0.0	0.0
1890-------	1928	7.0	5.4	3.9	2.6	1.8	1.2	0.7	0.3	0.2	0.0	0.1	0.0
1891-------	1929	6.4	5.4	3.6	2.6	1.8	1.2	0.6	0.4	0.1	0.1	0.1	0.0
1892-------	1930	6.4	5.0	3.5	2.5	1.7	1.1	0.6	0.3	0.2	0.1	0.0	0.0
1893-------	1931	6.0	4.7	3.3	2.4	1.6	1.0	0.5	0.3	0.2	0.1	0.0	0.0
1894-------	1932	5.6	4.5	3.2	2.3	1.4	0.9	0.6	0.3	0.2	0.1	0.0	0.0
1895-------	1933	5.3	4.4	3.1	2.1	1.4	1.0	0.5	0.3	0.1	0.0	0.0	0.0
1896-------	1934	5.2	4.1	2.9	2.1	1.4	0.9	0.5	0.2	0.1	0.0	0.0	0.0
1897-------	1935	4.9	3.8	2.8	2.0	1.3	0.8	0.4	0.3	0.1	0.0	0.0	0.0
1898-------	1936	4.6	3.7	2.7	2.0	1.3	0.8	0.6	0.3	0.1	0.1	0.0	0.0
1899-------	1937	4.4	3.7	2.7	1.9	1.3	0.9	0.6	0.3	0.2	0.1	0.0	0.0
1900-------	1938	4.4	3.5	2.6	1.9	1.3	0.9	0.6	0.3	0.2	0.0	0.0	0.0
1901-------	1939	4.1	3.4	2.5	1.8	1.4	1.0	0.6	0.3	0.1	0.0	0.0	0.0
1902-------	1940	4.0	3.2	2.4	2.0	1.5	0.9	0.6	0.3	0.1	0.0	0.0	0.0
1903-------	1941	3.8	3.2	2.6	2.1	1.4	1.0	0.6	0.3	0.1	0.0	0.0	0.0
1904-------	1942	3.9	3.5	2.7	2.0	1.4	1.0	0.5	0.3	0.1	0.0	0.0	0.0
1905-------	1943	4.3	3.6	2.8	2.1	1.5	0.9	0.5	0.3	0.1	0.0	0.0	0.0
1906-------	1944	4.4	3.7	2.8	2.1	1.4	0.8	0.5	0.3	0.1	0.1	0.0	0.0
1907-------	1945	4.4	3.7	2.9	2.0	1.3	0.9	0.5	0.3	0.2	0.1	0.0	0.0
1908-------	1946	4.4	3.7	2.6	1.9	1.4	0.9	0.6	0.3	0.2	0.1	0.0	0.0
1909-------	1947	4.5	3.5	2.6	2.0	1.4	1.0	0.6	0.3	0.2	0.1	0.0	0.0
1910-------	1948	4.2	3.5	2.7	2.0	1.5	1.0	0.6	0.3	0.2	0.1	0.0	0.0
1911-------	1949	4.3	3.6	2.7	2.2	1.5	1.1	0.7	0.3	0.2	0.0	0.0	0.0
1912-------	1950	4.3	3.7	3.0	2.3	1.7	1.2	0.6	0.3	0.1	0.1	0.0	0.0
1913-------	1951	4.5	4.0	3.1	2.5	1.8	1.1	0.6	0.3	0.2	0.1	0.0	0.0
1914-------	1952	5.0	4.3	3.5	2.7	1.8	1.2	0.7	0.4	0.2	0.1	0.0	0.0
1915-------	1953	5.3	4.6	3.7	2.7	1.9	1.2	0.7	0.3	0.2	0.1	0.0	0.0
1916-------	1954	5.6	4.8	3.7	2.8	1.9	1.2	0.7	0.4	0.2	0.1	0.0	0.0
1917-------	1955	5.9	5.0	3.8	2.9	1.9	1.2	0.7	0.3	0.2	0.0	0.0	0.0
1918-------	1956	6.1	5.0	3.8	2.8	2.0	1.3	0.6	0.3	0.1	0.0	0.0	0.0
1919-------	1957	6.4	5.2	4.0	2.9	2.0	1.2	0.7	0.3	0.1	0.0	0.0	0.0
1920-------	1958	6.5	5.3	4.1	3.0	1.9	1.2	0.6	0.3	0.1	0.0	0.0	0.0
1921-------	1959	6.8	5.4	4.1	2.8	1.9	1.1	0.6	0.3	0.1	0.0	0.0	0.0
1922-------	1960	6.8	5.5	3.9	2.8	1.8	1.1	0.6	0.3	0.1	0.0	0.0	0.0
1923-------	1961	6.9	5.2	3.8	2.7	1.7	1.0	0.5	0.2	0.1	0.0	0.0	0.0
1924-------	1962	6.6	5.1	3.7	2.5	1.5	0.9	0.4	0.2	0.1	0.0	0.0	0.0
1925-------	1963	6.4	4.9	3.5	2.2	1.4	0.8	0.5	0.2	0.0	0.0	0.0	
1926-------	1964	6.1	4.6	3.0	2.0	1.2	0.8	0.4	0.1	0.1	0.0		
1927-------	1965	5.7	4.0	2.7	1.8	1.2	0.7	0.3	0.1	0.1			
1928-------	1966	5.1	3.5	2.5	1.7	1.0	0.6	0.2	0.1				
1929-------	1967	4.7	3.4	2.4	1.5	0.9	0.5	0.2					
1930-------	1968	4.2	3.2	2.2	1.3	0.7	0.4						
1931-------	1969	4.1	3.1	1.8	1.1	0.6							
1932-------	1970	3.9	2.6	1.6	1.0								
1933-------	1971	3.3	2.2	1.4									
1934-------	1972	2.8	1.9										
1935-------	1973	2.4											

TABLE 4B. CENTRAL BIRTH RATES FOR WHITE WOMEN DURING EACH YEAR 1917-73 BY AGE AND LIVE-BIRTH ORDER FOR EACH COHORT FROM 1868 TO 1959--CON.

LIVE-BIRTH ORDER AND COHORT	DIAGONAL LINE FOR CALENDAR YEAR	CURRENT AGE 14	15	16	17	18	19	20	21	22	23	24	25
SIXTH BIRTHS													
1892-------													4.1
1893-------												2.3	3.8
1894-------											1.2	2.1	3.7
1895-------										0.5	1.0	2.1	3.7
1896-------									0.3	0.5	1.1	2.2	4.1
1897-------								0.1	0.3	0.5	1.2	2.4	3.8
1898-------							*	0.1	0.2	0.5	1.3	2.3	3.9
1899-------						*	*	0.1	0.3	0.6	1.2	2.3	3.8
1900-------					*	*	*	0.1	0.3	0.5	1.3	2.3	3.6
1901-------				*	*	*	*	0.1	0.2	0.5	1.2	2.2	3.5
1902-------			*	*	*	*	*	0.1	0.3	0.6	1.2	2.1	3.5
1903-------	1917	*	*	*	*	*	*	0.1	0.3	0.5	1.2	2.1	3.2
1904-------	1918	*	*	*	*	*	*	0.1	0.2	0.6	1.2	2.0	3.2
1905-------	1919	*	*	*	*	*	*	0.1	0.3	0.5	1.1	1.9	3.1
1906-------	1920	*	*	*	*	*	*	0.1	0.3	0.6	1.0	1.8	2.8
1907-------	1921	*	*	*	*	*	*	0.1	0.3	0.5	1.0	1.7	2.7
1908-------	1922	*	*	*	*	*	*	0.1	0.2	0.5	0.9	1.6	2.3
1909-------	1923	*	*	*	*	*	*	0.1	0.2	0.5	0.9	1.4	2.3
1910-------	1924	*	*	*	*	*	*	0.1	0.2	0.4	0.8	1.4	2.3
1911-------	1925	*	*	*	*	*	*	0.1	0.2	0.4	0.8	1.4	2.3
1912-------	1926	*	*	*	*	*	*	0.1	0.2	0.4	0.8	1.3	2.1
1913-------	1927	*	*	*	*	*	*	0.1	0.2	0.3	0.7	1.3	2.1
1914-------	1928	*	*	*	*	*	*	0.1	0.2	0.3	0.7	1.3	1.9
1915-------	1929	*	*	*	*	*	*	0.1	0.2	0.4	0.7	1.2	1.9
1916-------	1930	*	*	*	*	*	*	0.1	0.2	0.3	0.6	1.3	1.9
1917-------	1931	*	*	*	*	*	*	0.1	0.2	0.3	0.8	1.2	2.0
1918-------	1932	*	*	*	*	*	*	0.1	0.1	0.4	0.7	1.3	2.1
1919-------	1933	*	*	*	*	*	*	0.1	0.2	0.4	0.7	1.4	2.2
1920-------	1934	*	*	*	*	*	*	0.1	0.2	0.3	0.8	1.4	2.1
1921-------	1935	*	*	*	*	*	*	0.1	0.2	0.4	0.8	1.3	2.2
1922-------	1936	*	*	*	*	*	*	0.1	0.2	0.4	0.8	1.4	2.0
1923-------	1937	*	*	*	*	*	*	0.1	0.2	0.4	0.8	1.3	2.1
1924-------	1938	*	*	*	*	*	*	0.1	0.2	0.4	0.7	1.4	2.1
1925-------	1939	*	*	*	*	*	*	0.1	0.2	0.4	0.8	1.4	2.1
1926-------	1940	*	*	*	*	*	*	0.1	0.2	0.4	0.9	1.4	2.2
1927-------	1941	*	*	*	*	*	*	0.1	0.2	0.5	0.8	1.5	2.4
1928-------	1942	*	*	*	*	*	*	0.1	0.2	0.4	0.9	1.6	2.6
1929-------	1943	*	*	*	*	*	*	0.1	0.2	0.5	1.0	1.8	3.1
1930-------	1944	*	*	*	*	*	*	0.1	0.2	0.5	1.1	2.1	3.4
1931-------	1945	*	*	*	*	*	*	0.1	0.3	0.6	1.4	2.5	3.8
1932-------	1946	*	*	*	*	*	*	0.1	0.3	0.7	1.6	2.7	4.2
1933-------	1947	*	*	*	*	*	*	0.1	0.3	0.8	1.7	2.9	4.4
1934-------	1948	*	*	*	*	*	*	0.1	0.4	0.9	1.8	3.1	4.8
1935-------	1949	*	*	*	*	*	*	0.1	0.4	1.0	1.9	3.3	5.0
1936-------	1950	*	*	*	*	*	*	0.1	0.4	1.0	2.0	3.5	5.2
1937-------	1951	*	*	*	*	*	*	0.1	0.4	1.1	2.1	3.6	5.3
1938-------	1952	*	*	*	*	*	*	0.2	0.5	1.1	2.1	3.7	5.1
1939-------	1953	*	*	*	*	*	*	0.2	0.5	1.2	2.3	3.5	4.6
1940-------	1954	*	*	*	*	*	*	0.2	0.5	1.2	2.2	3.2	3.8
1941-------	1955	*	*	*	*	*	*	0.2	0.5	1.1	1.9	2.6	3.0
1942-------	1956	*	*	*	*	*	*	0.2	0.4	1.0	1.5	2.0	2.4
1943-------	1957	*	*	*	*	*	*	0.1	0.4	0.8	1.1	1.5	1.9
1944-------	1958	*	*	*	*	*	*	0.1	0.3	0.6	0.9	1.3	1.7
1945-------	1959	*	*	*	*	*	*	0.1	0.3	0.5	0.8	1.2	1.5
1946-------	1960	*	*	*	*	*	*	0.1	0.2	0.4	0.7	1.0	1.2
1947-------	1961	*	*	*	*	*	*	0.1	0.2	0.4	0.6	0.8	0.9
1948-------	1962	*	*	*	*	*	*	0.1	0.2	0.3	0.4	0.5	0.6
1949-------	1963	*	*	*	*	*	*	0.1	0.1	0.2	0.3	0.4	
1950-------	1964	*	*	*	*	*	*	0.1	0.1	0.2	0.2		
1951-------	1965	*	*	*	*	*	*	0.0	0.1	0.1			
1952-------	1966	*	*	*	*	*	*	0.0	0.1				
1953-------	1967	*	*	*	*	*	*	0.0					
1954-------	1968	*	*	*	*	*	*						
1955-------	1969	*	*	*	*	*							
1956-------	1970	*	*	*	*								
1957-------	1971	*	*	*									
1958-------	1972	*	*										
1959-------	1973	*											

TABLE 4B. CENTRAL BIRTH RATES FOR WHITE WOMEN DURING EACH YEAR 1917-73 BY AGE AND LIVE-BIRTH ORDER FOR EACH COHORT FROM 1868 TO 1959--CON.

LIVE-BIRTH ORDER AND COHORT	DIAGONAL LINE FOR CALENDAR YEAR	CURRENT AGE 26	27	28	29	30	31	32	33	34	35	36	37
SIXTH BIRTHS--CON.													
1880-------													12.4
1881-------												13.4	12.1
1882-------											14.6	13.0	11.7
1883-------										15.4	14.3	12.6	11.5
1884-------									16.1	15.1	13.7	12.4	11.3
1885-------								15.8	16.0	14.4	13.5	12.2	10.5
1886-------							15.9	15.8	15.2	14.2	13.5	11.5	10.2
1887-------						15.0	16.0	15.1	14.9	14.3	12.6	11.2	10.1
1888-------					14.5	14.8	15.2	14.6	15.1	13.3	12.4	11.0	9.5
1889-------				11.9	14.1	14.0	14.7	14.8	13.9	13.1	12.1	10.4	9.0
1890-------			9.4	11.3	13.3	13.7	14.9	13.7	13.8	12.8	11.4	9.8	8.8
1891-------	1917	6.3	8.9	10.7	13.1	14.1	13.7	13.6	13.4	12.0	10.8	9.7	8.0
1892-------	1918	6.0	8.4	10.6	13.7	12.8	13.6	13.2	12.5	11.3	10.5	8.7	7.4
1893-------	1919	5.6	8.3	11.3	12.3	12.7	13.2	12.3	11.7	11.1	9.5	8.1	7.2
1894-------	1920	5.6	8.9	10.1	12.4	12.4	12.4	11.5	11.4	10.0	8.9	7.8	6.8
1895-------	1921	6.1	8.1	10.3	12.1	11.7	11.8	11.4	10.5	9.3	8.6	7.5	6.4
1896-------	1922	5.6	8.3	10.0	11.3	11.3	11.3	10.3	9.7	9.0	8.0	7.0	6.0
1897-------	1923	5.7	8.1	9.3	10.9	10.8	10.5	9.5	9.5	8.4	7.7	6.6	5.9
1898-------	1924	5.6	7.4	9.1	10.5	10.0	9.9	9.6	8.9	8.2	7.3	6.5	5.6
1899-------	1925	5.3	7.4	8.9	9.9	9.6	9.9	9.1	8.9	7.8	7.2	6.1	5.2
1900-------	1926	5.2	7.2	8.3	9.3	9.4	9.3	8.8	8.2	7.7	6.7	5.8	4.9
1901-------	1927	5.1	6.7	7.6	9.0	8.7	8.9	8.0	8.0	7.0	6.2	5.3	4.7
1902-------	1928	4.7	6.1	7.5	8.3	8.3	8.1	7.7	7.3	6.5	5.8	5.0	4.4
1903-------	1929	4.5	6.1	7.0	8.1	7.5	7.8	7.1	6.7	6.0	5.5	4.7	4.1
1904-------	1930	4.4	5.7	6.9	7.2	7.5	7.3	6.7	6.4	5.8	5.1	4.5	4.0
1905-------	1931	4.2	5.5	6.0	7.2	7.0	6.7	6.3	6.2	5.3	4.9	4.2	4.0
1906-------	1932	3.9	4.8	6.0	6.7	6.4	6.4	6.1	5.6	5.1	4.6	4.2	4.0
1907-------	1933	3.4	4.8	5.7	6.2	6.2	6.2	5.5	5.4	4.8	4.6	4.3	4.1
1908-------	1934	3.4	4.6	5.3	6.0	5.9	5.6	5.3	5.0	4.8	4.7	4.4	4.0
1909-------	1935	3.4	4.4	5.2	5.7	5.4	5.4	5.0	5.0	5.0	4.8	4.3	3.9
1910-------	1936	3.2	4.2	4.9	5.3	5.3	5.1	4.8	5.3	5.1	4.6	4.2	3.8
1911-------	1937	3.1	4.0	4.6	5.2	5.1	4.8	5.2	5.3	4.8	4.5	4.1	3.6
1912-------	1938	3.0	3.7	4.5	5.0	4.7	5.2	5.2	5.1	4.8	4.5	3.9	3.6
1913-------	1939	2.7	3.6	4.4	4.6	5.0	5.2	5.0	5.0	4.7	4.2	3.9	3.6
1914-------	1940	2.7	3.6	4.0	4.9	5.0	5.1	5.0	4.8	4.4	4.3	3.9	3.8
1915-------	1941	2.7	3.4	4.3	4.9	4.9	5.1	4.7	4.6	4.5	4.3	4.2	3.8
1916-------	1942	2.7	3.7	4.3	4.7	4.9	4.8	4.6	4.7	4.5	4.5	4.2	4.0
1917-------	1943	2.9	3.7	4.2	4.7	4.6	4.7	4.6	4.7	4.6	4.5	4.3	4.2
1918-------	1944	2.9	3.6	4.1	4.5	4.6	4.7	4.7	4.7	4.8	4.6	4.5	4.4
1919-------	1945	2.9	3.6	4.1	4.5	4.7	4.8	4.8	5.1	5.0	5.1	5.0	4.7
1920-------	1946	2.9	3.5	4.1	4.7	4.7	4.9	5.2	5.3	5.6	5.5	5.3	5.0
1921-------	1947	2.8	3.6	4.3	4.6	4.9	5.3	5.4	5.9	5.9	5.8	5.7	5.2
1922-------	1948	2.8	3.7	4.1	4.8	5.0	5.3	5.8	6.1	6.1	6.2	5.7	5.4
1923-------	1949	2.9	3.5	4.4	4.9	5.3	5.8	6.2	6.5	6.6	6.4	6.1	5.4
1924-------	1950	2.8	3.8	4.5	5.2	5.8	6.4	6.7	7.1	6.9	6.6	6.2	5.8
1925-------	1951	3.0	4.0	4.9	5.8	6.4	7.0	7.2	7.3	7.2	6.9	6.5	5.5
1926-------	1952	3.2	4.3	5.4	6.3	6.9	7.4	7.5	7.7	7.5	7.2	6.4	5.5
1927-------	1953	3.6	4.7	5.8	6.9	7.3	7.7	8.1	8.1	7.9	7.2	6.4	5.3
1928-------	1954	3.9	5.1	6.3	7.1	7.7	8.5	8.5	8.5	7.9	7.1	6.2	4.9
1929-------	1955	4.3	5.7	6.7	7.7	8.6	9.0	9.1	8.6	8.0	7.0	5.7	4.4
1930-------	1956	4.7	6.2	7.3	8.5	9.1	9.5	9.2	8.8	7.8	6.5	5.1	4.2
1931-------	1957	5.3	6.7	8.0	9.2	9.7	9.6	9.3	8.7	7.2	5.8	4.8	3.8
1932-------	1958	5.7	7.2	8.6	9.6	9.8	9.7	9.1	7.8	6.4	5.3	4.4	3.5
1933-------	1959	6.1	7.8	9.0	9.8	9.8	9.4	8.2	6.8	5.8	4.9	4.1	3.3
1934-------	1960	6.5	8.1	9.3	9.8	9.4	8.3	7.0	6.1	5.1	4.7	3.8	3.0
1935-------	1961	6.8	8.2	9.0	9.2	8.3	7.2	6.2	5.3	5.1	4.3	3.4	2.6
1936-------	1962	6.9	7.9	8.5	7.9	7.0	6.3	5.4	5.2	4.7	3.9	2.9	2.1
1937-------	1963	6.5	7.4	7.2	6.7	6.1	5.5	5.3	4.9	4.2	3.2	2.4	
1938-------	1964	6.0	6.2	5.9	5.7	5.2	5.3	4.9	4.3	3.4	2.6		
1939-------	1965	5.0	5.0	5.0	4.9	5.1	4.9	4.4	3.5	2.8			
1940-------	1966	4.0	4.3	4.3	4.7	4.7	4.3	3.4	2.9				
1941-------	1967	3.3	3.6	4.0	4.2	4.0	3.2	2.8					
1942-------	1968	2.7	3.2	3.5	3.4	2.9	2.6						
1943-------	1969	2.4	2.8	2.9	2.5	2.2							
1944-------	1970	2.1	2.3	2.1	1.9								
1945-------	1971	1.8	1.7	1.7									
1946-------	1972	1.3	1.3										
1947-------	1973	1.0											

TABLE 4B. CENTRAL BIRTH RATES FOR WHITE WOMEN DURING EACH YEAR 1917-73 BY AGE AND LIVE-BIRTH ORDER FOR EACH COHORT FROM 1868 TO 1959--CON.

LIVE-BIRTH ORDER AND COHORT	DIAGONAL LINE FOR CALENDAR YEAR	CURRENT AGE											
		38	39	40	41	42	43	44	45	46	47	48	49
SIXTH BIRTHS--CON.													
1868-------													0.0
1869-------												0.1	0.0
1870-------											0.2	0.1	0.0
1871-------										0.5	0.2	0.1	0.0
1872-------									0.9	0.6	0.2	0.1	0.0
1873-------								1.5	0.9	0.5	0.2	0.1	0.0
1874-------							2.4	1.5	0.9	0.6	0.2	0.1	0.0
1875-------						3.3	2.3	1.4	0.9	0.5	0.2	0.1	0.0
1876-------					4.8	3.2	2.2	1.5	0.9	0.4	0.2	0.1	0.0
1877-------				6.4	4.7	3.1	2.3	1.4	0.7	0.5	0.2	0.1	0.0
1878-------			8.9	6.3	4.6	3.2	2.3	1.3	0.8	0.4	0.2	0.1	0.0
1879-------	1917	10.5	8.8	6.2	4.6	3.2	2.1	1.3	0.7	0.4	0.2	0.1	0.0
1880-------	1918	10.3	8.5	6.1	4.6	2.9	2.1	1.3	0.7	0.4	0.2	0.1	0.0
1881-------	1919	10.0	8.4	6.0	4.2	2.9	2.0	1.2	0.7	0.4	0.2	0.1	0.0
1882-------	1920	9.8	8.2	5.5	4.2	2.8	1.9	1.1	0.6	0.3	0.2	0.1	0.0
1883-------	1921	9.6	7.6	5.4	4.0	2.6	1.8	1.0	0.6	0.3	0.2	0.1	0.0
1884-------	1922	8.9	7.4	5.3	3.7	2.5	1.7	1.0	0.5	0.3	0.2	0.1	0.0
1885-------	1923	8.6	7.3	5.0	3.6	2.4	1.6	0.9	0.5	0.3	0.1	0.1	0.0
1886-------	1924	8.5	6.9	4.7	3.5	2.2	1.5	0.9	0.5	0.3	0.1	0.0	0.0
1887-------	1925	8.2	6.5	4.7	3.2	2.1	1.6	0.9	0.5	0.3	0.1	0.0	0.0
1888-------	1926	7.6	6.3	4.3	3.1	2.2	1.4	0.8	0.5	0.2	0.1	0.0	0.0
1889-------	1927	7.5	5.9	4.0	3.1	2.0	1.4	0.9	0.4	0.2	0.1	0.0	0.0
1890-------	1928	6.8	5.4	4.1	2.8	1.9	1.4	0.8	0.4	0.2	0.1	0.0	0.0
1891-------	1929	6.3	5.5	3.7	2.8	1.8	1.3	0.7	0.4	0.2	0.1	0.0	0.0
1892-------	1930	6.4	5.0	3.7	2.6	1.8	1.2	0.7	0.4	0.2	0.1	0.0	0.0
1893-------	1931	5.9	4.9	3.4	2.5	1.6	1.1	0.7	0.4	0.2	0.1	0.0	0.0
1894-------	1932	5.6	4.5	3.3	2.3	1.5	1.0	0.6	0.3	0.2	0.1	0.0	0.0
1895-------	1933	5.2	4.4	3.0	2.2	1.5	1.0	0.6	0.3	0.2	0.0	0.0	0.0
1896-------	1934	5.2	4.1	2.8	2.0	1.5	1.0	0.5	0.3	0.1	0.0	0.0	0.0
1897-------	1935	4.7	3.7	2.7	2.0	1.4	0.8	0.5	0.3	0.1	0.0	0.0	0.0
1898-------	1936	4.4	3.5	2.7	2.0	1.3	0.8	0.6	0.3	0.1	0.1	0.0	0.0
1899-------	1937	4.3	3.5	2.5	1.8	1.2	0.9	0.6	0.3	0.2	0.1	0.0	0.0
1900-------	1938	4.2	3.3	2.4	1.7	1.2	0.9	0.6	0.3	0.2	0.1	0.0	0.0
1901-------	1939	3.8	3.1	2.2	1.6	1.3	0.9	0.5	0.3	0.2	0.0	0.0	0.0
1902-------	1940	3.6	2.9	2.2	1.8	1.3	0.9	0.5	0.3	0.1	0.1	0.0	0.0
1903-------	1941	3.4	2.9	2.3	1.8	1.3	0.9	0.6	0.2	0.1	0.0	0.0	0.0
1904-------	1942	3.5	3.0	2.3	1.9	1.2	0.9	0.4	0.2	0.1	0.0	0.0	0.0
1905-------	1943	3.5	3.0	2.4	1.7	1.2	0.8	0.4	0.2	0.1	0.0	0.0	0.0
1906-------	1944	3.6	3.1	2.3	1.7	1.2	0.7	0.4	0.2	0.1	0.1	0.0	0.0
1907-------	1945	3.5	2.9	2.2	1.6	1.0	0.8	0.4	0.2	0.1	0.0	0.0	0.0
1908-------	1946	3.4	2.8	2.0	1.5	1.1	0.7	0.4	0.2	0.1	0.0	0.0	0.0
1909-------	1947	3.3	2.6	2.0	1.5	1.1	0.8	0.5	0.2	0.1	0.0	0.0	0.0
1910-------	1948	3.1	2.6	2.0	1.6	1.1	0.8	0.5	0.2	0.1	0.0	0.0	0.0
1911-------	1949	3.1	2.6	2.1	1.6	1.2	0.8	0.5	0.3	0.1	0.1	0.0	0.0
1912-------	1950	3.1	2.7	2.2	1.7	1.3	0.9	0.5	0.3	0.1	0.1	0.0	0.0
1913-------	1951	3.2	2.9	2.2	1.9	1.3	0.9	0.6	0.3	0.2	0.0	0.0	0.0
1914-------	1952	3.4	2.9	2.5	1.9	1.3	0.9	0.5	0.3	0.1	0.0	0.0	0.0
1915-------	1953	3.6	3.2	2.5	1.9	1.4	0.9	0.6	0.3	0.1	0.0	0.0	0.0
1916-------	1954	3.7	3.3	2.5	2.1	1.4	1.0	0.6	0.3	0.1	0.0	0.0	0.0
1917-------	1955	3.9	3.4	2.8	2.1	1.5	1.0	0.6	0.3	0.1	0.1	0.0	0.0
1918-------	1956	4.0	3.5	2.8	2.1	1.5	0.9	0.5	0.2	0.1	0.1	0.0	0.0
1919-------	1957	4.3	3.7	2.9	2.2	1.5	1.0	0.5	0.3	0.1	0.0	0.0	0.0
1920-------	1958	4.4	3.8	3.0	2.2	1.5	0.9	0.6	0.2	0.1	0.0	0.0	0.0
1921-------	1959	4.6	3.8	3.0	2.1	1.5	1.0	0.5	0.2	0.1	0.0	0.0	0.0
1922-------	1960	4.6	3.9	2.9	2.2	1.5	0.8	0.5	0.2	0.1	0.0	0.0	0.0
1923-------	1961	4.9	3.8	3.0	2.1	1.3	0.8	0.4	0.2	0.1	0.0	0.0	0.0
1924-------	1962	4.6	3.8	2.9	2.0	1.2	0.7	0.4	0.2	0.1	0.0	0.0	0.0
1925-------	1963	4.7	3.7	2.7	1.8	1.1	0.7	0.4	0.2	0.1	0.0	0.0	
1926-------	1964	4.5	3.5	2.4	1.5	1.0	0.6	0.3	0.2	0.0	0.0		
1927-------	1965	4.2	3.1	2.1	1.5	0.9	0.5	0.3	0.1	0.0			
1928-------	1966	3.7	2.8	2.0	1.3	0.8	0.5	0.2	0.1				
1929-------	1967	3.6	2.6	1.8	1.2	0.7	0.4	0.2					
1930-------	1968	3.1	2.4	1.7	1.1	0.7	0.4						
1931-------	1969	2.9	2.3	1.6	1.0	0.6							
1932-------	1970	2.8	2.1	1.3	0.8								
1933-------	1971	2.5	1.7	1.1									
1934-------	1972	2.2	1.5										
1935-------	1973	1.8											

TABLE 4B. CENTRAL BIRTH RATES FOR WHITE WOMEN DURING EACH YEAR 1917-73 BY AGE AND LIVE-BIRTH ORDER FOR EACH COHORT FROM 1868 TO 1959--CON.

LIVE-BIRTH ORDER AND COHORT	DIAGONAL LINE FOR CALENDAR YEAR	CURRENT AGE 14	15	16	17	18	19	20	21	22	23	24	25
SEVENTH BIRTHS													
1892-------													1.2
1893-------												0.7	1.1
1894-------											0.3	0.6	1.1
1895-------										0.2	0.3	0.6	1.1
1896-------									0.1	0.2	0.3	0.6	1.2
1897-------								0.1	0.1	0.2	0.3	0.6	1.1
1898-------							*	0.1	0.1	0.2	0.3	0.6	1.2
1899-------						*	*	0.0	0.1	0.2	0.3	0.7	1.2
1900-------					*	*	*	0.0	0.1	0.2	0.3	0.7	1.1
1901-------				*	*	*	*	0.0	0.1	0.2	0.3	0.6	1.1
1902-------			*	*	*	*	*	0.1	0.1	0.2	0.3	0.6	1.0
1903-------	1917	*	*	*	*	*	*	0.1	0.1	0.1	0.3	0.6	1.0
1904-------	1918	*	*	*	*	*	*	0.1	0.1	0.2	0.3	0.5	0.9
1905-------	1919	*	*	*	*	*	*	0.1	0.1	0.2	0.3	0.5	1.0
1906-------	1920	*	*	*	*	*	*	0.0	0.1	0.1	0.3	0.5	0.9
1907-------	1921	*	*	*	*	*	*	0.1	0.1	0.1	0.3	0.5	0.8
1908-------	1922	*	*	*	*	*	*	0.0	0.0	0.1	0.2	0.4	0.7
1909-------	1923	*	*	*	*	*	*	0.0	0.1	0.1	0.2	0.4	0.7
1910-------	1924	*	*	*	*	*	*	0.1	0.1	0.1	0.2	0.4	0.7
1911-------	1925	*	*	*	*	*	*	0.0	0.0	0.1	0.2	0.4	0.7
1912-------	1926	*	*	*	*	*	*	0.0	0.0	0.1	0.2	0.3	0.6
1913-------	1927	*	*	*	*	*	*	0.0	0.1	0.1	0.2	0.4	0.6
1914-------	1928	*	*	*	*	*	*	0.0	0.0	0.1	0.2	0.3	0.6
1915-------	1929	*	*	*	*	*	*	0.0	0.0	0.1	0.2	0.3	0.7
1916-------	1930	*	*	*	*	*	*	0.0	0.0	0.1	0.2	0.4	0.6
1917-------	1931	*	*	*	*	*	*	0.0	0.0	0.1	0.2	0.3	0.6
1918-------	1932	*	*	*	*	*	*	0.0	0.0	0.1	0.2	0.4	0.7
1919-------	1933	*	*	*	*	*	*	0.0	0.0	0.1	0.2	0.4	0.7
1920-------	1934	*	*	*	*	*	*	0.0	0.0	0.1	0.2	0.4	0.6
1921-------	1935	*	*	*	*	*	*	0.0	0.0	0.1	0.2	0.4	0.7
1922-------	1936	*	*	*	*	*	*	0.0	0.0	0.1	0.2	0.4	0.6
1923-------	1937	*	*	*	*	*	*	0.0	0.0	0.1	0.2	0.4	0.7
1924-------	1938	*	*	*	*	*	*	0.0	0.0	0.1	0.2	0.4	0.7
1925-------	1939	*	*	*	*	*	*	0.0	0.1	0.1	0.2	0.4	0.7
1926-------	1940	*	*	*	*	*	*	0.0	0.0	0.1	0.2	0.4	0.8
1927-------	1941	*	*	*	*	*	*	0.0	0.0	0.1	0.2	0.4	0.7
1928-------	1942	*	*	*	*	*	*	0.0	0.1	0.1	0.2	0.4	0.8
1929-------	1943	*	*	*	*	*	*	0.1	0.0	0.1	0.2	0.5	0.9
1930-------	1944	*	*	*	*	*	*	0.0	0.1	0.1	0.3	0.6	1.1
1931-------	1945	*	*	*	*	*	*	0.0	0.0	0.2	0.3	0.7	1.3
1932-------	1946	*	*	*	*	*	*	0.0	0.1	0.1	0.3	0.8	1.4
1933-------	1947	*	*	*	*	*	*	0.0	0.0	0.1	0.4	0.9	1.4
1934-------	1948	*	*	*	*	*	*	0.0	0.0	0.2	0.5	0.9	1.6
1935-------	1949	*	*	*	*	*	*	0.0	0.1	0.2	0.5	1.0	1.7
1936-------	1950	*	*	*	*	*	*	0.0	0.1	0.2	0.5	1.0	1.7
1937-------	1951	*	*	*	*	*	*	0.0	0.1	0.2	0.6	1.0	1.7
1938-------	1952	*	*	*	*	*	*	0.0	0.1	0.3	0.5	1.0	1.7
1939-------	1953	*	*	*	*	*	*	0.0	0.1	0.3	0.5	1.0	1.5
1940-------	1954	*	*	*	*	*	*	0.1	0.1	0.3	0.5	0.9	1.3
1941-------	1955	*	*	*	*	*	*	0.0	0.1	0.2	0.5	0.7	1.0
1942-------	1956	*	*	*	*	*	*	0.0	0.1	0.2	0.4	0.6	0.8
1943-------	1957	*	*	*	*	*	*	0.0	0.0	0.1	0.3	0.5	0.6
1944-------	1958	*	*	*	*	*	*	0.0	0.0	0.1	0.2	0.3	0.6
1945-------	1959	*	*	*	*	*	*	0.0	0.0	0.1	0.2	0.3	0.5
1946-------	1960	*	*	*	*	*	*	0.0	0.0	0.1	0.2	0.3	0.4
1947-------	1961	*	*	*	*	*	*	0.0	0.0	0.1	0.1	0.2	0.2
1948-------	1962	*	*	*	*	*	*	0.0	0.0	0.0	0.1	0.1	0.2
1949-------	1963	*	*	*	*	*	*	0.0	0.0	0.0	0.1	0.1	
1950-------	1964	*	*	*	*	*	*	0.0	0.0	0.0	0.1		
1951-------	1965	*	*	*	*	*	*	0.0	0.0	0.0			
1952-------	1966	*	*	*	*	*	*	0.0	0.0				
1953-------	1967	*	*	*	*	*	*	0.0					
1954-------	1968	*	*	*	*	*	*						
1955-------	1969	*	*	*	*	*							
1956-------	1970	*	*	*	*								
1957-------	1971	*	*	*									
1958-------	1972	*	*										
1959-------	1973	*											

TABLE 4B. CENTRAL BIRTH RATES FOR WHITE WOMEN DURING EACH YEAR 1917-73 BY AGE AND LIVE-BIRTH ORDER FOR EACH COHORT FROM 1868 TO 1959--CON.

LIVE-BIRTH ORDER AND COHORT	DIAGONAL LINE FOR CALENDAR YEAR	CURRENT AGE											
		26	27	28	29	30	31	32	33	34	35	36	37
SEVENTH BIRTHS--CON.													
1880-------													11.8
1881-------												12.2	11.5
1882-------											12.6	11.8	11.3
1883-------										12.4	12.3	11.7	11.1
1884-------									12.3	12.2	12.0	11.5	10.9
1885-------								11.0	12.2	11.8	11.8	11.4	10.1
1886-------							10.2	11.1	11.6	11.6	11.9	10.5	9.8
1887-------						8.4	10.3	10.5	11.5	11.9	11.0	10.3	9.7
1888-------					7.3	8.3	9.7	10.4	11.8	10.9	10.8	10.1	8.9
1889-------				5.1	7.0	7.9	9.6	10.7	10.8	10.8	10.6	9.5	8.6
1890-------			3.5	4.7	6.7	7.8	9.8	9.8	10.8	10.6	9.9	8.9	8.2
1891-------	1917	2.1	3.2	4.6	6.6	8.1	9.0	9.7	10.6	10.1	9.5	8.7	7.7
1892-------	1918	1.9	3.2	4.6	6.9	7.4	8.9	9.5	9.9	9.5	9.1	7.9	6.9
1893-------	1919	1.9	3.1	4.8	6.4	7.3	8.7	9.0	9.3	9.2	8.3	7.2	6.6
1894-------	1920	1.9	3.3	4.5	6.5	7.2	8.1	8.5	9.1	8.3	7.6	7.0	6.3
1895-------	1921	2.0	3.1	4.7	6.3	6.8	7.8	8.3	8.2	7.7	7.4	6.6	6.1
1896-------	1922	1.9	3.3	4.5	5.9	6.7	7.6	7.5	7.6	7.4	6.9	6.3	5.5
1897-------	1923	2.0	3.1	4.3	5.8	6.3	7.0	6.9	7.2	6.8	6.5	5.9	5.3
1898-------	1924	1.9	3.0	4.2	5.6	6.0	6.4	6.7	6.8	6.5	6.2	5.7	5.0
1899-------	1925	1.9	3.0	4.1	5.3	5.5	6.4	6.3	6.7	6.3	6.1	5.4	4.7
1900-------	1926	1.8	2.9	3.8	4.8	5.5	5.9	6.3	6.3	6.2	5.8	5.0	4.5
1901-------	1927	1.7	2.7	3.5	4.6	5.1	5.8	5.7	6.1	5.8	5.3	4.6	4.2
1902-------	1928	1.6	2.4	3.4	4.3	4.9	5.2	5.5	5.7	5.3	4.9	4.5	3.8
1903-------	1929	1.5	2.4	3.2	4.2	4.4	5.1	5.2	5.3	4.9	4.7	3.9	3.5
1904-------	1930	1.5	2.3	3.1	3.7	4.3	4.9	4.8	5.0	4.8	4.2	3.8	3.4
1905-------	1931	1.4	2.2	2.8	3.7	4.1	4.5	4.6	4.7	4.3	4.0	3.6	3.2
1906-------	1932	1.3	1.9	2.7	3.6	3.8	4.3	4.4	4.3	4.1	3.8	3.4	3.4
1907-------	1933	1.2	1.9	2.7	3.3	3.6	4.1	4.0	4.1	3.8	3.6	3.5	3.2
1908-------	1934	1.1	1.9	2.4	3.2	3.6	3.7	3.7	3.8	3.7	3.7	3.4	3.2
1909-------	1935	1.2	1.8	2.4	3.1	3.2	3.5	3.5	3.7	3.8	3.6	3.4	3.0
1910-------	1936	1.1	1.7	2.4	2.8	3.2	3.3	3.5	3.8	3.8	3.5	3.2	2.9
1911-------	1937	1.1	1.7	2.1	2.8	3.0	3.2	3.6	3.9	3.6	3.4	3.0	2.7
1912-------	1938	1.1	1.5	2.2	2.6	2.8	3.2	3.6	3.6	3.5	3.2	2.9	2.7
1913-------	1939	0.9	1.6	2.1	2.4	2.8	3.2	3.3	3.4	3.2	3.0	2.9	2.6
1914-------	1940	1.0	1.5	1.9	2.5	2.9	3.2	3.2	3.3	3.1	3.1	2.8	2.6
1915-------	1941	0.9	1.5	2.0	2.6	2.8	3.0	3.1	3.1	3.2	3.0	2.7	2.7
1916-------	1942	1.0	1.5	2.0	2.5	2.7	2.9	2.9	3.2	3.0	2.9	2.9	2.7
1917-------	1943	1.0	1.5	2.0	2.4	2.7	2.9	3.0	3.1	3.1	3.0	2.9	2.9
1918-------	1944	1.0	1.4	1.9	2.4	2.6	2.9	2.9	3.2	3.1	3.1	3.1	2.8
1919-------	1945	1.0	1.5	2.0	2.4	2.7	2.9	3.1	3.2	3.2	3.3	3.1	3.1
1920-------	1946	1.1	1.5	2.0	2.5	2.7	3.0	3.1	3.3	3.3	3.4	3.3	3.1
1921-------	1947	1.1	1.5	2.1	2.5	2.7	2.9	3.2	3.4	3.6	3.6	3.5	3.3
1922-------	1948	1.1	1.6	2.1	2.4	2.7	3.0	3.2	3.6	3.7	3.7	3.5	3.5
1923-------	1949	1.1	1.6	2.0	2.5	2.7	3.1	3.5	3.7	3.9	3.9	3.8	3.6
1924-------	1950	1.1	1.6	2.1	2.5	3.0	3.4	3.8	4.1	4.1	4.2	3.9	3.8
1925-------	1951	1.1	1.6	2.1	2.8	3.2	3.6	4.0	4.3	4.4	4.3	4.2	3.7
1926-------	1952	1.1	1.7	2.4	3.0	3.5	4.0	4.2	4.4	4.6	4.6	4.1	3.7
1927-------	1953	1.2	1.9	2.5	3.2	3.8	4.2	4.4	4.7	4.9	4.5	4.1	3.7
1928-------	1954	1.4	2.0	2.7	3.5	3.9	4.4	4.8	5.0	4.8	4.5	4.2	3.3
1929-------	1955	1.5	2.3	3.1	3.8	4.4	4.8	5.2	5.1	5.0	4.6	3.7	3.1
1930-------	1956	1.7	2.5	3.3	4.1	4.7	5.1	5.3	5.3	4.9	4.1	3.4	2.8
1931-------	1957	2.0	2.8	3.6	4.5	5.0	5.4	5.4	5.3	4.5	3.8	3.0	2.5
1932-------	1958	2.1	3.0	3.9	4.6	5.1	5.4	5.3	4.7	4.1	3.4	2.8	2.4
1933-------	1959	2.3	3.3	4.2	4.8	5.2	5.2	4.7	4.2	3.6	3.0	2.7	2.3
1934-------	1960	2.4	3.4	4.1	4.8	4.9	4.6	4.1	3.7	3.2	2.9	2.5	2.0
1935-------	1961	2.6	3.4	4.1	4.5	4.3	3.9	3.6	3.2	3.0	2.7	2.2	1.7
1936-------	1962	2.5	3.3	3.8	3.9	3.6	3.4	3.1	3.0	2.7	2.4	1.8	1.4
1937-------	1963	2.5	3.1	3.2	3.3	3.1	2.9	2.9	2.7	2.4	1.9	1.5	
1938-------	1964	2.2	2.6	2.7	2.7	2.6	2.8	2.6	2.4	1.9	1.6		
1939-------	1965	1.9	2.1	2.3	2.3	2.5	2.5	2.2	1.9	1.6			
1940-------	1966	1.5	1.7	1.9	2.1	2.2	2.0	1.8	1.6				
1941-------	1967	1.3	1.5	1.7	1.8	1.8	1.6	1.4					
1942-------	1968	1.0	1.3	1.4	1.5	1.3	1.2						
1943-------	1969	0.9	1.0	1.1	1.1	1.0							
1944-------	1970	0.7	0.8	0.9	0.8								
1945-------	1971	0.6	0.6	0.7									
1946-------	1972	0.4	0.5										
1947-------	1973	0.3											

TABLE 4B. CENTRAL BIRTH RATES FOR WHITE WOMEN DURING EACH YEAR 1917-73 BY AGE AND LIVE-BIRTH ORDER FOR EACH COHORT FROM 1868 TO 1959--CON.

LIVE-BIRTH ORDER AND COHORT	DIAGONAL LINE FOR CALENDAR YEAR	CURRENT AGE											
		38	39	40	41	42	43	44	45	46	47	48	49
SEVENTH BIRTHS--CON.													
1868-------													0.1
1869-------												0.1	0.1
1870-------											0.3	0.1	0.0
1871-------										0.6	0.3	0.1	0.1
1872-------									1.0	0.6	0.2	0.2	0.0
1873-------								1.7	1.0	0.5	0.3	0.1	0.0
1874-------							2.7	1.6	0.9	0.6	0.2	0.1	0.0
1875-------						3.5	2.7	1.5	1.0	0.5	0.2	0.1	0.0
1876-------					4.9	3.6	2.5	1.6	0.9	0.5	0.2	0.1	0.0
1877-------				6.3	4.9	3.4	2.6	1.5	0.9	0.5	0.2	0.1	0.0
1878-------			8.8	6.4	4.7	3.5	2.6	1.5	0.9	0.5	0.2	0.1	0.0
1879-------	1917	10.4	8.7	6.2	4.8	3.4	2.5	1.5	0.8	0.5	0.2	0.1	0.0
1880-------	1918	10.2	8.6	6.2	4.7	3.3	2.4	1.4	0.8	0.4	0.2	0.1	0.0
1881-------	1919	10.0	8.5	6.1	4.5	3.1	2.3	1.4	0.7	0.4	0.2	0.1	0.0
1882-------	1920	9.8	8.3	5.7	4.3	3.1	2.2	1.2	0.7	0.4	0.2	0.1	0.0
1883-------	1921	9.6	7.7	5.5	4.2	2.9	2.0	1.1	0.6	0.3	0.2	0.1	0.0
1884-------	1922	8.9	7.4	5.4	4.0	2.7	1.8	1.1	0.6	0.3	0.2	0.1	0.0
1885-------	1923	8.6	7.3	5.1	3.8	2.5	1.8	1.0	0.6	0.3	0.1	0.1	0.0
1886-------	1924	8.5	6.8	4.8	3.6	2.4	1.7	1.0	0.6	0.3	0.1	0.1	0.0
1887-------	1925	7.9	6.6	4.8	3.4	2.3	1.6	0.9	0.5	0.3	0.1	0.1	0.0
1888-------	1926	7.4	6.3	4.3	3.1	2.1	1.5	0.9	0.5	0.3	0.1	0.1	0.0
1889-------	1927	7.3	5.9	4.0	3.0	2.1	1.5	0.8	0.5	0.3	0.1	0.1	0.0
1890-------	1928	6.8	5.4	4.0	2.9	2.0	1.4	0.9	0.5	0.2	0.1	0.0	0.0
1891-------	1929	6.2	5.3	3.7	2.8	1.9	1.4	0.8	0.4	0.2	0.1	0.1	0.0
1892-------	1930	6.0	4.8	3.6	2.6	1.8	1.3	0.8	0.4	0.2	0.1	0.0	0.0
1893-------	1931	5.5	4.7	3.3	2.5	1.7	1.2	0.7	0.4	0.2	0.1	0.0	0.0
1894-------	1932	5.4	4.3	3.2	2.3	1.6	1.0	0.7	0.4	0.2	0.1	0.0	0.0
1895-------	1933	5.0	4.2	3.0	2.1	1.4	1.1	0.6	0.3	0.2	0.1	0.0	0.0
1896-------	1934	4.8	3.9	2.7	2.0	1.4	1.0	0.5	0.3	0.2	0.1	0.0	0.0
1897-------	1935	4.5	3.5	2.6	2.0	1.3	0.9	0.5	0.3	0.2	0.1	0.0	0.0
1898-------	1936	4.1	3.4	2.5	1.8	1.2	0.8	0.6	0.3	0.2	0.1	0.0	0.0
1899-------	1937	4.0	3.3	2.3	1.7	1.2	0.9	0.6	0.3	0.2	0.1	0.0	0.0
1900-------	1938	3.9	3.0	2.2	1.6	1.1	0.9	0.6	0.3	0.2	0.1	0.0	0.0
1901-------	1939	3.4	2.8	2.0	1.5	1.2	0.9	0.5	0.3	0.1	0.1	0.0	0.0
1902-------	1940	3.2	2.6	2.0	1.6	1.2	0.9	0.5	0.2	0.1	0.0	0.0	0.0
1903-------	1941	3.0	2.5	2.1	1.6	1.3	0.8	0.4	0.2	0.1	0.0	0.0	0.0
1904-------	1942	2.9	2.7	2.0	1.7	1.1	0.8	0.4	0.2	0.1	0.0	0.0	0.0
1905-------	1943	3.1	2.6	2.1	1.5	1.1	0.7	0.4	0.2	0.1	0.0	0.0	0.0
1906-------	1944	2.9	2.6	1.9	1.5	1.0	0.6	0.4	0.2	0.1	0.0	0.0	0.0
1907-------	1945	3.0	2.4	1.8	1.4	0.9	0.6	0.4	0.2	0.1	0.0	0.0	0.0
1908-------	1946	2.7	2.3	1.7	1.2	0.9	0.6	0.4	0.2	0.1	0.0	0.0	0.0
1909-------	1947	2.6	2.1	1.6	1.3	0.9	0.6	0.4	0.2	0.1	0.0	0.0	0.0
1910-------	1948	2.5	2.1	1.7	1.2	1.0	0.6	0.4	0.2	0.1	0.0	0.0	0.0
1911-------	1949	2.4	2.1	1.7	1.3	0.9	0.7	0.4	0.2	0.1	0.0	0.0	0.0
1912-------	1950	2.4	2.1	1.6	1.3	1.0	0.6	0.4	0.2	0.1	0.0	0.0	0.0
1913-------	1951	2.4	2.0	1.6	1.3	0.9	0.7	0.4	0.2	0.1	0.0	0.0	0.0
1914-------	1952	2.4	2.1	1.7	1.4	1.0	0.7	0.4	0.2	0.1	0.0	0.0	0.0
1915-------	1953	2.4	2.2	1.8	1.5	1.0	0.7	0.4	0.2	0.1	0.0	0.0	0.0
1916-------	1954	2.5	2.3	1.8	1.5	1.1	0.7	0.4	0.3	0.1	0.0	0.0	0.0
1917-------	1955	2.6	2.4	1.9	1.5	1.1	0.7	0.5	0.2	0.1	0.0	0.0	0.0
1918-------	1956	2.7	2.4	2.0	1.6	1.1	0.7	0.4	0.2	0.1	0.0	0.0	0.0
1919-------	1957	2.8	2.6	2.1	1.6	1.2	0.8	0.4	0.2	0.1	0.0	0.0	0.0
1920-------	1958	3.0	2.6	2.1	1.7	1.1	0.7	0.4	0.2	0.1	0.0	0.0	0.0
1921-------	1959	3.1	2.7	2.2	1.6	1.1	0.8	0.4	0.2	0.1	0.0	0.0	0.0
1922-------	1960	3.2	2.8	2.1	1.6	1.1	0.7	0.4	0.2	0.1	0.0	0.0	0.0
1923-------	1961	3.2	2.7	2.1	1.6	1.0	0.6	0.4	0.2	0.1	0.0	0.0	0.0
1924-------	1962	3.2	2.7	2.1	1.4	1.0	0.6	0.4	0.1	0.1	0.0	0.0	0.0
1925-------	1963	3.2	2.6	1.9	1.3	0.9	0.6	0.3	0.1	0.1	0.0	0.0	
1926-------	1964	3.2	2.4	1.8	1.2	0.8	0.5	0.2	0.1	0.0	0.0		
1927-------	1965	2.9	2.3	1.6	1.1	0.7	0.4	0.2	0.1	0.0			
1928-------	1966	2.7	2.1	1.5	1.0	0.7	0.4	0.2	0.1				
1929-------	1967	2.4	1.8	1.3	1.0	0.6	0.3	0.2					
1930-------	1968	2.2	1.7	1.3	0.8	0.5	0.3						
1931-------	1969	2.1	1.7	1.1	0.8	0.4							
1932-------	1970	2.0	1.4	1.0	0.6								
1933-------	1971	1.7	1.3	0.8									
1934-------	1972	1.5	1.0										
1935-------	1973	1.3											

TABLE 4B. CENTRAL BIRTH RATES FOR WHITE WOMEN DURING EACH YEAR 1917-73 BY AGE AND LIVE-BIRTH ORDER FOR EACH COHORT FROM 1868 TO 1959--CON.

LIVE-BIRTH ORDER AND COHORT	DIAGONAL LINE FOR CALENDAR YEAR	CURRENT AGE 14	15	16	17	18	19	20	21	22	23	24	25
EIGHTH AND HIGHER BIRTHS													
1892-------													0.6
1893-------												0.3	0.5
1894-------											0.2	0.3	0.5
1895-------										0.1	0.2	0.3	0.5
1896-------									0.0	0.1	0.2	0.3	0.5
1897-------								0.0	0.0	0.1	0.2	0.3	0.6
1898-------							*	0.0	0.0	0.1	0.2	0.4	0.6
1899-------						*	*	0.0	0.0	0.1	0.2	0.4	0.6
1900-------					*	*	*	0.0	0.0	0.1	0.2	0.4	0.6
1901-------				*	*	*	*	0.0	0.0	0.1	0.2	0.3	0.6
1902-------			*	*	*	*	*	0.0	0.0	0.1	0.2	0.4	0.5
1903-------	1917	*	*	*	*	*	*	0.0	0.0	0.1	0.2	0.3	0.5
1904-------	1918	*	*	*	*	*	*	0.0	0.0	0.1	0.2	0.3	0.5
1905-------	1919	*	*	*	*	*	*	0.0	0.0	0.1	0.2	0.3	0.5
1906-------	1920	*	*	*	*	*	*	0.0	0.0	0.1	0.2	0.3	0.4
1907-------	1921	*	*	*	*	*	*	0.0	0.0	0.1	0.2	0.2	0.4
1908-------	1922	*	*	*	*	*	*	0.0	0.0	0.1	0.1	0.2	0.3
1909-------	1923	*	*	*	*	*	*	0.0	0.0	0.1	0.1	0.2	0.3
1910-------	1924	*	*	*	*	*	*	0.0	0.0	0.1	0.1	0.2	0.3
1911-------	1925	*	*	*	*	*	*	0.0	0.0	0.1	0.1	0.2	0.4
1912-------	1926	*	*	*	*	*	*	0.0	0.0	0.0	0.1	0.2	0.3
1913-------	1927	*	*	*	*	*	*	0.0	0.0	0.1	0.1	0.2	0.3
1914-------	1928	*	*	*	*	*	*	0.0	0.0	0.1	0.1	0.1	0.2
1915-------	1929	*	*	*	*	*	*	0.0	0.0	0.0	0.1	0.1	0.3
1916-------	1930	*	*	*	*	*	*	0.0	0.0	0.0	0.1	0.2	0.3
1917-------	1931	*	*	*	*	*	*	0.0	0.0	0.0	0.1	0.2	0.3
1918-------	1932	*	*	*	*	*	*	0.0	0.0	0.1	0.1	0.2	0.3
1919-------	1933	*	*	*	*	*	*	0.0	0.0	0.1	0.1	0.2	0.3
1920-------	1934	*	*	*	*	*	*	0.0	0.0	0.0	0.1	0.2	0.3
1921-------	1935	*	*	*	*	*	*	0.0	0.0	0.0	0.1	0.2	0.3
1922-------	1936	*	*	*	*	*	*	0.0	0.0	0.0	0.1	0.2	0.3
1923-------	1937	*	*	*	*	*	*	0.0	0.0	0.0	0.1	0.1	0.2
1924-------	1938	*	*	*	*	*	*	0.0	0.0	0.0	0.1	0.1	0.4
1925-------	1939	*	*	*	*	*	*	0.0	0.0	0.0	0.1	0.2	0.3
1926-------	1940	*	*	*	*	*	*	0.0	0.0	0.0	0.1	0.2	0.3
1927-------	1941	*	*	*	*	*	*	0.0	0.0	0.1	0.1	0.2	0.3
1928-------	1942	*	*	*	*	*	*	0.0	0.0	0.0	0.1	0.2	0.4
1929-------	1943	*	*	*	*	*	*	0.0	0.0	0.0	0.1	0.2	0.4
1930-------	1944	*	*	*	*	*	*	0.0	0.0	0.0	0.1	0.2	0.4
1931-------	1945	*	*	*	*	*	*	0.0	0.0	0.1	0.1	0.2	0.5
1932-------	1946	*	*	*	*	*	*	0.0	0.0	0.0	0.1	0.3	0.5
1933-------	1947	*	*	*	*	*	*	0.0	0.0	0.0	0.1	0.3	0.6
1934-------	1948	*	*	*	*	*	*	0.0	0.0	0.1	0.2	0.3	0.6
1935-------	1949	*	*	*	*	*	*	0.0	0.0	0.1	0.2	0.3	0.7
1936-------	1950	*	*	*	*	*	*	0.0	0.0	0.1	0.1	0.3	0.7
1937-------	1951	*	*	*	*	*	*	0.0	0.0	0.0	0.2	0.4	0.7
1938-------	1952	*	*	*	*	*	*	0.0	0.0	0.1	0.2	0.3	0.6
1939-------	1953	*	*	*	*	*	*	0.0	0.0	0.1	0.2	0.4	0.6
1940-------	1954	*	*	*	*	*	*	0.0	0.0	0.1	0.2	0.3	0.5
1941-------	1955	*	*	*	*	*	*	0.0	0.0	0.1	0.2	0.3	0.4
1942-------	1956	*	*	*	*	*	*	0.0	0.0	0.1	0.1	0.2	0.3
1943-------	1957	*	*	*	*	*	*	0.0	0.0	0.0	0.1	0.2	0.2
1944-------	1958	*	*	*	*	*	*	0.0	0.0	0.0	0.1	0.1	0.2
1945-------	1959	*	*	*	*	*	*	0.0	0.0	0.0	0.0	0.1	0.2
1946-------	1960	*	*	*	*	*	*	0.0	0.0	0.0	0.1	0.1	0.2
1947-------	1961	*	*	*	*	*	*	0.0	0.0	0.1	0.1	0.1	0.1
1948-------	1962	*	*	*	*	*	*	0.0	0.1	0.0	0.0	0.1	0.1
1949-------	1963	*	*	*	*	*	*	0.1	0.0	0.0	0.0	0.0	
1950-------	1964	*	*	*	*	*	*	0.0	0.0	0.0	0.0		
1951-------	1965	*	*	*	*	*	*	0.0	0.0	0.0			
1952-------	1966	*	*	*	*	*	*	0.0	0.0				
1953-------	1967	*	*	*	*	*	*	0.0					
1954-------	1968	*	*	*	*	*	*						
1955-------	1969	*	*	*	*	*							
1956-------	1970	*	*	*	*								
1957-------	1971	*	*	*									
1958-------	1972	*	*										
1959-------	1973	*											

TABLE 4B. CENTRAL BIRTH RATES FOR WHITE WOMEN DURING EACH YEAR 1917-73 BY AGE AND LIVE-BIRTH ORDER FOR EACH COHORT FROM 1868 TO 1959--CON.

LIVE-BIRTH ORDER AND COHORT	DIAGONAL LINE FOR CALENDAR YEAR	CURRENT AGE											
		26	27	28	29	30	31	32	33	34	35	36	37
EIGHTH AND HIGHER BIRTHS--CON.													
1880-------													28.4
1881-------												25.0	27.8
1882-------											22.1	24.4	27.4
1883-------										18.3	21.8	24.0	27.1
1884-------									14.8	18.3	21.4	23.9	27.6
1885-------								11.4	15.0	17.9	21.3	24.3	25.6
1886-------							8.8	11.6	14.7	17.9	22.0	22.7	25.7
1887-------						6.3	9.0	11.4	14.7	18.8	20.6	22.9	25.5
1888-------					4.8	6.3	8.8	11.4	15.6	17.4	20.8	22.6	24.2
1889-------				2.9	4.6	6.0	8.8	12.0	14.3	17.7	20.4	21.6	23.1
1890-------			1.8	2.7	4.4	6.1	9.2	11.0	14.7	17.3	19.4	20.2	22.6
1891-------	1917	1.0	1.6	2.5	4.5	6.4	8.5	11.3	14.2	16.6	18.3	20.2	20.5
1892-------	1918	0.9	1.5	2.6	4.7	5.9	8.7	10.9	13.7	15.4	17.9	17.9	18.7
1893-------	1919	0.8	1.6	2.7	4.3	6.0	8.4	10.5	12.8	15.1	16.1	16.5	17.7
1894-------	1920	0.9	1.6	2.6	4.5	5.9	8.0	9.9	12.4	13.8	14.9	15.8	16.6
1895-------	1921	0.9	1.6	2.8	4.5	5.7	7.7	9.7	11.5	12.8	14.5	14.8	15.9
1896-------	1922	0.9	1.7	2.8	4.4	5.4	7.6	9.0	10.7	12.4	13.3	14.0	14.2
1897-------	1923	1.0	1.7	2.6	4.1	5.5	7.1	8.4	10.3	11.3	12.7	12.7	13.8
1898-------	1924	1.0	1.7	2.6	4.1	5.1	6.6	8.1	9.6	10.8	11.5	12.4	13.4
1899-------	1925	1.0	1.7	2.5	3.9	4.8	6.4	7.6	9.5	10.0	11.5	12.4	12.7
1900-------	1926	1.0	1.5	2.3	3.6	4.6	6.0	7.5	8.5	10.0	11.6	11.6	12.3
1901-------	1927	0.9	1.4	2.2	3.3	4.3	5.8	6.6	8.5	9.9	10.6	11.2	11.6
1902-------	1928	0.8	1.4	2.1	3.1	4.0	5.1	6.5	8.1	9.0	10.0	10.4	10.4
1903-------	1929	0.8	1.3	2.0	3.0	3.6	5.1	6.3	7.6	8.5	9.5	9.3	9.8
1904-------	1930	0.8	1.3	1.9	2.7	3.6	5.0	6.0	7.3	8.2	8.6	8.9	9.2
1905-------	1931	0.7	1.2	1.7	2.7	3.7	4.7	5.8	7.0	7.4	8.3	8.3	8.6
1906-------	1932	0.6	1.0	1.6	2.8	3.3	4.6	5.5	6.4	7.3	7.7	7.8	8.6
1907-------	1933	0.6	1.0	1.7	2.5	3.3	4.3	5.0	6.3	6.8	7.1	7.8	8.4
1908-------	1934	0.5	1.0	1.6	2.4	3.1	3.9	5.0	5.9	6.3	7.2	7.6	8.0
1909-------	1935	0.6	1.0	1.5	2.3	2.8	3.9	4.6	5.4	6.3	7.0	7.3	7.5
1910-------	1936	0.6	0.9	1.5	2.0	2.8	3.6	4.3	5.5	6.2	6.8	7.0	7.1
1911-------	1937	0.6	0.9	1.4	2.1	2.7	3.4	4.4	5.4	6.1	6.5	6.7	6.8
1912-------	1938	0.5	0.8	1.4	2.0	2.6	3.5	4.4	5.3	5.7	6.2	6.2	6.8
1913-------	1939	0.5	0.9	1.4	1.9	2.6	3.5	4.3	4.9	5.5	5.7	6.2	6.3
1914-------	1940	0.5	0.8	1.3	1.9	2.6	3.3	4.0	4.8	5.2	5.9	6.0	6.2
1915-------	1941	0.5	0.8	1.3	1.9	2.4	3.3	3.9	4.6	5.3	5.6	5.9	6.2
1916-------	1942	0.4	0.8	1.3	1.8	2.5	3.1	3.7	4.7	5.1	5.5	5.8	5.8
1917-------	1943	0.5	0.8	1.2	1.9	2.4	3.1	3.9	4.5	5.0	5.4	5.6	5.8
1918-------	1944	0.4	0.8	1.2	1.8	2.4	3.3	3.8	4.5	4.9	5.3	5.5	5.7
1919-------	1945	0.5	0.8	1.2	1.9	2.6	3.2	3.8	4.6	5.0	5.4	5.6	5.9
1920-------	1946	0.5	0.8	1.3	2.1	2.5	3.2	3.9	4.6	5.1	5.4	5.7	6.1
1921-------	1947	0.5	0.9	1.5	2.0	2.6	3.3	3.9	4.7	5.2	5.6	5.9	6.0
1922-------	1948	0.5	1.0	1.4	2.0	2.5	3.2	4.0	4.6	5.2	5.8	5.8	6.2
1923-------	1949	0.6	0.9	1.3	2.0	2.5	3.4	4.0	4.8	5.4	5.8	6.2	6.4
1924-------	1950	0.5	0.9	1.4	2.0	2.7	3.4	4.2	5.1	5.6	6.1	6.5	6.6
1925-------	1951	0.5	0.9	1.4	2.1	2.8	3.7	4.5	5.2	6.0	6.5	6.8	6.7
1926-------	1952	0.6	1.0	1.5	2.3	3.0	3.9	4.6	5.6	6.2	6.8	6.8	6.8
1927-------	1953	0.6	1.0	1.6	2.4	3.2	4.2	5.1	5.9	6.7	6.9	6.9	6.7
1928-------	1954	0.6	1.1	1.8	2.6	3.6	4.5	5.4	6.3	6.8	7.0	6.9	6.4
1929-------	1955	0.7	1.3	2.0	3.0	3.9	4.9	5.9	6.7	7.0	6.9	6.6	5.6
1930-------	1956	0.9	1.4	2.3	3.3	4.2	5.2	6.1	6.8	6.9	6.6	5.7	5.1
1931-------	1957	0.9	1.6	2.5	3.5	4.6	5.5	6.2	6.7	6.4	5.8	5.3	4.6
1932-------	1958	1.0	1.7	2.6	3.7	4.6	5.5	6.1	6.0	5.7	5.2	4.7	4.3
1933-------	1959	1.1	1.8	2.8	3.8	4.6	5.3	5.3	5.3	5.0	4.6	4.3	3.9
1934-------	1960	1.2	1.9	2.9	3.8	4.4	4.6	4.7	4.5	4.3	4.3	3.9	3.5
1935-------	1961	1.2	2.0	2.8	3.6	3.8	4.0	4.0	3.9	4.0	3.9	3.5	2.8
1936-------	1962	1.2	1.9	2.6	3.0	3.2	3.3	3.4	3.6	3.6	3.4	2.8	2.4
1937-------	1963	1.2	1.7	2.2	2.4	2.7	2.9	3.1	3.2	3.1	2.6	2.2	
1938-------	1964	1.1	1.5	1.7	2.1	2.3	2.5	2.6	2.7	2.3	2.1		
1939-------	1965	0.9	1.2	1.5	1.7	2.0	2.2	2.2	2.0	1.9			
1940-------	1966	0.7	1.0	1.2	1.5	1.8	1.8	1.7	1.6				
1941-------	1967	0.6	0.8	1.1	1.4	1.4	1.4	1.4					
1942-------	1968	0.5	0.7	0.9	1.0	1.0	1.0						
1943-------	1969	0.4	0.6	0.6	0.7	0.7							
1944-------	1970	0.4	0.4	0.4	0.5								
1945-------	1971	0.3	0.3	0.4									
1946-------	1972	0.2	0.2										
1947-------	1973	0.1											

TABLE 4B. CENTRAL BIRTH RATES FOR WHITE WOMEN DURING EACH YEAR 1917-73 BY AGE AND LIVE-BIRTH ORDER FOR EACH COHORT FROM 1868 TO 1959--CON.

LIVE-BIRTH ORDER AND COHORT	DIAGONAL LINE FOR CALENDAR YEAR	CURRENT AGE											
		38	39	40	41	42	43	44	45	46	47	48	49
EIGHTH AND HIGHER BIRTHS--CON.													
1868-------													0.5
1869-------												1.2	0.5
1870-------											2.3	1.2	0.5
1871-------										4.2	2.3	1.1	0.5
1872-------									6.8	4.2	2.2	1.2	0.5
1873-------								10.3	6.7	4.0	2.3	1.2	0.5
1874-------							14.4	10.0	6.5	4.2	2.3	1.1	0.5
1875-------						17.1	14.0	9.8	6.6	4.2	2.1	1.0	0.5
1876-------					21.6	16.6	13.7	9.9	6.7	3.8	1.9	1.0	0.4
1877-------				24.5	21.1	16.3	13.9	10.1	6.2	3.5	1.9	0.9	0.3
1878-------			29.6	24.2	20.9	16.6	14.1	9.4	5.9	3.6	1.8	0.8	0.4
1879-------	1917	29.1	29.2	23.9	21.1	16.8	13.2	9.2	6.0	3.5	1.6	0.8	0.3
1880-------	1918	28.6	28.9	24.0	21.3	15.6	13.0	9.3	5.8	3.3	1.6	0.7	0.3
1881-------	1919	28.3	28.7	24.2	19.7	15.3	13.1	8.9	5.4	3.1	1.5	0.7	0.3
1882-------	1920	27.9	29.0	22.3	19.3	15.4	12.5	8.2	5.1	2.9	1.4	0.6	0.3
1883-------	1921	28.4	26.7	21.9	19.4	14.9	11.7	8.0	4.8	2.7	1.3	0.7	0.3
1884-------	1922	26.2	26.5	21.9	18.4	13.9	11.4	7.3	4.4	2.5	1.3	0.6	0.3
1885-------	1923	26.1	26.3	20.8	17.3	13.8	10.5	6.7	4.2	2.4	1.2	0.6	0.3
1886-------	1924	25.9	24.8	19.4	16.9	12.6	9.5	6.5	4.0	2.2	1.1	0.6	0.2
1887-------	1925	24.8	23.5	19.3	15.9	11.5	9.4	6.2	3.7	2.1	1.1	0.5	0.2
1888-------	1926	23.4	22.8	17.8	14.4	11.3	8.7	5.8	3.5	2.0	1.0	0.5	0.2
1889-------	1927	23.1	21.3	16.5	14.0	10.6	8.4	5.5	3.5	1.9	0.9	0.5	0.2
1890-------	1928	21.0	19.5	15.8	13.1	10.1	7.8	5.4	3.2	1.7	0.9	0.5	0.2
1891-------	1929	19.4	18.7	14.9	12.3	9.4	7.7	5.1	3.0	1.6	0.8	0.4	0.1
1892-------	1930	18.4	17.3	13.7	11.3	9.3	7.2	4.6	2.7	1.6	0.7	0.3	0.1
1893-------	1931	17.1	16.2	12.7	11.2	8.5	6.4	4.1	2.6	1.4	0.6	0.3	0.1
1894-------	1932	16.2	14.8	12.6	10.4	7.7	5.9	4.0	2.3	1.2	0.6	0.2	0.1
1895-------	1933	14.9	14.5	11.8	9.5	7.3	5.7	3.6	2.2	1.2	0.5	0.2	0.1
1896-------	1934	14.5	13.8	10.7	8.9	6.9	5.1	3.3	1.9	1.1	0.5	0.2	0.1
1897-------	1935	13.7	12.6	10.2	8.6	6.3	4.8	3.0	2.0	1.0	0.5	0.2	0.1
1898-------	1936	12.7	11.9	9.9	7.8	6.1	4.4	3.2	2.0	1.0	0.5	0.2	0.1
1899-------	1937	12.4	11.7	9.0	7.5	5.7	4.4	3.0	1.8	1.0	0.5	0.2	0.1
1900-------	1938	11.9	10.6	8.6	7.1	5.4	4.4	3.0	1.8	0.9	0.5	0.2	0.1
1901-------	1939	10.6	9.9	8.0	6.5	5.4	4.3	2.9	1.6	0.9	0.4	0.2	0.1
1902-------	1940	10.1	9.2	7.6	6.6	5.5	4.2	2.6	1.6	0.8	0.4	0.2	0.1
1903-------	1941	9.3	8.8	7.6	6.6	5.3	3.8	2.6	1.4	0.8	0.3	0.1	0.1
1904-------	1942	8.9	8.8	7.4	6.3	4.8	3.8	2.3	1.3	0.7	0.3	0.1	0.1
1905-------	1943	8.9	8.5	7.1	5.8	4.6	3.3	2.1	1.2	0.6	0.3	0.1	0.1
1906-------	1944	8.7	8.1	6.7	5.6	4.1	3.1	1.9	1.2	0.6	0.3	0.1	0.1
1907-------	1945	8.2	7.6	6.3	5.0	4.0	2.9	2.0	1.1	0.5	0.3	0.1	0.0
1908-------	1946	7.7	7.1	5.7	4.9	3.7	2.8	1.8	1.0	0.5	0.2	0.1	0.1
1909-------	1947	7.2	6.7	5.7	4.6	3.6	2.8	1.6	1.0	0.5	0.3	0.1	0.0
1910-------	1948	6.8	6.7	5.4	4.5	3.4	2.5	1.7	0.9	0.5	0.2	0.1	0.1
1911-------	1949	6.9	6.3	5.2	4.2	3.3	2.6	1.6	1.0	0.5	0.2	0.1	0.1
1912-------	1950	6.5	6.0	4.9	4.1	3.3	2.4	1.6	0.9	0.5	0.2	0.1	0.1
1913-------	1951	6.2	5.9	4.8	4.1	3.1	2.4	1.5	0.9	0.4	0.2	0.1	0.0
1914-------	1952	6.2	5.5	4.7	3.9	3.1	2.3	1.5	0.8	0.4	0.2	0.1	0.0
1915-------	1953	5.8	5.4	4.6	3.9	3.1	2.2	1.4	0.8	0.4	0.2	0.1	0.0
1916-------	1954	5.7	5.4	4.6	3.8	3.0	2.2	1.4	0.8	0.4	0.2	0.1	0.0
1917-------	1955	5.8	5.4	4.6	3.7	3.0	2.2	1.4	0.8	0.4	0.2	0.0	0.0
1918-------	1956	5.7	5.5	4.4	3.8	3.0	2.2	1.4	0.7	0.3	0.1	0.1	0.0
1919-------	1957	6.0	5.3	4.8	3.9	3.0	2.2	1.4	0.7	0.4	0.2	0.0	0.0
1920-------	1958	5.8	5.7	4.7	3.9	3.0	2.2	1.3	0.7	0.3	0.1	0.0	0.0
1921-------	1959	6.1	5.6	4.8	4.0	3.0	2.1	1.2	0.7	0.3	0.1	0.0	0.0
1922-------	1960	6.0	5.6	4.8	3.9	2.9	1.9	1.2	0.6	0.3	0.1	0.0	0.0
1923-------	1961	6.2	5.7	4.8	3.8	2.7	1.8	1.1	0.5	0.2	0.1	0.0	0.0
1924-------	1962	6.3	5.8	4.8	3.6	2.5	1.7	1.0	0.5	0.2	0.1	0.0	0.0
1925-------	1963	6.4	5.7	4.4	3.3	2.3	1.5	0.9	0.4	0.2	0.1	0.0	
1926-------	1964	6.4	5.4	4.1	2.9	2.1	1.4	0.8	0.4	0.2	0.1		
1927-------	1965	5.9	4.8	3.6	2.7	1.9	1.2	0.7	0.4	0.2			
1928-------	1966	5.3	4.2	3.3	2.5	1.8	1.1	0.6	0.3				
1929-------	1967	4.8	3.9	3.1	2.4	1.6	1.0	0.6					
1930-------	1968	4.3	3.6	2.9	2.0	1.4	0.9						
1931-------	1969	4.1	3.4	2.5	1.8	1.3							
1932-------	1970	3.7	3.0	2.2	1.6								
1933-------	1971	3.3	2.5	1.9									
1934-------	1972	2.8	2.2										
1935-------	1973	2.3											

TABLE 4C. CENTRAL BIRTH RATES FOR ALL OTHER WOMEN DURING EACH YEAR 1917-73 BY AGE AND LIVE-BIRTH ORDER FOR EACH COHORT FROM 1868 TO 1959

LIVE-BIRTH ORDER AND COHORT	DIAGONAL LINE FOR CALENDAR YEAR	CURRENT AGE											
		14	15	16	17	18	19	20	21	22	23	24	25
TOTAL BIRTHS													
1892-------													169.1
1893-------												180.4	166.3
1894-------											188.6	178.9	166.1
1895-------										181.7	188.6	174.2	178.2
1896-------									186.9	181.4	179.2	185.3	183.3
1897-------								179.6	186.3	172.2	189.6	190.9	170.0
1898-------							173.5	177.7	177.7	186.6	197.0	181.6	170.2
1899-------						139.9	168.8	167.3	193.3	188.4	186.1	179.0	175.9
1900-------					105.4	134.7	158.9	185.4	193.6	178.3	187.0	188.4	173.4
1901-------				62.9	100.7	125.3	177.0	187.9	180.1	175.2	195.0	180.8	165.0
1902-------			34.5	60.9	94.7	143.2	185.5	175.8	179.2	187.4	185.5	170.8	147.9
1903-------	1917	12.8	32.9	56.8	108.9	152.6	169.8	176.2	189.0	180.6	176.6	156.5	133.4
1904-------	1918	12.1	30.6	65.7	114.0	137.7	173.2	185.4	184.0	177.5	164.7	144.8	128.2
1905-------	1919	11.2	35.5	67.9	101.6	144.3	182.4	180.7	180.2	164.5	152.0	138.1	127.0
1906-------	1920	13.0	36.7	60.1	106.6	152.4	177.8	178.3	169.2	152.5	144.9	139.2	123.5
1907-------	1921	13.6	32.7	63.5	113.3	152.7	175.3	167.0	157.9	146.0	146.9	132.8	122.8
1908-------	1922	12.3	34.9	67.7	116.8	150.1	165.1	156.1	153.6	147.9	141.3	133.3	117.3
1909-------	1923	13.2	37.3	72.3	116.2	142.6	156.6	153.9	156.6	146.0	144.9	130.2	123.3
1910-------	1924	14.3	40.0	72.0	112.0	135.0	154.0	156.9	153.4	150.0	140.2	136.2	121.0
1911-------	1925	15.6	41.6	71.7	107.1	131.9	157.9	153.5	158.8	142.9	147.6	135.3	120.2
1912-------	1926	16.4	40.6	67.2	103.0	134.2	151.9	157.3	147.4	148.9	144.9	131.2	122.6
1913-------	1927	16.1	38.2	64.5	105.0	130.9	155.0	147.3	155.1	149.2	142.1	136.4	124.4
1914-------	1928	14.7	36.2	65.7	101.7	132.2	145.7	154.9	156.0	147.4	149.0	138.4	125.8
1915-------	1929	14.2	37.1	64.1	102.3	124.4	153.5	156.2	153.7	153.7	149.7	140.0	129.5
1916-------	1930	14.5	35.6	65.1	95.7	131.1	155.2	153.0	160.2	153.6	151.3	145.1	133.6
1917-------	1931	13.9	36.2	60.5	101.5	134.6	151.7	160.2	159.8	154.2	158.0	150.6	138.1
1918-------	1932	14.2	34.2	63.5	105.8	131.8	159.6	161.3	157.5	157.9	162.1	154.4	143.8
1919-------	1933	13.6	35.4	68.2	106.0	141.6	163.7	162.0	163.0	163.4	167.4	158.3	142.5
1920-------	1934	13.9	39.2	68.5	113.6	145.5	164.5	168.1	166.0	167.4	169.6	154.3	137.2
1921-------	1935	15.5	39.6	74.3	117.0	147.6	170.2	174.0	170.3	168.8	163.4	146.6	153.7
1922-------	1936	14.8	41.3	75.0	114.5	148.4	173.5	172.3	171.8	162.2	150.6	163.5	163.4
1923-------	1937	15.7	42.3	72.5	113.4	154.2	172.7	175.0	165.3	152.4	172.0	177.5	171.1
1924-------	1938	16.4	41.4	72.6	118.3	156.5	176.0	166.5	157.2	177.6	193.1	190.7	180.2
1925-------	1939	16.8	42.7	77.0	126.0	160.0	164.9	159.6	181.4	203.0	206.7	198.8	188.7
1926-------	1940	17.0	45.2	83.5	128.6	147.1	158.3	181.5	211.9	216.9	214.8	206.5	198.0
1927-------	1941	17.9	48.2	84.9	117.6	142.2	172.1	212.9	224.7	223.4	218.5	213.3	202.8
1928-------	1942	18.2	49.0	77.2	114.5	149.2	203.2	224.9	229.6	224.6	223.9	214.3	207.8
1929-------	1943	18.5	44.9	76.8	116.8	179.0	215.2	230.0	231.0	231.2	227.6	223.2	216.6
1930-------	1944	17.1	44.6	76.2	139.4	188.6	217.7	228.8	235.3	231.8	231.4	230.4	220.0
1931-------	1945	17.5	44.4	92.7	148.9	192.4	217.9	233.9	236.2	238.6	243.8	237.6	231.1
1932-------	1946	16.4	53.0	98.8	150.8	191.9	221.7	231.6	239.4	249.3	250.7	247.8	233.8
1933-------	1947	20.4	57.6	101.6	152.6	196.3	219.3	239.1	254.9	261.0	264.9	255.8	236.2
1934-------	1948	22.1	59.8	103.0	156.0	194.0	226.0	253.4	266.7	276.9	272.7	258.2	243.5
1935-------	1949	22.6	60.0	105.3	153.6	198.8	235.9	262.2	281.2	284.3	275.2	263.6	240.6
1936-------	1950	23.2	61.5	102.5	155.9	205.3	239.5	273.7	286.1	282.6	275.9	258.1	238.6
1937-------	1951	24.3	58.7	102.9	158.4	205.2	248.3	277.3	281.2	280.2	269.0	254.5	233.2
1938-------	1952	22.1	58.0	104.8	155.8	210.2	246.9	268.9	277.6	272.4	263.3	245.2	222.2
1939-------	1953	22.0	60.7	103.6	160.5	209.6	241.5	268.7	273.6	272.3	255.5	238.2	213.0
1940-------	1954	23.8	58.8	105.3	160.1	205.9	240.5	264.7	272.8	264.3	248.2	228.2	194.2
1941-------	1955	22.7	60.6	106.3	154.7	203.5	235.3	260.7	265.3	255.9	239.2	208.4	177.3
1942-------	1956	22.7	60.6	100.8	153.1	197.4	229.4	254.5	258.2	247.5	219.1	190.7	162.5
1943-------	1957	23.0	56.4	100.2	147.5	192.2	222.8	249.0	250.2	230.8	202.3	175.0	150.5
1944-------	1958	21.5	57.5	97.2	146.3	188.8	222.0	245.8	238.1	215.3	187.5	164.0	151.1
1945-------	1959	22.3	55.4	96.2	142.3	187.2	221.2	235.3	224.6	201.2	177.5	164.0	157.6
1946-------	1960	21.3	55.0	93.7	141.4	189.3	214.2	225.7	212.1	191.5	178.2	169.7	149.1
1947-------	1961	21.2	52.9	93.3	142.8	183.7	208.7	217.0	202.7	190.1	180.6	161.7	133.3
1948-------	1962	20.1	52.3	93.0	139.5	180.3	202.0	206.8	200.4	191.8	171.8	142.4	124.4
1949-------	1963	19.9	52.3	92.4	138.4	176.2	196.1	204.5	201.0	181.7	150.6	132.6	
1950-------	1964	19.9	52.6	92.0	136.8	172.7	195.5	206.6	188.9	159.8	140.6		
1951-------	1965	20.4	52.7	93.3	135.4	172.9	197.7	194.9	169.3	149.3			
1952-------	1966	20.5	54.2	92.2	134.9	175.8	187.9	176.9	157.8				
1953-------	1967	21.3	54.3	91.8	139.3	169.1	175.0	165.6					
1954-------	1968	21.9	54.4	96.3	135.8	161.5	164.0						
1955-------	1969	22.4	58.0	95.3	133.7	152.3							
1956-------	1970	23.8	57.6	95.6	126.5								
1957-------	1971	23.6	58.2	91.9									
1958-------	1972	24.1	57.0										
1959-------	1973	24.5											

TABLE 4C. CENTRAL BIRTH RATES FOR ALL OTHER WOMEN DURING EACH YEAR 1917-73 BY AGE AND LIVE-BIRTH ORDER FOR EACH COHORT FROM 1868 TO 1959--CON.

LIVE-BIRTH ORDER AND COHORT	DIAGONAL LINE FOR CALENDAR YEAR	CURRENT AGE											
		26	27	28	29	30	31	32	33	34	35	36	37
TOTAL BIRTHS--CON.													
1880-------													100.7
1881-------												112.4	102.8
1882-------											116.1	113.8	108.8
1883-------										112.5	115.1	117.1	110.3
1884-------									101.1	109.2	115.3	116.1	102.5
1885-------								95.8	96.5	107.1	112.6	106.5	94.4
1886-------							111.5	92.0	93.2	103.7	106.7	98.2	87.8
1887-------						113.0	109.0	89.4	90.1	102.8	99.0	92.2	86.6
1888-------					133.9	110.2	107.4	87.6	95.4	96.5	94.8	91.9	87.2
1889-------				130.5	130.0	111.5	107.1	93.5	91.0	94.5	96.3	95.2	84.8
1890-------			143.2	125.8	134.1	114.9	114.3	89.6	90.9	97.6	99.0	91.6	80.9
1891-------	1917	149.9	138.8	131.8	141.2	122.6	109.9	89.7	95.1	99.8	96.3	86.3	70.9
1892-------	1918	145.9	144.4	142.3	149.7	115.9	109.6	93.5	97.9	96.8	88.3	75.0	66.3
1893-------	1919	150.6	156.9	149.9	139.4	114.7	113.5	95.7	94.3	88.6	78.0	71.7	66.7
1894-------	1920	163.9	162.6	136.6	137.2	119.1	112.5	92.6	88.2	78.4	75.3	70.2	63.7
1895-------	1921	167.9	148.3	134.2	143.1	116.4	108.2	86.4	78.0	75.8	73.7	66.7	64.3
1896-------	1922	153.4	144.9	140.5	138.3	113.6	99.6	76.2	74.1	74.4	69.4	66.2	59.1
1897-------	1923	149.1	151.5	136.0	132.8	103.2	91.0	71.2	73.8	70.8	68.3	61.1	59.7
1898-------	1924	158.5	149.0	132.4	124.7	95.6	86.7	73.7	72.4	70.9	65.6	62.8	55.7
1899-------	1925	158.0	147.5	128.4	117.4	93.8	90.9	75.0	77.2	72.2	71.6	62.3	56.7
1900-------	1926	155.1	139.7	115.9	114.1	96.9	89.6	77.6	76.6	75.5	68.1	61.2	58.9
1901-------	1927	141.4	122.9	109.5	111.9	92.5	87.5	73.0	76.8	68.2	63.5	60.4	57.0
1902-------	1928	124.6	114.1	106.3	104.9	87.2	79.6	70.0	66.4	62.0	60.3	56.5	54.2
1903-------	1929	117.5	110.4	101.7	101.9	81.0	78.6	63.0	61.8	60.2	57.9	53.7	52.3
1904-------	1930	115.8	109.3	101.5	98.5	83.0	74.9	61.5	62.8	59.6	56.9	53.0	53.1
1905-------	1931	114.4	108.3	97.5	98.9	79.6	71.4	61.8	63.3	58.8	56.6	53.5	51.4
1906-------	1932	113.6	104.0	98.9	93.8	76.5	72.2	62.9	63.0	59.5	57.5	52.5	53.5
1907-------	1933	107.3	105.7	93.2	90.2	76.9	72.4	62.9	64.7	61.3	58.6	55.0	54.5
1908-------	1934	109.7	99.5	90.5	91.3	76.6	71.7	64.7	66.8	63.7	62.0	56.5	55.5
1909-------	1935	108.1	100.4	94.4	93.3	77.4	74.5	67.6	69.6	67.9	64.2	61.0	57.2
1910-------	1936	107.6	103.6	97.1	93.3	79.6	77.5	70.3	74.6	70.6	68.6	62.5	59.0
1911-------	1937	110.8	106.9	98.2	95.5	82.5	78.7	75.4	77.9	73.8	69.9	65.6	60.7
1912-------	1938	112.2	106.8	100.0	98.4	85.9	84.8	79.0	78.8	73.8	72.3	65.1	61.5
1913-------	1939	112.6	109.2	103.1	99.3	91.7	88.9	79.9	81.1	77.5	73.0	66.5	62.8
1914-------	1940	115.0	112.8	105.1	105.6	95.6	89.9	83.5	85.1	78.8	74.6	68.7	66.6
1915-------	1941	118.2	113.6	110.7	109.2	95.3	94.1	87.6	86.7	81.2	76.3	72.0	65.6
1916-------	1942	121.0	120.1	113.7	108.2	100.4	98.2	89.1	88.8	82.5	80.2	71.3	67.6
1917-------	1943	127.5	122.5	110.9	114.8	105.3	101.4	92.6	91.3	85.8	80.1	73.7	70.2
1918-------	1944	129.1	119.1	120.3	121.1	110.4	105.9	96.9	96.0	89.9	83.8	77.6	71.2
1919-------	1945	127.1	133.5	131.1	130.9	118.5	112.4	104.9	104.0	95.3	90.2	81.6	75.6
1920-------	1946	141.6	143.5	139.6	136.3	122.8	119.7	110.2	107.4	100.8	92.2	83.7	76.2
1921-------	1947	152.1	150.0	144.0	139.2	130.1	123.6	113.7	112.0	102.0	94.7	84.4	73.2
1922-------	1948	155.9	152.2	145.8	144.4	130.8	125.7	117.4	111.7	102.5	93.7	80.3	72.6
1923-------	1949	162.0	158.1	153.4	148.2	135.8	131.4	119.1	115.6	105.0	91.4	81.2	71.6
1924-------	1950	171.8	168.4	161.4	157.5	146.5	136.8	125.3	119.3	104.3	95.8	81.3	73.1
1925-------	1951	181.9	178.3	171.0	167.3	150.2	143.5	129.6	118.5	108.0	93.9	83.5	70.9
1926-------	1952	190.4	187.2	181.2	171.4	156.2	146.6	128.5	121.9	106.1	95.4	80.0	67.5
1927-------	1953	196.9	193.3	181.3	176.6	159.5	144.8	130.1	118.2	106.2	92.1	76.2	66.0
1928-------	1954	201.4	194.0	183.5	176.4	154.4	145.0	126.7	117.8	102.0	85.3	73.8	60.8
1929-------	1955	205.2	200.8	187.5	173.7	158.0	143.9	129.6	116.2	97.5	85.8	69.5	55.3
1930-------	1956	211.7	201.1	183.8	175.2	155.7	143.7	124.8	109.9	95.6	78.3	62.5	50.6
1931-------	1957	215.9	200.7	187.3	172.6	157.0	138.3	120.6	108.5	87.9	71.2	56.5	45.7
1932-------	1958	215.6	203.3	183.0	174.6	149.3	135.0	115.3	98.9	79.1	64.1	51.9	43.1
1933-------	1959	220.6	201.3	189.8	167.7	148.0	131.6	108.1	89.1	72.5	60.2	49.9	42.1
1934-------	1960	219.9	207.0	184.9	166.9	143.6	123.1	98.2	82.4	67.5	58.6	49.2	39.4
1935-------	1961	222.9	202.9	181.7	163.0	134.1	111.0	91.2	76.5	65.7	56.4	45.8	35.3
1936-------	1962	218.3	196.4	174.0	150.3	120.6	101.2	82.7	73.9	63.6	53.1	40.5	30.6
1937-------	1963	210.2	186.6	161.1	133.2	109.7	92.2	80.7	71.6	60.2	45.9	35.9	
1938-------	1964	197.6	171.2	140.4	119.2	99.1	90.1	80.0	67.6	51.1	41.0		
1939-------	1965	183.4	152.5	129.1	111.3	98.8	91.0	76.7	59.3	47.7			
1940-------	1966	164.3	141.3	120.6	110.6	100.0	87.3	67.1	54.3				
1941-------	1967	151.1	130.7	118.8	111.3	97.3	75.9	61.0					
1942-------	1968	139.6	128.6	120.9	107.4	84.4	69.5						
1943-------	1969	138.1	133.3	116.5	94.5	77.9							
1944-------	1970	144.8	126.8	103.5	88.1								
1945-------	1971	137.7	113.1	96.4									
1946-------	1972	122.9	106.3										
1947-------	1973	115.2											

TABLE 4C. CENTRAL BIRTH RATES FOR ALL OTHER WOMEN DURING EACH YEAR 1917-73 BY AGE AND LIVE-BIRTH ORDER FOR EACH COHORT FROM 1868 TO 1959--CON.

LIVE-BIRTH ORDER AND COHORT	DIAGONAL LINE FOR CALENDAR YEAR	CURRENT AGE											
		38	39	40	41	42	43	44	45	46	47	48	49
TOTAL BIRTHS--CON.													
1868-------													4.9
1869-------												8.2	9.2
1870-------											11.8	14.8	4.5
1871-------										18.2	21.7	7.4	5.3
1872-------									21.0	33.7	10.7	9.0	3.8
1873-------								24.0	34.4	16.8	13.2	6.3	3.6
1874-------							26.0	33.8	19.4	20.6	9.4	5.7	3.8
1875-------						30.4	28.6	21.9	22.7	14.8	8.8	6.3	3.4
1876-------					44.3	33.8	23.9	24.3	17.6	13.5	9.3	5.8	2.7
1877-------				56.1	50.1	28.5	24.4	21.3	16.1	15.0	8.7	4.7	2.9
1878-------			81.7	60.9	43.3	29.5	25.7	19.5	17.6	14.5	6.9	5.2	2.5
1879-------	1917	88.6	85.6	58.1	45.8	31.6	23.4	20.6	17.0	13.3	8.1	4.5	3.1
1880-------	1918	90.0	87.3	61.4	49.5	28.9	23.9	20.5	16.1	14.3	6.6	4.7	3.1
1881-------	1919	96.8	91.7	63.5	45.4	29.4	23.9	20.5	16.9	12.0	7.0	4.9	2.7
1882-------	1920	100.0	90.9	59.1	45.2	29.0	24.6	20.4	15.2	11.7	7.2	4.3	2.7
1883-------	1921	94.8	84.2	57.1	43.7	30.2	24.2	18.6	14.0	11.1	6.3	4.2	2.6
1884-------	1922	87.8	79.8	55.2	42.8	28.4	21.2	16.7	12.8	10.8	5.5	4.3	2.5
1885-------	1923	81.8	77.1	54.3	40.9	24.4	18.5	14.6	12.6	9.6	5.4	3.7	2.8
1886-------	1924	79.9	74.6	50.3	36.5	21.1	16.6	14.5	11.4	9.6	4.4	4.1	2.7
1887-------	1925	80.7	70.6	46.8	31.3	20.1	16.4	13.7	11.8	8.1	4.7	3.7	2.6
1888-------	1926	75.8	66.0	39.8	29.9	19.7	15.5	14.5	10.0	7.6	4.2	3.6	2.1
1889-------	1927	72.8	58.7	40.0	31.1	18.9	16.7	12.6	9.6	7.2	4.3	3.4	2.2
1890-------	1928	63.4	56.4	41.1	29.0	20.2	15.3	13.0	9.2	6.8	4.0	3.3	2.0
1891-------	1929	60.9	58.8	38.3	30.4	19.1	16.4	12.0	8.8	6.8	3.8	3.0	1.7
1892-------	1930	62.5	54.7	39.9	28.6	19.5	15.5	11.3	8.8	6.2	3.6	2.9	1.4
1893-------	1931	58.8	55.8	37.0	28.4	18.7	14.6	11.0	7.7	5.6	3.3	2.3	1.3
1894-------	1932	59.8	51.7	36.5	27.8	17.6	14.2	10.2	7.0	5.7	2.9	1.8	0.9
1895-------	1933	55.0	51.6	35.0	25.5	17.3	13.0	9.1	7.2	4.7	2.8	1.4	0.9
1896-------	1934	55.0	47.5	32.1	25.0	16.4	11.8	9.6	6.1	4.5	2.4	1.4	1.1
1897-------	1935	50.3	44.0	31.9	24.0	15.0	12.4	8.5	7.1	4.2	2.0	1.7	1.2
1898-------	1936	48.5	44.6	33.1	22.9	16.4	12.2	10.2	7.3	4.0	2.8	1.7	0.9
1899-------	1937	52.1	47.4	31.0	24.4	16.2	13.4	9.8	6.3	4.3	2.4	1.6	1.0
1900-------	1938	53.7	45.5	32.1	24.8	16.4	13.9	9.6	6.6	4.1	2.2	1.5	0.8
1901-------	1939	49.9	43.6	31.5	22.2	16.5	13.6	9.4	5.9	3.6	2.0	1.4	0.6
1902-------	1940	47.9	43.4	30.3	23.5	16.8	13.6	8.8	5.3	3.1	1.7	1.2	0.5
1903-------	1941	47.7	42.0	31.3	23.3	17.2	13.0	8.1	4.6	2.8	1.5	1.2	0.4
1904-------	1942	47.3	43.5	31.3	24.4	17.1	12.5	7.5	4.7	2.9	1.6	1.0	0.6
1905-------	1943	49.3	43.7	32.3	24.0	16.7	11.6	7.9	4.7	2.6	1.2	0.9	0.6
1906-------	1944	49.8	44.5	31.2	23.7	15.8	12.3	7.4	4.4	2.5	1.4	1.0	0.4
1907-------	1945	49.8	42.3	31.5	22.4	16.1	11.8	7.0	4.2	2.5	1.1	1.0	0.3
1908-------	1946	48.0	42.4	29.9	23.1	15.2	11.6	6.8	4.2	2.3	1.2	0.5	0.4
1909-------	1947	51.0	43.3	32.4	23.8	17.3	12.4	8.2	4.5	2.3	1.1	0.8	0.4
1910-------	1948	51.8	45.9	33.2	26.6	17.3	13.3	7.9	4.6	2.4	1.4	1.0	0.4
1911-------	1949	54.4	46.7	36.0	25.8	18.6	13.5	8.3	4.5	2.6	1.3	0.7	0.4
1912-------	1950	54.6	48.6	34.8	26.9	18.9	13.7	8.3	4.9	2.4	1.3	0.8	0.4
1913-------	1951	56.9	48.0	36.1	27.0	18.8	14.2	8.4	4.8	2.6	1.2	0.6	0.2
1914-------	1952	57.6	49.8	37.3	26.8	19.7	14.6	8.2	4.7	2.5	0.9	0.6	0.2
1915-------	1953	58.5	50.8	36.7	28.3	19.7	13.3	8.1	4.4	2.2	1.1	0.5	0.1
1916-------	1954	61.1	50.4	38.3	28.0	18.7	13.2	8.0	4.1	2.3	1.1	0.5	0.1
1917-------	1955	61.2	52.5	37.5	27.6	19.2	12.9	7.9	4.2	2.3	1.1	0.3	0.2
1918-------	1956	63.2	51.8	37.5	27.6	19.4	13.4	7.5	4.3	2.1	0.9	0.4	0.1
1919-------	1957	64.7	53.0	39.6	28.7	20.2	13.6	8.0	4.3	2.2	1.0	0.3	0.2
1920-------	1958	64.1	53.8	39.2	28.9	19.6	13.5	8.3	4.3	2.0	0.8	0.3	0.1
1921-------	1959	63.7	52.0	39.1	27.8	19.3	13.2	7.5	3.8	1.7	0.7	0.4	0.1
1922-------	1960	61.8	51.3	36.5	26.6	18.5	12.0	6.9	3.6	1.7	0.9	0.2	0.1
1923-------	1961	61.7	49.0	35.4	26.3	17.1	11.2	6.3	3.1	1.5	0.7	0.3	0.1
1924-------	1962	59.4	47.3	36.3	24.9	16.5	10.5	5.9	2.9	1.5	0.5	0.2	0.0
1925-------	1963	58.6	48.0	33.9	23.9	15.4	9.5	5.7	3.1	1.4	0.5	0.1	
1926-------	1964	57.5	45.2	31.6	21.7	13.9	9.4	5.2	2.9	1.2	0.3		
1927-------	1965	53.4	40.7	29.0	19.2	13.1	8.4	4.9	2.4	1.2			
1928-------	1966	47.0	36.9	25.3	18.2	12.2	7.8	3.9	1.9				
1929-------	1967	44.1	33.2	24.1	16.9	11.4	6.4	3.5					
1930-------	1968	39.4	31.0	22.5	15.8	9.4	5.5						
1931-------	1969	36.6	29.4	21.1	13.6	8.5							
1932-------	1970	35.8	27.5	18.3	11.8								
1933-------	1971	33.2	23.5	15.8									
1934-------	1972	29.2	20.5										
1935-------	1973	26.0											

TABLE 4C. CENTRAL BIRTH RATES FOR ALL OTHER WOMEN DURING EACH YEAR 1917-73 BY AGE AND LIVE-BIRTH ORDER FOR EACH COHORT FROM 1868 TO 1959--CON.

LIVE-BIRTH ORDER AND COHORT	DIAGONAL LINE FOR CALENDAR YEAR	CURRENT AGE											
		14	15	16	17	18	19	20	21	22	23	24	25
FIRST BIRTHS													
1892-------													28.5
1893-------												35.9	29.7
1894-------											45.9	36.9	26.9
1895-------										56.0	46.7	33.6	32.3
1896-------									73.8	57.0	42.7	40.1	29.5
1897-------								89.6	75.2	52.1	50.7	37.1	25.3
1898-------							106.3	89.9	69.3	62.4	47.7	32.1	24.0
1899-------						101.1	104.0	82.5	82.0	58.0	41.0	30.4	24.8
1900-------					85.8	97.7	96.4	97.8	76.8	50.2	39.4	32.5	25.4
1901-------				55.8	82.4	90.5	113.6	94.5	66.3	48.1	42.9	32.7	23.0
1902-------			32.4	54.2	77.1	107.2	113.2	82.4	63.9	52.6	42.2	29.5	20.1
1903-------	1917	12.8	31.0	50.4	90.8	108.9	98.7	82.4	69.5	52.4	38.4	26.2	17.6
1904-------	1918	12.1	28.8	59.2	92.1	95.3	101.5	88.6	68.3	50.3	34.8	23.3	17.1
1905-------	1919	11.2	33.6	59.9	80.4	100.7	108.5	86.9	65.4	44.0	31.7	22.8	17.9
1906-------	1920	13.0	34.4	52.4	85.1	107.2	107.0	82.9	59.5	40.5	30.6	24.0	17.0
1907-------	1921	13.6	30.5	55.6	90.8	108.4	101.4	76.1	55.2	39.7	32.0	22.4	17.4
1908-------	1922	12.3	32.6	59.6	93.8	103.2	94.7	69.8	54.2	41.2	30.9	23.4	15.8
1909-------	1923	13.2	35.0	63.3	91.7	97.1	88.9	69.6	56.2	40.8	32.1	21.5	17.7
1910-------	1924	14.3	37.4	63.0	87.0	91.6	87.1	71.8	54.8	41.6	29.3	23.8	16.9
1911-------	1925	15.6	38.9	61.6	83.8	89.2	90.4	69.9	55.9	38.0	31.8	23.2	16.7
1912-------	1926	16.4	37.6	58.2	80.0	92.2	86.5	70.9	50.7	40.9	31.2	22.5	17.0
1913-------	1927	16.1	35.6	55.6	82.8	89.4	87.8	65.7	54.8	41.1	30.4	22.9	17.5
1914-------	1928	14.7	33.7	57.2	79.5	90.3	81.4	70.9	54.5	39.2	31.2	23.1	18.1
1915-------	1929	14.2	34.6	55.5	80.4	84.1	87.7	70.0	52.0	40.5	30.5	23.5	18.1
1916-------	1930	14.5	33.0	56.6	74.6	90.1	87.4	65.8	54.1	39.7	30.5	23.2	19.2
1917-------	1931	13.9	33.8	52.6	79.5	91.0	82.9	69.1	53.3	39.6	30.1	24.6	21.6
1918-------	1932	14.2	31.8	55.0	82.6	86.8	87.2	69.3	52.0	38.7	31.2	28.4	22.0
1919-------	1933	13.6	32.8	58.8	81.4	93.6	89.5	68.4	52.5	40.7	36.6	28.0	21.2
1920-------	1934	13.9	36.3	58.6	87.4	96.1	87.7	67.4	54.1	43.9	35.4	26.4	20.6
1921-------	1935	15.5	36.4	63.3	89.8	93.9	85.0	69.7	54.4	42.5	33.0	25.6	26.0
1922-------	1936	14.8	38.1	64.1	85.8	88.0	85.9	69.1	53.0	39.7	31.0	31.9	32.2
1923-------	1937	15.7	39.1	61.2	81.6	90.3	86.8	68.2	50.0	38.2	39.2	40.4	29.7
1924-------	1938	16.4	38.1	59.7	84.6	94.1	86.6	63.3	48.8	48.6	51.0	37.7	28.8
1925-------	1939	16.8	38.5	63.1	87.8	94.5	79.3	62.5	59.9	63.3	47.3	35.7	27.7
1926-------	1940	17.0	40.8	65.2	88.3	85.2	77.1	73.6	77.5	58.5	44.2	34.0	27.6
1927-------	1941	17.9	41.3	65.6	79.7	83.1	86.1	93.6	72.0	54.0	41.4	32.9	27.0
1928-------	1942	18.2	41.7	59.2	77.7	88.2	107.5	88.3	66.4	49.8	39.5	31.9	26.5
1929-------	1943	18.5	38.1	59.0	79.6	110.4	104.8	82.4	61.6	48.7	39.1	32.6	27.8
1930-------	1944	17.1	38.0	57.9	97.4	110.0	97.8	76.4	60.9	48.3	39.9	33.8	26.9
1931-------	1945	17.5	37.3	71.0	100.5	104.3	92.7	77.3	60.8	50.4	43.2	34.1	27.8
1932-------	1946	16.4	44.3	74.7	97.1	101.2	95.1	76.3	64.2	54.1	43.7	35.2	27.7
1933-------	1947	20.4	48.0	74.5	96.7	104.6	92.6	81.5	69.3	56.3	45.9	35.9	26.3
1934-------	1948	22.1	49.2	75.6	99.4	101.8	97.7	87.4	71.3	58.8	46.5	34.3	26.8
1935-------	1949	22.6	49.9	77.8	97.5	105.3	104.5	88.7	74.5	59.1	44.8	34.4	26.7
1936-------	1950	23.2	51.4	75.9	99.1	110.5	102.9	91.8	74.5	56.8	43.7	33.8	26.4
1937-------	1951	24.3	49.3	76.6	101.9	108.4	106.8	92.0	70.8	55.7	43.4	32.7	25.3
1938-------	1952	22.1	49.1	78.1	98.9	110.7	105.7	87.4	69.7	55.2	42.1	31.4	25.7
1939-------	1953	22.0	51.4	76.4	101.5	109.8	101.1	86.9	69.9	55.1	40.9	32.8	25.0
1940-------	1954	23.8	49.1	77.3	101.3	105.8	100.4	86.6	70.6	54.5	42.2	32.9	25.9
1941-------	1955	22.7	50.3	78.2	95.4	104.8	98.8	86.5	70.4	54.9	42.8	33.3	26.7
1942-------	1956	22.7	51.1	72.8	95.2	101.9	97.7	86.8	71.0	56.8	43.3	34.5	27.1
1943-------	1957	23.0	46.8	73.3	91.8	100.2	96.8	87.3	72.3	57.0	44.2	34.5	29.7
1944-------	1958	21.5	47.9	70.3	91.0	98.5	98.1	89.7	73.0	58.2	44.6	36.5	30.2
1945-------	1959	22.3	46.0	70.0	88.1	99.4	101.0	89.6	74.6	58.3	46.2	37.2	32.9
1946-------	1960	21.3	45.7	67.8	88.9	102.6	100.2	92.8	75.1	60.3	48.2	40.7	32.0
1947-------	1961	21.2	43.7	67.9	90.6	101.7	104.2	93.4	77.7	62.4	50.6	39.6	32.2
1948-------	1962	20.1	43.5	68.0	90.4	104.7	104.8	95.9	79.7	64.0	48.6	38.6	30.9
1949-------	1963	19.9	43.5	69.1	92.1	105.3	107.1	97.0	79.5	60.4	45.3	35.9	
1950-------	1964	19.9	44.3	69.6	93.1	107.6	109.2	98.4	74.8	54.8	42.2		
1951-------	1965	20.4	44.7	71.4	95.3	109.9	111.1	93.4	68.4	51.0			
1952-------	1966	20.5	46.4	72.5	97.1	113.3	106.7	86.2	63.7				
1953-------	1967	21.3	47.3	73.4	101.0	110.0	101.7	80.7					
1954-------	1968	21.9	47.8	77.6	99.5	107.7	95.3						
1955-------	1969	22.4	51.2	77.2	100.7	102.1							
1956-------	1970	23.8	51.0	79.1	95.8								
1957-------	1971	23.6	52.4	76.6									
1958-------	1972	24.1	51.5										
1959-------	1973	24.5											

TABLE 4C. CENTRAL BIRTH RATES FOR ALL OTHER WOMEN DURING EACH YEAR 1917-73 BY AGE AND LIVE-BIRTH ORDER FOR EACH COHORT FROM 1868 TO 1959--CON.

LIVE-BIRTH ORDER AND COHORT	DIAGONAL LINE FOR CALENDAR YEAR	CURRENT AGE											
		26	27	28	29	30	31	32	33	34	35	36	37
FIRST BIRTHS--CON.													
1880-------													3.1
1881-------												3.7	4.0
1882-------											4.5	4.7	3.5
1883-------										4.8	5.3	4.1	3.9
1884-------									5.1	5.4	4.6	4.4	3.7
1885-------								5.5	5.6	4.7	5.0	4.1	3.3
1886-------							7.6	6.0	4.9	5.1	4.6	3.7	2.7
1887-------						9.4	8.4	5.3	5.4	4.7	4.1	3.1	2.8
1888-------					12.8	10.2	7.6	5.9	5.0	4.3	3.6	3.2	2.8
1889-------				14.5	13.8	9.3	8.6	5.5	4.6	3.9	3.7	3.7	2.5
1890-------			17.9	15.4	12.6	10.9	8.0	5.1	4.4	4.0	4.2	3.1	2.8
1891-------	1917	21.7	19.0	14.0	15.0	10.0	7.4	4.9	4.3	4.4	3.2	3.4	2.0
1892-------	1918	23.0	17.3	17.1	13.7	9.1	7.1	4.8	4.7	3.4	3.5	2.4	1.8
1893-------	1919	20.9	21.1	15.4	12.1	8.6	7.0	5.0	3.5	3.8	2.7	2.3	2.0
1894-------	1920	25.3	18.9	13.2	11.3	8.5	7.1	4.3	3.9	3.0	2.7	2.3	1.8
1895-------	1921	22.7	16.2	12.2	11.2	8.1	6.0	4.1	3.3	2.9	2.6	2.2	1.8
1896-------	1922	19.4	14.9	12.2	10.8	7.1	5.3	3.5	3.1	2.9	2.5	2.0	1.5
1897-------	1923	17.9	15.0	11.8	9.2	6.4	5.1	3.2	3.4	2.8	2.3	1.9	1.7
1898-------	1924	18.2	15.1	10.5	8.8	5.9	4.7	3.8	3.1	2.5	2.2	1.8	1.4
1899-------	1925	19.3	14.0	10.8	8.3	5.8	5.4	3.7	3.3	2.8	2.3	2.0	1.7
1900-------	1926	17.9	13.3	9.1	8.1	6.4	5.1	3.7	3.2	2.8	2.5	2.1	1.7
1901-------	1927	16.1	11.4	9.0	8.3	6.2	5.2	3.5	3.4	2.7	2.4	2.1	1.7
1902-------	1928	13.6	10.8	9.2	8.0	5.9	4.4	3.4	2.9	2.5	2.2	1.9	1.8
1903-------	1929	13.0	11.2	8.8	7.7	5.0	4.4	3.0	2.7	2.4	2.2	2.0	1.8
1904-------	1930	13.8	10.8	8.8	6.7	5.3	4.2	3.0	2.8	2.6	2.4	2.0	2.0
1905-------	1931	13.1	10.7	7.8	7.0	5.1	4.2	3.1	3.0	2.7	2.4	2.2	2.1
1906-------	1932	13.4	9.8	8.2	7.0	5.2	4.2	3.4	3.2	2.8	2.7	2.5	2.2
1907-------	1933	12.0	10.4	8.2	7.1	5.0	4.6	3.6	3.3	3.1	3.0	2.7	2.5
1908-------	1934	13.0	10.2	8.2	6.8	5.5	4.8	3.8	3.8	3.6	3.3	3.1	2.6
1909-------	1935	12.9	10.2	8.2	7.4	5.9	5.1	4.3	4.3	4.1	3.7	3.3	3.0
1910-------	1936	12.6	10.5	8.6	7.7	6.1	5.8	4.8	5.0	4.5	4.0	3.7	3.3
1911-------	1937	12.9	11.0	9.0	7.9	6.7	6.0	5.6	5.4	4.7	4.6	4.4	3.5
1912-------	1938	13.6	11.4	9.2	8.6	7.5	7.0	6.0	5.5	5.2	5.4	4.2	3.8
1913-------	1939	14.2	11.7	9.9	9.7	8.3	7.5	6.1	6.1	6.5	5.1	4.3	3.7
1914-------	1940	14.5	12.6	11.6	10.6	8.8	7.5	6.8	7.6	5.9	5.4	4.5	3.9
1915-------	1941	15.5	13.8	12.2	10.9	8.7	8.7	8.6	7.0	6.3	5.4	4.7	3.6
1916-------	1942	16.3	14.6	12.3	10.7	10.1	10.4	7.7	7.5	6.1	5.5	4.4	4.0
1917-------	1943	17.2	14.6	12.1	12.8	12.2	9.9	8.5	7.0	6.4	5.3	4.5	3.5
1918-------	1944	17.1	14.2	14.6	15.1	11.9	10.4	8.2	7.3	6.2	5.2	4.3	3.6
1919-------	1945	16.8	18.0	18.2	15.4	12.4	10.2	8.7	7.3	6.2	5.5	4.5	3.6
1920-------	1946	21.3	22.1	18.1	15.1	12.2	10.4	8.2	7.6	6.2	5.2	4.1	3.1
1921-------	1947	26.4	21.2	17.4	14.6	12.0	10.2	8.6	7.2	6.0	4.9	3.8	3.2
1922-------	1948	24.6	20.1	16.6	14.2	11.8	9.9	8.3	6.9	5.4	4.3	3.6	2.9
1923-------	1949	23.5	19.3	16.4	14.3	11.2	10.1	7.8	6.6	5.2	4.3	3.6	2.6
1924-------	1950	22.7	19.6	17.0	13.9	12.2	9.5	7.7	6.2	5.0	4.4	3.2	2.6
1925-------	1951	23.3	20.0	16.8	14.5	11.1	9.4	7.1	6.1	5.1	4.0	3.0	2.4
1926-------	1952	23.4	19.7	16.8	13.3	10.7	8.6	6.9	5.8	4.6	3.7	2.8	2.5
1927-------	1953	22.8	19.6	15.4	12.7	10.0	8.2	6.6	5.4	4.3	3.4	2.9	2.3
1928-------	1954	22.7	18.2	14.6	12.4	9.5	8.0	6.1	5.0	4.0	3.3	2.7	2.1
1929-------	1955	21.8	18.2	14.3	11.7	9.6	7.6	6.1	4.8	3.8	3.1	2.6	2.1
1930-------	1956	22.1	17.4	14.0	11.6	9.2	7.4	5.6	4.7	3.8	3.1	2.7	1.9
1931-------	1957	21.3	16.8	13.7	11.3	8.9	7.0	5.6	4.6	3.7	3.2	2.3	2.2
1932-------	1958	20.8	16.9	13.6	11.0	8.5	7.0	5.5	4.5	4.0	2.7	2.7	2.1
1933-------	1959	20.9	16.8	13.4	10.4	8.5	6.8	5.5	4.7	3.4	3.3	2.6	2.1
1934-------	1960	20.9	16.9	13.0	10.8	8.3	7.0	5.6	4.3	4.0	3.3	2.6	2.1
1935-------	1961	20.9	16.4	13.2	10.6	8.6	7.1	5.3	5.0	4.0	3.2	2.5	1.8
1936-------	1962	20.4	16.3	12.8	11.0	8.5	6.6	6.0	5.1	4.0	3.1	2.4	1.9
1937-------	1963	20.3	15.6	13.7	11.0	8.2	7.6	6.4	5.1	3.7	3.2	2.5	
1938-------	1964	19.6	16.8	13.4	10.4	9.4	8.0	6.3	4.9	4.1	3.2		
1939-------	1965	20.8	17.0	13.4	12.4	10.2	8.3	6.4	5.3	4.0			
1940-------	1966	21.3	17.4	15.5	13.1	10.4	8.3	6.6	5.0				
1941-------	1967	21.9	19.4	16.3	13.5	10.7	8.6	6.4					
1942-------	1968	23.9	20.2	17.0	14.0	10.8	8.5						
1943-------	1969	24.6	21.7	17.6	14.1	11.3							
1944-------	1970	26.9	21.6	17.3	14.4								
1945-------	1971	26.0	21.3	18.0									
1946-------	1972	26.2	21.9										
1947-------	1973	26.2											

TABLE 4C. CENTRAL BIRTH RATES FOR ALL OTHER WOMEN DURING EACH YEAR 1917-73 BY AGE AND LIVE-BIRTH ORDER FOR EACH COHORT FROM 1868 TO 1959--CON.

LIVE-BIRTH ORDER AND COHORT	DIAGONAL LINE FOR CALENDAR YEAR	CURRENT AGE											
		38	39	40	41	42	43	44	45	46	47	48	49
FIRST BIRTHS--CON.													
1868-------													0.1
1869-------												0.3	0.3
1870-------											0.4	0.5	0.1
1871-------										0.5	0.6	0.2	0.1
1872-------									0.5	0.8	0.2	0.2	0.1
1873-------								0.4	0.7	0.3	0.3	0.2	0.1
1874-------							0.4	0.7	0.3	0.4	0.3	0.2	0.1
1875-------						0.4	0.6	0.3	0.4	0.4	0.3	0.2	0.1
1876-------					0.7	0.8	0.3	0.5	0.4	0.4	0.2	0.2	0.1
1877-------				1.2	1.4	0.4	0.5	0.4	0.4	0.3	0.3	0.2	0.1
1878-------			2.0	2.0	0.7	0.6	0.4	0.4	0.3	0.4	0.3	0.2	0.1
1879-------	1917	2.4	2.9	1.4	1.2	0.5	0.4	0.4	0.4	0.3	0.3	0.1	0.1
1880-------	1918	3.1	2.3	1.8	1.0	0.6	0.5	0.4	0.3	0.5	0.3	0.1	0.1
1881-------	1919	2.8	2.8	1.7	1.1	0.6	0.4	0.4	0.5	0.4	0.2	0.1	0.0
1882-------	1920	3.2	2.6	1.7	1.2	0.5	0.4	0.5	0.4	0.3	0.1	0.1	0.1
1883-------	1921	3.0	2.5	1.6	0.9	0.5	0.4	0.4	0.4	0.1	0.1	0.1	0.1
1884-------	1922	2.7	2.2	1.4	0.9	0.5	0.4	0.4	0.2	0.2	0.1	0.1	0.1
1885-------	1923	2.2	2.1	1.2	0.9	0.5	0.3	0.2	0.2	0.2	0.1	0.1	0.1
1886-------	1924	2.3	1.8	1.2	0.9	0.4	0.3	0.2	0.3	0.1	0.1	0.1	0.1
1887-------	1925	2.2	1.8	1.2	0.7	0.4	0.3	0.3	0.2	0.2	0.1	0.1	0.1
1888-------	1926	2.1	1.9	1.0	0.6	0.3	0.3	0.2	0.2	0.2	0.1	0.1	0.2
1889-------	1927	2.3	1.5	0.9	0.6	0.3	0.3	0.2	0.2	0.1	0.1	0.2	0.0
1890-------	1928	1.7	1.3	1.0	0.6	0.4	0.2	0.2	0.2	0.1	0.1	0.1	0.0
1891-------	1929	1.5	1.6	0.8	0.6	0.3	0.3	0.2	0.2	0.2	0.1	0.0	0.0
1892-------	1930	1.8	1.3	0.8	0.5	0.3	0.2	0.2	0.2	0.2	0.1	0.1	0.0
1893-------	1931	1.5	1.2	0.7	0.5	0.3	0.2	0.2	0.2	0.1	0.1	0.0	0.1
1894-------	1932	1.5	1.1	0.6	0.5	0.3	0.2	0.2	0.1	0.2	0.1	0.1	0.0
1895-------	1933	1.3	1.1	0.7	0.5	0.3	0.2	0.1	0.2	0.1	0.1	0.0	0.0
1896-------	1934	1.4	1.0	0.6	0.4	0.3	0.2	0.2	0.1	0.1	0.0	0.0	0.0
1897-------	1935	1.1	1.0	0.6	0.4	0.3	0.2	0.1	0.1	0.1	0.0	0.0	0.1
1898-------	1936	1.3	0.9	0.6	0.4	0.3	0.2	0.1	0.1	0.1	0.0	0.1	0.1
1899-------	1937	1.3	1.1	0.7	0.6	0.3	0.2	0.1	0.1	0.1	0.1	0.1	0.1
1900-------	1938	1.4	1.2	0.8	0.5	0.4	0.2	0.2	0.1	0.1	0.1	0.1	0.0
1901-------	1939	1.4	1.2	0.8	0.5	0.4	0.3	0.2	0.1	0.1	0.1	0.0	0.0
1902-------	1940	1.4	1.2	0.8	0.5	0.5	0.3	0.2	0.1	0.1	0.0	0.0	0.0
1903-------	1941	1.5	1.2	0.9	0.6	0.5	0.3	0.2	0.1	0.1	0.0	0.0	0.0
1904-------	1942	1.7	1.3	1.0	0.8	0.5	0.3	0.1	0.1	0.1	0.0	0.0	0.1
1905-------	1943	1.8	1.4	1.1	0.8	0.5	0.3	0.3	0.2	0.0	0.0	0.1	0.0
1906-------	1944	2.0	1.6	1.2	0.8	0.6	0.4	0.2	0.1	0.1	0.1	0.0	0.0
1907-------	1945	2.1	1.8	1.3	0.9	0.7	0.4	0.2	0.2	0.1	0.0	0.0	0.0
1908-------	1946	2.2	1.9	1.3	1.1	0.5	0.4	0.3	0.1	0.1	0.0	0.0	0.0
1909-------	1947	2.6	1.9	1.6	1.0	0.7	0.5	0.3	0.2	0.0	0.0	0.0	0.0
1910-------	1948	2.7	2.4	1.6	1.2	0.6	0.5	0.2	0.1	0.1	0.0	0.1	0.0
1911-------	1949	2.9	2.4	1.7	1.0	0.8	0.4	0.3	0.1	0.0	0.1	0.0	0.0
1912-------	1950	2.9	2.4	1.5	1.0	0.7	0.5	0.2	0.1	0.1	0.1	0.1	0.0
1913-------	1951	3.0	2.3	1.6	1.0	0.8	0.4	0.3	0.2	0.1	0.1	0.0	0.0
1914-------	1952	2.9	2.4	1.6	1.0	0.7	0.5	0.2	0.2	0.1	0.0	0.0	0.0
1915-------	1953	3.3	2.3	1.4	1.1	0.6	0.4	0.3	0.1	0.1	0.0	0.0	0.0
1916-------	1954	2.8	2.1	1.6	1.0	0.5	0.5	0.2	0.1	0.0	0.1	0.0	0.0
1917-------	1955	2.9	2.2	1.4	0.9	0.7	0.4	0.2	0.1	0.1	0.0	0.0	0.0
1918-------	1956	2.8	2.0	1.3	0.9	0.6	0.4	0.2	0.1	0.0	0.0	0.0	0.0
1919-------	1957	2.6	2.0	1.3	0.9	0.6	0.4	0.2	0.1	0.1	0.0	0.0	0.0
1920-------	1958	2.5	1.7	1.4	0.8	0.6	0.3	0.2	0.1	0.0	0.0	0.0	0.0
1921-------	1959	2.3	1.8	1.1	0.7	0.5	0.4	0.2	0.1	0.0	0.0	0.1	0.0
1922-------	1960	2.2	1.7	1.0	0.7	0.5	0.3	0.1	0.0	0.0	0.1	0.0	0.0
1923-------	1961	2.1	1.5	1.0	0.8	0.5	0.2	0.1	0.0	0.1	0.0	0.0	0.0
1924-------	1962	1.9	1.4	1.0	0.7	0.4	0.3	0.1	0.1	0.0	0.0	0.0	0.0
1925-------	1963	2.1	1.5	1.1	0.7	0.4	0.2	0.2	0.1	0.0	0.0	0.0	
1926-------	1964	1.9	1.5	1.0	0.6	0.4	0.3	0.1	0.1	0.0	0.0		
1927-------	1965	1.9	1.3	1.0	0.6	0.4	0.2	0.1	0.1	0.1			
1928-------	1966	1.7	1.2	1.0	0.7	0.4	0.2	0.1	0.1				
1929-------	1967	1.7	1.4	1.0	0.5	0.3	0.2	0.2					
1930-------	1968	1.8	1.3	0.8	0.6	0.3	0.2						
1931-------	1969	1.6	1.2	0.8	0.4	0.4							
1932-------	1970	1.7	1.2	0.7	0.5								
1933-------	1971	1.5	1.0	0.7									
1934-------	1972	1.4	1.0										
1935-------	1973	1.4											

TABLE 4C. CENTRAL BIRTH RATES FOR ALL OTHER WOMEN DURING EACH YEAR 1917-73 BY AGE AND LIVE-BIRTH ORDER FOR EACH COHORT FROM 1868 TO 1959--CON.

LIVE-BIRTH ORDER AND COHORT	DIAGONAL LINE FOR CALENDAR YEAR	CURRENT AGE											
		14	15	16	17	18	19	20	21	22	23	24	25
SECOND BIRTHS													
1892-------													34.1
1893-------												42.7	31.8
1894-------											52.0	40.0	33.4
1895-------										56.1	48.8	40.7	36.2
1896-------									61.1	52.6	48.4	43.4	35.7
1897-------								57.7	57.3	52.3	51.0	43.2	35.7
1898-------							49.5	54.5	57.4	55.6	51.7	44.2	33.6
1899-------						31.7	46.6	53.2	60.2	55.5	52.4	41.2	31.9
1900-------					16.9	30.0	45.0	55.9	60.6	56.8	49.9	40.6	31.6
1901-------				6.4	15.7	27.9	46.4	59.2	61.7	53.7	49.9	38.4	30.6
1902-------			2.0	6.1	15.0	29.1	52.9	60.1	59.1	54.4	46.4	37.0	25.9
1903-------	1917	*	1.8	5.7	15.5	35.9	52.4	57.8	59.3	52.5	45.3	32.8	23.0
1904-------	1918	*	1.7	5.9	19.0	34.6	50.9	58.6	57.5	51.5	41.0	29.7	22.0
1905-------	1919	*	1.8	7.2	18.3	34.2	52.1	56.2	57.4	47.6	37.0	28.7	22.5
1906-------	1920	*	2.2	6.9	18.1	35.6	49.5	57.4	53.6	42.9	36.1	29.3	22.7
1907-------	1921	*	2.1	7.0	18.9	34.9	52.3	53.7	48.9	42.1	36.6	29.1	22.5
1908-------	1922	*	2.2	7.2	19.5	36.7	49.1	50.0	48.5	42.3	36.6	29.4	21.1
1909-------	1923	*	2.2	8.0	20.7	35.6	46.4	49.9	49.3	42.7	37.9	28.3	21.9
1910-------	1924	*	2.4	8.0	21.1	33.5	46.8	50.7	48.8	44.6	35.9	29.1	22.2
1911-------	1925	*	2.6	9.1	19.4	33.6	47.4	49.5	51.5	41.9	37.2	28.8	22.4
1912-------	1926	*	2.8	8.0	19.5	33.2	45.6	52.0	48.1	43.0	36.6	29.0	22.7
1913-------	1927	*	2.4	7.9	18.9	32.7	47.2	49.2	49.7	42.6	37.0	30.0	22.9
1914-------	1928	*	2.3	7.6	18.8	33.1	45.3	50.3	49.7	43.7	38.7	29.9	22.9
1915-------	1929	*	2.4	7.7	18.6	31.7	46.1	51.2	50.2	45.3	38.2	30.2	22.9
1916-------	1930	*	2.4	7.6	17.8	32.1	47.4	51.8	52.2	44.8	38.7	29.7	24.2
1917-------	1931	*	2.3	7.1	18.5	34.4	48.2	54.0	51.8	45.2	37.9	31.2	25.4
1918-------	1932	*	2.2	7.6	19.8	35.1	50.7	54.3	51.3	43.9	39.0	32.5	27.0
1919-------	1933	*	2.4	8.5	20.8	37.7	51.5	55.5	51.1	45.6	40.5	33.7	25.8
1920-------	1934	*	2.7	8.9	22.2	38.6	53.4	57.2	52.2	46.1	41.4	31.4	24.8
1921-------	1935	*	3.0	9.8	22.8	41.5	56.8	59.8	52.3	47.1	37.9	29.9	31.4
1922-------	1936	*	3.0	9.8	23.9	44.5	58.9	56.3	53.7	43.4	35.1	37.8	33.6
1923-------	1937	*	3.0	10.1	25.6	47.3	55.7	58.5	49.9	40.3	44.6	41.1	37.8
1924-------	1938	*	3.1	11.3	27.3	45.4	58.4	54.5	47.1	51.4	50.3	47.3	39.5
1925-------	1939	*	3.8	12.2	30.5	48.0	54.4	51.6	57.0	58.3	57.4	48.7	39.9
1926-------	1940	*	3.9	15.8	32.3	44.5	52.2	59.4	64.7	66.8	59.0	48.0	39.3
1927-------	1941	*	6.4	16.7	29.9	42.9	56.0	66.9	74.7	68.0	57.1	47.0	38.0
1928-------	1942	*	6.7	15.5	29.2	44.4	62.9	77.8	76.6	65.6	55.2	44.4	37.4
1929-------	1943	*	6.2	15.4	29.5	50.4	73.7	81.4	74.8	64.2	53.0	44.7	38.2
1930-------	1944	*	6.1	15.6	33.4	58.5	78.2	79.8	72.7	60.6	52.5	45.6	38.6
1931-------	1945	*	6.4	18.6	38.9	64.0	78.5	78.7	69.5	62.1	55.0	47.3	39.8
1932-------	1946	*	7.8	20.7	42.7	64.6	77.2	75.1	70.4	65.2	58.0	49.6	40.9
1933-------	1947	*	8.6	23.3	44.0	64.4	75.9	77.3	74.8	69.3	62.1	51.7	40.8
1934-------	1948	*	9.4	23.3	43.9	63.3	77.1	80.7	80.1	74.8	63.4	51.4	41.7
1935-------	1949	*	9.1	23.3	43.2	64.5	78.2	86.0	85.4	75.5	63.1	51.3	40.1
1936-------	1950	*	9.0	22.4	43.9	64.8	82.6	90.4	84.5	74.6	61.8	49.4	38.9
1937-------	1951	*	8.5	22.2	43.5	66.9	85.9	89.6	83.1	72.5	59.3	48.1	38.2
1938-------	1952	*	7.9	22.7	43.9	68.6	84.3	86.8	82.0	69.5	58.1	46.1	37.5
1939-------	1953	*	8.4	23.0	45.3	68.4	82.7	87.1	79.4	70.0	56.3	46.2	36.6
1940-------	1954	*	8.8	23.6	45.0	67.9	82.6	84.6	79.3	67.8	56.4	44.9	35.2
1941-------	1955	*	9.2	23.6	45.3	66.4	80.1	82.3	76.2	66.6	55.2	43.6	34.6
1942-------	1956	*	8.6	23.5	43.8	64.3	76.8	79.5	75.4	65.9	52.9	42.3	35.0
1943-------	1957	*	8.5	22.5	42.3	61.3	73.8	78.1	73.8	62.8	51.2	42.4	33.7
1944-------	1958	*	8.6	22.5	41.3	60.4	73.4	76.7	70.2	60.3	50.4	40.8	37.4
1945-------	1959	*	8.4	21.7	40.7	59.4	72.0	73.3	67.2	58.6	48.3	43.8	40.8
1946-------	1960	*	8.3	21.6	39.8	58.8	68.9	69.3	65.1	56.6	51.2	47.7	40.4
1947-------	1961	*	8.2	21.0	39.6	55.9	65.2	67.1	61.6	57.9	54.4	47.4	38.0
1948-------	1962	*	7.8	20.9	37.3	52.9	62.2	63.4	62.6	60.8	54.4	43.0	38.3
1949-------	1963	*	7.9	19.5	36.1	50.4	58.7	63.3	64.9	60.3	48.2	42.8	
1950-------	1964	*	7.4	19.1	34.6	47.7	58.3	65.0	63.5	53.6	47.5		
1951-------	1965	*	7.3	18.7	32.0	46.7	59.6	63.1	57.5	52.3			
1952-------	1966	*	7.0	17.1	30.6	47.2	57.0	57.8	55.0				
1953-------	1967	*	6.5	15.9	31.4	45.1	52.4	55.0					
1954-------	1968	*	6.1	16.4	29.9	41.8	49.3						
1955-------	1969	*	6.3	15.9	27.5	39.3							
1956-------	1970	*	6.1	14.6	25.7								
1957-------	1971	*	5.4	13.7									
1958-------	1972	*	5.2										
1959-------	1973	*											

TABLE 4C. CENTRAL BIRTH RATES FOR ALL OTHER WOMEN DURING EACH YEAR 1917-73 BY AGE AND LIVE-BIRTH ORDER FOR EACH COHORT FROM 1868 TO 1959--CON.

LIVE-BIRTH ORDER AND COHORT	DIAGONAL LINE FOR CALENDAR YEAR	CURRENT AGE 26	27	28	29	30	31	32	33	34	35	36	37
SECOND BIRTHS--CON.													
1880-------													4.3
1881-------												5.3	4.8
1882-------											6.0	5.7	4.7
1883-------										6.7	6.3	5.5	5.1
1884-------									7.1	6.8	6.0	5.9	4.4
1885-------								7.8	7.2	6.6	6.3	5.0	4.5
1886-------							10.0	7.8	7.0	6.7	5.7	5.1	4.0
1887-------						12.0	10.1	7.8	7.0	6.5	5.7	4.6	3.5
1888-------					16.1	11.7	10.2	7.8	7.5	6.4	5.1	4.1	2.9
1889-------				18.2	15.4	12.3	10.4	8.4	7.3	5.8	4.7	3.9	2.9
1890-------			21.9	17.0	16.6	13.1	11.2	8.2	6.5	5.6	4.9	3.6	2.8
1891-------	1917	25.6	20.4	18.7	18.2	13.6	11.1	7.4	6.5	5.4	4.4	3.4	2.1
1892-------	1918	23.8	22.5	20.9	18.3	13.5	9.9	7.3	6.4	5.1	4.0	2.7	2.6
1893-------	1919	26.2	25.0	20.5	18.1	12.2	9.8	6.9	6.1	4.4	3.3	3.2	2.3
1894-------	1920	29.0	24.4	20.2	16.4	11.6	9.3	6.7	5.2	3.8	3.6	2.8	2.3
1895-------	1921	28.3	24.1	18.5	15.4	10.7	9.0	5.6	4.4	3.8	3.2	2.7	2.0
1896-------	1922	27.9	22.0	17.0	14.4	10.5	7.3	4.8	4.3	3.6	3.2	2.4	2.0
1897-------	1923	25.5	20.3	16.3	13.8	8.4	6.4	4.7	4.2	3.5	2.8	2.5	1.8
1898-------	1924	23.9	20.3	15.3	11.5	7.5	6.3	4.6	4.0	3.2	2.9	2.3	1.8
1899-------	1925	25.0	19.9	14.3	10.6	7.8	6.9	4.6	4.2	3.6	3.2	2.6	2.0
1900-------	1926	24.2	17.9	12.4	10.7	8.5	6.5	4.8	4.3	3.8	3.2	2.5	2.1
1901-------	1927	21.3	15.3	12.2	11.2	7.7	6.5	4.7	4.4	3.9	2.9	2.6	2.3
1902-------	1928	18.2	14.5	12.2	9.9	7.3	5.8	4.5	4.2	3.2	2.9	2.5	2.3
1903-------	1929	17.3	14.4	11.2	9.8	6.9	5.9	4.4	3.7	3.2	2.9	2.6	2.2
1904-------	1930	17.7	14.0	11.3	9.5	7.3	5.7	4.2	3.7	3.3	3.0	2.5	2.5
1905-------	1931	17.6	14.1	11.0	9.7	6.9	5.5	4.3	4.0	3.4	3.0	2.8	2.5
1906-------	1932	17.4	13.3	11.2	9.1	6.8	5.9	4.5	4.1	3.6	3.4	2.9	2.8
1907-------	1933	16.4	13.4	10.6	9.2	7.1	5.7	4.7	4.4	4.0	3.7	3.3	3.0
1908-------	1934	16.4	13.1	10.7	9.6	7.0	5.9	5.0	4.9	4.6	4.1	3.6	3.1
1909-------	1935	16.7	13.7	11.3	9.6	7.2	6.3	5.6	5.6	5.1	4.4	3.8	3.8
1910-------	1936	16.9	14.1	11.9	9.5	7.5	7.0	6.3	6.2	5.5	4.9	4.4	4.1
1911-------	1937	17.3	14.6	11.7	9.8	8.2	7.7	7.0	6.7	5.7	5.4	5.1	4.5
1912-------	1938	17.8	14.3	11.9	10.6	9.2	8.5	7.6	6.9	6.4	6.2	5.4	4.5
1913-------	1939	17.4	14.7	12.7	11.8	10.2	9.2	7.6	7.9	7.3	6.6	5.6	4.5
1914-------	1940	17.9	15.7	13.8	13.0	10.8	9.4	8.9	8.9	7.8	7.0	5.5	4.7
1915-------	1941	19.0	16.4	15.2	13.4	11.0	10.9	10.1	9.3	8.3	6.5	5.7	5.0
1916-------	1942	19.3	18.1	15.4	13.2	12.7	12.0	10.5	9.8	7.9	7.1	6.1	5.1
1917-------	1943	21.1	18.2	14.9	15.6	14.1	13.1	10.8	9.5	8.4	7.4	6.2	5.4
1918-------	1944	21.0	17.1	17.8	17.4	15.7	13.2	11.2	9.9	9.0	7.7	6.5	5.3
1919-------	1945	20.5	21.7	21.1	19.7	16.3	13.8	12.1	11.0	9.4	7.9	6.8	5.2
1920-------	1946	25.7	24.8	22.9	20.6	16.5	15.0	12.8	11.1	9.1	8.2	6.3	5.1
1921-------	1947	28.6	26.6	24.3	20.2	17.6	15.6	12.8	11.0	9.6	7.8	6.2	5.1
1922-------	1948	30.9	27.7	23.5	20.6	17.7	15.1	12.8	11.0	9.3	7.5	6.1	4.2
1923-------	1949	32.1	27.8	23.5	20.7	17.7	15.6	12.6	11.3	9.1	7.3	5.2	4.3
1924-------	1950	32.9	27.9	24.2	21.5	18.7	15.4	12.8	10.8	8.9	6.7	5.4	4.5
1925-------	1951	32.7	28.8	25.2	21.8	18.1	15.0	12.6	10.4	8.2	6.7	5.4	4.3
1926-------	1952	33.1	29.6	25.3	21.7	17.2	15.2	11.8	10.0	8.3	6.3	5.3	3.9
1927-------	1953	33.0	28.4	24.7	20.8	17.6	13.9	11.4	9.8	7.5	6.5	5.0	3.6
1928-------	1954	32.5	28.2	23.8	20.5	15.8	13.5	11.3	9.0	7.5	5.8	4.4	3.6
1929-------	1955	32.5	28.4	23.7	18.9	15.7	13.5	10.7	8.9	7.2	5.5	4.5	3.3
1930-------	1956	32.9	28.2	22.1	18.9	15.8	13.1	10.4	8.7	6.4	5.4	4.1	3.3
1931-------	1957	33.4	26.8	22.4	19.1	15.4	12.3	10.4	7.8	6.6	5.1	4.3	3.3
1932-------	1958	32.9	27.2	22.2	18.9	14.6	12.5	9.3	8.1	6.1	5.3	4.0	3.4
1933-------	1959	33.2	26.8	22.4	17.9	14.6	12.0	9.7	7.6	6.4	5.2	4.4	3.3
1934-------	1960	32.4	27.0	22.0	17.9	14.3	12.0	9.3	7.6	6.5	5.3	4.3	3.2
1935-------	1961	32.4	26.6	21.4	17.8	14.4	11.7	9.3	8.2	6.6	5.4	4.1	3.6
1936-------	1962	31.6	25.5	20.9	17.6	14.2	11.6	9.8	8.3	6.8	5.3	4.4	3.1
1937-------	1963	30.7	25.3	20.9	17.5	14.0	11.9	10.2	8.7	6.8	5.6	4.1	
1938-------	1964	30.0	24.3	20.8	17.3	14.2	12.7	11.0	8.9	6.8	5.5		
1939-------	1965	29.3	24.5	20.8	17.7	15.8	14.0	11.4	9.0	7.2			
1940-------	1966	28.8	25.0	21.2	19.2	17.1	14.7	11.5	9.3				
1941-------	1967	29.0	25.0	22.7	20.8	18.0	14.6	11.9					
1942-------	1968	28.9	26.6	24.7	21.3	17.9	14.8						
1943-------	1969	31.5	29.3	25.1	21.6	18.2							
1944-------	1970	34.7	29.6	25.0	21.7								
1945-------	1971	34.6	28.6	25.0									
1946-------	1972	33.0	29.0										
1947-------	1973	33.2											

TABLE 4C. CENTRAL BIRTH RATES FOR ALL OTHER WOMEN DURING EACH YEAR 1917-73 BY AGE AND LIVE-BIRTH ORDER FOR EACH COHORT FROM 1868 TO 1959--CON.

LIVE-BIRTH ORDER AND COHORT	DIAGONAL LINE FOR CALENDAR YEAR	CURRENT AGE											
		38	39	40	41	42	43	44	45	46	47	48	49
SECOND BIRTHS--CON.													
1868-------													0.2
1869-------												0.3	0.1
1870-------											0.3	0.1	0.1
1871-------										0.6	0.1	0.1	0.2
1872-------									0.6	0.2	0.1	0.3	0.1
1873-------								0.7	0.3	0.3	0.3	0.1	0.1
1874-------							0.5	0.5	0.4	0.6	0.1	0.1	0.1
1875-------						0.7	0.7	0.5	0.7	0.2	0.1	0.1	0.1
1876-------					1.0	1.0	0.7	0.8	0.2	0.1	0.1	0.1	0.1
1877-------				1.6	1.3	1.0	0.7	0.5	0.2	0.3	0.1	0.2	0.1
1878-------			2.8	1.9	1.4	1.0	0.8	0.4	0.4	0.3	0.2	0.2	0.1
1879-------	1917	3.6	3.1	1.9	1.3	1.2	0.7	0.5	0.3	0.4	0.1	0.2	0.0
1880-------	1918	3.9	3.1	2.0	1.6	1.0	0.6	0.4	0.4	0.3	0.2	0.1	0.1
1881-------	1919	3.9	3.5	2.1	1.4	1.0	0.5	0.5	0.2	0.3	0.2	0.1	0.0
1882-------	1920	4.4	3.3	2.0	1.3	0.7	0.6	0.4	0.3	0.3	0.2	0.1	0.1
1883-------	1921	3.9	3.2	1.8	1.0	0.7	0.3	0.3	0.3	0.3	0.1	0.1	0.0
1884-------	1922	3.9	2.9	1.5	1.0	0.5	0.4	0.3	0.3	0.2	0.1	0.1	0.0
1885-------	1923	3.5	2.4	1.4	1.0	0.4	0.4	0.2	0.2	0.1	0.1	0.1	0.0
1886-------	1924	3.0	2.1	1.4	0.8	0.5	0.2	0.2	0.1	0.1	0.1	0.0	0.1
1887-------	1925	2.4	2.1	1.1	0.8	0.4	0.2	0.2	0.2	0.2	0.0	0.1	0.1
1888-------	1926	2.3	1.8	1.1	0.7	0.3	0.3	0.2	0.2	0.1	0.1	0.2	0.1
1889-------	1927	2.2	1.7	1.0	0.6	0.3	0.3	0.2	0.2	0.1	0.1	0.1	0.1
1890-------	1928	1.8	1.6	1.0	0.5	0.4	0.3	0.2	0.1	0.1	0.1	0.1	0.1
1891-------	1929	2.0	1.5	0.9	0.6	0.3	0.2	0.2	0.1	0.1	0.1	0.1	0.0
1892-------	1930	1.9	1.6	0.9	0.5	0.3	0.3	0.2	0.2	0.1	0.1	0.0	0.0
1893-------	1931	1.9	1.4	0.8	0.6	0.4	0.2	0.2	0.1	0.1	0.0	0.1	0.0
1894-------	1932	1.6	1.3	0.8	0.6	0.3	0.2	0.1	0.1	0.0	0.0	0.0	0.0
1895-------	1933	1.6	1.2	0.7	0.5	0.3	0.2	0.1	0.0	0.1	0.1	0.0	0.0
1896-------	1934	1.4	1.0	0.8	0.5	0.3	0.2	0.1	0.1	0.1	0.1	0.0	0.0
1897-------	1935	1.3	1.1	0.9	0.5	0.3	0.2	0.1	0.2	0.1	0.0	0.0	0.0
1898-------	1936	1.4	1.3	0.8	0.5	0.3	0.2	0.2	0.2	0.1	0.0	0.0	0.0
1899-------	1937	1.7	1.4	0.7	0.6	0.3	0.3	0.2	0.1	0.1	0.0	0.0	0.1
1900-------	1938	1.8	1.4	0.8	0.6	0.4	0.3	0.2	0.1	0.1	0.0	0.1	0.0
1901-------	1939	1.8	1.4	0.9	0.7	0.4	0.3	0.2	0.2	0.0	0.1	0.1	0.0
1902-------	1940	1.7	1.5	1.1	0.7	0.4	0.4	0.3	0.1	0.1	0.1	0.1	0.0
1903-------	1941	1.9	1.6	1.1	0.7	0.5	0.4	0.2	0.1	0.1	0.0	0.1	0.0
1904-------	1942	2.1	1.8	1.2	0.8	0.5	0.4	0.2	0.2	0.1	0.1	0.0	0.0
1905-------	1943	2.3	1.9	1.2	0.9	0.6	0.4	0.3	0.1	0.1	0.0	0.0	0.0
1906-------	1944	2.4	1.8	1.4	1.0	0.6	0.5	0.2	0.1	0.1	0.0	0.1	0.0
1907-------	1945	2.4	2.3	1.5	1.0	0.7	0.5	0.2	0.1	0.1	0.0	0.0	0.0
1908-------	1946	2.9	2.3	1.5	1.1	0.7	0.4	0.3	0.2	0.1	0.0	0.0	0.0
1909-------	1947	3.1	2.4	1.7	1.3	0.9	0.6	0.3	0.2	0.0	0.0	0.0	0.0
1910-------	1948	3.3	2.7	1.9	1.5	0.9	0.5	0.3	0.1	0.1	0.0	0.1	0.0
1911-------	1949	3.6	2.8	2.3	1.4	0.9	0.6	0.3	0.2	0.1	0.1	0.0	0.0
1912-------	1950	3.6	3.2	2.1	1.5	0.9	0.7	0.3	0.2	0.1	0.0	0.0	0.0
1913-------	1951	3.9	3.0	2.2	1.5	1.0	0.6	0.4	0.2	0.1	0.0	0.0	0.0
1914-------	1952	4.1	3.2	2.2	1.6	0.9	0.6	0.3	0.1	0.1	0.0	0.0	0.0
1915-------	1953	4.0	3.2	2.2	1.4	0.9	0.6	0.3	0.1	0.1	0.0	0.0	0.0
1916-------	1954	4.3	3.1	2.1	1.4	1.0	0.6	0.3	0.1	0.1	0.0	0.0	0.0
1917-------	1955	4.0	3.1	2.1	1.4	1.0	0.5	0.3	0.1	0.1	0.0	0.0	0.0
1918-------	1956	4.1	3.1	2.0	1.3	0.8	0.5	0.2	0.2	0.0	0.0	0.0	0.0
1919-------	1957	4.1	3.0	2.0	1.2	0.8	0.5	0.3	0.1	0.0	0.0	0.0	0.0
1920-------	1958	4.2	2.8	1.7	1.2	0.8	0.5	0.3	0.1	0.1	0.0	0.0	0.0
1921-------	1959	3.5	2.6	1.8	1.3	0.8	0.5	0.3	0.1	0.1	0.0	0.0	0.0
1922-------	1960	3.5	2.7	1.9	1.2	0.7	0.5	0.2	0.1	0.1	0.0	0.0	0.0
1923-------	1961	3.6	2.7	1.7	1.1	0.7	0.5	0.2	0.1	0.0	0.0	0.0	0.0
1924-------	1962	3.4	2.4	1.7	1.1	0.7	0.3	0.3	0.1	0.0	0.0	0.0	0.0
1925-------	1963	3.3	2.3	1.6	1.1	0.7	0.5	0.3	0.1	0.0	0.0	0.0	
1926-------	1964	3.0	2.4	1.5	1.1	0.7	0.5	0.2	0.1	0.0	0.0		
1927-------	1965	2.9	2.1	1.7	0.9	0.8	0.4	0.2	0.1	0.0			
1928-------	1966	2.5	2.0	1.3	1.1	0.6	0.4	0.2	0.1				
1929-------	1967	2.7	1.9	1.4	0.9	0.7	0.4	0.2					
1930-------	1968	2.5	1.8	1.3	0.9	0.6	0.3						
1931-------	1969	2.6	1.9	1.3	1.0	0.5							
1932-------	1970	2.5	1.8	1.3	0.8								
1933-------	1971	2.5	1.8	1.2									
1934-------	1972	2.5	1.7										
1935-------	1973	2.3											

TABLE 4C. CENTRAL BIRTH RATES FOR ALL OTHER WOMEN DURING EACH YEAR 1917-73 BY AGE AND LIVE-BIRTH ORDER FOR EACH COHORT FROM 1868 TO 1959--CON.

LIVE-BIRTH ORDER AND COHORT	DIAGONAL LINE FOR CALENDAR YEAR	CURRENT AGE											
		14	15	16	17	18	19	20	21	22	23	24	25
THIRD BIRTHS													
1892-------													36.9
1893-------												41.4	38.2
1894-------											43.9	43.3	36.9
1895-------										39.6	46.4	40.9	38.9
1896-------									33.8	41.8	43.0	42.3	41.1
1897-------								23.4	35.7	38.8	43.6	45.2	37.3
1898-------							14.4	24.7	33.3	39.7	47.7	42.2	38.9
1899-------						6.2	15.0	23.0	33.7	42.8	44.1	43.5	41.0
1900-------					2.4	6.3	14.2	23.4	36.6	40.0	46.9	46.8	36.9
1901-------				0.6	2.4	5.9	14.1	25.1	33.7	41.9	49.8	41.8	33.0
1902-------			0.1	0.6	2.3	6.2	15.8	24.1	36.4	45.7	44.1	37.6	30.6
1903-------	1917	*	0.1	0.6	2.4	6.8	15.1	26.1	39.1	40.7	40.9	36.4	28.4
1904-------	1918	*	0.1	0.6	2.6	6.7	16.8	27.8	35.5	39.3	39.9	33.7	26.5
1905-------	1919	*	0.1	0.7	2.6	8.0	17.6	25.5	34.2	38.9	36.7	31.5	26.5
1906-------	1920	*	0.1	0.7	3.0	8.1	16.8	25.6	33.9	36.0	34.8	31.3	25.5
1907-------	1921	*	0.1	0.8	3.1	7.7	17.1	25.5	32.2	34.0	34.6	30.0	26.0
1908-------	1922	*	0.1	0.8	3.0	8.5	17.1	24.6	31.0	33.9	33.0	30.5	25.3
1909-------	1923	*	0.1	0.9	3.2	8.4	16.8	23.5	31.5	33.2	34.7	30.8	25.9
1910-------	1924	*	0.2	0.9	3.4	8.2	16.0	24.0	30.6	34.7	34.7	31.9	24.9
1911-------	1925	*	0.1	0.9	3.4	7.7	16.0	23.6	32.1	34.1	36.1	30.7	24.4
1912-------	1926	*	0.2	0.9	3.1	7.3	15.8	24.1	30.1	35.2	34.4	29.6	25.4
1913-------	1927	*	0.2	0.9	2.8	7.3	16.1	22.5	31.3	34.5	33.7	31.5	26.2
1914-------	1928	*	0.2	0.8	2.9	7.4	15.1	23.5	31.4	34.0	35.5	32.5	26.1
1915-------	1929	*	0.1	0.8	2.9	7.2	15.8	24.1	31.1	36.1	36.8	32.4	26.5
1916-------	1930	*	0.2	0.8	2.8	7.6	16.3	24.2	32.9	37.2	36.7	33.3	27.1
1917-------	1931	*	0.1	0.7	3.1	7.8	16.5	25.8	33.8	36.9	38.4	34.2	27.1
1918-------	1932	*	0.2	0.8	3.0	8.4	17.5	26.3	33.0	38.4	38.8	33.5	27.9
1919-------	1933	*	0.2	0.8	3.3	8.8	18.2	26.6	35.0	39.1	38.5	34.1	28.1
1920-------	1934	*	0.2	0.9	3.5	9.1	18.9	29.6	35.1	38.8	38.9	33.6	26.2
1921-------	1935	*	0.2	1.0	3.8	10.4	22.5	30.4	36.6	39.3	38.0	30.9	28.8
1922-------	1936	*	0.2	1.0	4.2	13.2	22.8	31.1	37.2	38.5	34.1	33.2	30.9
1923-------	1937	*	0.2	1.1	5.3	13.8	23.6	31.7	36.7	35.2	36.6	35.3	34.6
1924-------	1938	*	0.2	1.4	5.5	14.1	24.1	31.5	33.8	38.3	39.5	41.0	37.3
1925-------	1939	*	0.3	1.5	6.7	14.4	24.0	28.9	36.6	41.3	46.1	44.1	40.8
1926-------	1940	*	0.4	2.3	6.9	14.2	21.9	31.5	40.2	47.9	50.1	48.5	43.2
1927-------	1941	*	0.5	2.4	6.8	13.1	23.2	34.3	45.9	52.8	54.4	50.5	42.7
1928-------	1942	*	0.6	2.3	6.4	13.7	25.4	39.0	50.9	57.3	56.1	49.0	42.8
1929-------	1943	*	0.6	2.2	6.6	15.0	28.5	44.1	56.0	59.4	55.7	49.1	42.6
1930-------	1944	*	0.5	2.4	7.3	16.7	32.9	48.5	58.1	58.5	54.0	49.7	42.8
1931-------	1945	*	0.6	2.8	8.2	20.1	36.4	50.7	57.5	57.0	56.0	50.6	44.7
1932-------	1946	*	0.8	3.1	9.6	21.5	38.1	50.2	55.9	59.3	57.4	52.9	46.0
1933-------	1947	*	0.9	3.4	10.2	22.4	38.3	50.2	58.8	61.5	60.4	55.0	46.7
1934-------	1948	*	1.1	3.7	10.9	23.3	38.3	52.6	61.0	65.5	62.8	56.1	47.7
1935-------	1949	*	0.9	3.8	11.0	23.3	40.0	53.5	64.5	68.5	64.9	56.9	46.6
1936-------	1950	*	1.0	3.8	10.9	24.2	40.5	56.0	67.4	68.2	63.6	55.3	45.8
1937-------	1951	*	0.9	3.6	11.1	24.1	41.7	58.5	66.5	67.1	62.4	54.1	43.6
1938-------	1952	*	0.9	3.6	11.1	24.7	42.7	57.1	64.5	65.8	60.6	51.7	41.7
1939-------	1953	*	0.8	3.7	11.7	25.2	42.9	56.7	64.3	64.0	58.7	50.0	40.7
1940-------	1954	*	0.8	3.9	11.8	25.7	42.5	56.1	62.3	63.1	55.6	47.5	37.1
1941-------	1955	*	1.0	3.9	11.9	25.8	41.6	54.0	60.6	58.9	52.9	43.1	34.6
1942-------	1956	*	0.8	4.0	12.0	24.7	40.4	52.1	56.7	55.8	47.7	39.3	32.2
1943-------	1957	*	1.0	3.9	11.3	24.3	38.5	49.4	53.8	50.7	43.4	36.0	29.9
1944-------	1958	*	0.9	3.9	11.8	23.7	37.0	47.3	49.5	46.1	39.2	34.1	30.9
1945-------	1959	*	0.9	4.0	11.5	22.6	35.8	43.7	44.8	41.0	37.4	34.6	32.8
1946-------	1960	*	0.9	3.8	10.8	22.4	33.3	39.4	39.8	38.1	37.2	36.1	32.5
1947-------	1961	*	0.9	3.9	10.7	20.7	29.4	35.4	36.4	37.2	37.6	35.4	28.2
1948-------	1962	*	0.9	3.6	10.0	18.3	26.6	30.8	34.2	37.7	36.1	30.0	26.5
1949-------	1963	*	0.8	3.4	8.7	16.6	23.4	29.2	34.8	35.6	30.9	28.1	
1950-------	1964	*	0.8	3.0	7.9	14.3	21.8	29.4	31.8	30.3	29.1		
1951-------	1965	*	0.7	2.9	7.0	13.5	21.3	26.6	28.0	28.5			
1952-------	1966	*	0.7	2.3	6.3	12.8	19.2	23.4	26.2				
1953-------	1967	*	0.5	2.2	6.1	11.8	16.9	21.6					
1954-------	1968	*	0.5	2.1	5.7	10.2	15.7						
1955-------	1969	*	0.5	2.0	4.9	9.4							
1956-------	1970	*	0.5	1.7	4.5								
1957-------	1971	*	0.4	1.5									
1958-------	1972	*	0.3										
1959-------	1973	*											

TABLE 4C. CENTRAL BIRTH RATES FOR ALL OTHER WOMEN DURING EACH YEAR 1917-73 BY AGE AND LIVE-BIRTH ORDER FOR EACH COHORT FROM 1868 TO 1959--CON.

LIVE-BIRTH ORDER AND COHORT	DIAGONAL LINE FOR CALENDAR YEAR	CURRENT AGE											
		26	27	28	29	30	31	32	33	34	35	36	37
THIRD BIRTHS--CON.													
1880-------													5.8
1881-------												7.3	6.8
1882-------											7.7	8.3	6.5
1883-------										8.1	8.5	7.7	7.6
1884-------									8.7	8.7	8.0	8.9	6.4
1885-------								9.5	8.9	8.2	8.9	7.5	6.2
1886-------							12.7	9.8	8.8	8.8	7.7	7.2	5.7
1887-------						14.5	13.2	9.7	9.2	8.1	7.4	6.7	5.7
1888-------					19.1	15.1	13.3	10.2	9.0	7.8	7.0	6.8	5.0
1889-------				21.7	19.7	15.2	14.2	10.1	8.7	7.6	7.3	6.0	4.7
1890-------			26.3	22.2	19.8	16.4	14.1	9.9	8.6	8.1	7.1	5.8	4.2
1891-------	1917	30.3	27.0	22.1	21.5	16.7	13.8	9.8	9.4	7.9	6.9	5.1	3.4
1892-------	1918	31.0	26.8	24.3	22.2	15.8	13.6	10.7	8.9	7.9	5.7	4.3	3.2
1893-------	1919	30.8	29.3	25.3	20.4	15.6	14.8	9.7	8.8	6.4	5.1	4.3	3.2
1894-------	1920	33.4	30.5	22.6	20.3	16.8	12.9	9.2	7.4	5.7	4.9	4.0	3.2
1895-------	1921	34.7	27.1	22.7	21.8	15.1	11.4	8.3	6.4	5.6	4.5	3.7	3.1
1896-------	1922	30.9	27.2	24.1	19.4	13.2	10.7	6.9	6.0	5.2	4.3	3.6	2.8
1897-------	1923	31.0	29.0	21.6	17.6	12.1	8.9	6.3	5.6	4.8	4.0	3.3	2.7
1898-------	1924	33.8	26.0	20.4	15.7	10.4	8.4	6.3	5.7	4.7	3.8	3.3	2.6
1899-------	1925	30.9	25.1	18.7	14.5	10.5	8.7	6.4	6.0	4.8	4.4	3.6	2.9
1900-------	1926	28.6	22.9	16.4	14.1	10.7	8.5	6.7	5.9	5.2	4.3	3.5	3.1
1901-------	1927	26.6	20.1	15.6	14.0	9.8	8.4	6.4	6.1	4.8	3.9	3.6	2.8
1902-------	1928	23.4	18.1	15.0	12.7	9.2	8.0	6.2	5.1	4.4	4.0	3.4	2.7
1903-------	1929	21.5	17.9	14.4	12.3	9.3	7.8	5.6	4.9	4.4	4.0	3.2	2.6
1904-------	1930	21.3	18.0	14.2	12.6	9.0	7.7	5.6	5.2	4.5	3.9	3.2	2.8
1905-------	1931	21.3	17.9	14.2	12.1	9.1	7.1	5.5	5.2	4.5	3.9	3.4	3.0
1906-------	1932	21.3	17.3	14.0	11.9	8.6	7.3	5.8	5.3	4.5	4.2	3.4	3.4
1907-------	1933	20.6	17.3	13.3	11.3	8.6	7.5	5.9	5.3	4.9	4.3	3.9	3.7
1908-------	1934	20.5	16.2	12.9	11.5	8.9	7.5	5.9	5.7	5.2	4.9	4.2	3.8
1909-------	1935	20.0	16.0	13.5	12.1	8.9	7.6	6.5	6.3	5.8	5.2	4.6	4.4
1910-------	1936	19.4	16.7	14.3	12.0	9.0	8.3	7.0	7.0	6.1	5.5	5.1	4.7
1911-------	1937	20.5	17.7	14.1	11.9	9.6	8.6	7.7	7.4	6.5	6.2	5.6	4.8
1912-------	1938	21.1	17.4	14.0	12.5	10.2	9.5	8.1	7.8	6.9	6.5	5.8	5.0
1913-------	1939	20.8	17.4	14.5	13.1	11.0	10.1	8.5	8.4	7.5	7.0	6.1	5.4
1914-------	1940	20.8	18.0	15.3	13.9	11.6	10.1	9.5	8.9	8.3	7.5	6.4	6.0
1915-------	1941	21.4	18.3	16.0	14.6	11.4	11.5	10.0	9.8	9.0	7.7	7.3	5.9
1916-------	1942	21.4	19.2	16.8	14.0	13.0	12.1	10.8	10.4	9.1	8.7	6.5	6.4
1917-------	1943	22.3	20.0	15.8	15.9	14.0	13.0	11.6	10.8	9.8	8.3	7.5	6.5
1918-------	1944	23.1	18.6	18.1	17.0	15.0	14.2	12.5	11.5	10.3	9.0	8.1	6.4
1919-------	1945	22.0	21.8	19.8	19.0	17.0	15.5	13.4	13.0	11.0	9.7	8.1	6.7
1920-------	1946	24.7	23.4	22.0	20.8	18.1	16.4	14.5	13.6	11.6	9.9	8.0	6.8
1921-------	1947	27.1	25.8	23.7	21.7	19.1	17.0	15.4	13.3	11.6	9.8	8.4	6.5
1922-------	1948	28.9	26.9	24.6	22.8	19.2	18.1	15.0	13.6	11.5	9.9	8.0	6.5
1923-------	1949	31.0	28.9	26.5	23.1	20.0	17.7	15.3	13.8	11.8	9.6	7.7	6.2
1924-------	1950	34.3	31.8	27.2	24.6	21.0	18.4	16.0	14.0	11.7	9.5	7.6	6.2
1925-------	1951	37.1	32.3	28.1	25.2	21.0	19.0	16.0	13.7	11.1	9.1	7.6	6.2
1926-------	1952	37.1	33.0	28.8	25.4	21.5	19.0	15.2	13.4	10.7	9.2	7.4	5.5
1927-------	1953	37.1	32.6	28.9	25.5	21.8	17.7	14.8	12.6	10.6	8.9	6.5	5.4
1928-------	1954	36.4	32.8	28.2	25.5	19.7	17.5	14.3	12.2	10.2	8.0	6.5	5.1
1929-------	1955	37.2	32.9	29.0	23.7	19.9	17.1	14.5	11.8	9.6	8.0	6.2	4.8
1930-------	1956	37.6	33.2	27.1	23.5	19.8	17.2	13.4	11.5	9.4	7.4	5.9	4.8
1931-------	1957	39.0	32.2	27.4	23.1	20.1	16.0	13.3	11.3	8.9	7.3	5.4	4.3
1932-------	1958	38.0	32.7	27.1	23.7	18.9	15.8	12.9	10.6	8.8	6.6	5.5	4.3
1933-------	1959	39.4	32.0	27.5	22.8	18.9	15.7	12.4	10.5	7.9	6.9	5.4	4.5
1934-------	1960	38.8	32.5	27.1	22.7	18.0	15.2	12.1	9.6	8.2	7.0	5.6	4.2
1935-------	1961	38.1	31.7	26.6	22.0	17.4	14.2	11.5	9.7	8.3	7.0	5.4	4.1
1936-------	1962	37.2	30.4	25.3	20.8	16.3	13.8	11.1	10.1	8.6	6.7	5.2	3.8
1937-------	1963	35.7	29.7	24.1	19.3	16.0	13.2	11.7	10.3	8.4	6.3	5.0	
1938-------	1964	34.5	27.9	21.7	18.5	15.3	14.0	12.4	10.2	7.5	6.2		
1939-------	1965	32.4	25.6	21.2	17.8	16.3	14.9	12.5	9.4	7.7			
1940-------	1966	29.6	24.8	20.1	19.0	17.5	14.9	11.5	9.1				
1941-------	1967	28.2	22.6	21.2	20.5	17.8	13.7	10.9					
1942-------	1968	26.0	24.0	23.0	20.5	15.7	13.1						
1943-------	1969	27.0	26.1	23.1	17.9	15.2							
1944-------	1970	29.2	26.0	20.4	17.7								
1945-------	1971	29.3	22.9	19.8									
1946-------	1972	25.4	22.3										
1947-------	1973	24.3											

TABLE 4C. CENTRAL BIRTH RATES FOR ALL OTHER WOMEN DURING EACH YEAR 1917-73 BY AGE AND LIVE-BIRTH ORDER FOR EACH COHORT FROM 1868 TO 1959--CON.

LIVE-BIRTH ORDER AND COHORT	DIAGONAL LINE FOR CALENDAR YEAR	CURRENT AGE											
		38	39	40	41	42	43	44	45	46	47	48	49
THIRD BIRTHS--CON.													
1868-------													0.1
1869-------												0.2	0.2
1870-------											0.4	0.4	0.1
1871-------										0.7	0.7	0.2	0.1
1872-------									0.7	1.3	0.3	0.3	0.1
1873-------								0.6	1.3	0.5	0.5	0.1	0.1
1874-------							0.5	1.0	0.6	0.8	0.3	0.1	0.1
1875-------						0.7	0.8	0.5	0.9	0.5	0.3	0.1	0.1
1876-------					1.2	1.1	0.6	0.8	0.6	0.5	0.2	0.2	0.1
1877-------				1.8	1.9	0.7	0.8	0.6	0.6	0.4	0.3	0.2	0.2
1878-------			3.2	2.6	1.3	1.0	0.8	0.6	0.5	0.6	0.2	0.3	0.0
1879-------	1917	4.5	4.0	2.1	1.9	1.1	0.7	0.5	0.7	0.5	0.4	0.1	0.1
1880-------	1918	5.3	3.6	2.8	2.1	1.0	0.8	0.6	0.6	0.5	0.1	0.1	0.1
1881-------	1919	5.1	4.5	2.8	1.9	1.1	0.7	0.7	0.6	0.4	0.2	0.1	0.0
1882-------	1920	6.0	4.2	2.7	2.0	1.0	0.7	0.6	0.4	0.2	0.1	0.0	0.1
1883-------	1921	5.2	4.0	2.6	1.7	1.0	0.6	0.5	0.2	0.3	0.1	0.2	0.1
1884-------	1922	5.1	3.8	2.4	1.5	0.8	0.6	0.3	0.3	0.3	0.2	0.2	0.1
1885-------	1923	4.6	3.6	2.5	1.3	0.8	0.4	0.3	0.4	0.3	0.1	0.1	0.1
1886-------	1924	4.6	3.6	2.0	1.2	0.5	0.4	0.3	0.2	0.2	0.1	0.2	0.1
1887-------	1925	4.3	3.0	1.7	0.9	0.6	0.3	0.3	0.2	0.2	0.2	0.1	0.1
1888-------	1926	3.8	2.6	1.4	1.0	0.5	0.3	0.3	0.2	0.2	0.1	0.1	0.0
1889-------	1927	3.4	2.3	1.5	1.0	0.4	0.4	0.3	0.2	0.1	0.1	0.1	0.1
1890-------	1928	2.7	2.2	1.5	0.7	0.5	0.4	0.3	0.2	0.2	0.1	0.1	0.1
1891-------	1929	2.7	2.2	1.1	0.9	0.5	0.4	0.2	0.2	0.1	0.1	0.1	0.1
1892-------	1930	2.6	1.9	1.3	0.9	0.5	0.4	0.3	0.2	0.1	0.1	0.1	0.1
1893-------	1931	2.4	2.0	1.2	0.8	0.5	0.3	0.2	0.1	0.1	0.1	0.1	0.0
1894-------	1932	2.5	1.9	1.2	0.8	0.4	0.4	0.2	0.1	0.1	0.1	0.1	0.0
1895-------	1933	2.2	1.8	1.2	0.7	0.4	0.2	0.2	0.1	0.1	0.1	0.0	0.0
1896-------	1934	2.2	1.8	1.1	0.7	0.4	0.2	0.2	0.1	0.1	0.0	0.1	0.0
1897-------	1935	2.1	1.8	1.0	0.7	0.4	0.2	0.2	0.2	0.1	0.1	0.1	0.0
1898-------	1936	2.2	1.7	1.2	0.7	0.4	0.2	0.3	0.2	0.1	0.1	0.1	0.1
1899-------	1937	2.4	1.9	1.2	0.7	0.4	0.3	0.2	0.2	0.1	0.1	0.1	0.1
1900-------	1938	2.4	1.9	1.2	0.8	0.4	0.3	0.3	0.2	0.2	0.1	0.1	0.1
1901-------	1939	2.3	1.8	1.2	0.8	0.4	0.4	0.3	0.2	0.1	0.1	0.1	0.0
1902-------	1940	2.2	1.8	1.2	0.8	0.5	0.4	0.2	0.1	0.1	0.1	0.0	0.1
1903-------	1941	2.3	2.0	1.3	0.9	0.6	0.4	0.3	0.2	0.1	0.0	0.1	0.0
1904-------	1942	2.4	2.2	1.4	1.0	0.6	0.5	0.3	0.2	0.1	0.1	0.0	0.0
1905-------	1943	2.8	2.4	1.6	0.9	0.8	0.5	0.3	0.2	0.1	0.0	0.1	0.0
1906-------	1944	3.0	2.4	1.4	1.2	0.8	0.5	0.3	0.2	0.1	0.1	0.0	0.0
1907-------	1945	3.0	2.4	1.8	1.2	0.8	0.5	0.3	0.2	0.2	0.0	0.1	0.0
1908-------	1946	3.2	2.7	1.8	1.2	0.7	0.6	0.3	0.2	0.1	0.1	0.1	0.0
1909-------	1947	3.7	2.9	1.9	1.3	1.0	0.7	0.4	0.1	0.1	0.1	0.0	0.0
1910-------	1948	3.8	3.0	2.1	1.6	1.1	0.7	0.3	0.3	0.1	0.1	0.1	0.0
1911-------	1949	4.1	3.4	2.3	1.7	1.1	0.7	0.5	0.2	0.1	0.1	0.0	0.0
1912-------	1950	4.4	3.4	2.4	1.7	1.2	0.8	0.3	0.2	0.1	0.0	0.0	0.0
1913-------	1951	4.6	3.9	2.5	1.9	1.1	0.7	0.4	0.2	0.1	0.0	0.0	0.0
1914-------	1952	4.9	3.8	2.7	1.8	1.2	0.9	0.4	0.2	0.2	0.0	0.0	0.0
1915-------	1953	5.1	3.7	2.7	1.9	1.2	0.6	0.4	0.3	0.1	0.0	0.0	0.0
1916-------	1954	5.1	3.9	2.8	1.8	1.0	0.7	0.5	0.2	0.1	0.0	0.0	0.0
1917-------	1955	5.1	4.1	2.6	1.6	1.3	0.7	0.4	0.2	0.1	0.0	0.0	0.0
1918-------	1956	5.3	3.8	2.5	1.9	1.1	0.8	0.3	0.2	0.1	0.0	0.0	0.0
1919-------	1957	5.3	3.8	2.9	1.8	1.3	0.6	0.4	0.2	0.1	0.1	0.0	0.0
1920-------	1958	5.4	4.0	2.7	2.0	1.0	0.7	0.4	0.2	0.1	0.0	0.0	0.0
1921-------	1959	5.3	3.9	2.9	1.8	1.1	0.8	0.4	0.2	0.1	0.0	0.0	0.0
1922-------	1960	5.0	3.9	2.6	1.6	1.2	0.6	0.4	0.3	0.1	0.1	0.0	0.0
1923-------	1961	5.0	3.8	2.4	1.7	1.0	0.7	0.5	0.2	0.1	0.0	0.0	0.0
1924-------	1962	4.9	3.4	2.6	1.5	1.0	0.7	0.3	0.2	0.1	0.1	0.0	0.0
1925-------	1963	4.6	3.6	2.3	1.6	1.0	0.6	0.4	0.2	0.1	0.0	0.0	
1926-------	1964	4.5	3.3	2.3	1.6	0.9	0.6	0.3	0.2	0.1	0.0		
1927-------	1965	4.2	3.0	2.3	1.2	0.8	0.5	0.2	0.1	0.1			
1928-------	1966	3.8	3.3	1.8	1.3	0.8	0.4	0.3	0.1				
1929-------	1967	4.0	2.5	1.9	1.2	0.6	0.4	0.2					
1930-------	1968	3.4	2.6	1.6	1.1	0.7	0.3						
1931-------	1969	3.3	2.5	1.8	1.1	0.7							
1932-------	1970	3.4	2.5	1.7	1.0								
1933-------	1971	3.3	2.3	1.5									
1934-------	1972	3.1	2.1										
1935-------	1973	2.9											

TABLE 4C. CENTRAL BIRTH RATES FOR ALL OTHER WOMEN DURING EACH YEAR 1917-73 BY AGE AND LIVE-BIRTH ORDER FOR EACH COHORT FROM 1868 TO 1959--CON.

LIVE-BIRTH ORDER AND COHORT	DIAGONAL LINE FOR CALENDAR YEAR	CURRENT AGE											
		14	15	16	17	18	19	20	21	22	23	24	25
FOURTH BIRTHS													
1892-------													30.2
1893-------												30.0	29.8
1894-------											26.8	30.0	29.8
1895-------										19.1	27.4	29.2	31.8
1896-------									12.7	19.5	25.8	30.2	33.6
1897-------								6.6	12.9	18.4	25.9	32.8	31.1
1898-------							3.3	6.6	12.3	18.7	29.1	31.1	31.6
1899-------						0.9	3.2	6.4	12.3	20.7	27.5	31.1	33.3
1900-------					0.3	0.7	3.3	6.3	13.7	19.7	28.4	33.3	34.2
1901-------				0.1	0.2	1.0	2.9	6.9	12.7	19.8	29.4	33.9	33.0
1902-------			0.0	0.0	0.3	0.7	3.6	6.9	13.5	21.5	30.1	32.4	28.7
1903-------	1917	*	0.0	0.1	0.2	1.0	3.6	7.3	14.3	22.5	29.1	29.1	26.4
1904-------	1918	*	0.0	0.0	0.3	1.1	4.0	7.7	15.5	22.6	26.7	27.4	25.5
1905-------	1919	*	0.0	0.1	0.3	1.4	4.2	8.6	15.4	21.0	25.0	26.1	24.8
1906-------	1920	*	0.0	0.1	0.4	1.5	4.5	8.7	14.4	19.7	23.6	26.1	24.3
1907-------	1921	*	0.0	0.1	0.5	1.7	4.5	8.1	13.7	18.5	24.4	24.9	24.6
1908-------	1922	*	0.0	0.1	0.5	1.7	4.2	8.1	13.1	18.9	22.8	25.1	23.8
1909-------	1923	*	0.0	0.1	0.6	1.5	4.5	7.7	13.0	18.3	23.2	25.3	25.0
1910-------	1924	*	0.0	0.1	0.5	1.7	4.1	7.3	12.8	18.5	23.3	26.0	24.6
1911-------	1925	*	0.0	0.1	0.5	1.4	4.1	7.5	13.2	18.3	24.6	26.3	24.1
1912-------	1926	*	0.0	0.1	0.4	1.5	4.0	7.4	12.3	19.0	24.5	24.8	24.3
1913-------	1927	*	0.0	0.1	0.5	1.5	3.9	7.1	13.2	19.6	23.4	25.7	24.4
1914-------	1928	*	0.0	0.1	0.5	1.4	3.9	7.4	13.7	19.1	24.7	26.1	24.6
1915-------	1929	*	0.0	0.1	0.4	1.4	3.9	7.8	13.6	19.9	24.9	26.3	25.8
1916-------	1930	*	0.0	0.1	0.5	1.3	4.1	8.0	13.9	20.0	25.3	28.6	25.9
1917-------	1931	*	0.0	0.1	0.4	1.4	4.1	8.0	14.1	20.2	28.4	28.9	25.7
1918-------	1932	*	0.0	0.1	0.4	1.5	4.2	8.3	14.1	22.7	28.5	28.1	26.8
1919-------	1933	*	0.0	0.1	0.5	1.5	4.5	8.3	16.0	22.8	27.9	29.0	26.9
1920-------	1934	*	0.0	0.1	0.5	1.7	4.5	10.0	15.8	23.6	28.4	29.2	25.6
1921-------	1935	*	0.0	0.2	0.6	1.8	5.9	10.1	17.7	24.0	28.9	27.4	26.6
1922-------	1936	*	0.0	0.1	0.6	2.7	5.9	11.4	18.1	24.5	26.3	27.8	26.3
1923-------	1937	*	0.0	0.1	0.9	2.8	6.6	11.9	18.6	22.6	27.0	27.6	27.6
1924-------	1938	*	0.0	0.2	0.9	2.9	6.9	12.3	17.5	23.3	27.2	30.1	30.6
1925-------	1939	*	0.1	0.2	1.0	3.1	7.2	11.7	17.8	23.6	30.0	33.4	33.8
1926-------	1940	*	0.1	0.2	1.1	3.2	7.1	11.8	18.6	26.3	33.3	36.6	37.6
1927-------	1941	*	0.0	0.2	1.2	3.1	6.8	12.5	20.7	29.6	35.9	41.0	40.1
1928-------	1942	*	0.0	0.2	1.2	2.9	7.4	14.0	23.2	31.8	41.0	42.8	40.8
1929-------	1943	*	0.0	0.2	1.1	3.2	8.2	15.7	25.3	36.7	43.5	45.0	42.2
1930-------	1944	*	0.0	0.3	1.3	3.4	8.8	17.2	28.9	39.2	44.3	45.0	41.8
1931-------	1945	*	0.1	0.3	1.3	4.0	10.3	19.5	31.7	40.0	44.6	45.4	43.4
1932-------	1946	*	0.1	0.3	1.4	4.6	11.3	21.5	31.3	40.1	45.3	46.9	43.1
1933-------	1947	*	0.1	0.4	1.7	4.9	12.5	22.1	32.2	41.7	47.8	47.6	44.2
1934-------	1948	*	0.1	0.4	1.8	5.6	12.9	22.8	33.7	44.3	48.4	48.8	46.4
1935-------	1949	*	0.1	0.4	1.9	5.7	13.2	23.6	35.8	45.1	49.8	50.7	45.6
1936-------	1950	*	0.1	0.4	2.0	5.8	13.5	24.9	36.6	46.5	51.7	49.5	44.7
1937-------	1951	*	0.0	0.5	1.9	5.8	13.9	25.7	37.6	47.2	49.7	49.0	43.8
1938-------	1952	*	0.1	0.4	1.9	6.2	14.2	26.1	38.1	44.9	48.7	47.0	40.5
1939-------	1953	*	0.1	0.5	2.0	6.2	14.8	26.5	36.4	45.8	46.9	44.2	38.5
1940-------	1954	*	0.1	0.5	2.0	6.5	15.0	25.6	36.9	42.9	44.2	41.8	34.3
1941-------	1955	*	0.1	0.6	2.1	6.5	14.8	26.1	34.7	40.9	41.4	36.8	30.5
1942-------	1956	*	0.1	0.5	2.1	6.5	14.5	24.5	33.1	37.7	36.2	31.9	26.5
1943-------	1957	*	0.1	0.5	2.1	6.4	13.7	23.2	30.4	33.6	31.3	27.3	23.9
1944-------	1958	*	0.1	0.5	2.2	6.2	13.5	21.9	27.5	28.5	26.4	24.6	23.0
1945-------	1959	*	0.1	0.5	2.0	5.8	12.4	19.8	23.5	24.4	24.0	23.6	23.2
1946-------	1960	*	0.1	0.5	1.9	5.5	11.8	16.8	20.1	21.6	22.7	23.0	21.4
1947-------	1961	*	0.1	0.5	1.9	5.4	9.9	14.8	17.5	19.8	21.6	21.0	17.6
1948-------	1962	*	0.1	0.5	1.8	4.4	8.4	12.0	15.5	18.7	19.2	17.1	15.2
1949-------	1963	*	0.1	0.4	1.5	3.9	6.9	10.7	14.7	16.4	16.2	15.0	
1950-------	1964	*	0.1	0.3	1.2	3.1	6.2	10.2	12.8	14.1	13.8		
1951-------	1965	*	0.0	0.3	1.1	2.8	5.7	8.8	10.9	12.0			
1952-------	1966	*	0.1	0.3	0.9	2.5	5.0	7.2	9.4				
1953-------	1967	*	0.0	0.3	0.8	2.2	4.0	6.4					
1954-------	1968	*	0.0	0.2	0.7	1.8	3.7						
1955-------	1969	*	0.0	0.2	0.6	1.5							
1956-------	1970	*	0.0	0.2	0.5								
1957-------	1971	*	0.0	0.1									
1958-------	1972	*	0.0										
1959-------	1973	*											

TABLE 4C. CENTRAL BIRTH RATES FOR ALL OTHER WOMEN DURING EACH YEAR 1917-73 BY AGE AND LIVE-BIRTH ORDER FOR EACH COHORT FROM 1868 TO 1959--CON.

LIVE-BIRTH ORDER AND COHORT	DIAGONAL LINE FOR CALENDAR YEAR	CURRENT AGE											
		26	27	28	29	30	31	32	33	34	35	36	37
FOURTH BIRTHS--CON.													
1880-------													6.8
1881-------												8.8	7.2
1882-------											10.1	9.2	7.6
1883-------										10.5	10.3	9.6	8.1
1884-------									10.5	10.6	10.5	9.9	7.4
1885-------								10.6	10.3	10.6	10.7	9.0	6.7
1886-------							13.9	10.4	10.4	10.7	10.0	8.1	6.1
1887-------						15.9	13.8	10.5	10.4	10.3	9.1	7.5	6.1
1888-------					20.6	15.6	14.1	10.7	10.5	9.6	8.7	7.5	6.3
1889-------				21.8	20.1	16.2	14.5	11.0	10.1	9.5	8.9	7.4	6.1
1890-------			24.9	21.1	20.9	17.2	15.0	10.6	10.2	9.8	8.2	7.3	5.3
1891-------	1917	26.7	24.0	22.0	22.8	17.9	14.5	10.7	10.7	8.9	8.7	6.5	4.9
1892-------	1918	25.8	25.0	24.4	23.6	16.9	14.6	11.2	10.3	9.6	7.4	5.5	4.5
1893-------	1919	26.7	27.8	25.3	22.0	16.8	15.2	11.4	10.8	8.3	6.3	5.3	4.3
1894-------	1920	29.6	28.6	23.1	21.6	17.7	15.2	11.4	9.3	7.2	6.5	5.0	4.2
1895-------	1921	30.4	26.1	22.5	23.0	17.3	14.7	9.9	8.1	7.3	5.9	5.0	3.9
1896-------	1922	27.8	25.5	24.3	22.7	16.7	12.9	8.5	7.9	6.4	5.8	4.5	3.9
1897-------	1923	27.1	27.4	24.8	21.3	14.7	11.2	8.0	7.0	6.4	5.3	4.3	3.7
1898-------	1924	29.9	28.6	23.6	19.6	13.3	10.7	7.8	7.2	6.2	5.1	4.4	3.5
1899-------	1925	31.1	28.1	21.9	18.0	12.7	10.9	8.1	7.6	6.2	5.6	4.4	3.8
1900-------	1926	30.8	25.4	19.8	16.7	13.2	10.8	8.5	7.4	6.6	5.4	4.7	3.8
1901-------	1927	26.9	22.5	18.0	16.6	12.5	10.8	7.9	7.4	6.2	5.5	4.4	3.9
1902-------	1928	24.3	20.4	17.6	16.0	12.0	9.9	7.5	6.9	5.7	4.7	4.2	3.7
1903-------	1929	23.0	19.8	17.4	15.5	11.4	9.4	7.4	6.1	5.2	4.7	4.1	3.5
1904-------	1930	22.0	20.1	17.4	15.2	11.4	9.6	6.6	6.0	5.3	4.7	4.0	3.4
1905-------	1931	22.1	20.1	16.6	15.1	11.0	8.7	6.6	6.2	5.4	4.5	3.9	3.6
1906-------	1932	22.7	19.2	17.0	14.3	10.6	8.9	6.9	6.4	5.2	4.5	4.2	3.8
1907-------	1933	21.2	19.8	15.8	13.8	10.5	9.0	7.1	6.2	5.4	5.2	4.4	4.1
1908-------	1934	21.9	18.5	15.3	13.7	10.6	9.1	6.9	6.5	6.2	5.5	4.7	4.3
1909-------	1935	21.4	18.6	15.5	14.3	10.9	9.0	7.3	7.2	6.7	5.9	5.2	4.6
1910-------	1936	21.2	18.7	16.4	14.3	10.8	9.5	7.7	7.9	7.1	6.2	5.4	4.7
1911-------	1937	21.3	19.3	16.4	14.3	11.1	9.2	8.4	8.3	7.1	6.5	5.9	4.9
1912-------	1938	21.3	19.2	16.5	14.4	11.3	10.0	8.9	8.2	7.5	7.0	5.7	5.1
1913-------	1939	21.3	19.4	16.5	14.0	12.1	10.6	9.0	9.1	8.0	7.0	6.0	5.6
1914-------	1940	21.6	19.4	16.4	15.0	12.6	11.1	10.1	9.1	8.1	7.2	6.8	6.2
1915-------	1941	21.5	19.0	17.3	15.3	12.6	11.8	9.8	9.4	8.4	8.1	7.0	6.2
1916-------	1942	21.9	20.1	17.5	15.3	13.2	11.8	10.1	9.8	9.3	8.4	7.5	6.5
1917-------	1943	23.2	20.3	16.9	15.9	13.7	12.4	10.9	10.7	9.6	8.6	7.6	6.9
1918-------	1944	23.2	19.6	17.9	16.9	14.5	13.3	11.9	11.6	10.3	9.2	8.2	7.1
1919-------	1945	22.6	21.2	19.4	18.6	15.6	14.5	13.3	12.8	11.2	10.2	8.8	7.2
1920-------	1946	23.8	22.0	20.6	19.2	16.8	16.3	14.6	13.2	12.0	10.4	8.8	8.0
1921-------	1947	24.0	23.1	21.3	20.4	18.7	17.0	14.8	14.1	12.4	10.7	9.2	7.2
1922-------	1948	24.5	24.0	22.9	22.1	19.2	17.4	15.6	14.2	12.3	10.7	8.4	6.9
1923-------	1949	26.8	26.4	25.2	23.2	20.4	18.8	16.0	14.6	12.5	10.2	8.3	7.4
1924-------	1950	30.2	29.3	27.0	25.2	22.1	19.3	16.5	15.0	12.0	10.2	8.7	7.5
1925-------	1951	33.4	31.4	29.0	26.8	22.5	19.8	17.0	14.4	12.0	10.5	9.0	7.1
1926-------	1952	35.6	33.1	30.4	27.1	22.7	19.9	16.5	13.9	12.1	10.6	8.1	6.2
1927-------	1953	36.6	34.6	30.2	27.3	22.5	19.7	15.8	14.0	12.3	9.6	7.4	6.5
1928-------	1954	37.8	33.9	30.1	26.0	22.0	18.8	15.6	14.1	11.4	8.8	7.4	5.6
1929-------	1955	37.7	34.6	29.7	25.8	22.3	18.7	16.4	13.7	10.6	9.1	7.0	5.5
1930-------	1956	38.1	33.7	28.8	26.2	21.0	18.8	15.2	12.8	10.2	8.4	6.4	5.2
1931-------	1957	38.3	33.8	29.6	24.5	21.9	17.6	14.9	12.5	9.9	7.5	6.1	4.4
1932-------	1958	38.7	34.4	28.0	25.5	20.1	17.7	13.9	11.8	8.7	7.2	5.5	4.7
1933-------	1959	39.8	33.9	30.1	24.6	20.4	16.9	13.6	10.6	8.8	6.9	5.7	4.9
1934-------	1960	39.6	34.8	28.9	24.0	19.6	16.1	12.5	10.6	8.1	7.0	5.9	4.4
1935-------	1961	40.1	34.1	27.9	23.6	18.4	15.1	12.6	9.6	8.3	7.2	5.6	4.3
1936-------	1962	38.7	32.1	26.8	21.8	17.2	13.8	10.9	9.7	8.5	6.9	5.1	3.7
1937-------	1963	36.9	30.4	25.0	19.3	15.4	12.6	11.1	9.9	8.1	5.8	4.6	
1938-------	1964	33.9	28.2	21.0	17.4	14.1	13.1	11.6	9.2	6.8	5.7		
1939-------	1965	31.7	24.1	19.9	16.5	14.8	13.4	10.9	8.0	6.7			
1940-------	1966	27.4	22.6	18.5	17.0	15.3	13.0	9.5	7.8				
1941-------	1967	24.7	20.9	18.5	17.1	15.0	10.9	8.8					
1942-------	1968	22.4	20.3	19.1	16.8	12.7	10.1						
1943-------	1969	21.6	21.0	18.1	14.3	11.4							
1944-------	1970	22.3	19.5	15.8	12.9								
1945-------	1971	20.8	16.9	14.0									
1946-------	1972	17.6	14.9										
1947-------	1973	15.4											

TABLE 4C. CENTRAL BIRTH RATES FOR ALL OTHER WOMEN DURING EACH YEAR 1917-73 BY AGE AND LIVE-BIRTH ORDER FOR EACH COHORT FROM 1868 TO 1959--CON.

LIVE-BIRTH ORDER AND COHORT	DIAGONAL LINE FOR CALENDAR YEAR	CURRENT AGE											
		38	39	40	41	42	43	44	45	46	47	48	49
FOURTH BIRTHS--CON.													
1868-------													0.2
1869-------												0.4	0.5
1870-------											0.4	0.9	0.1
1871-------										0.7	1.0	0.3	0.2
1872-------									0.7	1.8	0.3	0.4	0.2
1873-------								0.9	1.6	0.6	0.4	0.3	0.1
1874-------							1.0	1.6	0.6	0.8	0.3	0.2	0.1
1875-------						1.2	0.9	0.8	0.9	0.7	0.2	0.2	0.1
1876-------					2.1	1.1	0.8	1.0	0.8	0.5	0.2	0.3	0.1
1877-------				3.1	2.0	1.1	1.0	0.9	0.6	0.5	0.3	0.2	0.2
1878-------			4.8	3.1	2.0	1.3	1.1	0.7	0.6	0.6	0.3	0.3	0.0
1879-------	1917	5.6	4.9	3.2	2.5	1.4	0.8	0.7	0.7	0.5	0.4	0.1	0.1
1880-------	1918	5.9	5.2	3.8	2.6	1.0	0.9	0.9	0.6	0.7	0.2	0.1	0.1
1881-------	1919	6.3	5.9	3.8	2.0	1.1	1.1	0.6	0.9	0.5	0.2	0.2	0.1
1882-------	1920	6.9	5.7	3.2	2.1	1.4	0.8	1.0	0.7	0.5	0.2	0.2	0.0
1883-------	1921	6.4	5.0	3.2	2.6	1.4	1.0	0.8	0.6	0.4	0.2	0.1	0.2
1884-------	1922	5.8	4.8	3.5	2.4	1.0	1.0	0.7	0.4	0.4	0.1	0.3	0.2
1885-------	1923	5.3	4.9	3.2	1.8	1.1	0.7	0.5	0.5	0.4	0.2	0.2	0.1
1886-------	1924	5.2	4.4	2.7	1.6	0.9	0.6	0.5	0.4	0.3	0.2	0.1	0.1
1887-------	1925	5.1	4.3	2.2	1.4	0.7	0.6	0.5	0.3	0.3	0.2	0.1	0.2
1888-------	1926	5.1	3.4	1.8	1.3	0.7	0.5	0.5	0.4	0.3	0.1	0.2	0.0
1889-------	1927	4.3	3.3	1.9	1.4	0.7	0.6	0.5	0.4	0.3	0.2	0.1	0.1
1890-------	1928	3.9	3.2	2.1	1.3	0.7	0.5	0.5	0.3	0.2	0.1	0.1	0.1
1891-------	1929	3.6	3.3	1.9	1.1	0.7	0.6	0.4	0.3	0.2	0.1	0.1	0.1
1892-------	1930	3.7	3.1	1.9	1.3	0.8	0.5	0.4	0.3	0.2	0.1	0.1	0.1
1893-------	1931	3.6	3.0	1.9	1.2	0.7	0.5	0.4	0.2	0.2	0.1	0.1	0.1
1894-------	1932	3.5	2.9	1.7	1.2	0.7	0.5	0.3	0.2	0.2	0.1	0.1	0.0
1895-------	1933	3.2	2.6	1.6	1.0	0.7	0.4	0.2	0.2	0.1	0.1	0.0	0.0
1896-------	1934	3.0	2.4	1.4	1.1	0.6	0.4	0.3	0.2	0.2	0.0	0.0	0.1
1897-------	1935	2.9	2.3	1.5	0.9	0.5	0.4	0.3	0.3	0.1	0.0	0.1	0.1
1898-------	1936	2.8	2.3	1.5	0.9	0.6	0.4	0.4	0.3	0.1	0.1	0.1	0.0
1899-------	1937	2.9	2.6	1.4	1.0	0.6	0.6	0.4	0.2	0.2	0.1	0.1	0.0
1900-------	1938	3.4	2.5	1.5	1.1	0.7	0.7	0.4	0.3	0.2	0.1	0.0	0.1
1901-------	1939	3.2	2.4	1.5	1.0	0.8	0.7	0.4	0.3	0.1	0.1	0.1	0.0
1902-------	1940	3.0	2.4	1.5	1.2	0.8	0.5	0.4	0.2	0.1	0.1	0.0	0.0
1903-------	1941	2.9	2.4	1.6	1.2	0.8	0.6	0.4	0.2	0.1	0.1	0.0	0.0
1904-------	1942	3.0	2.5	1.7	1.3	0.9	0.6	0.3	0.2	0.2	0.0	0.1	0.0
1905-------	1943	3.2	2.6	1.9	1.3	0.9	0.6	0.4	0.3	0.1	0.0	0.0	0.1
1906-------	1944	3.4	2.9	2.0	1.4	0.9	0.7	0.5	0.3	0.1	0.1	0.1	0.0
1907-------	1945	3.5	2.9	2.0	1.5	0.9	0.7	0.5	0.2	0.1	0.1	0.1	0.0
1908-------	1946	3.5	2.8	2.0	1.4	0.9	0.8	0.3	0.2	0.2	0.1	0.0	0.0
1909-------	1947	3.7	3.2	2.2	1.4	1.1	0.7	0.5	0.3	0.2	0.0	0.0	0.1
1910-------	1948	4.0	3.3	2.2	1.8	1.0	0.8	0.5	0.3	0.1	0.0	0.1	0.0
1911-------	1949	4.2	3.4	2.5	1.9	1.2	1.0	0.6	0.2	0.1	0.1	0.0	0.0
1912-------	1950	4.5	3.8	2.9	1.9	1.5	0.9	0.5	0.3	0.1	0.1	0.0	0.0
1913-------	1951	4.9	3.9	2.8	2.3	1.4	0.8	0.4	0.2	0.2	0.0	0.0	0.0
1914-------	1952	5.1	4.2	3.3	2.1	1.3	0.9	0.4	0.4	0.1	0.0	0.0	0.0
1915-------	1953	5.3	4.7	3.2	2.0	1.4	0.8	0.6	0.3	0.1	0.1	0.0	0.0
1916-------	1954	5.8	4.5	3.0	2.1	1.4	0.9	0.5	0.3	0.1	0.0	0.0	0.0
1917-------	1955	5.8	4.3	3.0	2.3	1.3	0.8	0.6	0.3	0.1	0.1	0.0	0.0
1918-------	1956	5.6	4.5	3.2	2.1	1.5	1.0	0.4	0.2	0.1	0.0	0.0	0.0
1919-------	1957	6.3	4.7	3.3	2.3	1.6	0.9	0.5	0.2	0.1	0.0	0.1	0.0
1920-------	1958	5.9	4.7	3.3	2.3	1.4	0.9	0.4	0.3	0.1	0.1	0.0	0.0
1921-------	1959	5.7	4.6	3.2	2.3	1.5	0.8	0.5	0.3	0.1	0.0	0.0	0.0
1922-------	1960	5.9	4.5	3.1	2.2	1.3	0.9	0.5	0.2	0.1	0.1	0.0	0.0
1923-------	1961	5.9	4.4	3.3	2.2	1.4	0.8	0.4	0.3	0.1	0.0	0.0	0.0
1924-------	1962	5.7	4.3	3.0	2.1	1.3	0.7	0.4	0.2	0.1	0.0	0.0	0.0
1925-------	1963	5.3	4.2	2.9	2.0	1.2	0.7	0.4	0.2	0.1	0.0	0.0	
1926-------	1964	5.0	3.9	2.6	1.6	1.1	0.7	0.4	0.2	0.1	0.0		
1927-------	1965	4.7	3.5	2.3	1.7	1.1	0.7	0.4	0.2	0.1			
1928-------	1966	4.3	3.2	2.3	1.7	1.1	0.5	0.3	0.1				
1929-------	1967	4.2	3.0	2.4	1.7	1.0	0.5	0.2					
1930-------	1968	3.6	3.3	2.2	1.4	0.8	0.4						
1931-------	1969	3.8	3.1	2.1	1.2	0.7							
1932-------	1970	3.8	2.7	1.8	1.1								
1933-------	1971	3.4	2.5	1.6									
1934-------	1972	3.4	2.2										
1935-------	1973	2.9											

TABLE 4C. CENTRAL BIRTH RATES FOR ALL OTHER WOMEN DURING EACH YEAR 1917-73 BY AGE AND LIVE-BIRTH ORDER FOR EACH COHORT FROM 1868 TO 1959--CON.

LIVE-BIRTH ORDER AND COHORT	DIAGONAL LINE FOR CALENDAR YEAR	CURRENT AGE											
		14	15	16	17	18	19	20	21	22	23	24	25
FIFTH BIRTHS													
1892-------													19.3
1893-------												16.3	18.1
1894-------											11.7	15.3	19.6
1895-------										6.8	11.1	16.3	19.8
1896-------									3.7	6.5	11.5	16.3	21.2
1897-------								1.5	3.5	6.7	11.2	17.6	20.0
1898-------							*	1.4	3.7	6.6	12.4	17.3	20.8
1899-------						*	*	1.5	3.6	7.2	12.5	17.8	22.0
1900-------					*	*	*	1.5	4.0	7.3	13.2	19.0	21.3
1901-------				*	*	*	*	1.6	3.9	7.4	13.6	17.9	21.6
1902-------			*	*	*	*	*	1.6	4.3	8.2	12.9	18.0	21.4
1903-------	1917	*	*	*	*	*	*	1.8	4.5	7.6	13.0	17.9	18.7
1904-------	1918	*	*	*	*	*	*	1.8	4.6	8.5	13.3	16.6	18.9
1905-------	1919	*	*	*	*	*	*	2.3	5.1	8.2	12.6	16.4	17.8
1906-------	1920	*	*	*	*	*	*	2.4	5.1	8.2	12.3	15.8	17.1
1907-------	1921	*	*	*	*	*	*	2.4	5.2	7.6	11.7	14.8	17.0
1908-------	1922	*	*	*	*	*	*	2.4	4.6	7.6	11.0	14.4	16.5
1909-------	1923	*	*	*	*	*	*	2.1	4.6	7.1	10.6	14.2	17.4
1910-------	1924	*	*	*	*	*	*	2.2	4.3	7.0	10.7	14.9	17.0
1911-------	1925	*	*	*	*	*	*	2.0	4.3	7.0	11.3	15.1	16.9
1912-------	1926	*	*	*	*	*	*	2.1	4.3	7.1	11.4	14.4	17.2
1913-------	1927	*	*	*	*	*	*	2.0	4.2	7.5	10.9	15.0	17.7
1914-------	1928	*	*	*	*	*	*	2.0	4.7	7.6	11.7	15.4	18.0
1915-------	1929	*	*	*	*	*	*	2.2	4.8	7.8	12.0	16.0	18.8
1916-------	1930	*	*	*	*	*	*	2.3	4.9	7.7	12.6	17.2	19.5
1917-------	1931	*	*	*	*	*	*	2.3	4.6	8.1	14.3	18.2	19.3
1918-------	1932	*	*	*	*	*	*	2.1	4.9	9.1	15.3	18.0	20.1
1919-------	1933	*	*	*	*	*	*	2.2	5.7	9.8	14.7	18.6	20.3
1920-------	1934	*	*	*	*	*	*	2.7	6.0	10.1	15.2	18.9	19.6
1921-------	1935	*	*	*	*	*	*	2.8	6.7	10.4	15.6	18.1	20.2
1922-------	1936	*	*	*	*	*	*	3.4	6.9	10.7	14.6	18.0	19.6
1923-------	1937	*	*	*	*	*	*	3.6	7.2	10.5	14.8	17.9	20.4
1924-------	1938	*	*	*	*	*	*	3.8	7.0	10.4	14.9	18.7	21.6
1925-------	1939	*	*	*	*	*	*	3.6	7.1	10.7	15.5	20.2	23.5
1926-------	1940	*	*	*	*	*	*	3.7	7.5	11.1	17.1	22.1	25.9
1927-------	1941	*	*	*	*	*	*	4.0	7.9	12.5	18.3	24.3	28.3
1928-------	1942	*	*	*	*	*	*	4.2	9.0	13.5	20.2	26.3	30.7
1929-------	1943	*	*	*	*	*	*	4.8	9.6	15.1	22.6	29.5	33.1
1930-------	1944	*	*	*	*	*	*	5.1	10.8	17.0	25.6	31.2	34.0
1931-------	1945	*	*	*	*	*	*	5.9	12.1	19.9	27.1	32.6	35.1
1932-------	1946	*	*	*	*	*	*	6.5	12.8	20.0	27.7	32.8	35.3
1933-------	1947	*	*	*	*	*	*	6.1	14.1	20.9	28.4	34.5	36.2
1934-------	1948	*	*	*	*	*	*	7.3	14.7	21.9	30.2	35.3	36.9
1935-------	1949	*	*	*	*	*	*	7.8	15.2	23.2	31.0	36.3	36.4
1936-------	1950	*	*	*	*	*	*	8.1	16.5	23.7	31.7	35.8	36.9
1937-------	1951	*	*	*	*	*	*	8.7	17.0	24.2	31.0	35.7	36.5
1938-------	1952	*	*	*	*	*	*	8.8	16.5	23.5	30.6	34.9	33.6
1939-------	1953	*	*	*	*	*	*	8.7	16.4	23.7	30.2	32.8	31.7
1940-------	1954	*	*	*	*	*	*	8.7	16.7	22.9	28.4	30.7	27.8
1941-------	1955	*	*	*	*	*	*	8.9	16.6	22.0	26.3	26.3	23.4
1942-------	1956	*	*	*	*	*	*	8.7	15.5	19.6	22.6	22.2	19.1
1943-------	1957	*	*	*	*	*	*	8.3	14.0	17.3	18.7	18.3	15.9
1944-------	1958	*	*	*	*	*	*	7.6	12.7	14.2	15.6	15.2	15.0
1945-------	1959	*	*	*	*	*	*	6.8	10.4	12.4	13.1	14.0	14.6
1946-------	1960	*	*	*	*	*	*	5.8	8.7	10.0	11.7	12.8	12.6
1947-------	1961	*	*	*	*	*	*	4.8	7.0	8.6	10.2	11.0	9.8
1948-------	1962	*	*	*	*	*	*	3.7	6.0	7.1	8.7	8.6	8.0
1949-------	1963	*	*	*	*	*	*	3.2	5.1	6.3	6.8	6.9	
1950-------	1964	*	*	*	*	*	*	2.7	4.4	5.1	5.5		
1951-------	1965	*	*	*	*	*	*	2.3	3.4	4.0			
1952-------	1966	*	*	*	*	*	*	1.8	2.7				
1953-------	1967	*	*	*	*	*	*	1.4					
1954-------	1968	*	*	*	*	*	*						
1955-------	1969	*	*	*	*	*							
1956-------	1970	*	*	*	*								
1957-------	1971	*	*	*									
1958-------	1972	*	*										
1959-------	1973	*											

TABLE 4C. CENTRAL BIRTH RATES FOR ALL OTHER WOMEN DURING EACH YEAR 1917-73 BY AGE AND LIVE-BIRTH ORDER FOR EACH COHORT FROM 1868 TO 1959--CON.

LIVE-BIRTH ORDER AND COHORT	DIAGONAL LINE FOR CALENDAR YEAR	CURRENT AGE											
		26	27	28	29	30	31	32	33	34	35	36	37
FIFTH BIRTHS--CON.													
1880-------													8.1
1881-------												10.4	7.8
1882-------											11.6	10.0	8.4
1883-------										12.5	11.2	10.5	8.6
1884-------									11.8	12.1	11.4	10.4	8.2
1885-------								12.0	11.6	12.1	11.0	9.9	7.7
1886-------							14.4	11.8	11.3	11.4	10.8	9.3	6.7
1887-------						15.2	14.3	11.7	10.5	11.7	10.2	8.2	7.1
1888-------					18.4	14.9	14.4	10.9	11.4	11.1	9.4	8.7	7.0
1889-------				18.8	17.6	15.6	13.6	12.0	10.9	10.6	9.9	8.5	6.7
1890-------			19.8	17.2	19.0	15.3	15.0	11.5	11.0	11.0	9.6	8.6	6.5
1891-------	1917	19.8	18.6	19.1	19.2	16.7	14.5	11.7	11.1	10.7	9.6	7.5	5.9
1892-------	1918	18.6	20.6	19.7	20.7	15.9	14.7	11.8	11.4	10.4	8.7	7.1	5.8
1893-------	1919	20.5	21.3	21.1	19.4	16.0	14.7	11.9	10.7	9.6	8.2	6.9	5.9
1894-------	1920	21.0	22.6	19.4	19.5	16.5	14.6	11.9	10.3	8.9	7.8	6.9	5.3
1895-------	1921	22.3	20.8	19.6	20.5	16.3	15.0	11.0	9.8	8.4	7.9	6.3	5.0
1896-------	1922	20.5	21.0	21.0	19.8	16.6	13.9	10.1	8.9	8.7	6.8	6.2	4.8
1897-------	1923	20.7	22.5	20.2	19.6	15.7	13.0	9.4	9.3	7.7	6.9	5.7	4.8
1898-------	1924	22.8	21.7	20.0	19.9	14.7	12.7	9.9	8.3	7.8	6.6	5.7	4.4
1899-------	1925	21.7	22.2	21.1	18.9	15.1	13.0	9.4	9.3	8.0	7.1	5.6	4.6
1900-------	1926	22.7	23.1	19.7	19.0	14.7	12.1	10.1	9.3	8.1	6.8	5.5	4.8
1901-------	1927	22.5	20.3	19.1	17.9	13.7	12.2	9.5	9.2	7.5	6.4	5.4	4.6
1902-------	1928	19.8	19.8	17.8	16.5	13.5	11.4	9.2	7.9	6.8	5.9	5.1	4.1
1903-------	1929	19.5	18.4	16.8	16.5	12.5	11.3	8.2	7.6	6.7	5.8	4.6	4.4
1904-------	1930	18.3	17.9	17.0	16.3	12.9	10.5	7.9	7.7	6.7	5.5	4.9	4.6
1905-------	1931	17.9	17.9	16.8	16.2	12.4	10.2	8.2	7.8	6.4	5.8	5.1	4.5
1906-------	1932	18.0	17.9	16.9	15.3	11.6	10.2	8.1	7.5	6.7	5.9	5.0	4.6
1907-------	1933	17.4	18.0	16.0	14.6	11.8	9.9	7.9	7.9	6.8	5.9	5.1	4.6
1908-------	1934	17.7	16.8	15.4	14.7	11.3	9.5	8.3	7.8	6.8	6.2	5.1	4.7
1909-------	1935	17.3	17.2	16.0	14.5	11.1	10.2	8.3	7.9	7.2	6.3	5.7	4.9
1910-------	1936	17.6	17.6	15.7	14.3	11.5	10.1	8.6	8.4	7.3	6.9	5.7	5.1
1911-------	1937	18.0	17.6	15.8	14.5	11.6	10.3	9.1	8.6	8.0	6.8	6.0	5.4
1912-------	1938	17.8	17.5	15.7	14.7	12.1	10.9	9.4	9.1	7.6	6.9	6.3	5.4
1913-------	1939	17.9	17.5	16.2	14.7	12.8	11.3	9.7	8.9	8.0	7.4	6.3	5.7
1914-------	1940	18.0	18.1	16.2	15.5	13.1	11.7	9.4	9.2	8.3	7.5	6.7	6.2
1915-------	1941	18.4	17.8	17.0	15.9	13.1	11.4	10.0	9.5	8.5	7.8	7.0	6.1
1916-------	1942	18.6	18.7	17.3	15.7	13.1	11.6	10.2	9.7	8.9	8.4	7.1	6.7
1917-------	1943	19.4	18.9	17.1	15.8	13.1	12.0	10.5	10.5	9.3	8.5	7.7	7.2
1918-------	1944	19.5	18.9	17.3	15.7	13.7	12.6	11.4	10.8	10.1	8.9	8.2	7.2
1919-------	1945	19.9	19.5	17.6	16.9	14.9	13.9	12.3	12.3	10.7	10.3	8.7	7.6
1920-------	1946	20.2	19.4	18.8	17.8	15.6	14.8	13.8	12.9	12.3	10.5	9.2	8.2
1921-------	1947	19.9	20.3	19.2	18.4	17.2	16.2	14.5	14.5	12.3	10.8	9.4	8.0
1922-------	1948	20.5	20.4	19.7	19.7	17.8	16.9	15.3	14.1	12.4	10.8	9.1	7.9
1923-------	1949	21.1	21.7	21.0	20.7	18.9	17.5	15.4	14.5	12.7	10.7	8.9	7.2
1924-------	1950	23.2	23.1	23.3	22.7	20.3	18.6	16.5	15.1	12.6	11.1	8.5	7.7
1925-------	1951	24.9	26.4	25.5	24.7	21.5	20.2	17.4	14.8	13.0	10.5	9.1	7.4
1926-------	1952	27.9	28.7	28.1	25.6	22.7	20.3	16.5	15.4	12.6	10.6	8.8	7.1
1927-------	1953	30.6	30.9	28.2	26.5	23.0	19.3	17.2	14.6	12.1	10.2	8.5	6.6
1928-------	1954	32.3	31.0	28.1	26.3	21.5	19.8	16.2	14.3	12.0	9.6	7.6	6.2
1929-------	1955	33.0	32.1	29.1	25.4	22.5	19.1	16.0	14.3	11.3	9.2	7.6	5.8
1930-------	1956	33.8	31.9	27.9	25.8	21.7	18.9	15.9	13.1	10.8	8.7	6.8	5.3
1931-------	1957	34.1	31.4	28.7	25.4	21.4	18.2	15.0	13.0	10.2	7.9	6.2	5.0
1932-------	1958	34.1	32.2	28.1	25.5	20.6	17.9	14.3	11.9	9.2	7.4	5.9	5.0
1933-------	1959	35.0	31.6	28.8	24.4	20.8	17.2	13.6	10.9	8.6	7.2	5.8	4.6
1934-------	1960	34.5	32.6	28.3	24.4	19.8	16.1	12.5	10.1	8.0	7.0	5.7	4.5
1935-------	1961	35.5	31.9	28.0	23.5	18.3	14.6	11.7	9.2	8.1	7.0	5.3	3.9
1936-------	1962	35.1	31.2	26.1	21.1	16.1	13.4	10.1	9.2	8.1	6.2	4.9	3.6
1937-------	1963	33.6	28.5	23.1	18.3	14.6	11.6	10.3	9.3	7.2	5.7	4.3	
1938-------	1964	30.5	25.2	19.6	15.9	12.7	11.5	10.4	8.4	6.7	5.0		
1939-------	1965	27.0	21.6	17.2	14.0	12.8	11.6	9.6	7.5	5.9			
1940-------	1966	23.0	18.7	15.1	14.1	12.9	11.1	8.4	6.7				
1941-------	1967	19.4	15.9	14.9	14.0	12.2	9.1	7.2					
1942-------	1968	16.3	15.2	14.8	12.9	9.8	7.9						
1943-------	1969	15.2	15.2	13.5	10.4	8.1							
1944-------	1970	15.0	13.7	10.7	8.8								
1945-------	1971	13.7	10.9	8.8									
1946-------	1972	10.7	9.0										
1947-------	1973	8.6											

TABLE 4C. CENTRAL BIRTH RATES FOR ALL OTHER WOMEN DURING EACH YEAR 1917-73 BY AGE AND LIVE-BIRTH ORDER FOR EACH COHORT FROM 1868 TO 1959--CON.

LIVE-BIRTH ORDER AND COHORT	DIAGONAL LINE FOR CALENDAR YEAR	CURRENT AGE											
		38	39	40	41	42	43	44	45	46	47	48	49
FIFTH BIRTHS--CON.													
1868-------													0.2
1869-------												0.4	0.2
1870-------											0.5	0.5	0.2
1871-------										0.9	0.7	0.3	0.2
1872-------									1.0	1.2	0.4	0.4	0.1
1873-------								1.1	1.1	0.8	0.6	0.3	0.1
1874-------							1.2	1.2	0.9	1.0	0.4	0.3	0.2
1875-------						1.5	1.2	1.0	1.0	0.6	0.4	0.4	0.2
1876-------					2.5	1.6	1.1	1.1	0.7	0.6	0.5	0.3	0.2
1877-------				3.6	2.8	1.4	1.2	0.8	0.7	0.9	0.5	0.2	0.1
1878-------			5.8	3.8	2.6	1.6	1.1	0.8	0.9	0.9	0.2	0.3	0.1
1879-------	1917	6.7	5.8	3.8	3.0	1.5	1.0	1.0	0.9	0.7	0.4	0.2	0.2
1880-------	1918	6.5	6.1	4.2	2.8	1.3	1.1	1.1	0.8	0.6	0.4	0.2	0.2
1881-------	1919	7.1	6.6	4.0	2.5	1.4	1.2	1.1	0.6	0.6	0.4	0.3	0.2
1882-------	1920	7.4	6.4	3.8	2.5	1.5	1.3	0.8	0.7	0.5	0.4	0.2	0.1
1883-------	1921	7.2	6.0	3.6	2.7	1.8	1.1	0.8	0.6	0.5	0.3	0.3	0.2
1884-------	1922	6.8	5.4	3.8	2.2	1.4	1.0	0.7	0.6	0.5	0.3	0.2	0.1
1885-------	1923	5.9	5.7	3.0	2.3	1.3	0.9	0.7	0.6	0.7	0.2	0.1	0.1
1886-------	1924	6.2	4.6	3.1	1.9	1.1	0.7	0.8	0.7	0.4	0.2	0.2	0.2
1887-------	1925	6.0	4.7	2.8	1.9	0.9	0.9	0.7	0.5	0.3	0.2	0.2	0.1
1888-------	1926	5.4	4.5	2.7	1.6	1.1	0.7	0.6	0.4	0.3	0.2	0.1	0.2
1889-------	1927	5.5	4.2	2.4	1.9	0.9	0.8	0.5	0.4	0.3	0.2	0.2	0.1
1890-------	1928	4.8	3.9	2.8	1.7	1.1	0.7	0.6	0.4	0.3	0.1	0.1	0.1
1891-------	1929	4.7	4.6	2.6	1.8	0.9	0.7	0.6	0.4	0.3	0.1	0.2	0.1
1892-------	1930	5.2	3.9	2.4	1.6	0.9	0.7	0.5	0.3	0.1	0.2	0.2	0.1
1893-------	1931	4.6	3.4	2.3	1.5	1.0	0.7	0.5	0.2	0.2	0.2	0.1	0.1
1894-------	1932	4.1	3.5	2.2	1.6	0.9	0.6	0.3	0.3	0.2	0.2	0.1	0.0
1895-------	1933	4.1	3.4	2.3	1.4	0.7	0.4	0.3	0.3	0.2	0.1	0.0	0.1
1896-------	1934	3.9	3.3	2.0	1.1	0.7	0.4	0.3	0.2	0.2	0.1	0.1	0.0
1897-------	1935	3.7	3.0	1.8	1.2	0.7	0.5	0.3	0.3	0.2	0.1	0.1	0.1
1898-------	1936	3.5	3.0	2.1	1.3	0.8	0.5	0.5	0.3	0.2	0.2	0.1	0.0
1899-------	1937	4.0	3.2	2.0	1.4	0.8	0.7	0.5	0.4	0.2	0.1	0.1	0.0
1900-------	1938	4.0	3.0	2.1	1.4	0.8	0.6	0.5	0.3	0.2	0.1	0.1	0.0
1901-------	1939	3.5	3.1	2.1	1.2	0.7	0.7	0.4	0.3	0.2	0.1	0.1	0.1
1902-------	1940	3.6	3.1	1.9	1.2	0.8	0.7	0.5	0.2	0.1	0.1	0.1	0.0
1903-------	1941	3.8	3.0	1.9	1.3	1.0	0.7	0.3	0.2	0.2	0.1	0.1	0.0
1904-------	1942	3.7	3.0	2.0	1.5	0.9	0.6	0.4	0.2	0.1	0.1	0.1	0.0
1905-------	1943	3.9	3.1	2.3	1.4	1.0	0.6	0.4	0.2	0.1	0.1	0.0	0.0
1906-------	1944	3.8	3.3	1.9	1.5	0.9	0.6	0.4	0.2	0.1	0.1	0.0	0.1
1907-------	1945	4.0	3.1	2.2	1.4	0.9	0.7	0.4	0.2	0.1	0.0	0.1	0.0
1908-------	1946	3.9	3.2	2.1	1.6	1.0	0.7	0.3	0.2	0.1	0.1	0.0	0.0
1909-------	1947	4.2	3.4	2.4	1.7	1.1	0.7	0.6	0.2	0.2	0.1	0.0	0.0
1910-------	1948	4.3	3.6	2.4	1.9	1.1	1.0	0.5	0.3	0.2	0.1	0.0	0.0
1911-------	1949	4.4	3.5	2.8	1.8	1.5	0.9	0.5	0.3	0.2	0.0	0.0	0.1
1912-------	1950	4.5	4.0	2.7	2.1	1.4	0.9	0.5	0.4	0.1	0.1	0.1	0.0
1913-------	1951	4.9	4.1	3.0	2.0	1.4	1.1	0.6	0.3	0.2	0.1	0.0	0.0
1914-------	1952	5.1	4.4	3.1	2.2	1.5	1.1	0.5	0.3	0.2	0.0	0.1	0.0
1915-------	1953	5.6	4.5	3.2	2.5	1.6	0.9	0.6	0.3	0.1	0.1	0.1	0.0
1916-------	1954	5.9	4.6	3.5	2.4	1.4	1.1	0.5	0.3	0.2	0.1	0.1	0.0
1917-------	1955	5.8	4.9	3.3	2.3	1.7	1.0	0.5	0.3	0.1	0.1	0.0	0.0
1918-------	1956	6.1	4.8	3.4	2.4	1.7	1.0	0.5	0.3	0.2	0.1	0.0	0.0
1919-------	1957	6.4	5.1	3.5	2.6	1.5	1.1	0.6	0.3	0.2	0.1	0.0	0.0
1920-------	1958	6.6	5.1	3.5	2.2	1.8	1.1	0.6	0.3	0.2	0.1	0.0	0.0
1921-------	1959	6.4	4.8	3.4	2.5	1.6	0.9	0.6	0.3	0.1	0.0	0.1	0.0
1922-------	1960	5.9	4.7	3.2	2.5	1.5	1.0	0.5	0.3	0.1	0.1	0.0	0.0
1923-------	1961	6.3	4.5	3.3	2.4	1.5	0.8	0.4	0.3	0.1	0.1	0.0	0.0
1924-------	1962	5.9	4.4	3.3	2.3	1.4	0.8	0.5	0.2	0.1	0.0	0.0	0.0
1925-------	1963	5.7	4.4	3.1	2.1	1.2	0.7	0.5	0.2	0.1	0.1	0.0	
1926-------	1964	5.5	4.1	3.1	1.7	1.2	0.9	0.4	0.3	0.1	0.0		
1927-------	1965	5.2	4.0	2.4	1.6	1.2	0.7	0.5	0.2	0.1			
1928-------	1966	4.9	3.4	2.2	1.7	1.1	0.6	0.4	0.2				
1929-------	1967	4.2	3.0	2.2	1.7	0.9	0.6	0.3					
1930-------	1968	3.9	3.2	2.4	1.3	0.9	0.5						
1931-------	1969	3.9	3.0	1.9	1.2	0.8							
1932-------	1970	3.8	2.8	1.8	1.2								
1933-------	1971	3.7	2.4	1.7									
1934-------	1972	3.1	2.3										
1935-------	1973	2.9											

TABLE 4C. CENTRAL BIRTH RATES FOR ALL OTHER WOMEN DURING EACH YEAR 1917-73 BY AGE AND LIVE-BIRTH ORDER FOR EACH COHORT FROM 1868 TO 1959--CON.

LIVE-BIRTH ORDER AND COHORT	DIAGONAL LINE FOR CALENDAR YEAR	CURRENT AGE											
		14	15	16	17	18	19	20	21	22	23	24	25
SIXTH BIRTHS													
1892-------													11.5
1893-------												8.4	11.1
1894-------											5.2	8.2	11.0
1895-------										2.6	5.3	7.9	11.4
1896-------									1.2	2.6	4.8	8.1	12.4
1897-------								0.5	1.2	2.4	4.8	9.0	11.9
1898-------							*	0.4	1.1	2.4	5.6	8.9	12.0
1899-------						*	*	0.4	1.1	2.8	5.6	8.9	13.1
1900-------					*	*	*	0.4	1.3	2.8	5.9	9.8	12.9
1901-------				*	*	*	*	0.4	1.2	2.8	6.1	9.3	13.4
1902-------			*	*	*	*	*	0.5	1.4	3.3	6.0	9.4	11.4
1903-------	1917	*	*	*	*	*	*	0.5	1.6	3.2	5.9	7.9	10.5
1904-------	1918	*	*	*	*	*	*	0.6	1.8	3.2	5.3	8.0	10.5
1905-------	1919	*	*	*	*	*	*	0.8	1.9	3.0	5.4	7.6	10.0
1906-------	1920	*	*	*	*	*	*	0.9	1.8	3.2	4.7	7.5	9.8
1907-------	1921	*	*	*	*	*	*	0.8	1.8	2.6	4.6	7.1	8.7
1908-------	1922	*	*	*	*	*	*	0.8	1.5	2.5	4.5	6.3	8.8
1909-------	1923	*	*	*	*	*	*	0.7	1.4	2.6	4.0	6.3	9.1
1910-------	1924	*	*	*	*	*	*	0.7	1.5	2.4	4.1	6.4	8.9
1911-------	1925	*	*	*	*	*	*	0.7	1.3	2.4	4.3	6.8	9.1
1912-------	1926	*	*	*	*	*	*	0.6	1.4	2.4	4.4	6.7	9.4
1913-------	1927	*	*	*	*	*	*	0.6	1.3	2.6	4.3	6.9	9.3
1914-------	1928	*	*	*	*	*	*	0.5	1.4	2.5	4.6	7.1	9.5
1915-------	1929	*	*	*	*	*	*	0.6	1.4	2.7	4.7	7.2	10.0
1916-------	1930	*	*	*	*	*	*	0.6	1.5	2.8	4.8	7.9	10.3
1917-------	1931	*	*	*	*	*	*	0.7	1.5	2.8	5.5	8.3	10.9
1918-------	1932	*	*	*	*	*	*	0.7	1.5	3.3	6.0	8.6	11.3
1919-------	1933	*	*	*	*	*	*	0.7	1.8	3.6	6.0	9.1	11.7
1920-------	1934	*	*	*	*	*	*	0.9	1.9	3.4	6.6	9.3	11.6
1921-------	1935	*	*	*	*	*	*	0.9	1.9	3.7	6.6	9.0	11.8
1922-------	1936	*	*	*	*	*	*	0.8	2.1	3.8	6.1	9.0	11.6
1923-------	1937	*	*	*	*	*	*	0.9	2.1	3.8	6.3	9.3	11.7
1924-------	1938	*	*	*	*	*	*	0.9	2.1	3.8	6.5	9.5	12.8
1925-------	1939	*	*	*	*	*	*	1.0	2.1	3.9	6.6	10.3	13.2
1926-------	1940	*	*	*	*	*	*	1.0	2.3	4.1	7.3	10.7	14.5
1927-------	1941	*	*	*	*	*	*	1.1	2.3	4.5	7.4	11.5	15.7
1928-------	1942	*	*	*	*	*	*	1.1	2.4	4.5	8.1	12.7	17.4
1929-------	1943	*	*	*	*	*	*	1.1	2.5	5.0	9.4	14.1	19.0
1930-------	1944	*	*	*	*	*	*	1.2	2.7	5.9	10.2	15.8	20.5
1931-------	1945	*	*	*	*	*	*	1.2	3.3	6.6	11.9	17.1	22.9
1932-------	1946	*	*	*	*	*	*	1.4	3.6	7.6	12.3	18.7	22.5
1933-------	1947	*	*	*	*	*	*	1.4	4.2	7.9	13.2	18.9	22.9
1934-------	1948	*	*	*	*	*	*	1.9	4.3	8.0	14.1	19.6	23.6
1935-------	1949	*	*	*	*	*	*	1.9	4.3	9.1	14.4	20.3	24.5
1936-------	1950	*	*	*	*	*	*	1.9	4.9	9.1	15.3	20.5	24.7
1937-------	1951	*	*	*	*	*	*	2.2	4.7	9.4	15.2	20.8	24.6
1938-------	1952	*	*	*	*	*	*	2.1	5.0	9.4	15.1	20.5	22.5
1939-------	1953	*	*	*	*	*	*	2.1	5.2	9.6	14.7	18.7	21.3
1940-------	1954	*	*	*	*	*	*	2.2	5.2	9.4	13.8	17.9	18.3
1941-------	1955	*	*	*	*	*	*	2.2	5.1	8.8	13.1	14.9	14.9
1942-------	1956	*	*	*	*	*	*	2.3	4.8	8.1	10.6	12.5	12.6
1943-------	1957	*	*	*	*	*	*	2.0	4.3	6.6	9.1	10.1	9.7
1944-------	1958	*	*	*	*	*	*	2.0	3.8	5.8	7.5	7.8	8.4
1945-------	1959	*	*	*	*	*	*	1.7	3.2	4.5	5.7	6.7	7.6
1946-------	1960	*	*	*	*	*	*	1.3	2.4	3.5	4.9	6.0	6.2
1947-------	1961	*	*	*	*	*	*	1.1	1.8	3.0	4.2	4.8	4.6
1948-------	1962	*	*	*	*	*	*	0.7	1.6	2.5	3.3	3.4	3.5
1949-------	1963	*	*	*	*	*	*	0.7	1.4	2.0	2.3	2.6	
1950-------	1964	*	*	*	*	*	*	0.6	1.1	1.4	1.8		
1951-------	1965	*	*	*	*	*	*	0.5	0.8	1.1			
1952-------	1966	*	*	*	*	*	*	0.3	0.6				
1953-------	1967	*	*	*	*	*	*	0.3					
1954-------	1968	*	*	*	*	*	*						
1955-------	1969	*	*	*	*	*							
1956-------	1970	*	*	*	*								
1957-------	1971	*	*	*									
1958-------	1972	*	*										
1959-------	1973	*											

TABLE 4C. CENTRAL BIRTH RATES FOR ALL OTHER WOMEN DURING EACH YEAR 1917-73 BY AGE AND LIVE-BIRTH ORDER FOR EACH COHORT FROM 1868 TO 1959--CON.

LIVE-BIRTH ORDER AND COHORT	DIAGONAL LINE FOR CALENDAR YEAR	CURRENT AGE											
		26	27	28	29	30	31	32	33	34	35	36	37
SIXTH BIRTHS--CON.													
1880-------													10.4
1881-------												13.0	12.3
1882-------											14.6	15.1	11.7
1883-------										15.2	16.1	14.0	11.2
1884-------									14.7	15.8	14.6	13.1	10.6
1885-------								14.2	14.4	14.1	13.6	12.3	9.3
1886-------							16.5	13.8	12.8	13.2	13.3	10.8	9.0
1887-------						15.9	16.3	12.4	12.0	13.6	11.9	10.5	8.3
1888-------					18.0	15.6	14.8	11.8	13.3	12.3	11.8	9.8	8.4
1889-------				16.0	17.5	14.7	14.3	13.2	12.4	12.5	11.5	10.0	8.8
1890-------			15.8	15.3	17.2	14.8	16.1	12.3	12.8	12.7	11.5	10.7	7.9
1891-------	1917	13.6	15.2	15.7	17.7	16.4	15.0	12.8	13.5	12.8	12.0	9.1	7.2
1892-------	1918	13.0	15.5	16.6	19.3	15.4	15.6	13.4	13.3	12.3	10.1	8.4	6.7
1893-------	1919	13.2	16.4	17.9	18.2	15.6	16.3	13.1	12.6	10.7	9.4	8.0	7.2
1894-------	1920	13.9	17.5	16.8	18.1	16.7	15.6	12.6	11.7	10.0	9.2	7.8	6.5
1895-------	1921	14.8	16.5	16.4	19.7	16.1	14.7	12.1	10.6	9.9	8.9	7.7	7.2
1896-------	1922	14.0	16.1	18.4	18.3	15.8	14.0	10.9	10.3	9.4	8.4	7.9	5.9
1897-------	1923	13.6	18.0	16.8	18.3	14.5	13.4	10.1	10.4	9.1	8.7	6.7	5.8
1898-------	1924	15.5	16.7	17.8	17.4	14.1	12.8	10.8	9.9	9.6	7.9	6.9	5.5
1899-------	1925	15.1	17.9	17.2	16.8	13.7	13.6	10.8	11.1	9.3	8.6	6.8	5.6
1900-------	1926	15.9	17.1	15.7	16.8	14.5	13.5	11.5	10.7	9.7	8.0	6.6	5.6
1901-------	1927	14.1	15.1	14.9	16.4	14.0	13.2	10.7	10.5	8.6	7.3	6.3	5.6
1902-------	1928	12.7	14.4	14.5	15.4	13.2	12.2	10.0	9.1	7.9	6.9	6.0	5.3
1903-------	1929	12.2	13.4	14.2	15.2	12.3	11.5	9.0	8.5	7.3	6.6	5.7	5.1
1904-------	1930	11.8	13.6	14.2	14.7	12.2	11.0	8.8	8.3	7.3	6.5	5.5	5.1
1905-------	1931	12.0	13.4	13.6	14.4	11.9	10.5	8.9	8.4	7.1	6.3	5.6	4.8
1906-------	1932	11.0	13.1	13.7	13.7	11.4	10.6	8.9	8.3	7.0	6.3	5.3	4.9
1907-------	1933	10.8	13.3	12.7	13.2	11.6	10.6	8.8	8.2	7.1	6.4	5.5	5.0
1908-------	1934	11.1	12.0	12.5	13.4	11.1	10.4	8.7	8.3	7.4	6.8	5.6	5.2
1909-------	1935	10.6	12.2	13.0	13.4	11.2	10.4	8.9	8.5	7.9	7.0	6.1	5.1
1910-------	1936	10.9	12.6	13.3	13.4	11.2	10.6	9.1	9.0	8.2	7.2	6.1	5.4
1911-------	1937	11.1	13.3	13.5	13.6	11.4	10.5	9.7	9.4	8.1	7.2	6.3	5.5
1912-------	1938	11.3	13.4	13.8	13.8	11.7	11.3	10.1	9.1	8.1	7.4	6.3	5.8
1913-------	1939	11.4	13.8	14.0	13.3	12.3	11.7	9.7	9.2	8.2	7.2	6.5	5.8
1914-------	1940	11.8	14.0	13.6	13.8	12.9	11.6	9.8	9.5	8.1	7.5	6.4	6.2
1915-------	1941	11.9	13.5	13.9	14.5	12.6	11.2	9.8	9.5	8.5	7.4	7.0	6.2
1916-------	1942	12.4	13.8	14.7	14.4	12.1	11.3	10.3	9.7	8.3	8.0	7.1	6.5
1917-------	1943	12.6	14.5	14.2	13.8	12.1	11.9	10.3	9.8	9.1	8.4	7.5	6.9
1918-------	1944	13.2	14.4	14.2	14.0	12.7	11.9	10.6	10.6	9.8	9.1	8.1	7.1
1919-------	1945	13.3	14.7	14.5	14.9	13.6	12.9	12.0	11.7	10.4	9.7	8.5	7.7
1920-------	1946	13.6	14.6	15.3	15.4	14.3	14.0	12.4	11.8	11.3	10.1	8.8	8.0
1921-------	1947	13.5	15.2	15.6	16.3	15.1	14.2	12.7	13.0	11.6	10.4	9.3	7.5
1922-------	1948	13.5	15.3	16.2	16.9	15.2	14.7	14.0	12.9	11.7	10.7	8.6	8.0
1923-------	1949	14.2	16.0	17.2	17.1	16.5	15.6	14.1	13.7	12.2	10.2	9.1	7.6
1924-------	1950	14.9	17.6	18.0	19.0	17.5	16.8	15.4	14.4	11.9	11.2	8.8	7.4
1925-------	1951	16.5	18.7	19.8	20.3	19.0	18.3	16.2	14.3	12.8	10.6	8.8	7.4
1926-------	1952	17.8	20.5	22.0	22.2	20.6	18.8	16.2	15.0	12.1	10.6	8.7	6.8
1927-------	1953	19.5	22.5	22.9	23.4	20.9	19.0	16.2	13.9	12.4	10.5	8.0	6.6
1928-------	1954	21.1	23.6	23.9	23.8	20.9	18.7	15.3	14.1	11.8	9.2	7.8	6.4
1929-------	1955	22.5	24.9	25.2	23.9	21.0	18.2	15.9	14.0	10.9	9.5	7.5	5.7
1930-------	1956	24.3	25.9	25.2	23.9	20.7	18.3	15.6	12.6	11.2	8.6	6.5	5.2
1931-------	1957	24.8	26.0	25.3	23.5	20.7	18.1	14.4	13.3	9.6	7.5	6.1	5.0
1932-------	1958	24.9	25.6	24.6	23.7	19.9	16.9	14.4	11.2	8.5	7.1	5.7	4.0
1933-------	1959	25.0	25.8	25.8	22.2	19.0	16.6	12.7	10.1	8.1	6.5	4.9	4.2
1934-------	1960	25.8	27.3	24.3	21.6	18.6	15.3	11.8	9.4	7.5	6.2	5.0	4.2
1935-------	1961	27.0	26.1	23.5	21.6	17.1	13.7	10.5	8.6	7.2	6.0	5.1	3.7
1936-------	1962	26.5	25.0	23.4	19.2	15.2	12.0	9.2	8.2	6.9	5.9	4.3	3.2
1937-------	1963	24.8	23.9	20.0	16.3	13.1	10.2	8.6	7.7	6.8	4.8	3.8	
1938-------	1964	23.1	20.5	16.7	13.9	11.0	9.6	8.5	7.4	5.3	4.2		
1939-------	1965	20.2	16.7	14.2	12.2	10.0	9.7	8.1	6.1	4.8			
1940-------	1966	16.4	14.6	12.5	11.0	10.2	8.7	6.7	5.2				
1941-------	1967	13.7	12.2	11.0	10.5	8.9	7.1	5.6					
1942-------	1968	11.0	10.8	10.1	9.2	7.2	5.7						
1943-------	1969	9.7	9.7	8.7	7.2	5.6							
1944-------	1970	8.9	8.3	7.1	5.7								
1945-------	1971	7.3	6.7	5.5									
1946-------	1972	5.8	5.2										
1947-------	1973	4.4											

TABLE 4C. CENTRAL BIRTH RATES FOR ALL OTHER WOMEN DURING EACH YEAR 1917-73 BY AGE AND LIVE-BIRTH ORDER FOR EACH COHORT FROM 1868 TO 1959--CON.

LIVE-BIRTH ORDER AND COHORT	DIAGONAL LINE FOR CALENDAR YEAR	CURRENT AGE											
		38	39	40	41	42	43	44	45	46	47	48	49
SIXTH BIRTHS--CON.													
1868-------													0.4
1869-------												0.5	1.2
1870-------											0.6	1.4	0.3
1871-------										1.0	1.8	0.4	0.4
1872-------									1.2	3.1	0.5	0.5	0.2
1873-------								1.6	3.2	0.9	0.6	0.3	0.3
1874-------							1.7	3.3	1.1	1.1	0.3	0.3	0.3
1875-------						2.2	2.0	1.4	1.3	0.6	0.4	0.4	0.3
1876-------					3.5	2.6	1.5	1.6	0.8	0.6	0.5	0.4	0.2
1877-------				5.0	4.2	1.9	1.5	1.3	0.8	0.9	0.5	0.3	0.2
1878-------			7.6	5.9	3.2	2.0	1.6	1.2	1.1	0.9	0.3	0.3	0.1
1879-------	1917	8.7	9.0	5.1	3.3	2.2	1.5	1.4	1.1	0.7	0.5	0.3	0.2
1880-------	1918	10.3	8.2	5.2	3.7	2.0	1.4	1.4	0.9	1.0	0.6	0.3	0.3
1881-------	1919	9.9	8.3	5.4	3.5	1.9	1.5	1.1	1.1	0.8	0.4	0.4	0.2
1882-------	1920	9.7	8.3	5.0	3.1	1.9	1.5	1.3	0.9	0.7	0.5	0.2	0.2
1883-------	1921	9.4	7.5	4.7	3.1	2.0	1.6	0.9	0.9	0.9	0.3	0.3	0.1
1884-------	1922	8.3	7.1	4.5	3.3	1.9	1.2	1.1	1.0	0.7	0.4	0.3	0.1
1885-------	1923	8.0	6.6	4.5	2.9	1.5	1.1	1.1	0.8	0.6	0.4	0.2	0.2
1886-------	1924	7.3	6.7	3.9	2.5	1.3	1.0	1.0	0.6	0.8	0.2	0.3	0.3
1887-------	1925	7.5	5.7	3.6	2.1	1.3	1.0	0.7	0.9	0.5	0.3	0.3	0.2
1888-------	1926	6.9	5.5	3.1	2.0	1.2	0.9	1.0	0.6	0.6	0.2	0.2	0.2
1889-------	1927	6.5	5.1	3.0	2.1	1.3	0.9	0.7	0.6	0.4	0.2	0.3	0.2
1890-------	1928	5.9	4.8	3.0	2.3	1.3	0.8	0.7	0.5	0.3	0.3	0.2	0.2
1891-------	1929	5.5	5.1	3.2	2.3	1.1	0.8	0.6	0.4	0.4	0.2	0.2	0.1
1892-------	1930	6.0	4.9	3.5	2.0	1.1	0.8	0.5	0.4	0.3	0.2	0.2	0.1
1893-------	1931	5.7	5.3	2.9	2.0	1.1	0.8	0.5	0.3	0.3	0.2	0.1	0.1
1894-------	1932	6.2	4.4	2.9	1.9	1.1	0.7	0.5	0.3	0.3	0.1	0.1	0.0
1895-------	1933	4.9	4.3	2.7	1.7	1.0	0.7	0.5	0.3	0.2	0.2	0.1	0.0
1896-------	1934	4.9	3.8	2.4	1.6	0.9	0.7	0.5	0.2	0.3	0.1	0.1	0.1
1897-------	1935	4.4	3.6	2.5	1.5	1.0	0.7	0.4	0.5	0.2	0.1	0.1	0.1
1898-------	1936	4.4	3.6	2.4	1.6	1.0	0.7	0.6	0.4	0.3	0.2	0.1	0.1
1899-------	1937	4.5	3.9	2.3	1.6	1.0	0.7	0.6	0.4	0.3	0.2	0.1	0.0
1900-------	1938	4.9	3.8	2.3	1.6	0.9	0.8	0.6	0.4	0.3	0.1	0.1	0.1
1901-------	1939	4.5	3.5	2.3	1.3	1.0	0.8	0.5	0.4	0.2	0.1	0.1	0.0
1902-------	1940	4.2	3.5	2.2	1.5	1.0	0.7	0.5	0.3	0.2	0.1	0.1	0.0
1903-------	1941	4.2	3.5	2.3	1.5	1.1	0.8	0.5	0.3	0.2	0.1	0.1	0.0
1904-------	1942	4.2	3.6	2.4	1.8	1.1	0.8	0.4	0.3	0.2	0.1	0.0	0.1
1905-------	1943	4.4	3.7	2.6	1.7	1.1	0.6	0.5	0.3	0.2	0.0	0.1	0.1
1906-------	1944	4.5	3.7	2.5	1.6	0.9	0.7	0.5	0.3	0.1	0.1	0.1	0.0
1907-------	1945	4.5	3.4	2.5	1.5	1.1	0.8	0.4	0.2	0.2	0.1	0.1	0.0
1908-------	1946	4.1	3.5	2.3	1.6	1.1	0.6	0.5	0.2	0.1	0.1	0.0	0.1
1909-------	1947	4.4	3.5	2.5	1.8	1.1	0.9	0.5	0.3	0.2	0.1	0.1	0.1
1910-------	1948	4.5	3.7	2.7	1.9	1.3	0.9	0.5	0.3	0.2	0.1	0.1	0.0
1911-------	1949	4.8	4.0	2.8	2.0	1.4	0.9	0.6	0.3	0.1	0.1	0.1	0.0
1912-------	1950	4.9	4.0	2.8	2.2	1.3	1.0	0.7	0.3	0.2	0.1	0.0	0.1
1913-------	1951	5.0	3.9	3.1	2.2	1.5	1.1	0.5	0.3	0.2	0.1	0.1	0.0
1914-------	1952	5.1	4.3	3.2	2.2	1.6	1.1	0.6	0.4	0.1	0.1	0.1	0.0
1915-------	1953	5.2	4.6	3.4	2.4	1.7	1.0	0.6	0.3	0.2	0.1	0.0	0.0
1916-------	1954	5.6	4.8	3.5	2.3	1.5	1.0	0.7	0.3	0.2	0.1	0.0	0.0
1917-------	1955	6.1	4.9	3.3	2.2	1.4	1.1	0.6	0.3	0.2	0.1	0.0	0.0
1918-------	1956	6.2	4.7	3.0	2.2	1.6	1.0	0.6	0.3	0.2	0.1	0.0	0.0
1919-------	1957	6.4	4.7	3.5	2.4	1.7	1.0	0.5	0.4	0.2	0.0	0.0	0.0
1920-------	1958	6.2	5.4	3.6	2.7	1.6	1.0	0.8	0.4	0.1	0.0	0.0	0.0
1921-------	1959	6.8	5.1	3.9	2.3	1.5	1.1	0.6	0.3	0.1	0.1	0.0	0.0
1922-------	1960	6.4	5.2	3.3	2.4	1.6	1.1	0.6	0.3	0.1	0.0	0.0	0.0
1923-------	1961	6.2	4.6	3.3	2.2	1.6	1.0	0.5	0.2	0.1	0.1	0.0	0.0
1924-------	1962	5.9	4.7	3.2	2.4	1.5	0.9	0.5	0.2	0.2	0.0	0.0	0.0
1925-------	1963	5.8	4.4	3.1	2.2	1.3	0.8	0.5	0.3	0.1	0.0	0.0	
1926-------	1964	5.5	4.2	3.0	2.1	1.2	0.8	0.5	0.2	0.1	0.0		
1927-------	1965	5.2	4.1	2.9	1.8	1.2	0.7	0.4	0.2	0.1			
1928-------	1966	4.7	3.7	2.4	1.7	1.1	0.7	0.3	0.1				
1929-------	1967	4.4	3.4	2.3	1.6	1.0	0.5	0.3					
1930-------	1968	4.3	2.9	2.3	1.5	0.9	0.6						
1931-------	1969	3.4	3.0	2.1	1.3	0.8							
1932-------	1970	3.6	2.7	1.8	1.2								
1933-------	1971	3.4	2.3	1.5									
1934-------	1972	3.1	2.0										
1935-------	1973	2.5											

TABLE 4C. CENTRAL BIRTH RATES FOR ALL OTHER WOMEN DURING EACH YEAR 1917-73 BY AGE AND LIVE-BIRTH ORDER FOR EACH COHORT FROM 1868 TO 1959--CON.

LIVE-BIRTH ORDER AND COHORT	DIAGONAL LINE FOR CALENDAR YEAR	CURRENT AGE											
		14	15	16	17	18	19	20	21	22	23	24	25
SEVENTH BIRTHS													
1892-------													5.1
1893-------												3.5	4.4
1894-------											2.0	2.9	5.1
1895-------										1.0	1.6	3.4	4.6
1896-------									0.4	0.8	1.9	2.9	5.7
1897-------								0.2	0.3	1.0	1.5	3.4	5.1
1898-------							*	0.1	0.4	0.8	1.6	3.4	5.4
1899-------						*	*	0.2	0.3	0.8	1.8	3.6	5.8
1900-------					*	*	*	0.1	0.4	0.9	2.1	3.8	6.3
1901-------				*	*	*	*	0.1	0.4	1.0	2.1	4.0	5.8
1902-------			*	*	*	*	*	0.1	0.4	1.1	2.3	3.9	5.3
1903-------	1917	*	*	*	*	*	*	0.2	0.5	1.1	2.2	3.4	4.9
1904-------	1918	*	*	*	*	*	*	0.2	0.6	1.2	2.1	3.4	4.4
1905-------	1919	*	*	*	*	*	*	0.3	0.5	1.1	2.0	2.9	4.4
1906-------	1920	*	*	*	*	*	*	0.3	0.6	1.2	1.6	3.0	4.2
1907-------	1921	*	*	*	*	*	*	0.3	0.6	0.9	1.7	2.7	3.9
1908-------	1922	*	*	*	*	*	*	0.3	0.5	0.9	1.5	2.5	3.5
1909-------	1923	*	*	*	*	*	*	0.3	0.4	0.8	1.4	2.3	3.7
1910-------	1924	*	*	*	*	*	*	0.2	0.4	0.7	1.4	2.5	3.9
1911-------	1925	*	*	*	*	*	*	0.2	0.3	0.7	1.4	2.6	4.0
1912-------	1926	*	*	*	*	*	*	0.1	0.3	0.8	1.5	2.5	4.1
1913-------	1927	*	*	*	*	*	*	0.1	0.4	0.8	1.5	2.7	3.9
1914-------	1928	*	*	*	*	*	*	0.2	0.4	0.8	1.7	2.7	4.0
1915-------	1929	*	*	*	*	*	*	0.2	0.4	0.9	1.7	2.7	4.4
1916-------	1930	*	*	*	*	*	*	0.2	0.5	0.9	1.7	3.2	4.4
1917-------	1931	*	*	*	*	*	*	0.2	0.5	0.9	2.2	3.1	4.9
1918-------	1932	*	*	*	*	*	*	0.2	0.5	1.2	2.1	3.3	5.3
1919-------	1933	*	*	*	*	*	*	0.2	0.6	1.1	2.0	3.7	5.2
1920-------	1934	*	*	*	*	*	*	0.2	0.6	1.0	2.4	3.5	5.5
1921-------	1935	*	*	*	*	*	*	0.2	0.5	1.2	2.2	3.7	5.4
1922-------	1936	*	*	*	*	*	*	0.2	0.6	1.1	2.2	3.6	5.5
1923-------	1937	*	*	*	*	*	*	0.2	0.6	1.2	2.3	3.7	5.7
1924-------	1938	*	*	*	*	*	*	0.2	0.7	1.2	2.4	4.0	5.7
1925-------	1939	*	*	*	*	*	*	0.3	0.6	1.2	2.5	4.0	6.0
1926-------	1940	*	*	*	*	*	*	0.3	0.7	1.4	2.5	4.3	6.2
1927-------	1941	*	*	*	*	*	*	0.3	0.8	1.4	2.6	4.0	7.1
1928-------	1942	*	*	*	*	*	*	0.3	0.7	1.4	2.6	4.8	7.6
1929-------	1943	*	*	*	*	*	*	0.3	0.8	1.4	3.0	5.5	8.7
1930-------	1944	*	*	*	*	*	*	0.4	0.8	1.6	3.4	6.3	9.7
1931-------	1945	*	*	*	*	*	*	0.4	0.9	1.9	4.2	7.0	11.1
1932-------	1946	*	*	*	*	*	*	0.4	0.8	2.2	4.4	8.0	11.4
1933-------	1947	*	*	*	*	*	*	0.3	1.1	2.4	5.0	8.0	11.4
1934-------	1948	*	*	*	*	*	*	0.5	1.1	2.7	4.9	8.2	12.5
1935-------	1949	*	*	*	*	*	*	0.5	1.1	2.6	4.9	9.0	12.8
1936-------	1950	*	*	*	*	*	*	0.4	1.2	2.6	5.6	9.2	12.9
1937-------	1951	*	*	*	*	*	*	0.4	1.1	2.9	5.6	9.4	12.7
1938-------	1952	*	*	*	*	*	*	0.4	1.3	3.0	5.7	8.8	12.3
1939-------	1953	*	*	*	*	*	*	0.5	1.4	3.0	5.5	8.7	11.6
1940-------	1954	*	*	*	*	*	*	0.6	1.3	2.8	5.3	8.0	9.8
1941-------	1955	*	*	*	*	*	*	0.5	1.3	2.8	5.0	7.0	7.8
1942-------	1956	*	*	*	*	*	*	0.4	1.3	2.5	4.2	5.4	6.3
1943-------	1957	*	*	*	*	*	*	0.5	1.1	2.1	3.1	4.4	4.7
1944-------	1958	*	*	*	*	*	*	0.4	1.0	1.6	2.8	3.3	3.9
1945-------	1959	*	*	*	*	*	*	0.3	0.6	1.5	2.0	2.7	3.6
1946-------	1960	*	*	*	*	*	*	0.2	0.6	1.1	1.6	2.3	2.5
1947-------	1961	*	*	*	*	*	*	0.3	0.6	0.8	1.4	1.7	1.9
1948-------	1962	*	*	*	*	*	*	0.2	0.5	0.7	1.0	1.1	1.4
1949-------	1963	*	*	*	*	*	*	0.2	0.4	0.5	0.6	0.9	
1950-------	1964	*	*	*	*	*	*	0.2	0.3	0.3	0.5		
1951-------	1965	*	*	*	*	*	*	0.1	0.2	0.3			
1952-------	1966	*	*	*	*	*	*	0.1	0.1				
1953-------	1967	*	*	*	*	*	*	0.1					
1954-------	1968	*	*	*	*	*	*						
1955-------	1969	*	*	*	*	*							
1956-------	1970	*	*	*	*								
1957-------	1971	*	*	*									
1958-------	1972	*	*										
1959-------	1973	*											

TABLE 4C. CENTRAL BIRTH RATES FOR ALL OTHER WOMEN DURING EACH YEAR 1917-73 BY AGE AND LIVE-BIRTH ORDER FOR EACH COHORT FROM 1868 TO 1959--CON.

LIVE-BIRTH ORDER AND COHORT	DIAGONAL LINE FOR CALENDAR YEAR	CURRENT AGE											
		26	27	28	29	30	31	32	33	34	35	36	37
SEVENTH BIRTHS--CON.													
1880-------													12.7
1881-------												14.7	12.1
1882-------											15.1	13.8	13.0
1883-------										14.9	14.1	14.4	11.7
1884-------									13.8	13.8	14.2	12.8	10.6
1885-------								13.1	12.8	13.4	12.5	11.4	10.7
1886-------							14.5	12.2	12.0	11.9	11.7	11.5	10.1
1887-------						12.8	13.6	11.5	10.9	11.9	11.6	11.0	10.1
1888-------					13.1	11.9	13.1	10.6	11.8	11.7	11.4	11.1	10.2
1889-------				10.1	12.0	12.0	12.1	11.5	11.4	11.7	11.5	11.4	9.9
1890-------			9.1	9.0	12.8	11.3	13.3	11.2	11.7	11.9	12.0	11.0	9.0
1891-------	1917	7.0	8.1	10.4	12.0	13.0	12.9	11.5	11.9	12.3	12.0	10.4	7.9
1892-------	1918	6.2	9.3	9.8	14.4	12.2	13.3	11.8	12.3	12.3	10.8	8.9	7.4
1893-------	1919	7.1	8.8	12.5	13.1	12.4	13.5	11.9	12.4	11.4	9.6	8.4	7.1
1894-------	1920	6.7	11.1	10.8	13.3	12.9	13.3	12.1	11.8	9.7	9.1	8.1	7.2
1895-------	1921	8.5	9.6	11.0	14.1	12.9	13.7	12.0	10.0	9.6	9.0	8.0	7.4
1896-------	1922	7.4	9.8	12.0	13.9	13.5	13.1	9.8	9.6	9.5	8.9	8.4	6.7
1897-------	1923	7.5	10.7	11.5	13.8	12.7	11.6	9.3	9.8	9.5	8.9	7.5	6.8
1898-------	1924	8.3	10.3	11.4	13.8	11.6	10.9	9.9	10.2	9.6	8.8	7.7	6.7
1899-------	1925	8.1	10.0	11.9	12.8	11.0	11.6	10.6	10.6	10.0	9.1	7.8	6.6
1900-------	1926	8.1	10.3	10.7	12.1	11.4	12.1	10.7	10.9	9.9	8.7	7.4	6.5
1901-------	1927	7.5	9.1	9.6	11.7	11.4	11.4	10.3	10.3	8.8	8.1	7.3	6.5
1902-------	1928	6.7	8.2	9.8	11.5	10.7	10.6	9.5	8.8	8.0	7.7	6.8	6.1
1903-------	1929	6.1	8.2	9.3	11.2	10.0	10.5	8.3	8.1	8.1	7.2	6.4	5.6
1904-------	1930	6.3	8.0	9.3	10.8	10.3	9.6	8.2	8.4	7.9	6.9	6.0	5.9
1905-------	1931	6.0	7.8	9.0	10.9	9.5	9.0	8.2	8.8	7.6	6.7	6.2	5.4
1906-------	1932	5.6	7.4	8.8	9.9	9.0	9.2	8.7	8.3	7.5	6.8	5.8	5.6
1907-------	1933	5.1	7.1	8.2	9.3	9.4	9.5	8.3	8.6	7.7	6.8	6.0	5.8
1908-------	1934	5.2	6.9	7.8	9.7	9.4	9.0	8.6	8.6	7.5	7.1	6.3	5.4
1909-------	1935	5.3	6.9	8.6	10.2	9.2	9.4	8.7	8.6	7.7	7.4	6.3	5.7
1910-------	1936	5.2	7.3	8.7	10.1	9.6	9.4	8.6	8.8	8.0	7.4	6.6	5.7
1911-------	1937	5.7	7.4	9.0	10.5	9.7	9.7	8.8	9.1	8.4	7.5	6.6	5.7
1912-------	1938	5.4	7.4	9.4	10.6	9.8	10.0	9.2	9.2	8.1	7.3	6.4	5.8
1913-------	1939	5.5	7.8	9.6	10.1	10.2	10.4	9.5	9.0	8.1	7.4	6.5	6.1
1914-------	1940	5.8	8.0	8.9	10.5	10.5	10.4	9.4	9.2	8.3	7.5	6.8	6.0
1915-------	1941	5.9	7.8	9.3	10.9	10.3	10.3	9.5	9.2	8.3	7.6	6.9	6.0
1916-------	1942	6.4	8.2	9.6	10.9	10.4	10.5	9.6	9.2	8.4	7.8	6.8	6.5
1917-------	1943	6.7	8.4	9.7	10.8	10.6	10.5	9.5	9.4	8.7	7.9	7.3	6.7
1918-------	1944	6.9	8.9	9.9	11.1	10.7	10.7	9.9	10.1	9.0	8.2	7.4	7.2
1919-------	1945	7.2	8.9	10.1	11.5	11.4	11.2	11.1	10.5	9.4	8.7	8.0	7.8
1920-------	1946	7.1	9.1	10.5	12.0	11.6	12.0	10.8	10.7	10.1	8.9	8.9	7.8
1921-------	1947	7.1	9.4	10.9	12.1	12.4	11.9	11.2	11.4	10.0	10.2	8.8	7.5
1922-------	1948	7.4	9.4	10.9	12.5	12.0	12.4	12.2	11.2	11.0	10.1	8.2	7.6
1923-------	1949	7.5	9.6	11.6	13.0	12.8	13.2	12.1	12.2	11.3	9.6	8.6	7.4
1924-------	1950	7.9	10.3	12.2	14.0	14.1	13.8	13.2	13.1	11.1	10.5	8.6	7.5
1925-------	1951	8.1	11.3	13.5	15.1	14.8	15.3	14.2	13.0	12.1	10.0	8.7	7.1
1926-------	1952	9.2	12.4	14.9	16.0	16.5	16.2	14.3	14.2	11.7	10.4	8.0	6.8
1927-------	1953	10.3	13.6	15.3	18.0	17.5	16.6	15.2	13.5	12.0	9.6	8.0	6.7
1928-------	1954	11.1	14.2	16.9	18.1	17.8	17.0	14.6	13.6	10.7	9.0	7.6	6.0
1929-------	1955	12.1	15.9	17.3	19.1	18.1	16.9	15.0	12.7	10.4	9.2	6.9	5.5
1930-------	1956	13.5	15.9	18.4	19.2	18.0	16.2	14.0	12.0	10.8	8.1	6.4	5.1
1931-------	1957	14.3	17.2	18.8	19.3	17.7	15.9	13.6	12.3	9.3	7.3	5.7	4.4
1932-------	1958	14.6	17.5	18.4	18.7	17.0	15.3	13.2	10.9	8.3	6.4	5.0	4.2
1933-------	1959	15.3	17.5	18.9	18.1	16.3	14.9	11.9	9.2	7.4	5.8	4.9	4.0
1934-------	1960	15.7	17.8	18.3	18.2	15.8	13.7	9.9	8.6	6.6	5.8	4.7	4.1
1935-------	1961	15.9	17.9	18.5	17.1	14.5	11.0	9.5	7.4	6.3	5.3	4.7	3.3
1936-------	1962	15.9	18.0	16.9	15.6	11.8	10.1	7.8	6.9	5.9	5.3	3.7	2.7
1937-------	1963	15.5	16.6	15.3	12.8	10.5	8.4	7.3	6.5	5.6	4.1	3.2	
1938-------	1964	14.4	14.2	12.4	10.5	8.4	7.8	6.7	6.0	4.2	3.6		
1939-------	1965	12.3	11.7	10.5	8.7	7.5	7.1	6.3	4.7	3.9			
1940-------	1966	10.1	9.6	8.4	7.4	6.8	6.6	4.7	4.0				
1941-------	1967	8.2	7.6	6.6	6.8	6.3	4.8	4.0					
1942-------	1968	6.3	6.0	6.1	6.0	4.6	3.9						
1943-------	1969	5.0	5.7	5.4	4.4	3.7							
1944-------	1970	4.6	4.5	3.8	3.3								
1945-------	1971	3.6	3.3	2.9									
1946-------	1972	2.6	2.4										
1947-------	1973	2.0											

TABLE 4C. CENTRAL BIRTH RATES FOR ALL OTHER WOMEN DURING EACH YEAR 1917-73 BY AGE AND LIVE-BIRTH ORDER FOR EACH COHORT FROM 1868 TO 1959--CON.

LIVE-BIRTH ORDER AND COHORT	DIAGONAL LINE FOR CALENDAR YEAR	CURRENT AGE											
		38	39	40	41	42	43	44	45	46	47	48	49
SEVENTH BIRTHS--CON.													
1868-------													0.5
1869-------												0.6	0.9
1870-------											0.9	0.9	0.5
1871-------										1.4	1.5	0.6	0.5
1872-------									1.7	2.4	0.9	0.6	0.3
1873-------								1.7	2.7	1.4	0.9	0.3	0.4
1874-------							1.5	2.4	1.7	1.4	0.5	0.4	0.4
1875-------						2.0	1.8	1.7	1.7	0.8	0.7	0.5	0.3
1876-------				*	3.5	2.3	1.6	1.7	1.1	1.1	0.8	0.4	0.1
1877-------				5.3	4.1	2.2	1.5	1.4	1.3	1.2	0.6	0.2	0.3
1878-------			8.7	5.7	3.9	2.0	1.8	1.5	1.5	1.1	0.4	0.5	0.1
1879-------	1917	10.5	8.8	5.8	3.6	2.4	1.6	1.6	1.3	1.1	0.7	0.3	0.1
1880-------	1918	10.0	9.3	5.4	4.5	2.2	1.6	1.5	1.3	1.1	0.3	0.3	0.3
1881-------	1919	10.9	8.6	6.0	4.0	2.2	1.6	1.7	1.3	0.8	0.5	0.4	0.2
1882-------	1920	10.0	8.7	5.7	4.0	2.2	1.8	1.3	1.0	1.0	0.5	0.2	0.2
1883-------	1921	9.2	8.6	5.5	3.9	2.1	1.7	1.3	1.1	0.7	0.5	0.3	0.2
1884-------	1922	9.4	8.2	5.4	3.1	2.0	1.5	1.2	0.8	0.7	0.3	0.3	0.1
1885-------	1923	8.9	8.0	4.4	3.4	1.8	1.4	0.9	0.9	0.7	0.3	0.3	0.2
1886-------	1924	8.8	7.0	4.7	3.1	1.5	1.1	1.1	0.9	0.7	0.3	0.3	0.1
1887-------	1925	8.6	7.1	4.1	2.4	1.5	1.4	1.1	0.8	0.7	0.3	0.2	0.2
1888-------	1926	8.1	6.3	3.1	2.4	1.7	1.2	1.0	0.8	0.5	0.3	0.3	0.1
1889-------	1927	7.3	5.2	3.5	2.8	1.6	1.1	0.9	0.6	0.5	0.3	0.2	0.2
1890-------	1928	6.4	5.3	3.9	2.5	1.5	1.2	0.8	0.6	0.5	0.3	0.3	0.2
1891-------	1929	6.3	5.7	3.5	2.5	1.6	1.1	0.8	0.6	0.5	0.3	0.3	0.1
1892-------	1930	6.4	5.3	3.6	2.4	1.4	1.1	0.7	0.6	0.5	0.3	0.2	0.1
1893-------	1931	6.1	5.4	3.3	2.3	1.3	1.0	0.7	0.5	0.4	0.2	0.2	0.1
1894-------	1932	6.3	5.0	3.4	2.2	1.3	1.0	0.7	0.4	0.4	0.2	0.1	0.1
1895-------	1933	5.7	5.2	3.0	2.2	1.3	0.9	0.6	0.5	0.3	0.2	0.1	0.1
1896-------	1934	6.0	4.6	2.9	2.0	1.2	0.7	0.7	0.3	0.3	0.2	0.1	0.1
1897-------	1935	5.5	4.4	2.6	1.8	1.0	0.9	0.5	0.4	0.3	0.2	0.1	0.1
1898-------	1936	5.1	4.0	2.8	1.6	1.2	0.8	0.6	0.4	0.3	0.2	0.1	0.1
1899-------	1937	5.3	4.5	2.6	1.8	1.2	0.8	0.6	0.4	0.3	0.2	0.1	0.1
1900-------	1938	5.7	4.3	2.7	1.8	1.1	0.9	0.6	0.4	0.3	0.1	0.1	0.1
1901-------	1939	5.3	4.0	2.6	1.7	1.1	0.8	0.6	0.3	0.2	0.1	0.1	0.0
1902-------	1940	4.9	4.0	2.5	1.9	1.1	0.9	0.5	0.3	0.2	0.1	0.1	0.0
1903-------	1941	5.0	3.7	2.6	1.8	1.3	0.8	0.5	0.3	0.2	0.1	0.1	0.0
1904-------	1942	4.5	3.9	2.6	1.9	1.3	0.9	0.5	0.3	0.2	0.1	0.1	0.0
1905-------	1943	4.6	4.0	2.7	2.0	1.2	0.8	0.5	0.3	0.2	0.1	0.0	0.1
1906-------	1944	4.8	3.9	2.8	1.9	1.1	0.9	0.5	0.3	0.2	0.0	0.1	0.0
1907-------	1945	4.7	3.8	2.5	1.7	1.1	0.9	0.5	0.4	0.1	0.1	0.1	0.0
1908-------	1946	4.5	3.6	2.5	1.8	1.2	0.8	0.5	0.3	0.1	0.1	0.0	0.0
1909-------	1947	4.7	3.8	2.7	1.9	1.3	0.8	0.6	0.3	0.2	0.0	0.1	0.0
1910-------	1948	4.7	4.1	2.8	2.1	1.3	1.0	0.5	0.4	0.1	0.1	0.0	0.1
1911-------	1949	5.0	4.1	3.0	2.0	1.4	1.0	0.6	0.3	0.2	0.1	0.1	0.0
1912-------	1950	5.0	4.1	2.7	2.2	1.5	1.0	0.6	0.3	0.1	0.1	0.1	0.0
1913-------	1951	5.0	3.9	3.0	2.2	1.4	1.1	0.5	0.3	0.2	0.1	0.0	0.0
1914-------	1952	4.9	4.4	3.1	2.1	1.6	1.0	0.5	0.4	0.2	0.1	0.0	0.0
1915-------	1953	5.4	4.4	3.1	2.5	1.4	1.0	0.6	0.4	0.2	0.1	0.0	0.0
1916-------	1954	5.6	4.7	3.4	2.4	1.4	1.1	0.7	0.3	0.2	0.1	0.0	0.0
1917-------	1955	6.1	5.1	3.4	2.5	1.7	1.1	0.7	0.3	0.3	0.0	0.0	0.0
1918-------	1956	6.2	5.0	3.5	2.5	1.7	1.1	0.7	0.4	0.1	0.1	0.1	0.0
1919-------	1957	6.2	5.2	3.6	2.6	1.7	1.2	0.5	0.3	0.1	0.1	0.0	0.0
1920-------	1958	6.4	5.2	3.7	2.6	1.7	1.0	0.6	0.3	0.1	0.0	0.0	0.0
1921-------	1959	6.4	4.9	3.5	2.4	1.7	1.1	0.6	0.2	0.1	0.1	0.0	0.0
1922-------	1960	6.2	4.9	3.3	2.5	1.6	1.0	0.5	0.2	0.2	0.1	0.0	0.0
1923-------	1961	6.0	4.7	3.4	2.4	1.5	0.8	0.5	0.3	0.1	0.1	0.1	0.0
1924-------	1962	5.8	4.4	3.3	2.2	1.4	0.9	0.6	0.3	0.1	0.0	0.0	0.0
1925-------	1963	5.6	4.5	3.2	2.1	1.4	0.9	0.5	0.3	0.1	0.0	0.0	
1926-------	1964	5.7	4.3	2.8	2.0	1.3	0.8	0.4	0.2	0.1	0.0		
1927-------	1965	5.3	3.7	2.8	1.9	1.1	0.7	0.4	0.3	0.1			
1928-------	1966	4.5	3.6	2.6	1.6	1.0	0.6	0.4	0.1				
1929-------	1967	4.5	3.4	2.3	1.5	1.0	0.7	0.3					
1930-------	1968	4.0	3.0	2.1	1.5	0.9	0.4						
1931-------	1969	3.6	2.8	2.0	1.3	0.7							
1932-------	1970	3.5	2.7	1.6	1.0								
1933-------	1971	3.4	2.1	1.5									
1934-------	1972	2.6	1.9										
1935-------	1973	2.4											

TABLE 4C. CENTRAL BIRTH RATES FOR ALL OTHER WOMEN DURING EACH YEAR 1917-73 BY AGE AND LIVE-BIRTH ORDER FOR EACH COHORT FROM 1868 TO 1959--CON.

LIVE-BIRTH ORDER AND COHORT	DIAGONAL LINE FOR CALENDAR YEAR	CURRENT AGE											
		14	15	16	17	18	19	20	21	22	23	24	25
EIGHTH AND HIGHER BIRTHS													
1892-------													3.5
1893-------												2.2	3.2
1894-------											1.1	2.3	3.4
1895-------										0.5	1.3	2.2	3.2
1896-------									0.2	0.6	1.1	2.0	4.1
1897-------								0.1	0.2	0.5	0.9	2.6	3.6
1898-------							*	0.1	0.2	0.4	1.2	2.4	3.9
1899-------						*	*	0.1	0.1	0.6	1.2	2.5	4.0
1900-------					*	*	*	0.0	0.2	0.6	1.2	2.6	4.8
1901-------				*	*	*	*	0.1	0.2	0.5	1.2	2.8	4.6
1902-------			*	*	*	*	*	0.1	0.2	0.6	1.5	3.0	4.5
1903-------	1917	*	*	*	*	*	*	0.1	0.2	0.6	1.8	2.8	3.9
1904-------	1918	*	*	*	*	*	*	0.1	0.2	0.9	1.6	2.7	3.3
1905-------	1919	*	*	*	*	*	*	0.1	0.3	0.7	1.6	2.1	3.1
1906-------	1920	*	*	*	*	*	*	0.1	0.3	0.8	1.2	2.2	2.9
1907-------	1921	*	*	*	*	*	*	0.1	0.3	0.6	1.3	1.8	2.7
1908-------	1922	*	*	*	*	*	*	0.1	0.2	0.6	1.0	1.7	2.5
1909-------	1923	*	*	*	*	*	*	0.1	0.2	0.5	1.0	1.5	2.6
1910-------	1924	*	*	*	*	*	*	0.0	0.2	0.5	0.8	1.6	2.6
1911-------	1925	*	*	*	*	*	*	0.1	0.2	0.5	0.9	1.8	2.6
1912-------	1926	*	*	*	*	*	*	0.1	0.2	0.5	0.9	1.7	2.5
1913-------	1927	*	*	*	*	*	*	0.1	0.2	0.5	0.9	1.7	2.5
1914-------	1928	*	*	*	*	*	*	0.1	0.2	0.5	0.9	1.6	2.6
1915-------	1929	*	*	*	*	*	*	0.1	0.2	0.5	0.9	1.7	3.0
1916-------	1930	*	*	*	*	*	*	0.1	0.2	0.5	1.0	2.0	3.0
1917-------	1931	*	*	*	*	*	*	0.1	0.2	0.5	1.2	2.1	3.2
1918-------	1932	*	*	*	*	*	*	0.1	0.2	0.6	1.2	2.0	3.4
1919-------	1933	*	*	*	*	*	*	0.1	0.3	0.7	1.2	2.1	3.3
1920-------	1934	*	*	*	*	*	*	0.1	0.3	0.5	1.3	2.0	3.3
1921-------	1935	*	*	*	*	*	*	0.1	0.2	0.6	1.2	2.0	3.5
1922-------	1936	*	*	*	*	*	*	0.0	0.2	0.5	1.2	2.2	3.7
1923-------	1937	*	*	*	*	*	*	0.0	0.2	0.6	1.2	2.2	3.6
1924-------	1938	*	*	*	*	*	*	0.0	0.2	0.6	1.3	2.4	3.9
1925-------	1939	*	*	*	*	*	*	0.0	0.3	0.7	1.3	2.4	3.8
1926-------	1940	*	*	*	*	*	*	0.2	0.4	0.8	1.3	2.3	3.7
1927-------	1941	*	*	*	*	*	*	0.2	0.4	0.6	1.4	2.1	3.9
1928-------	1942	*	*	*	*	*	*	0.2	0.4	0.7	1.2	2.4	4.6
1929-------	1943	*	*	*	*	*	*	0.2	0.4	0.7	1.3	2.7	5.0
1930-------	1944	*	*	*	*	*	*	0.2	0.4	0.7	1.5	3.0	5.7
1931-------	1945	*	*	*	*	*	*	0.2	0.4	0.7	1.8	3.5	6.3
1932-------	1946	*	*	*	*	*	*	0.2	0.4	0.8	1.9	3.7	6.9
1933-------	1947	*	*	*	*	*	*	0.2	0.4	1.0	2.1	4.2	7.7
1934-------	1948	*	*	*	*	*	*	0.2	0.5	0.9	2.4	4.5	7.9
1935-------	1949	*	*	*	*	*	*	0.2	0.4	1.2	2.3	4.7	7.9
1936-------	1950	*	*	*	*	*	*	0.2	0.5	1.1	2.5	4.6	8.3
1937-------	1951	*	*	*	*	*	*	0.2	0.4	1.2	2.4	4.7	8.5
1938-------	1952	*	*	*	*	*	*	0.2	0.5	1.1	2.4	4.8	8.4
1939-------	1953	*	*	*	*	*	*	0.2	0.6	1.1	2.3	4.8	7.6
1940-------	1954	*	*	*	*	*	*	0.3	0.5	0.9	2.3	4.5	5.8
1941-------	1955	*	*	*	*	*	*	0.2	0.4	1.0	2.5	3.4	4.8
1942-------	1956	*	*	*	*	*	*	0.2	0.4	1.1	1.6	2.6	3.7
1943-------	1957	*	*	*	*	*	*	0.2	0.5	0.7	1.3	2.0	3.0
1944-------	1958	*	*	*	*	*	*	0.2	0.4	0.6	1.0	1.7	2.3
1945-------	1959	*	*	*	*	*	*	0.1	0.3	0.5	0.8	1.4	2.1
1946-------	1960	*	*	*	*	*	*	0.1	0.3	0.3	0.7	1.1	1.5
1947-------	1961	*	*	*	*	*	*	0.1	0.1	0.4	0.6	0.8	1.0
1948-------	1962	*	*	*	*	*	*	0.1	0.3	0.3	0.5	0.6	0.6
1949-------	1963	*	*	*	*	*	*	0.2	0.2	0.2	0.3	0.4	
1950-------	1964	*	*	*	*	*	*	0.1	0.2	0.2	0.2		
1951-------	1965	*	*	*	*	*	*	0.1	0.1	0.1			
1952-------	1966	*	*	*	*	*	*	0.1	0.1				
1953-------	1967	*	*	*	*	*	*	0.1					
1954-------	1968	*	*	*	*	*	*						
1955-------	1969	*	*	*	*	*							
1956-------	1970	*	*	*	*								
1957-------	1971	*	*	*									
1958-------	1972	*	*										
1959-------	1973	*											

TABLE 4C. CENTRAL BIRTH RATES FOR ALL OTHER WOMEN DURING EACH YEAR 1917-73 BY AGE AND LIVE-BIRTH ORDER FOR EACH COHORT FROM 1868 TO 1959--CON.

LIVE-BIRTH ORDER AND COHORT	DIAGONAL LINE FOR CALENDAR YEAR	CURRENT AGE											
		26	27	28	29	30	31	32	33	34	35	36	37
EIGHTH AND HIGHER BIRTHS--CON.													
1880-------													49.5
1881-------												49.2	47.8
1882-------											46.5	47.0	53.4
1883-------										39.8	43.3	51.3	54.1
1884-------									29.4	36.0	46.0	50.7	51.2
1885-------								23.1	25.7	37.4	44.6	47.3	46.0
1886-------							21.9	20.2	26.0	35.9	42.9	42.5	43.5
1887-------						17.3	19.3	20.5	24.7	36.0	39.0	40.6	43.0
1888-------					15.8	15.2	19.9	19.7	26.9	33.3	37.8	40.7	44.6
1889-------				9.9	13.9	16.2	19.4	21.8	25.6	32.9	38.8	44.3	43.2
1890-------			7.5	8.6	15.2	15.9	21.6	20.8	25.7	34.5	41.5	41.5	42.4
1891-------	1917	5.2	6.5	9.8	14.8	18.3	20.7	20.9	27.7	37.4	39.5	40.9	37.5
1892-------	1918	4.5	7.4	9.5	17.5	17.1	20.8	22.5	30.6	35.8	38.1	35.7	34.3
1893-------	1919	5.2	7.2	11.9	16.1	17.5	22.2	25.8	29.4	34.0	33.4	33.3	34.7
1894-------	1920	5.0	9.0	10.5	16.7	18.4	24.5	24.4	28.6	30.1	31.5	33.3	33.2
1895-------	1921	6.2	7.9	11.3	17.4	19.9	23.7	23.4	25.4	28.3	31.7	31.1	33.9
1896-------	1922	5.5	8.4	11.5	19.0	20.2	22.4	21.7	24.0	28.7	29.5	31.2	31.5
1897-------	1923	5.8	8.6	13.0	19.2	18.7	21.4	20.2	24.1	27.0	29.4	29.2	32.4
1898-------	1924	6.1	10.3	13.4	18.0	18.1	20.2	20.6	24.0	27.3	28.3	30.7	29.8
1899-------	1925	6.8	10.3	12.5	17.5	17.2	20.8	21.4	25.1	27.5	31.3	29.5	29.5
1900-------	1926	6.9	9.7	12.1	16.6	17.5	21.0	21.6	24.9	29.4	29.2	28.9	31.3
1901-------	1927	6.4	9.1	11.1	15.8	17.2	19.8	20.0	25.5	25.7	27.0	28.7	29.6
1902-------	1928	5.9	7.9	10.2	14.9	15.4	17.3	19.7	21.5	23.5	26.0	26.6	28.2
1903-------	1929	4.9	7.1	9.6	13.7	13.6	17.8	17.1	20.2	22.9	24.5	25.1	27.1
1904-------	1930	4.6	6.9	9.3	12.7	14.6	16.6	17.2	20.7	22.0	24.0	24.9	26.8
1905-------	1931	4.4	6.4	8.5	13.5	13.7	16.2	17.0	19.9	21.7	24.0	24.3	25.5
1906-------	1932	4.2	6.0	9.1	12.6	13.3	15.9	16.6	19.9	22.2	23.7	23.4	26.2
1907-------	1933	3.8	6.4	8.4	11.7	12.9	15.6	16.6	20.8	22.3	23.3	24.1	25.8
1908-------	1934	3.9	5.8	7.7	11.9	12.8	15.5	17.5	21.2	22.4	24.1	23.9	26.4
1909-------	1935	3.9	5.6	8.3	11.8	13.0	16.5	18.0	21.2	23.4	24.3	26.0	25.7
1910-------	1936	3.8	6.1	8.2	12.0	13.9	16.8	18.2	22.3	23.9	26.5	25.5	26.0
1911-------	1937	4.0	6.0	8.7	13.0	14.2	16.7	19.1	23.0	25.3	25.7	25.7	26.4
1912-------	1938	3.9	6.2	9.5	13.2	14.1	17.6	19.7	23.0	24.0	25.6	25.0	26.1
1913-------	1939	4.1	6.9	9.7	12.6	14.8	18.1	19.8	22.5	23.9	25.3	25.2	26.0
1914-------	1940	4.6	7.0	9.3	13.3	15.3	18.1	19.6	22.7	24.0	25.0	25.6	27.4
1915-------	1941	4.6	7.0	9.8	13.7	15.6	18.3	19.8	23.0	23.9	25.8	26.4	26.6
1916-------	1942	4.7	7.4	10.1	14.0	15.8	18.5	19.9	22.7	24.5	26.3	25.8	25.9
1917-------	1943	5.0	7.6	10.2	14.2	15.5	18.6	20.5	23.6	24.5	25.7	25.4	27.1
1918-------	1944	5.1	7.4	10.5	13.9	16.2	19.6	21.2	24.2	25.2	26.5	26.8	27.3
1919-------	1945	4.8	7.7	10.4	14.9	17.3	20.4	22.0	25.4	27.0	28.2	28.2	29.8
1920-------	1946	5.2	8.1	11.4	15.4	17.7	20.8	23.1	26.5	28.2	29.0	29.6	29.2
1921-------	1947	5.5	8.4	11.6	15.5	18.0	21.5	23.7	27.5	28.5	30.1	29.3	28.2
1922-------	1948	5.6	8.4	11.4	15.6	17.9	21.2	24.2	27.8	28.9	29.7	28.3	28.6
1923-------	1949	5.8	8.4	12.0	16.1	18.3	22.9	25.8	28.9	30.2	29.5	29.8	28.9
1924-------	1950	5.7	8.8	12.5	16.6	20.6	25.0	27.2	30.7	31.1	32.2	30.5	29.7
1925-------	1951	5.9	9.4	13.1	18.9	22.2	26.5	29.1	31.8	33.7	32.5	31.9	29.0
1926-------	1952	6.3	10.2	14.9	20.1	24.3	28.6	31.1	34.2	34.0	34.0	30.9	28.7
1927-------	1953	7.0	11.1	15.7	22.4	26.2	30.4	32.9	34.4	35.0	33.4	29.9	28.3
1928-------	1954	7.5	12.1	17.9	23.8	27.2	31.7	33.3	35.5	34.4	31.6	29.8	25.8
1929-------	1955	8.4	13.8	19.2	25.2	28.9	32.8	35.0	36.0	33.7	32.2	27.2	22.6
1930-------	1956	9.4	14.9	20.3	26.1	29.5	33.8	34.7	34.5	33.0	28.6	23.7	19.8
1931-------	1957	10.7	16.5	21.4	26.4	30.9	33.2	33.4	33.7	29.7	25.4	20.4	17.1
1932-------	1958	11.6	16.8	21.0	27.6	29.7	31.9	31.8	29.9	25.5	21.4	17.6	15.4
1933-------	1959	12.0	16.9	22.9	27.3	29.5	31.5	28.7	25.5	21.9	18.4	16.2	14.5
1934-------	1960	12.2	18.1	23.0	27.3	29.2	27.7	24.5	22.2	18.6	17.0	15.4	12.7
1935-------	1961	13.0	18.2	22.6	26.8	25.4	23.6	20.8	18.8	16.9	15.3	13.1	10.6
1936-------	1962	12.9	17.9	21.8	23.2	21.3	19.9	17.8	16.4	14.8	13.7	10.5	8.6
1937-------	1963	12.7	16.6	19.0	18.7	17.9	16.7	15.1	14.1	13.6	10.4	8.4	
1938-------	1964	11.6	14.1	14.8	15.3	14.0	13.4	13.1	12.6	9.7	7.6		
1939-------	1965	9.7	11.3	11.9	12.0	11.4	12.0	11.5	9.3	7.5			
1940-------	1966	7.7	8.6	9.3	9.8	9.8	10.0	8.2	7.2				
1941-------	1967	6.0	7.1	7.6	8.1	8.4	7.1	6.2					
1942-------	1968	4.8	5.5	6.1	6.7	5.7	5.5						
1943-------	1969	3.5	4.6	5.0	4.6	4.4							
1944-------	1970	3.2	3.6	3.4	3.6								
1945-------	1971	2.4	2.5	2.4									
1946-------	1972	1.6	1.6										
1947-------	1973	1.1											

TABLE 4C. CENTRAL BIRTH RATES FOR ALL OTHER WOMEN DURING EACH YEAR 1917-73 BY AGE AND LIVE-BIRTH ORDER FOR EACH COHORT FROM 1868 TO 1959--CON.

LIVE-BIRTH ORDER AND COHORT	DIAGONAL LINE FOR CALENDAR YEAR	CURRENT AGE											
		38	39	40	41	42	43	44	45	46	47	48	49
EIGHTH AND HIGHER BIRTHS--CON.													
1868-------													3.2
1869-------												5.5	5.8
1870-------											8.3	10.1	3.1
1871-------										12.4	15.3	5.3	3.6
1872-------									14.6	22.9	8.0	6.3	2.7
1873-------								17.0	23.5	12.0	9.6	4.7	2.4
1874-------							19.2	23.1	13.8	14.5	7.2	4.1	2.5
1875-------						21.7	20.6	15.7	15.8	11.0	6.4	4.4	2.2
1876-------					29.8	23.3	17.3	16.8	13.0	9.7	6.8	3.9	1.8
1877-------				34.5	32.4	19.8	17.2	15.4	11.5	10.5	6.1	3.2	1.7
1878-------			46.8	35.9	28.2	20.0	18.1	13.9	12.3	9.7	5.0	3.1	2.0
1879-------	1917	46.6	47.1	34.8	29.0	21.3	16.7	14.5	11.6	9.1	5.3	3.2	2.3
1880-------	1918	45.0	49.5	36.2	31.2	19.8	17.0	14.2	11.2	9.6	4.5	3.5	1.9
1881-------	1919	50.8	51.5	37.7	29.0	20.1	16.9	14.4	11.7	8.2	4.9	3.3	2.0
1882-------	1920	52.4	51.7	35.0	29.0	19.8	17.5	14.5	10.8	8.2	5.2	3.3	1.9
1883-------	1921	50.5	47.4	34.1	27.8	20.7	17.5	13.6	9.9	7.9	4.7	2.8	1.7
1884-------	1922	45.8	45.4	32.7	28.4	20.3	15.1	12.0	9.2	7.8	4.0	2.8	1.8
1885-------	1923	43.4	43.8	34.1	27.3	17.0	13.3	10.7	9.0	6.6	4.0	2.6	2.0
1886-------	1924	42.5	44.4	31.3	24.5	14.9	12.3	10.4	8.2	7.0	3.2	2.9	1.7
1887-------	1925	44.6	41.9	30.1	21.1	14.3	11.7	9.9	8.7	5.7	3.4	2.6	1.6
1888-------	1926	42.1	40.0	25.6	20.3	13.9	11.3	10.7	7.2	5.4	3.1	2.4	1.3
1889-------	1927	41.3	35.4	25.8	20.7	13.4	12.3	9.3	7.0	5.4	3.1	2.2	1.4
1890-------	1928	36.2	34.1	25.8	19.4	14.3	11.2	9.7	6.9	5.1	2.9	2.3	1.2
1891-------	1929	34.6	34.8	24.3	20.6	13.7	12.3	9.0	6.6	5.0	2.8	2.0	1.2
1892-------	1930	34.9	32.7	25.5	19.4	14.2	11.5	8.5	6.6	4.7	2.5	2.0	0.9
1893-------	1931	33.0	34.1	23.9	19.5	13.4	10.9	8.3	6.1	4.2	2.4	1.6	0.8
1894-------	1932	34.1	31.6	23.7	19.0	12.6	10.6	7.9	5.5	4.3	2.1	1.2	0.8
1895-------	1933	32.0	32.0	22.8	17.5	12.6	10.0	7.1	5.6	3.6	1.9	1.2	0.7
1896-------	1934	32.2	29.6	20.9	17.6	12.0	9.0	7.3	4.9	3.2	1.9	1.0	0.8
1897-------	1935	29.3	26.8	21.0	17.0	10.8	9.3	6.6	5.1	3.1	1.5	1.2	0.7
1898-------	1936	27.8	27.8	21.7	15.9	11.8	9.2	7.5	5.4	2.8	2.0	1.1	0.5
1899-------	1937	30.0	28.8	20.1	16.7	11.6	9.8	7.2	4.5	3.0	1.6	1.0	0.6
1900-------	1938	30.1	27.4	20.7	17.0	11.7	10.1	6.8	4.8	2.7	1.6	0.9	0.4
1901-------	1939	27.9	26.2	20.1	15.0	11.7	9.6	6.8	4.1	2.7	1.3	0.8	0.5
1902-------	1940	26.9	25.9	19.1	15.7	11.7	9.7	6.2	4.0	2.2	1.1	0.8	0.4
1903-------	1941	26.1	24.6	19.6	15.3	11.4	9.0	5.7	3.2	1.8	1.1	0.7	0.4
1904-------	1942	25.7	25.2	19.0	15.3	11.3	8.4	5.3	3.2	1.9	1.1	0.7	0.4
1905-------	1943	26.3	24.6	18.9	15.0	10.6	7.8	5.2	3.1	1.8	1.0	0.6	0.3
1906-------	1944	25.9	24.9	18.0	14.3	10.0	8.0	4.8	2.9	1.7	0.9	0.6	0.3
1907-------	1945	25.6	22.6	17.7	13.2	9.9	7.3	4.5	2.7	1.6	0.8	0.5	0.3
1908-------	1946	23.7	22.4	16.4	13.3	9.1	7.3	4.3	2.8	1.5	0.7	0.4	0.3
1909-------	1947	24.6	22.2	17.4	13.4	10.1	7.5	5.0	2.9	1.4	0.8	0.6	0.2
1910-------	1948	24.5	23.1	17.5	14.6	10.0	7.9	5.1	2.8	1.5	1.0	0.5	0.3
1911-------	1949	25.4	23.1	18.6	14.0	10.3	8.0	4.9	2.9	1.8	0.7	0.5	0.3
1912-------	1950	24.8	23.7	17.7	14.3	10.4	7.9	5.2	3.1	1.6	0.8	0.5	0.3
1913-------	1951	25.6	23.0	17.9	13.9	10.2	8.4	5.3	3.1	1.5	0.8	0.5	0.2
1914-------	1952	25.5	23.1	18.1	13.8	10.9	8.5	5.3	2.7	1.5	0.7	0.4	0.2
1915-------	1953	24.6	23.4	17.5	14.5	10.9	8.0	4.7	2.6	1.3	0.7	0.4	0.1
1916-------	1954	26.0	22.7	18.4	14.6	10.5	7.3	4.6	2.5	1.4	0.7	0.4	0.1
1917-------	1955	25.4	23.9	18.4	14.4	10.1	7.3	4.6	2.6	1.3	0.8	0.3	0.2
1918-------	1956	26.9	23.9	18.6	14.3	10.4	7.6	4.6	2.6	1.4	0.6	0.3	0.1
1919-------	1957	27.4	24.5	19.5	14.9	11.0	7.9	5.0	2.7	1.4	0.7	0.2	0.2
1920-------	1958	26.9	24.9	19.3	15.1	10.7	8.0	5.0	2.6	1.3	0.6	0.3	0.1
1921-------	1959	27.3	24.3	19.3	14.5	10.6	7.6	4.3	2.3	1.1	0.5	0.2	0.1
1922-------	1960	26.7	23.7	18.1	13.5	10.1	6.6	4.1	2.2	1.0	0.4	0.2	0.1
1923-------	1961	26.6	22.8	17.0	13.5	8.9	6.4	3.7	1.7	0.9	0.4	0.2	0.1
1924-------	1962	25.9	22.3	18.2	12.6	8.8	5.9	3.2	1.6	0.9	0.4	0.2	0.0
1925-------	1963	26.2	23.1	16.6	12.1	8.2	5.1	2.9	1.7	0.9	0.4	0.1	
1926-------	1964	26.4	21.5	15.3	11.0	7.1	4.8	2.9	1.6	0.7	0.3		
1927-------	1965	24.0	19.0	13.6	9.5	6.5	4.5	2.7	1.2	0.6			
1928-------	1966	20.6	16.5	11.7	8.4	6.1	4.4	1.9	1.1				
1929-------	1967	18.4	14.6	10.6	7.8	5.9	3.1	1.8					
1930-------	1968	15.9	12.9	9.8	7.5	4.3	2.8						
1931-------	1969	14.4	11.9	9.1	6.1	3.9							
1932-------	1970	13.5	11.1	7.6	5.0								
1933-------	1971	12.0	9.1	6.1									
1934-------	1972	10.0	7.3										
1935-------	1973	8.7											

TABLE 5A. CUMULATIVE BIRTH RATES FOR ALL WOMEN AS OF THE BEGINNING OF EACH YEAR 1917-74 BY AGE AND LIVE-BIRTH ORDER FOR GROUPS OF COHORTS FROM 1867-71 TO 1955-59

(RATES ARE SIMPLE AVERAGES OF THE RATES FOR SINGLE COHORTS IN TABLE 6A)

EXACT AGE AND COHORT	AS OF JANUARY 1	TOTAL	LIVE-BIRTH ORDER							
			1	2	3	4	5	6	7	8 AND HIGHER
15-19 YEARS										
1898-1902----------	1917	65.5	55.8	8.7	1.0	0.1	*	*	*	*
1899-1903----------	1918	66.8	57.2	8.5	1.0	0.1	*	*	*	*
1900-1904----------	1919	66.5	57.1	8.3	1.0	0.1	*	*	*	*
1901-1905----------	1920	62.0	53.1	7.9	0.9	0.1	*	*	*	*
1902-1906----------	1921	67.3	58.2	8.0	1.0	0.1	*	*	*	*
1903-1907----------	1922	73.0	63.2	8.7	1.0	0.1	*	*	*	*
1904-1908----------	1923	71.6	61.3	9.2	1.0	0.1	*	*	*	*
1905-1909----------	1924	70.4	59.7	9.5	1.1	0.1	*	*	*	*
1906-1910----------	1925	71.6	61.0	9.3	1.2	0.1	*	*	*	*
1907-1911----------	1926	71.9	61.5	9.2	1.1	0.1	*	*	*	*
1908-1912----------	1927	71.8	61.2	9.4	1.1	0.1	*	*	*	*
1909-1913----------	1928	71.5	60.8	9.5	1.1	0.1	*	*	*	*
1910-1914----------	1929	69.8	59.4	9.2	1.1	0.1	*	*	*	*
1911-1915----------	1930	67.9	57.8	8.9	1.1	0.1	*	*	*	*
1912-1916----------	1931	67.7	57.9	8.7	1.0	0.1	*	*	*	*
1913-1917----------	1932	65.5	56.0	8.4	1.0	0.1	*	*	*	*
1914-1918----------	1933	63.1	54.0	8.1	0.9	0.1	*	*	*	*
1915-1919----------	1934	59.5	50.9	7.6	0.9	0.1	*	*	*	*
1916-1920----------	1935	59.1	50.8	7.3	0.9	0.1	*	*	*	*
1917-1921----------	1936	59.8	51.6	7.2	0.9	0.1	*	*	*	*
1918-1922----------	1937	60.1	51.6	7.5	0.9	0.1	*	*	*	*
1919-1923----------	1938	62.3	53.3	8.0	0.9	0.1	*	*	*	*
1920-1924----------	1939	64.6	55.1	8.4	1.0	0.1	*	*	*	*
1921-1925----------	1940	64.3	54.5	8.6	1.1	0.1	*	*	*	*
1922-1926----------	1941	64.0	53.2	9.2	1.4	0.2	*	*	*	*
1923-1927----------	1942	65.8	54.5	9.6	1.5	0.2	*	*	*	*
1924-1928----------	1943	69.3	57.5	10.1	1.5	0.2	*	*	*	*
1925-1929----------	1944	71.2	58.6	10.7	1.7	0.2	*	*	*	*
1926-1930----------	1945	67.7	55.4	10.4	1.7	0.2	*	*	*	*
1927-1931----------	1946	63.8	52.4	9.7	1.5	0.2	*	*	*	*
1928-1932----------	1947	65.9	54.3	9.9	1.5	0.2	*	*	*	*
1929-1933----------	1948	79.2	66.4	11.0	1.6	0.2	*	*	*	*
1930-1934----------	1949	88.7	73.4	13.2	1.9	0.2	*	*	*	*
1931-1935----------	1950	94.8	76.4	15.7	2.4	0.3	*	*	*	*
1932-1936----------	1951	97.1	77.2	16.9	2.7	0.3	*	*	*	*
1933-1937----------	1952	101.6	80.6	17.7	2.9	0.4	*	*	*	*
1934-1938----------	1953	102.7	81.3	17.9	3.1	0.4	*	*	*	*
1935-1939----------	1954	104.3	82.5	18.2	3.2	0.4	*	*	*	*
1936-1940----------	1955	106.3	84.2	18.4	3.2	0.5	*	*	*	*
1937-1941----------	1956	107.1	84.5	18.9	3.2	0.5	*	*	*	*
1938-1942----------	1957	110.4	86.7	19.8	3.4	0.5	*	*	*	*
1939-1943----------	1958	113.7	89.1	20.5	3.6	0.5	*	*	*	*
1940-1944----------	1959	113.1	88.0	20.9	3.7	0.5	*	*	*	*
1941-1945----------	1960	110.8	85.8	20.7	3.8	0.5	*	*	*	*
1942-1946----------	1961	107.1	82.8	20.1	3.7	0.5	*	*	*	*
1943-1947----------	1962	104.2	80.7	19.4	3.6	0.5	*	*	*	*
1944-1948----------	1963	101.3	78.3	19.0	3.5	0.5	*	*	*	*
1945-1949----------	1964	97.9	75.9	18.1	3.4	0.5	*	*	*	*
1946-1950----------	1965	93.8	73.4	16.8	3.1	0.5	*	*	*	*
1947-1951----------	1966	89.4	71.0	15.2	2.8	0.4	*	*	*	*
1948-1952----------	1967	86.7	70.2	13.8	2.4	0.3	*	*	*	*
1949-1953----------	1968	84.9	69.2	13.3	2.1	0.3	*	*	*	*
1950-1954----------	1969	84.1	69.5	12.5	1.9	0.2	*	*	*	*
1951-1955----------	1970	84.4	70.4	12.0	1.8	0.2	*	*	*	*
1952-1956----------	1971	87.3	73.5	11.9	1.7	0.2	*	*	*	*
1953-1957----------	1972	87.8	74.3	11.7	1.6	0.2	*	*	*	*
1954-1958----------	1973	87.8	75.1	11.2	1.4	0.1	*	*	*	*
1955-1959----------	1974	87.4	75.3	10.7	1.3	0.1	*	*	*	*

TABLE 5A. CUMULATIVE BIRTH RATES FOR ALL WOMEN AS OF THE BEGINNING OF EACH YEAR 1917-74 BY AGE AND LIVE-BIRTH ORDER FOR GROUPS OF COHORTS FROM 1867-71 TO 1955-59--CON.

(RATES ARE SIMPLE AVERAGES OF THE RATES FOR SINGLE COHORTS IN TABLE 6A)

EXACT AGE AND COHORT	AS OF JANUARY 1	TOTAL	LIVE-BIRTH ORDER							
			1	2	3	4	5	6	7	8 AND HIGHER
20-24 YEARS										
1893-1897----------	1917	612.2	370.6	159.8	58.2	17.7	4.4	1.3	0.3	0.0
1894-1898----------	1918	615.6	376.1	160.7	57.0	16.4	3.9	1.1	0.3	0.1
1895-1899----------	1919	618.9	381.4	160.4	56.3	15.8	3.5	1.1	0.3	0.1
1896-1900----------	1920	602.0	368.9	158.1	54.9	15.3	3.4	1.0	0.3	0.1
1897-1901----------	1921	604.7	375.7	155.3	53.8	15.1	3.4	1.0	0.3	0.1
1898-1902----------	1922	613.1	385.7	153.3	53.5	15.5	3.6	1.1	0.3	0.1
1899-1903----------	1923	613.0	387.2	154.2	51.5	15.0	3.6	1.1	0.3	0.1
1900-1904----------	1924	615.5	387.0	156.9	51.4	14.9	3.7	1.1	0.4	0.1
1901-1905----------	1925	622.3	390.5	158.6	52.9	15.0	3.7	1.1	0.4	0.1
1902-1906----------	1926	623.6	390.9	158.2	53.7	15.5	3.7	1.1	0.4	0.1
1903-1907----------	1927	618.4	387.4	156.5	53.0	15.9	3.9	1.2	0.4	0.1
1904-1908----------	1928	608.7	381.9	153.5	51.9	15.8	3.9	1.2	0.4	0.1
1905-1909----------	1929	593.9	373.9	149.1	50.3	15.1	3.8	1.2	0.4	0.1
1906-1910----------	1930	577.4	364.8	144.8	48.4	14.3	3.6	1.1	0.3	0.1
1907-1911----------	1931	566.0	359.0	141.5	46.9	13.8	3.4	1.0	0.3	0.1
1908-1912----------	1932	551.7	351.1	137.7	45.1	13.2	3.2	1.0	0.3	0.1
1909-1913----------	1933	537.1	342.4	134.1	43.6	12.7	3.0	0.9	0.3	0.1
1910-1914----------	1934	518.4	331.4	129.1	41.8	12.1	2.9	0.8	0.2	0.1
1911-1915----------	1935	508.8	326.8	125.7	40.6	11.8	2.8	0.8	0.2	0.1
1912-1916----------	1936	501.5	325.2	121.8	39.0	11.5	2.8	0.8	0.3	0.1
1913-1917----------	1937	496.5	324.1	119.7	37.7	11.2	2.7	0.7	0.3	0.1
1914-1918----------	1938	496.8	325.0	119.7	37.3	11.0	2.7	0.7	0.3	0.1
1915-1919----------	1939	501.9	328.1	121.4	37.7	10.9	2.7	0.7	0.3	0.1
1916-1920----------	1940	503.7	328.9	122.6	37.8	10.7	2.6	0.7	0.3	0.1
1917-1921----------	1941	510.8	330.8	125.4	39.2	11.3	2.9	0.8	0.3	0.1
1918-1922----------	1942	524.6	338.9	129.0	40.7	11.7	3.0	0.9	0.3	0.1
1919-1923----------	1943	551.9	358.6	134.3	42.3	12.3	3.1	0.9	0.3	0.1
1920-1924----------	1944	570.2	367.1	140.5	44.6	13.2	3.4	1.0	0.3	0.1
1921-1925----------	1945	569.9	364.9	140.3	45.9	13.9	3.5	1.0	0.3	0.1
1922-1926----------	1946	555.0	357.6	134.6	44.2	13.7	3.5	1.0	0.3	0.1
1923-1927----------	1947	578.1	374.0	141.3	44.2	13.7	3.5	1.0	0.3	0.1
1924-1928----------	1948	625.8	410.9	151.1	45.4	13.5	3.5	1.0	0.3	0.1
1925-1929----------	1949	661.3	429.8	164.5	48.2	13.8	3.6	1.0	0.3	0.1
1926-1930----------	1950	693.9	440.3	180.1	53.0	15.0	3.9	1.1	0.3	0.2
1927-1931----------	1951	719.7	444.2	193.7	59.4	16.6	4.1	1.1	0.4	0.2
1928-1932----------	1952	753.5	454.8	206.6	66.7	19.0	4.6	1.2	0.4	0.2
1929-1933----------	1953	786.4	465.7	218.4	73.2	21.6	5.4	1.4	0.4	0.3
1930-1934----------	1954	816.6	475.7	230.0	78.6	23.9	6.1	1.5	0.5	0.3
1931-1935----------	1955	848.2	487.8	240.7	84.3	26.0	6.8	1.8	0.5	0.3
1932-1936----------	1956	874.9	497.9	249.9	89.1	27.7	7.3	2.1	0.6	0.3
1933-1937----------	1957	903.2	509.1	259.4	94.1	29.6	7.8	2.3	0.6	0.3
1934-1938----------	1958	928.2	518.7	268.0	98.7	31.1	8.4	2.4	0.6	0.3
1935-1939----------	1959	944.0	523.4	274.1	102.0	32.4	8.7	2.5	0.6	0.3
1936-1940----------	1960	955.9	525.1	279.5	105.0	33.7	9.0	2.6	0.7	0.3
1937-1941----------	1961	961.2	523.6	282.0	107.9	34.7	9.3	2.7	0.7	0.3
1938-1942----------	1962	957.4	518.7	280.7	109.1	35.7	9.5	2.7	0.7	0.3
1939-1943----------	1963	941.6	509.3	275.3	108.0	35.5	9.7	2.8	0.7	0.3
1940-1944----------	1964	914.6	497.5	266.4	103.8	34.0	9.3	2.6	0.7	0.3
1941-1945----------	1965	880.2	485.6	254.2	97.0	31.4	8.6	2.4	0.7	0.3
1942-1946----------	1966	833.0	470.4	237.6	87.0	27.6	7.4	2.1	0.6	0.3
1943-1947----------	1967	787.1	458.5	220.2	76.3	23.6	6.1	1.7	0.5	0.2
1944-1948----------	1968	745.9	446.2	205.3	67.2	20.2	5.1	1.4	0.4	0.1
1945-1949----------	1969	709.8	436.3	191.4	59.1	17.3	4.2	1.1	0.3	0.1
1946-1950----------	1970	684.3	429.8	181.3	53.3	15.0	3.5	1.0	0.3	0.1
1947-1951----------	1971	668.3	426.4	174.8	49.5	13.3	3.0	0.8	0.3	0.2
1948-1952----------	1972	647.3	418.1	167.9	45.9	11.8	2.6	0.6	0.2	0.2
1949-1953----------	1973	615.1	402.9	157.9	41.2	10.2	2.2	0.5	0.1	0.1
1950-1954----------	1974	583.5	387.1	148.5	36.9	8.7	1.8	0.4	0.1	0.0

TABLE 5A. CUMULATIVE BIRTH RATES FOR ALL WOMEN AS OF THE BEGINNING OF EACH YEAR 1917-74 BY AGE AND LIVE-BIRTH ORDER FOR GROUPS OF COHORTS FROM 1867-71 TO 1955-59--CON.

(RATES ARE SIMPLE AVERAGES OF THE RATES FOR SINGLE COHORTS IN TABLE 6A)

EXACT AGE AND COHORT	AS OF JANUARY 1	TOTAL	LIVE-BIRTH ORDER							
			1	2	3	4	5	6	7	8 AND HIGHER
25-29 YEARS										
1888-1892----------	1917	1,477.9	625.5	406.8	232.9	120.6	55.0	23.5	8.7	4.8
1889-1893----------	1918	1,480.1	631.0	408.9	232.6	118.8	53.5	22.6	8.2	4.5
1890-1894----------	1919	1,481.9	638.2	410.0	231.6	116.9	51.8	21.6	7.6	4.2
1891-1895----------	1920	1,470.2	636.6	408.8	228.5	114.2	50.1	20.6	7.4	4.0
1892-1896----------	1921	1,467.8	642.7	407.1	225.7	112.2	49.0	20.0	7.2	3.9
1893-1897----------	1922	1,469.1	650.0	404.0	223.5	111.0	48.9	20.2	7.4	4.1
1894-1898----------	1923	1,459.9	652.6	402.1	218.4	108.1	47.5	19.8	7.3	4.1
1895-1899----------	1924	1,452.1	652.8	400.8	214.2	105.8	47.0	19.8	7.4	4.3
1896-1900----------	1925	1,445.6	652.5	398.5	211.9	104.1	46.7	20.0	7.5	4.4
1897-1901----------	1926	1,435.8	651.1	395.2	209.3	102.4	45.9	19.8	7.5	4.6
1898-1902----------	1927	1,424.9	649.2	391.4	206.2	101.2	45.0	19.7	7.5	4.7
1899-1903----------	1928	1,413.2	647.7	386.4	202.8	100.1	44.7	19.4	7.4	4.7
1900-1904----------	1929	1,395.2	644.9	380.0	198.2	97.9	43.7	18.7	7.2	4.6
1901-1905----------	1930	1,372.0	640.4	373.0	192.5	94.8	42.5	17.8	6.7	4.3
1902-1906----------	1931	1,349.1	635.2	366.1	187.1	91.9	41.2	17.1	6.4	4.1
1903-1907----------	1932	1,319.8	626.6	357.8	180.9	88.5	39.5	16.5	6.2	3.8
1904-1908----------	1933	1,284.9	614.4	348.0	174.4	85.0	37.9	15.8	5.9	3.5
1905-1909----------	1934	1,245.2	599.7	337.5	167.7	81.1	35.7	14.8	5.5	3.2
1906-1910----------	1935	1,213.2	587.5	329.0	162.2	78.0	34.1	14.1	5.2	3.1
1907-1911----------	1936	1,184.8	578.1	320.9	156.5	75.0	32.7	13.5	5.0	3.1
1908-1912----------	1937	1,159.8	571.3	313.5	150.9	72.1	31.3	13.0	4.8	2.9
1909-1913----------	1938	1,143.5	568.7	308.2	146.3	69.6	30.4	12.6	4.8	2.9
1910-1914----------	1939	1,136.0	570.1	305.8	143.0	67.7	29.6	12.3	4.7	2.8
1911-1915----------	1940	1,132.9	573.3	305.2	140.5	65.8	28.8	12.0	4.6	2.7
1912-1916----------	1941	1,135.8	577.6	306.6	139.4	64.7	28.2	11.8	4.7	2.8
1913-1917----------	1942	1,148.2	586.4	310.4	139.8	64.3	28.1	11.7	4.7	2.8
1914-1918----------	1943	1,177.8	604.2	319.5	142.1	64.6	28.2	11.7	4.7	2.8
1915-1919----------	1944	1,215.8	618.5	334.6	147.7	66.4	29.0	12.0	4.8	2.8
1916-1920----------	1945	1,241.6	625.4	344.8	152.9	68.3	29.9	12.5	4.9	2.9
1917-1921----------	1946	1,258.2	630.3	351.6	156.0	69.3	30.3	12.8	5.0	2.9
1918-1922----------	1947	1,299.4	651.2	365.7	159.9	70.9	30.7	13.0	5.1	2.9
1919-1923----------	1948	1,355.8	682.2	384.2	165.3	71.9	30.9	13.1	5.2	3.0
1920-1924----------	1949	1,397.6	700.8	400.9	170.7	72.5	31.1	13.2	5.3	3.1
1921-1925----------	1950	1,439.1	714.2	419.7	177.8	74.1	31.3	13.4	5.4	3.2
1922-1926----------	1951	1,479.7	722.4	439.1	187.2	76.8	31.9	13.5	5.5	3.3
1923-1927----------	1952	1,531.0	732.4	460.3	200.1	81.7	33.5	14.1	5.6	3.3
1924-1928----------	1953	1,586.8	741.0	481.3	215.7	88.4	36.1	14.9	5.9	3.5
1925-1929----------	1954	1,641.7	747.2	501.1	231.7	96.4	39.3	16.0	6.3	3.7
1926-1930----------	1955	1,698.8	752.8	520.2	248.8	105.5	43.3	17.5	6.8	3.9
1927-1931----------	1956	1,758.2	759.8	538.5	266.3	114.9	47.6	19.3	7.5	4.3
1928-1932----------	1957	1,821.2	768.9	557.1	284.1	124.5	51.9	21.4	8.4	4.9
1929-1933----------	1958	1,889.3	780.6	576.8	302.4	134.6	56.6	23.6	9.3	5.4
1930-1934----------	1959	1,950.3	791.1	593.9	318.6	144.0	60.9	25.5	10.2	6.1
1931-1935----------	1960	2,005.5	800.1	608.7	333.6	153.1	64.9	27.4	11.1	6.6
1932-1936----------	1961	2,048.1	806.0	619.3	345.9	160.8	68.3	29.0	11.8	7.0
1933-1937----------	1962	2,079.2	809.3	625.9	355.1	167.2	71.6	30.4	12.3	7.4
1934-1938----------	1963	2,092.3	809.0	627.6	359.8	170.9	73.5	31.3	12.6	7.6
1935-1939----------	1964	2,090.3	806.6	625.9	360.3	171.9	74.1	31.3	12.6	7.6
1936-1940----------	1965	2,073.6	803.0	621.1	356.7	169.6	72.8	30.7	12.3	7.4
1937-1941----------	1966	2,029.4	795.9	610.4	345.6	162.0	68.7	28.7	11.4	6.7
1938-1942----------	1967	1,963.3	787.5	594.8	327.4	149.6	62.3	25.7	10.2	5.8
1939-1943----------	1968	1,885.3	777.2	576.3	305.6	135.1	55.0	22.4	8.8	4.9
1940-1944----------	1969	1,802.9	767.4	556.1	281.7	120.0	47.4	19.0	7.3	4.0
1941-1945----------	1970	1,725.3	755.9	536.5	259.9	106.8	40.9	16.0	6.0	3.3
1942-1946----------	1971	1,657.0	745.8	518.2	240.8	95.6	35.5	13.5	4.9	2.7
1943-1947----------	1972	1,587.0	734.3	497.8	221.6	85.1	30.7	11.3	4.0	2.2
1944-1948----------	1973	1,511.5	720.8	475.9	200.6	74.1	25.9	9.2	3.2	1.8
1945-1949----------	1974	1,436.4	704.8	454.2	180.7	63.9	21.5	7.4	2.5	1.4

TABLE 5A. CUMULATIVE BIRTH RATES FOR ALL WOMEN AS OF THE BEGINNING OF EACH YEAR 1917-74 BY AGE AND LIVE-BIRTH ORDER FOR GROUPS OF COHORTS FROM 1867-71 TO 1955-59--CON.

(RATES ARE SIMPLE AVERAGES OF THE RATES FOR SINGLE COHORTS IN TABLE 6A)

EXACT AGE AND COHORT	AS OF JANUARY 1	TOTAL	LIVE-BIRTH ORDER							
			1	2	3	4	5	6	7	8 AND HIGHER
30-34 YEARS										
1883-1887----------	1917	2,291.2	728.4	559.1	390.9	260.0	163.1	95.0	51.3	43.3
1884-1888----------	1918	2,277.3	729.5	557.8	389.0	257.1	160.1	93.5	49.5	40.8
1885-1889----------	1919	2,266.3	732.3	557.2	387.0	254.0	157.2	92.0	47.8	38.8
1886-1890----------	1920	2,253.6	734.2	557.3	384.9	250.5	153.5	89.8	46.1	37.3
1887-1891----------	1921	2,244.9	738.3	558.5	382.9	247.1	150.1	87.4	44.5	36.1
1888-1892----------	1922	2,240.8	743.5	560.2	380.7	244.0	147.0	85.8	43.6	36.0
1889-1893----------	1923	2,229.6	748.7	561.1	377.1	239.2	143.0	83.1	42.2	35.2
1890-1894----------	1924	2,217.4	753.4	560.8	372.6	234.0	139.5	80.9	41.3	34.9
1891-1895----------	1925	2,204.8	757.7	559.3	368.1	228.8	136.2	79.2	40.8	34.7
1892-1896----------	1926	2,187.6	761.2	556.5	362.3	223.1	132.5	77.3	40.0	34.7
1893-1897----------	1927	2,166.0	763.0	552.6	355.8	217.3	128.5	75.3	39.2	34.3
1894-1898----------	1928	2,142.5	763.2	548.3	348.5	211.5	124.8	73.4	38.6	34.2
1895-1899----------	1929	2,114.0	761.6	542.5	340.7	205.6	121.2	71.4	37.4	33.6
1896-1900----------	1930	2,080.9	758.3	535.1	332.5	199.6	117.6	69.0	36.1	32.7
1897-1901----------	1931	2,049.1	755.3	527.6	324.5	194.0	114.3	66.9	34.8	31.7
1898-1902----------	1932	2,016.3	752.3	519.7	316.4	188.5	110.7	64.6	33.5	30.6
1899-1903----------	1933	1,983.5	749.6	511.4	308.0	182.8	107.3	62.5	32.4	29.5
1900-1904----------	1934	1,943.9	745.2	501.7	298.9	176.7	103.2	59.6	30.9	27.7
1901-1905----------	1935	1,905.9	740.4	492.8	290.1	170.8	99.2	56.9	29.4	26.3
1902-1906----------	1936	1,864.7	734.0	483.2	281.0	164.6	94.9	54.1	27.9	25.0
1903-1907----------	1937	1,821.9	725.9	473.5	271.9	158.1	90.7	51.4	26.5	23.9
1904-1908----------	1938	1,778.2	716.8	463.4	262.6	151.6	86.5	49.0	25.3	23.0
1905-1909----------	1939	1,738.8	708.8	455.0	254.2	145.3	82.5	46.7	24.2	22.1
1906-1910----------	1940	1,704.5	702.8	448.2	246.7	139.5	78.6	44.4	23.1	21.2
1907-1911----------	1941	1,681.3	699.9	444.8	241.0	134.8	75.4	42.6	22.2	20.6
1908-1912----------	1942	1,667.1	700.8	443.4	236.5	131.0	72.7	41.0	21.6	20.1
1909-1913----------	1943	1,669.2	708.0	447.0	234.7	128.4	70.7	39.7	21.0	19.7
1910-1914----------	1944	1,686.7	716.9	456.1	236.9	127.6	69.9	39.0	20.7	19.6
1911-1915----------	1945	1,709.8	724.8	466.9	241.5	128.1	69.6	38.7	20.6	19.6
1912-1916----------	1946	1,736.4	731.8	480.1	247.4	129.2	69.5	38.4	20.5	19.5
1913-1917----------	1947	1,775.8	744.2	497.0	255.5	131.3	69.9	38.3	20.3	19.3
1914-1918----------	1948	1,821.2	759.9	514.8	264.5	133.9	70.5	38.2	20.3	19.1
1915-1919----------	1949	1,863.0	773.3	531.5	273.0	136.4	71.1	38.3	20.3	19.1
1916-1920----------	1950	1,906.5	786.5	548.2	281.7	139.6	72.0	38.6	20.5	19.4
1917-1921----------	1951	1,954.3	799.7	566.3	292.1	143.5	73.1	39.1	20.7	19.8
1918-1922----------	1952	2,005.4	812.3	584.7	304.2	148.5	74.6	39.8	21.1	20.2
1919-1923----------	1953	2,064.2	825.1	604.3	319.3	155.3	77.2	40.8	21.5	20.7
1920-1924----------	1954	2,121.6	834.9	622.8	335.6	163.2	80.3	41.9	21.9	21.0
1921-1925----------	1955	2,182.3	842.7	641.2	353.3	172.8	84.4	43.7	22.6	21.6
1922-1926----------	1956	2,241.2	847.5	657.5	371.4	183.4	89.5	46.0	23.6	22.3
1923-1927----------	1957	2,305.0	851.8	673.3	390.6	195.9	95.8	49.1	25.0	23.5
1924-1928----------	1958	2,369.6	854.6	687.5	410.1	209.4	103.0	52.7	27.0	25.3
1925-1929----------	1959	2,431.3	856.3	699.8	428.9	223.2	110.4	56.5	29.0	27.2
1926-1930----------	1960	2,493.2	857.6	711.3	447.1	237.4	118.4	60.7	31.1	29.6
1927-1931----------	1961	2,559.0	860.7	723.5	465.3	251.8	126.9	65.3	33.5	32.0
1928-1932----------	1962	2,625.8	865.3	735.7	482.9	266.1	135.3	69.9	36.0	34.6
1929-1933----------	1963	2,688.4	871.1	747.3	498.7	278.9	143.1	74.2	38.2	36.9
1930-1934----------	1964	2,741.2	876.7	757.2	511.9	289.7	149.6	77.7	39.9	38.5
1931-1935----------	1965	2,781.8	882.7	764.7	521.9	297.7	154.2	80.1	41.1	39.4
1932-1936----------	1966	2,796.9	886.2	768.2	526.5	300.7	155.5	80.3	40.8	38.7
1933-1937----------	1967	2,788.1	887.8	768.2	525.7	298.7	153.3	78.4	39.3	36.7
1934-1938----------	1968	2,756.8	886.7	765.1	519.8	292.0	148.0	74.7	37.0	33.5
1935-1939----------	1969	2,709.1	885.2	759.8	509.6	281.4	140.1	69.5	33.8	29.7
1936-1940----------	1970	2,651.4	882.3	753.1	496.7	268.3	130.9	63.8	30.4	25.9
1937-1941----------	1971	2,585.1	878.5	744.6	480.8	253.2	121.0	57.7	27.0	22.3
1938-1942----------	1972	2,506.8	873.4	733.9	460.4	235.5	109.8	51.4	23.6	18.8
1939-1943----------	1973	2,414.9	866.6	720.5	435.2	215.0	97.6	44.6	20.0	15.4
1940-1944----------	1974	2,314.4	858.0	704.5	406.9	193.3	85.0	37.8	16.5	12.4

TABLE 5A. CUMULATIVE BIRTH RATES FOR ALL WOMEN AS OF THE BEGINNING OF EACH YEAR 1917-74 BY AGE AND LIVE-BIRTH ORDER FOR GROUPS OF COHORTS FROM 1867-71 TO 1955-59--CON.

(RATES ARE SIMPLE AVERAGES OF THE RATES FOR SINGLE COHORTS IN TABLE 6A)

EXACT AGE AND COHORT	AS OF JANUARY 1	TOTAL	LIVE-BIRTH ORDER 1	2	3	4	5	6	7	8 AND HIGHER
35-39 YEARS										
1878-1882----------	1917	3,001.1	766.2	630.5	485.6	362.7	264.3	188.5	125.8	177.4
1879-1883----------	1918	2,966.7	766.1	628.2	481.4	357.9	259.4	183.6	122.7	167.4
1880-1884----------	1919	2,934.3	766.4	626.4	477.4	353.1	254.3	178.8	119.2	158.7
1881-1885----------	1920	2,902.6	766.6	624.7	473.3	347.8	248.9	173.8	115.6	151.9
1882-1886----------	1921	2,873.7	767.3	622.7	469.6	342.8	243.7	169.3	112.0	146.3
1883-1887----------	1922	2,850.2	768.6	620.9	466.5	338.5	239.1	165.5	108.6	142.5
1884-1888----------	1923	2,826.6	770.1	619.7	463.7	333.9	234.1	161.9	105.1	138.1
1885-1889----------	1924	2,805.5	772.2	619.4	461.2	329.3	228.8	158.0	101.8	134.8
1886-1890----------	1925	2,788.7	775.3	620.1	459.2	324.9	223.7	154.2	98.9	132.4
1887-1891----------	1926	2,771.8	779.1	621.2	456.5	320.1	218.4	150.3	96.0	130.2
1888-1892----------	1927	2,751.8	783.2	622.3	452.8	314.4	212.6	146.0	93.2	127.3
1889-1893----------	1928	2,728.6	787.7	622.2	448.2	308.0	206.4	141.3	90.3	124.5
1890-1894----------	1929	2,697.9	791.7	620.5	442.0	300.5	199.9	136.3	87.1	119.9
1891-1895----------	1930	2,662.1	794.9	617.2	434.4	292.1	193.3	131.4	83.9	114.9
1892-1896----------	1931	2,624.5	797.5	613.0	426.1	283.5	186.9	126.6	80.6	110.3
1893-1897----------	1932	2,583.4	798.8	607.7	417.0	274.7	180.4	121.8	77.4	105.6
1894-1898----------	1933	2,541.1	798.2	601.9	407.4	265.8	174.0	117.5	74.5	101.8
1895-1899----------	1934	2,497.7	796.3	595.1	397.6	257.7	168.2	113.5	71.7	97.6
1896-1900----------	1935	2,454.3	792.8	587.0	388.0	250.3	162.9	109.8	69.2	94.3
1897-1901----------	1936	2,410.1	789.2	578.5	378.2	242.8	157.6	105.9	66.7	91.2
1898-1902----------	1937	2,365.4	786.2	570.0	368.4	235.3	152.1	101.8	63.9	87.7
1899-1903----------	1938	2,321.9	784.3	561.9	358.7	227.7	146.6	97.3	61.0	84.4
1900-1904----------	1939	2,276.5	782.1	553.6	348.8	220.1	140.7	92.6	58.0	80.6
1901-1905----------	1940	2,229.7	779.6	545.8	339.0	212.3	134.5	87.7	54.8	76.0
1902-1906----------	1941	2,183.9	775.7	538.5	329.6	204.6	128.5	83.1	51.8	72.1
1903-1907----------	1942	2,141.4	770.8	531.9	321.2	197.3	123.0	79.1	49.2	68.9
1904-1908----------	1943	2,102.3	765.9	526.2	313.4	190.5	117.9	75.6	46.8	66.0
1905-1909----------	1944	2,073.7	762.3	523.6	308.2	185.1	113.5	72.4	44.9	63.7
1906-1910----------	1945	2,055.4	760.0	523.7	305.3	181.1	109.9	70.0	43.4	62.0
1907-1911----------	1946	2,050.3	760.3	527.5	305.2	178.7	107.5	68.1	42.3	60.7
1908-1912----------	1947	2,055.9	764.0	534.0	307.1	177.6	105.8	66.5	41.4	59.5
1909-1913----------	1948	2,073.1	771.5	543.5	311.4	177.8	104.7	65.3	40.5	58.4
1910-1914----------	1949	2,094.7	779.9	554.5	316.8	178.5	103.8	64.2	39.7	57.3
1911-1915----------	1950	2,123.4	789.8	567.5	323.8	180.0	103.5	63.4	39.0	56.4
1912-1916----------	1951	2,154.0	798.8	581.0	331.6	182.5	103.6	62.7	38.5	55.3
1913-1917----------	1952	2,191.4	807.8	595.9	341.4	186.5	104.6	62.6	38.0	54.6
1914-1918----------	1953	2,232.0	815.8	611.0	352.5	191.5	106.2	62.8	38.0	54.2
1915-1919----------	1954	2,280.4	825.4	627.0	365.0	198.1	108.9	63.6	38.3	54.1
1916-1920----------	1955	2,334.7	835.9	643.2	378.8	205.9	112.4	65.0	39.0	54.5
1917-1921----------	1956	2,394.8	847.3	660.3	394.0	214.8	116.5	66.9	39.7	55.3
1918-1922----------	1957	2,454.6	857.4	676.2	409.3	224.1	121.1	69.2	40.8	56.5
1919-1923----------	1958	2,518.7	867.5	692.1	425.6	234.8	126.6	72.0	42.1	58.0
1920-1924----------	1959	2,579.2	875.1	706.4	441.6	245.7	132.5	75.1	43.5	59.3
1921-1925----------	1960	2,639.0	880.3	719.2	457.6	257.2	139.3	78.7	45.4	61.3
1922-1926----------	1961	2,696.1	883.0	730.6	473.0	269.1	146.4	82.7	47.6	63.7
1923-1927----------	1962	2,757.0	885.4	741.6	488.9	281.9	154.5	87.3	50.3	67.1
1924-1928----------	1963	2,813.4	886.0	750.7	503.7	294.4	162.6	92.1	53.1	70.8
1925-1929----------	1964	2,867.8	885.6	759.0	518.2	306.9	170.8	96.9	55.9	74.5
1926-1930----------	1965	2,921.2	885.6	767.0	532.3	319.3	178.8	101.6	58.6	78.0
1927-1931----------	1966	2,973.8	887.6	775.6	546.1	331.1	186.2	106.0	60.8	80.4
1928-1932----------	1967	3,020.5	891.1	784.4	558.6	341.3	192.4	109.2	62.3	81.2
1929-1933----------	1968	3,061.5	896.2	793.3	569.9	349.9	197.0	111.5	63.1	80.6
1930-1934----------	1969	3,088.1	901.6	800.7	578.2	355.3	199.2	112.1	62.8	78.2
1931-1935----------	1970	3,099.6	906.3	806.0	583.2	357.6	199.3	111.1	61.6	74.5
1932-1936----------	1971	3,091.2	909.1	808.2	584.1	355.9	196.7	108.3	59.2	69.7
1933-1937----------	1972	3,064.6	910.1	807.7	580.8	350.5	191.5	104.0	56.0	64.0
1934-1938----------	1973	3,016.9	909.0	804.6	572.9	340.5	183.1	97.9	51.8	57.1
1935-1939----------	1974	2,954.4	906.9	799.7	561.2	327.0	172.4	90.5	47.0	49.7

TABLE 5A. CUMULATIVE BIRTH RATES FOR ALL WOMEN AS OF THE BEGINNING OF EACH YEAR 1917-74 BY AGE AND LIVE-BIRTH ORDER FOR GROUPS OF COHORTS FROM 1867-71 TO 1955-59--CON.

(RATES ARE SIMPLE AVERAGES OF THE RATES FOR SINGLE COHORTS IN TABLE 6A)

EXACT AGE AND COHORT	AS OF JANUARY 1	TOTAL	LIVE-BIRTH ORDER							
			1	2	3	4	5	6	7	8 AND HIGHER
40-44 YEARS										
1873-1877----------	1917	3,560.6	785.9	667.9	538.9	425.4	330.7	255.0	188.9	367.9
1874-1878----------	1918	3,514.0	783.9	663.9	533.2	419.0	324.3	249.6	183.7	356.4
1875-1879----------	1919	3,469.3	782.1	660.0	527.9	413.0	318.5	244.5	178.8	344.5
1876-1880----------	1920	3,426.6	780.7	656.5	522.9	407.4	313.0	239.6	174.1	332.4
1877-1881----------	1921	3,386.6	779.8	653.4	518.3	402.1	307.6	234.7	170.0	320.7
1878-1882----------	1922	3,349.6	779.5	650.8	513.9	397.0	302.4	229.7	166.4	309.9
1879-1883----------	1923	3,310.5	779.7	648.5	509.7	391.7	296.8	223.9	162.4	297.8
1880-1884----------	1924	3,272.1	780.0	646.7	505.5	386.2	290.9	217.8	157.9	287.1
1881-1885----------	1925	3,233.9	780.3	645.0	501.2	380.5	284.6	211.5	153.0	277.8
1882-1886----------	1926	3,196.7	780.8	642.9	497.1	374.9	278.3	205.6	148.0	269.1
1883-1887----------	1927	3,161.3	781.6	640.7	493.4	369.5	272.2	200.1	143.0	260.8
1884-1888----------	1928	3,130.0	783.0	639.2	490.3	364.4	266.2	195.3	138.2	253.4
1885-1889----------	1929	3,098.9	784.9	638.5	487.2	359.1	259.9	190.0	133.5	245.8
1886-1890----------	1930	3,068.5	787.8	638.7	484.3	353.5	253.3	184.5	128.8	237.6
1887-1891----------	1931	3,039.1	791.2	639.2	480.9	347.5	246.7	179.2	124.4	230.0
1888-1892----------	1932	3,005.6	795.1	639.8	476.2	340.5	239.5	173.4	119.9	221.2
1889-1893----------	1933	2,968.0	799.1	639.1	470.5	332.8	231.9	167.2	115.3	212.1
1890-1894----------	1934	2,925.7	802.7	637.0	463.4	324.2	224.3	160.9	110.8	202.4
1891-1895----------	1935	2,881.0	805.7	633.3	455.2	315.1	216.7	155.0	106.5	193.5
1892-1896----------	1936	2,832.1	807.8	628.5	446.0	305.4	209.0	148.9	102.0	184.5
1893-1897----------	1937	2,781.4	808.7	622.7	436.3	295.7	201.5	143.0	97.6	175.9
1894-1898----------	1938	2,729.7	808.0	616.6	426.1	286.1	194.0	137.4	93.5	168.0
1895-1899----------	1939	2,682.1	806.5	610.1	416.3	277.5	187.6	132.6	89.9	161.6
1896-1900----------	1940	2,632.7	803.5	602.2	406.4	269.4	181.5	127.9	86.4	155.4
1897-1901----------	1941	2,583.2	800.4	594.3	396.5	261.3	175.4	123.1	82.9	149.3
1898-1902----------	1942	2,534.3	798.0	586.4	386.8	253.4	169.2	118.1	79.2	143.2
1899-1903----------	1943	2,487.7	797.1	579.3	377.4	245.6	163.1	112.9	75.5	136.8
1900-1904----------	1944	2,441.7	796.2	572.5	368.3	238.0	156.9	107.7	71.7	130.4
1901-1905----------	1945	2,397.5	795.1	566.5	359.8	230.7	150.7	102.5	68.1	124.1
1902-1906----------	1946	2,357.2	792.8	561.4	352.3	224.1	145.0	97.9	64.9	118.8
1903-1907----------	1947	2,321.7	789.6	557.7	346.3	218.0	140.0	93.9	62.1	114.1
1904-1908----------	1948	2,289.3	785.7	554.8	341.1	212.6	135.4	90.3	59.5	109.9
1905-1909----------	1949	2,263.2	782.7	553.8	337.6	208.1	131.2	86.9	57.2	105.7
1906-1910----------	1950	2,246.1	781.4	555.2	335.8	204.5	127.7	84.0	55.2	102.3
1907-1911----------	1951	2,241.1	782.6	559.4	336.3	202.5	125.3	81.9	53.7	99.4
1908-1912----------	1952	2,244.0	785.5	565.2	338.3	201.7	123.5	80.2	52.6	97.0
1909-1913----------	1953	2,258.0	791.0	573.7	342.7	202.4	122.6	79.0	51.6	95.0
1910-1914----------	1954	2,280.4	798.3	584.4	349.0	204.2	122.4	78.2	50.8	93.1
1911-1915----------	1955	2,312.4	807.3	597.3	357.5	207.6	123.2	77.9	50.2	91.4
1912-1916----------	1956	2,347.0	815.8	610.6	366.8	211.9	124.6	78.0	49.8	89.5
1913-1917----------	1957	2,387.4	823.9	625.0	377.9	217.5	126.8	78.3	49.7	88.3
1914-1918----------	1958	2,429.8	831.0	639.0	389.4	224.0	129.5	79.2	50.1	87.6
1915-1919----------	1959	2,480.1	839.8	654.1	402.1	231.6	133.3	80.7	50.8	87.7
1916-1920----------	1960	2,534.3	849.3	669.0	415.3	239.9	137.6	82.8	51.9	88.5
1917-1921----------	1961	2,594.7	859.9	684.6	429.8	249.3	142.7	85.5	53.1	89.8
1918-1922----------	1962	2,653.0	869.2	698.9	443.9	258.7	147.9	88.5	54.6	91.3
1919-1923----------	1963	2,714.2	878.6	713.2	458.7	268.8	153.7	91.7	56.2	93.3
1920-1924----------	1964	2,771.0	885.3	725.9	473.0	278.9	159.7	95.1	58.0	95.1
1921-1925----------	1965	2,826.2	890.0	737.4	487.3	289.4	166.1	98.7	59.9	97.4
1922-1926----------	1966	2,877.3	892.3	747.5	500.9	299.8	172.6	102.4	62.0	99.8
1923-1927----------	1967	2,929.3	894.3	757.1	514.6	310.7	179.5	106.4	64.3	102.4
1924-1928----------	1968	2,976.2	894.5	765.2	527.6	321.5	186.1	110.2	66.5	104.6
1925-1929----------	1969	3,020.3	894.2	772.5	540.2	332.1	192.7	113.9	68.5	106.2
1926-1930----------	1970	3,060.6	893.6	779.5	552.4	342.2	198.9	117.2	70.0	106.8
1927-1931----------	1971	3,101.7	895.1	787.4	564.4	352.1	204.6	120.3	71.3	106.5
1928-1932----------	1972	3,138.0	898.1	795.5	575.5	360.5	209.2	122.4	71.9	104.9
1929-1933----------	1973	3,169.7	902.9	803.8	585.4	367.5	212.6	123.6	71.9	102.0
1930-1934----------	1974	3,187.7	907.7	810.7	592.7	371.5	213.6	123.2	70.8	97.5

TABLE 5A. CUMULATIVE BIRTH RATES FOR ALL WOMEN AS OF THE BEGINNING OF EACH YEAR 1917-74 BY AGE AND LIVE-BIRTH ORDER FOR GROUPS OF COHORTS FROM 1867-71 TO 1955-59--CON.

(RATES ARE SIMPLE AVERAGES OF THE RATES FOR SINGLE COHORTS IN TABLE 6A)

EXACT AGE AND COHORT	AS OF JANUARY 1	TOTAL	LIVE-BIRTH ORDER							
			1	2	3	4	5	6	7	8 AND HIGHER
45-49 YEARS										
1868-1872----------	1917	3,914.1	799.8	692.5	572.6	464.6	370.1	292.6	224.1	497.8
1869-1873----------	1918	3,863.8	797.5	688.4	567.0	458.3	364.0	287.2	219.3	482.1
1870-1874----------	1919	3,814.2	795.1	684.1	561.4	451.9	357.9	281.9	214.6	467.3
1871-1875----------	1920	3,763.0	792.6	679.8	555.5	445.2	351.6	276.3	209.8	452.2
1872-1876----------	1921	3,712.4	790.3	675.5	549.7	438.5	345.1	270.5	204.6	438.2
1873-1877----------	1922	3,661.8	788.2	671.2	543.7	431.8	338.5	264.4	199.0	425.0
1874-1878----------	1923	3,613.6	786.3	667.1	538.0	425.3	332.1	258.7	193.7	412.4
1875-1879----------	1924	3,567.6	784.5	663.4	532.7	419.3	326.1	253.5	188.6	399.5
1876-1880----------	1925	3,523.9	783.1	659.8	527.7	413.7	320.5	248.5	183.8	386.8
1877-1881----------	1926	3,481.8	782.2	656.7	523.0	408.2	315.1	243.3	179.4	373.9
1878-1882----------	1927	3,441.2	781.8	654.1	518.6	402.9	309.5	237.9	175.4	361.0
1879-1883----------	1928	3,399.8	781.9	651.7	514.2	397.6	303.7	231.9	171.1	347.7
1880-1884----------	1929	3,358.4	782.2	649.8	509.8	392.0	297.5	225.5	166.2	335.4
1881-1885----------	1930	3,315.5	782.5	647.9	505.3	385.9	290.8	218.7	160.8	323.6
1882-1886----------	1931	3,274.1	783.0	645.8	501.1	380.0	284.3	212.4	155.3	312.2
1883-1887----------	1932	3,234.6	783.7	643.4	497.3	374.4	277.9	206.5	149.9	301.5
1884-1888----------	1933	3,198.9	784.9	641.8	494.0	369.1	271.7	201.3	144.7	291.4
1885-1889----------	1934	3,164.6	786.8	641.0	490.9	363.6	265.1	195.8	139.7	281.7
1886-1890----------	1935	3,132.0	789.6	641.1	487.8	357.9	258.4	190.3	134.8	272.1
1887-1891----------	1936	3,099.5	792.9	641.5	484.2	351.8	251.6	184.7	130.1	262.7
1888-1892----------	1937	3,063.3	796.8	642.0	479.4	344.6	244.2	178.7	125.3	252.3
1889-1893----------	1938	3,022.6	800.7	641.2	473.5	336.7	236.5	172.1	120.4	241.5
1890-1894----------	1939	2,977.5	804.2	638.9	466.4	328.0	228.6	165.6	115.5	230.3
1891-1895----------	1940	2,929.6	807.2	635.3	458.0	318.7	220.8	159.3	110.9	219.4
1892-1896----------	1941	2,878.1	809.4	630.4	448.8	308.9	212.9	153.0	106.2	208.5
1893-1897----------	1942	2,825.0	810.3	624.7	439.1	299.1	205.1	146.8	101.5	198.4
1894-1898----------	1943	2,772.1	809.7	618.7	428.9	289.4	197.6	141.1	97.3	189.4
1895-1899----------	1944	2,722.9	808.2	612.3	419.1	280.8	191.0	136.2	93.5	181.8
1896-1900----------	1945	2,673.5	805.4	604.7	409.4	272.8	184.9	131.4	89.9	175.0
1897-1901----------	1946	2,624.0	802.5	596.9	399.7	264.8	178.9	126.6	86.3	168.3
1898-1902----------	1947	2,576.0	800.4	589.3	390.2	257.2	172.9	121.7	82.6	161.7
1899-1903----------	1948	2,530.1	799.7	582.5	381.2	249.6	166.9	116.5	78.9	154.8
1900-1904----------	1949	2,484.4	799.0	576.1	372.4	242.1	160.7	111.2	75.1	147.8
1901-1905----------	1950	2,439.6	798.0	570.4	364.2	234.8	154.5	105.9	71.2	140.6
1902-1906----------	1951	2,398.2	795.9	565.5	356.8	228.3	148.7	101.1	67.8	134.1
1903-1907----------	1952	2,361.8	792.8	561.9	350.9	222.3	143.7	97.0	64.8	128.4
1904-1908----------	1953	2,327.5	788.7	558.8	345.6	216.8	139.0	93.2	62.1	123.3
1905-1909----------	1954	2,301.2	785.7	557.8	342.1	212.4	134.8	89.9	59.8	118.7
1906-1910----------	1955	2,284.4	784.4	559.2	340.5	209.0	131.5	87.1	57.9	114.8
1907-1911----------	1956	2,279.8	785.5	563.5	341.3	207.3	129.2	85.0	56.4	111.6
1908-1912----------	1957	2,283.2	788.3	569.3	343.5	206.7	127.7	83.5	55.3	108.9
1909-1913----------	1958	2,297.5	793.7	577.8	348.1	207.6	127.0	82.4	54.3	106.6
1910-1914----------	1959	2,320.7	800.9	588.4	354.7	209.6	127.1	81.8	53.6	104.6
1911-1915----------	1960	2,352.7	809.8	601.2	363.1	213.2	128.0	81.8	53.0	102.6
1912-1916----------	1961	2,387.0	818.1	614.4	372.3	217.6	129.5	81.8	52.7	100.6
1913-1917----------	1962	2,427.2	826.1	628.5	383.2	223.4	131.8	82.3	52.7	99.2
1914-1918----------	1963	2,468.9	833.0	642.4	394.6	229.7	134.6	83.2	53.1	98.3
1915-1919----------	1964	2,519.0	841.6	657.3	407.2	237.3	138.4	84.8	53.9	98.5
1916-1920----------	1965	2,572.9	851.0	672.0	420.2	245.6	142.8	87.0	55.0	99.3
1917-1921----------	1966	2,632.4	861.5	687.4	434.4	254.8	147.7	89.6	56.3	100.7
1918-1922----------	1967	2,688.8	870.7	701.4	448.2	263.8	152.7	92.4	57.7	101.9
1919-1923----------	1968	2,748.4	880.1	715.4	462.7	273.6	158.3	95.6	59.2	103.5
1920-1924----------	1969	2,803.4	886.9	727.9	476.7	283.5	164.0	98.8	60.8	104.8
1921-1925----------	1970	2,856.1	891.4	739.4	490.6	293.6	170.1	102.1	62.6	106.3
1922-1926----------	1971	2,904.5	893.6	749.3	503.9	303.6	176.2	105.5	64.5	107.9
1923-1927----------	1972	2,954.2	895.5	758.8	517.4	314.2	182.7	109.2	66.6	109.8
1924-1928----------	1973	2,998.8	895.7	766.8	530.0	324.5	189.1	112.8	68.5	111.4
1925-1929----------	1974	3,040.6	895.1	774.0	542.4	334.8	195.4	116.2	70.3	112.4

TABLE 5A. CUMULATIVE BIRTH RATES FOR ALL WOMEN AS OF THE BEGINNING OF EACH YEAR 1917-74 BY AGE AND LIVE-BIRTH ORDER FOR GROUPS OF COHORTS FROM 1867-71 TO 1955-59--CON.

(RATES ARE SIMPLE AVERAGES OF THE RATES FOR SINGLE COHORTS IN TABLE 6A)

EXACT AGE AND COHORT	AS OF JANUARY 1	TOTAL	LIVE-BIRTH ORDER							
			1	2	3	4	5	6	7	8 AND HIGHER
50-54 YEARS										
1863-1867----------	1917	---	---	---	---	---	---	---	---	---
1864-1868----------	1918	---	---	---	---	---	---	---	---	---
1865-1869----------	1919	---	---	---	---	---	---	---	---	---
1866-1870----------	1920	---	---	---	---	---	---	---	---	---
1867-1871----------	1921	3,974.8	802.2	696.7	578.3	471.3	376.8	298.9	229.8	520.8
1868-1872----------	1922	3,925.5	800.0	692.8	572.9	465.2	370.7	293.5	225.1	505.3
1869-1873----------	1923	3,875.4	797.7	688.7	567.4	458.9	364.7	288.1	220.2	489.7
1870-1874----------	1924	3,824.9	795.3	684.4	561.7	452.5	358.5	282.7	215.5	474.3
1871-1875----------	1925	3,773.5	792.8	680.0	555.8	445.8	352.2	277.1	210.7	459.1
1872-1876----------	1926	3,722.0	790.5	675.6	549.9	439.0	345.6	271.2	205.4	444.8
1873-1877----------	1927	3,671.0	788.3	671.4	544.0	432.2	339.0	265.1	199.9	431.1
1874-1878----------	1928	3,622.5	786.4	667.3	538.3	425.7	332.6	259.4	194.5	418.3
1875-1879----------	1929	3,575.8	784.6	663.6	532.9	419.6	326.6	254.1	189.3	405.1
1876-1880----------	1930	3,531.9	783.2	660.0	528.0	414.0	321.0	249.0	184.5	392.2
1877-1881----------	1931	3,489.6	782.3	656.9	523.3	408.6	315.5	243.9	180.1	379.0
1878-1882----------	1932	3,448.5	782.0	654.2	518.8	403.3	309.9	238.5	176.0	365.8
1879-1883----------	1933	3,406.3	782.0	651.8	514.4	397.8	304.0	232.4	171.6	352.3
1880-1884----------	1934	3,364.6	782.3	649.9	510.0	392.2	297.9	226.0	166.7	339.6
1881-1885----------	1935	3,321.6	782.6	648.0	505.5	386.2	291.2	219.2	161.3	327.6
1882-1886----------	1936	3,279.7	783.0	645.9	501.3	380.3	284.6	212.8	155.8	316.0
1883-1887----------	1937	3,240.2	783.8	643.5	497.5	374.7	278.2	206.9	150.4	305.2
1884-1888----------	1938	3,204.0	785.0	641.8	494.1	369.4	272.0	201.7	145.2	294.8
1885-1889----------	1939	3,169.5	786.9	641.0	491.0	363.8	265.4	196.2	140.2	285.0
1886-1890----------	1940	3,136.8	789.6	641.1	487.9	358.2	258.7	190.7	135.3	275.3
1887-1891----------	1941	3,103.9	793.0	641.6	484.3	352.0	251.8	185.0	130.5	265.7
1888-1892----------	1942	3,067.2	796.8	642.1	479.4	344.8	244.4	179.0	125.7	255.0
1889-1893----------	1943	3,026.2	800.8	641.2	473.6	336.9	236.7	172.3	120.7	244.0
1890-1894----------	1944	2,980.8	804.3	639.0	466.4	328.1	228.8	165.8	115.8	232.6
1891-1895----------	1945	2,932.6	807.3	635.3	458.1	318.8	221.0	159.5	111.2	221.4
1892-1896----------	1946	2,880.8	809.5	630.5	448.9	309.0	213.0	153.1	106.4	210.4
1893-1897----------	1947	2,827.6	810.4	624.8	439.2	299.2	205.2	147.0	101.7	200.1
1894-1898----------	1948	2,774.9	809.8	618.8	429.0	289.6	197.7	141.3	97.5	191.2
1895-1899----------	1949	2,725.6	808.3	612.4	419.2	281.0	191.2	136.3	93.7	183.5
1896-1900----------	1950	2,675.9	805.4	604.7	409.5	272.9	185.1	131.6	90.1	176.6
1897-1901----------	1951	2,626.6	802.6	597.0	399.8	265.0	179.1	126.8	86.5	169.8
1898-1902----------	1952	2,578.4	800.5	589.4	390.3	257.3	173.1	121.8	82.8	163.2
1899-1903----------	1953	2,532.3	799.8	582.6	381.3	249.7	167.1	116.7	79.0	156.1
1900-1904----------	1954	2,486.3	799.1	576.2	372.5	242.2	160.8	111.4	75.2	148.9
1901-1905----------	1955	2,441.4	798.1	570.5	364.3	235.0	154.6	106.0	71.3	141.6
1902-1906----------	1956	2,400.0	796.0	565.6	356.9	228.4	148.9	101.2	67.9	135.1
1903-1907----------	1957	2,363.6	792.9	562.0	351.0	222.5	143.8	97.1	64.9	129.4
1904-1908----------	1958	2,329.1	788.8	558.8	345.7	217.0	139.1	93.3	62.2	124.2
1905-1909----------	1959	2,303.0	785.8	557.9	342.2	212.6	135.0	90.0	59.9	119.6
1906-1910----------	1960	2,285.8	784.4	559.3	340.6	209.2	131.7	87.1	57.9	115.6
1907-1911----------	1961	2,281.5	785.6	563.5	341.5	207.4	129.4	85.1	56.5	112.5
1908-1912----------	1962	2,285.0	788.4	569.4	343.7	206.9	127.9	83.6	55.3	109.8
1909-1913----------	1963	2,299.5	793.8	577.9	348.3	207.8	127.2	82.6	54.4	107.5
1910-1914----------	1964	2,322.5	801.0	588.5	354.8	209.8	127.3	82.0	53.7	105.4
1911-1915----------	1965	2,354.3	809.9	601.3	363.2	213.4	128.2	81.9	53.1	103.3
1912-1916----------	1966	2,388.6	818.1	614.4	372.5	217.8	129.7	82.0	52.8	101.3
1913-1917----------	1967	2,428.7	826.1	628.6	383.4	223.5	132.0	82.5	52.8	99.8
1914-1918----------	1968	2,470.3	833.0	642.5	394.7	229.8	134.8	83.4	53.2	98.9
1915-1919----------	1969	2,520.1	841.6	657.3	407.3	237.4	138.6	84.9	54.0	99.0
1916-1920----------	1970	2,574.0	851.0	672.0	420.3	245.7	142.9	87.1	55.1	99.9
1917-1921----------	1971	2,633.5	861.5	687.5	434.5	254.9	147.8	89.7	56.4	101.2
1918-1922----------	1972	2,689.9	870.7	701.5	448.3	263.9	152.8	92.5	57.8	102.4
1919-1923----------	1973	2,749.3	880.1	715.5	462.8	273.7	158.4	95.6	59.3	103.9
1920-1924----------	1974	2,804.2	886.9	728.0	476.8	283.6	164.1	98.8	60.9	105.1

TABLE 5B. CUMULATIVE BIRTH RATES FOR WHITE WOMEN AS OF THE BEGINNING OF EACH YEAR 1917-74 BY AGE AND LIVE-BIRTH ORDER FOR GROUPS OF COHORTS FROM 1867-71 TO 1955-59

(RATES ARE SIMPLE AVERAGES OF THE RATES FOR SINGLE COHORTS IN TABLE 6B)

EXACT AGE AND COHORT	AS OF JANUARY 1	TOTAL	LIVE-BIRTH ORDER							
			1	2	3	4	5	6	7	8 AND HIGHER
15-19 YEARS										
1898-1902----------	1917	54.6	47.0	6.9	0.7	0.0	*	*	*	*
1899-1903----------	1918	54.9	47.3	6.9	0.7	0.0	*	*	*	*
1900-1904----------	1919	54.3	46.7	6.9	0.7	0.0	*	*	*	*
1901-1905----------	1920	49.8	42.5	6.6	0.7	0.0	*	*	*	*
1902-1906----------	1921	54.4	47.2	6.5	0.7	0.0	*	*	*	*
1903-1907----------	1922	59.8	52.2	6.9	0.7	0.0	*	*	*	*
1904-1908----------	1923	59.2	50.9	7.5	0.7	0.1	*	*	*	*
1905-1909----------	1924	57.9	49.2	7.8	0.8	0.1	*	*	*	*
1906-1910----------	1925	58.6	50.2	7.5	0.8	0.1	*	*	*	*
1907-1911----------	1926	58.5	50.2	7.4	0.8	0.1	*	*	*	*
1908-1912----------	1927	58.0	49.5	7.6	0.8	0.1	*	*	*	*
1909-1913----------	1928	57.9	49.4	7.6	0.8	0.1	*	*	*	*
1910-1914----------	1929	56.6	48.4	7.3	0.8	0.1	*	*	*	*
1911-1915----------	1930	55.2	47.3	7.1	0.7	0.1	*	*	*	*
1912-1916----------	1931	55.6	47.8	7.0	0.7	0.1	*	*	*	*
1913-1917----------	1932	53.7	46.1	6.8	0.7	0.1	*	*	*	*
1914-1918----------	1933	51.0	44.0	6.4	0.6	0.0	*	*	*	*
1915-1919----------	1934	47.7	41.2	5.9	0.6	0.0	*	*	*	*
1916-1920----------	1935	47.2	41.1	5.6	0.5	0.0	*	*	*	*
1917-1921----------	1936	47.6	41.7	5.4	0.5	0.0	*	*	*	*
1918-1922----------	1937	47.6	41.5	5.6	0.5	0.0	*	*	*	*
1919-1923----------	1938	49.0	42.5	5.9	0.6	0.0	*	*	*	*
1920-1924----------	1939	50.5	43.8	6.1	0.6	0.0	*	*	*	*
1921-1925----------	1940	50.0	43.0	6.3	0.7	0.0	*	*	*	*
1922-1926----------	1941	49.3	41.7	6.7	0.8	0.1	*	*	*	*
1923-1927----------	1942	50.5	42.9	6.7	0.8	0.1	*	*	*	*
1924-1928----------	1943	53.5	45.7	6.9	0.8	0.1	*	*	*	*
1925-1929----------	1944	54.7	46.5	7.2	0.9	0.1	*	*	*	*
1926-1930----------	1945	51.1	43.4	6.8	0.8	0.1	*	*	*	*
1927-1931----------	1946	47.3	40.5	6.0	0.7	0.1	*	*	*	*
1928-1932----------	1947	49.6	42.7	6.2	0.7	0.0	*	*	*	*
1929-1933----------	1948	62.4	54.6	7.0	0.8	0.0	*	*	*	*
1930-1934----------	1949	70.7	61.0	8.7	0.9	0.1	*	*	*	*
1931-1935----------	1950	75.4	63.4	10.7	1.2	0.1	*	*	*	*
1932-1936----------	1951	76.7	63.6	11.6	1.4	0.1	*	*	*	*
1933-1937----------	1952	80.7	66.8	12.3	1.5	0.1	*	*	*	*
1934-1938----------	1953	82.1	67.6	12.7	1.6	0.2	*	*	*	*
1935-1939----------	1954	83.7	68.8	13.1	1.7	0.1	*	*	*	*
1936-1940----------	1955	85.7	70.4	13.4	1.7	0.2	*	*	*	*
1937-1941----------	1956	86.6	70.8	13.8	1.8	0.2	*	*	*	*
1938-1942----------	1957	90.1	73.3	14.7	1.9	0.2	*	*	*	*
1939-1943----------	1958	93.8	76.1	15.4	2.1	0.2	*	*	*	*
1940-1944----------	1959	93.8	75.5	15.9	2.2	0.2	*	*	*	*
1941-1945----------	1960	92.1	73.7	15.9	2.3	0.2	*	*	*	*
1942-1946----------	1961	89.0	71.0	15.5	2.3	0.2	*	*	*	*
1943-1947----------	1962	86.5	69.1	15.0	2.2	0.2	*	*	*	*
1944-1948----------	1963	83.6	66.7	14.5	2.2	0.2	*	*	*	*
1945-1949----------	1964	80.4	64.4	13.7	2.1	0.2	*	*	*	*
1946-1950----------	1965	76.0	61.6	12.4	1.8	0.2	*	*	*	*
1947-1951----------	1966	71.1	58.7	10.7	1.5	0.2	*	*	*	*
1948-1952----------	1967	67.9	57.2	9.4	1.2	0.1	*	*	*	*
1949-1953----------	1968	65.0	55.2	8.7	1.0	0.1	*	*	*	*
1950-1954----------	1969	63.7	54.7	8.0	0.9	0.1	*	*	*	*
1951-1955----------	1970	63.8	55.1	7.8	0.8	0.1	*	*	*	*
1952-1956----------	1971	66.3	57.6	7.8	0.8	0.1	*	*	*	*
1953-1957----------	1972	66.6	58.0	7.7	0.8	0.1	*	*	*	*
1954-1958----------	1973	66.2	58.3	7.2	0.7	0.0	*	*	*	*
1955-1959----------	1974	66.1	58.4	7.0	0.7	0.0	*	*	*	*

TABLE 5B. CUMULATIVE BIRTH RATES FOR WHITE WOMEN AS OF THE BEGINNING OF EACH YEAR 1917-74 BY AGE AND LIVE-BIRTH ORDER FOR GROUPS OF COHORTS FROM 1867-71 TO 1955-59--CON.

(RATES ARE SIMPLE AVERAGES OF THE RATES FOR SINGLE COHORTS IN TABLE 6B)

EXACT AGE AND COHORT	AS OF JANUARY 1	TOTAL	LIVE-BIRTH ORDER							
			1	2	3	4	5	6	7	8 AND HIGHER
20-24 YEARS										
1893-1897----------	1917	567.4	350.8	148.1	50.6	14.0	3.1	0.7	0.1	0.0
1894-1898----------	1918	574.4	356.6	149.8	50.6	13.4	3.0	0.7	0.2	0.1
1895-1899----------	1919	579.6	361.6	150.5	50.5	13.2	2.8	0.7	0.2	0.1
1896-1900----------	1920	562.0	347.1	148.8	49.5	12.9	2.7	0.7	0.2	0.1
1897-1901----------	1921	564.1	353.1	145.9	48.6	12.8	2.7	0.7	0.2	0.1
1898-1902----------	1922	571.5	363.3	143.4	47.9	13.0	2.9	0.7	0.2	0.1
1899-1903----------	1923	570.5	364.5	144.0	45.7	12.5	2.8	0.7	0.2	0.1
1900-1904----------	1924	572.6	364.4	146.9	45.2	12.3	2.8	0.7	0.2	0.1
1901-1905----------	1925	578.8	367.9	148.5	46.3	12.2	2.8	0.7	0.3	0.1
1902-1906----------	1926	579.3	368.0	147.9	47.1	12.4	2.8	0.7	0.3	0.1
1903-1907----------	1927	573.4	364.2	146.1	46.5	12.7	2.9	0.7	0.2	0.1
1904-1908----------	1928	564.5	359.0	143.2	45.5	12.8	2.9	0.7	0.3	0.1
1905-1909----------	1929	550.4	351.4	139.0	44.0	12.2	2.8	0.7	0.2	0.1
1906-1910----------	1930	535.0	342.7	134.9	42.3	11.5	2.6	0.7	0.2	0.1
1907-1911----------	1931	524.3	337.2	131.6	41.0	11.1	2.5	0.6	0.2	0.1
1908-1912----------	1932	510.1	329.6	127.6	39.2	10.6	2.3	0.6	0.1	0.1
1909-1913----------	1933	494.8	320.7	123.6	37.4	10.1	2.2	0.6	0.1	0.1
1910-1914----------	1934	475.8	309.9	118.3	35.5	9.4	2.0	0.5	0.1	0.1
1911-1915----------	1935	466.1	305.6	114.8	34.2	9.0	1.9	0.5	0.1	0.0
1912-1916----------	1936	459.0	304.6	110.6	32.7	8.6	1.9	0.5	0.1	0.0
1913-1917----------	1937	454.5	304.2	108.3	31.2	8.3	1.8	0.5	0.1	0.1
1914-1918----------	1938	454.2	305.5	107.9	30.5	8.0	1.7	0.5	0.1	0.0
1915-1919----------	1939	459.0	309.0	109.4	30.5	7.8	1.7	0.5	0.1	0.0
1916-1920----------	1940	459.8	309.4	110.1	30.5	7.6	1.7	0.4	0.1	0.0
1917-1921----------	1941	465.0	310.8	112.4	31.5	7.9	1.8	0.5	0.1	0.0
1918-1922----------	1942	477.7	319.2	115.4	32.5	8.1	1.8	0.5	0.1	0.1
1919-1923----------	1943	505.8	340.5	120.5	33.8	8.5	1.9	0.5	0.1	0.0
1920-1924----------	1944	523.5	349.7	126.4	35.7	9.1	2.0	0.5	0.1	0.0
1921-1925----------	1945	522.1	347.5	125.7	36.6	9.6	2.1	0.5	0.1	0.0
1922-1926----------	1946	505.7	339.8	119.2	34.7	9.3	2.1	0.5	0.1	0.0
1923-1927----------	1947	529.6	357.8	125.7	34.3	9.2	2.0	0.5	0.1	0.0
1924-1928----------	1948	578.4	396.8	135.1	35.1	8.8	2.0	0.5	0.1	0.0
1925-1929----------	1949	611.6	415.8	147.3	37.1	8.8	2.0	0.5	0.1	0.0
1926-1930----------	1950	641.4	426.1	162.0	40.9	9.6	2.1	0.6	0.1	0.0
1927-1931----------	1951	664.1	429.7	174.8	46.1	10.6	2.3	0.5	0.1	0.0
1928-1932----------	1952	696.1	440.9	187.5	52.3	12.2	2.5	0.6	0.1	0.0
1929-1933----------	1953	727.8	452.6	199.4	58.0	14.2	2.9	0.6	0.1	0.0
1930-1934----------	1954	757.7	462.7	211.6	63.3	15.9	3.3	0.7	0.2	0.0
1931-1935----------	1955	788.3	474.6	222.6	68.7	17.7	3.8	0.8	0.1	0.0
1932-1936----------	1956	813.6	484.1	231.9	73.3	19.1	4.2	0.9	0.1	0.0
1933-1937----------	1957	840.4	495.0	241.1	78.0	20.6	4.5	1.0	0.2	0.0
1934-1938----------	1958	864.8	504.5	249.7	82.5	21.9	4.8	1.1	0.2	0.1
1935-1939----------	1959	880.6	509.4	256.2	85.5	23.0	5.1	1.1	0.2	0.1
1936-1940----------	1960	893.9	511.7	262.3	89.0	24.1	5.4	1.2	0.2	0.0
1937-1941----------	1961	901.5	510.8	265.7	92.3	25.3	5.7	1.3	0.3	0.1
1938-1942----------	1962	899.7	506.5	265.1	94.1	26.4	5.9	1.3	0.3	0.1
1939-1943----------	1963	885.0	496.9	260.0	93.5	26.6	6.2	1.4	0.3	0.1
1940-1944----------	1964	858.3	484.4	251.2	89.7	25.4	5.9	1.3	0.3	0.1
1941-1945----------	1965	823.1	471.5	238.5	83.1	23.1	5.4	1.2	0.2	0.1
1942-1946----------	1966	774.3	454.6	221.0	73.2	19.8	4.5	1.0	0.2	0.0
1943-1947----------	1967	727.3	441.0	202.7	62.7	16.4	3.6	0.8	0.1	0.0
1944-1948----------	1968	685.2	426.6	187.2	54.1	13.7	2.9	0.6	0.1	0.0
1945-1949----------	1969	648.5	414.3	172.9	46.7	11.5	2.4	0.6	0.1	0.0
1946-1950----------	1970	621.7	405.1	162.4	41.6	9.9	2.0	0.5	0.1	0.1
1947-1951----------	1971	603.7	399.3	155.4	38.2	8.6	1.7	0.4	0.0	0.1
1948-1952----------	1972	580.2	388.2	147.7	35.0	7.5	1.5	0.3	0.0	0.0
1949-1953----------	1973	546.3	370.4	137.4	30.7	6.4	1.2	0.2	0.0	0.0
1950-1954----------	1974	514.0	352.5	128.0	27.0	5.3	1.0	0.2	0.0	0.0

TABLE 5B. CUMULATIVE BIRTH RATES FOR WHITE WOMEN AS OF THE BEGINNING OF EACH YEAR 1917-74 BY AGE AND LIVE-BIRTH ORDER FOR GROUPS OF COHORTS FROM 1867-71 TO 1955-59--CON.

(RATES ARE SIMPLE AVERAGES OF THE RATES FOR SINGLE COHORTS IN TABLE 6B)

EXACT AGE AND COHORT	AS OF JANUARY 1	TOTAL	LIVE-BIRTH ORDER							
			1	2	3	4	5	6	7	8 AND HIGHER
25-29 YEARS										
1888-1892----------	1917	1,421.4	617.6	398.6	220.8	110.0	47.6	18.0	6.0	2.8
1889-1893----------	1918	1,427.2	623.3	400.9	220.8	108.8	46.9	17.8	5.9	2.8
1890-1894----------	1919	1,432.3	630.6	402.3	220.2	107.6	46.0	17.3	5.6	2.7
1891-1895----------	1920	1,421.7	627.9	401.3	217.4	105.5	44.8	16.7	5.5	2.6
1892-1896----------	1921	1,419.8	633.4	399.7	214.8	103.7	44.0	16.2	5.4	2.6
1893-1897----------	1922	1,421.0	640.5	397.0	212.6	102.5	43.8	16.5	5.5	2.6
1894-1898----------	1923	1,414.0	643.3	395.7	208.0	100.0	42.6	16.2	5.5	2.7
1895-1899----------	1924	1,407.4	643.4	395.2	204.1	97.9	42.1	16.2	5.6	2.9
1896-1900----------	1925	1,400.0	642.9	393.6	201.5	95.8	41.5	16.2	5.6	2.9
1897-1901----------	1926	1,388.1	641.3	390.4	198.7	93.4	40.3	15.7	5.4	2.9
1898-1902----------	1927	1,375.6	639.3	386.4	195.5	91.6	39.1	15.3	5.4	3.0
1899-1903----------	1928	1,363.3	637.4	381.6	192.3	90.5	38.5	15.0	5.2	2.8
1900-1904----------	1929	1,346.6	634.9	375.6	188.0	88.4	37.5	14.5	5.0	2.7
1901-1905----------	1930	1,325.2	630.9	368.8	182.7	85.6	36.2	13.8	4.7	2.5
1902-1906----------	1931	1,304.5	626.2	362.2	177.7	83.0	35.1	13.3	4.5	2.5
1903-1907----------	1932	1,276.3	617.7	354.0	171.7	79.7	33.7	12.8	4.4	2.3
1904-1908----------	1933	1,241.4	605.3	344.0	165.3	76.3	32.0	12.2	4.1	2.2
1905-1909----------	1934	1,200.9	590.1	333.1	158.3	72.4	29.9	11.3	3.8	2.0
1906-1910----------	1935	1,167.8	577.6	324.1	152.5	69.3	28.4	10.6	3.5	1.8
1907-1911----------	1936	1,138.4	568.3	315.3	146.4	66.1	27.0	10.1	3.4	1.8
1908-1912----------	1937	1,112.5	561.9	307.1	140.4	63.0	25.5	9.7	3.2	1.7
1909-1913----------	1938	1,095.5	560.0	301.2	135.3	60.3	24.4	9.4	3.2	1.7
1910-1914----------	1939	1,088.1	562.7	298.5	131.7	58.1	23.4	9.0	3.1	1.6
1911-1915----------	1940	1,084.8	567.1	297.8	128.8	55.9	22.3	8.6	2.8	1.5
1912-1916----------	1941	1,088.1	572.8	299.4	127.4	54.4	21.6	8.3	2.8	1.4
1913-1917----------	1942	1,101.3	583.1	303.4	127.4	53.8	21.3	8.1	2.8	1.4
1914-1918----------	1943	1,132.4	603.1	313.0	129.4	53.8	21.1	7.9	2.7	1.4
1915-1919----------	1944	1,172.2	618.6	329.1	135.1	55.4	21.7	8.1	2.8	1.4
1916-1920----------	1945	1,197.2	625.5	339.6	140.3	57.0	22.3	8.3	2.8	1.4
1917-1921----------	1946	1,212.2	629.9	346.2	143.2	57.8	22.5	8.4	2.8	1.4
1918-1922----------	1947	1,254.5	652.4	360.7	146.9	59.0	22.8	8.5	2.8	1.4
1919-1923----------	1948	1,313.1	685.9	380.0	152.0	59.6	22.8	8.5	2.9	1.4
1920-1924----------	1949	1,354.3	705.8	396.7	156.7	59.7	22.7	8.4	2.9	1.4
1921-1925----------	1950	1,394.7	719.7	415.5	163.1	60.8	22.6	8.5	3.0	1.5
1922-1926----------	1951	1,432.4	727.9	434.8	171.5	62.5	22.7	8.5	3.0	1.5
1923-1927----------	1952	1,480.6	737.8	456.0	183.5	66.4	23.7	8.7	3.0	1.5
1924-1928----------	1953	1,532.3	746.1	477.0	198.4	71.9	25.4	9.0	3.0	1.5
1925-1929----------	1954	1,583.0	751.9	496.8	213.8	78.6	27.6	9.6	3.1	1.6
1926-1930----------	1955	1,637.1	757.7	516.3	230.6	86.5	30.4	10.5	3.4	1.7
1927-1931----------	1956	1,694.1	765.2	535.2	248.1	95.0	33.6	11.5	3.7	1.8
1928-1932----------	1957	1,755.5	774.7	554.5	266.2	104.0	37.1	12.8	4.2	2.0
1929-1933----------	1958	1,822.1	786.6	574.7	284.9	113.9	40.9	14.2	4.7	2.2
1930-1934----------	1959	1,881.5	796.9	592.3	301.4	123.0	44.7	15.6	5.2	2.4
1931-1935----------	1960	1,933.9	804.8	606.9	316.4	131.9	48.3	17.1	5.8	2.7
1932-1936----------	1961	1,974.5	809.4	617.5	329.1	139.7	51.4	18.3	6.2	2.9
1933-1937----------	1962	2,003.5	811.4	623.8	338.6	146.0	54.6	19.4	6.6	3.1
1934-1938----------	1963	2,015.8	810.3	625.3	343.6	149.9	56.5	20.2	6.8	3.2
1935-1939----------	1964	2,014.3	807.4	623.5	344.5	151.2	57.2	20.4	6.9	3.2
1936-1940----------	1965	1,999.8	803.9	618.8	341.3	149.4	56.5	20.1	6.7	3.1
1937-1941----------	1966	1,957.4	796.6	607.7	330.2	142.2	53.0	18.7	6.2	2.8
1938-1942----------	1967	1,892.9	787.7	591.4	311.7	130.3	47.5	16.5	5.4	2.4
1939-1943----------	1968	1,816.7	776.5	572.0	289.4	116.5	41.5	14.1	4.6	2.1
1940-1944----------	1969	1,736.6	765.4	550.8	265.4	102.4	35.3	11.8	3.8	1.7
1941-1945----------	1970	1,660.6	752.3	529.9	243.4	90.3	30.3	9.9	3.1	1.4
1942-1946----------	1971	1,592.9	740.1	510.3	224.2	80.3	26.0	8.3	2.6	1.1
1943-1947----------	1972	1,522.1	726.1	488.2	204.7	70.8	22.3	7.0	2.1	0.9
1944-1948----------	1973	1,444.4	709.5	464.2	183.3	60.8	18.6	5.7	1.6	0.7
1945-1949----------	1974	1,367.2	690.3	440.7	163.0	51.5	15.2	4.6	1.3	0.6

TABLE 5B. CUMULATIVE BIRTH RATES FOR WHITE WOMEN AS OF THE BEGINNING OF EACH YEAR 1917-74 BY AGE AND LIVE-BIRTH ORDER FOR GROUPS OF COHORTS FROM 1867-71 TO 1955-59--CON.

(RATES ARE SIMPLE AVERAGES OF THE RATES FOR SINGLE COHORTS IN TABLE 6B)

EXACT AGE AND COHORT	AS OF JANUARY 1	TOTAL	LIVE-BIRTH ORDER							
			1	2	3	4	5	6	7	8 AND HIGHER
30-34 YEARS										
1883-1887----------	1917	2,235.1	726.8	558.2	383.7	250.3	153.6	86.1	44.0	32.4
1884-1888----------	1918	2,224.3	728.0	557.3	382.0	247.7	151.0	84.7	42.6	31.0
1885-1889----------	1919	2,217.0	731.0	557.2	380.2	245.0	148.5	83.4	41.5	30.2
1886-1890----------	1920	2,207.5	732.8	557.8	378.2	241.9	145.4	81.7	40.2	29.5
1887-1891----------	1921	2,202.1	736.9	559.3	376.4	238.9	142.7	79.8	39.1	29.0
1888-1892----------	1922	2,200.5	742.2	561.1	374.4	236.4	140.4	78.4	38.5	29.1
1889-1893----------	1923	2,190.0	747.4	561.7	370.4	231.6	136.9	76.2	37.4	28.4
1890-1894----------	1924	2,178.2	752.0	561.2	365.8	226.5	133.6	74.3	36.6	28.2
1891-1895----------	1925	2,164.6	756.0	559.7	361.1	221.2	130.3	72.5	35.9	27.9
1892-1896----------	1926	2,146.5	759.2	557.3	355.3	215.3	126.5	70.5	35.0	27.4
1893-1897----------	1927	2,124.3	760.8	554.4	348.8	209.2	122.1	68.3	34.0	26.7
1894-1898----------	1928	2,102.2	761.4	551.2	342.2	203.4	118.1	66.4	33.2	26.3
1895-1899----------	1929	2,074.4	759.9	546.4	334.9	197.4	114.1	64.1	32.0	25.6
1896-1900----------	1930	2,040.4	756.5	539.6	326.8	191.0	109.9	61.5	30.6	24.5
1897-1901----------	1931	2,007.9	753.6	532.4	318.8	185.1	106.1	59.2	29.2	23.5
1898-1902----------	1932	1,974.4	750.8	524.7	310.7	179.2	102.2	56.7	27.8	22.3
1899-1903----------	1933	1,941.1	747.8	516.5	302.5	173.3	98.6	54.5	26.6	21.3
1900-1904----------	1934	1,902.4	743.8	506.8	293.4	167.3	94.3	51.7	25.2	19.9
1901-1905----------	1935	1,865.9	739.4	498.0	284.8	161.6	90.3	49.1	23.9	18.8
1902-1906----------	1936	1,826.6	733.5	488.6	275.8	155.5	86.1	46.5	22.6	18.0
1903-1907----------	1937	1,785.1	725.8	479.0	266.7	149.1	81.9	43.9	21.5	17.2
1904-1908----------	1938	1,741.3	716.9	468.9	257.2	142.4	77.6	41.5	20.3	16.5
1905-1909----------	1939	1,701.5	709.2	460.2	248.4	135.8	73.6	39.3	19.3	15.7
1906-1910----------	1940	1,666.5	703.6	453.1	240.4	129.7	69.6	37.1	18.2	14.8
1907-1911----------	1941	1,642.4	701.4	449.3	234.1	124.6	66.2	35.3	17.3	14.2
1908-1912----------	1942	1,627.5	703.5	447.7	229.1	120.4	63.3	33.6	16.4	13.5
1909-1913----------	1943	1,629.8	712.4	451.3	227.0	117.4	61.0	32.1	15.7	12.9
1910-1914----------	1944	1,648.3	722.9	461.1	229.2	116.4	59.8	31.2	15.2	12.5
1911-1915----------	1945	1,672.7	732.2	472.9	234.0	116.6	59.1	30.7	14.9	12.3
1912-1916----------	1946	1,700.8	740.3	487.3	240.2	117.5	58.7	30.2	14.6	12.0
1913-1917----------	1947	1,742.0	754.1	505.2	248.5	119.5	58.8	29.9	14.3	11.7
1914-1918----------	1948	1,788.7	771.1	524.0	257.6	121.8	59.1	29.6	14.1	11.4
1915-1919----------	1949	1,830.4	785.0	541.2	266.1	124.0	59.4	29.4	14.0	11.3
1916-1920----------	1950	1,872.2	798.3	558.2	274.6	126.6	59.8	29.4	13.9	11.4
1917-1921----------	1951	1,917.9	811.4	576.5	284.8	129.9	60.4	29.4	14.0	11.5
1918-1922----------	1952	1,967.2	824.3	595.2	296.8	134.2	61.4	29.6	14.1	11.6
1919-1923----------	1953	2,025.0	837.6	615.3	312.0	140.6	63.2	30.2	14.3	11.8
1920-1924----------	1954	2,080.7	847.9	633.9	328.3	147.9	65.7	30.8	14.4	11.8
1921-1925----------	1955	2,138.1	855.6	652.2	345.9	156.9	68.9	31.9	14.7	12.0
1922-1926----------	1956	2,192.8	860.1	668.2	363.8	166.8	73.1	33.5	15.2	12.1
1923-1927----------	1957	2,250.8	863.8	683.3	382.6	178.4	78.4	35.7	16.0	12.6
1924-1928----------	1958	2,308.6	865.8	696.7	401.9	191.1	84.5	38.2	17.1	13.3
1925-1929----------	1959	2,364.5	866.8	708.4	420.6	204.2	90.9	41.1	18.3	14.2
1926-1930----------	1960	2,422.4	868.1	719.8	439.0	218.1	98.0	44.3	19.7	15.4
1927-1931----------	1961	2,485.7	871.5	732.1	457.6	232.5	105.8	48.1	21.4	16.7
1928-1932----------	1962	2,550.8	876.1	744.5	475.9	247.0	113.8	52.0	23.3	18.2
1929-1933----------	1963	2,612.0	881.7	756.1	492.2	260.2	121.4	55.8	25.1	19.5
1930-1934----------	1964	2,662.4	886.6	765.5	505.5	271.1	127.7	59.0	26.5	20.5
1931-1935----------	1965	2,699.4	891.1	772.0	515.4	279.1	132.2	61.1	27.5	21.0
1932-1936----------	1966	2,711.2	892.9	774.6	519.5	281.8	133.4	61.3	27.2	20.5
1933-1937----------	1967	2,700.1	893.1	773.5	517.9	279.3	131.2	59.6	26.2	19.3
1934-1938----------	1968	2,669.0	891.1	769.7	511.6	272.3	126.1	56.4	24.3	17.5
1935-1939----------	1969	2,623.7	889.1	763.9	500.8	261.5	118.8	52.0	22.1	15.5
1936-1940----------	1970	2,570.4	886.0	756.9	487.6	248.6	110.5	47.5	19.8	13.5
1937-1941----------	1971	2,508.7	882.0	748.0	471.4	233.7	101.6	42.8	17.5	11.7
1938-1942----------	1972	2,434.2	876.4	736.7	450.3	216.2	91.6	37.8	15.2	10.0
1939-1943----------	1973	2,345.5	868.6	722.5	424.1	196.2	80.7	32.4	12.8	8.2
1940-1944----------	1974	2,247.3	858.5	705.2	394.8	175.0	69.5	27.2	10.5	6.6

TABLE 5B. CUMULATIVE BIRTH RATES FOR WHITE WOMEN AS OF THE BEGINNING OF EACH YEAR 1917-74 BY AGE AND LIVE-BIRTH ORDER FOR GROUPS OF COHORTS FROM 1867-71 TO 1955-59--CON.

(RATES ARE SIMPLE AVERAGES OF THE RATES FOR SINGLE COHORTS IN TABLE 6B)

EXACT AGE AND COHORT	AS OF JANUARY 1	TOTAL	LIVE-BIRTH ORDER							
			1	2	3	4	5	6	7	8 AND HIGHER
35-39 YEARS										
1878-1882----------	1917	2,928.2	765.0	630.7	480.7	354.6	254.7	177.6	115.6	149.2
1879-1883----------	1918	2,898.0	765.1	628.8	476.8	350.0	250.2	173.2	112.6	141.3
1880-1884----------	1919	2,870.5	765.7	627.5	473.1	345.6	245.7	168.8	109.5	134.6
1881-1885----------	1920	2,842.6	766.2	626.2	469.2	340.6	240.7	164.2	106.3	129.2
1882-1886----------	1921	2,817.6	767.1	624.7	465.7	335.9	236.0	160.1	103.2	124.9
1883-1887----------	1922	2,798.7	768.7	623.3	463.0	332.0	231.7	156.9	100.6	122.5
1884-1888----------	1923	2,779.4	770.5	622.6	460.4	327.7	227.1	153.5	97.7	119.9
1885-1889----------	1924	2,762.7	772.9	622.9	458.1	323.4	222.3	150.0	95.0	118.1
1886-1890----------	1925	2,749.8	776.2	624.3	456.2	319.3	217.8	146.7	92.6	116.7
1887-1891----------	1926	2,734.9	780.0	625.9	453.8	314.9	212.9	142.9	89.9	114.6
1888-1892----------	1927	2,715.6	784.2	627.1	450.3	309.5	207.5	138.6	87.0	111.4
1889-1893----------	1928	2,691.7	788.4	626.7	445.2	303.0	201.6	134.2	84.2	108.4
1890-1894----------	1929	2,661.1	792.3	624.9	438.9	295.4	195.2	129.3	81.1	104.0
1891-1895----------	1930	2,624.5	795.3	621.6	431.2	286.8	188.5	124.3	77.7	99.1
1892-1896----------	1931	2,586.3	797.8	617.9	422.9	278.0	181.7	119.4	74.3	94.3
1893-1897----------	1932	2,545.6	799.0	613.7	414.0	269.0	174.8	114.5	70.9	89.7
1894-1898----------	1933	2,504.7	799.0	609.0	405.1	260.2	168.2	109.9	67.8	85.5
1895-1899----------	1934	2,461.1	797.0	603.2	395.7	251.9	161.8	105.6	64.8	81.1
1896-1900----------	1935	2,415.4	793.5	595.7	386.0	243.9	155.8	101.5	61.9	77.1
1897-1901----------	1936	2,369.3	790.0	587.5	376.1	235.8	149.9	97.2	59.0	73.8
1898-1902----------	1937	2,323.7	787.2	579.2	366.3	227.9	143.9	92.8	56.1	70.3
1899-1903----------	1938	2,279.9	785.3	571.2	356.6	220.1	137.9	88.3	53.3	67.2
1900-1904----------	1939	2,236.2	783.8	563.3	346.9	212.4	131.9	83.6	50.4	63.9
1901-1905----------	1940	2,192.1	782.1	555.9	337.2	204.7	125.7	78.9	47.4	60.2
1902-1906----------	1941	2,148.5	779.0	549.0	327.9	197.0	119.7	74.5	44.6	56.8
1903-1907----------	1942	2,107.0	774.9	542.9	319.4	189.7	114.0	70.4	42.0	53.7
1904-1908----------	1943	2,068.3	770.6	537.5	311.5	182.7	108.7	66.8	39.7	50.8
1905-1909----------	1944	2,040.0	767.6	535.2	306.1	177.0	104.2	63.6	37.8	48.5
1906-1910----------	1945	2,021.4	766.0	535.6	303.0	172.7	100.5	61.0	36.2	46.4
1907-1911----------	1946	2,016.2	767.2	539.7	303.0	170.0	97.8	59.0	34.9	44.6
1908-1912----------	1947	2,021.5	771.9	546.6	304.9	168.5	95.8	57.2	33.6	43.0
1909-1913----------	1948	2,038.9	780.8	556.5	309.3	168.4	94.2	55.7	32.5	41.5
1910-1914----------	1949	2,060.7	790.6	568.0	314.9	168.8	92.8	54.2	31.5	39.9
1911-1915----------	1950	2,090.3	801.8	581.9	322.0	170.2	92.0	53.1	30.5	38.8
1912-1916----------	1951	2,122.0	812.0	596.2	330.0	172.5	91.8	52.2	29.7	37.6
1913-1917----------	1952	2,158.8	821.5	611.6	339.7	176.2	92.3	51.8	29.1	36.6
1914-1918----------	1953	2,198.7	829.9	627.0	350.8	180.9	93.6	51.7	28.8	36.0
1915-1919----------	1954	2,245.5	839.5	643.3	363.4	187.2	95.8	52.0	28.8	35.5
1916-1920----------	1955	2,296.7	849.8	659.5	377.2	194.5	98.6	52.8	29.0	35.3
1917-1921----------	1956	2,353.9	861.0	676.3	392.4	203.0	102.1	54.1	29.5	35.5
1918-1922----------	1957	2,410.8	871.1	692.2	407.9	211.9	106.1	55.8	30.1	35.7
1919-1923----------	1958	2,472.9	881.6	708.3	424.4	222.3	111.0	58.0	30.9	36.4
1920-1924----------	1959	2,530.6	889.4	722.2	440.3	232.9	116.4	60.5	32.0	36.9
1921-1925----------	1960	2,586.1	894.5	734.4	456.1	244.1	122.5	63.4	33.3	37.8
1922-1926----------	1961	2,637.3	896.7	744.9	471.0	255.5	128.9	66.5	34.8	39.0
1923-1927----------	1962	2,690.9	898.3	754.8	486.4	267.4	136.1	70.4	36.7	40.8
1924-1928----------	1963	2,739.5	898.0	762.8	500.7	279.1	143.3	74.2	38.6	42.8
1925-1929----------	1964	2,787.7	896.9	770.2	514.8	291.1	150.6	78.4	40.6	45.1
1926-1930----------	1965	2,837.1	896.9	777.8	528.8	303.3	157.9	82.4	42.8	47.2
1927-1931----------	1966	2,888.0	899.2	786.3	542.8	315.1	165.0	86.1	44.6	48.9
1928-1932----------	1967	2,934.0	902.8	795.1	555.7	325.4	170.9	88.9	45.9	49.3
1929-1933----------	1968	2,973.5	907.5	803.6	567.0	334.0	175.3	90.8	46.5	48.8
1930-1934----------	1969	2,998.5	912.0	810.4	575.0	339.3	177.3	91.2	46.1	47.2
1931-1935----------	1970	3,007.1	915.1	814.5	579.3	341.1	177.1	90.1	45.1	44.8
1932-1936----------	1971	2,995.7	916.1	815.5	579.3	338.7	174.2	87.4	43.0	41.5
1933-1937----------	1972	2,967.1	915.6	813.7	574.9	332.5	168.8	83.4	40.3	37.9
1934-1938----------	1973	2,920.5	913.5	809.6	566.3	322.0	160.6	77.9	36.9	33.7
1935-1939----------	1974	2,860.9	910.9	804.1	553.7	308.0	150.3	71.4	33.2	29.3

TABLE 5B. CUMULATIVE BIRTH RATES FOR WHITE WOMEN AS OF THE BEGINNING OF EACH YEAR 1917-74 BY AGE AND LIVE-BIRTH ORDER FOR GROUPS OF COHORTS FROM 1867-71 TO 1955-59--CON.

(RATES ARE SIMPLE AVERAGES OF THE RATES FOR SINGLE COHORTS IN TABLE 6B)

EXACT AGE AND COHORT	AS OF JANUARY 1	TOTAL	LIVE-BIRTH ORDER							
			1	2	3	4	5	6	7	8 AND HIGHER
40-44 YEARS										
1873-1877----------	1917	3,465.3	783.9	666.8	534.0	417.5	320.8	243.4	177.3	321.6
1874-1878----------	1918	3,422.9	782.2	663.2	528.6	411.3	314.8	238.3	172.5	312.0
1875-1879----------	1919	3,381.5	780.5	659.7	523.5	405.5	309.2	233.3	167.9	301.9
1876-1880----------	1920	3,342.6	779.3	656.5	518.7	400.1	304.0	228.6	163.6	291.8
1877-1881----------	1921	3,306.3	778.6	653.8	514.2	395.0	298.9	223.9	159.7	282.2
1878-1882----------	1922	3,272.5	778.5	651.5	509.9	389.9	293.9	219.1	156.2	273.5
1879-1883----------	1923	3,236.8	778.8	649.6	505.8	384.8	288.6	213.6	152.3	263.3
1880-1884----------	1924	3,202.5	779.4	648.3	501.7	379.6	283.1	207.9	148.1	254.4
1881-1885----------	1925	3,169.1	780.1	647.1	497.8	374.2	277.3	202.1	143.7	246.8
1882-1886----------	1926	3,136.7	780.9	645.6	494.1	369.0	271.4	196.6	139.2	239.9
1883-1887----------	1927	3,106.5	782.1	643.8	490.8	364.1	265.8	191.8	134.9	233.2
1884-1888----------	1928	3,080.1	783.8	643.0	488.1	359.3	260.2	187.3	130.7	227.7
1885-1889----------	1929	3,053.5	786.1	643.0	485.2	354.2	254.4	182.4	126.6	221.6
1886-1890----------	1930	3,027.0	789.1	643.9	482.5	349.1	248.3	177.3	122.3	214.5
1887-1891----------	1931	3,000.2	792.6	645.0	479.4	343.5	242.1	172.1	118.2	207.3
1888-1892----------	1932	2,967.9	796.5	645.7	474.9	336.8	235.2	166.4	113.7	198.7
1889-1893----------	1933	2,929.8	800.4	644.8	468.7	328.9	227.9	160.3	109.2	189.6
1890-1894----------	1934	2,886.4	803.8	642.4	461.4	320.1	220.2	154.1	104.6	179.8
1891-1895----------	1935	2,840.6	806.6	638.7	453.1	310.8	212.5	148.0	100.1	170.8
1892-1896----------	1936	2,791.3	808.6	634.3	444.0	301.0	204.5	141.8	95.4	161.7
1893-1897----------	1937	2,740.4	809.4	629.7	434.4	291.0	196.5	135.7	90.8	152.9
1894-1898----------	1938	2,690.4	809.3	624.7	424.9	281.5	188.8	129.9	86.5	144.8
1895-1899----------	1939	2,641.8	807.7	619.3	415.5	272.6	181.7	124.7	82.5	137.8
1896-1900----------	1940	2,590.3	804.7	612.2	405.7	263.8	174.8	119.6	78.6	130.9
1897-1901----------	1941	2,538.4	801.9	604.4	395.7	255.1	168.0	114.3	74.6	124.4
1898-1902----------	1942	2,488.5	799.9	596.8	385.9	246.8	161.3	109.0	70.8	118.0
1899-1903----------	1943	2,441.6	799.0	590.1	376.5	238.7	154.8	103.6	67.1	111.8
1900-1904----------	1944	2,397.3	798.9	583.7	367.6	231.1	148.4	98.4	63.4	105.8
1901-1905----------	1945	2,356.3	798.7	578.3	359.4	224.0	142.2	93.3	60.0	100.4
1902-1906----------	1946	2,318.9	797.5	573.9	352.2	217.5	136.4	88.9	57.0	95.5
1903-1907----------	1947	2,285.6	795.3	571.0	346.4	211.5	131.3	84.8	54.3	91.0
1904-1908----------	1948	2,254.4	792.2	568.7	341.3	206.0	126.5	81.2	51.7	86.8
1905-1909----------	1949	2,228.3	789.7	568.2	337.7	201.1	122.2	77.7	49.3	82.4
1906-1910----------	1950	2,210.9	789.0	569.8	335.9	197.3	118.4	74.7	47.2	78.6
1907-1911----------	1951	2,204.7	791.0	574.2	336.2	194.9	115.6	72.2	45.4	75.2
1908-1912----------	1952	2,206.3	794.8	580.2	338.1	193.6	113.4	70.2	43.8	72.2
1909-1913----------	1953	2,219.3	801.3	588.8	342.5	194.0	112.0	68.7	42.5	69.5
1910-1914----------	1954	2,241.5	809.8	599.9	349.0	195.5	111.3	67.5	41.4	67.1
1911-1915----------	1955	2,273.8	820.0	613.5	357.6	198.7	111.6	66.9	40.4	65.1
1912-1916----------	1956	2,309.1	829.5	627.4	367.3	202.9	112.7	66.6	39.7	63.0
1913-1917----------	1957	2,349.3	838.2	642.2	378.4	208.4	114.5	66.6	39.4	61.6
1914-1918----------	1958	2,390.5	845.6	656.4	389.8	214.6	117.0	67.1	39.5	60.5
1915-1919----------	1959	2,438.7	854.3	671.6	402.6	221.9	120.2	68.3	39.9	59.9
1916-1920----------	1960	2,489.6	863.6	686.4	415.7	229.8	123.9	69.8	40.5	59.9
1917-1921----------	1961	2,546.3	873.9	701.6	430.1	238.7	128.3	71.9	41.5	60.3
1918-1922----------	1962	2,601.7	883.3	715.8	444.3	247.8	133.0	74.1	42.5	60.9
1919-1923----------	1963	2,660.5	892.9	730.1	459.1	257.7	138.3	76.8	43.7	61.9
1920-1924----------	1964	2,714.3	899.9	742.3	473.2	267.5	143.9	79.6	45.0	62.9
1921-1925----------	1965	2,765.0	904.4	753.1	487.1	277.4	149.7	82.6	46.5	64.2
1922-1926----------	1966	2,810.2	906.2	762.3	500.2	287.2	155.5	85.6	47.9	65.3
1923-1927----------	1967	2,854.8	907.3	770.7	513.3	297.2	161.4	88.9	49.4	66.6
1924-1928----------	1968	2,894.5	906.7	777.6	525.6	307.2	167.1	91.8	50.9	67.6
1925-1929----------	1969	2,932.0	905.6	783.8	537.6	317.1	172.7	94.8	52.2	68.2
1926-1930----------	1970	2,969.2	905.0	790.4	549.6	326.9	178.2	97.4	53.3	68.4
1927-1931----------	1971	3,008.6	906.7	798.1	561.8	336.5	183.5	99.8	54.2	68.0
1928-1932----------	1972	3,045.1	909.8	806.3	573.0	345.0	187.9	101.6	54.7	66.8
1929-1933----------	1973	3,075.6	914.2	814.2	582.8	351.9	190.9	102.4	54.6	64.6
1930-1934----------	1974	3,092.0	918.1	820.3	589.6	355.7	191.6	101.8	53.5	61.4

TABLE 5B. CUMULATIVE BIRTH RATES FOR WHITE WOMEN AS OF THE BEGINNING OF EACH YEAR 1917-74 BY AGE AND LIVE-BIRTH ORDER FOR GROUPS OF COHORTS FROM 1867-71 TO 1955-59--CON.

(RATES ARE SIMPLE AVERAGES OF THE RATES FOR SINGLE COHORTS IN TABLE 6B)

EXACT AGE AND COHORT	AS OF JANUARY 1	TOTAL	LIVE-BIRTH ORDER							
			1	2	3	4	5	6	7	8 AND HIGHER
45-49 YEARS										
1868-1872----------	1917	3,793.3	796.9	690.0	566.5	455.6	359.0	279.6	210.7	434.9
1869-1873----------	1918	3,747.3	794.7	686.2	561.2	449.6	353.2	274.4	206.2	421.8
1870-1874----------	1919	3,701.6	792.5	682.2	555.7	443.4	347.4	269.3	201.8	409.3
1871-1875----------	1920	3,655.3	790.2	678.1	550.1	437.0	341.4	264.1	197.3	397.1
1872-1876----------	1921	3,609.3	788.1	674.0	544.5	430.5	335.2	258.6	192.6	385.8
1873-1877----------	1922	3,563.8	786.2	670.1	538.9	424.1	328.9	252.9	187.5	375.2
1874-1878----------	1923	3,520.1	784.5	666.5	533.5	417.8	322.7	247.6	182.6	364.9
1875-1879----------	1924	3,477.6	782.9	663.0	528.4	412.0	317.0	242.5	177.8	354.0
1876-1880----------	1925	3,437.7	781.7	659.8	523.6	406.6	311.6	237.6	173.4	343.4
1877-1881----------	1926	3,399.3	781.0	657.0	519.0	401.3	306.4	232.6	169.3	332.7
1878-1882----------	1927	3,361.8	780.8	654.7	514.6	396.0	301.0	227.4	165.3	322.0
1879-1883----------	1928	3,323.8	781.1	652.8	510.3	390.8	295.6	221.6	161.0	310.6
1880-1884----------	1929	3,286.4	781.6	651.4	506.2	385.4	289.8	215.5	156.4	300.1
1881-1885----------	1930	3,248.6	782.3	650.1	502.2	379.6	283.6	209.3	151.4	290.1
1882-1886----------	1931	3,212.1	783.1	648.5	498.3	374.2	277.5	203.4	146.5	280.6
1883-1887----------	1932	3,178.8	784.2	646.6	494.9	369.1	271.7	198.4	141.9	272.0
1884-1888----------	1933	3,147.9	785.8	645.7	491.9	364.2	265.8	193.5	137.2	263.8
1885-1889----------	1934	3,118.1	788.0	645.6	489.0	358.9	259.8	188.4	132.8	255.6
1886-1890----------	1935	3,089.2	790.9	646.5	486.2	353.7	253.5	183.1	128.3	247.0
1887-1891----------	1936	3,059.3	794.4	647.5	482.9	347.9	247.1	177.6	123.9	238.0
1888-1892----------	1937	3,024.1	798.2	648.1	478.2	341.0	240.1	171.6	119.2	227.7
1889-1893----------	1938	2,982.8	802.0	647.0	471.9	333.0	232.4	165.3	114.4	216.8
1890-1894----------	1939	2,936.6	805.4	644.4	464.5	324.1	224.5	158.8	109.4	205.5
1891-1895----------	1940	2,888.0	808.2	640.7	456.1	314.7	216.7	152.4	104.6	194.6
1892-1896----------	1941	2,836.0	810.2	636.3	447.0	304.7	208.5	146.0	99.7	183.6
1893-1897----------	1942	2,782.8	811.0	631.8	437.4	294.6	200.3	139.6	94.8	173.3
1894-1898----------	1943	2,731.3	811.0	627.0	427.9	285.0	192.4	133.7	90.3	164.0
1895-1899----------	1944	2,681.6	809.7	621.7	418.5	276.1	185.3	128.4	86.1	155.8
1896-1900----------	1945	2,629.1	806.8	614.7	408.8	267.3	178.3	123.1	82.0	148.1
1897-1901----------	1946	2,577.5	804.2	607.2	399.0	258.8	171.6	117.8	78.0	140.9
1898-1902----------	1947	2,528.3	802.4	599.9	389.5	250.6	165.1	112.5	74.2	134.1
1899-1903----------	1948	2,482.8	801.8	593.6	380.7	242.8	158.7	107.3	70.4	127.5
1900-1904----------	1949	2,439.0	802.0	587.6	372.2	235.4	152.3	101.9	66.7	120.9
1901-1905----------	1950	2,397.5	802.0	582.5	364.2	228.4	146.1	96.7	63.1	114.5
1902-1906----------	1951	2,359.0	800.9	578.3	357.0	221.9	140.3	92.1	59.8	108.7
1903-1907----------	1952	2,324.8	798.8	575.4	351.3	216.0	135.1	87.9	57.0	103.3
1904-1908----------	1953	2,291.5	795.4	572.9	346.1	210.4	130.2	84.1	54.2	98.2
1905-1909----------	1954	2,265.0	792.8	572.4	342.5	205.6	126.0	80.6	51.8	93.3
1906-1910----------	1955	2,247.4	792.1	574.0	340.8	201.9	122.3	77.7	49.7	88.9
1907-1911----------	1956	2,241.7	794.0	578.5	341.4	199.8	119.7	75.3	47.9	85.1
1908-1912----------	1957	2,243.6	797.7	584.5	343.6	198.7	117.7	73.4	46.3	81.7
1909-1913----------	1958	2,257.1	804.1	593.1	348.2	199.4	116.5	72.0	45.0	78.8
1910-1914----------	1959	2,279.9	812.5	604.1	354.9	201.2	116.0	71.0	44.0	76.2
1911-1915----------	1960	2,312.2	822.6	617.6	363.5	204.5	116.5	70.5	43.1	73.9
1912-1916----------	1961	2,347.3	831.8	631.3	373.0	208.9	117.7	70.4	42.5	71.7
1913-1917----------	1962	2,387.2	840.4	645.9	383.9	214.5	119.6	70.6	42.3	70.0
1914-1918----------	1963	2,427.5	847.5	659.9	395.2	220.6	122.1	71.0	42.4	68.8
1915-1919----------	1964	2,475.5	856.1	674.9	407.8	227.9	125.4	72.2	42.9	68.3
1916-1920----------	1965	2,525.9	865.4	689.5	420.8	235.6	129.1	73.8	43.5	68.2
1917-1921----------	1966	2,581.8	875.6	704.5	434.9	244.4	133.4	75.9	44.5	68.6
1918-1922----------	1967	2,635.6	884.9	718.4	448.7	253.1	137.9	78.0	45.5	69.1
1919-1923----------	1968	2,692.6	894.4	732.4	463.2	262.7	143.0	80.6	46.6	69.7
1920-1924----------	1969	2,744.7	901.4	744.5	477.0	272.2	148.3	83.2	47.8	70.3
1921-1925----------	1970	2,793.1	905.8	755.1	490.6	281.8	153.8	85.9	49.1	71.0
1922-1926----------	1971	2,835.4	907.4	764.1	503.2	291.1	159.1	88.6	50.3	71.6
1923-1927----------	1972	2,877.9	908.5	772.4	516.0	300.8	164.7	91.6	51.6	72.3
1924-1928----------	1973	2,915.2	907.9	779.2	528.1	310.2	170.0	94.2	52.8	72.8
1925-1929----------	1974	2,950.9	906.6	785.3	539.9	319.8	175.5	96.9	53.9	73.0

TABLE 5B. CUMULATIVE BIRTH RATES FOR WHITE WOMEN AS OF THE BEGINNING OF EACH YEAR 1917-74 BY AGE AND LIVE-BIRTH ORDER FOR GROUPS OF COHORTS FROM 1867-71 TO 1955-59--CON.

(RATES ARE SIMPLE AVERAGES OF THE RATES FOR SINGLE COHORTS IN TABLE 6B)

EXACT AGE AND COHORT	AS OF JANUARY 1	TOTAL	LIVE-BIRTH ORDER							
			1	2	3	4	5	6	7	8 AND HIGHER
50-54 YEARS										
1863-1867----------	1917	---	---	---	---	---	---	---	---	---
1864-1868----------	1918	---	---	---	---	---	---	---	---	---
1865-1869----------	1919	---	---	---	---	---	---	---	---	---
1866-1870----------	1920	---	---	---	---	---	---	---	---	---
1867-1871----------	1921	3,848.1	799.1	694.0	572.0	462.1	365.4	285.4	216.0	454.1
1868-1872----------	1922	3,802.0	797.0	690.2	566.7	456.1	359.6	280.2	211.5	440.7
1869-1873----------	1923	3,755.8	794.8	686.3	561.4	450.1	353.7	275.0	206.9	427.6
1870-1874----------	1924	3,709.8	792.5	682.3	555.9	443.8	347.9	269.9	202.5	415.0
1871-1875----------	1925	3,663.6	790.3	678.2	550.3	437.4	341.9	264.7	198.0	402.8
1872-1876----------	1926	3,617.4	788.2	674.2	544.7	430.9	335.7	259.2	193.2	391.3
1873-1877----------	1927	3,571.3	786.3	670.3	539.1	424.4	329.3	253.5	188.1	380.3
1874-1878----------	1928	3,527.4	784.6	666.6	533.8	418.2	323.1	248.1	183.2	369.8
1875-1879----------	1929	3,484.8	783.0	663.1	528.7	412.4	317.4	243.0	178.4	358.8
1876-1880----------	1930	3,444.4	781.8	659.9	523.8	406.9	312.1	238.1	173.9	347.9
1877-1881----------	1931	3,405.5	781.1	657.1	519.2	401.6	306.7	233.1	169.8	336.9
1878-1882----------	1932	3,367.9	780.9	654.8	514.8	396.3	301.4	227.9	165.8	326.0
1879-1883----------	1933	3,329.3	781.2	652.9	510.5	391.0	295.9	222.0	161.5	314.3
1880-1884----------	1934	3,291.6	781.7	651.5	506.4	385.6	290.1	215.9	156.8	303.6
1881-1885----------	1935	3,253.8	782.4	650.2	502.3	379.9	283.9	209.7	151.9	293.5
1882-1886----------	1936	3,217.0	783.2	648.6	498.5	374.4	277.8	203.8	146.9	283.8
1883-1887----------	1937	3,183.3	784.3	646.7	495.0	369.3	272.0	198.7	142.3	275.0
1884-1888----------	1938	3,151.9	785.8	645.7	492.0	364.4	266.1	193.7	137.6	266.6
1885-1889----------	1939	3,122.0	788.0	645.7	489.1	359.1	260.0	188.7	133.1	258.3
1886-1890----------	1940	3,092.9	790.9	646.6	486.3	353.9	253.7	183.4	128.6	249.5
1887-1891----------	1941	3,062.5	794.4	647.5	482.9	348.1	247.3	177.8	124.2	240.3
1888-1892----------	1942	3,027.1	798.2	648.1	478.3	341.2	240.3	171.8	119.4	229.8
1889-1893----------	1943	2,985.7	802.0	647.0	472.0	333.1	232.7	165.5	114.6	218.8
1890-1894----------	1944	2,939.5	805.5	644.5	464.6	324.2	224.8	159.0	109.7	207.2
1891-1895----------	1945	2,890.4	808.3	640.8	456.2	314.8	216.8	152.6	104.8	196.1
1892-1896----------	1946	2,838.2	810.3	636.4	447.1	304.8	208.6	146.1	99.9	185.0
1893-1897----------	1947	2,784.9	811.1	631.8	437.5	294.7	200.4	139.7	95.0	174.7
1894-1898----------	1948	2,733.7	811.1	627.1	428.0	285.2	192.6	133.8	90.5	165.4
1895-1899----------	1949	2,683.8	809.8	621.8	418.6	276.3	185.4	128.5	86.3	157.1
1896-1900----------	1950	2,631.5	806.9	614.8	408.9	267.5	178.5	123.3	82.2	149.4
1897-1901----------	1951	2,579.6	804.2	607.3	399.2	258.9	171.8	117.9	78.2	142.1
1898-1902----------	1952	2,530.3	802.5	600.0	389.7	250.7	165.2	112.7	74.3	135.2
1899-1903----------	1953	2,484.6	801.9	593.7	380.8	242.9	158.8	107.4	70.5	128.6
1900-1904----------	1954	2,440.5	802.0	587.7	372.3	235.5	152.4	102.0	66.7	121.9
1901-1905----------	1955	2,399.0	802.1	582.6	364.3	228.5	146.2	96.8	63.1	115.4
1902-1906----------	1956	2,360.5	801.0	578.4	357.1	222.0	140.4	92.2	59.9	109.5
1903-1907----------	1957	2,326.0	798.8	575.4	351.4	216.2	135.2	88.0	57.0	104.0
1904-1908----------	1958	2,293.0	795.4	573.0	346.2	210.6	130.4	84.2	54.3	98.9
1905-1909----------	1959	2,266.4	792.9	572.4	342.6	205.7	126.2	80.7	51.9	94.0
1906-1910----------	1960	2,248.9	792.1	574.1	340.9	202.1	122.5	77.8	49.8	89.6
1907-1911----------	1961	2,243.2	794.1	578.6	341.5	199.9	119.9	75.4	48.0	85.8
1908-1912----------	1962	2,245.2	797.8	584.6	343.7	198.9	117.9	73.5	46.4	82.4
1909-1913----------	1963	2,258.6	804.2	593.2	348.3	199.6	116.6	72.2	45.1	79.4
1910-1914----------	1964	2,281.5	812.6	604.2	355.0	201.4	116.2	71.2	44.1	76.8
1911-1915----------	1965	2,313.5	822.6	617.7	363.6	204.7	116.7	70.6	43.2	74.4
1912-1916----------	1966	2,348.7	831.9	631.4	373.1	209.1	117.9	70.5	42.6	72.2
1913-1917----------	1967	2,388.5	840.4	646.0	384.0	214.7	119.8	70.7	42.4	70.5
1914-1918----------	1968	2,428.7	847.6	659.9	395.3	220.7	122.3	71.2	42.5	69.2
1915-1919----------	1969	2,476.6	856.2	674.9	407.9	228.0	125.5	72.4	43.0	68.7
1916-1920----------	1970	2,526.7	865.4	689.5	420.8	235.7	129.2	73.9	43.6	68.6
1917-1921----------	1971	2,582.7	875.6	704.5	435.0	244.5	133.5	76.0	44.6	69.0
1918-1922----------	1972	2,636.4	884.9	718.4	448.8	253.2	138.0	78.1	45.6	69.4
1919-1923----------	1973	2,693.5	894.5	732.4	463.3	262.8	143.1	80.7	46.7	70.0
1920-1924----------	1974	2,745.4	901.5	744.5	477.1	272.2	148.4	83.2	47.9	70.6

TABLE 5C. CUMULATIVE BIRTH RATES FOR ALL OTHER WOMEN AS OF THE BEGINNING OF EACH YEAR 1917-74 BY AGE AND LIVE-BIRTH ORDER FOR GROUPS OF COHORTS FROM 1867-71 TO 1955-59

(RATES ARE SIMPLE AVERAGES OF THE RATES FOR SINGLE COHORTS IN TABLE 6C)

EXACT AGE AND COHORT	AS OF JANUARY 1	TOTAL	LIVE-BIRTH ORDER							
			1	2	3	4	5	6	7	8 AND HIGHER
15-19 YEARS										
1898-1902----------	1917	133.8	110.3	19.8	3.2	0.5	*	*	*	*
1899-1903----------	1918	140.3	118.1	19.0	2.8	0.4	*	*	*	*
1900-1904----------	1919	141.8	120.8	18.0	2.7	0.3	*	*	*	*
1901-1905----------	1920	137.8	118.0	16.9	2.6	0.3	*	*	*	*
1902-1906----------	1921	144.8	125.0	16.9	2.6	0.3	*	*	*	*
1903-1907----------	1922	152.8	130.4	19.3	2.8	0.3	*	*	*	*
1904-1908----------	1923	149.0	125.8	19.9	2.9	0.4	*	*	*	*
1905-1909----------	1924	149.4	125.7	20.0	3.2	0.5	*	*	*	*
1906-1910----------	1925	154.3	129.9	20.5	3.4	0.5	*	*	*	*
1907-1911----------	1926	160.1	135.2	20.9	3.4	0.6	*	*	*	*
1908-1912----------	1927	164.2	138.1	21.9	3.6	0.6	*	*	*	*
1909-1913----------	1928	164.4	137.6	22.5	3.7	0.6	*	*	*	*
1910-1914----------	1929	160.6	134.4	21.9	3.7	0.6	*	*	*	*
1911-1915----------	1930	155.7	130.2	21.5	3.5	0.5	*	*	*	*
1912-1916----------	1931	153.5	128.7	21.0	3.3	0.5	*	*	*	*
1913-1917----------	1932	150.5	126.1	20.6	3.2	0.6	*	*	*	*
1914-1918----------	1933	149.5	125.2	20.6	3.2	0.5	*	*	*	*
1915-1919----------	1934	145.2	121.5	20.0	3.2	0.5	*	*	*	*
1916-1920----------	1935	145.8	122.0	20.0	3.3	0.5	*	*	*	*
1917-1921----------	1936	150.1	125.1	21.1	3.4	0.5	*	*	*	*
1918-1922----------	1937	152.8	126.5	22.2	3.6	0.5	*	*	*	*
1919-1923----------	1938	160.2	132.0	23.8	3.8	0.6	*	*	*	*
1920-1924----------	1939	166.5	137.1	24.8	4.0	0.6	*	*	*	*
1921-1925----------	1940	169.0	137.8	26.0	4.5	0.7	*	*	*	*
1922-1926----------	1941	168.9	135.0	27.6	5.4	0.9	*	*	*	*
1923-1927----------	1942	172.7	136.2	29.5	5.9	1.1	*	*	*	*
1924-1928----------	1943	179.5	139.9	31.9	6.6	1.1	*	*	*	*
1925-1929----------	1944	186.7	143.0	35.3	7.2	1.2	*	*	*	*
1926-1930----------	1945	183.0	138.8	35.6	7.4	1.2	*	*	*	*
1927-1931----------	1946	177.8	134.5	35.0	7.1	1.2	*	*	*	*
1928-1932----------	1947	176.3	132.9	35.0	7.2	1.2	*	*	*	*
1929-1933----------	1948	191.6	144.6	37.9	7.8	1.3	*	*	*	*
1930-1934----------	1949	207.5	154.5	42.9	8.7	1.4	*	*	*	*
1931-1935----------	1950	219.8	160.0	48.1	10.1	1.6	*	*	*	*
1932-1936----------	1951	226.7	163.2	50.7	11.0	1.8	*	*	*	*
1933-1937----------	1952	233.3	167.9	51.7	11.7	2.0	*	*	*	*
1934-1938----------	1953	233.8	168.4	51.1	12.1	2.2	*	*	*	*
1935-1939----------	1954	234.2	169.2	50.8	12.0	2.2	*	*	*	*
1936-1940----------	1955	236.9	171.7	50.7	12.2	2.3	*	*	*	*
1937-1941----------	1956	236.4	170.8	51.2	12.1	2.3	*	*	*	*
1938-1942----------	1957	238.3	171.2	52.3	12.4	2.4	*	*	*	*
1939-1943----------	1958	240.0	172.1	52.8	12.7	2.4	*	*	*	*
1940-1944----------	1959	236.7	168.4	52.8	13.0	2.5	*	*	*	*
1941-1945----------	1960	233.1	165.6	52.0	13.0	2.5	*	*	*	*
1942-1946----------	1961	227.4	161.6	50.6	12.7	2.5	*	*	*	*
1943-1947----------	1962	222.7	158.5	49.1	12.6	2.5	*	*	*	*
1944-1948----------	1963	218.4	155.1	48.3	12.5	2.5	*	*	*	*
1945-1949----------	1964	214.9	153.2	47.4	12.0	2.3	*	*	*	*
1946-1950----------	1965	213.6	152.9	46.8	11.7	2.2	*	*	*	*
1947-1951----------	1966	211.2	152.8	45.1	11.1	2.2	*	*	*	*
1948-1952----------	1967	209.1	154.1	43.2	10.0	1.8	*	*	*	*
1949-1953----------	1968	208.6	156.3	41.6	9.1	1.6	*	*	*	*
1950-1954----------	1969	208.0	159.2	39.5	8.0	1.3	*	*	*	*
1951-1955----------	1970	208.6	162.5	37.6	7.3	1.2	*	*	*	*
1952-1956----------	1971	212.2	167.5	36.9	6.8	1.0	*	*	*	*
1953-1957----------	1972	213.0	169.8	35.9	6.4	0.9	*	*	*	*
1954-1958----------	1973	212.4	172.0	34.0	5.7	0.7	*	*	*	*
1955-1959----------	1974	208.8	171.2	31.9	5.1	0.6	*	*	*	*

TABLE 5C. CUMULATIVE BIRTH RATES FOR ALL OTHER WOMEN AS OF THE BEGINNING OF EACH YEAR 1917-74 BY AGE AND LIVE-BIRTH ORDER FOR GROUPS OF COHORTS FROM 1867-71 TO 1955-59--CON.

(RATES ARE SIMPLE AVERAGES OF THE RATES FOR SINGLE COHORTS IN TABLE 6C)

EXACT AGE AND COHORT	AS OF JANUARY 1	TOTAL	LIVE-BIRTH ORDER							
			1	2	3	4	5	6	7	8 AND HIGHER
20-24 YEARS										
1893-1897----------	1917	908.5	498.3	235.5	110.6	42.9	13.9	5.1	1.6	0.5
1894-1898----------	1918	887.8	501.6	231.3	101.4	36.9	10.7	3.9	1.4	0.6
1895-1899----------	1919	876.3	507.1	224.6	96.7	33.7	9.0	3.4	1.1	0.7
1896-1900----------	1920	861.6	506.8	218.6	91.7	31.3	8.5	3.0	1.1	0.6
1897-1901----------	1921	865.9	517.9	216.1	89.1	30.2	8.2	2.9	1.0	0.5
1898-1902----------	1922	878.0	526.0	216.8	90.5	31.2	8.7	3.2	1.0	0.6
1899-1903----------	1923	881.6	527.7	219.3	89.6	31.2	8.9	3.3	1.0	0.6
1900-1904----------	1924	884.1	525.9	220.5	91.6	31.7	9.3	3.4	1.1	0.6
1901-1905----------	1925	895.8	528.9	222.9	95.7	33.0	9.7	3.7	1.2	0.7
1902-1906----------	1926	902.1	531.9	223.3	95.9	35.1	9.9	3.9	1.4	0.7
1903-1907----------	1927	903.3	532.1	223.6	94.6	36.3	10.3	4.1	1.4	0.9
1904-1908----------	1928	894.4	527.1	220.5	93.8	36.0	10.7	4.0	1.4	0.9
1905-1909----------	1929	876.8	518.2	214.7	91.7	35.0	10.8	4.1	1.4	0.9
1906-1910----------	1930	858.0	508.7	210.0	89.2	33.7	10.5	3.8	1.3	0.8
1907-1911----------	1931	846.5	502.3	207.7	87.9	33.1	10.1	3.5	1.2	0.7
1908-1912----------	1932	834.2	495.1	205.8	86.4	32.2	9.6	3.4	1.1	0.6
1909-1913----------	1933	829.3	490.2	206.4	86.6	32.0	9.3	3.2	1.0	0.6
1910-1914----------	1934	816.0	480.7	204.3	85.7	31.6	9.2	3.1	0.9	0.5
1911-1915----------	1935	811.0	476.1	203.3	85.7	32.0	9.3	3.1	0.9	0.6
1912-1916----------	1936	805.9	471.7	202.3	85.3	32.3	9.5	3.2	1.0	0.6
1913-1917----------	1937	802.4	467.0	203.2	85.3	32.5	9.6	3.2	1.0	0.6
1914-1918----------	1938	808.2	465.6	206.8	87.5	33.2	10.1	3.3	1.1	0.6
1915-1919----------	1939	817.9	467.6	210.9	90.4	33.8	10.1	3.4	1.1	0.6
1916-1920----------	1940	830.3	471.8	215.9	92.6	34.4	10.3	3.5	1.2	0.6
1917-1921----------	1941	849.4	477.1	221.7	96.7	36.8	11.2	3.9	1.3	0.7
1918-1922----------	1942	870.0	482.4	229.2	101.1	38.8	12.1	4.3	1.4	0.7
1919-1923----------	1943	890.0	488.4	235.8	105.6	41.0	12.8	4.4	1.3	0.7
1920-1924----------	1944	906.5	490.5	242.3	110.0	43.4	13.6	4.6	1.4	0.7
1921-1925----------	1945	912.0	487.5	244.7	113.3	45.6	14.2	4.7	1.4	0.6
1922-1926----------	1946	904.1	481.7	243.1	112.4	45.8	14.3	4.7	1.5	0.6
1923-1927----------	1947	918.1	486.8	250.2	113.7	46.1	14.3	4.8	1.5	0.7
1924-1928----------	1948	957.4	508.3	263.0	117.6	46.7	14.5	4.9	1.6	0.8
1925-1929----------	1949	1,007.2	525.3	283.6	126.3	49.2	15.1	5.1	1.7	0.9
1926-1930----------	1950	1,055.8	535.8	304.3	137.9	53.4	16.4	5.4	1.7	0.9
1927-1931----------	1951	1,098.2	540.8	321.3	151.7	58.3	17.8	5.6	1.8	0.9
1928-1932----------	1952	1,137.1	544.9	334.4	164.5	65.0	19.6	6.0	1.8	0.9
1929-1933----------	1953	1,169.3	549.9	342.5	173.6	71.8	21.9	6.7	2.0	0.9
1930-1934----------	1954	1,197.0	557.8	348.6	178.8	76.7	24.4	7.5	2.2	1.0
1931-1935----------	1955	1,230.3	571.4	355.9	184.2	80.2	26.4	8.6	2.5	1.1
1932-1936----------	1956	1,262.8	585.0	364.8	189.1	83.1	27.6	9.3	2.7	1.2
1933-1937----------	1957	1,300.9	599.2	376.4	195.5	86.9	28.9	9.8	3.0	1.2
1934-1938----------	1958	1,331.0	608.6	384.6	202.3	89.9	30.7	10.5	3.1	1.3
1935-1939----------	1959	1,345.9	611.0	388.4	206.6	92.7	32.0	10.9	3.0	1.3
1936-1940----------	1960	1,349.6	608.8	389.0	207.9	95.1	32.8	11.3	3.3	1.4
1937-1941----------	1961	1,340.8	603.9	385.7	207.3	94.9	32.7	11.5	3.4	1.4
1938-1942----------	1962	1,326.4	597.2	380.8	204.7	94.7	32.5	11.6	3.5	1.4
1939-1943----------	1963	1,306.7	590.3	373.6	201.2	92.9	32.3	11.6	3.5	1.3
1940-1944----------	1964	1,282.3	583.9	366.1	195.2	89.9	31.3	11.2	3.4	1.3
1941-1945----------	1965	1,254.6	579.2	357.6	187.7	85.6	29.5	10.5	3.2	1.3
1942-1946----------	1966	1,221.5	576.1	348.0	178.2	79.5	26.6	9.2	2.8	1.1
1943-1947----------	1967	1,187.0	576.1	337.4	167.2	72.0	23.2	8.0	2.2	0.9
1944-1948----------	1968	1,153.1	578.1	327.0	154.9	64.0	19.8	6.7	1.9	0.7
1945-1949----------	1969	1,119.7	583.0	314.7	142.1	56.2	16.5	5.2	1.5	0.5
1946-1950----------	1970	1,095.6	590.1	305.2	130.9	49.6	13.9	4.2	1.2	0.5
1947-1951----------	1971	1,081.8	598.6	299.2	122.8	44.4	11.7	3.5	1.1	0.5
1948-1952----------	1972	1,063.6	602.6	293.1	114.6	39.3	9.9	2.9	0.8	0.4
1949-1953----------	1973	1,033.5	600.6	282.3	105.0	34.3	8.2	2.2	0.6	0.3
1950-1954----------	1974	1,000.4	594.2	271.1	96.2	29.8	6.7	1.7	0.4	0.3

TABLE 5C. CUMULATIVE BIRTH RATES FOR ALL OTHER WOMEN AS OF THE BEGINNING OF EACH YEAR 1917-74 BY AGE AND LIVE-BIRTH ORDER FOR GROUPS OF COHORTS FROM 1867-71 TO 1955-59--CON.

(RATES ARE SIMPLE AVERAGES OF THE RATES FOR SINGLE COHORTS IN TABLE 6C)

EXACT AGE AND COHORT	AS OF JANUARY 1	TOTAL	LIVE-BIRTH ORDER							
			1	2	3	4	5	6	7	8 AND HIGHER
25-29 YEARS										
1888-1892----------	1917	1,881.8	672.3	461.6	316.6	203.9	114.3	62.5	29.4	21.2
1889-1893----------	1918	1,851.4	675.7	459.1	314.0	195.2	105.6	57.2	26.2	18.4
1890-1894----------	1919	1,820.7	681.4	454.5	310.3	185.9	96.8	52.5	23.2	16.1
1891-1895----------	1920	1,797.1	685.7	450.6	305.0	178.0	91.3	49.2	22.0	15.3
1892-1896----------	1921	1,787.9	694.6	447.9	301.3	173.3	87.7	47.5	20.9	14.7
1893-1897----------	1922	1,786.5	701.5	443.1	299.1	171.0	86.6	47.5	21.9	15.8
1894-1898----------	1923	1,763.4	702.3	438.5	289.8	165.3	83.6	46.5	21.5	15.9
1895-1899----------	1924	1,745.9	702.3	432.2	283.5	161.5	82.8	46.0	21.4	16.2
1896-1900----------	1925	1,743.2	702.7	425.7	282.3	161.8	84.5	47.5	22.1	16.6
1897-1901----------	1926	1,742.1	703.2	420.7	280.0	164.0	85.5	48.1	22.7	17.9
1898-1902----------	1927	1,740.8	701.7	417.2	277.1	166.3	87.0	49.6	23.0	18.9
1899-1903----------	1928	1,729.6	701.2	411.5	272.0	165.0	88.3	49.3	23.2	19.1
1900-1904----------	1929	1,701.5	696.2	403.6	264.8	161.2	87.0	47.5	22.5	18.7
1901-1905----------	1930	1,664.0	689.0	394.7	255.8	155.8	85.0	45.3	20.9	17.5
1902-1906----------	1931	1,629.2	681.6	386.3	247.9	151.0	82.7	43.4	20.1	16.2
1903-1907----------	1932	1,594.8	672.7	377.9	240.7	147.1	80.2	41.9	19.3	15.0
1904-1908----------	1933	1,564.8	663.5	370.3	235.0	144.2	78.5	40.6	18.6	14.1
1905-1909----------	1934	1,535.1	653.5	363.8	230.5	141.1	76.6	39.1	17.5	13.0
1906-1910----------	1935	1,514.4	644.8	359.4	227.9	139.6	75.4	38.0	16.7	12.6
1907-1911----------	1936	1,497.3	637.1	356.9	226.0	138.4	74.0	36.8	16.1	12.0
1908-1912----------	1937	1,483.6	629.3	355.5	224.2	137.5	73.3	36.4	15.8	11.6
1909-1913----------	1938	1,478.4	622.9	355.5	224.1	137.6	73.7	36.7	16.2	11.7
1910-1914----------	1939	1,475.8	616.5	355.9	224.9	138.4	74.4	37.4	16.5	11.8
1911-1915----------	1940	1,475.5	611.5	356.3	226.1	139.3	75.4	38.1	16.8	12.0
1912-1916----------	1941	1,478.5	606.6	357.3	228.0	140.9	76.8	39.0	17.3	12.6
1913-1917----------	1942	1,491.3	604.4	360.8	231.9	143.6	79.2	40.2	18.0	13.2
1914-1918----------	1943	1,509.5	605.4	366.0	236.4	146.5	81.7	41.4	18.6	13.5
1915-1919----------	1944	1,538.4	611.3	373.8	241.7	150.3	84.6	43.0	19.5	14.2
1916-1920----------	1945	1,569.8	619.3	381.7	247.1	154.2	87.4	45.0	20.4	14.7
1917-1921----------	1946	1,596.3	627.4	389.0	250.9	157.1	89.5	46.4	21.2	14.8
1918-1922----------	1947	1,627.7	636.5	399.6	256.2	160.1	91.2	47.4	21.7	15.0
1919-1923----------	1948	1,665.5	649.4	412.6	262.8	163.0	92.3	48.1	22.0	15.3
1920-1924----------	1949	1,706.7	659.9	428.1	271.7	166.3	93.6	48.7	22.5	15.9
1921-1925----------	1950	1,755.2	669.7	446.8	283.3	171.3	95.3	49.6	22.9	16.3
1922-1926----------	1951	1,813.0	679.3	466.6	298.1	179.3	98.5	51.1	23.5	16.6
1923-1927----------	1952	1,887.3	691.2	487.9	317.2	191.5	104.2	54.0	24.4	16.9
1924-1928----------	1953	1,968.0	702.4	509.0	337.1	206.4	112.3	57.5	25.8	17.5
1925-1929----------	1954	2,049.9	711.1	528.5	356.8	222.4	122.6	62.1	27.9	18.5
1926-1930----------	1955	2,125.3	716.7	544.3	374.1	238.0	133.9	67.8	30.5	20.0
1927-1931----------	1956	2,192.5	721.2	558.1	389.2	251.1	144.2	73.7	33.3	21.7
1928-1932----------	1957	2,258.2	727.7	571.4	402.6	262.4	153.0	80.1	36.9	24.1
1929-1933----------	1958	2,327.5	738.9	586.9	416.1	272.2	160.8	85.9	40.1	26.6
1930-1934----------	1959	2,391.9	752.0	601.7	428.2	280.4	166.9	90.6	42.9	29.2
1931-1935----------	1960	2,459.7	767.9	617.6	441.2	289.6	172.7	94.1	45.3	31.3
1932-1936----------	1961	2,513.7	782.4	630.3	451.7	296.7	176.6	96.8	46.8	32.4
1933-1937----------	1962	2,559.9	794.1	639.4	459.9	303.5	180.7	100.0	48.3	34.0
1934-1938----------	1963	2,578.6	798.6	642.2	463.1	306.3	182.8	101.7	49.1	34.8
1935-1939----------	1964	2,573.0	798.9	640.4	461.3	304.8	182.1	101.1	49.4	35.0
1936-1940----------	1965	2,543.6	795.1	635.2	455.1	299.0	177.9	98.9	48.3	34.1
1937-1941----------	1966	2,489.8	790.3	626.7	444.2	289.0	169.5	93.3	45.4	31.4
1938-1942----------	1967	2,413.3	785.4	616.1	428.6	273.5	157.1	84.8	40.7	27.1
1939-1943----------	1968	2,328.6	781.6	604.9	410.6	255.8	142.7	75.2	35.3	22.5
1940-1944----------	1969	2,237.0	780.3	592.0	389.5	235.7	126.5	65.2	29.5	18.3
1941-1945----------	1970	2,151.0	780.2	580.1	369.2	215.9	111.5	55.4	24.0	14.7
1942-1946----------	1971	2,082.7	784.2	571.5	351.7	198.1	98.5	47.1	19.8	11.8
1943-1947----------	1972	2,022.7	789.8	563.5	335.7	181.5	86.7	39.7	16.3	9.5
1944-1948----------	1973	1,959.7	796.7	554.2	317.0	164.0	74.7	32.8	12.9	7.4
1945-1949----------	1974	1,895.3	802.1	543.5	297.9	146.6	63.3	26.4	10.0	5.5

TABLE 5C. CUMULATIVE BIRTH RATES FOR ALL OTHER WOMEN AS OF THE BEGINNING OF EACH YEAR 1917-74 BY AGE AND LIVE-BIRTH ORDER FOR GROUPS OF COHORTS FROM 1867-71 TO 1955-59--CON.

(RATES ARE SIMPLE AVERAGES OF THE RATES FOR SINGLE COHORTS IN TABLE 6C)

EXACT AGE AND COHORT	AS OF JANUARY 1	TOTAL	LIVE-BIRTH ORDER							
			1	2	3	4	5	6	7	8 AND HIGHER
30-34 YEARS										
1883-1887----------	1917	2,718.2	733.0	561.9	442.9	332.5	236.7	171.9	110.1	129.1
1884-1888----------	1918	2,672.5	732.1	556.9	436.6	328.2	230.9	165.5	104.2	118.1
1885-1889----------	1919	2,627.9	732.9	552.3	431.3	323.6	224.3	158.7	97.9	106.9
1886-1890----------	1920	2,585.8	733.9	548.4	426.4	318.3	217.2	150.9	92.0	98.7
1887-1891----------	1921	2,545.9	736.6	545.6	422.0	311.5	208.1	143.6	86.3	92.2
1888-1892----------	1922	2,517.0	739.8	544.4	417.7	303.2	199.5	139.1	83.2	90.1
1889-1893----------	1923	2,495.0	743.5	543.6	417.1	296.2	191.9	134.1	80.4	88.2
1890-1894----------	1924	2,476.4	747.5	541.5	414.4	289.4	185.8	130.8	79.2	87.8
1891-1895----------	1925	2,464.2	751.6	537.9	411.4	283.7	181.4	129.6	79.2	89.4
1892-1896----------	1926	2,451.6	755.3	531.7	406.1	278.7	178.3	128.6	79.7	93.2
1893-1897----------	1927	2,433.6	757.1	522.8	399.2	274.5	176.3	127.5	80.3	95.9
1894-1898----------	1928	2,399.6	755.1	512.2	387.1	267.9	173.9	125.8	80.4	97.2
1895-1899----------	1929	2,366.4	753.3	501.1	376.1	262.5	172.8	124.6	79.3	96.7
1896-1900----------	1930	2,336.8	751.2	491.0	366.7	258.4	172.7	123.6	77.7	95.5
1897-1901----------	1931	2,309.1	748.8	482.0	358.2	254.3	172.5	122.7	76.3	94.3
1898-1902----------	1932	2,279.1	744.7	473.7	349.9	250.2	171.1	121.1	75.4	93.0
1899-1903----------	1933	2,244.5	742.2	465.0	340.7	244.8	168.6	118.8	73.9	90.5
1900-1904----------	1934	2,199.1	736.2	455.8	331.0	238.4	164.8	115.1	71.7	86.1
1901-1905----------	1935	2,147.6	728.3	446.2	320.7	231.1	160.1	110.6	68.8	81.8
1902-1906----------	1936	2,095.7	719.2	436.4	311.2	224.9	155.6	106.2	65.6	76.6
1903-1907----------	1937	2,048.4	709.6	427.1	302.9	219.2	151.6	102.5	62.6	72.9
1904-1908----------	1938	2,008.1	699.5	418.6	296.0	214.4	148.5	99.9	60.6	70.6
1905-1909----------	1939	1,975.9	690.6	412.5	291.0	210.9	145.7	97.5	59.3	68.4
1906-1910----------	1940	1,952.3	682.3	408.8	287.9	208.9	143.2	95.8	58.3	67.1
1907-1911----------	1941	1,940.3	675.6	407.5	286.7	207.9	142.0	95.0	58.3	67.3
1908-1912----------	1942	1,936.1	669.6	407.7	286.7	207.8	141.6	95.3	58.9	68.5
1909-1913----------	1943	1,941.3	665.6	409.9	288.3	208.8	142.5	96.4	59.9	69.9
1910-1914----------	1944	1,952.2	662.4	413.0	290.9	210.6	144.4	98.1	60.9	71.9
1911-1915----------	1945	1,968.9	660.7	417.1	294.5	213.1	147.1	100.2	62.2	74.0
1912-1916----------	1946	1,986.8	658.8	421.7	298.8	216.1	150.3	102.0	63.4	75.7
1913-1917----------	1947	2,015.5	660.3	429.5	305.7	220.8	153.7	103.6	64.7	77.2
1914-1918----------	1948	2,051.8	665.5	439.4	313.4	225.9	157.4	105.5	66.2	78.5
1915-1919----------	1949	2,098.7	675.1	452.2	322.7	231.6	161.4	107.9	67.8	80.0
1916-1920----------	1950	2,155.0	688.5	466.9	333.1	238.4	165.7	110.8	69.7	81.9
1917-1921----------	1951	2,218.2	703.3	483.5	345.2	246.1	170.5	113.9	71.5	84.2
1918-1922----------	1952	2,281.1	715.5	500.3	357.6	254.5	175.4	117.5	73.8	86.5
1919-1923----------	1953	2,346.9	726.2	518.0	371.5	263.9	181.3	121.3	75.8	88.9
1920-1924----------	1954	2,415.2	735.0	535.9	387.0	274.7	188.0	125.4	78.0	91.2
1921-1925----------	1955	2,495.6	744.2	555.9	404.2	288.1	196.8	130.9	81.3	94.2
1922-1926----------	1956	2,586.0	753.2	576.7	423.2	303.6	207.4	138.0	85.3	98.6
1923-1927----------	1957	2,692.5	763.9	598.2	444.3	321.6	221.0	147.4	91.2	104.9
1924-1928----------	1958	2,800.1	772.9	618.5	465.6	339.7	235.4	157.4	97.8	112.8
1925-1929----------	1959	2,898.4	779.5	635.9	484.6	356.7	248.9	167.2	104.4	121.2
1926-1930----------	1960	2,982.8	782.4	649.5	500.9	371.0	261.3	176.5	111.1	130.1
1927-1931----------	1961	3,055.3	785.2	661.7	514.8	383.2	271.5	184.0	116.9	138.0
1928-1932----------	1962	3,121.5	790.1	673.4	527.3	393.6	279.5	190.6	121.5	145.5
1929-1933----------	1963	3,188.0	799.7	687.1	539.2	402.9	286.7	196.1	124.9	151.4
1930-1934----------	1964	3,247.8	812.0	701.3	550.8	410.6	292.0	199.4	126.9	154.8
1931-1935----------	1965	3,304.9	827.2	715.2	561.9	417.7	296.1	202.0	128.3	156.5
1932-1936----------	1966	3,338.9	841.2	726.3	569.7	422.0	297.3	201.5	127.3	153.6
1933-1937----------	1967	3,347.6	852.4	733.7	573.9	423.2	295.5	198.6	123.6	146.7
1934-1938----------	1968	3,316.4	856.7	734.9	572.1	418.4	288.8	192.2	117.8	135.5
1935-1939----------	1969	3,254.0	858.0	732.6	565.3	408.4	277.3	181.9	109.4	121.1
1936-1940----------	1970	3,169.9	856.9	727.7	554.6	394.5	262.7	168.9	99.5	105.1
1937-1941----------	1971	3,074.8	854.8	721.6	541.5	378.3	246.1	154.4	88.6	89.5
1938-1942----------	1972	2,971.6	853.0	714.7	525.7	359.3	227.3	139.1	77.6	74.9
1939-1943----------	1973	2,862.9	853.3	707.6	507.2	337.7	207.2	122.9	66.2	60.8
1940-1944----------	1974	2,750.9	854.2	699.9	486.7	314.0	185.9	106.6	55.3	48.3

TABLE 5C. CUMULATIVE BIRTH RATES FOR ALL OTHER WOMEN AS OF THE BEGINNING OF EACH YEAR 1917-74 BY AGE AND LIVE-BIRTH ORDER FOR GROUPS OF COHORTS FROM 1867-71 TO 1955-59--CON.

(RATES ARE SIMPLE AVERAGES OF THE RATES FOR SINGLE COHORTS IN TABLE 6C)

EXACT AGE AND COHORT	AS OF JANUARY 1	TOTAL	LIVE-BIRTH ORDER							
			1	2	3	4	5	6	7	8 AND HIGHER
35-39 YEARS										
1878-1882----------	1917	3,579.4	771.4	626.6	521.3	425.8	338.4	275.5	207.6	412.7
1879-1883----------	1918	3,505.5	768.3	620.3	514.3	416.9	329.2	269.5	203.0	384.0
1880-1884----------	1919	3,434.9	765.7	614.2	508.0	407.7	319.3	265.0	197.4	357.6
1881-1885----------	1920	3,370.0	762.7	607.8	501.0	398.7	309.8	258.8	191.6	339.6
1882-1886----------	1921	3,308.0	760.6	602.1	494.8	391.3	301.2	250.6	183.3	324.1
1883-1887----------	1922	3,242.9	759.1	596.1	487.6	384.7	293.4	240.6	173.2	308.2
1884-1888----------	1923	3,178.4	757.8	590.8	481.0	379.4	286.3	230.3	164.1	288.7
1885-1889----------	1924	3,116.8	757.1	585.7	474.9	373.6	278.0	220.3	155.6	271.6
1886-1890----------	1925	3,066.4	757.7	581.2	469.8	367.8	270.0	211.2	148.8	259.9
1887-1891----------	1926	3,027.1	759.4	577.4	464.6	360.3	261.2	204.2	144.0	256.0
1888-1892----------	1927	2,993.2	761.5	574.6	459.5	351.5	251.8	199.2	140.9	254.2
1889-1893----------	1928	2,967.7	764.7	572.0	457.9	343.9	243.6	193.7	137.9	254.0
1890-1894----------	1929	2,935.0	767.6	568.1	453.4	335.6	236.2	188.7	135.1	250.3
1891-1895----------	1930	2,899.9	770.2	562.7	446.9	327.5	230.0	184.3	132.9	245.4
1892-1896----------	1931	2,862.1	772.2	554.5	438.3	319.4	225.2	180.4	130.7	241.4
1893-1897----------	1932	2,818.3	773.0	543.3	428.3	311.5	220.6	176.7	128.5	236.4
1894-1898----------	1933	2,767.8	770.0	531.3	414.1	302.5	216.1	173.8	126.8	233.2
1895-1899----------	1934	2,726.7	768.0	520.0	402.1	295.9	214.0	171.6	125.5	229.6
1896-1900----------	1935	2,698.0	766.1	509.9	392.6	291.6	213.5	170.7	124.8	228.8
1897-1901----------	1936	2,665.5	763.4	500.9	383.9	287.2	212.4	169.0	123.1	225.6
1898-1902----------	1937	2,626.4	759.1	492.3	375.2	282.6	210.3	166.1	120.6	220.2
1899-1903----------	1938	2,580.6	756.1	483.5	365.6	276.1	206.5	161.5	117.2	214.1
1900-1904----------	1939	2,523.5	749.9	474.0	355.3	268.8	201.3	155.8	113.0	205.4
1901-1905----------	1940	2,456.6	741.7	464.0	344.2	260.3	194.8	149.2	107.9	194.5
1902-1906----------	1941	2,397.2	732.8	454.2	334.4	253.1	189.6	143.7	103.5	185.9
1903-1907----------	1942	2,349.3	723.8	445.6	326.5	247.3	185.7	139.6	100.4	180.4
1904-1908----------	1943	2,310.6	714.9	438.1	320.2	243.1	182.6	136.6	98.0	177.1
1905-1909----------	1944	2,284.9	707.3	433.6	316.4	240.6	180.2	134.4	96.6	175.8
1906-1910----------	1945	2,271.6	700.8	431.8	315.0	239.9	178.5	133.3	96.2	176.1
1907-1911----------	1946	2,273.0	696.0	432.8	315.8	240.8	178.3	133.6	96.8	178.9
1908-1912----------	1947	2,282.3	692.1	435.6	318.2	242.5	179.1	135.0	98.1	181.7
1909-1913----------	1948	2,302.6	690.7	440.5	322.3	245.6	181.4	137.2	99.8	185.1
1910-1914----------	1949	2,324.7	689.4	446.3	327.0	249.0	184.5	139.5	101.3	187.7
1911-1915----------	1950	2,350.8	689.6	453.1	333.0	252.8	188.0	141.7	102.8	189.8
1912-1916----------	1951	2,379.6	689.9	460.5	340.2	257.8	192.0	143.8	104.2	191.2
1913-1917----------	1952	2,421.3	693.0	470.5	350.0	264.5	197.1	146.2	106.0	194.0
1914-1918----------	1953	2,469.8	697.9	482.1	360.5	272.1	202.7	149.5	108.2	196.8
1915-1919----------	1954	2,533.9	708.1	496.5	373.0	281.2	209.4	154.2	111.3	200.2
1916-1920----------	1955	2,610.1	721.1	513.0	386.5	291.8	217.4	160.0	114.8	205.5
1917-1921----------	1956	2,693.5	735.9	531.5	401.2	303.0	225.9	166.1	118.6	211.3
1918-1922----------	1957	2,773.4	747.5	549.0	415.6	313.9	234.1	172.1	122.9	218.3
1919-1923----------	1958	2,853.6	757.2	566.5	430.7	325.9	242.7	178.5	127.1	225.0
1920-1924----------	1959	2,931.9	764.9	584.3	446.7	338.1	251.5	184.6	131.2	230.6
1921-1925----------	1960	3,020.1	772.7	602.9	464.2	351.7	261.6	192.3	136.4	238.3
1922-1926----------	1961	3,116.9	780.3	622.2	482.7	367.3	272.9	201.0	142.5	248.0
1923-1927----------	1962	3,227.4	789.6	642.4	502.6	385.2	286.4	210.7	149.8	260.7
1924-1928----------	1963	3,331.7	797.3	660.9	522.0	402.0	299.8	220.3	156.5	272.9
1925-1929----------	1964	3,424.4	802.8	676.9	539.3	417.5	312.5	228.9	162.6	283.9
1926-1930----------	1965	3,497.4	804.6	689.0	553.8	430.1	322.6	236.5	167.8	293.0
1927-1931----------	1966	3,554.8	806.6	699.6	566.0	440.6	330.7	242.4	171.5	297.4
1928-1932----------	1967	3,595.3	810.9	709.6	576.4	447.8	335.9	245.8	172.9	296.0
1929-1933----------	1968	3,635.0	820.0	722.5	586.8	454.9	340.0	247.6	173.0	290.2
1930-1934----------	1969	3,664.2	832.4	735.7	596.6	459.6	342.1	247.6	171.1	279.1
1931-1935----------	1970	3,689.4	847.7	749.8	606.1	464.4	342.9	245.5	167.9	265.1
1932-1936----------	1971	3,696.2	862.0	760.9	613.1	466.7	341.2	241.5	162.5	248.3
1933-1937----------	1972	3,683.5	873.4	768.9	616.8	466.4	336.8	235.7	156.1	229.4
1934-1938----------	1973	3,631.4	878.5	771.1	614.8	459.8	327.6	226.4	146.9	206.3
1935-1939----------	1974	3,551.5	880.2	770.1	608.2	448.7	314.3	213.6	135.6	180.8

TABLE 5C. CUMULATIVE BIRTH RATES FOR ALL OTHER WOMEN AS OF THE BEGINNING OF EACH YEAR 1917-74 BY AGE AND LIVE-BIRTH ORDER FOR GROUPS OF COHORTS FROM 1867-71 TO 1955-59--CON.

(RATES ARE SIMPLE AVERAGES OF THE RATES FOR SINGLE COHORTS IN TABLE 6C)

EXACT AGE AND COHORT	AS OF JANUARY 1	TOTAL	LIVE-BIRTH ORDER							
			1	2	3	4	5	6	7	8 AND HIGHER
40-44 YEARS										
1873-1877----------	1917	4,400.5	801.7	677.2	579.2	493.4	415.3	356.7	290.3	786.7
1874-1878----------	1918	4,301.3	797.1	669.3	570.1	483.6	404.7	346.4	279.8	750.3
1875-1879----------	1919	4,209.1	793.2	661.8	561.9	474.2	394.4	337.1	270.2	716.3
1876-1880----------	1920	4,117.9	789.1	654.6	554.0	465.5	384.5	327.8	261.6	680.8
1877-1881----------	1921	4,037.2	786.0	648.0	547.4	457.9	375.5	320.2	254.5	647.7
1878-1882----------	1922	3,966.6	783.2	642.1	541.6	450.9	367.0	314.4	249.2	618.2
1879-1883----------	1923	3,896.6	780.7	636.2	535.6	442.6	357.9	309.0	243.9	590.7
1880-1884----------	1924	3,824.1	777.8	629.9	529.3	433.4	348.0	302.5	237.5	565.7
1881-1885----------	1925	3,746.3	774.4	622.9	522.1	424.0	337.8	294.4	229.6	541.1
1882-1886----------	1926	3,665.4	771.3	615.8	514.3	415.0	327.8	284.2	219.5	517.5
1883-1887----------	1927	3,583.2	768.9	608.8	505.9	407.0	318.5	271.9	208.4	493.8
1884-1888----------	1928	3,503.9	767.0	602.1	498.1	400.4	309.9	260.1	197.8	468.5
1885-1889----------	1929	3,429.2	766.1	595.9	490.7	393.6	301.1	248.5	187.7	445.6
1886-1890----------	1930	3,364.4	766.4	590.6	484.1	386.3	292.0	238.3	179.2	427.5
1887-1891----------	1931	3,309.2	767.4	586.1	477.7	377.7	282.4	230.0	172.9	415.0
1888-1892----------	1932	3,258.0	768.9	582.7	471.0	367.4	272.0	223.3	167.9	404.8
1889-1893----------	1933	3,220.7	771.3	579.7	468.7	358.9	263.1	217.3	163.5	398.2
1890-1894----------	1934	3,181.4	774.0	575.7	463.8	350.2	255.0	211.9	160.1	390.7
1891-1895----------	1935	3,141.6	776.3	569.8	456.9	341.6	248.2	207.1	157.5	384.2
1892-1896----------	1936	3,095.3	777.8	561.2	448.0	332.8	242.2	202.2	154.8	376.3
1893-1897----------	1937	3,042.9	778.3	549.6	437.5	324.2	236.9	197.4	151.9	367.1
1894-1898----------	1938	2,982.8	775.1	537.4	422.9	314.6	231.7	192.9	149.1	359.1
1895-1899----------	1939	2,939.4	773.2	526.2	411.1	307.9	229.4	190.4	147.5	353.7
1896-1900----------	1940	2,906.0	771.4	516.3	401.8	303.6	228.6	189.1	146.0	349.2
1897-1901----------	1941	2,871.5	768.9	507.5	393.1	299.4	227.5	187.1	143.9	344.1
1898-1902----------	1942	2,830.5	764.6	499.2	384.4	294.6	225.3	183.9	141.0	337.5
1899-1903----------	1943	2,779.5	761.8	490.6	374.7	288.0	221.2	178.8	136.9	327.5
1900-1904----------	1944	2,718.6	755.9	481.4	364.4	280.6	215.6	172.7	132.1	315.9
1901-1905----------	1945	2,650.5	748.0	471.9	353.8	272.2	209.5	165.9	126.5	302.7
1902-1906----------	1946	2,592.5	739.7	462.7	344.6	265.3	204.6	160.6	122.1	292.9
1903-1907----------	1947	2,545.8	731.3	454.7	337.4	260.3	200.8	156.6	119.0	285.7
1904-1908----------	1948	2,509.7	723.1	448.0	332.0	256.7	198.0	153.9	116.8	281.2
1905-1909----------	1949	2,485.4	716.2	444.2	329.1	254.9	195.9	151.8	115.4	277.9
1906-1910----------	1950	2,475.9	710.6	443.5	328.5	255.0	194.8	150.8	115.0	277.7
1907-1911----------	1951	2,481.0	706.7	445.7	330.5	256.4	195.0	151.5	115.9	279.3
1908-1912----------	1952	2,496.5	703.7	449.6	333.8	259.0	196.6	153.5	117.4	282.9
1909-1913----------	1953	2,522.5	702.5	455.3	339.0	263.1	199.8	156.2	119.4	287.2
1910-1914----------	1954	2,551.0	701.5	461.7	344.8	267.7	203.8	159.3	121.4	290.8
1911-1915----------	1955	2,582.5	701.8	468.8	351.9	273.0	208.3	162.1	123.3	293.3
1912-1916----------	1956	2,616.1	702.0	476.8	359.8	279.0	213.4	165.1	125.2	294.8
1913-1917----------	1957	2,661.6	704.9	487.0	370.0	286.3	219.5	168.5	127.8	297.6
1914-1918----------	1958	2,715.9	709.6	498.9	381.2	294.6	226.1	172.8	131.0	301.7
1915-1919----------	1959	2,786.0	719.4	513.4	393.9	304.6	233.8	178.3	135.0	307.6
1916-1920----------	1960	2,866.5	732.1	529.6	407.6	315.6	242.6	184.7	139.7	314.6
1917-1921----------	1961	2,952.7	746.4	547.5	422.4	327.1	251.7	191.4	144.2	322.0
1918-1922----------	1962	3,031.3	757.3	564.4	436.8	338.1	259.8	197.9	148.2	328.8
1919-1923----------	1963	3,108.2	766.5	581.3	451.5	349.6	268.0	204.0	152.1	335.2
1920-1924----------	1964	3,184.3	773.7	598.4	467.1	361.7	276.4	210.2	156.1	340.7
1921-1925----------	1965	3,268.4	781.0	616.8	484.1	375.3	285.9	217.0	160.7	347.6
1922-1926----------	1966	3,360.1	788.3	635.8	502.0	390.1	297.0	225.1	166.3	355.5
1923-1927----------	1967	3,461.3	797.3	655.3	521.1	406.7	309.6	233.9	172.5	364.9
1924-1928----------	1968	3,553.4	804.8	673.0	539.6	422.0	321.5	242.3	178.1	372.1
1925-1929----------	1969	3,632.4	810.0	688.5	556.0	436.6	332.7	249.7	183.0	375.9
1926-1930----------	1970	3,688.2	811.7	700.2	569.6	448.0	341.5	255.7	186.5	375.0
1927-1931----------	1971	3,728.6	813.4	710.3	580.9	457.4	348.3	260.0	188.5	369.8
1928-1932----------	1972	3,755.4	817.5	720.3	590.6	463.8	352.3	262.0	188.5	360.4
1929-1933----------	1973	3,783.6	826.7	733.0	600.6	470.2	355.7	262.5	187.4	347.5
1930-1934----------	1974	3,802.4	838.8	746.1	610.1	474.4	357.0	261.4	184.4	330.2

TABLE 5C. CUMULATIVE BIRTH RATES FOR ALL OTHER WOMEN AS OF THE BEGINNING OF EACH YEAR 1917-74 BY AGE AND LIVE-BIRTH ORDER FOR GROUPS OF COHORTS FROM 1867-71 TO 1955-59--CON.

(RATES ARE SIMPLE AVERAGES OF THE RATES FOR SINGLE COHORTS IN TABLE 6C)

EXACT AGE AND COHORT	AS OF JANUARY 1	TOTAL	LIVE-BIRTH ORDER							
			1	2	3	4	5	6	7	8 AND HIGHER
45-49 YEARS										
1868-1872----------	1917	5,038.1	826.1	716.5	627.0	547.8	471.8	412.3	346.8	1,089.8
1869-1873----------	1918	4,940.0	822.2	710.0	618.9	538.7	462.5	403.6	338.3	1,045.8
1870-1874----------	1919	4,849.5	818.2	702.9	610.7	529.7	453.0	396.2	330.1	1,008.7
1871-1875----------	1920	4,743.3	813.6	695.5	601.6	519.4	442.8	386.6	320.7	963.1
1872-1876----------	1921	4,638.6	808.9	688.1	592.5	509.1	432.4	376.6	310.7	920.3
1873-1877----------	1922	4,529.8	804.2	680.3	583.2	498.7	421.4	365.8	299.7	876.5
1874-1878----------	1923	4,424.9	799.8	672.5	574.1	488.6	410.7	354.9	289.1	835.2
1875-1879----------	1924	4,325.8	795.5	665.0	565.6	479.1	400.4	344.7	279.2	796.3
1876-1880----------	1925	4,235.0	791.7	657.7	558.1	470.6	390.6	335.6	270.6	760.1
1877-1881----------	1926	4,152.6	788.4	651.2	551.5	462.8	381.4	327.9	263.6	725.8
1878-1882----------	1927	4,079.7	785.8	645.1	545.7	455.7	372.8	322.0	258.2	694.4
1879-1883----------	1928	4,007.8	783.2	638.9	539.5	447.6	363.7	316.4	252.5	666.0
1880-1884----------	1929	3,931.9	780.1	632.3	532.7	438.5	353.6	309.7	245.7	639.3
1881-1885----------	1930	3,849.0	776.5	625.1	525.2	428.5	343.0	301.3	237.1	612.3
1882-1886----------	1931	3,760.2	773.2	617.8	516.9	419.0	332.5	290.5	226.6	583.7
1883-1887----------	1932	3,669.2	770.7	610.5	508.3	410.4	323.0	277.5	214.8	554.0
1884-1888----------	1933	3,583.1	768.5	603.6	500.1	403.4	314.1	265.3	203.7	524.4
1885-1889----------	1934	3,505.4	767.5	597.2	492.7	396.5	305.0	253.5	193.6	499.4
1886-1890----------	1935	3,439.0	767.8	591.9	486.0	389.2	295.8	243.2	185.1	480.0
1887-1891----------	1936	3,381.6	768.7	587.4	479.4	380.5	286.1	234.7	178.5	466.3
1888-1892----------	1937	3,329.3	770.2	584.0	472.9	370.1	275.5	227.7	173.2	455.7
1889-1893----------	1938	3,288.9	772.5	580.9	470.4	361.5	266.4	221.4	168.5	447.3
1890-1894----------	1939	3,248.0	775.2	576.9	465.5	352.7	258.2	215.7	165.0	438.8
1891-1895----------	1940	3,204.3	777.5	570.9	458.4	343.8	251.1	210.7	162.1	429.8
1892-1896----------	1941	3,154.8	779.0	562.2	449.4	335.0	244.8	205.6	159.2	419.6
1893-1897----------	1942	3,099.4	779.4	550.5	438.9	326.2	239.3	200.6	155.9	408.6
1894-1898----------	1943	3,037.8	776.1	538.4	424.2	316.6	234.2	196.1	153.0	399.2
1895-1899----------	1944	2,993.6	774.1	527.3	412.5	309.9	232.0	193.7	151.2	392.9
1896-1900----------	1945	2,960.9	772.4	517.5	403.2	305.7	231.4	192.4	149.8	388.5
1897-1901----------	1946	2,926.4	769.9	508.8	394.7	301.7	230.3	190.4	147.6	383.0
1898-1902----------	1947	2,885.1	765.8	500.6	386.0	297.1	228.1	187.2	144.7	375.6
1899-1903----------	1948	2,833.8	763.1	492.0	376.5	290.6	223.9	182.2	140.7	364.8
1900-1904----------	1949	2,771.5	757.3	483.0	366.3	283.1	218.4	176.0	135.7	351.7
1901-1905----------	1950	2,702.5	749.5	473.6	355.8	274.8	212.4	169.3	130.2	336.9
1902-1906----------	1951	2,642.5	741.2	464.4	346.7	268.0	207.3	163.8	125.8	325.3
1903-1907----------	1952	2,594.6	732.9	456.6	339.7	263.0	203.6	159.8	122.6	316.4
1904-1908----------	1953	2,556.9	724.8	449.9	334.3	259.5	200.7	156.9	120.3	310.5
1905-1909----------	1954	2,533.7	718.1	446.3	331.5	257.8	198.8	155.0	119.0	307.2
1906-1910----------	1955	2,525.5	712.5	445.8	331.2	258.0	197.9	154.3	118.7	307.1
1907-1911----------	1956	2,532.7	708.7	448.1	333.4	259.8	198.5	155.1	119.8	309.3
1908-1912----------	1957	2,549.1	705.6	452.1	336.9	262.6	200.3	157.3	121.3	313.0
1909-1913----------	1958	2,576.9	704.4	457.9	342.2	266.8	203.8	160.3	123.6	317.9
1910-1914----------	1959	2,606.1	703.4	464.4	348.1	271.6	207.9	163.5	125.5	321.7
1911-1915----------	1960	2,638.0	703.8	471.5	355.1	276.8	212.5	166.5	127.5	324.3
1912-1916----------	1961	2,671.9	704.0	479.4	363.1	282.8	217.7	169.5	129.6	325.8
1913-1917----------	1962	2,716.2	706.7	489.5	373.2	290.1	223.7	172.8	132.3	327.9
1914-1918----------	1963	2,769.7	711.3	501.2	384.3	298.5	230.3	177.0	135.6	331.5
1915-1919----------	1964	2,840.5	721.1	515.6	397.1	308.5	238.2	182.6	139.8	337.6
1916-1920----------	1965	2,921.6	733.7	531.7	410.8	319.6	247.0	189.3	144.4	345.1
1917-1921----------	1966	3,007.4	747.8	549.7	425.6	331.1	256.0	196.0	148.8	352.4
1918-1922----------	1967	3,084.2	758.6	566.5	439.9	341.9	264.2	202.3	152.7	358.1
1919-1923----------	1968	3,159.1	767.8	583.4	454.6	353.4	272.2	208.3	156.3	363.1
1920-1924----------	1969	3,232.9	774.9	600.3	470.1	365.4	280.4	214.4	160.2	367.2
1921-1925----------	1970	3,314.1	782.2	618.8	487.0	378.8	289.7	221.0	164.7	371.9
1922-1926----------	1971	3,402.5	789.4	637.6	504.8	393.4	300.5	228.8	170.0	378.0
1923-1927----------	1972	3,500.6	798.4	657.2	523.7	409.7	312.8	237.4	176.1	385.3
1924-1928----------	1973	3,589.3	805.9	674.8	541.9	424.9	324.6	245.5	181.3	390.4
1925-1929----------	1974	3,665.8	811.1	690.2	558.2	439.5	335.7	252.7	185.9	392.5

TABLE 5C. CUMULATIVE BIRTH RATES FOR ALL OTHER WOMEN AS OF THE BEGINNING OF EACH YEAR 1917-74 BY AGE AND LIVE-BIRTH ORDER FOR GROUPS OF COHORTS FROM 1867-71 TO 1955-59--CON.

(RATES ARE SIMPLE AVERAGES OF THE RATES FOR SINGLE COHORTS IN TABLE 6C)

EXACT AGE AND COHORT	AS OF JANUARY 1	TOTAL	LIVE-BIRTH ORDER							
			1	2	3	4	5	6	7	8 AND HIGHER
50-54 YEARS										
1863-1867----------	1917	---	---	---	---	---	---	---	---	---
1864-1868----------	1918	---	---	---	---	---	---	---	---	---
1865-1869----------	1919	---	---	---	---	---	---	---	---	---
1866-1870----------	1920	---	---	---	---	---	---	---	---	---
1867-1871----------	1921	5,167.1	830.7	723.5	635.6	557.9	482.2	423.1	357.7	1,156.4
1868-1872----------	1922	5,074.8	827.1	717.2	628.1	549.4	473.2	415.0	349.6	1,115.2
1869-1873----------	1923	4,978.9	823.1	710.5	620.1	540.4	464.0	406.7	341.2	1,072.9
1870-1874----------	1924	4,877.7	818.9	703.5	611.6	530.7	454.3	397.7	332.3	1,028.7
1871-1875----------	1925	4,770.8	814.3	696.1	602.5	520.5	444.1	388.0	322.7	982.6
1872-1876----------	1926	4,661.6	809.6	688.4	593.2	510.0	433.5	377.8	312.3	936.8
1873-1877----------	1927	4,552.1	804.9	680.7	583.9	499.5	422.6	367.1	301.5	891.9
1874-1878----------	1928	4,446.7	800.4	673.0	574.8	489.4	411.8	356.3	290.8	850.2
1875-1879----------	1929	4,346.3	796.1	665.5	566.4	480.0	401.4	345.9	280.7	810.3
1876-1880----------	1930	4,254.7	792.3	658.3	558.8	471.4	391.5	336.8	272.0	773.6
1877-1881----------	1931	4,172.4	789.1	651.6	552.2	463.6	382.4	329.3	265.0	739.2
1878-1882----------	1932	4,098.0	786.3	645.5	546.1	456.4	373.7	323.2	259.4	707.4
1879-1883----------	1933	4,025.6	783.6	639.3	539.8	448.2	364.6	317.6	253.8	678.7
1880-1884----------	1934	3,949.0	780.4	632.6	533.2	439.1	354.5	310.9	246.9	651.4
1881-1885----------	1935	3,865.0	776.9	625.4	525.6	429.1	343.8	302.3	238.2	623.7
1882-1886----------	1936	3,775.3	773.6	618.0	517.4	419.6	333.3	291.5	227.6	594.3
1883-1887----------	1937	3,683.6	771.0	610.7	508.7	411.0	323.6	278.5	215.8	564.3
1884-1888----------	1938	3,596.5	768.9	603.9	500.5	404.0	314.6	266.2	204.6	533.8
1885-1889----------	1939	3,518.5	767.9	597.5	493.1	397.0	305.6	254.4	194.5	508.5
1886-1890----------	1940	3,451.4	768.1	592.2	486.3	389.7	296.4	244.0	186.0	488.7
1887-1891----------	1941	3,393.2	769.0	587.7	479.7	380.9	286.6	235.4	179.4	474.5
1888-1892----------	1942	3,340.4	770.5	584.2	473.2	370.5	276.0	228.4	174.1	463.5
1889-1893----------	1943	3,298.9	772.7	581.1	470.7	361.9	266.8	221.9	169.3	454.5
1890-1894----------	1944	3,256.9	775.4	577.0	465.7	353.0	258.6	216.2	165.7	445.3
1891-1895----------	1945	3,212.5	777.7	571.0	458.6	344.1	251.5	211.1	162.7	435.8
1892-1896----------	1946	3,162.0	779.1	562.3	449.5	335.2	245.2	206.0	159.7	425.0
1893-1897----------	1947	3,106.1	779.5	550.6	439.0	326.4	239.6	201.0	156.4	413.6
1894-1898----------	1948	3,044.5	776.2	538.5	424.4	316.8	234.5	196.5	153.5	404.1
1895-1899----------	1949	3,000.1	774.3	527.4	412.7	310.1	232.3	194.1	151.7	397.5
1896-1900----------	1950	2,967.7	772.6	517.6	403.5	306.0	231.7	192.9	150.3	393.1
1897-1901----------	1951	2,932.7	770.2	508.9	395.0	302.0	230.7	190.8	148.0	387.1
1898-1902----------	1952	2,890.8	766.0	500.8	386.3	297.3	228.4	187.6	145.1	379.3
1899-1903----------	1953	2,838.6	763.2	492.2	376.7	290.8	224.2	182.5	141.0	368.0
1900-1904----------	1954	2,776.0	757.3	483.1	366.5	283.3	218.7	176.3	136.0	354.8
1901-1905----------	1955	2,706.7	749.6	473.7	355.9	274.9	212.6	169.6	130.5	339.9
1902-1906----------	1956	2,646.7	741.3	464.6	346.8	268.2	207.5	164.1	126.1	328.1
1903-1907----------	1957	2,598.2	733.0	456.6	339.8	263.2	203.8	160.0	122.8	319.0
1904-1908----------	1958	2,560.6	724.9	450.0	334.5	259.7	200.9	157.2	120.5	312.9
1905-1909----------	1959	2,537.4	718.2	446.4	331.7	258.1	199.0	155.3	119.2	309.5
1906-1910----------	1960	2,529.1	712.5	445.9	331.4	258.2	198.1	154.6	119.0	309.4
1907-1911----------	1961	2,536.4	708.8	448.2	333.6	260.0	198.7	155.4	120.0	311.7
1908-1912----------	1962	2,552.8	705.7	452.2	337.0	262.7	200.5	157.6	121.6	315.5
1909-1913----------	1963	2,580.5	704.6	458.0	342.3	267.0	204.0	160.6	123.8	320.2
1910-1914----------	1964	2,609.7	703.6	464.5	348.2	271.7	208.1	163.8	125.8	324.0
1911-1915----------	1965	2,641.2	703.9	471.5	355.2	276.9	212.8	166.7	127.8	326.4
1912-1916----------	1966	2,674.8	704.0	479.4	363.1	282.9	218.0	169.8	129.8	327.8
1913-1917----------	1967	2,719.4	706.8	489.6	373.3	290.2	224.0	173.1	132.5	329.9
1914-1918----------	1968	2,772.6	711.4	501.3	384.3	298.6	230.6	177.2	135.8	333.4
1915-1919----------	1969	2,843.5	721.2	515.7	397.2	308.6	238.5	182.8	140.0	339.5
1916-1920----------	1970	2,924.2	733.8	531.8	410.9	319.7	247.2	189.4	144.5	346.9
1917-1921----------	1971	3,009.9	747.9	549.7	425.7	331.2	256.2	196.2	148.9	354.1
1918-1922----------	1972	3,086.4	758.7	566.5	440.0	342.0	264.4	202.4	152.8	359.6
1919-1923----------	1973	3,161.3	767.9	583.4	454.7	353.5	272.4	208.5	156.5	364.4
1920-1924----------	1974	3,234.7	775.0	600.3	470.2	365.5	280.5	214.5	160.4	368.3

TABLE 6A. CUMULATIVE BIRTH RATES FOR ALL WOMEN AS OF THE BEGINNING OF EACH YEAR 1917-74 BY AGE AND LIVE-BIRTH ORDER FOR EACH COHORT FROM 1867 TO 1959

LIVE-BIRTH ORDER AND COHORT	DIAGONAL LINE FOR JANUARY 1	EXACT AGE											
		15	16	17	18	19	20	21	22	23	24	25	26
TOTAL BIRTHS													
1891-------													1,304.6
1892-------												1,129.4	1,310.2
1893-------											958.2	1,141.4	1,320.1
1894-------										772.4	957.9	1,139.5	1,302.7
1895-------									599.2	774.5	958.7	1,122.6	1,298.3
1896-------								436.7	604.0	778.5	941.8	1,120.0	1,299.5
1897-------							294.5	443.0	610.1	763.1	942.5	1,124.2	1,293.9
1898-------						176.2	298.8	447.0	592.4	764.6	948.0	1,121.2	1,293.1
1899-------					93.1	179.3	300.4	428.5	593.3	766.5	938.2	1,111.4	1,282.6
1900-------				40.6	94.8	178.8	284.0	432.2	597.6	759.3	932.5	1,107.6	1,271.8
1901-------			14.4	41.4	93.8	167.5	291.3	443.2	596.5	757.9	934.0	1,102.7	1,260.7
1902-------	1917	3.4	14.9	41.4	88.1	178.6	310.5	453.6	608.2	775.7	945.0	1,107.5	1,261.0
1903-------	1918	3.5	14.9	38.5	96.3	195.0	317.9	461.5	620.0	782.7	947.5	1,106.2	1,252.4
1904-------	1919	3.6	13.4	42.4	104.2	194.8	317.4	463.7	616.7	775.6	935.2	1,086.0	1,226.5
1905-------	1920	3.0	15.0	45.5	101.1	192.2	318.0	458.1	606.6	760.0	910.8	1,054.6	1,194.4
1906-------	1921	3.6	16.3	43.5	99.4	194.1	314.9	451.2	596.1	741.0	885.1	1,028.4	1,161.2
1907-------	1922	3.8	15.0	42.3	100.8	192.9	310.9	444.5	582.4	721.8	865.9	1,002.2	1,130.4
1908-------	1923	3.4	14.8	43.7	101.9	191.9	307.5	434.6	567.3	706.9	843.2	974.2	1,094.1
1909-------	1924	3.5	15.6	45.1	102.2	190.1	300.3	422.1	555.8	688.9	820.8	944.2	1,068.7
1910-------	1925	3.7	16.1	44.8	101.3	185.1	290.4	413.5	540.1	668.4	792.4	920.0	1,041.4
1911-------	1926	3.9	16.4	45.9	99.9	180.4	288.0	405.4	529.0	650.6	780.1	906.6	1,028.6
1912-------	1927	3.9	16.8	44.5	96.9	179.2	280.6	394.6	510.4	636.8	765.0	891.3	1,015.9
1913-------	1928	4.1	16.1	43.3	97.0	174.4	272.9	379.2	500.5	627.0	755.0	884.9	1,013.9
1914-------	1929	3.7	15.4	43.2	93.1	167.9	259.3	371.2	493.0	619.8	752.2	886.7	1,014.3
1915-------	1930	3.7	15.7	41.8	90.1	159.4	255.6	368.2	489.9	620.8	757.5	890.0	1,023.0
1916-------	1931	3.8	15.0	40.0	84.4	156.9	253.5	365.4	490.0	623.9	757.2	893.9	1,034.8
1917-------	1932	3.5	14.3	37.3	83.9	157.1	252.2	366.2	493.8	624.0	761.1	906.5	1,065.6
1918-------	1933	3.3	13.2	37.4	84.8	156.6	254.3	371.2	494.2	627.6	772.8	939.1	1,101.6
1919-------	1934	3.2	13.6	38.8	85.9	161.2	262.7	377.1	506.0	650.2	820.1	988.0	1,137.3
1920-------	1935	3.4	14.7	39.7	89.5	167.6	266.4	385.9	523.8	687.5	856.3	1,009.9	1,149.3
1921-------	1936	3.7	15.0	41.9	93.7	170.1	272.9	400.5	552.6	713.0	867.5	1,009.7	1,188.9
1922-------	1937	3.5	15.2	42.4	91.5	168.3	275.3	412.6	561.8	709.8	849.9	1,034.4	1,230.8
1923-------	1938	3.7	15.6	41.4	90.7	170.9	287.0	423.1	561.4	696.5	881.4	1,086.4	1,270.8
1924-------	1939	3.8	15.2	41.4	93.5	180.5	296.6	421.2	548.1	728.3	937.8	1,132.1	1,318.9
1925-------	1940	3.7	15.6	43.6	98.6	186.0	290.1	405.6	572.4	780.1	978.8	1,175.1	1,362.1
1926-------	1941	3.8	16.5	45.7	101.3	178.3	274.9	421.9	619.8	817.1	1,017.1	1,212.4	1,410.1
1927-------	1942	4.1	17.4	47.1	96.3	168.6	286.4	466.9	656.7	854.7	1,052.2	1,258.5	1,461.3
1928-------	1943	4.1	17.5	43.6	90.0	174.0	324.6	500.0	690.0	885.4	1,095.4	1,306.4	1,511.5
1929-------	1944	4.2	16.2	41.4	93.2	204.8	354.4	531.0	718.9	928.8	1,145.4	1,362.0	1,574.3
1930-------	1945	3.8	15.6	42.2	112.5	226.3	376.5	550.1	752.7	968.7	1,190.2	1,415.2	1,631.5
1931-------	1946	3.9	16.1	53.3	127.8	243.3	391.7	580.7	789.6	1,012.8	1,246.1	1,477.1	1,702.5
1932-------	1947	3.8	20.1	60.3	135.6	249.3	410.0	602.4	817.6	1,051.8	1,291.4	1,532.4	1,764.0
1933-------	1948	5.2	23.5	64.8	139.8	263.0	425.3	624.9	851.2	1,092.7	1,343.1	1,591.0	1,821.5
1934-------	1949	5.8	24.6	66.0	146.2	268.8	437.4	645.7	878.2	1,130.8	1,388.5	1,635.3	1,867.7
1935-------	1950	5.7	24.5	67.9	146.9	273.4	446.6	658.6	901.7	1,160.6	1,416.3	1,663.8	1,895.6
1936-------	1951	5.8	25.2	67.7	149.2	278.8	453.6	675.6	924.3	1,180.4	1,435.9	1,682.7	1,911.5
1937-------	1952	6.0	24.9	68.4	151.1	280.9	464.6	691.8	937.8	1,194.3	1,450.1	1,694.0	1,914.6
1938-------	1953	5.7	24.8	69.4	151.7	288.2	476.0	700.6	948.6	1,205.0	1,457.0	1,691.3	1,903.0
1939-------	1954	5.8	25.9	70.6	157.8	298.3	484.6	712.6	959.6	1,212.9	1,455.8	1,681.4	1,884.7
1940-------	1955	6.3	26.2	73.0	162.3	300.4	488.0	712.2	955.4	1,199.9	1,432.8	1,648.1	1,831.6
1941-------	1956	6.1	27.0	74.9	161.2	297.3	479.2	698.3	932.5	1,165.4	1,386.8	1,580.5	1,751.2
1942-------	1957	6.2	27.0	72.4	156.1	287.3	463.7	673.7	896.2	1,116.5	1,315.0	1,496.3	1,660.9
1943-------	1958	6.1	25.6	69.4	149.6	276.7	445.8	646.3	856.1	1,053.2	1,239.4	1,413.5	1,574.7
1944-------	1959	5.8	25.1	67.7	146.8	269.4	432.7	623.0	811.9	997.5	1,175.7	1,344.4	1,506.9
1945-------	1960	6.0	25.2	67.5	143.8	262.8	418.1	590.1	768.0	943.9	1,114.4	1,282.4	1,445.4
1946-------	1961	6.0	24.8	65.1	138.5	251.9	394.3	557.8	726.1	894.9	1,066.1	1,236.2	1,387.4
1947-------	1962	5.5	22.9	61.5	131.6	237.0	373.1	527.4	688.9	856.7	1,027.9	1,184.7	1,317.9
1948-------	1963	5.1	21.8	58.8	125.2	227.0	356.5	505.4	665.5	832.9	990.0	1,126.4	1,251.5
1949-------	1964	5.1	21.8	57.8	122.6	220.1	345.3	492.0	651.2	804.2	939.5	1,066.1	
1950-------	1965	5.2	21.7	57.2	120.4	216.1	340.6	487.7	632.2	763.1	888.2		
1951-------	1966	5.2	21.6	56.9	119.5	215.2	341.2	475.1	599.7	720.5			
1952-------	1967	5.3	21.8	57.0	120.1	218.4	334.5	451.7	566.7				
1953-------	1968	5.3	22.0	57.8	124.4	216.8	321.8	430.6					
1954-------	1969	5.7	23.1	61.9	126.1	213.2	311.7						
1955-------	1970	6.0	25.2	63.5	127.0	210.1							
1956-------	1971	6.6	25.8	65.1	126.6								
1957-------	1972	6.7	26.8	65.6									
1958-------	1973	7.1	27.3										
1959-------	1974	7.4											

TABLE 6A. CUMULATIVE BIRTH RATES FOR ALL WOMEN AS OF THE BEGINNING OF EACH YEAR 1917-74 BY AGE AND LIVE-BIRTH ORDER FOR EACH COHORT FROM 1867 TO 1959--CON.

LIVE-BIRTH ORDER AND COHORT	DIAGONAL LINE FOR JANUARY 1	EXACT AGE											
		27	28	29	30	31	32	33	34	35	36	37	38
TOTAL BIRTHS--CON.													
1879-------													3,138.3
1880-------												3,006.7	3,102.0
1881-------											2,869.7	2,971.0	3,065.2
1882-------										2,728.0	2,837.6	2,937.7	3,030.9
1883-------									2,585.5	2,700.2	2,808.4	2,907.0	2,999.6
1884-------								2,441.1	2,562.1	2,675.2	2,780.7	2,878.9	2,971.6
1885-------							2,294.9	2,417.2	2,536.9	2,646.1	2,751.3	2,850.0	2,936.2
1886-------						2,144.5	2,279.0	2,400.9	2,516.0	2,625.6	2,732.5	2,824.8	2,910.1
1887-------					1,989.8	2,134.7	2,269.3	2,386.6	2,502.5	2,614.6	2,714.9	2,806.6	2,891.4
1888-------				1,827.4	1,993.6	2,137.7	2,266.8	2,385.0	2,503.5	2,608.8	2,708.4	2,799.2	2,880.8
1889-------			1,652.0	1,822.7	1,986.8	2,123.6	2,254.1	2,374.8	2,486.4	2,591.0	2,689.8	2,777.8	2,856.2
1890-------	1917	1,476.3	1,650.9	1,819.8	1,975.0	2,115.0	2,248.4	2,362.6	2,474.3	2,578.8	2,673.8	2,757.6	2,833.7
1891-------	1918	1,475.7	1,649.3	1,807.2	1,967.5	2,110.1	2,236.5	2,350.5	2,461.9	2,563.0	2,654.0	2,735.9	2,806.4
1892-------	1919	1,480.4	1,641.3	1,805.6	1,967.6	2,100.8	2,226.0	2,339.2	2,446.1	2,541.7	2,629.2	2,703.8	2,768.4
1893-------	1920	1,476.9	1,645.5	1,811.0	1,961.4	2,092.9	2,217.5	2,326.5	2,427.3	2,519.8	2,600.6	2,670.2	2,733.8
1894-------	1921	1,469.8	1,641.2	1,794.9	1,943.8	2,074.8	2,194.8	2,299.0	2,397.5	2,483.4	2,559.4	2,628.1	2,688.5
1895-------	1922	1,469.0	1,629.4	1,782.2	1,930.4	2,057.1	2,172.6	2,274.5	2,366.9	2,448.3	2,523.9	2,589.2	2,647.1
1896-------	1923	1,460.2	1,619.7	1,771.1	1,913.7	2,036.0	2,148.2	2,243.4	2,330.4	2,410.9	2,481.7	2,544.1	2,597.6
1897-------	1924	1,453.9	1,612.7	1,758.2	1,895.3	2,013.3	2,118.9	2,209.0	2,295.1	2,370.5	2,439.0	2,496.9	2,550.2
1898-------	1925	1,454.2	1,606.8	1,746.6	1,878.6	1,989.9	2,090.8	2,181.0	2,262.5	2,335.4	2,399.2	2,457.3	2,508.3
1899-------	1926	1,439.4	1,587.6	1,724.5	1,851.0	1,959.0	2,060.8	2,147.9	2,229.4	2,299.6	2,365.6	2,422.9	2,472.6
1900-------	1927	1,422.0	1,566.1	1,695.0	1,815.6	1,923.6	2,020.5	2,105.4	2,181.9	2,253.5	2,317.6	2,372.8	2,421.8
1901-------	1928	1,408.0	1,543.4	1,666.0	1,785.5	1,888.4	1,982.0	2,061.2	2,138.5	2,207.0	2,267.8	2,321.3	2,369.3
1902-------	1929	1,399.1	1,527.6	1,649.4	1,762.7	1,860.2	1,946.3	2,025.7	2,098.8	2,163.4	2,222.1	2,274.5	2,320.3
1903-------	1930	1,385.3	1,513.8	1,630.9	1,739.6	1,830.9	1,918.8	1,994.9	2,065.3	2,128.8	2,187.3	2,237.9	2,282.9
1904-------	1931	1,359.5	1,483.0	1,596.1	1,698.9	1,793.3	1,878.9	1,953.5	2,023.8	2,087.7	2,145.1	2,196.0	2,241.5
1905-------	1932	1,321.8	1,440.7	1,547.0	1,652.6	1,744.2	1,827.4	1,902.0	1,972.7	2,035.4	2,092.8	2,144.1	2,191.3
1906-------	1933	1,283.5	1,395.4	1,504.3	1,606.8	1,696.2	1,779.6	1,854.9	1,924.7	1,988.4	2,046.4	2,099.0	2,150.5
1907-------	1934	1,245.7	1,360.9	1,467.2	1,567.2	1,657.5	1,742.5	1,817.5	1,888.6	1,953.5	2,015.3	2,073.1	2,126.1
1908-------	1935	1,212.2	1,323.9	1,427.5	1,527.8	1,619.6	1,703.6	1,780.3	1,852.6	1,922.8	1,990.4	2,050.3	2,104.9
1909-------	1936	1,184.7	1,295.1	1,400.8	1,504.4	1,596.1	1,683.1	1,762.6	1,842.6	1,919.3	1,988.3	2,051.2	2,107.8
1910-------	1937	1,156.4	1,268.8	1,378.1	1,480.5	1,575.7	1,665.6	1,751.7	1,838.7	1,916.2	1,988.2	2,053.7	2,111.1
1911-------	1938	1,146.9	1,264.2	1,372.6	1,479.3	1,578.5	1,674.0	1,767.8	1,854.2	1,934.7	2,010.6	2,077.5	2,131.6
1912-------	1939	1,137.9	1,253.0	1,365.6	1,476.5	1,584.0	1,688.1	1,781.1	1,869.9	1,954.9	2,031.6	2,093.8	2,146.7
1913-------	1940	1,134.7	1,254.6	1,373.2	1,494.5	1,609.6	1,712.2	1,807.8	1,903.1	1,989.8	2,061.4	2,122.5	2,175.1
1914-------	1941	1,140.9	1,268.6	1,400.6	1,529.3	1,640.9	1,746.4	1,851.1	1,949.0	2,030.0	2,100.9	2,162.1	2,216.4
1915-------	1942	1,157.6	1,299.5	1,437.9	1,560.6	1,674.0	1,791.0	1,899.0	1,990.2	2,070.4	2,141.6	2,204.9	2,261.1
1916-------	1943	1,184.1	1,331.8	1,461.0	1,583.4	1,710.4	1,831.2	1,930.8	2,020.6	2,100.8	2,173.8	2,238.7	2,295.1
1917-------	1944	1,219.6	1,356.4	1,483.7	1,623.7	1,757.0	1,869.2	1,968.2	2,058.5	2,141.1	2,216.0	2,281.8	2,339.9
1918-------	1945	1,243.4	1,374.9	1,522.5	1,670.1	1,792.7	1,903.9	2,003.0	2,095.8	2,180.8	2,256.4	2,323.5	2,380.9
1919-------	1946	1,273.2	1,433.1	1,593.7	1,732.1	1,856.7	1,969.9	2,074.7	2,172.9	2,260.4	2,339.5	2,407.7	2,466.8
1920-------	1947	1,318.2	1,492.6	1,642.7	1,782.5	1,908.5	2,027.1	2,136.8	2,236.4	2,326.6	2,405.5	2,474.1	2,533.6
1921-------	1948	1,375.1	1,538.4	1,690.2	1,831.7	1,963.8	2,088.0	2,198.8	2,301.5	2,392.0	2,471.7	2,541.3	2,599.4
1922-------	1949	1,403.5	1,566.6	1,718.7	1,865.2	2,001.9	2,126.0	2,238.9	2,340.5	2,430.7	2,510.7	2,577.7	2,634.8
1923-------	1950	1,445.1	1,609.5	1,769.0	1,921.2	2,058.4	2,185.7	2,298.4	2,400.9	2,492.6	2,570.5	2,637.3	2,693.5
1924-------	1951	1,495.2	1,669.4	1,835.4	1,989.2	2,131.0	2,258.6	2,372.9	2,477.4	2,566.8	2,644.7	2,710.9	2,766.9
1925-------	1952	1,548.3	1,728.6	1,896.0	2,053.9	2,195.2	2,324.3	2,440.1	2,541.7	2,630.6	2,707.8	2,773.7	2,826.9
1926-------	1953	1,602.1	1,783.6	1,955.3	2,113.3	2,256.0	2,386.0	2,498.7	2,599.3	2,687.1	2,763.1	2,825.4	2,876.6
1927-------	1954	1,655.5	1,840.4	2,011.8	2,171.5	2,315.7	2,442.9	2,554.9	2,654.3	2,741.2	2,813.7	2,874.0	2,924.0
1928-------	1955	1,709.5	1,895.3	2,068.2	2,229.3	2,370.8	2,497.9	2,608.7	2,707.0	2,789.4	2,859.1	2,917.7	2,963.5
1929-------	1956	1,775.2	1,965.3	2,143.0	2,302.6	2,445.6	2,572.4	2,684.1	2,779.1	2,859.8	2,928.6	2,982.8	3,024.6
1930-------	1957	1,837.8	2,032.5	2,208.1	2,369.1	2,511.4	2,637.8	2,744.8	2,837.6	2,916.8	2,979.9	3,028.9	3,067.2
1931-------	1958	1,916.2	2,110.2	2,287.8	2,448.5	2,590.9	2,712.7	2,817.4	2,908.3	2,980.8	3,037.9	3,083.1	3,118.4
1932-------	1959	1,976.2	2,172.1	2,349.4	2,509.1	2,645.4	2,764.1	2,865.7	2,948.7	3,013.8	3,065.9	3,107.7	3,140.6
1933-------	1960	2,035.4	2,230.9	2,407.5	2,560.5	2,692.8	2,807.9	2,900.7	2,974.7	3,034.7	3,083.5	3,123.0	3,154.3
1934-------	1961	2,081.4	2,275.5	2,445.4	2,594.1	2,722.9	2,828.0	2,911.1	2,979.2	3,034.7	3,081.4	3,119.1	3,147.7
1935-------	1962	2,107.0	2,294.2	2,458.5	2,603.5	2,720.0	2,814.0	2,890.5	2,953.8	3,007.6	3,052.1	3,086.4	3,111.3
1936-------	1963	2,116.2	2,296.9	2,456.7	2,587.3	2,692.4	2,778.9	2,850.1	2,911.9	2,963.7	3,004.2	3,033.8	3,055.6
1937-------	1964	2,111.5	2,286.0	2,429.7	2,548.0	2,645.9	2,728.1	2,798.9	2,859.1	2,906.3	2,941.1	2,967.3	
1938-------	1965	2,092.1	2,249.3	2,379.3	2,489.6	2,582.6	2,664.5	2,734.5	2,789.4	2,830.5	2,861.6		
1939-------	1966	2,056.0	2,199.7	2,323.2	2,430.3	2,524.9	2,607.5	2,672.5	2,721.3	2,758.8			
1940-------	1967	1,989.0	2,126.1	2,247.2	2,356.6	2,452.6	2,529.1	2,586.5	2,631.1				
1941-------	1968	1,902.3	2,037.6	2,161.3	2,272.6	2,362.2	2,430.1	2,483.3					
1942-------	1969	1,810.5	1,949.6	2,076.0	2,180.0	2,259.6	2,323.1						
1943-------	1970	1,726.4	1,867.0	1,984.8	2,076.9	2,151.5							
1944-------	1971	1,660.1	1,791.0	1,895.7	1,983.0								
1945-------	1972	1,587.5	1,703.6	1,802.8									
1946-------	1973	1,513.6	1,624.4										
1947-------	1974	1,437.2											

TABLE 6A. CUMULATIVE BIRTH RATES FOR ALL WOMEN AS OF THE BEGINNING OF EACH YEAR 1917-74 BY AGE AND LIVE-BIRTH ORDER FOR EACH COHORT FROM 1867 TO 1959--CON.

LIVE-BIRTH ORDER AND COHORT	DIAGONAL LINE FOR JANUARY 1	EXACT AGE											
		39	40	41	42	43	44	45	46	47	48	49	50
TOTAL BIRTHS--CON.													
1867-------													4,071.7
1868-------												4,023.2	4,024.3
1869-------											3,972.3	3,974.6	3,976.0
1870-------										3,918.2	3,922.3	3,925.1	3,926.2
1871-------									3,860.0	3,867.5	3,872.6	3,874.7	3,876.0
1872-------								3,796.8	3,808.5	3,817.6	3,821.5	3,823.9	3,824.9
1873-------							3,728.5	3,746.3	3,759.1	3,766.4	3,770.8	3,772.8	3,773.7
1874-------						3,653.4	3,678.8	3,697.2	3,708.4	3,716.3	3,720.2	3,722.1	3,723.0
1875-------					3,569.9	3,602.1	3,627.2	3,644.1	3,656.0	3,663.1	3,666.6	3,668.5	3,669.4
1876-------				3,477.1	3,521.3	3,553.4	3,577.8	3,595.1	3,606.2	3,612.8	3,616.4	3,618.2	3,618.9
1877-------			3,374.0	3,429.8	3,474.4	3,505.4	3,530.0	3,547.0	3,557.3	3,563.9	3,567.3	3,569.0	3,569.7
1878-------	1917	3,262.9	3,338.0	3,394.0	3,437.2	3,468.5	3,493.6	3,509.7	3,520.1	3,526.5	3,529.5	3,531.2	3,531.8
1879-------	1918	3,222.6	3,297.8	3,352.7	3,396.8	3,428.7	3,452.1	3,468.1	3,478.4	3,484.6	3,487.6	3,489.0	3,489.5
1880-------	1919	3,185.6	3,259.9	3,315.4	3,359.7	3,389.5	3,412.7	3,428.6	3,438.5	3,444.5	3,447.3	3,448.8	3,449.5
1881-------	1920	3,148.1	3,222.5	3,278.4	3,319.7	3,349.3	3,372.5	3,387.6	3,396.8	3,402.2	3,404.8	3,406.1	3,406.7
1882-------	1921	3,113.4	3,188.0	3,239.8	3,280.4	3,309.9	3,332.1	3,346.3	3,355.0	3,360.2	3,362.9	3,364.1	3,364.5
1883-------	1922	3,082.2	3,151.2	3,202.1	3,242.4	3,270.6	3,291.6	3,305.0	3,313.2	3,318.0	3,320.5	3,321.6	3,322.0
1884-------	1923	3,048.1	3,115.9	3,166.2	3,205.0	3,231.9	3,251.8	3,264.4	3,272.0	3,276.5	3,278.7	3,279.9	3,280.4
1885-------	1924	3,011.4	3,078.3	3,126.8	3,163.5	3,189.3	3,207.9	3,219.4	3,226.8	3,231.1	3,233.1	3,234.3	3,234.8
1886-------	1925	2,984.9	3,049.0	3,094.4	3,129.7	3,153.6	3,170.5	3,181.9	3,188.9	3,193.1	3,195.0	3,196.1	3,196.8
1887-------	1926	2,963.9	3,025.1	3,070.0	3,103.0	3,125.3	3,142.3	3,153.0	3,159.6	3,163.4	3,165.2	3,166.2	3,166.8
1888-------	1927	2,949.4	3,008.7	3,050.1	3,080.5	3,102.5	3,118.3	3,128.5	3,134.6	3,138.1	3,139.8	3,140.8	3,141.3
1889-------	1928	2,923.9	2,979.5	3,018.5	3,049.0	3,070.0	3,085.6	3,095.4	3,101.3	3,104.9	3,106.5	3,107.4	3,107.8
1890-------	1929	2,896.1	2,947.7	2,986.5	3,015.1	3,035.3	3,050.1	3,059.6	3,065.3	3,068.6	3,070.1	3,071.1	3,071.5
1891-------	1930	2,864.3	2,915.5	2,951.6	2,979.1	2,998.2	3,012.8	3,021.6	3,026.8	3,029.7	3,031.1	3,032.0	3,032.2
1892-------	1931	2,825.7	2,873.0	2,907.4	2,933.1	2,951.8	2,965.2	2,973.4	2,978.3	2,981.2	2,982.4	2,983.1	2,983.3
1893-------	1932	2,787.4	2,832.7	2,865.0	2,890.2	2,907.5	2,919.9	2,927.4	2,932.1	2,934.7	2,935.8	2,936.2	2,936.4
1894-------	1933	2,739.6	2,781.6	2,813.5	2,837.3	2,853.4	2,864.9	2,872.5	2,876.8	2,879.2	2,880.3	2,880.6	2,880.8
1895-------	1934	2,694.9	2,736.6	2,766.8	2,789.1	2,804.5	2,815.8	2,822.7	2,826.7	2,829.0	2,829.9	2,830.2	2,830.3
1896-------	1935	2,644.9	2,684.3	2,712.5	2,733.7	2,748.9	2,759.3	2,765.7	2,769.5	2,771.7	2,772.4	2,772.7	2,772.9
1897-------	1936	2,595.1	2,632.0	2,659.3	2,680.2	2,694.3	2,704.4	2,710.5	2,714.4	2,716.4	2,717.2	2,717.5	2,717.6
1898-------	1937	2,550.7	2,586.5	2,613.6	2,633.5	2,647.4	2,657.1	2,664.0	2,668.2	2,670.3	2,671.4	2,671.7	2,671.9
1899-------	1938	2,515.0	2,551.2	2,577.5	2,597.1	2,610.8	2,620.8	2,627.6	2,631.5	2,633.8	2,634.8	2,635.1	2,635.3
1900-------	1939	2,464.1	2,498.7	2,524.6	2,544.1	2,557.6	2,568.1	2,575.0	2,579.0	2,581.2	2,582.2	2,582.5	2,582.6
1901-------	1940	2,409.5	2,442.8	2,468.0	2,486.4	2,500.6	2,511.4	2,518.2	2,522.0	2,524.1	2,524.9	2,525.2	2,525.3
1902-------	1941	2,359.5	2,392.5	2,417.8	2,438.0	2,453.0	2,463.9	2,470.5	2,474.1	2,475.8	2,476.5	2,476.7	2,476.8
1903-------	1942	2,321.7	2,355.6	2,382.6	2,403.4	2,418.8	2,429.5	2,436.0	2,439.3	2,441.0	2,441.6	2,441.8	2,441.9
1904-------	1943	2,282.3	2,318.7	2,346.4	2,368.1	2,383.0	2,393.6	2,399.4	2,402.6	2,404.2	2,404.7	2,404.9	2,405.0
1905-------	1944	2,235.3	2,272.4	2,301.1	2,322.5	2,337.6	2,347.4	2,353.3	2,356.3	2,357.7	2,358.2	2,358.4	2,358.5
1906-------	1945	2,195.5	2,233.7	2,262.4	2,283.8	2,297.8	2,307.3	2,312.7	2,315.7	2,317.1	2,317.6	2,317.8	2,317.9
1907-------	1946	2,172.5	2,211.4	2,240.6	2,260.9	2,274.6	2,283.9	2,289.4	2,292.4	2,293.8	2,294.3	2,294.4	2,294.5
1908-------	1947	2,152.0	2,190.6	2,217.7	2,237.4	2,250.5	2,259.6	2,265.1	2,268.0	2,269.6	2,270.1	2,270.2	2,270.3
1909-------	1948	2,155.7	2,192.3	2,219.3	2,238.8	2,252.4	2,261.9	2,267.6	2,270.5	2,272.0	2,272.5	2,272.7	2,272.8
1910-------	1949	2,156.3	2,192.8	2,219.8	2,239.8	2,253.8	2,263.4	2,269.1	2,271.9	2,273.4	2,273.9	2,274.1	2,274.2
1911-------	1950	2,176.3	2,212.4	2,240.0	2,260.5	2,274.7	2,284.5	2,290.3	2,293.3	2,294.8	2,295.4	2,295.5	2,295.6
1912-------	1951	2,190.9	2,227.6	2,255.7	2,276.4	2,291.2	2,301.0	2,306.7	2,309.7	2,311.1	2,311.7	2,311.8	2,311.9
1913-------	1952	2,220.2	2,257.9	2,286.3	2,307.6	2,322.2	2,332.1	2,337.7	2,340.5	2,342.0	2,342.6	2,342.7	2,342.8
1914-------	1953	2,263.4	2,301.6	2,330.9	2,352.1	2,367.0	2,376.9	2,382.5	2,385.5	2,387.0	2,387.5	2,387.6	2,387.7
1915-------	1954	2,308.5	2,347.7	2,377.1	2,398.8	2,413.7	2,423.2	2,428.9	2,431.7	2,433.1	2,433.7	2,433.8	2,433.8
1916-------	1955	2,343.3	2,382.5	2,411.4	2,433.0	2,447.2	2,456.8	2,462.3	2,465.3	2,466.8	2,467.1	2,467.2	2,467.2
1917-------	1956	2,388.4	2,427.7	2,457.3	2,478.3	2,492.7	2,502.0	2,507.6	2,510.4	2,511.6	2,512.0	2,512.1	2,512.1
1918-------	1957	2,429.0	2,468.2	2,496.7	2,517.5	2,531.6	2,541.0	2,546.2	2,548.7	2,549.9	2,550.1	2,550.2	2,550.2
1919-------	1958	2,516.2	2,555.1	2,584.2	2,605.1	2,619.6	2,628.8	2,634.1	2,636.6	2,637.6	2,637.8	2,637.9	2,637.9
1920-------	1959	2,581.8	2,620.8	2,649.6	2,670.8	2,684.8	2,693.6	2,698.6	2,701.0	2,702.0	2,702.2	2,702.3	2,702.3
1921-------	1960	2,647.5	2,685.6	2,714.5	2,734.7	2,748.3	2,757.0	2,761.7	2,764.0	2,764.9	2,765.1	2,765.2	2,765.2
1922-------	1961	2,681.7	2,719.4	2,746.5	2,765.8	2,778.6	2,786.4	2,790.8	2,793.0	2,793.8	2,794.0	2,794.0	2,794.0
1923-------	1962	2,740.1	2,775.8	2,801.8	2,820.6	2,832.7	2,839.9	2,844.0	2,845.9	2,846.6	2,846.7	2,846.7	2,846.7
1924-------	1963	2,811.1	2,845.7	2,871.5	2,889.0	2,900.0	2,906.7	2,910.4	2,912.2	2,913.0	2,913.1	2,913.1	2,913.1
1925-------	1964	2,869.7	2,903.8	2,927.8	2,943.8	2,953.8	2,959.9	2,963.2	2,964.9	2,965.6	2,965.7	2,965.7	
1926-------	1965	2,918.6	2,950.3	2,971.9	2,986.5	2,995.8	3,001.4	3,004.5	3,005.9	3,006.4	3,006.5		
1927-------	1966	2,962.7	2,991.0	3,010.7	3,023.9	3,032.3	3,037.3	3,039.7	3,040.8	3,041.2			
1928-------	1967	2,998.1	3,023.7	3,041.5	3,053.5	3,061.3	3,065.7	3,067.8	3,068.8				
1929-------	1968	3,056.7	3,080.4	3,097.2	3,108.6	3,115.3	3,119.3	3,121.3					
1930-------	1969	3,096.5	3,118.5	3,134.3	3,144.1	3,150.0	3,153.4						
1931-------	1970	3,145.7	3,166.7	3,180.4	3,189.1	3,194.5							
1932-------	1971	3,166.5	3,184.9	3,196.9	3,204.6								
1933-------	1972	3,177.3	3,193.2	3,203.8									
1934-------	1973	3,168.1	3,182.2										
1935-------	1974	3,129.1											

TABLE 6A. CUMULATIVE BIRTH RATES FOR ALL WOMEN AS OF THE BEGINNING OF EACH YEAR 1917-74 BY AGE AND LIVE-BIRTH ORDER FOR EACH COHORT FROM 1867 TO 1959--CON.

LIVE-BIRTH ORDER AND COHORT	DIAGONAL LINE FOR JANUARY 1	EXACT AGE											
		15	16	17	18	19	20	21	22	23	24	25	26
FIRST BIRTHS													
1891-------													597.2
1892-------												557.4	605.2
1893-------											507.3	564.2	612.8
1894-------										445.9	513.2	570.7	608.8
1895-------									377.1	451.7	519.3	563.8	613.6
1896-------								300.8	383.8	458.9	510.6	569.4	620.9
1897-------							221.7	307.1	390.9	448.6	517.5	578.0	624.3
1898-------						143.1	224.9	310.6	375.7	452.9	523.7	577.9	623.1
1899-------					81.0	146.7	227.4	295.8	381.4	459.6	521.5	573.8	619.8
1900-------				37.4	83.0	146.9	213.6	302.9	389.4	457.7	517.8	571.8	615.9
1901-------			13.9	38.3	82.4	137.3	223.6	316.0	391.7	458.1	521.1	573.4	616.0
1902-------	1917	3.4	14.3	38.3	76.9	148.2	239.9	321.9	395.9	466.0	526.9	577.2	619.2
1903-------	1918	3.5	14.4	35.5	85.1	162.0	243.3	323.7	401.1	469.0	527.9	577.7	618.6
1904-------	1919	3.6	12.9	39.4	92.0	159.9	239.7	324.0	398.6	464.5	522.1	570.2	609.8
1905-------	1920	3.0	14.5	42.3	88.5	155.9	240.2	320.7	392.4	456.4	511.6	557.6	598.5
1906-------	1921	3.6	15.7	40.1	86.2	158.2	239.1	316.6	386.9	447.9	500.7	548.1	587.2
1907-------	1922	3.8	14.4	38.8	87.9	157.7	235.7	311.6	378.5	437.5	492.0	537.3	574.7
1908-------	1923	3.4	14.2	40.3	89.0	156.4	232.5	304.7	369.5	430.1	481.5	524.7	559.8
1909-------	1924	3.5	15.0	41.5	88.7	154.3	227.0	296.2	362.9	420.2	469.6	510.1	547.8
1910-------	1925	3.7	15.5	41.1	87.7	150.6	219.9	291.2	354.0	408.9	454.9	498.4	537.7
1911-------	1926	3.9	15.7	42.0	86.6	146.8	218.6	286.1	346.9	398.7	448.7	494.4	535.3
1912-------	1927	3.9	16.1	40.8	84.1	146.4	213.7	278.9	336.0	392.2	444.5	491.6	534.8
1913-------	1928	4.1	15.4	39.7	84.4	142.5	207.8	269.2	331.5	390.3	443.5	493.1	538.7
1914-------	1929	3.7	14.8	39.8	81.2	137.4	198.3	264.9	329.6	389.0	444.9	496.9	542.4
1915-------	1930	3.7	15.1	38.5	78.6	130.8	196.6	265.1	329.5	391.1	449.1	500.2	547.4
1916-------	1931	3.8	14.4	36.8	73.7	129.4	196.3	263.6	329.6	392.9	449.0	500.9	553.8
1917-------	1932	3.5	13.7	34.3	73.5	130.0	194.8	263.5	331.2	392.3	448.7	507.3	571.9
1918-------	1933	3.3	12.7	34.5	74.5	129.1	195.7	265.9	330.6	392.1	455.5	527.8	585.3
1919-------	1934	3.2	13.1	35.8	74.9	132.2	201.4	269.3	336.5	406.8	486.4	551.1	599.7
1920-------	1935	3.4	14.1	36.4	77.8	137.1	203.3	272.4	347.6	432.6	503.8	559.8	605.8
1921-------	1936	3.7	14.3	38.2	81.2	137.9	204.3	280.5	368.0	444.0	507.3	560.7	628.4
1922-------	1937	3.5	14.5	38.7	78.9	133.5	204.3	291.0	370.4	439.0	498.9	576.3	653.9
1923-------	1938	3.7	14.9	37.7	76.9	134.8	214.8	296.3	368.6	434.0	519.9	610.0	672.4
1924-------	1939	3.8	14.5	37.2	79.0	143.6	221.0	294.2	363.4	456.1	558.4	631.8	688.8
1925-------	1940	3.7	14.6	39.0	83.1	147.2	215.5	286.0	381.1	494.2	578.4	645.4	697.5
1926-------	1941	3.8	15.5	40.5	84.6	140.4	205.7	298.3	418.1	512.2	589.2	650.7	705.0
1927-------	1942	4.1	16.0	41.1	79.7	132.9	214.8	335.6	437.4	523.4	594.1	658.5	711.8
1928-------	1943	4.1	16.1	38.1	74.8	138.1	248.3	354.3	447.8	527.3	602.3	666.0	716.8
1929-------	1944	4.2	14.9	36.2	77.8	165.7	266.9	365.7	453.0	538.9	614.1	675.7	726.3
1930-------	1945	3.8	14.3	36.9	95.4	180.2	275.3	368.0	463.2	549.5	622.6	685.0	734.5
1931-------	1946	3.9	14.7	47.0	106.8	188.0	278.6	381.0	476.9	562.1	637.5	699.6	749.0
1932-------	1947	3.8	18.5	52.7	110.6	188.8	288.7	390.9	487.6	576.2	652.0	714.4	763.1
1933-------	1948	5.2	21.5	55.6	112.6	198.4	297.2	401.9	502.3	591.7	668.6	730.4	775.9
1934-------	1949	5.8	22.3	56.4	117.6	201.8	304.1	412.8	513.7	605.7	682.4	740.7	784.2
1935-------	1950	5.7	22.3	58.2	118.2	205.0	310.2	418.8	524.2	616.4	689.4	745.5	787.5
1936-------	1951	5.8	23.0	58.2	120.0	209.1	313.4	427.3	533.3	621.6	692.0	746.6	787.6
1937-------	1952	6.0	22.8	59.0	121.9	210.0	319.8	435.3	537.6	623.7	693.1	746.6	785.6
1938-------	1953	5.7	22.8	59.8	121.8	214.3	326.3	438.3	539.0	623.9	691.9	742.6	781.0
1939-------	1954	5.8	23.7	60.5	126.0	221.2	330.1	441.6	540.8	624.2	688.9	738.9	777.8
1940-------	1955	6.3	23.9	62.4	129.5	221.4	329.3	438.3	536.3	616.4	679.8	730.3	768.3
1941-------	1956	6.1	24.6	64.0	127.8	217.6	321.9	429.1	523.7	601.8	665.8	714.8	755.6
1942-------	1957	6.2	24.7	61.6	123.3	209.7	312.2	415.8	508.1	586.5	648.2	700.9	742.6
1943-------	1958	6.1	23.3	59.0	118.0	202.6	301.5	403.0	494.0	568.0	632.6	685.0	729.7
1944-------	1959	5.8	22.9	57.5	115.9	197.5	294.8	394.0	479.5	555.5	618.5	672.5	717.6
1945-------	1960	6.0	22.9	57.2	113.1	193.3	287.5	380.1	466.1	539.3	602.7	657.1	703.6
1946-------	1961	6.0	22.5	54.9	109.4	187.0	276.3	369.9	453.3	527.5	592.8	650.0	695.2
1947-------	1962	5.5	20.7	52.1	104.8	178.9	268.4	358.2	442.1	517.4	584.5	638.5	680.6
1948-------	1963	5.1	19.8	50.3	101.5	175.7	261.7	351.9	436.0	512.4	574.3	623.0	663.9
1949-------	1964	5.1	19.8	49.7	100.4	171.6	257.2	346.3	430.3	499.1	553.1	598.9	
1950-------	1965	5.2	19.8	49.7	99.5	171.0	256.4	346.2	421.5	480.9	531.3		
1951-------	1966	5.2	19.9	49.6	99.8	171.7	258.7	339.6	404.9	459.8			
1952-------	1967	5.3	20.1	50.3	101.4	176.1	255.8	327.1	387.3				
1953-------	1968	5.3	20.5	51.4	105.8	175.9	248.6	314.6					
1954-------	1969	5.7	21.6	55.3	107.8	174.6	242.6						
1955-------	1970	6.0	23.6	57.0	109.7	173.4							
1956-------	1971	6.6	24.2	58.9	110.1								
1957-------	1972	6.7	25.3	59.7									
1958-------	1973	7.1	25.9										
1959-------	1974	7.4											

TABLE 6A. CUMULATIVE BIRTH RATES FOR ALL WOMEN AS OF THE BEGINNING OF EACH YEAR 1917-74 BY AGE AND LIVE-BIRTH ORDER FOR EACH COHORT FROM 1867 TO 1959--CON.

LIVE-BIRTH ORDER AND COHORT	DIAGONAL LINE FOR JANUARY 1	EXACT AGE											
		27	28	29	30	31	32	33	34	35	36	37	38
FIRST BIRTHS--CON.													
1879-------													770.7
1880-------												765.8	769.7
1881-------											761.6	766.4	770.5
1882-------										757.1	763.2	768.2	772.2
1883-------									750.2	757.4	763.7	768.6	772.8
1884-------								740.6	749.3	756.8	762.8	767.9	772.3
1885-------							729.7	739.8	749.1	756.0	762.4	767.8	771.9
1886-------						717.9	731.1	742.0	750.3	758.0	764.7	769.7	773.6
1887-------					703.7	720.8	735.0	744.7	754.1	761.9	768.2	773.1	777.1
1888-------				683.7	706.6	724.7	737.4	748.4	757.8	765.3	771.4	776.4	780.4
1889-------			659.0	686.8	710.8	726.2	740.6	751.6	760.8	768.1	774.3	779.3	783.0
1890-------	1917	630.2	663.5	692.5	712.3	730.7	745.1	755.9	764.8	772.2	778.3	782.9	786.8
1891-------	1918	635.5	670.2	693.3	717.8	736.5	750.6	761.1	770.1	777.5	783.2	788.0	791.7
1892-------	1919	645.0	672.5	701.9	726.7	744.1	757.7	768.2	777.0	783.8	789.6	794.1	797.5
1893-------	1920	644.4	679.4	709.6	732.2	748.9	762.5	772.9	781.1	787.9	793.4	797.6	801.1
1894-------	1921	649.4	685.7	712.8	734.5	751.3	764.7	774.6	783.0	789.5	794.7	799.0	802.4
1895-------	1922	655.9	688.7	714.7	736.6	753.1	766.0	775.9	783.9	790.3	795.8	800.1	803.3
1896-------	1923	659.3	690.9	717.1	738.4	754.3	767.1	776.6	784.5	791.2	796.5	800.5	803.5
1897-------	1924	661.3	693.2	718.5	738.9	754.5	766.9	776.3	784.6	791.0	796.0	799.7	802.7
1898-------	1925	660.7	691.4	715.6	735.5	750.6	762.9	772.8	780.6	786.5	791.1	794.9	798.0
1899-------	1926	656.4	686.2	710.3	730.0	745.2	758.2	767.8	775.5	781.4	786.4	790.6	794.0
1900-------	1927	651.0	680.2	703.5	722.8	738.7	751.2	760.5	767.8	774.0	779.3	783.6	787.1
1901-------	1928	651.0	679.4	702.3	722.4	737.9	750.1	758.9	766.7	773.2	778.7	783.2	786.9
1902-------	1929	652.8	680.6	704.4	724.0	738.8	750.0	759.4	767.5	774.2	779.9	784.7	788.6
1903-------	1930	651.8	680.8	704.3	723.0	736.8	749.0	758.9	767.4	774.5	780.7	785.9	790.0
1904-------	1931	644.3	672.6	694.9	712.6	727.8	740.9	751.5	760.6	768.5	775.2	780.7	785.2
1905-------	1932	631.8	658.6	679.6	698.9	715.0	728.7	740.0	749.9	758.3	765.3	771.4	777.0
1906-------	1933	618.9	644.4	667.3	687.6	704.5	719.1	731.4	741.9	750.7	758.4	765.3	771.2
1907-------	1934	604.7	632.2	656.4	677.6	695.9	711.9	725.0	736.0	745.7	755.2	762.6	768.4
1908-------	1935	591.8	620.7	645.6	668.2	687.9	704.7	718.4	730.4	742.5	752.1	759.4	765.4
1909-------	1936	581.5	611.3	638.2	662.8	683.5	701.3	716.5	731.9	743.8	752.8	760.2	767.3
1910-------	1937	572.7	604.6	633.5	658.7	680.6	700.2	718.2	733.0	743.7	752.8	761.7	769.5
1911-------	1938	572.6	607.0	636.4	663.1	687.3	709.2	726.6	739.3	750.1	761.2	771.1	777.6
1912-------	1939	574.4	608.9	639.9	669.5	696.9	717.9	732.8	745.5	758.8	770.9	779.0	785.0
1913-------	1940	578.6	615.1	649.9	683.9	709.2	727.3	742.1	758.1	772.8	782.7	790.1	795.7
1914-------	1941	584.7	625.9	666.9	697.6	719.0	736.6	755.8	773.7	785.6	794.7	801.6	807.0
1915-------	1942	594.9	643.8	680.1	705.7	726.4	750.0	771.7	785.9	796.7	805.1	811.8	817.1
1916-------	1943	610.8	654.0	683.7	708.2	736.5	762.9	779.8	792.6	802.4	810.5	817.0	822.0
1917-------	1944	622.2	657.5	686.1	720.5	752.4	773.2	788.4	799.9	809.5	817.4	823.5	828.3
1918-------	1945	626.5	659.9	700.3	738.7	763.5	782.0	795.6	807.0	816.3	823.5	829.2	833.6
1919-------	1946	639.0	687.7	733.7	764.1	786.6	803.5	817.2	828.4	837.1	844.1	849.5	853.7
1920-------	1947	663.5	719.0	755.3	782.8	803.2	820.1	833.5	843.8	852.1	858.6	863.7	867.7
1921-------	1948	694.5	738.5	771.3	796.2	816.6	833.0	845.3	855.3	863.0	869.1	873.9	877.6
1922-------	1949	706.2	745.7	775.5	800.5	820.2	835.2	847.1	856.2	863.4	869.2	873.7	877.1
1923-------	1950	719.7	755.9	786.1	810.3	828.7	843.4	854.3	863.0	870.0	875.4	879.6	882.8
1924-------	1951	732.4	769.7	799.2	821.7	839.4	852.8	863.2	871.6	878.0	883.1	887.0	890.0
1925-------	1952	742.7	779.0	806.6	828.2	844.6	857.4	867.4	875.2	881.3	886.1	889.8	892.5
1926-------	1953	749.0	783.0	809.3	829.6	845.1	857.4	866.7	874.0	879.7	884.1	887.4	889.9
1927-------	1954	753.7	786.3	811.2	830.5	845.6	857.1	865.9	872.7	878.0	882.1	885.2	888.0
1928-------	1955	757.3	788.4	812.2	831.1	845.2	856.1	864.3	870.7	875.6	879.4	882.8	885.5
1929-------	1956	765.5	795.8	819.4	837.1	850.4	860.7	868.5	874.4	879.0	883.2	886.5	889.0
1930-------	1957	773.1	802.9	825.0	841.6	854.2	863.9	871.1	876.7	881.8	885.8	888.9	891.1
1931-------	1958	787.2	815.2	835.9	851.7	863.6	872.5	879.3	885.4	890.1	893.8	896.5	898.9
1932-------	1959	798.7	825.1	844.8	859.6	870.5	879.1	886.4	892.1	896.5	899.8	902.8	904.8
1933-------	1960	809.6	834.7	853.3	866.9	877.5	886.5	893.4	898.8	902.8	906.4	909.0	911.0
1934-------	1961	816.4	840.2	857.7	871.1	882.4	891.0	897.6	902.5	906.9	910.1	912.6	914.4
1935-------	1962	818.6	841.4	858.4	872.7	883.3	891.7	897.7	903.1	907.0	910.1	912.4	914.1
1936-------	1963	817.6	839.7	857.9	871.4	881.9	889.6	896.3	901.2	905.2	908.1	910.3	911.9
1937-------	1964	814.8	837.9	855.4	869.1	879.2	887.8	894.2	899.3	903.0	905.8	907.9	
1938-------	1965	811.0	833.6	851.2	864.6	875.7	884.1	890.7	895.4	899.1	901.8		
1939-------	1966	807.2	830.4	848.0	862.9	874.1	882.9	889.3	894.1	897.7			
1940-------	1967	799.2	822.9	842.8	857.7	869.4	877.9	884.1	888.8				
1941-------	1968	787.4	814.1	834.2	850.2	861.8	870.2	876.6					
1942-------	1969	777.9	805.2	826.7	842.4	853.8	862.6						
1943-------	1970	765.5	794.0	815.3	830.6	842.5							
1944-------	1971	754.7	782.8	803.4	819.5								
1945-------	1972	739.7	766.8	788.1									
1946-------	1973	730.0	758.0										
1947-------	1974	715.3											

TABLE 6A. CUMULATIVE BIRTH RATES FOR ALL WOMEN AS OF THE BEGINNING OF EACH YEAR 1917-74 BY AGE AND LIVE-BIRTH ORDER FOR EACH COHORT FROM 1867 TO 1959--CON.

LIVE-BIRTH ORDER AND COHORT	DIAGONAL LINE FOR JANUARY 1	EXACT AGE 39	40	41	42	43	44	45	46	47	48	49	50
FIRST BIRTHS--CON.													
1867-------													806.6
1868-------												804.4	804.4
1869-------											802.2	802.3	802.3
1870-------										799.9	800.0	800.1	800.1
1871-------									797.5	797.6	797.7	797.7	797.7
1872-------								794.9	795.1	795.3	795.4	795.4	795.4
1873-------							792.1	792.4	792.6	792.7	792.8	792.8	792.8
1874-------						789.0	789.5	789.9	790.1	790.2	790.3	790.4	790.4
1875-------					785.8	786.5	787.0	787.3	787.5	787.6	787.7	787.7	787.7
1876-------				782.8	783.9	784.7	785.3	785.6	785.8	785.9	786.0	786.0	786.0
1877-------			779.8	781.4	782.6	783.4	784.0	784.3	784.5	784.6	784.7	784.8	784.8
1878-------	1917	775.8	778.2	779.9	781.1	781.9	782.5	782.8	783.0	783.1	783.2	783.2	783.2
1879-------	1918	773.7	776.3	778.0	779.3	780.1	780.7	781.0	781.2	781.3	781.3	781.3	781.3
1880-------	1919	772.9	775.5	777.3	778.6	779.4	780.0	780.3	780.5	780.6	780.6	780.6	780.6
1881-------	1920	773.6	776.3	778.2	779.4	780.2	780.8	781.1	781.3	781.4	781.4	781.5	781.5
1882-------	1921	775.5	778.3	780.0	781.2	782.0	782.5	782.8	783.0	783.1	783.2	783.2	783.2
1883-------	1922	776.2	778.8	780.5	781.7	782.4	782.9	783.2	783.4	783.5	783.6	783.6	783.6
1884-------	1923	775.5	778.0	779.7	780.9	781.7	782.2	782.5	782.7	782.8	782.8	782.8	782.8
1885-------	1924	774.9	777.4	779.1	780.2	780.9	781.4	781.7	781.9	782.0	782.0	782.0	782.0
1886-------	1925	776.7	779.2	780.8	781.9	782.6	783.0	783.3	783.5	783.6	783.6	783.6	783.6
1887-------	1926	780.2	782.5	784.1	785.2	785.9	786.3	786.6	786.7	786.8	786.8	786.8	786.8
1888-------	1927	783.3	785.7	787.2	788.2	788.9	789.3	789.5	789.6	789.6	789.6	789.6	789.6
1889-------	1928	786.0	788.3	789.8	790.8	791.5	791.9	792.1	792.2	792.3	792.3	792.3	792.3
1890-------	1929	789.7	791.9	793.4	794.4	795.0	795.4	795.6	795.8	795.9	795.9	795.9	795.9
1891-------	1930	794.4	796.6	798.0	799.0	799.6	800.0	800.2	800.3	800.3	800.3	800.3	800.3
1892-------	1931	800.3	802.4	803.8	804.7	805.3	805.7	805.9	806.0	806.1	806.1	806.1	806.1
1893-------	1932	803.8	805.8	807.0	807.9	808.4	808.8	809.0	809.1	809.2	809.2	809.2	809.2
1894-------	1933	804.9	806.7	807.9	808.7	809.2	809.6	809.8	809.9	810.0	810.0	810.0	810.0
1895-------	1934	805.6	807.4	808.6	809.5	810.1	810.5	810.7	810.8	810.9	810.9	810.9	810.9
1896-------	1935	805.8	807.6	808.9	809.8	810.4	810.8	811.0	811.1	811.2	811.2	811.2	811.2
1897-------	1936	805.1	807.0	808.3	809.2	809.8	810.2	810.4	810.5	810.6	810.6	810.6	810.6
1898-------	1937	800.5	802.4	803.7	804.6	805.2	805.6	805.8	806.0	806.1	806.1	806.1	806.1
1899-------	1938	796.6	798.6	800.1	801.1	801.8	802.2	802.5	802.7	802.8	802.8	802.8	802.8
1900-------	1939	789.9	792.1	793.6	794.7	795.4	795.9	796.2	796.4	796.5	796.5	796.5	796.5
1901-------	1940	789.9	792.1	793.8	795.0	795.8	796.4	796.8	797.0	797.1	797.1	797.1	797.1
1902-------	1941	791.7	794.2	796.2	797.6	798.6	799.3	799.7	799.9	800.0	800.0	800.0	800.0
1903-------	1942	793.4	796.5	798.7	800.3	801.3	802.0	802.4	802.6	802.7	802.7	802.7	802.7
1904-------	1943	789.5	792.8	795.1	796.7	797.8	798.5	798.8	799.0	799.1	799.1	799.1	799.1
1905-------	1944	781.6	784.9	787.3	789.1	790.3	791.0	791.4	791.6	791.7	791.7	791.7	791.7
1906-------	1945	775.7	779.2	782.0	784.0	785.1	785.8	786.2	786.4	786.5	786.5	786.5	786.5
1907-------	1946	773.1	777.2	780.3	782.1	783.2	783.9	784.3	784.5	784.6	784.6	784.6	784.6
1908-------	1947	770.9	775.3	778.1	779.9	780.9	781.5	781.9	782.1	782.2	782.2	782.2	782.2
1909-------	1948	773.3	777.2	779.8	781.5	782.5	783.2	783.6	783.8	783.9	783.9	783.9	783.9
1910-------	1949	774.7	778.4	780.9	782.5	783.6	784.3	784.7	784.9	785.0	785.0	785.0	785.0
1911-------	1950	782.3	785.7	788.1	789.7	790.8	791.4	791.8	792.0	792.1	792.1	792.1	792.1
1912-------	1951	789.4	792.7	795.1	796.7	797.7	798.3	798.6	798.8	798.8	798.8	798.8	798.8
1913-------	1952	800.0	803.3	805.5	807.0	808.0	808.6	808.9	809.0	809.1	809.1	809.1	809.1
1914-------	1953	811.2	814.3	816.5	817.9	818.8	819.4	819.7	819.9	820.0	820.0	820.0	820.0
1915-------	1954	821.1	824.1	826.1	827.4	828.3	828.8	829.1	829.2	829.3	829.3	829.3	829.3
1916-------	1955	825.8	828.6	830.4	831.7	832.5	833.0	833.2	833.3	833.3	833.3	833.3	833.3
1917-------	1956	831.9	834.4	836.2	837.4	838.1	838.5	838.7	838.8	838.8	838.8	838.8	838.8
1918-------	1957	836.9	839.4	841.0	842.1	842.8	843.2	843.4	843.5	843.5	843.5	843.5	843.5
1919-------	1958	856.9	859.2	860.8	861.8	862.4	862.8	863.0	863.1	863.1	863.1	863.1	863.1
1920-------	1959	870.6	872.7	874.2	875.2	875.8	876.1	876.3	876.4	876.4	876.4	876.4	876.4
1921-------	1960	880.3	882.3	883.7	884.6	885.2	885.6	885.8	885.9	885.9	885.9	885.9	885.9
1922-------	1961	879.6	881.5	882.7	883.5	884.1	884.5	884.7	884.8	884.8	884.8	884.8	884.8
1923-------	1962	885.2	886.9	888.1	889.1	889.7	890.0	890.2	890.3	890.3	890.3	890.3	890.3
1924-------	1963	892.2	893.8	895.1	896.0	896.5	896.8	897.0	897.1	897.1	897.1	897.1	897.1
1925-------	1964	894.5	896.3	897.5	898.3	898.7	899.0	899.1	899.2	899.2	899.2	899.2	
1926-------	1965	892.2	893.9	895.0	895.7	896.2	896.4	896.5	896.6	896.6	896.6		
1927-------	1966	890.2	891.7	892.7	893.5	893.9	894.1	894.2	894.2	894.2			
1928-------	1967	887.5	888.8	889.9	890.5	890.9	891.1	891.2	891.2				
1929-------	1968	890.7	892.2	893.1	893.7	894.0	894.2	894.3					
1930-------	1969	893.0	894.2	895.1	895.6	895.9	896.1						
1931-------	1970	900.5	901.7	902.5	903.0	903.3							
1932-------	1971	906.4	907.4	908.1	908.6								
1933-------	1972	912.4	913.4	914.1									
1934-------	1973	915.7	916.6										
1935-------	1974	915.3											

TABLE 6A. CUMULATIVE BIRTH RATES FOR ALL WOMEN AS OF THE BEGINNING OF EACH YEAR 1917-74 BY AGE AND LIVE-BIRTH ORDER FOR EACH COHORT FROM 1867 TO 1959--CON.

LIVE-BIRTH ORDER AND COHORT	DIAGONAL LINE FOR JANUARY 1	EXACT AGE											
		15	16	17	18	19	20	21	22	23	24	25	26
SECOND BIRTHS													
1891-------													368.7
1892-------												321.6	371.2
1893-------											269.3	323.4	372.0
1894-------										211.7	269.8	322.7	369.6
1895-------									155.7	212.2	268.9	319.7	366.6
1896-------								102.9	156.5	211.7	265.8	316.1	362.5
1897-------							59.3	104.0	156.5	209.4	262.5	312.3	360.4
1898-------						28.9	61.0	105.0	155.6	207.9	260.8	313.3	362.7
1899-------					11.0	28.5	60.0	102.0	151.5	202.8	257.9	310.9	358.5
1900-------				3.0	10.7	27.8	57.8	99.1	147.7	201.1	257.0	308.5	353.5
1901-------			0.5	2.9	10.3	26.3	55.7	97.4	147.9	202.0	256.5	305.4	348.7
1902-------	1917	*	0.6	2.9	10.1	26.4	57.9	102.2	153.9	207.3	258.7	305.9	347.3
1903-------	1918	*	0.5	2.8	10.1	28.7	62.1	107.3	157.7	209.0	259.3	304.6	344.3
1904-------	1919	*	0.5	2.8	11.0	30.6	64.4	107.8	156.0	206.3	254.3	297.4	335.9
1905-------	1920	*	0.5	3.0	11.5	31.5	63.8	105.2	152.6	200.8	246.0	287.6	325.9
1906-------	1921	*	0.6	3.2	11.9	30.9	61.9	103.0	149.1	194.4	238.2	279.3	316.2
1907-------	1922	*	0.6	3.3	11.6	30.3	61.5	101.8	145.4	189.4	232.7	272.5	308.4
1908-------	1923	*	0.6	3.2	11.7	30.7	61.4	99.5	141.7	185.1	226.7	265.1	298.9
1909-------	1924	*	0.6	3.4	12.2	31.0	60.0	96.8	138.5	180.5	221.0	257.4	292.1
1910-------	1925	*	0.6	3.5	12.3	29.8	57.8	94.1	134.0	174.8	213.0	250.0	283.2
1911-------	1926	*	0.7	3.7	12.0	29.1	57.0	92.0	131.4	170.0	209.1	244.8	278.4
1912-------	1927	*	0.7	3.5	11.6	28.5	55.1	89.6	126.4	165.6	203.0	239.2	273.9
1913-------	1928	*	0.7	3.4	11.4	27.7	53.7	85.5	122.8	160.5	198.6	236.1	272.8
1914-------	1929	*	0.6	3.2	10.8	26.6	50.5	82.5	118.4	156.9	196.5	235.9	272.7
1915-------	1930	*	0.6	3.1	10.4	24.9	48.7	79.8	116.6	156.6	197.8	237.0	275.5
1916-------	1931	*	0.6	3.0	9.7	23.9	47.1	79.0	116.8	157.9	198.4	238.6	278.9
1917-------	1932	*	0.6	2.8	9.4	23.5	47.5	80.0	118.9	159.1	200.2	242.0	287.8
1918-------	1933	*	0.5	2.7	9.3	23.9	48.4	81.8	119.6	160.5	202.6	250.7	302.0
1919-------	1934	*	0.5	2.8	9.9	25.2	50.6	83.9	123.3	165.8	215.1	268.1	314.9
1920-------	1935	*	0.6	3.1	10.6	26.4	52.0	87.3	127.6	173.8	227.0	274.6	317.7
1921-------	1936	*	0.7	3.5	11.3	27.7	55.6	91.8	133.0	182.7	230.0	273.0	330.3
1922-------	1937	*	0.7	3.5	11.3	29.2	57.0	92.2	136.9	181.6	223.1	281.6	344.7
1923-------	1938	*	0.7	3.5	12.1	30.1	57.5	95.6	136.2	175.3	233.1	297.8	361.5
1924-------	1939	*	0.7	3.9	12.7	30.8	60.2	94.8	130.3	185.1	249.2	316.3	383.1
1925-------	1940	*	0.9	4.2	13.5	32.4	58.9	89.3	137.3	197.7	265.6	336.1	403.5
1926-------	1941	*	0.9	4.7	14.5	31.4	54.8	93.6	146.7	212.6	284.1	354.8	424.0
1927-------	1942	*	1.3	5.4	14.3	29.6	57.2	100.5	160.8	230.7	302.0	374.5	443.7
1928-------	1943	*	1.3	5.0	13.2	30.0	61.4	112.4	177.0	246.7	320.0	392.8	462.5
1929-------	1944	*	1.2	4.7	13.4	32.9	71.1	126.9	191.8	263.9	338.5	413.5	483.7
1930-------	1945	*	1.2	4.8	14.9	39.1	81.7	137.9	205.2	279.2	356.5	432.8	502.5
1931-------	1946	*	1.3	5.7	18.4	46.3	89.9	148.7	218.5	296.6	376.9	453.8	524.9
1932-------	1947	*	1.5	6.9	21.7	50.3	95.4	155.9	229.3	310.6	392.5	472.1	544.3
1933-------	1948	*	1.8	8.2	23.5	53.2	99.9	163.9	240.6	324.5	409.8	491.3	562.0
1934-------	1949	*	2.1	8.6	24.5	54.8	103.8	169.9	249.8	337.5	425.3	505.8	575.5
1935-------	1950	*	2.0	8.6	24.6	56.0	105.6	174.4	257.5	347.8	435.2	514.8	582.8
1936-------	1951	*	2.0	8.4	24.9	56.7	108.5	180.2	265.5	355.3	442.3	520.6	586.1
1937-------	1952	*	1.9	8.3	24.9	57.9	112.2	185.7	271.2	361.5	447.4	523.1	585.4
1938-------	1953	*	1.8	8.5	25.6	60.3	115.5	189.5	276.7	365.9	449.4	521.5	581.9
1939-------	1954	*	2.0	9.0	27.2	62.8	119.2	195.2	281.0	368.3	448.1	518.1	576.8
1940-------	1955	*	2.1	9.4	28.0	64.3	121.8	195.9	279.5	363.4	440.7	508.2	563.1
1941-------	1956	*	2.2	9.7	28.6	64.5	119.9	191.3	271.5	351.9	425.6	488.3	541.8
1942-------	1957	*	2.1	9.6	27.9	62.6	115.2	183.4	259.6	335.2	402.9	463.4	517.9
1943-------	1958	*	2.1	9.2	26.9	59.7	110.0	174.2	245.0	313.4	377.7	438.7	493.7
1944-------	1959	*	2.0	9.0	26.1	57.9	105.5	165.1	228.2	292.2	356.3	416.7	473.8
1945-------	1960	*	2.1	9.1	25.9	55.9	100.0	152.7	210.9	273.1	334.7	395.5	453.3
1946-------	1961	*	2.1	9.0	24.7	52.3	90.9	138.6	194.5	254.0	316.4	378.5	433.3
1947-------	1962	*	2.0	8.3	22.6	46.9	81.6	127.2	179.8	239.3	302.2	360.5	411.2
1948-------	1963	*	1.8	7.5	20.1	42.0	75.2	117.8	170.2	229.8	288.6	341.3	390.7
1949-------	1964	*	1.8	7.1	18.9	40.0	70.6	112.5	164.8	220.4	272.3	322.5	
1950-------	1965	*	1.7	6.7	18.1	37.7	68.1	110.2	159.0	207.5	256.6		
1951-------	1966	*	1.6	6.6	17.1	36.5	67.2	106.7	149.3	195.0			
1952-------	1967	*	1.6	6.1	16.4	35.8	64.7	99.5	139.5				
1953-------	1968	*	1.4	5.8	16.3	34.9	60.8	93.6					
1954-------	1969	*	1.4	6.0	16.2	33.3	57.9						
1955-------	1970	*	1.5	6.0	15.5	31.9							
1956-------	1971	*	1.5	5.7	14.8								
1957-------	1972	*	1.4	5.5									
1958-------	1973	*	1.3										
1959-------	1974	*											

TABLE 6A. CUMULATIVE BIRTH RATES FOR ALL WOMEN AS OF THE BEGINNING OF EACH YEAR 1917-74 BY AGE AND LIVE-BIRTH ORDER FOR EACH COHORT FROM 1867 TO 1959--CON.

LIVE-BIRTH ORDER AND COHORT	DIAGONAL LINE FOR JANUARY 1	EXACT AGE											
		27	28	29	30	31	32	33	34	35	36	37	38
SECOND BIRTHS--CON.													
1879-------													640.4
1880-------												631.0	637.2
1881-------											621.4	629.2	635.5
1882-------										610.6	620.2	628.1	634.4
1883-------									597.5	609.0	618.6	626.4	632.7
1884-------								582.3	596.3	607.7	617.2	625.1	631.6
1885-------							563.4	579.8	593.6	604.9	614.6	622.8	629.0
1886-------						540.0	560.3	576.6	590.4	602.0	612.0	619.8	626.1
1887-------					512.4	537.6	557.9	574.1	588.3	600.2	609.9	617.8	624.0
1888-------				483.3	515.2	540.2	560.3	577.0	591.4	603.2	613.0	620.8	626.8
1889-------			449.3	486.0	517.7	542.3	563.0	579.9	594.4	606.1	615.8	623.4	629.2
1890-------	1917	411.2	452.0	488.6	519.6	544.7	565.8	582.9	597.3	609.0	618.6	626.0	631.8
1891-------	1918	411.8	452.5	488.0	519.3	544.4	565.6	582.5	596.9	608.5	617.7	625.0	630.5
1892-------	1919	414.0	453.3	488.7	519.5	544.6	565.5	582.4	596.5	607.5	616.4	623.2	628.4
1893-------	1920	413.4	452.7	487.1	518.0	542.9	563.8	580.1	593.5	604.2	612.7	619.3	624.7
1894-------	1921	411.4	450.0	484.9	515.8	540.4	560.6	576.5	589.7	600.1	608.3	615.1	620.2
1895-------	1922	407.9	447.3	482.5	512.8	536.8	556.8	572.4	585.3	595.4	603.9	610.4	615.3
1896-------	1923	404.8	444.6	478.8	508.3	531.8	551.1	566.2	578.6	588.9	596.9	603.1	607.7
1897-------	1924	403.3	442.1	475.5	504.3	526.9	545.5	560.1	572.6	582.4	590.2	596.0	600.7
1898-------	1925	404.8	442.2	474.1	501.3	522.8	540.9	555.6	567.5	576.9	584.2	590.2	594.9
1899-------	1926	399.5	435.7	466.6	492.9	514.3	532.8	547.3	559.3	568.5	576.3	582.5	587.3
1900-------	1927	392.4	427.0	456.2	481.8	503.4	521.2	535.3	546.6	556.3	564.2	570.4	575.3
1901-------	1928	386.4	419.3	447.8	473.7	494.6	511.9	525.2	537.1	546.8	554.7	561.1	566.2
1902-------	1929	383.0	414.7	443.3	468.0	487.8	503.9	517.9	529.7	539.4	547.4	554.1	559.5
1903-------	1930	379.0	411.1	438.8	462.6	481.5	498.7	512.6	524.5	534.5	543.1	550.1	555.8
1904-------	1931	370.8	401.8	428.4	451.2	471.4	488.5	502.6	514.9	525.6	534.7	542.4	548.6
1905-------	1932	359.7	389.5	414.9	438.7	458.5	475.6	490.2	503.4	514.6	524.3	532.5	539.5
1906-------	1933	348.6	377.0	403.4	426.8	446.7	464.4	480.1	493.9	506.0	516.3	525.2	533.5
1907-------	1934	339.4	368.8	394.6	418.1	438.7	457.7	474.1	489.0	501.9	513.8	524.4	533.4
1908-------	1935	330.6	359.0	384.8	408.8	430.5	450.1	467.8	483.5	498.5	512.3	523.8	533.5
1909-------	1936	322.8	351.2	377.7	403.2	425.8	447.2	466.2	484.8	502.1	516.5	529.0	539.5
1910-------	1937	313.8	343.1	371.3	397.3	421.7	444.4	465.9	487.2	504.8	520.4	533.8	544.4
1911-------	1938	310.3	341.6	370.3	398.2	424.1	449.2	473.8	494.9	513.8	530.6	544.0	553.9
1912-------	1939	307.6	339.0	369.5	398.9	428.5	457.3	481.6	504.2	524.6	541.4	553.9	563.3
1913-------	1940	306.8	340.2	372.5	406.7	440.4	468.8	495.1	519.6	540.0	555.5	567.5	576.8
1914-------	1941	309.0	344.6	382.6	421.6	454.1	484.8	513.6	538.3	557.1	572.1	583.9	593.3
1915-------	1942	314.0	354.9	398.3	435.2	469.9	503.5	532.5	555.1	573.4	588.2	600.1	609.6
1916-------	1943	321.5	368.1	408.2	446.6	484.8	519.0	545.5	567.5	585.6	600.4	612.3	621.3
1917-------	1944	336.3	379.4	420.3	463.4	503.1	535.0	561.3	583.3	601.5	616.3	627.7	636.7
1918-------	1945	346.9	389.2	435.8	481.3	518.3	549.8	576.0	597.9	615.9	630.0	641.1	649.6
1919-------	1946	357.9	408.9	460.0	503.4	540.9	572.7	599.5	621.6	639.1	653.2	664.0	672.3
1920-------	1947	371.8	428.0	477.1	521.3	559.1	591.4	618.1	639.5	656.8	670.1	680.4	688.2
1921-------	1948	390.5	445.4	495.9	540.6	578.9	611.3	637.0	658.1	674.3	687.0	696.7	704.0
1922-------	1949	404.1	460.4	511.1	555.8	594.2	625.2	650.2	669.8	685.2	697.2	706.1	712.6
1923-------	1950	423.2	480.1	531.5	576.5	613.2	643.5	666.9	685.6	700.2	711.1	719.2	725.3
1924-------	1951	445.8	504.0	555.8	599.2	635.4	663.8	686.0	703.6	716.8	726.9	734.6	740.4
1925-------	1952	467.6	526.0	576.1	618.6	652.2	679.0	699.9	715.9	728.2	737.8	745.1	750.4
1926-------	1953	488.4	545.7	594.9	635.0	666.9	692.3	711.5	726.4	738.0	746.9	753.4	758.3
1927-------	1954	507.8	563.8	610.6	649.1	679.7	703.1	720.8	734.8	745.6	753.6	759.8	764.4
1928-------	1955	525.8	579.9	625.1	662.1	690.4	712.2	729.0	742.0	751.8	759.4	765.2	769.4
1929-------	1956	545.8	599.1	643.6	678.2	705.1	725.9	741.8	754.0	763.3	770.6	775.9	779.8
1930-------	1957	564.4	617.2	659.0	692.2	717.9	737.6	752.4	763.9	772.9	779.5	784.4	788.1
1931-------	1958	587.4	638.0	678.3	710.1	734.4	752.6	766.6	777.6	785.7	791.9	796.6	800.1
1932-------	1959	604.7	653.9	692.7	722.8	745.3	762.6	776.0	786.2	793.8	799.6	804.0	807.4
1933-------	1960	620.8	667.9	704.7	732.4	753.7	770.3	782.8	792.2	799.5	805.2	809.5	812.8
1934-------	1961	632.6	677.8	712.4	739.2	759.8	775.7	787.4	796.5	803.5	809.1	813.4	816.4
1935-------	1962	637.6	680.3	713.6	739.6	759.2	773.9	785.2	794.2	801.3	806.9	810.9	813.9
1936-------	1963	638.5	679.8	712.5	737.3	756.0	770.4	781.8	791.0	798.1	803.3	807.2	810.0
1937-------	1964	636.0	676.6	707.5	731.4	750.0	764.9	776.6	785.9	792.7	797.8	801.6	
1938-------	1965	631.4	669.6	699.7	723.5	742.5	757.9	770.0	779.0	785.7	790.8		
1939-------	1966	623.3	660.6	691.0	715.6	735.8	752.0	764.1	773.1	780.0			
1940-------	1967	608.4	646.2	677.6	704.3	725.8	742.0	754.2	763.4				
1941-------	1968	587.9	627.0	661.0	689.5	711.1	727.6	740.0					
1942-------	1969	565.6	608.2	644.8	673.2	695.3	712.1						
1943-------	1970	543.9	588.5	624.1	652.4	674.7							
1944-------	1971	525.7	568.7	603.5	632.1								
1945-------	1972	502.6	543.5	578.7									
1946-------	1973	479.9	521.5										
1947-------	1974	457.5											

TABLE 6A. CUMULATIVE BIRTH RATES FOR ALL WOMEN AS OF THE BEGINNING OF EACH YEAR 1917-74 BY AGE AND LIVE-BIRTH ORDER FOR EACH COHORT FROM 1867 TO 1959--CON.

LIVE-BIRTH ORDER AND COHORT	DIAGONAL LINE FOR JANUARY 1	EXACT AGE											
		15	16	17	18	19	20	21	22	23	24	25	26
THIRD BIRTHS													
1891-------													195.4
1892-------												155.7	194.5
1893-------											120.2	158.4	196.6
1894-------										82.0	118.0	155.9	192.0
1895-------									50.5	80.3	116.3	152.2	188.6
1896-------								26.6	49.3	79.2	113.3	149.2	186.2
1897-------							11.6	26.1	48.9	77.3	111.1	147.6	181.6
1898-------						3.8	11.3	25.9	47.7	76.1	110.7	144.5	179.6
1899-------					1.0	3.7	11.3	25.2	46.8	75.4	106.7	141.4	177.4
1900-------				0.2	1.0	3.7	10.9	24.6	46.4	72.4	105.3	141.7	176.1
1901-------			0.0	0.2	1.0	3.5	10.4	24.2	43.7	70.6	105.4	140.5	172.7
1902-------	1917	*	0.0	0.2	1.0	3.6	11.0	23.9	44.8	74.1	107.5	140.3	171.4
1903-------	1918	*	0.0	0.2	1.0	3.9	10.8	24.7	47.1	75.6	107.2	139.1	168.5
1904-------	1919	*	0.0	0.2	1.1	3.8	11.4	25.9	47.4	74.5	105.0	135.0	162.7
1905-------	1920	*	0.0	0.2	1.0	4.2	12.0	25.9	46.4	72.6	101.2	129.5	156.8
1906-------	1921	*	0.0	0.2	1.2	4.4	11.9	25.3	45.3	70.0	97.1	124.9	150.5
1907-------	1922	*	0.0	0.2	1.2	4.3	11.7	25.0	44.3	67.8	94.3	120.4	145.4
1908-------	1923	*	0.0	0.2	1.1	4.2	11.6	24.4	42.6	65.5	90.4	115.7	139.2
1909-------	1924	*	0.0	0.2	1.2	4.3	11.5	23.6	41.5	63.4	87.7	111.8	135.6
1910-------	1925	*	0.0	0.2	1.2	4.2	10.9	22.7	39.7	60.9	84.1	108.3	130.5
1911-------	1926	*	0.0	0.2	1.2	4.0	10.6	22.0	38.6	58.9	82.3	105.2	126.8
1912-------	1927	*	0.0	0.2	1.1	3.8	10.1	21.1	36.7	56.8	78.8	100.8	122.2
1913-------	1928	*	0.0	0.2	1.1	3.7	9.8	20.0	35.5	54.7	75.7	97.8	119.9
1914-------	1929	*	0.0	0.2	1.0	3.5	9.1	19.3	34.2	52.7	74.0	96.7	118.3
1915-------	1930	*	0.0	0.2	1.0	3.3	8.9	18.8	33.2	52.1	74.1	96.4	118.9
1916-------	1931	*	0.0	0.2	0.9	3.2	8.7	18.3	33.0	52.3	73.8	97.0	120.0
1917-------	1932	*	0.0	0.2	0.9	3.2	8.5	18.4	33.5	52.4	74.9	98.5	122.3
1918-------	1933	*	0.0	0.2	0.9	3.2	8.8	19.1	33.8	53.6	76.3	100.8	127.6
1919-------	1934	*	0.0	0.2	1.0	3.4	9.3	19.5	35.2	55.3	79.3	106.4	133.1
1920-------	1935	*	0.0	0.2	1.0	3.6	9.6	21.1	36.9	57.6	83.6	110.2	134.6
1921-------	1936	*	0.0	0.2	1.1	4.0	11.2	22.8	38.9	61.1	86.4	110.2	137.4
1922-------	1937	*	0.0	0.2	1.2	4.9	12.0	23.4	40.7	62.6	84.4	110.5	139.9
1923-------	1938	*	0.0	0.2	1.5	5.2	12.4	24.7	42.0	60.8	84.8	113.1	144.7
1924-------	1939	*	0.0	0.3	1.6	5.3	13.0	25.3	40.1	60.8	86.8	117.9	152.1
1925-------	1940	*	0.1	0.4	1.8	5.6	13.2	23.6	39.8	62.2	91.0	124.8	161.8
1926-------	1941	*	0.1	0.5	2.0	5.7	12.1	23.5	41.0	65.9	97.5	134.2	174.7
1927-------	1942	*	0.1	0.6	2.1	5.3	12.1	24.3	43.9	71.8	106.4	146.4	189.5
1928-------	1943	*	0.1	0.5	1.8	5.1	12.5	26.4	48.9	79.8	117.6	159.7	204.3
1929-------	1944	*	0.1	0.5	1.8	5.4	13.9	30.4	55.8	89.9	129.7	174.0	221.4
1930-------	1945	*	0.1	0.5	2.0	6.2	16.6	35.3	63.4	99.0	140.7	188.0	237.8
1931-------	1946	*	0.1	0.6	2.4	7.9	19.7	40.5	69.9	107.5	152.8	202.8	255.8
1932-------	1947	*	0.1	0.7	3.0	9.0	21.9	43.6	74.2	114.8	162.4	215.9	271.3
1933-------	1948	*	0.2	0.9	3.3	9.9	23.6	46.2	79.4	122.1	173.4	229.4	285.7
1934-------	1949	*	0.2	0.9	3.6	10.5	24.6	48.9	83.8	129.6	183.4	240.7	298.7
1935-------	1950	*	0.2	1.0	3.7	10.8	25.7	50.7	87.5	135.4	190.2	249.2	307.7
1936-------	1951	*	0.2	1.0	3.8	11.2	26.4	52.7	91.5	140.1	196.0	255.5	313.5
1937-------	1952	*	0.2	1.0	3.8	11.2	27.2	54.9	93.9	143.5	200.5	259.7	315.4
1938-------	1953	*	0.2	1.0	3.8	11.7	28.5	56.3	96.4	147.3	203.9	260.9	313.9
1939-------	1954	*	0.2	1.0	4.1	12.3	29.3	58.6	100.1	150.6	205.5	259.6	309.5
1940-------	1955	*	0.2	1.1	4.3	12.7	30.7	60.4	100.9	150.1	201.7	251.9	295.7
1941-------	1956	*	0.2	1.1	4.3	13.2	31.1	59.9	99.0	144.4	191.5	234.6	273.0
1942-------	1957	*	0.2	1.1	4.4	12.9	30.0	57.1	92.7	133.5	173.1	210.2	246.4
1943-------	1958	*	0.2	1.1	4.2	12.4	28.4	53.2	85.0	118.9	152.6	187.1	221.1
1944-------	1959	*	0.2	1.1	4.3	12.1	26.9	49.4	76.1	104.9	135.9	167.9	202.3
1945-------	1960	*	0.2	1.1	4.3	11.7	25.4	44.3	66.8	92.8	121.0	152.7	187.0
1946-------	1961	*	0.2	1.1	3.9	10.8	22.4	38.2	58.0	81.1	108.6	140.1	170.8
1947-------	1962	*	0.2	1.0	3.7	9.5	19.0	32.8	50.3	72.6	99.6	127.8	152.8
1948-------	1963	*	0.2	0.9	3.2	8.0	16.4	28.4	45.1	66.9	91.2	114.0	136.1
1949-------	1964	*	0.2	0.9	2.9	7.3	14.7	26.3	42.7	62.7	82.5	102.7	
1950-------	1965	*	0.2	0.8	2.6	6.5	13.7	25.1	40.1	56.3	74.0		
1951-------	1966	*	0.1	0.7	2.4	6.2	13.1	23.5	35.8	50.4			
1952-------	1967	*	0.1	0.6	2.1	5.7	12.0	20.7	31.9				
1953-------	1968	*	0.1	0.6	2.1	5.3	10.7	18.6					
1954-------	1969	*	0.1	0.6	2.0	4.8	9.8						
1955-------	1970	*	0.1	0.5	1.7	4.3							
1956-------	1971	*	0.1	0.5	1.6								
1957-------	1972	*	0.1	0.4									
1958-------	1973	*	0.1										
1959-------	1974	*											

TABLE 6A. CUMULATIVE BIRTH RATES FOR ALL WOMEN AS OF THE BEGINNING OF EACH YEAR 1917-74 BY AGE AND LIVE-BIRTH ORDER FOR EACH COHORT FROM 1867 TO 1959--CON.

LIVE-BIRTH ORDER AND COHORT	DIAGONAL LINE FOR JANUARY 1	EXACT AGE											
		39	40	41	42	43	44	45	46	47	48	49	50
SECOND BIRTHS--CON.													
1867-------													704.6
1868-------												700.7	700.7
1869-------											696.7	696.8	696.8
1870-------										692.7	692.8	692.8	692.8
1871-------									688.4	688.6	688.7	688.7	688.8
1872-------								684.0	684.3	684.5	684.6	684.7	684.7
1873-------							679.1	679.6	679.9	680.1	680.2	680.2	680.2
1874-------						673.6	674.3	674.8	675.1	675.3	675.3	675.3	675.3
1875-------					668.0	669.1	669.9	670.4	670.7	670.8	670.9	670.9	670.9
1876-------				662.4	664.1	665.2	666.0	666.5	666.7	666.8	666.9	666.9	666.9
1877-------			656.4	658.9	660.7	661.8	662.6	663.0	663.2	663.4	663.5	663.5	663.5
1878-------	1917	649.2	652.9	655.4	657.2	658.3	659.1	659.5	659.8	660.0	660.0	660.1	660.1
1879-------	1918	645.2	649.0	651.6	653.4	654.6	655.4	655.9	656.2	656.3	656.4	656.4	656.4
1880-------	1919	642.1	645.9	648.5	650.3	651.4	652.1	652.6	652.8	653.0	653.1	653.1	653.1
1881-------	1920	640.4	644.2	646.9	648.7	649.8	650.5	650.9	651.1	651.2	651.3	651.3	651.3
1882-------	1921	639.3	643.2	645.7	647.4	648.5	649.3	649.7	649.9	650.0	650.1	650.1	650.1
1883-------	1922	637.8	641.5	644.0	645.7	646.8	647.5	647.9	648.1	648.2	648.3	648.3	648.3
1884-------	1923	636.4	640.1	642.6	644.3	645.3	645.9	646.3	646.5	646.6	646.6	646.6	646.6
1885-------	1924	633.8	637.5	639.9	641.6	642.6	643.3	643.6	643.8	643.9	643.9	643.9	643.9
1886-------	1925	630.9	634.4	636.8	638.3	639.3	639.9	640.2	640.4	640.5	640.5	640.5	640.5
1887-------	1926	628.6	632.1	634.4	635.9	636.8	637.4	637.7	637.9	638.0	638.0	638.0	638.0
1888-------	1927	631.2	634.6	636.8	638.2	639.1	639.6	639.9	640.1	640.2	640.2	640.2	640.2
1889-------	1928	633.7	637.0	639.1	640.5	641.4	642.0	642.3	642.4	642.5	642.5	642.5	642.5
1890-------	1929	636.1	639.3	641.4	642.8	643.6	644.1	644.3	644.4	644.5	644.5	644.5	644.5
1891-------	1930	634.6	637.8	639.8	641.1	641.9	642.4	642.6	642.7	642.7	642.7	642.7	642.7
1892-------	1931	632.6	635.6	637.5	638.8	639.5	640.0	640.2	640.3	640.4	640.4	640.4	640.4
1893-------	1932	628.6	631.5	633.4	634.6	635.3	635.8	636.0	636.1	636.1	636.1	636.1	636.1
1894-------	1933	623.9	626.6	628.4	629.6	630.3	630.7	631.0	631.1	631.1	631.1	631.1	631.1
1895-------	1934	618.9	621.7	623.5	624.7	625.4	625.9	626.1	626.2	626.3	626.3	626.3	626.3
1896-------	1935	611.4	614.0	615.7	616.9	617.7	618.1	618.3	618.5	618.6	618.6	618.6	618.6
1897-------	1936	604.3	606.9	608.7	610.0	610.7	611.2	611.5	611.7	611.8	611.8	611.8	611.8
1898-------	1937	598.4	601.1	603.0	604.2	605.0	605.5	605.8	606.0	606.1	606.1	606.1	606.1
1899-------	1938	591.0	593.9	595.9	597.3	598.1	598.6	598.9	599.1	599.2	599.2	599.2	599.2
1900-------	1939	579.2	582.2	584.4	585.8	586.7	587.3	587.7	587.9	588.0	588.0	588.0	588.0
1901-------	1940	570.3	573.5	575.7	577.2	578.2	578.9	579.3	579.5	579.6	579.7	579.7	579.7
1902-------	1941	563.8	567.1	569.6	571.4	572.6	573.3	573.8	574.0	574.1	574.1	574.1	574.1
1903-------	1942	560.4	564.2	567.1	569.1	570.4	571.3	571.8	572.0	572.1	572.1	572.1	572.1
1904-------	1943	553.9	558.4	561.6	563.9	565.3	566.2	566.7	566.9	567.0	567.0	567.0	567.0
1905-------	1944	545.7	550.5	554.0	556.4	558.0	558.9	559.4	559.6	559.7	559.7	559.7	559.7
1906-------	1945	540.2	545.4	549.2	551.8	553.3	554.2	554.7	554.9	555.0	555.0	555.0	555.0
1907-------	1946	540.7	546.5	550.5	553.0	554.5	555.4	555.8	556.0	556.1	556.1	556.1	556.1
1908-------	1947	541.4	547.3	551.0	553.4	554.8	555.6	556.1	556.3	556.4	556.4	556.4	556.4
1909-------	1948	547.5	553.0	556.7	559.1	560.5	561.4	561.9	562.1	562.2	562.2	562.2	562.2
1910-------	1949	552.0	557.4	561.1	563.6	565.2	566.1	566.6	566.8	566.9	566.9	566.9	566.9
1911-------	1950	561.2	566.6	570.4	572.9	574.4	575.3	575.8	576.0	576.1	576.1	576.1	576.1
1912-------	1951	570.5	576.0	579.7	582.2	583.8	584.7	585.2	585.4	585.5	585.5	585.5	585.5
1913-------	1952	584.0	589.4	593.2	595.7	597.2	598.1	598.5	598.7	598.8	598.8	598.8	598.8
1914-------	1953	600.7	606.1	609.8	612.2	613.7	614.5	614.9	615.1	615.2	615.2	615.2	615.2
1915-------	1954	616.7	622.0	625.6	628.0	629.4	630.2	630.6	630.8	630.9	630.9	630.9	630.9
1916-------	1955	628.3	633.4	636.8	639.0	640.3	641.1	641.5	641.7	641.8	641.8	641.8	641.8
1917-------	1956	643.4	648.3	651.6	653.7	655.0	655.7	656.1	656.3	656.4	656.4	656.4	656.4
1918-------	1957	655.9	660.6	663.6	665.5	666.7	667.4	667.8	668.0	668.0	668.0	668.0	668.0
1919-------	1958	678.4	682.8	685.6	687.4	688.5	689.1	689.5	689.6	689.6	689.6	689.6	689.6
1920-------	1959	693.9	697.9	700.5	702.3	703.4	704.0	704.3	704.4	704.4	704.4	704.4	704.4
1921-------	1960	709.2	712.8	715.4	717.0	718.0	718.5	718.8	718.9	718.9	718.9	718.9	718.9
1922-------	1961	717.4	721.0	723.3	724.8	725.6	726.1	726.3	726.4	726.4	726.4	726.4	726.4
1923-------	1962	729.9	733.0	735.1	736.4	737.2	737.7	737.9	738.0	738.0	738.0	738.0	738.0
1924-------	1963	744.5	747.4	749.4	750.7	751.4	751.8	752.0	752.1	752.1	752.1	752.1	752.1
1925-------	1964	754.2	757.0	758.9	760.1	760.8	761.2	761.4	761.5	761.5	761.5	761.5	
1926-------	1965	761.9	764.5	766.1	767.2	767.9	768.3	768.5	768.6	768.6	768.6		
1927-------	1966	767.7	770.0	771.6	772.6	773.2	773.5	773.6	773.7	773.7			
1928-------	1967	772.3	774.4	775.9	776.9	777.5	777.8	778.0	778.1				
1929-------	1968	782.7	784.8	786.2	787.1	787.6	787.9	788.0					
1930-------	1969	790.8	792.8	794.1	794.9	795.4	795.6						
1931-------	1970	802.7	804.6	805.8	806.5	806.9							
1932-------	1971	809.9	811.6	812.7	813.4								
1933-------	1972	815.0	816.5	817.5									
1934-------	1973	818.6	820.1										
1935-------	1974	816.0											

TABLE 6A. CUMULATIVE BIRTH RATES FOR ALL WOMEN AS OF THE BEGINNING OF EACH YEAR 1917-74 BY AGE AND LIVE-BIRTH ORDER FOR EACH COHORT FROM 1867 TO 1959--CON.

LIVE-BIRTH ORDER AND COHORT	DIAGONAL LINE FOR JANUARY 1	EXACT AGE											
		27	28	29	30	31	32	33	34	35	36	37	38
THIRD BIRTHS--CON.													
1879-------													500.4
1880-------												487.3	496.0
1881-------											472.5	483.1	491.9
1882-------										455.8	468.6	479.2	487.8
1883-------									437.2	452.2	464.9	475.3	484.1
1884-------								416.0	433.6	448.3	460.7	471.3	480.2
1885-------							393.0	412.3	429.5	443.8	456.4	467.1	475.5
1886-------						368.1	391.0	409.9	426.7	441.3	454.1	464.3	472.7
1887-------					340.3	367.1	389.6	408.2	425.3	440.2	452.5	462.8	471.3
1888-------				308.3	340.8	367.2	389.2	408.0	425.3	439.5	451.8	462.1	470.2
1889-------			271.7	307.0	339.0	364.4	386.7	405.8	422.4	436.6	449.1	459.0	467.0
1890-------	1917	233.6	270.6	305.6	336.1	361.8	384.4	402.7	419.4	434.0	445.9	455.6	463.3
1891-------	1918	232.4	269.0	301.9	332.7	358.6	380.3	398.7	415.9	429.9	441.5	450.8	458.1
1892-------	1919	231.0	265.4	298.4	329.2	353.3	374.9	393.7	410.1	423.6	434.6	443.4	450.2
1893-------	1920	230.9	265.5	298.4	326.6	350.5	372.6	390.6	406.2	419.1	429.5	437.8	444.5
1894-------	1921	226.8	261.6	291.5	319.5	344.0	365.2	382.6	397.6	409.9	419.8	428.1	434.6
1895-------	1922	223.9	255.7	285.5	314.1	337.6	357.9	374.7	389.0	400.7	410.7	418.6	424.9
1896-------	1923	218.6	250.4	280.6	308.0	330.6	350.2	366.0	379.7	391.4	400.9	408.6	414.5
1897-------	1924	214.1	246.5	275.5	301.7	323.3	341.7	356.8	370.3	381.4	390.6	397.8	403.7
1898-------	1925	213.2	244.3	271.9	296.7	317.0	334.7	349.7	362.5	373.2	381.8	389.1	394.8
1899-------	1926	210.0	239.6	266.1	289.7	309.3	326.9	341.5	354.2	364.4	373.4	380.7	386.4
1900-------	1927	206.5	235.0	259.7	282.1	301.4	318.2	332.1	344.0	354.5	363.2	370.2	375.9
1901-------	1928	202.4	228.8	252.1	274.0	292.5	308.5	321.7	333.8	343.9	352.3	359.2	364.8
1902-------	1929	198.9	223.7	246.5	267.1	284.5	299.6	312.8	324.2	333.8	342.0	348.8	354.4
1903-------	1930	194.5	219.0	240.8	260.7	277.2	292.3	304.9	316.0	325.6	333.8	340.7	346.4
1904-------	1931	188.4	211.7	232.9	251.8	268.6	283.1	295.4	306.5	316.1	324.5	331.6	337.6
1905-------	1932	181.2	204.0	223.9	243.0	258.9	272.9	285.1	296.2	305.9	314.5	321.9	328.5
1906-------	1933	174.2	195.6	215.8	233.8	249.2	263.1	275.4	286.6	296.6	305.5	313.5	321.3
1907-------	1934	167.8	189.5	208.5	225.9	241.2	255.3	267.7	279.3	289.7	299.5	309.0	317.5
1908-------	1935	161.7	181.8	200.0	217.0	232.4	246.4	259.2	271.2	282.6	294.2	304.6	313.8
1909-------	1936	156.7	176.1	194.2	211.6	227.1	241.7	255.1	268.3	281.9	294.4	305.8	315.6
1910-------	1937	150.8	170.0	188.5	205.7	221.8	237.0	251.6	267.3	281.9	295.6	307.7	317.8
1911-------	1938	147.2	167.1	185.3	203.2	219.8	236.1	253.4	270.2	286.0	300.6	313.0	322.6
1912-------	1939	143.0	162.3	181.2	199.5	217.7	237.0	255.5	273.4	290.2	305.0	316.8	326.3
1913-------	1940	140.2	160.3	179.7	200.0	221.3	241.8	261.4	280.6	297.9	312.2	324.0	333.7
1914-------	1941	139.5	160.3	181.9	205.4	227.7	249.4	270.7	290.6	307.4	321.6	333.7	344.0
1915-------	1942	140.7	163.1	187.9	212.1	235.1	258.7	280.8	300.2	317.0	331.8	344.7	355.8
1916-------	1943	142.6	168.3	193.4	217.7	242.5	266.9	288.4	307.7	325.1	340.7	354.4	365.6
1917-------	1944	148.1	174.0	198.7	225.1	251.4	275.4	297.2	317.5	336.0	352.7	366.7	378.5
1918-------	1945	153.7	178.4	204.9	232.8	258.5	283.0	305.7	327.1	346.8	363.9	378.5	390.0
1919-------	1946	157.9	185.2	214.3	242.5	269.6	295.7	320.5	343.9	364.4	382.2	396.6	408.3
1920-------	1947	161.7	191.6	221.2	250.9	279.8	308.0	334.7	359.0	380.1	397.7	412.1	423.5
1921-------	1948	167.5	198.4	229.9	261.9	293.4	324.1	352.0	376.8	397.9	415.4	429.6	440.5
1922-------	1949	171.1	204.0	237.7	272.1	306.1	337.9	366.2	390.9	411.7	428.9	442.3	452.6
1923-------	1950	178.4	213.6	250.3	287.8	323.0	355.4	383.7	408.2	428.9	445.3	458.1	467.9
1924-------	1951	188.5	227.4	267.4	306.3	342.7	375.3	403.6	428.2	447.9	463.6	475.8	485.3
1925-------	1952	201.8	243.9	285.4	325.6	362.1	394.9	423.2	446.4	465.0	479.9	491.7	500.4
1926-------	1953	217.8	261.1	304.4	345.1	381.7	414.3	441.1	463.2	481.0	495.3	506.0	514.1
1927-------	1954	233.9	279.3	323.3	364.6	401.5	432.8	458.6	479.7	496.8	509.9	519.9	527.6
1928-------	1955	250.9	297.4	341.9	383.5	419.2	449.6	474.3	494.6	510.2	522.5	532.0	538.9
1929-------	1956	270.0	318.3	364.2	404.9	440.2	469.6	493.8	512.6	527.6	539.4	548.1	554.4
1930-------	1957	288.5	338.3	383.4	424.1	458.5	487.3	509.8	527.9	542.2	552.9	560.8	566.7
1931-------	1958	308.9	358.5	404.2	444.3	478.3	505.3	526.9	544.3	557.5	567.2	574.6	579.9
1932-------	1959	324.8	375.2	420.8	460.4	492.4	518.2	538.9	554.8	566.7	575.8	582.6	587.6
1933-------	1960	340.5	391.3	436.2	473.5	503.9	528.9	547.9	562.3	573.4	581.9	588.3	593.1
1934-------	1961	354.1	404.2	446.8	482.4	511.9	534.8	552.0	565.4	575.9	584.2	590.5	594.9
1935-------	1962	362.1	409.9	450.7	485.4	512.3	533.0	549.2	562.0	572.3	580.3	586.0	589.9
1936-------	1963	366.0	411.8	451.2	482.7	507.2	526.8	542.1	555.0	565.2	572.5	577.6	581.2
1937-------	1964	365.6	409.5	445.1	473.8	497.2	516.0	531.9	544.7	554.0	560.5	565.2	
1938-------	1965	361.4	400.8	433.1	460.3	482.8	502.4	518.5	530.3	538.6	544.7		
1939-------	1966	351.9	387.4	418.3	445.0	468.7	488.9	503.8	514.4	522.3			
1940-------	1967	333.3	367.2	397.4	425.3	449.9	468.5	481.8	491.9				
1941-------	1968	308.8	341.6	373.2	402.2	424.9	441.4	454.1					
1942-------	1969	280.7	315.0	347.6	374.3	394.2	410.0						
1943-------	1970	256.4	291.3	321.1	344.0	362.7							
1944-------	1971	237.8	269.4	294.4	315.6								
1945-------	1972	219.0	245.1	267.9									
1946-------	1973	196.9	220.5										
1947-------	1974	176.1											

TABLE 6A. CUMULATIVE BIRTH RATES FOR ALL WOMEN AS OF THE BEGINNING OF EACH YEAR 1917-74 BY AGE AND LIVE-BIRTH ORDER FOR EACH COHORT FROM 1867 TO 1959--CON.

LIVE-BIRTH ORDER AND COHORT	DIAGONAL LINE FOR JANUARY 1	EXACT AGE											
		39	40	41	42	43	44	45	46	47	48	49	50
THIRD BIRTHS--CON.													
1867-------													589.0
1868-------												583.6	583.6
1869-------											578.3	578.3	578.3
1870-------										572.8	572.9	573.0	573.0
1871-------									567.1	567.3	567.5	567.5	567.5
1872-------								561.1	561.5	561.9	562.0	562.1	562.1
1873-------							554.5	555.2	555.7	555.9	556.1	556.1	556.1
1874-------						547.2	548.3	549.0	549.4	549.7	549.8	549.8	549.8
1875-------					539.4	541.0	542.1	542.8	543.3	543.5	543.6	543.6	543.6
1876-------				531.2	533.6	535.3	536.4	537.1	537.5	537.7	537.8	537.8	537.8
1877-------			522.2	525.7	528.4	530.0	531.1	531.8	532.2	532.4	532.5	532.5	532.5
1878-------	1917	512.0	517.3	521.0	523.5	525.1	526.2	526.9	527.3	527.5	527.6	527.7	527.7
1879-------	1918	507.3	512.8	516.3	518.9	520.5	521.6	522.3	522.7	523.0	523.1	523.1	523.1
1880-------	1919	502.9	508.3	512.0	514.6	516.2	517.3	518.0	518.4	518.6	518.7	518.8	518.8
1881-------	1920	498.7	504.2	507.9	510.3	511.9	513.0	513.6	513.9	514.1	514.2	514.2	514.2
1882-------	1921	494.8	500.4	503.9	506.3	507.9	508.9	509.5	509.8	510.0	510.1	510.1	510.1
1883-------	1922	491.1	496.3	499.8	502.2	503.7	504.7	505.2	505.5	505.7	505.7	505.8	505.8
1884-------	1923	486.8	492.0	495.5	497.9	499.3	500.2	500.7	501.0	501.1	501.2	501.2	501.2
1885-------	1924	482.1	487.3	490.7	492.9	494.3	495.2	495.7	496.0	496.2	496.3	496.3	496.3
1886-------	1925	479.4	484.4	487.6	489.9	491.3	492.1	492.6	492.9	493.0	493.1	493.1	493.1
1887-------	1926	477.7	482.6	485.8	487.9	489.2	490.0	490.5	490.8	490.9	490.9	490.9	490.9
1888-------	1927	476.4	481.2	484.2	486.2	487.5	488.3	488.7	488.9	489.0	489.1	489.1	489.1
1889-------	1928	473.1	477.6	480.6	482.7	484.0	484.8	485.2	485.4	485.5	485.5	485.5	485.5
1890-------	1929	469.1	473.4	476.5	478.4	479.6	480.4	480.8	481.0	481.1	481.1	481.1	481.1
1891-------	1930	463.6	467.9	470.6	472.4	473.5	474.3	474.7	474.9	475.0	475.0	475.0	475.0
1892-------	1931	455.6	459.6	462.2	464.0	465.1	465.8	466.2	466.4	466.5	466.5	466.5	466.5
1893-------	1932	449.6	453.4	455.9	457.6	458.7	459.3	459.6	459.8	459.9	459.9	459.9	459.9
1894-------	1933	439.5	443.2	445.7	447.4	448.4	449.0	449.4	449.6	449.7	449.7	449.7	449.7
1895-------	1934	429.6	433.2	435.7	437.3	438.2	438.8	439.2	439.4	439.5	439.5	439.5	439.5
1896-------	1935	419.1	422.6	425.0	426.5	427.5	428.1	428.5	428.7	428.8	428.8	428.8	428.8
1897-------	1936	408.2	411.7	414.0	415.6	416.6	417.2	417.6	417.8	417.9	417.9	417.9	417.9
1898-------	1937	399.2	402.6	405.0	406.6	407.6	408.2	408.6	408.8	408.9	408.9	408.9	408.9
1899-------	1938	390.9	394.4	396.9	398.5	399.6	400.3	400.7	400.9	401.0	401.0	401.0	401.0
1900-------	1939	380.5	384.0	386.5	388.2	389.3	390.1	390.6	390.9	391.0	391.1	391.1	391.1
1901-------	1940	369.4	372.9	375.5	377.2	378.4	379.3	379.8	380.1	380.2	380.2	380.2	380.2
1902-------	1941	359.0	362.6	365.3	367.3	368.7	369.7	370.2	370.4	370.5	370.5	370.5	370.5
1903-------	1942	351.1	355.0	358.1	360.4	362.0	363.0	363.5	363.8	363.9	363.9	363.9	363.9
1904-------	1943	342.8	347.4	350.8	353.3	354.9	356.0	356.6	356.9	357.0	357.0	357.0	357.0
1905-------	1944	334.6	339.6	343.4	346.0	347.7	348.8	349.4	349.6	349.7	349.7	349.7	349.7
1906-------	1945	327.9	333.3	337.1	339.8	341.5	342.5	343.0	343.3	343.4	343.4	343.4	343.4
1907-------	1946	324.8	330.5	334.6	337.3	338.9	339.9	340.5	340.8	340.9	340.9	340.9	340.9
1908-------	1947	321.4	327.3	331.2	333.8	335.4	336.5	337.1	337.4	337.5	337.5	337.5	337.5
1909-------	1948	323.5	329.1	333.0	335.6	337.3	338.4	339.0	339.3	339.4	339.4	339.4	339.4
1910-------	1949	325.2	330.9	334.9	337.7	339.6	340.8	341.5	341.8	341.9	342.0	342.0	342.0
1911-------	1950	330.1	335.8	340.0	343.0	344.9	346.2	346.9	347.2	347.4	347.5	347.5	347.5
1912-------	1951	333.9	339.9	344.4	347.5	349.6	350.8	351.5	351.8	352.0	352.0	352.0	352.0
1913-------	1952	341.7	348.1	352.7	356.0	358.1	359.4	360.1	360.4	360.5	360.5	360.5	360.5
1914-------	1953	352.7	359.3	364.1	367.4	369.5	370.8	371.5	371.8	371.9	371.9	371.9	371.9
1915-------	1954	364.6	371.4	376.3	379.7	381.8	383.0	383.7	384.0	384.1	384.2	384.2	384.2
1916-------	1955	374.6	381.5	386.2	389.5	391.4	392.6	393.3	393.6	393.8	393.8	393.8	393.8
1917-------	1956	387.6	394.5	399.3	402.4	404.3	405.5	406.1	406.4	406.5	406.5	406.5	406.5
1918-------	1957	399.0	405.6	410.1	413.1	414.9	416.0	416.6	416.9	417.0	417.0	417.0	417.0
1919-------	1958	417.3	423.8	428.3	431.2	433.1	434.1	434.7	435.0	435.1	435.1	435.1	435.1
1920-------	1959	432.1	438.4	442.7	445.6	447.3	448.3	448.8	449.0	449.1	449.1	449.1	449.1
1921-------	1960	448.7	454.7	458.9	461.5	463.1	464.0	464.5	464.7	464.8	464.8	464.8	464.8
1922-------	1961	460.4	466.1	469.9	472.4	473.9	474.8	475.2	475.4	475.5	475.5	475.5	475.5
1923-------	1962	475.4	480.7	484.2	486.6	488.0	488.8	489.2	489.4	489.4	489.4	489.4	489.4
1924-------	1963	492.2	497.1	500.5	502.6	503.8	504.5	504.9	505.0	505.1	505.1	505.1	505.1
1925-------	1964	506.8	511.5	514.5	516.4	517.5	518.1	518.4	518.5	518.6	518.6	518.6	
1926-------	1965	520.2	524.5	527.3	529.1	530.1	530.7	531.0	531.1	531.2	531.2		
1927-------	1966	533.1	536.9	539.5	541.0	542.0	542.5	542.7	542.8	542.8			
1928-------	1967	543.9	547.5	549.7	551.1	551.9	552.3	552.5	552.6				
1929-------	1968	559.1	562.2	564.3	565.6	566.3	566.7	566.9					
1930-------	1969	570.9	573.8	575.7	576.9	577.5	577.8						
1931-------	1970	583.7	586.5	588.2	589.2	589.8							
1932-------	1971	591.3	593.7	595.2	596.1								
1933-------	1972	596.4	598.5	599.8									
1934-------	1973	597.9	599.8										
1935-------	1974	592.6											

TABLE 6A. CUMULATIVE BIRTH RATES FOR ALL WOMEN AS OF THE BEGINNING OF EACH YEAR 1917-74 BY AGE AND LIVE-BIRTH ORDER FOR EACH COHORT FROM 1867 TO 1959--CON.

LIVE-BIRTH ORDER AND COHORT	DIAGONAL LINE FOR JANUARY 1	EXACT AGE											
		15	16	17	18	19	20	21	22	23	24	25	26
FOURTH BIRTHS													
1891-------													90.2
1892-------												63.6	88.2
1893-------											43.8	64.5	88.9
1894-------										24.8	40.9	61.6	85.2
1895-------									12.6	23.0	39.3	59.5	83.4
1896-------								5.4	11.5	22.0	37.9	58.3	82.7
1897-------							1.9	4.9	11.1	21.4	37.3	58.4	81.0
1898-------						0.4	1.6	4.7	10.8	21.2	38.0	57.7	80.4
1899-------					0.1	0.4	1.7	4.7	10.9	21.8	37.2	56.9	79.2
1900-------				0.0	0.1	0.4	1.7	4.7	11.2	21.2	36.9	56.6	78.5
1901-------			0.0	0.0	0.1	0.4	1.6	4.7	10.4	20.3	35.9	55.4	76.8
1902-------	1917	*	0.0	0.0	0.1	0.4	1.7	4.7	10.7	21.1	36.7	56.0	77.0
1903-------	1918	*	0.0	0.0	0.1	0.4	1.7	4.8	11.0	21.8	37.6	56.6	76.1
1904-------	1919	*	0.0	0.0	0.1	0.5	1.9	5.0	11.5	22.5	37.9	55.4	73.8
1905-------	1920	*	0.0	0.0	0.1	0.6	2.0	5.3	11.9	22.5	36.6	53.1	70.9
1906-------	1921	*	0.0	0.0	0.1	0.6	2.0	5.3	11.6	21.2	34.4	50.5	67.2
1907-------	1922	*	0.0	0.0	0.1	0.6	2.0	5.1	10.9	20.0	33.0	48.0	64.2
1908-------	1923	*	0.0	0.0	0.1	0.6	2.0	5.0	10.5	19.6	31.7	46.2	61.3
1909-------	1924	*	0.0	0.0	0.1	0.5	1.8	4.6	10.1	18.6	30.4	44.0	59.5
1910-------	1925	*	0.0	0.0	0.1	0.5	1.8	4.6	9.7	17.9	29.0	42.9	57.3
1911-------	1926	*	0.0	0.0	0.1	0.5	1.8	4.4	9.4	17.2	28.5	41.7	55.6
1912-------	1927	*	0.0	0.0	0.1	0.5	1.7	4.2	8.9	16.7	27.5	40.1	53.6
1913-------	1928	*	0.0	0.0	0.1	0.5	1.6	3.9	8.6	16.2	26.5	38.9	52.2
1914-------	1929	*	0.0	0.0	0.1	0.4	1.4	3.8	8.5	15.8	26.0	38.2	51.0
1915-------	1930	*	0.0	0.0	0.1	0.4	1.4	3.8	8.3	15.6	25.7	37.6	50.9
1916-------	1931	*	0.0	0.0	0.1	0.4	1.4	3.8	8.3	15.5	25.4	38.1	51.3
1917-------	1932	*	0.0	0.0	0.1	0.4	1.4	3.7	8.1	15.1	26.0	38.6	51.8
1918-------	1933	*	0.0	0.0	0.1	0.4	1.4	3.7	8.0	15.8	26.7	39.2	53.7
1919-------	1934	*	0.0	0.0	0.1	0.4	1.4	3.7	8.5	16.4	27.3	40.8	55.4
1920-------	1935	*	0.0	0.0	0.1	0.5	1.5	4.2	9.0	17.2	28.9	42.6	56.3
1921-------	1936	*	0.0	0.0	0.1	0.5	1.8	4.5	9.8	18.5	30.4	43.1	57.7
1922-------	1937	*	0.0	0.0	0.1	0.7	2.0	5.0	10.7	19.6	30.2	43.4	57.5
1923-------	1938	*	0.0	0.0	0.2	0.8	2.3	5.5	11.4	19.4	30.4	43.1	57.5
1924-------	1939	*	0.0	0.0	0.2	0.8	2.4	5.8	11.1	19.3	30.0	43.3	59.1
1925-------	1940	*	0.0	0.0	0.2	0.8	2.5	5.6	10.9	18.9	30.2	45.0	62.1
1926-------	1941	*	0.0	0.0	0.2	0.8	2.3	5.4	10.7	19.3	32.0	48.0	67.1
1927-------	1942	*	0.0	0.0	0.2	0.8	2.3	5.4	11.2	21.0	34.7	52.7	73.8
1928-------	1943	*	0.0	0.0	0.2	0.8	2.4	5.8	12.5	23.2	39.0	58.7	81.1
1929-------	1944	*	0.0	0.0	0.2	0.8	2.5	6.6	14.1	26.7	44.2	65.6	90.0
1930-------	1945	*	0.0	0.0	0.2	0.8	2.9	7.5	16.4	30.3	49.0	72.0	97.9
1931-------	1946	*	0.0	0.0	0.2	1.1	3.5	8.9	18.9	34.0	54.3	78.8	107.0
1932-------	1947	*	0.0	0.0	0.3	1.2	4.0	10.1	20.5	36.5	57.9	84.4	114.5
1933-------	1948	*	0.0	0.1	0.4	1.5	4.6	11.1	22.4	39.5	62.6	90.9	122.2
1934-------	1949	*	0.0	0.1	0.5	1.7	4.9	11.8	23.7	42.0	66.5	95.8	129.0
1935-------	1950	*	0.0	0.1	0.4	1.6	5.1	12.3	24.9	43.9	69.1	99.7	133.8
1936-------	1951	*	0.0	0.1	0.5	1.8	5.3	12.9	26.0	45.8	72.1	103.6	138.0
1937-------	1952	*	0.0	0.1	0.5	1.8	5.4	13.3	27.0	47.4	74.4	106.4	140.2
1938-------	1953	*	0.0	0.1	0.5	1.9	5.7	13.9	28.1	49.1	76.5	107.7	139.5
1939-------	1954	*	0.0	0.1	0.5	2.0	6.0	14.5	29.0	50.5	77.3	106.7	136.3
1940-------	1955	*	0.0	0.1	0.5	2.0	6.2	14.9	29.8	50.5	75.4	102.2	127.2
1941-------	1956	*	0.0	0.1	0.5	2.0	6.3	15.2	29.3	48.4	70.7	93.1	113.6
1942-------	1957	*	0.0	0.1	0.5	2.1	6.3	14.5	27.3	44.1	62.3	80.2	98.0
1943-------	1958	*	0.0	0.1	0.5	2.0	5.9	13.4	24.7	38.5	53.1	68.6	84.5
1944-------	1959	*	0.0	0.1	0.5	1.9	5.5	12.2	21.6	32.8	45.5	59.2	74.6
1945-------	1960	*	0.0	0.1	0.5	1.9	5.2	11.0	18.8	28.5	39.7	52.8	67.5
1946-------	1961	*	0.0	0.1	0.5	1.8	4.7	9.4	15.9	24.1	34.5	46.7	59.4
1947-------	1962	*	0.0	0.1	0.5	1.7	4.1	8.0	13.4	20.8	30.3	40.9	50.7
1948-------	1963	*	0.0	0.1	0.4	1.3	3.2	6.4	11.3	18.1	26.4	34.6	42.8
1949-------	1964	*	0.0	0.1	0.4	1.2	2.8	5.8	10.5	16.6	23.3	30.3	
1950-------	1965	*	0.0	0.0	0.2	0.9	2.4	5.2	9.2	14.2	19.8		
1951-------	1966	*	0.0	0.0	0.2	0.8	2.2	4.6	8.0	12.2			
1952-------	1967	*	0.0	0.0	0.2	0.8	2.0	3.9	6.7				
1953-------	1968	*	0.0	0.0	0.2	0.7	1.7	3.4					
1954-------	1969	*	0.0	0.0	0.1	0.5	1.4						
1955-------	1970	*	0.0	0.0	0.1	0.5							
1956-------	1971	*	0.0	0.0	0.1								
1957-------	1972	*	0.0	0.0									
1958-------	1973	*	0.0										
1959-------	1974	*											

TABLE 6A. CUMULATIVE BIRTH RATES FOR ALL WOMEN AS OF THE BEGINNING OF EACH YEAR 1917-74 BY AGE AND LIVE-BIRTH ORDER FOR EACH COHORT FROM 1867 TO 1959--CON.

LIVE-BIRTH ORDER AND COHORT	DIAGONAL LINE FOR JANUARY 1	EXACT AGE											
		27	28	29	30	31	32	33	34	35	36	37	38
FOURTH BIRTHS--CON.													
1879-------													380.1
1880-------												365.0	375.4
1881-------											347.5	359.7	370.1
1882-------										327.9	342.3	354.5	364.6
1883-------									307.3	323.6	337.8	349.6	359.6
1884-------								284.8	303.1	319.0	332.8	344.5	354.6
1885-------							261.2	280.4	298.2	313.6	327.3	339.2	348.6
1886-------						236.5	258.3	277.1	294.3	309.6	323.6	334.7	344.1
1887-------					210.2	234.4	255.8	274.0	291.2	307.0	319.9	331.0	340.4
1888-------				181.2	209.2	233.1	253.8	271.9	289.6	304.0	316.9	327.9	337.2
1889-------			149.5	178.1	205.7	228.6	249.2	267.9	284.0	298.4	311.2	322.0	330.9
1890-------	1917	118.6	146.9	175.2	201.8	224.7	246.0	263.0	279.1	293.5	305.8	316.2	324.7
1891-------	1918	116.4	144.5	171.7	198.3	221.6	240.9	257.9	273.9	287.7	299.7	309.6	317.6
1892-------	1919	114.1	141.0	168.3	195.0	216.1	235.3	252.1	267.5	280.9	292.3	301.5	308.8
1893-------	1920	113.7	140.7	167.7	191.8	212.5	231.6	247.9	262.7	275.5	286.1	294.6	301.9
1894-------	1921	110.3	137.3	161.9	185.4	205.8	224.2	239.9	254.2	266.1	276.0	284.5	291.5
1895-------	1922	108.8	133.6	157.5	180.7	200.3	218.0	233.1	246.4	257.5	267.3	275.4	282.0
1896-------	1923	106.1	130.2	153.6	175.8	194.7	211.7	225.7	238.0	248.9	258.2	265.9	272.2
1897-------	1924	103.9	127.6	150.0	171.4	189.5	205.3	218.4	230.5	240.8	249.7	257.0	263.3
1898-------	1925	103.3	126.4	148.2	168.8	185.6	200.4	213.4	224.9	234.7	243.1	250.4	256.3
1899-------	1926	101.7	124.4	145.7	165.0	181.0	195.8	208.3	219.6	229.2	237.8	244.8	250.5
1900-------	1927	100.5	122.7	142.4	160.3	176.1	190.1	202.2	213.0	222.7	230.9	237.6	243.1
1901-------	1928	98.5	118.8	136.9	154.4	169.3	182.7	194.1	204.8	213.8	221.5	227.9	233.5
1902-------	1929	96.9	115.6	133.3	149.8	163.9	176.4	187.6	197.6	206.1	213.4	219.8	225.1
1903-------	1930	94.6	112.8	129.7	145.4	158.8	171.3	181.8	191.1	199.2	206.5	212.7	217.8
1904-------	1931	91.9	109.4	125.8	141.0	154.4	166.2	176.0	185.0	193.0	200.1	206.1	211.3
1905-------	1932	88.1	105.0	120.7	135.8	148.4	159.4	169.0	177.8	185.5	192.4	198.5	203.9
1906-------	1933	83.9	99.9	115.2	129.2	141.0	151.7	161.0	169.6	177.3	184.3	190.5	196.7
1907-------	1934	79.8	95.7	110.0	123.1	134.6	145.0	154.1	162.6	170.4	177.6	184.6	191.1
1908-------	1935	76.9	91.6	105.0	117.6	128.8	138.9	148.0	156.6	164.7	172.9	180.4	187.2
1909-------	1936	74.2	88.3	101.4	114.0	124.8	134.9	144.1	153.2	162.4	171.0	179.0	186.1
1910-------	1937	71.3	84.9	98.0	110.0	120.9	131.1	140.7	151.0	160.7	169.8	178.0	185.3
1911-------	1938	69.3	83.0	95.5	107.6	118.6	129.0	139.9	150.6	160.7	170.2	178.8	185.9
1912-------	1939	67.1	80.0	92.5	104.6	116.0	127.8	139.2	150.2	160.7	170.5	178.8	185.9
1913-------	1940	65.1	78.0	90.6	103.0	115.7	128.0	139.6	151.3	162.2	171.8	180.2	187.6
1914-------	1941	63.9	77.0	90.0	103.8	116.9	129.5	141.9	153.8	164.6	174.4	183.3	191.3
1915-------	1942	63.9	77.2	91.6	105.7	118.9	132.2	144.8	156.7	167.9	178.4	188.0	196.7
1916-------	1943	64.6	79.3	93.8	107.6	121.4	134.9	147.4	159.7	171.5	182.7	193.0	202.3
1917-------	1944	66.4	81.2	95.2	109.9	124.0	137.4	150.6	163.6	176.2	188.2	199.4	209.3
1918-------	1945	68.4	82.5	97.2	112.0	125.9	140.1	153.8	167.7	181.3	194.2	205.8	215.8
1919-------	1946	69.5	84.7	99.8	114.8	129.9	144.9	160.1	175.6	190.4	204.2	216.4	226.8
1920-------	1947	71.3	86.5	101.7	117.8	133.8	150.4	167.4	184.0	199.8	214.0	226.3	237.0
1921-------	1948	72.5	87.9	104.3	121.5	139.3	157.9	176.0	193.9	210.4	225.0	238.0	248.5
1922-------	1949	72.3	88.6	106.0	124.8	144.4	164.0	183.3	201.7	218.5	233.6	246.1	256.5
1923-------	1950	73.6	91.2	110.7	131.4	152.1	173.2	193.4	212.5	230.0	244.9	257.4	267.7
1924-------	1951	76.6	96.4	117.7	140.0	162.7	184.9	206.1	226.0	243.4	258.3	270.8	280.8
1925-------	1952	81.7	103.4	126.4	150.7	174.5	197.8	219.7	239.6	256.9	271.7	283.8	293.2
1926-------	1953	88.6	112.0	137.1	162.7	187.8	211.8	233.7	253.4	270.6	285.0	296.4	305.3
1927-------	1954	97.0	122.3	148.5	175.4	201.3	225.6	247.6	267.2	284.0	297.5	308.4	317.0
1928-------	1955	106.1	132.7	160.4	188.3	214.6	239.3	261.3	280.7	296.4	309.4	319.8	327.6
1929-------	1956	116.4	144.7	174.0	202.7	230.1	255.0	277.3	295.8	311.2	323.9	333.5	340.6
1930-------	1957	126.2	156.3	186.5	216.6	244.2	269.5	290.6	308.7	323.7	335.3	343.9	350.4
1931-------	1958	137.5	169.0	200.9	231.4	259.7	283.9	304.8	322.4	336.0	346.3	354.4	360.4
1932-------	1959	146.4	179.8	212.4	243.4	270.5	294.3	314.3	330.3	342.4	352.0	359.3	364.9
1933-------	1960	156.0	190.4	223.7	253.8	280.3	303.1	321.2	335.3	346.7	355.6	362.6	367.9
1934-------	1961	163.8	198.6	231.0	260.2	285.8	306.4	322.5	335.7	346.1	354.6	361.3	366.2
1935-------	1962	169.1	203.2	234.6	262.8	285.4	303.6	318.7	330.7	340.9	349.1	355.2	359.4
1936-------	1963	172.5	205.3	235.3	260.1	280.1	296.8	310.4	322.3	332.2	339.6	344.8	348.4
1937-------	1964	173.2	204.1	230.2	251.8	270.1	285.5	299.2	310.8	319.7	326.0	330.6	
1938-------	1965	170.3	196.9	219.2	238.9	255.9	271.4	284.9	295.4	303.0	308.6		
1939-------	1966	162.8	185.5	206.1	224.4	241.5	257.0	269.4	278.5	285.3			
1940-------	1967	149.3	169.7	188.7	207.2	224.4	238.5	248.9	256.9				
1941-------	1968	133.1	151.8	170.8	189.1	204.7	216.4	225.6					
1942-------	1969	115.6	134.2	152.8	169.3	181.9	192.1						
1943-------	1970	101.7	119.6	136.1	149.4	160.3							
1944-------	1971	91.2	107.0	120.2	131.5								
1945-------	1972	82.0	94.5	105.6									
1946-------	1973	70.6	80.9										
1947-------	1974	60.0											

TABLE 6A. CUMULATIVE BIRTH RATES FOR ALL WOMEN AS OF THE BEGINNING OF EACH YEAR 1917-74 BY AGE AND LIVE-BIRTH ORDER FOR EACH COHORT FROM 1867 TO 1959--CON.

LIVE-BIRTH ORDER AND COHORT	DIAGONAL LINE FOR JANUARY 1	EXACT AGE											
		39	40	41	42	43	44	45	46	47	48	49	50
FOURTH BIRTHS--CON.													
1867-------													483.2
1868-------												477.2	477.3
1869-------											471.2	471.3	471.4
1870-------										464.9	465.1	465.3	465.4
1871-------									458.4	458.7	458.9	459.0	459.1
1872-------								451.3	451.9	452.3	452.4	452.5	452.6
1873-------							443.7	444.7	445.3	445.6	445.8	445.9	446.0
1874-------						435.4	436.9	437.9	438.4	438.8	439.0	439.1	439.2
1875-------					426.3	428.5	429.9	430.8	431.4	431.7	431.8	431.9	432.0
1876-------				416.3	419.6	421.7	423.2	424.2	424.8	425.1	425.2	425.3	425.3
1877-------			405.3	410.0	413.2	415.3	416.8	417.7	418.2	418.5	418.6	418.7	418.7
1878-------	1917	393.2	400.0	404.7	408.0	410.1	411.6	412.5	413.0	413.3	413.4	413.5	413.5
1879-------	1918	388.5	395.3	399.9	403.3	405.4	406.8	407.7	408.2	408.5	408.6	408.7	408.7
1880-------	1919	383.9	390.6	395.3	398.6	400.6	402.0	402.9	403.4	403.7	403.9	404.0	404.0
1881-------	1920	378.4	385.2	389.9	393.0	395.0	396.4	397.2	397.7	398.0	398.1	398.1	398.1
1882-------	1921	372.8	379.6	384.0	387.1	389.1	390.4	391.2	391.7	392.0	392.1	392.1	392.1
1883-------	1922	367.9	374.2	378.5	381.6	383.6	384.9	385.6	386.0	386.2	386.3	386.3	386.3
1884-------	1923	362.3	368.5	372.8	375.9	377.8	379.0	379.7	380.1	380.3	380.4	380.5	380.5
1885-------	1924	356.2	362.4	366.7	369.5	371.3	372.4	373.1	373.5	373.7	373.8	373.9	373.9
1886-------	1925	351.7	357.8	361.7	364.4	366.1	367.2	367.9	368.3	368.5	368.6	368.6	368.6
1887-------	1926	348.0	353.8	357.6	360.2	361.8	362.9	363.5	363.8	364.0	364.1	364.1	364.1
1888-------	1927	344.4	349.9	353.5	355.9	357.5	358.5	359.1	359.4	359.6	359.7	359.8	359.8
1889-------	1928	337.8	343.1	346.5	349.0	350.5	351.5	352.1	352.4	352.6	352.7	352.7	352.7
1890-------	1929	331.2	336.1	339.6	341.9	343.4	344.4	345.0	345.3	345.5	345.6	345.7	345.7
1891-------	1930	323.6	328.6	331.9	334.2	335.6	336.6	337.1	337.4	337.6	337.7	337.7	337.7
1892-------	1931	314.9	319.6	322.7	324.8	326.2	327.1	327.6	327.9	328.1	328.1	328.1	328.1
1893-------	1932	307.7	312.1	315.1	317.2	318.5	319.3	319.8	320.1	320.2	320.2	320.2	320.2
1894-------	1933	296.9	301.1	304.1	306.1	307.3	308.1	308.6	308.9	309.0	309.0	309.0	309.0
1895-------	1934	287.2	291.4	294.2	296.1	297.4	298.2	298.7	298.9	299.0	299.0	299.0	299.0
1896-------	1935	277.4	281.3	284.0	285.9	287.1	287.9	288.3	288.5	288.6	288.6	288.6	288.6
1897-------	1936	268.2	272.0	274.7	276.5	277.7	278.5	278.9	279.1	279.2	279.3	279.3	279.3
1898-------	1937	260.9	264.5	267.0	268.9	270.1	270.9	271.4	271.7	271.9	272.0	272.0	272.0
1899-------	1938	255.0	258.6	261.2	263.0	264.2	265.0	265.5	265.8	266.0	266.1	266.1	266.1
1900-------	1939	247.7	251.2	253.7	255.5	256.7	257.6	258.2	258.5	258.7	258.7	258.7	258.7
1901-------	1940	237.9	241.2	243.7	245.5	246.8	247.8	248.4	248.7	248.8	248.8	248.8	248.8
1902-------	1941	229.3	232.7	235.3	237.3	238.7	239.7	240.3	240.6	240.7	240.7	240.7	240.7
1903-------	1942	222.0	225.6	228.5	230.6	232.1	233.1	233.7	234.0	234.1	234.2	234.2	234.2
1904-------	1943	215.8	219.9	222.9	225.2	226.7	227.7	228.2	228.5	228.7	228.7	228.7	228.7
1905-------	1944	209.0	213.3	216.6	218.9	220.5	221.5	222.1	222.4	222.5	222.6	222.6	222.6
1906-------	1945	202.1	206.7	210.0	212.4	213.9	214.9	215.4	215.7	215.8	215.9	215.9	215.9
1907-------	1946	196.8	201.4	204.9	207.3	208.8	209.8	210.4	210.7	210.9	211.0	211.0	211.0
1908-------	1947	192.9	197.6	200.9	203.2	204.7	205.7	206.3	206.6	206.8	206.9	206.9	206.9
1909-------	1948	192.1	196.7	200.0	202.3	204.0	205.1	205.8	206.1	206.3	206.4	206.4	206.4
1910-------	1949	191.2	195.8	199.2	201.7	203.4	204.6	205.2	205.5	205.7	205.7	205.7	205.7
1911-------	1950	191.8	196.5	200.2	202.9	204.7	205.9	206.6	206.9	207.0	207.1	207.1	207.1
1912-------	1951	191.9	196.9	200.9	203.7	205.7	207.0	207.7	208.1	208.3	208.4	208.4	208.4
1913-------	1952	194.1	199.6	203.8	206.9	208.9	210.2	210.9	211.2	211.4	211.5	211.5	211.5
1914-------	1953	198.4	204.2	208.7	211.8	213.9	215.2	215.9	216.3	216.5	216.5	216.5	216.5
1915-------	1954	204.3	210.6	215.2	218.4	220.6	221.9	222.7	223.1	223.2	223.3	223.3	223.3
1916-------	1955	210.3	216.6	221.1	224.5	226.6	228.0	228.7	229.1	229.3	229.3	229.3	229.3
1917-------	1956	217.5	224.0	228.9	232.2	234.4	235.7	236.5	236.9	237.0	237.0	237.0	237.0
1918-------	1957	224.0	230.6	235.3	238.6	240.7	242.0	242.7	243.0	243.1	243.1	243.1	243.1
1919-------	1958	235.4	241.9	246.6	249.9	252.1	253.4	254.1	254.4	254.5	254.5	254.5	254.5
1920-------	1959	245.4	252.0	256.7	260.0	262.1	263.3	264.0	264.3	264.4	264.4	264.4	264.4
1921-------	1960	256.9	263.4	268.1	271.3	273.2	274.4	275.0	275.3	275.4	275.4	275.4	275.4
1922-------	1961	264.8	271.1	275.5	278.4	280.2	281.2	281.8	282.1	282.2	282.2	282.2	282.2
1923-------	1962	275.7	281.6	285.7	288.5	290.2	291.2	291.8	292.0	292.1	292.1	292.1	292.1
1924-------	1963	288.4	294.0	298.0	300.6	302.2	303.2	303.7	303.9	304.0	304.0	304.0	304.0
1925-------	1964	300.4	305.9	309.6	311.9	313.4	314.2	314.6	314.8	314.9	314.9	314.9	
1926-------	1965	312.3	317.3	320.6	322.8	324.0	324.7	325.1	325.3	325.3	325.3		
1927-------	1966	323.3	327.8	330.8	332.7	333.8	334.5	334.8	334.9	334.9			
1928-------	1967	333.3	337.4	340.1	341.8	342.9	343.4	343.6	343.7				
1929-------	1968	345.8	349.5	352.1	353.7	354.6	355.1	355.3					
1930-------	1969	355.2	358.7	361.1	362.4	363.2	363.6						
1931-------	1970	364.9	368.2	370.2	371.4	372.1							
1932-------	1971	369.1	371.9	373.6	374.6								
1933-------	1972	371.6	374.0	375.5									
1934-------	1973	369.5	371.6										
1935-------	1974	362.2											

TABLE 6A. CUMULATIVE BIRTH RATES FOR ALL WOMEN AS OF THE BEGINNING OF EACH YEAR 1917-74 BY AGE AND LIVE-BIRTH ORDER FOR EACH COHORT FROM 1867 TO 1959--CON.

LIVE-BIRTH ORDER AND COHORT	DIAGONAL LINE FOR JANUARY 1	EXACT AGE											
		15	16	17	18	19	20	21	22	23	24	25	26
FIFTH BIRTHS													
1891-------													34.7
1892-------												21.1	33.5
1893-------											12.9	21.6	33.4
1894-------										5.9	11.4	19.7	31.3
1895-------									2.4	5.2	10.4	18.7	30.5
1896-------								0.7	2.1	4.8	10.0	18.5	30.9
1897-------							*	0.6	1.9	4.6	9.9	18.9	30.4
1898-------						*	*	0.5	1.8	4.6	10.3	18.7	30.6
1899-------					*	*	*	0.5	1.9	4.9	10.3	19.1	30.7
1900-------				*	*	*	*	0.6	2.1	4.9	10.7	19.3	30.4
1901-------			*	*	*	*	*	0.6	2.0	4.9	10.5	18.7	29.6
1902-------	1917	*	*	*	*	*	*	0.6	2.1	5.1	10.4	18.6	29.4
1903-------	1918	*	*	*	*	*	*	0.7	2.3	5.2	10.7	18.9	29.1
1904-------	1919	*	*	*	*	*	*	0.7	2.3	5.5	11.0	18.8	28.8
1905-------	1920	*	*	*	*	*	*	0.7	2.4	5.5	10.7	18.2	27.6
1906-------	1921	*	*	*	*	*	*	0.7	2.3	5.2	10.2	17.3	26.1
1907-------	1922	*	*	*	*	*	*	0.7	2.3	5.0	9.7	16.2	24.6
1908-------	1923	*	*	*	*	*	*	0.7	2.2	4.8	9.1	15.4	23.1
1909-------	1924	*	*	*	*	*	*	0.6	2.0	4.4	8.5	14.3	22.2
1910-------	1925	*	*	*	*	*	*	0.6	1.9	4.2	8.0	14.0	21.5
1911-------	1926	*	*	*	*	*	*	0.6	1.9	4.1	8.1	13.9	21.1
1912-------	1927	*	*	*	*	*	*	0.6	1.8	4.0	7.9	13.3	20.4
1913-------	1928	*	*	*	*	*	*	0.5	1.6	3.9	7.6	13.0	19.9
1914-------	1929	*	*	*	*	*	*	0.5	1.7	3.9	7.6	13.0	19.6
1915-------	1930	*	*	*	*	*	*	0.5	1.7	3.9	7.6	12.8	19.7
1916-------	1931	*	*	*	*	*	*	0.5	1.7	3.8	7.4	13.0	19.9
1917-------	1932	*	*	*	*	*	*	0.5	1.6	3.7	7.9	13.6	20.5
1918-------	1933	*	*	*	*	*	*	0.5	1.6	4.0	8.2	13.9	21.3
1919-------	1934	*	*	*	*	*	*	0.5	1.8	4.2	8.4	14.5	22.0
1920-------	1935	*	*	*	*	*	*	0.6	1.9	4.5	9.0	15.2	22.3
1921-------	1936	*	*	*	*	*	*	0.6	2.1	4.8	9.4	15.3	22.6
1922-------	1937	*	*	*	*	*	*	0.7	2.3	5.1	9.4	15.2	22.3
1923-------	1938	*	*	*	*	*	*	0.7	2.4	5.1	9.3	15.0	22.2
1924-------	1939	*	*	*	*	*	*	0.8	2.4	5.1	9.3	15.2	22.7
1925-------	1940	*	*	*	*	*	*	0.8	2.4	5.1	9.4	15.7	23.5
1926-------	1941	*	*	*	*	*	*	0.8	2.4	5.1	9.9	16.5	25.3
1927-------	1942	*	*	*	*	*	*	0.8	2.5	5.6	10.5	17.9	27.6
1928-------	1943	*	*	*	*	*	*	0.8	2.8	6.1	11.7	19.9	30.4
1929-------	1944	*	*	*	*	*	*	1.0	3.1	6.9	13.4	22.7	34.5
1930-------	1945	*	*	*	*	*	*	1.0	3.4	7.9	15.3	25.5	38.0
1931-------	1946	*	*	*	*	*	*	1.2	4.1	9.3	17.4	28.4	42.1
1932-------	1947	*	*	*	*	*	*	1.4	4.5	10.0	18.6	30.3	44.8
1933-------	1948	*	*	*	*	*	*	1.4	4.9	10.8	19.9	32.5	47.9
1934-------	1949	*	*	*	*	*	*	1.7	5.4	11.6	21.4	34.6	50.6
1935-------	1950	*	*	*	*	*	*	1.8	5.7	12.4	22.6	36.2	52.8
1936-------	1951	*	*	*	*	*	*	1.9	6.1	12.9	23.3	37.4	54.6
1937-------	1952	*	*	*	*	*	*	2.0	6.2	13.3	24.2	38.7	55.7
1938-------	1953	*	*	*	*	*	*	2.0	6.3	13.6	24.5	38.8	54.7
1939-------	1954	*	*	*	*	*	*	2.1	6.6	14.1	25.2	38.7	53.6
1940-------	1955	*	*	*	*	*	*	2.1	6.7	14.2	24.5	36.9	49.3
1941-------	1956	*	*	*	*	*	*	2.2	6.9	13.9	23.2	33.3	43.3
1942-------	1957	*	*	*	*	*	*	2.2	6.4	12.5	19.9	27.9	36.1
1943-------	1958	*	*	*	*	*	*	1.9	5.6	10.5	16.3	22.9	29.7
1944-------	1959	*	*	*	*	*	*	1.8	4.9	8.8	13.7	19.2	25.6
1945-------	1960	*	*	*	*	*	*	1.5	4.0	7.4	11.5	16.6	22.6
1946-------	1961	*	*	*	*	*	*	1.3	3.4	6.1	9.8	14.4	19.4
1947-------	1962	*	*	*	*	*	*	1.0	2.6	4.9	8.1	11.9	15.6
1948-------	1963	*	*	*	*	*	*	0.7	2.1	4.1	6.8	9.6	12.6
1949-------	1964	*	*	*	*	*	*	0.7	2.0	3.8	5.9	8.3	
1950-------	1965	*	*	*	*	*	*	0.7	1.8	3.2	5.0		
1951-------	1966	*	*	*	*	*	*	0.6	1.4	2.5			
1952-------	1967	*	*	*	*	*	*	0.4	1.1				
1953-------	1968	*	*	*	*	*	*	0.3					
1954-------	1969	*	*	*	*	*	*						
1955-------	1970	*	*	*	*	*							
1956-------	1971	*	*	*	*								
1957-------	1972	*	*	*									
1958-------	1973	*	*										
1959-------	1974	*											

TABLE 6A. CUMULATIVE BIRTH RATES FOR ALL WOMEN AS OF THE BEGINNING OF EACH YEAR 1917-74 BY AGE AND LIVE-BIRTH ORDER FOR EACH COHORT FROM 1867 TO 1959--CON.

LIVE-BIRTH ORDER AND COHORT	DIAGONAL LINE FOR JANUARY 1	EXACT AGE											
		27	28	29	30	31	32	33	34	35	36	37	38
FIFTH BIRTHS--CON.													
1879-------													282.6
1880-------												266.9	278.3
1881-------											248.3	261.1	272.3
1882-------										227.6	242.4	255.0	266.0
1883-------									207.0	223.1	237.6	250.0	260.9
1884-------								185.5	203.1	219.0	233.0	245.3	256.1
1885-------							163.4	181.2	198.6	213.7	227.6	239.8	249.8
1886-------						141.1	160.5	178.2	194.6	209.6	223.5	234.9	244.8
1887-------					118.5	138.6	158.0	174.7	191.0	206.0	218.9	230.1	239.8
1888-------				95.5	117.3	137.1	155.4	172.0	188.2	202.2	214.9	225.9	235.2
1889-------			72.3	92.7	113.9	132.7	150.8	167.3	182.4	196.2	208.7	219.3	228.3
1890-------	1917	51.5	70.0	89.7	110.2	129.0	147.1	162.5	177.6	191.3	203.1	213.2	221.7
1891-------	1918	49.9	67.8	87.1	107.6	126.5	143.4	158.8	173.6	186.6	197.8	207.4	215.4
1892-------	1919	48.2	65.7	85.0	105.8	123.1	139.8	154.8	168.7	180.8	191.4	200.3	207.7
1893-------	1920	47.8	65.3	85.0	103.8	120.9	137.2	151.5	164.4	176.1	186.0	194.3	201.6
1894-------	1921	45.8	63.9	81.6	100.3	117.1	132.6	146.0	158.6	169.5	179.0	187.3	194.2
1895-------	1922	45.6	62.0	79.8	98.1	114.1	128.7	141.8	153.7	164.0	173.3	181.1	187.6
1896-------	1923	44.7	61.2	78.5	95.7	110.8	125.1	137.3	148.3	158.3	166.9	174.3	180.4
1897-------	1924	44.3	60.5	76.7	92.7	107.4	120.7	132.1	142.9	152.2	160.6	167.5	173.6
1898-------	1925	44.4	59.6	74.9	90.9	104.8	117.4	128.6	138.7	147.8	155.5	162.3	167.9
1899-------	1926	43.9	58.6	74.2	89.5	102.8	115.3	126.0	136.1	144.7	152.6	159.1	164.5
1900-------	1927	43.4	58.3	73.0	87.4	100.4	112.1	122.6	132.1	140.7	148.1	154.3	159.5
1901-------	1928	42.6	56.4	70.2	84.1	96.2	107.5	117.2	126.6	134.6	141.5	147.3	152.4
1902-------	1929	41.4	54.5	67.8	80.7	92.2	102.6	112.1	120.6	127.9	134.4	140.0	144.7
1903-------	1930	40.7	53.3	65.7	78.0	88.7	99.0	107.7	115.7	122.7	129.0	134.2	138.8
1904-------	1931	39.9	51.7	63.8	75.4	86.1	95.6	103.8	111.5	118.3	124.2	129.3	133.8
1905-------	1932	38.0	49.4	60.6	72.2	82.1	91.1	99.1	106.6	113.0	118.7	123.7	128.2
1906-------	1933	36.1	46.6	57.7	68.5	77.8	86.5	94.1	101.1	107.3	112.9	117.9	122.8
1907-------	1934	33.8	44.4	54.8	64.9	73.9	82.2	89.4	96.1	102.2	107.8	113.2	118.2
1908-------	1935	32.4	42.3	52.0	61.7	70.3	78.0	84.9	91.5	97.7	103.8	109.3	114.4
1909-------	1936	31.0	40.4	50.0	59.4	67.5	75.0	81.9	88.6	95.3	101.5	107.3	112.5
1910-------	1937	29.9	39.1	48.4	57.2	65.1	72.5	79.5	86.8	93.6	100.1	105.9	111.0
1911-------	1938	29.4	38.4	47.2	55.9	63.8	71.2	78.8	86.2	93.3	99.8	105.6	110.6
1912-------	1939	28.4	36.8	45.4	54.0	61.8	69.9	77.6	85.1	92.1	98.5	104.1	109.1
1913-------	1940	27.4	35.7	44.3	52.6	61.1	69.3	77.0	84.5	91.4	97.7	103.3	108.5
1914-------	1941	27.1	35.4	43.7	52.8	61.3	69.4	77.1	84.6	91.5	97.9	103.8	109.3
1915-------	1942	27.2	35.3	44.3	53.4	61.8	70.0	77.8	85.2	92.2	98.9	105.2	111.1
1916-------	1943	27.4	36.2	45.3	54.2	62.8	70.9	78.5	86.0	93.2	100.3	107.0	113.4
1917-------	1944	28.6	37.5	46.3	55.3	63.7	71.7	79.4	87.2	94.9	102.4	109.6	116.3
1918-------	1945	29.4	37.8	46.7	55.5	63.8	71.9	79.9	88.1	96.3	104.2	111.9	118.8
1919-------	1946	29.9	38.7	47.6	56.5	65.2	73.9	82.7	91.9	100.8	109.6	117.7	125.0
1920-------	1947	30.4	39.1	48.1	57.3	66.4	75.7	85.5	95.3	105.0	114.2	122.7	130.5
1921-------	1948	30.7	39.5	48.7	58.2	68.0	78.4	88.8	99.4	109.7	119.5	128.6	136.5
1922-------	1949	30.3	39.1	48.4	58.6	69.2	80.2	91.2	102.4	113.2	123.4	132.4	140.5
1923-------	1950	30.4	39.6	49.7	60.8	72.2	84.0	95.9	107.8	119.2	129.5	138.9	147.0
1924-------	1951	31.4	41.5	52.8	65.0	77.5	90.3	103.0	115.6	127.3	138.1	147.6	155.8
1925-------	1952	33.0	44.3	56.5	69.8	83.2	96.9	110.5	123.4	135.5	146.5	156.2	164.1
1926-------	1953	35.9	48.0	61.4	75.5	89.8	104.4	118.2	131.5	143.8	154.8	164.1	171.7
1927-------	1954	39.1	52.3	66.5	81.5	96.7	111.4	125.8	139.5	152.0	162.7	171.8	179.1
1928-------	1955	43.0	57.0	71.9	87.8	103.4	119.0	133.8	147.7	159.8	170.2	178.9	185.6
1929-------	1956	47.9	62.9	79.1	95.8	112.5	128.8	144.2	158.0	170.0	180.1	188.2	194.4
1930-------	1957	52.5	68.7	85.7	103.4	120.8	137.6	152.8	166.4	178.0	187.4	194.7	200.3
1931-------	1958	57.8	74.8	92.9	111.4	129.4	146.2	161.3	174.4	185.2	193.6	200.2	205.4
1932-------	1959	61.3	79.4	98.3	117.6	135.5	152.2	166.7	178.9	188.4	196.0	202.1	207.0
1933-------	1960	65.3	84.1	104.0	123.2	141.0	156.9	170.2	180.8	189.5	196.6	202.5	207.1
1934-------	1961	68.7	88.6	108.3	127.1	144.1	158.4	170.0	179.7	187.6	194.5	200.1	204.4
1935-------	1962	71.9	91.6	110.9	128.9	143.8	156.3	166.8	175.5	183.3	189.8	194.9	198.5
1936-------	1963	73.3	92.4	110.6	126.1	139.1	150.4	159.7	168.2	175.6	181.5	185.7	188.8
1937-------	1964	73.7	91.5	107.0	120.3	132.0	142.0	151.2	159.4	166.0	170.9	174.5	
1938-------	1965	71.3	86.3	99.3	111.1	121.3	131.1	140.1	147.4	152.9	157.0		
1939-------	1966	67.6	80.1	91.5	101.9	112.1	121.7	129.7	135.8	140.5			
1940-------	1967	60.8	71.6	81.7	92.0	101.9	110.5	117.1	122.2				
1941-------	1968	53.0	62.3	72.1	81.9	90.7	97.5	103.0					
1942-------	1969	44.2	53.1	62.2	70.8	77.5	83.1						
1943-------	1970	37.3	45.5	53.5	60.0	65.5							
1944-------	1971	32.7	39.8	45.9	51.3								
1945-------	1972	28.7	34.2	39.1									
1946-------	1973	24.0	28.3										
1947-------	1974	19.1											

TABLE 6A. CUMULATIVE BIRTH RATES FOR ALL WOMEN AS OF THE BEGINNING OF EACH YEAR 1917-74 BY AGE AND LIVE-BIRTH ORDER FOR EACH COHORT FROM 1867 TO 1959--CON.

LIVE-BIRTH ORDER AND COHORT	DIAGONAL LINE FOR JANUARY 1	EXACT AGE											
		39	40	41	42	43	44	45	46	47	48	49	50
FIFTH BIRTHS--CON.													
1867-------													388.6
1868-------												382.6	382.7
1869-------											376.6	376.7	376.8
1870-------										370.4	370.6	370.7	370.8
1871-------									363.9	364.4	364.7	364.8	364.9
1872-------								357.0	357.7	358.2	358.4	358.5	358.5
1873-------							349.5	350.7	351.5	352.0	352.3	352.4	352.4
1874-------						341.4	343.2	344.4	345.1	345.6	345.8	345.9	345.9
1875-------					332.1	334.6	336.5	337.7	338.5	338.9	339.1	339.2	339.2
1876-------				321.3	325.1	327.7	329.5	330.7	331.4	331.8	332.0	332.1	332.2
1877-------			309.1	314.5	318.5	321.0	322.8	324.0	324.6	325.0	325.2	325.3	325.3
1878-------	1917	296.2	304.1	309.6	313.4	315.9	317.8	318.9	319.6	320.0	320.2	320.3	320.3
1879-------	1918	292.2	300.1	305.5	309.3	311.9	313.6	314.7	315.4	315.8	316.0	316.1	316.1
1880-------	1919	287.7	295.5	300.8	304.7	307.1	308.8	309.9	310.5	310.8	311.0	311.1	311.1
1881-------	1920	281.6	289.3	294.7	298.4	300.8	302.5	303.5	304.0	304.3	304.4	304.5	304.5
1882-------	1921	275.2	282.9	287.9	291.5	293.9	295.5	296.4	296.9	297.2	297.3	297.4	297.4
1883-------	1922	270.0	277.1	282.0	285.5	287.7	289.2	290.1	290.6	290.9	291.1	291.1	291.1
1884-------	1923	264.5	271.5	276.3	279.6	281.8	283.3	284.2	284.7	285.0	285.1	285.2	285.2
1885-------	1924	258.0	264.8	269.3	272.5	274.6	276.0	276.8	277.3	277.6	277.7	277.8	277.8
1886-------	1925	252.9	259.3	263.6	266.6	268.5	269.8	270.6	271.0	271.3	271.4	271.5	271.6
1887-------	1926	247.6	253.8	258.0	260.9	262.7	264.0	264.7	265.1	265.3	265.4	265.5	265.5
1888-------	1927	242.7	248.7	252.7	255.4	257.2	258.4	259.1	259.5	259.7	259.8	259.8	259.8
1889-------	1928	235.6	241.3	245.0	247.8	249.5	250.7	251.4	251.8	252.0	252.1	252.2	252.2
1890-------	1929	228.5	233.8	237.6	240.2	241.9	243.1	243.8	244.2	244.4	244.5	244.6	244.6
1891-------	1930	221.6	226.9	230.4	232.9	234.6	235.7	236.3	236.7	236.9	237.0	237.1	237.1
1892-------	1931	214.0	218.9	222.2	224.6	226.2	227.2	227.8	228.1	228.3	228.4	228.5	228.5
1893-------	1932	207.5	212.0	215.2	217.6	219.1	220.1	220.6	220.9	221.1	221.2	221.2	221.2
1894-------	1933	199.6	203.9	207.1	209.3	210.7	211.6	212.1	212.4	212.6	212.7	212.7	212.7
1895-------	1934	192.8	197.1	200.1	202.2	203.5	204.4	204.9	205.2	205.3	205.3	205.3	205.3
1896-------	1935	185.5	189.5	192.3	194.3	195.6	196.5	197.0	197.2	197.3	197.3	197.3	197.3
1897-------	1936	178.4	182.1	184.8	186.7	188.0	188.8	189.2	189.5	189.6	189.6	189.6	189.6
1898-------	1937	172.4	176.0	178.6	180.5	181.7	182.5	183.1	183.4	183.5	183.6	183.6	183.6
1899-------	1938	168.9	172.5	175.1	176.9	178.1	178.9	179.5	179.8	180.0	180.1	180.1	180.1
1900-------	1939	163.8	167.3	169.8	171.6	172.8	173.7	174.3	174.6	174.8	174.9	174.9	174.9
1901-------	1940	156.5	159.8	162.2	163.9	165.2	166.1	166.7	167.0	167.2	167.2	167.2	167.2
1902-------	1941	148.6	151.8	154.2	156.1	157.5	158.4	159.0	159.3	159.4	159.5	159.5	159.5
1903-------	1942	142.6	145.8	148.3	150.2	151.6	152.6	153.1	153.4	153.6	153.6	153.6	153.6
1904-------	1943	137.7	141.1	143.7	145.7	147.1	148.0	148.5	148.8	148.9	149.0	149.0	149.0
1905-------	1944	132.4	135.9	138.6	140.6	142.0	142.8	143.3	143.6	143.7	143.7	143.7	143.7
1906-------	1945	127.1	130.8	133.5	135.5	136.8	137.6	138.1	138.4	138.5	138.5	138.5	138.5
1907-------	1946	122.6	126.3	129.1	131.0	132.3	133.2	133.7	134.0	134.1	134.2	134.2	134.2
1908-------	1947	118.8	122.4	125.0	126.9	128.2	129.1	129.6	129.9	130.1	130.2	130.2	130.2
1909-------	1948	116.9	120.4	123.0	125.0	126.3	127.2	127.8	128.1	128.3	128.4	128.4	128.4
1910-------	1949	115.2	118.7	121.4	123.4	124.8	125.8	126.4	126.7	126.9	127.0	127.0	127.0
1911-------	1950	114.9	118.5	121.3	123.5	125.0	126.1	126.8	127.1	127.3	127.3	127.3	127.3
1912-------	1951	113.5	117.2	120.2	122.4	124.1	125.3	125.9	126.2	126.3	126.4	126.4	126.4
1913-------	1952	113.1	117.2	120.3	122.8	124.6	125.7	126.3	126.6	126.8	126.9	126.9	126.9
1914-------	1953	114.3	118.6	122.0	124.6	126.4	127.5	128.2	128.6	128.8	128.9	128.9	128.9
1915-------	1954	116.5	121.1	124.7	127.4	129.2	130.4	131.1	131.4	131.6	131.7	131.7	131.7
1916-------	1955	119.0	123.8	127.5	130.2	132.0	133.2	133.9	134.3	134.5	134.6	134.6	134.6
1917-------	1956	122.2	127.1	130.8	133.6	135.5	136.7	137.4	137.7	137.9	138.0	138.0	138.0
1918-------	1957	124.9	129.9	133.7	136.5	138.4	139.7	140.3	140.6	140.8	140.8	140.8	140.8
1919-------	1958	131.4	136.6	140.5	143.4	145.4	146.6	147.3	147.6	147.7	147.7	147.7	147.7
1920-------	1959	137.0	142.3	146.3	149.2	151.1	152.3	152.9	153.2	153.3	153.3	153.3	153.3
1921-------	1960	143.3	148.6	152.6	155.4	157.3	158.4	159.0	159.3	159.4	159.4	159.4	159.4
1922-------	1961	147.2	152.6	156.4	159.1	160.8	161.8	162.4	162.7	162.8	162.8	162.8	162.8
1923-------	1962	153.8	158.9	162.6	165.2	166.9	167.8	168.3	168.5	168.6	168.6	168.6	168.6
1924-------	1963	162.3	167.3	170.9	173.4	174.9	175.7	176.1	176.3	176.4	176.4	176.4	176.4
1925-------	1964	170.4	175.2	178.6	180.8	182.1	182.9	183.4	183.6	183.6	183.6	183.6	
1926-------	1965	177.7	182.2	185.2	187.2	188.4	189.2	189.6	189.7	189.8	189.8		
1927-------	1966	184.7	188.7	191.4	193.2	194.4	195.0	195.3	195.4	195.5			
1928-------	1967	190.7	194.2	196.6	198.3	199.3	199.9	200.1	200.2				
1929-------	1968	199.0	202.3	204.7	206.3	207.2	207.7	207.9					
1930-------	1969	204.5	207.7	210.0	211.3	212.0	212.4						
1931-------	1970	209.4	212.4	214.2	215.4	216.1							
1932-------	1971	210.8	213.4	215.0	216.0								
1933-------	1972	210.5	212.8	214.3									
1934-------	1973	207.3	209.3										
1935-------	1974	201.0											

TABLE 6A. CUMULATIVE BIRTH RATES FOR ALL WOMEN AS OF THE BEGINNING OF EACH YEAR 1917-74 BY AGE AND LIVE-BIRTH ORDER FOR EACH COHORT FROM 1867 TO 1959--CON.

LIVE-BIRTH ORDER AND COHORT	DIAGONAL LINE FOR JANUARY 1	EXACT AGE											
		15	16	17	18	19	20	21	22	23	24	25	26
SIXTH BIRTHS													
1891-------													12.4
1892-------												6.9	11.9
1893-------											3.8	6.8	11.5
1894-------										1.7	3.4	6.2	10.7
1895-------									0.7	1.5	3.1	5.9	10.5
1896-------								0.2	0.6	1.4	2.9	5.8	10.9
1897-------							*	0.2	0.6	1.3	2.9	6.1	10.8
1898-------						*	*	0.2	0.6	1.4	3.2	6.2	11.1
1899-------					*	*	*	0.2	0.6	1.5	3.3	6.4	11.4
1900-------				*	*	*	*	0.2	0.6	1.4	3.3	6.5	11.3
1901-------			*	*	*	*	*	0.2	0.6	1.4	3.2	6.3	11.1
1902-------	1917	*	*	*	*	*	*	0.2	0.6	1.5	3.3	6.3	10.8
1903-------	1918	*	*	*	*	*	*	0.2	0.6	1.5	3.3	6.2	10.3
1904-------	1919	*	*	*	*	*	*	0.2	0.7	1.6	3.3	6.1	10.2
1905-------	1920	*	*	*	*	*	*	0.2	0.7	1.6	3.3	5.9	9.8
1906-------	1921	*	*	*	*	*	*	0.2	0.7	1.6	3.1	5.6	9.3
1907-------	1922	*	*	*	*	*	*	0.2	0.7	1.5	2.9	5.3	8.7
1908-------	1923	*	*	*	*	*	*	0.2	0.6	1.3	2.7	4.9	8.0
1909-------	1924	*	*	*	*	*	*	0.2	0.6	1.3	2.5	4.5	7.7
1910-------	1925	*	*	*	*	*	*	0.2	0.6	1.2	2.4	4.4	7.5
1911-------	1926	*	*	*	*	*	*	0.2	0.5	1.1	2.3	4.4	7.5
1912-------	1927	*	*	*	*	*	*	0.2	0.5	1.1	2.3	4.3	7.3
1913-------	1928	*	*	*	*	*	*	0.1	0.4	1.0	2.2	4.1	7.0
1914-------	1929	*	*	*	*	*	*	0.1	0.4	1.0	2.1	4.0	6.8
1915-------	1930	*	*	*	*	*	*	0.1	0.4	1.0	2.1	4.0	6.9
1916-------	1931	*	*	*	*	*	*	0.1	0.4	1.0	2.1	4.1	7.0
1917-------	1932	*	*	*	*	*	*	0.1	0.4	1.0	2.3	4.3	7.4
1918-------	1933	*	*	*	*	*	*	0.1	0.4	1.1	2.4	4.5	7.7
1919-------	1934	*	*	*	*	*	*	0.1	0.5	1.2	2.5	4.8	8.1
1920-------	1935	*	*	*	*	*	*	0.2	0.6	1.3	2.8	5.2	8.4
1921-------	1936	*	*	*	*	*	*	0.2	0.6	1.4	2.9	5.1	8.4
1922-------	1937	*	*	*	*	*	*	0.2	0.6	1.4	2.8	5.1	8.3
1923-------	1938	*	*	*	*	*	*	0.2	0.6	1.4	2.8	5.1	8.3
1924-------	1939	*	*	*	*	*	*	0.2	0.6	1.4	2.9	5.2	8.6
1925-------	1940	*	*	*	*	*	*	0.2	0.6	1.4	2.9	5.4	8.9
1926-------	1941	*	*	*	*	*	*	0.2	0.6	1.4	3.0	5.5	9.2
1927-------	1942	*	*	*	*	*	*	0.2	0.6	1.5	3.1	5.8	9.9
1928-------	1943	*	*	*	*	*	*	0.2	0.7	1.6	3.4	6.4	10.9
1929-------	1944	*	*	*	*	*	*	0.2	0.7	1.7	3.8	7.2	12.3
1930-------	1945	*	*	*	*	*	*	0.2	0.7	1.9	4.2	8.1	13.7
1931-------	1946	*	*	*	*	*	*	0.2	0.8	2.2	5.0	9.4	15.7
1932-------	1947	*	*	*	*	*	*	0.3	1.0	2.6	5.6	10.5	17.1
1933-------	1948	*	*	*	*	*	*	0.3	1.2	3.0	6.3	11.4	18.3
1934-------	1949	*	*	*	*	*	*	0.4	1.3	3.2	6.7	12.1	19.4
1935-------	1950	*	*	*	*	*	*	0.4	1.4	3.5	7.1	12.7	20.4
1936-------	1951	*	*	*	*	*	*	0.4	1.4	3.5	7.3	13.1	20.9
1937-------	1952	*	*	*	*	*	*	0.4	1.4	3.6	7.5	13.4	21.3
1938-------	1953	*	*	*	*	*	*	0.4	1.5	3.8	7.7	13.6	21.0
1939-------	1954	*	*	*	*	*	*	0.5	1.6	3.9	7.8	13.4	20.2
1940-------	1955	*	*	*	*	*	*	0.4	1.6	3.9	7.6	12.8	18.6
1941-------	1956	*	*	*	*	*	*	0.5	1.6	3.7	7.1	11.3	15.9
1942-------	1957	*	*	*	*	*	*	0.5	1.5	3.4	6.1	9.5	13.3
1943-------	1958	*	*	*	*	*	*	0.4	1.3	2.8	5.0	7.7	10.7
1944-------	1959	*	*	*	*	*	*	0.3	1.1	2.4	4.2	6.3	8.9
1945-------	1960	*	*	*	*	*	*	0.3	1.0	2.0	3.4	5.4	7.7
1946-------	1961	*	*	*	*	*	*	0.3	0.8	1.6	2.9	4.5	6.3
1947-------	1962	*	*	*	*	*	*	0.2	0.6	1.3	2.3	3.6	4.9
1948-------	1963	*	*	*	*	*	*	0.1	0.5	1.0	1.8	2.7	3.7
1949-------	1964	*	*	*	*	*	*	0.2	0.5	1.0	1.6	2.3	
1950-------	1965	*	*	*	*	*	*	0.1	0.3	0.6	1.0		
1951-------	1966	*	*	*	*	*	*	0.1	0.3	0.5			
1952-------	1967	*	*	*	*	*	*	0.1	0.2				
1953-------	1968	*	*	*	*	*	*	0.1					
1954-------	1969	*	*	*	*	*	*						
1955-------	1970	*	*	*	*	*							
1956-------	1971	*	*	*	*								
1957-------	1972	*	*	*									
1958-------	1973	*	*										
1959-------	1974	*											

TABLE 6A. CUMULATIVE BIRTH RATES FOR ALL WOMEN AS OF THE BEGINNING OF EACH YEAR 1917-74 BY AGE AND LIVE-BIRTH ORDER FOR EACH COHORT FROM 1867 TO 1959--CON.

LIVE-BIRTH ORDER AND COHORT	DIAGONAL LINE FOR JANUARY 1	EXACT AGE											
		27	28	29	30	31	32	33	34	35	36	37	38
SIXTH BIRTHS--CON.													
1879-------													207.5
1880-------												191.2	203.4
1881-------											171.7	185.0	197.1
1882-------										150.8	165.4	178.6	190.3
1883-------									131.0	146.4	160.9	173.6	185.1
1884-------								112.6	128.6	143.8	157.6	170.1	181.3
1885-------							94.7	110.3	126.1	140.5	154.0	166.2	176.6
1886-------						76.7	92.7	108.3	123.3	137.3	150.7	162.1	172.2
1887-------					60.0	75.1	91.1	105.9	120.4	134.6	147.2	158.3	168.3
1888-------				46.0	61.0	75.9	91.0	105.3	120.2	133.4	145.7	156.6	166.0
1889-------			31.8	44.2	58.6	72.7	87.3	101.9	115.6	128.6	140.6	151.0	160.0
1890-------	1917	20.4	30.5	42.2	56.0	69.8	84.9	98.4	112.1	124.9	136.3	146.2	154.9
1891-------	1918	19.6	29.2	40.5	54.2	68.6	82.5	96.0	109.5	121.6	132.5	142.2	150.2
1892-------	1919	18.7	27.9	39.2	53.5	66.6	80.4	93.6	106.2	117.6	128.0	136.7	144.0
1893-------	1920	18.0	27.2	39.2	52.2	65.2	78.7	91.0	102.8	113.8	123.4	131.5	138.7
1894-------	1921	17.3	27.2	38.0	51.0	63.8	76.6	88.2	99.7	109.7	118.6	126.4	133.2
1895-------	1922	17.6	26.6	37.6	50.5	62.8	74.9	86.4	97.0	106.4	115.0	122.5	129.0
1896-------	1923	17.4	26.6	37.6	49.8	61.6	73.3	83.7	93.4	102.5	110.5	117.6	123.6
1897-------	1924	17.5	26.8	37.0	48.8	60.0	70.9	80.4	90.0	98.4	106.2	112.8	118.7
1898-------	1925	17.9	26.4	36.5	47.8	58.3	68.5	78.2	87.2	95.6	103.0	109.6	115.2
1899-------	1926	17.9	26.6	36.4	47.1	57.1	67.4	76.6	85.8	93.8	101.2	107.3	112.5
1900-------	1927	17.8	26.2	35.4	45.6	55.6	65.4	74.5	83.0	90.9	97.7	103.6	108.6
1901-------	1928	17.3	25.1	33.6	43.5	52.8	62.2	70.5	78.8	86.0	92.4	97.8	102.6
1902-------	1929	16.5	23.6	32.0	41.2	50.1	58.6	66.6	74.1	80.7	86.6	91.7	96.2
1903-------	1930	15.8	22.8	30.7	39.7	47.8	56.1	63.4	70.3	76.5	82.1	86.9	91.1
1904-------	1931	15.5	22.2	30.1	38.2	46.3	54.1	61.0	67.7	73.7	79.0	83.6	87.7
1905-------	1932	14.9	21.4	28.4	36.5	44.1	51.3	58.0	64.4	69.9	74.9	79.3	83.3
1906-------	1933	14.1	20.0	27.0	34.6	41.6	48.6	55.0	60.9	66.2	71.0	75.3	79.4
1907-------	1934	13.1	19.0	25.6	32.7	39.6	46.4	52.3	58.0	63.1	67.9	72.3	76.5
1908-------	1935	12.4	17.9	24.1	31.0	37.6	43.8	49.5	54.9	60.0	65.0	69.5	73.6
1909-------	1936	12.0	17.3	23.4	30.1	36.2	42.2	47.7	53.1	58.5	63.6	68.1	72.1
1910-------	1937	11.6	16.8	22.7	28.9	34.9	40.6	45.9	51.6	57.1	62.0	66.4	70.4
1911-------	1938	11.6	16.7	22.3	28.5	34.3	39.8	45.5	51.3	56.5	61.3	65.7	69.5
1912-------	1939	11.2	16.1	21.7	27.7	33.2	39.1	44.9	50.4	55.6	60.4	64.6	68.4
1913-------	1940	10.8	15.6	21.1	26.7	32.5	38.4	43.9	49.4	54.5	59.0	63.2	67.0
1914-------	1941	10.6	15.4	20.6	26.5	32.5	38.3	43.9	49.2	54.0	58.7	62.9	67.0
1915-------	1942	10.6	15.2	20.6	26.6	32.4	38.2	43.5	48.7	53.7	58.4	62.9	67.0
1916-------	1943	10.8	15.6	21.1	26.9	32.6	38.1	43.4	48.7	53.7	58.6	63.1	67.4
1917-------	1944	11.4	16.3	21.6	27.3	32.8	38.3	43.6	48.9	54.0	58.9	63.6	68.1
1918-------	1945	11.8	16.6	21.9	27.5	33.0	38.5	43.9	49.3	54.6	59.7	64.6	69.3
1919-------	1946	12.2	17.1	22.3	28.0	33.7	39.4	45.0	50.8	56.5	62.1	67.5	72.5
1920-------	1947	12.5	17.3	22.7	28.6	34.4	40.4	46.4	52.5	58.7	64.7	70.4	75.8
1921-------	1948	12.4	17.4	23.0	29.0	35.1	41.4	47.6	54.3	60.9	67.2	73.3	78.8
1922-------	1949	12.4	17.4	22.9	29.1	35.4	41.8	48.6	55.5	62.3	69.0	75.1	80.8
1923-------	1950	12.5	17.5	23.4	29.8	36.4	43.4	50.5	57.8	65.1	72.0	78.4	84.1
1924-------	1951	12.9	18.4	24.5	31.4	38.6	46.2	53.9	61.9	69.4	76.6	83.2	89.2
1925-------	1952	13.5	19.3	26.0	33.6	41.5	49.8	58.2	66.3	74.2	81.6	88.4	94.1
1926-------	1953	14.2	20.5	27.9	36.1	44.7	53.5	62.0	70.6	78.7	86.3	93.0	98.7
1927-------	1954	15.4	22.3	30.2	39.1	48.1	57.1	66.2	75.1	83.5	91.1	97.7	103.2
1928-------	1955	16.9	24.3	32.8	42.0	51.3	61.1	70.5	79.7	88.1	95.5	101.9	107.0
1929-------	1956	18.9	27.0	36.1	45.8	56.0	66.2	76.2	85.5	93.8	101.2	107.1	111.7
1930-------	1957	20.9	29.6	39.2	49.7	60.4	71.0	81.0	90.3	98.6	105.3	110.6	114.9
1931-------	1958	23.6	32.8	43.1	54.2	65.4	76.2	86.2	95.5	103.0	109.1	114.1	118.1
1932-------	1959	25.3	35.0	45.8	57.3	68.5	79.2	89.0	97.3	104.0	109.5	114.1	117.7
1933-------	1960	27.0	37.2	48.5	60.0	71.0	81.4	90.2	97.5	103.6	108.7	113.0	116.4
1934-------	1961	28.5	39.2	50.5	61.8	72.4	81.7	89.4	95.9	101.3	106.2	110.2	113.4
1935-------	1962	29.9	40.5	51.4	62.3	71.8	79.8	86.6	92.3	97.7	102.2	105.9	108.6
1936-------	1963	30.4	40.6	51.1	60.5	68.6	75.6	81.5	87.1	92.0	96.2	99.3	101.6
1937-------	1964	30.3	39.9	48.8	56.8	63.8	69.9	75.6	80.9	85.4	88.8	91.3	
1938-------	1965	29.3	37.4	44.7	51.5	57.5	63.3	68.7	73.4	77.1	79.9		
1939-------	1966	27.3	33.9	40.2	46.1	51.9	57.5	62.4	66.3	69.4			
1940-------	1967	24.3	30.0	35.4	41.0	46.4	51.3	55.2	58.4				
1941-------	1968	20.6	25.3	30.2	35.2	39.8	43.6	46.8					
1942-------	1969	17.1	21.3	25.7	29.9	33.4	36.4						
1943-------	1970	14.1	17.8	21.5	24.6	27.3							
1944-------	1971	11.9	15.0	17.8	20.3								
1945-------	1972	10.2	12.6	14.8									
1946-------	1973	8.1	10.0										
1947-------	1974	6.3											

TABLE 6A. CUMULATIVE BIRTH RATES FOR ALL WOMEN AS OF THE BEGINNING OF EACH YEAR 1917-74 BY AGE AND LIVE-BIRTH ORDER FOR EACH COHORT FROM 1867 TO 1959--CON.

LIVE-BIRTH ORDER AND COHORT	DIAGONAL LINE FOR JANUARY 1	EXACT AGE											
		39	40	41	42	43	44	45	46	47	48	49	50
SIXTH BIRTHS--CON.													
1867-------													309.5
1868-------												304.1	304.2
1869-------											298.6	298.8	298.9
1870-------										293.0	293.3	293.5	293.6
1871-------									287.0	287.6	288.0	288.2	288.3
1872-------								280.4	281.3	282.1	282.4	282.6	282.7
1873-------							273.4	274.9	276.0	276.6	276.9	277.0	277.0
1874-------						265.9	268.2	269.8	270.7	271.3	271.5	271.6	271.7
1875-------					256.9	260.1	262.3	263.7	264.6	265.1	265.3	265.5	265.6
1876-------				245.8	250.5	253.6	255.7	257.1	257.9	258.4	258.7	258.9	258.9
1877-------			233.0	239.3	243.9	246.9	249.0	250.4	251.2	251.7	251.9	252.0	252.1
1878-------	1917	221.3	230.1	236.3	240.7	243.7	245.9	247.2	248.0	248.5	248.7	248.8	248.8
1879-------	1918	217.8	226.6	232.6	237.1	240.2	242.2	243.5	244.2	244.6	244.8	244.9	244.9
1880-------	1919	213.7	222.2	228.2	232.7	235.5	237.5	238.8	239.6	240.1	240.3	240.4	240.5
1881-------	1920	207.0	215.4	221.4	225.5	228.3	230.3	231.5	232.2	232.6	232.8	232.9	233.0
1882-------	1921	200.1	208.4	213.9	218.0	220.7	222.6	223.8	224.5	224.9	225.1	225.2	225.2
1883-------	1922	194.7	202.3	207.7	211.7	214.2	216.0	217.0	217.6	218.0	218.2	218.3	218.3
1884-------	1923	190.1	197.5	202.7	206.4	208.9	210.6	211.6	212.2	212.5	212.7	212.8	212.8
1885-------	1924	185.1	192.3	197.2	200.8	203.1	204.6	205.5	206.0	206.3	206.4	206.5	206.5
1886-------	1925	180.6	187.5	192.1	195.5	197.6	199.0	199.9	200.4	200.7	200.8	200.9	201.0
1887-------	1926	176.4	182.8	187.4	190.5	192.5	194.0	194.9	195.4	195.7	195.8	195.9	196.0
1888-------	1927	173.5	179.8	184.0	186.9	188.9	190.3	191.2	191.7	192.0	192.1	192.2	192.3
1889-------	1928	167.4	173.2	177.1	180.1	182.1	183.5	184.3	184.8	185.1	185.3	185.4	185.4
1890-------	1929	161.7	167.0	171.0	173.8	175.7	177.0	177.8	178.2	178.5	178.6	178.7	178.7
1891-------	1930	156.4	161.9	165.6	168.3	170.0	171.3	172.0	172.4	172.6	172.7	172.8	172.8
1892-------	1931	150.3	155.3	158.9	161.4	163.1	164.2	164.9	165.3	165.5	165.6	165.6	165.6
1893-------	1932	144.6	149.5	152.8	155.2	156.8	157.9	158.5	158.9	159.1	159.2	159.2	159.2
1894-------	1933	138.9	143.4	146.7	149.0	150.5	151.5	152.1	152.4	152.6	152.7	152.7	152.7
1895-------	1934	134.2	138.6	141.6	143.7	145.1	146.1	146.7	147.0	147.2	147.3	147.3	147.3
1896-------	1935	128.8	132.9	135.7	137.6	139.0	139.9	140.4	140.7	140.9	140.9	140.9	140.9
1897-------	1936	123.4	127.1	129.7	131.7	133.0	133.8	134.3	134.6	134.7	134.7	134.7	134.7
1898-------	1937	119.6	123.1	125.7	127.6	128.8	129.6	130.2	130.5	130.6	130.7	130.7	130.7
1899-------	1938	116.8	120.4	122.9	124.7	125.9	126.8	127.4	127.7	127.9	128.0	128.0	128.0
1900-------	1939	112.8	116.2	118.6	120.4	121.6	122.5	123.0	123.3	123.5	123.6	123.6	123.6
1901-------	1940	106.5	109.6	111.9	113.5	114.8	115.7	116.2	116.5	116.7	116.8	116.8	116.8
1902-------	1941	99.9	102.9	105.1	106.9	108.2	109.1	109.6	109.9	110.0	110.1	110.1	110.1
1903-------	1942	94.6	97.6	99.9	101.7	103.0	103.9	104.5	104.7	104.8	104.9	104.9	104.9
1904-------	1943	91.3	94.4	96.7	98.6	99.8	100.7	101.1	101.3	101.4	101.4	101.4	101.4
1905-------	1944	87.0	90.1	92.5	94.3	95.5	96.3	96.7	96.9	97.0	97.0	97.0	97.0
1906-------	1945	83.1	86.2	88.5	90.1	91.2	91.9	92.3	92.5	92.6	92.7	92.7	92.7
1907-------	1946	80.1	83.1	85.3	86.9	88.0	88.8	89.2	89.4	89.5	89.5	89.5	89.5
1908-------	1947	77.1	80.0	82.0	83.5	84.6	85.3	85.7	85.9	86.0	86.0	86.0	86.0
1909-------	1948	75.6	78.3	80.4	82.0	83.1	83.9	84.4	84.6	84.7	84.7	84.7	84.7
1910-------	1949	73.7	76.4	78.5	80.1	81.2	82.0	82.5	82.7	82.8	82.8	82.8	82.8
1911-------	1950	72.8	75.6	77.8	79.5	80.8	81.6	82.1	82.4	82.5	82.6	82.6	82.6
1912-------	1951	71.7	74.6	76.9	78.7	80.0	80.9	81.4	81.7	81.8	81.9	81.9	81.9
1913-------	1952	70.4	73.4	75.8	77.7	79.0	79.9	80.5	80.8	81.0	81.0	81.0	81.0
1914-------	1953	70.5	73.6	76.2	78.2	79.6	80.6	81.1	81.4	81.5	81.6	81.6	81.6
1915-------	1954	70.8	74.2	76.9	78.9	80.4	81.3	81.9	82.2	82.4	82.5	82.5	82.5
1916-------	1955	71.3	74.8	77.5	79.6	81.0	82.0	82.6	82.9	83.1	83.1	83.1	83.1
1917-------	1956	72.2	75.7	78.5	80.5	82.0	83.0	83.6	83.9	84.0	84.1	84.1	84.1
1918-------	1957	73.5	77.1	79.9	82.0	83.5	84.5	85.1	85.3	85.5	85.5	85.5	85.5
1919-------	1958	77.0	80.8	83.8	86.0	87.6	88.6	89.1	89.4	89.5	89.5	89.5	89.5
1920-------	1959	80.4	84.4	87.4	89.7	91.2	92.1	92.7	93.0	93.1	93.1	93.1	93.1
1921-------	1960	83.7	87.7	90.8	93.0	94.5	95.5	96.0	96.2	96.3	96.3	96.3	96.3
1922-------	1961	85.7	89.8	92.8	95.0	96.5	97.4	97.9	98.1	98.2	98.2	98.2	98.2
1923-------	1962	89.2	93.1	96.1	98.2	99.6	100.4	100.8	101.0	101.1	101.1	101.1	101.1
1924-------	1963	94.0	97.9	100.8	102.8	104.1	104.8	105.2	105.4	105.5	105.5	105.5	105.5
1925-------	1964	98.9	102.7	105.5	107.4	108.5	109.2	109.6	109.8	109.9	109.9	109.9	
1926-------	1965	103.3	106.9	109.4	111.0	112.1	112.7	113.1	113.3	113.4	113.4		
1927-------	1966	107.6	110.8	113.0	114.5	115.4	116.0	116.3	116.4	116.4			
1928-------	1967	110.8	113.7	115.7	117.1	118.0	118.5	118.7	118.8				
1929-------	1968	115.4	118.1	120.0	121.3	122.0	122.4	122.6					
1930-------	1969	118.2	120.7	122.5	123.6	124.3	124.7						
1931-------	1970	121.1	123.5	125.1	126.1	126.7							
1932-------	1971	120.6	122.8	124.2	125.1								
1933-------	1972	119.0	120.8	122.0									
1934-------	1973	115.7	117.3										
1935-------	1974	110.5											

TABLE 6A. CUMULATIVE BIRTH RATES FOR ALL WOMEN AS OF THE BEGINNING OF EACH YEAR 1917-74 BY AGE AND LIVE-BIRTH ORDER FOR EACH COHORT FROM 1867 TO 1959--CON.

LIVE-BIRTH ORDER AND COHORT	DIAGONAL LINE FOR JANUARY 1	EXACT AGE											
		15	16	17	18	19	20	21	22	23	24	25	26
SEVENTH BIRTHS													
1891-------													4.0
1892-------												2.1	3.8
1893-------											0.9	1.9	3.4
1894-------										0.4	0.9	1.8	3.4
1895-------									0.2	0.5	1.0	1.9	3.4
1896-------								0.1	0.2	0.4	0.9	1.8	3.5
1897-------							*	0.1	0.2	0.4	0.9	1.9	3.5
1898-------						*	*	0.1	0.2	0.4	0.9	1.9	3.6
1899-------					*	*	*	0.1	0.2	0.4	0.9	1.9	3.6
1900-------				*	*	*	*	0.1	0.2	0.5	1.1	2.1	3.9
1901-------			*	*	*	*	*	0.1	0.2	0.5	1.0	2.0	3.7
1902-------	1917	*	*	*	*	*	*	0.1	0.2	0.5	1.1	2.1	3.7
1903-------	1918	*	*	*	*	*	*	0.1	0.2	0.5	1.0	1.9	3.4
1904-------	1919	*	*	*	*	*	*	0.1	0.2	0.5	1.0	1.9	3.3
1905-------	1920	*	*	*	*	*	*	0.1	0.2	0.5	1.0	1.8	3.2
1906-------	1921	*	*	*	*	*	*	0.1	0.2	0.5	0.9	1.7	3.0
1907-------	1922	*	*	*	*	*	*	0.1	0.2	0.4	0.8	1.6	2.8
1908-------	1923	*	*	*	*	*	*	0.1	0.2	0.4	0.8	1.5	2.5
1909-------	1924	*	*	*	*	*	*	0.1	0.2	0.4	0.8	1.4	2.5
1910-------	1925	*	*	*	*	*	*	0.1	0.2	0.4	0.7	1.3	2.4
1911-------	1926	*	*	*	*	*	*	0.1	0.2	0.4	0.7	1.4	2.5
1912-------	1927	*	*	*	*	*	*	0.0	0.1	0.3	0.7	1.3	2.4
1913-------	1928	*	*	*	*	*	*	0.0	0.1	0.3	0.6	1.2	2.2
1914-------	1929	*	*	*	*	*	*	0.1	0.2	0.4	0.8	1.4	2.4
1915-------	1930	*	*	*	*	*	*	0.1	0.2	0.4	0.8	1.4	2.5
1916-------	1931	*	*	*	*	*	*	0.1	0.2	0.4	0.8	1.5	2.6
1917-------	1932	*	*	*	*	*	*	0.0	0.1	0.3	0.7	1.4	2.5
1918-------	1933	*	*	*	*	*	*	0.1	0.2	0.4	0.8	1.5	2.7
1919-------	1934	*	*	*	*	*	*	0.1	0.2	0.4	0.8	1.6	2.8
1920-------	1935	*	*	*	*	*	*	0.1	0.2	0.4	0.9	1.6	2.8
1921-------	1936	*	*	*	*	*	*	0.1	0.2	0.4	0.8	1.6	2.8
1922-------	1937	*	*	*	*	*	*	0.1	0.2	0.4	0.8	1.6	2.8
1923-------	1938	*	*	*	*	*	*	0.1	0.2	0.4	0.8	1.6	2.9
1924-------	1939	*	*	*	*	*	*	0.1	0.2	0.4	0.9	1.7	3.0
1925-------	1940	*	*	*	*	*	*	0.1	0.2	0.4	0.9	1.8	3.2
1926-------	1941	*	*	*	*	*	*	0.1	0.2	0.4	0.9	1.8	3.2
1927-------	1942	*	*	*	*	*	*	0.1	0.2	0.5	1.0	1.9	3.4
1928-------	1943	*	*	*	*	*	*	0.1	0.2	0.5	1.0	2.0	3.7
1929-------	1944	*	*	*	*	*	*	0.1	0.2	0.5	1.1	2.2	4.1
1930-------	1945	*	*	*	*	*	*	0.1	0.2	0.5	1.2	2.5	4.7
1931-------	1946	*	*	*	*	*	*	0.1	0.3	0.7	1.5	3.0	5.5
1932-------	1947	*	*	*	*	*	*	0.1	0.3	0.7	1.6	3.3	6.0
1933-------	1948	*	*	*	*	*	*	0.1	0.3	0.8	1.8	3.6	6.4
1934-------	1949	*	*	*	*	*	*	0.1	0.3	0.8	1.9	3.8	6.9
1935-------	1950	*	*	*	*	*	*	0.1	0.3	0.8	1.9	4.0	7.2
1936-------	1951	*	*	*	*	*	*	0.1	0.3	0.8	2.0	4.1	7.3
1937-------	1952	*	*	*	*	*	*	0.1	0.3	0.9	2.1	4.2	7.4
1938-------	1953	*	*	*	*	*	*	0.1	0.4	1.0	2.2	4.3	7.4
1939-------	1954	*	*	*	*	*	*	0.1	0.4	1.0	2.2	4.2	7.1
1940-------	1955	*	*	*	*	*	*	0.1	0.4	1.0	2.2	4.0	6.4
1941-------	1956	*	*	*	*	*	*	0.1	0.4	1.0	2.1	3.6	5.5
1942-------	1957	*	*	*	*	*	*	0.1	0.4	0.9	1.8	3.0	4.6
1943-------	1958	*	*	*	*	*	*	0.1	0.3	0.7	1.4	2.4	3.6
1944-------	1959	*	*	*	*	*	*	0.1	0.3	0.6	1.1	1.8	2.8
1945-------	1960	*	*	*	*	*	*	0.1	0.3	0.6	1.0	1.6	2.5
1946-------	1961	*	*	*	*	*	*	0.1	0.2	0.4	0.8	1.4	2.0
1947-------	1962	*	*	*	*	*	*	0.0	0.1	0.3	0.6	1.0	1.4
1948-------	1963	*	*	*	*	*	*	0.1	0.2	0.4	0.6	0.8	1.1
1949-------	1964	*	*	*	*	*	*	0.1	0.2	0.3	0.4	0.6	
1950-------	1965	*	*	*	*	*	*	0.1	0.1	0.2	0.3		
1951-------	1966	*	*	*	*	*	*	0.0	0.0	0.1			
1952-------	1967	*	*	*	*	*	*	0.0	0.0				
1953-------	1968	*	*	*	*	*	*	0.0					
1954-------	1969	*	*	*	*	*	*						
1955-------	1970	*	*	*	*	*							
1956-------	1971	*	*	*	*								
1957-------	1972	*	*	*									
1958-------	1973	*	*										
1959-------	1974	*											

TABLE 6A. CUMULATIVE BIRTH RATES FOR ALL WOMEN AS OF THE BEGINNING OF EACH YEAR 1917-74 BY AGE AND LIVE-BIRTH ORDER FOR EACH COHORT FROM 1867 TO 1959--CON.

LIVE-BIRTH ORDER AND COHORT	DIAGONAL LINE FOR JANUARY 1	EXACT AGE											
		27	28	29	30	31	32	33	34	35	36	37	38
SEVENTH BIRTHS--CON.													
1879-------													141.4
1880-------												126.9	138.8
1881-------											111.1	123.5	135.0
1882-------										94.8	107.6	119.6	131.1
1883-------									78.9	91.6	104.1	116.0	127.2
1884-------								63.6	76.1	88.5	100.7	112.3	123.2
1885-------							49.8	61.1	73.4	85.3	97.1	108.5	118.6
1886-------						37.2	47.9	59.1	70.8	82.4	94.3	104.9	114.7
1887-------					26.9	35.8	46.4	57.1	68.5	80.4	91.4	101.8	111.5
1888-------				18.5	26.5	35.2	45.3	55.7	67.5	78.5	89.4	99.6	108.7
1889-------			11.9	17.6	25.1	33.5	43.3	54.1	64.9	75.8	86.5	96.2	104.9
1890-------	1917	7.1	11.2	16.4	23.8	31.9	42.1	52.0	62.9	73.7	83.8	93.0	101.3
1891-------	1918	6.6	10.4	15.7	22.9	31.5	40.9	50.8	61.6	71.9	81.7	90.6	98.3
1892-------	1919	6.2	10.1	15.3	23.0	30.9	40.3	50.1	60.3	70.1	79.4	87.4	94.3
1893-------	1920	5.9	9.7	15.3	22.4	30.3	39.5	48.8	58.4	67.9	76.3	83.6	90.3
1894-------	1921	5.8	10.0	15.2	22.4	30.2	38.9	47.8	57.2	65.7	73.4	80.5	86.9
1895-------	1922	6.1	10.0	15.4	22.5	30.0	38.5	47.2	55.6	63.5	71.1	77.8	84.0
1896-------	1923	6.0	10.0	15.3	22.1	29.5	37.7	45.5	53.3	60.9	68.0	74.5	80.1
1897-------	1924	6.1	10.1	15.3	22.0	29.1	36.6	43.8	51.3	58.4	65.2	71.2	76.7
1898-------	1925	6.3	10.2	15.2	21.7	28.3	35.3	42.4	49.6	56.5	63.0	68.9	74.1
1899-------	1926	6.3	10.1	15.1	21.2	27.4	34.4	41.2	48.4	55.1	61.6	67.3	72.2
1900-------	1927	6.5	10.3	14.9	20.5	26.7	33.3	40.1	46.9	53.6	59.8	65.1	69.8
1901-------	1928	6.1	9.6	13.8	19.3	25.2	31.7	38.0	44.6	50.8	56.4	61.3	65.8
1902-------	1929	6.0	9.1	13.2	18.4	24.0	29.8	35.8	41.9	47.5	52.7	57.4	61.4
1903-------	1930	5.5	8.6	12.6	17.7	22.8	28.5	34.1	39.7	45.0	50.0	54.2	58.0
1904-------	1931	5.4	8.4	12.3	16.9	21.9	27.3	32.6	38.1	43.2	47.7	51.8	55.5
1905-------	1932	5.2	8.1	11.7	16.2	21.0	26.1	31.2	36.4	41.1	45.4	49.3	52.8
1906-------	1933	4.9	7.5	10.9	15.3	19.8	24.7	29.6	34.4	38.9	43.0	46.7	50.3
1907-------	1934	4.5	7.0	10.4	14.4	18.7	23.4	27.9	32.5	36.8	40.8	44.6	48.1
1908-------	1935	4.1	6.6	9.7	13.7	18.0	22.3	26.6	30.9	35.0	39.1	42.8	46.3
1909-------	1936	4.2	6.6	9.7	13.7	17.6	21.8	25.9	30.2	34.5	38.6	42.3	45.6
1910-------	1937	4.0	6.4	9.5	13.2	17.1	21.1	25.2	29.6	33.9	37.9	41.5	44.7
1911-------	1938	4.1	6.5	9.4	13.2	17.0	20.9	25.1	29.5	33.7	37.5	41.0	44.1
1912-------	1939	4.0	6.2	9.3	12.9	16.5	20.5	24.7	29.0	33.0	36.6	39.9	43.0
1913-------	1940	3.7	6.0	9.0	12.3	16.0	20.0	24.1	28.1	31.9	35.4	38.7	41.7
1914-------	1941	4.0	6.3	9.0	12.4	16.1	20.1	24.0	27.9	31.6	35.2	38.4	41.4
1915-------	1942	4.1	6.3	9.1	12.6	16.3	20.2	24.0	27.8	31.5	35.0	38.2	41.3
1916-------	1943	4.2	6.5	9.4	12.9	16.5	20.3	24.0	27.8	31.5	35.0	38.3	41.5
1917-------	1944	4.2	6.5	9.3	12.7	16.3	20.0	23.7	27.5	31.2	34.7	38.1	41.4
1918-------	1945	4.4	6.7	9.6	13.0	16.5	20.3	24.0	27.9	31.6	35.3	38.9	42.2
1919-------	1946	4.5	6.9	9.8	13.2	16.9	20.7	24.7	28.7	32.6	36.6	40.3	43.9
1920-------	1947	4.6	7.0	10.0	13.6	17.3	21.3	25.3	29.4	33.5	37.5	41.4	45.1
1921-------	1948	4.6	7.1	10.2	13.8	17.6	21.6	25.7	30.0	34.3	38.6	42.7	46.5
1922-------	1949	4.6	7.1	10.2	13.8	17.6	21.7	26.0	30.4	34.9	39.4	43.5	47.4
1923-------	1950	4.8	7.3	10.4	14.1	18.0	22.3	26.7	31.4	36.2	40.7	45.1	49.1
1924-------	1951	4.9	7.5	10.8	14.7	19.0	23.6	28.5	33.7	38.6	43.5	48.0	52.2
1925-------	1952	5.2	7.9	11.4	15.7	20.3	25.3	30.6	35.9	41.2	46.2	50.9	55.0
1926-------	1953	5.3	8.3	12.2	16.8	21.9	27.3	32.7	38.3	43.8	49.1	53.7	57.8
1927-------	1954	5.7	9.0	13.1	18.1	23.6	29.3	35.0	40.8	46.6	51.8	56.4	60.5
1928-------	1955	6.3	9.9	14.4	19.7	25.4	31.4	37.4	43.5	49.1	54.2	58.8	62.4
1929-------	1956	7.0	11.0	15.9	21.6	27.7	34.1	40.6	46.7	52.4	57.6	61.7	65.1
1930-------	1957	7.9	12.1	17.3	23.3	29.7	36.3	42.7	48.9	54.6	59.2	63.0	66.1
1931-------	1958	9.1	13.7	19.3	25.7	32.4	39.2	45.7	51.9	57.0	61.3	64.7	67.4
1932-------	1959	9.7	14.7	20.6	27.1	33.8	40.5	46.9	52.4	57.0	60.8	63.9	66.5
1933-------	1960	10.5	15.7	21.9	28.5	35.2	41.7	47.4	52.2	56.3	59.7	62.7	65.2
1934-------	1961	11.2	16.6	22.7	29.3	35.7	41.5	46.3	50.7	54.3	57.6	60.4	62.6
1935-------	1962	11.6	16.9	23.0	29.2	34.9	39.7	44.1	47.9	51.3	54.4	56.9	58.8
1936-------	1963	11.6	16.9	22.5	27.9	32.6	36.9	40.6	44.1	47.3	50.1	52.2	53.8
1937-------	1964	11.6	16.5	21.3	25.8	29.9	33.6	37.1	40.3	43.2	45.4	47.2	
1938-------	1965	11.3	15.4	19.4	23.2	26.6	30.0	33.2	36.1	38.4	40.3		
1939-------	1966	10.4	13.8	17.2	20.4	23.5	26.6	29.4	31.7	33.6			
1940-------	1967	9.1	11.9	14.7	17.5	20.3	23.0	25.2	27.1				
1941-------	1968	7.7	10.0	12.3	14.7	17.1	19.1	20.9					
1942-------	1969	6.3	8.2	10.2	12.3	14.1	15.7						
1943-------	1970	5.0	6.6	8.3	9.8	11.2							
1944-------	1971	4.0	5.3	6.6	7.8								
1945-------	1972	3.5	4.5	5.5									
1946-------	1973	2.7	3.4										
1947-------	1974	1.9											

TABLE 6A. CUMULATIVE BIRTH RATES FOR ALL WOMEN AS OF THE BEGINNING OF EACH YEAR 1917-74 BY AGE AND LIVE-BIRTH ORDER FOR EACH COHORT FROM 1867 TO 1959--CON.

LIVE-BIRTH ORDER AND COHORT	DIAGONAL LINE FOR JANUARY 1	EXACT AGE											
		39	40	41	42	43	44	45	46	47	48	49	50
SEVENTH BIRTHS--CON.													
1867-------													239.2
1868-------												234.5	234.6
1869-------											229.6	229.8	229.9
1870-------										224.5	224.8	225.0	225.1
1871-------									219.0	219.7	220.1	220.3	220.4
1872-------								212.9	214.0	214.7	215.0	215.2	215.3
1873-------							206.4	208.1	209.2	209.8	210.1	210.3	210.4
1874-------						199.7	202.3	204.0	205.0	205.7	206.0	206.2	206.3
1875-------					191.1	194.5	197.1	198.7	199.8	200.4	200.7	200.9	201.0
1876-------				180.1	184.8	188.2	190.6	192.2	193.1	193.7	194.0	194.2	194.2
1877-------			167.2	173.4	178.2	181.4	183.9	185.4	186.3	186.9	187.2	187.3	187.4
1878-------	1917	154.8	163.6	169.9	174.5	177.8	180.3	181.8	182.7	183.2	183.4	183.6	183.7
1879-------	1918	151.8	160.5	166.6	171.3	174.6	176.9	178.4	179.3	179.8	180.1	180.2	180.2
1880-------	1919	148.9	157.5	163.6	168.3	171.4	173.7	175.1	176.0	176.5	176.7	176.8	176.9
1881-------	1920	145.1	153.6	159.6	164.0	167.1	169.3	170.7	171.5	172.0	172.2	172.3	172.4
1882-------	1921	140.9	149.2	154.9	159.2	162.2	164.3	165.5	166.2	166.6	166.8	166.9	166.9
1883-------	1922	136.8	144.6	150.1	154.3	157.1	159.1	160.2	160.9	161.3	161.5	161.6	161.6
1884-------	1923	132.1	139.6	144.9	148.9	151.5	153.3	154.4	155.0	155.4	155.6	155.7	155.8
1885-------	1924	127.2	134.5	139.6	143.4	145.8	147.6	148.6	149.2	149.5	149.7	149.8	149.9
1886-------	1925	123.2	130.1	134.9	138.5	140.8	142.4	143.4	144.0	144.4	144.6	144.7	144.8
1887-------	1926	119.5	126.1	130.8	134.1	136.3	137.9	138.8	139.4	139.7	139.9	140.0	140.1
1888-------	1927	116.2	122.5	126.7	129.7	131.8	133.3	134.2	134.7	135.0	135.1	135.2	135.3
1889-------	1928	112.3	118.2	122.2	125.2	127.2	128.7	129.6	130.1	130.4	130.5	130.6	130.7
1890-------	1929	108.0	113.4	117.4	120.2	122.2	123.6	124.4	124.9	125.1	125.2	125.3	125.4
1891-------	1930	104.5	109.8	113.4	116.2	118.1	119.4	120.2	120.6	120.8	120.9	121.0	121.0
1892-------	1931	100.4	105.2	108.8	111.4	113.2	114.4	115.1	115.5	115.7	115.8	115.9	115.9
1893-------	1932	95.9	100.7	104.0	106.5	108.1	109.2	109.9	110.3	110.5	110.6	110.6	110.6
1894-------	1933	92.4	96.7	99.9	102.2	103.8	104.8	105.5	105.9	106.1	106.2	106.2	106.2
1895-------	1934	89.0	93.3	96.3	98.5	99.9	100.9	101.5	101.8	102.0	102.1	102.1	102.1
1896-------	1935	85.0	89.0	91.7	93.7	95.1	96.0	96.5	96.8	97.0	97.1	97.1	97.1
1897-------	1936	81.3	84.9	87.5	89.4	90.7	91.6	92.1	92.4	92.6	92.7	92.7	92.7
1898-------	1937	78.3	81.8	84.4	86.2	87.4	88.2	88.8	89.1	89.3	89.4	89.4	89.4
1899-------	1938	76.3	79.7	82.1	83.8	85.0	85.9	86.5	86.8	87.0	87.1	87.1	87.1
1900-------	1939	73.8	76.9	79.2	80.9	82.0	82.9	83.5	83.8	84.0	84.1	84.1	84.1
1901-------	1940	69.4	72.3	74.4	75.9	77.1	78.0	78.5	78.8	79.0	79.1	79.1	79.1
1902-------	1941	64.8	67.6	69.6	71.2	72.4	73.3	73.8	74.1	74.2	74.2	74.2	74.2
1903-------	1942	61.3	64.0	66.1	67.7	69.0	69.8	70.3	70.5	70.6	70.6	70.6	70.6
1904-------	1943	58.6	61.4	63.5	65.2	66.3	67.1	67.5	67.7	67.8	67.8	67.8	67.8
1905-------	1944	56.0	58.7	60.8	62.4	63.5	64.2	64.6	64.8	64.9	64.9	64.9	64.9
1906-------	1945	53.4	56.1	58.1	59.6	60.6	61.3	61.7	61.9	62.0	62.0	62.0	62.0
1907-------	1946	51.2	53.8	55.7	57.1	58.0	58.6	59.0	59.2	59.3	59.3	59.3	59.3
1908-------	1947	49.2	51.6	53.4	54.7	55.6	56.2	56.6	56.8	56.9	56.9	56.9	56.9
1909-------	1948	48.5	50.8	52.5	53.8	54.8	55.5	55.9	56.1	56.2	56.2	56.2	56.2
1910-------	1949	47.4	49.7	51.5	52.9	53.9	54.6	55.0	55.2	55.3	55.3	55.3	55.3
1911-------	1950	46.8	49.1	50.9	52.3	53.3	54.0	54.4	54.6	54.7	54.7	54.7	54.7
1912-------	1951	45.7	48.0	49.8	51.2	52.2	52.9	53.3	53.5	53.6	53.6	53.6	53.6
1913-------	1952	44.4	46.6	48.4	49.8	50.8	51.5	51.9	52.1	52.2	52.3	52.3	52.3
1914-------	1953	44.1	46.5	48.4	49.8	50.9	51.7	52.1	52.3	52.4	52.4	52.4	52.4
1915-------	1954	44.1	46.5	48.4	50.0	51.1	51.9	52.3	52.5	52.6	52.6	52.6	52.6
1916-------	1955	44.4	46.9	48.9	50.5	51.6	52.4	52.8	53.1	53.2	53.2	53.2	53.2
1917-------	1956	44.4	47.1	49.2	50.8	52.0	52.7	53.2	53.4	53.5	53.5	53.5	53.5
1918-------	1957	45.2	47.9	50.0	51.6	52.7	53.5	53.9	54.1	54.2	54.2	54.2	54.2
1919-------	1958	47.1	49.9	52.1	53.8	55.0	55.8	56.2	56.4	56.5	56.5	56.5	56.5
1920-------	1959	48.4	51.3	53.6	55.4	56.6	57.4	57.8	58.0	58.1	58.1	58.1	58.1
1921-------	1960	49.9	52.9	55.3	57.0	58.2	59.0	59.4	59.6	59.7	59.7	59.7	59.7
1922-------	1961	50.9	53.9	56.2	57.9	59.0	59.7	60.1	60.3	60.4	60.4	60.4	60.4
1923-------	1962	52.7	55.6	57.8	59.4	60.5	61.1	61.5	61.7	61.8	61.8	61.8	61.8
1924-------	1963	55.7	58.6	60.8	62.3	63.3	63.9	64.3	64.5	64.6	64.6	64.6	64.6
1925-------	1964	58.5	61.4	63.5	64.9	65.8	66.4	66.7	66.9	67.0	67.0	67.0	
1926-------	1965	61.3	64.0	65.9	67.2	68.1	68.6	68.9	69.0	69.0	69.0		
1927-------	1966	63.7	66.1	67.9	69.1	69.8	70.3	70.5	70.6	70.7			
1928-------	1967	65.3	67.6	69.2	70.2	70.9	71.3	71.5	71.6				
1929-------	1968	67.8	69.8	71.2	72.2	72.8	73.2	73.4					
1930-------	1969	68.5	70.3	71.7	72.6	73.1	73.4						
1931-------	1970	69.7	71.5	72.7	73.5	73.9							
1932-------	1971	68.6	70.2	71.3	71.9								
1933-------	1972	67.1	68.5	69.4									
1934-------	1973	64.2	65.4										
1935-------	1974	60.2											

TABLE 6A. CUMULATIVE BIRTH RATES FOR ALL WOMEN AS OF THE BEGINNING OF EACH YEAR 1917-74 BY AGE AND LIVE-BIRTH ORDER FOR EACH COHORT FROM 1867 TO 1959--CON.

LIVE-BIRTH ORDER AND COHORT	DIAGONAL LINE FOR JANUARY 1	EXACT AGE											
		15	16	17	18	19	20	21	22	23	24	25	26
EIGHTH AND HIGHER BIRTHS													
1891-------													2.0
1892-------												1.0	1.9
1893-------											0.0	0.6	1.5
1894-------										0.0	0.3	0.9	1.7
1895-------									0.0	0.1	0.4	0.9	1.7
1896-------								0.0	0.0	0.1	0.4	0.9	1.9
1897-------							*	0.0	0.0	0.1	0.4	1.0	1.9
1898-------						*	*	0.0	0.0	0.1	0.4	1.0	2.0
1899-------					*	*	*	0.0	0.0	0.1	0.4	1.0	2.0
1900-------				*	*	*	*	0.0	0.0	0.1	0.4	1.1	2.2
1901-------			*	*	*	*	*	0.0	0.0	0.1	0.4	1.0	2.1
1902-------	1917	*	*	*	*	*	*	0.0	0.0	0.1	0.4	1.1	2.2
1903-------	1918	*	*	*	*	*	*	0.0	0.0	0.1	0.5	1.2	2.1
1904-------	1919	*	*	*	*	*	*	0.0	0.0	0.2	0.6	1.2	2.0
1905-------	1920	*	*	*	*	*	*	0.0	0.0	0.1	0.4	0.9	1.7
1906-------	1921	*	*	*	*	*	*	0.0	0.0	0.2	0.5	1.0	1.7
1907-------	1922	*	*	*	*	*	*	0.0	0.1	0.2	0.5	0.9	1.6
1908-------	1923	*	*	*	*	*	*	0.0	0.0	0.1	0.3	0.7	1.3
1909-------	1924	*	*	*	*	*	*	0.0	0.0	0.1	0.3	0.7	1.3
1910-------	1925	*	*	*	*	*	*	0.0	0.0	0.1	0.3	0.7	1.3
1911-------	1926	*	*	*	*	*	*	0.0	0.1	0.2	0.4	0.8	1.4
1912-------	1927	*	*	*	*	*	*	0.0	0.0	0.1	0.3	0.7	1.3
1913-------	1928	*	*	*	*	*	*	0.0	0.0	0.1	0.3	0.7	1.2
1914-------	1929	*	*	*	*	*	*	0.0	0.0	0.1	0.3	0.6	1.1
1915-------	1930	*	*	*	*	*	*	0.0	0.0	0.1	0.3	0.6	1.2
1916-------	1931	*	*	*	*	*	*	0.0	0.0	0.1	0.3	0.7	1.3
1917-------	1932	*	*	*	*	*	*	0.0	0.0	0.1	0.4	0.8	1.4
1918-------	1933	*	*	*	*	*	*	0.0	0.0	0.1	0.3	0.7	1.3
1919-------	1934	*	*	*	*	*	*	0.0	0.0	0.1	0.3	0.7	1.3
1920-------	1935	*	*	*	*	*	*	0.0	0.0	0.1	0.3	0.7	1.4
1921-------	1936	*	*	*	*	*	*	0.0	0.0	0.1	0.3	0.7	1.3
1922-------	1937	*	*	*	*	*	*	0.0	0.0	0.1	0.3	0.7	1.4
1923-------	1938	*	*	*	*	*	*	0.0	0.0	0.1	0.3	0.7	1.3
1924-------	1939	*	*	*	*	*	*	0.0	0.0	0.1	0.3	0.7	1.5
1925-------	1940	*	*	*	*	*	*	0.0	0.1	0.2	0.4	0.9	1.6
1926-------	1941	*	*	*	*	*	*	0.0	0.1	0.2	0.5	0.9	1.6
1927-------	1942	*	*	*	*	*	*	0.0	0.1	0.2	0.4	0.8	1.6
1928-------	1943	*	*	*	*	*	*	0.0	0.1	0.2	0.4	0.9	1.8
1929-------	1944	*	*	*	*	*	*	0.1	0.2	0.3	0.6	1.1	2.0
1930-------	1945	*	*	*	*	*	*	0.1	0.2	0.4	0.7	1.3	2.4
1931-------	1946	*	*	*	*	*	*	0.1	0.2	0.4	0.7	1.3	2.5
1932-------	1947	*	*	*	*	*	*	0.1	0.2	0.4	0.8	1.5	2.9
1933-------	1948	*	*	*	*	*	*	0.0	0.1	0.3	0.7	1.5	3.1
1934-------	1949	*	*	*	*	*	*	0.1	0.2	0.4	0.9	1.8	3.4
1935-------	1950	*	*	*	*	*	*	0.1	0.2	0.4	0.8	1.7	3.4
1936-------	1951	*	*	*	*	*	*	0.1	0.2	0.4	0.9	1.8	3.5
1937-------	1952	*	*	*	*	*	*	0.1	0.2	0.4	0.9	1.9	3.6
1938-------	1953	*	*	*	*	*	*	0.1	0.2	0.4	0.9	1.9	3.6
1939-------	1954	*	*	*	*	*	*	0.0	0.1	0.3	0.8	1.8	3.4
1940-------	1955	*	*	*	*	*	*	0.1	0.2	0.4	0.9	1.8	3.0
1941-------	1956	*	*	*	*	*	*	0.0	0.1	0.3	0.8	1.5	2.5
1942-------	1957	*	*	*	*	*	*	0.1	0.2	0.4	0.7	1.2	2.0
1943-------	1958	*	*	*	*	*	*	0.1	0.2	0.4	0.7	1.1	1.7
1944-------	1959	*	*	*	*	*	*	0.1	0.2	0.3	0.5	0.8	1.3
1945-------	1960	*	*	*	*	*	*	0.1	0.1	0.2	0.4	0.7	1.2
1946-------	1961	*	*	*	*	*	*	0.0	0.0	0.1	0.3	0.6	1.0
1947-------	1962	*	*	*	*	*	*	0.0	0.0	0.1	0.3	0.5	0.7
1948-------	1963	*	*	*	*	*	*	0.0	0.1	0.2	0.3	0.4	0.6
1949-------	1964	*	*	*	*	*	*	0.1	0.2	0.3	0.4	0.5	
1950-------	1965	*	*	*	*	*	*	0.1	0.2	0.2	0.2		
1951-------	1966	*	*	*	*	*	*	0.0	0.0	0.0			
1952-------	1967	*	*	*	*	*	*	0.0	0.0				
1953-------	1968	*	*	*	*	*	*	0.0					
1954-------	1969	*	*	*	*	*	*						
1955-------	1970	*	*	*	*	*							
1956-------	1971	*	*	*	*								
1957-------	1972	*	*	*									
1958-------	1973	*	*										
1959-------	1974	*											

TABLE 6A. CUMULATIVE BIRTH RATES FOR ALL WOMEN AS OF THE BEGINNING OF EACH YEAR 1917-74 BY AGE AND LIVE-BIRTH ORDER FOR EACH COHORT FROM 1867 TO 1959--CON.

LIVE-BIRTH ORDER AND COHORT	DIAGONAL LINE FOR JANUARY 1	EXACT AGE											
		27	28	29	30	31	32	33	34	35	36	37	38
EIGHTH AND HIGHER BIRTHS--CON.													
1879-------													215.2
1880-------												172.6	203.2
1881-------											135.6	163.0	192.8
1882-------										103.4	127.9	154.5	184.5
1883-------									76.4	96.9	120.8	147.5	177.2
1884-------								55.7	72.0	92.1	115.9	142.4	172.3
1885-------							39.7	52.3	68.4	88.3	111.9	138.6	166.2
1886-------						27.0	37.2	49.7	65.6	85.4	109.6	134.4	161.9
1887-------					17.8	25.3	35.5	47.9	63.7	84.3	106.9	131.7	159.0
1888-------				10.9	17.0	24.3	34.4	46.7	63.5	82.7	105.3	129.9	156.3
1889-------			6.5	10.3	16.0	23.2	33.2	46.3	61.9	81.2	103.6	127.6	152.9
1890-------	1917	3.7	6.2	9.6	15.2	22.4	33.0	45.2	61.1	80.2	102.0	124.5	149.2
1891-------	1918	3.5	5.7	9.0	14.7	22.4	32.3	44.7	60.4	79.3	99.9	122.3	144.6
1892-------	1919	3.2	5.4	8.8	14.9	22.1	32.1	44.3	59.8	77.4	97.5	117.2	137.5
1893-------	1920	2.8	5.0	8.7	14.4	21.7	31.6	43.7	58.2	75.3	93.2	111.5	131.0
1894-------	1921	3.0	5.5	9.0	14.9	22.2	32.0	43.4	57.5	72.9	89.6	107.2	125.5
1895-------	1922	3.2	5.5	9.2	15.1	22.4	31.8	43.0	56.0	70.5	86.8	103.3	121.0
1896-------	1923	3.3	5.8	9.6	15.6	22.7	32.0	42.4	54.6	68.8	83.8	99.6	115.6
1897-------	1924	3.4	5.9	9.7	15.5	22.6	31.3	41.1	52.9	65.9	80.5	94.9	110.8
1898-------	1925	3.6	6.3	10.2	15.9	22.5	30.7	40.3	51.5	64.2	77.5	91.9	107.1
1899-------	1926	3.7	6.4	10.1	15.6	21.9	30.0	39.2	50.5	62.5	76.3	90.6	105.2
1900-------	1927	3.9	6.4	9.9	15.1	21.3	29.0	38.1	48.5	60.8	74.4	88.0	102.5
1901-------	1928	3.7	6.0	9.3	14.1	19.9	27.4	35.6	46.1	57.9	70.3	83.5	97.1
1902-------	1929	3.6	5.8	8.9	13.5	18.9	25.4	33.5	43.2	53.8	65.7	78.0	90.4
1903-------	1930	3.4	5.4	8.3	12.5	17.3	23.9	31.5	40.6	50.8	62.1	73.2	85.0
1904-------	1931	3.3	5.2	7.9	11.8	16.8	23.2	30.6	39.5	49.3	59.7	70.5	81.8
1905-------	1932	2.9	4.7	7.2	11.3	16.2	22.3	29.4	38.0	47.1	57.3	67.5	78.1
1906-------	1933	2.8	4.4	7.0	11.0	15.6	21.5	28.3	36.3	45.4	55.0	64.6	75.3
1907-------	1934	2.6	4.3	6.9	10.5	14.9	20.6	27.0	35.1	43.7	52.7	62.4	72.9
1908-------	1935	2.3	4.0	6.3	9.8	14.1	19.4	25.9	33.6	41.8	51.0	60.5	70.7
1909-------	1936	2.3	3.9	6.2	9.6	13.6	19.0	25.2	32.5	40.8	49.9	59.5	69.1
1910-------	1937	2.3	3.9	6.2	9.5	13.6	18.7	24.7	32.2	40.5	49.6	58.7	68.0
1911-------	1938	2.4	3.9	6.2	9.6	13.6	18.6	24.7	32.2	40.6	49.4	58.3	67.4
1912-------	1939	2.2	3.7	6.1	9.4	13.4	18.6	24.8	32.1	39.9	48.3	56.7	65.7
1913-------	1940	2.1	3.7	6.1	9.3	13.4	18.6	24.6	31.5	39.1	47.1	55.5	64.1
1914-------	1941	2.1	3.7	5.9	9.2	13.3	18.3	24.1	30.9	38.2	46.3	54.5	63.1
1915-------	1942	2.2	3.7	6.0	9.3	13.2	18.2	23.9	30.6	38.0	45.8	54.0	62.5
1916-------	1943	2.2	3.8	6.1	9.3	13.3	18.2	23.8	30.6	37.8	45.6	53.6	61.6
1917-------	1944	2.4	4.0	6.2	9.5	13.3	18.2	24.0	30.6	37.8	45.4	53.2	61.3
1918-------	1945	2.3	3.8	6.1	9.3	13.2	18.3	24.1	30.8	38.0	45.6	53.5	61.6
1919-------	1946	2.3	3.9	6.2	9.6	13.9	19.1	25.0	32.0	39.5	47.5	55.7	64.3
1920-------	1947	2.4	4.1	6.6	10.2	14.5	19.8	25.9	32.9	40.6	48.7	57.1	65.8
1921-------	1948	2.4	4.2	6.9	10.5	14.9	20.3	26.4	33.7	41.5	49.9	58.5	67.0
1922-------	1949	2.5	4.3	6.9	10.5	14.8	20.0	26.3	33.6	41.5	50.0	58.5	67.3
1923-------	1950	2.5	4.3	6.9	10.5	14.8	20.5	27.0	34.6	43.0	51.6	60.6	69.6
1924-------	1951	2.7	4.5	7.2	10.9	15.7	21.7	28.6	36.8	45.4	54.6	63.9	73.2
1925-------	1952	2.8	4.8	7.6	11.7	16.8	23.2	30.6	39.0	48.3	58.0	67.8	77.2
1926-------	1953	2.9	5.0	8.1	12.5	18.1	25.0	32.8	41.9	51.5	61.6	71.4	80.8
1927-------	1954	2.9	5.1	8.4	13.2	19.2	26.5	35.0	44.5	54.7	65.0	74.8	84.2
1928-------	1955	3.2	5.7	9.5	14.8	21.3	29.2	38.1	48.1	58.4	68.5	78.3	87.1
1929-------	1956	3.7	6.5	10.7	16.5	23.6	32.1	41.7	52.1	62.5	72.6	81.8	89.6
1930-------	1957	4.3	7.4	12.0	18.2	25.7	34.6	44.4	54.8	65.0	74.5	82.6	89.6
1931-------	1958	4.7	8.2	13.2	19.7	27.7	36.8	46.6	56.8	66.3	74.7	82.0	88.2
1932-------	1959	5.3	9.0	14.0	20.9	28.9	38.0	47.5	56.7	65.0	72.4	78.9	84.7
1933-------	1960	5.7	9.6	15.2	22.2	30.2	39.1	47.6	55.6	62.9	69.4	75.4	80.8
1934-------	1961	6.1	10.3	16.0	23.0	30.8	38.5	45.9	52.8	59.1	65.1	70.6	75.4
1935-------	1962	6.2	10.4	15.9	22.6	29.3	36.0	42.2	48.1	53.8	59.3	64.2	68.1
1936-------	1963	6.3	10.4	15.6	21.3	26.9	32.4	37.7	43.0	48.1	52.9	56.7	59.9
1937-------	1964	6.3	10.0	14.4	19.0	23.7	28.4	33.1	37.8	42.3	45.9	49.0	
1938-------	1965	6.1	9.3	12.7	16.5	20.3	24.3	28.4	32.4	35.7	38.5		
1939-------	1966	5.5	8.0	10.9	14.0	17.3	20.9	24.4	27.4	30.0			
1940-------	1967	4.6	6.6	8.9	11.6	14.5	17.4	20.0	22.4				
1941-------	1968	3.8	5.5	7.5	9.8	12.1	14.3	16.3					
1942-------	1969	3.1	4.4	6.0	7.8	9.4	11.1						
1943-------	1970	2.5	3.7	4.9	6.1	7.3							
1944-------	1971	2.1	3.0	3.9	4.9								
1945-------	1972	1.8	2.4	3.1									
1946-------	1973	1.4	1.8										
1947-------	1974	1.0											

TABLE 6A. CUMULATIVE BIRTH RATES FOR ALL WOMEN AS OF THE BEGINNING OF EACH YEAR 1917-74 BY AGE AND LIVE-BIRTH ORDER FOR EACH COHORT FROM 1867 TO 1959--CON.

LIVE-BIRTH ORDER AND COHORT	DIAGONAL LINE FOR JANUARY 1	EXACT AGE											
		39	40	41	42	43	44	45	46	47	48	49	50
EIGHTH AND HIGHER BIRTHS--CON.													
1867-------													551.0
1868-------												536.1	536.8
1869-------											519.1	520.6	521.6
1870-------										500.0	502.8	504.7	505.4
1871-------									478.7	483.6	487.0	488.5	489.3
1872-------								455.2	462.7	468.6	471.3	472.9	473.6
1873-------							429.8	440.7	448.9	453.7	456.6	458.1	458.8
1874-------						401.2	416.1	427.4	434.6	439.7	442.5	443.8	444.4
1875-------					370.3	387.8	402.4	412.7	420.2	425.1	427.5	428.8	429.4
1876-------				337.2	359.7	377.0	391.1	401.7	409.0	413.4	415.8	417.0	417.6
1877-------			301.0	326.6	348.9	365.6	379.8	390.4	397.1	401.4	403.7	404.9	405.4
1878-------	1917	260.4	291.8	317.2	338.8	355.7	370.2	380.1	386.7	390.9	393.0	394.0	394.5
1879-------	1918	246.1	277.2	302.2	324.2	341.4	354.9	364.6	371.2	375.3	377.3	378.3	378.8
1880-------	1919	233.5	264.4	289.7	311.9	327.9	341.3	351.0	357.3	361.2	363.0	364.0	364.5
1881-------	1920	223.3	254.3	279.8	300.4	316.2	329.7	339.1	345.1	348.6	350.4	351.3	351.7
1882-------	1921	214.8	246.0	269.5	289.7	305.6	318.6	327.4	333.0	336.4	338.2	339.1	339.5
1883-------	1922	207.7	236.4	259.5	279.7	295.1	307.3	315.8	321.1	324.2	325.8	326.6	327.0
1884-------	1923	200.4	228.7	251.7	271.1	285.6	297.3	305.0	309.8	312.8	314.3	315.1	315.5
1885-------	1924	194.1	222.1	244.3	262.6	276.7	287.4	294.4	299.1	301.9	303.3	304.1	304.5
1886-------	1925	189.5	216.3	236.9	254.6	267.4	277.1	284.0	288.4	291.1	292.4	293.2	293.6
1887-------	1926	185.9	211.4	231.9	248.3	260.1	269.8	276.3	280.5	283.0	284.3	285.0	285.4
1888-------	1927	181.7	206.3	225.0	240.0	251.6	260.6	266.8	270.7	273.0	274.2	274.9	275.2
1889-------	1928	178.0	200.8	218.2	232.9	243.8	252.5	258.4	262.2	264.5	265.6	266.2	266.5
1890-------	1929	171.8	192.8	209.6	223.4	233.9	242.1	247.9	251.5	253.6	254.7	255.3	255.6
1891-------	1930	165.6	186.0	201.9	215.0	224.9	233.1	238.5	241.8	243.8	244.8	245.4	245.6
1892-------	1931	157.6	176.4	191.3	203.4	213.2	220.8	225.7	228.8	230.6	231.5	232.0	232.2
1893-------	1932	149.7	167.7	181.6	193.6	202.6	209.5	214.0	216.9	218.6	219.4	219.8	220.0
1894-------	1933	143.5	160.0	173.7	185.0	193.2	199.6	204.0	206.6	208.1	208.9	209.2	209.4
1895-------	1934	137.6	153.9	166.8	177.1	184.9	191.0	194.9	197.4	198.8	199.5	199.8	199.9
1896-------	1935	131.9	147.4	159.2	169.0	176.5	182.0	185.7	188.0	189.3	189.9	190.2	190.4
1897-------	1936	126.2	140.3	151.6	161.1	167.8	173.1	176.5	178.8	180.0	180.6	180.9	181.0
1898-------	1937	121.4	135.0	146.2	154.9	161.6	166.6	170.3	172.7	173.9	174.6	174.9	175.1
1899-------	1938	119.5	133.1	143.3	151.8	158.1	163.1	166.6	168.7	169.9	170.5	170.8	171.0
1900-------	1939	116.4	128.8	138.8	147.0	153.1	158.1	161.5	163.6	164.7	165.3	165.6	165.7
1901-------	1940	109.6	121.4	130.8	138.2	144.3	149.2	152.5	154.4	155.5	156.0	156.3	156.4
1902-------	1941	102.4	113.6	122.5	130.2	136.3	141.1	144.1	145.9	146.9	147.4	147.6	147.7
1903-------	1942	96.3	106.9	115.9	123.4	129.4	133.8	136.7	138.3	139.2	139.6	139.8	139.9
1904-------	1943	92.7	103.3	112.1	119.5	125.1	129.4	132.0	133.5	134.3	134.7	134.9	135.0
1905-------	1944	89.0	99.4	107.9	114.8	120.1	123.9	126.4	127.8	128.5	128.9	129.1	129.2
1906-------	1945	86.0	96.0	104.0	110.6	115.4	119.1	121.3	122.6	123.3	123.6	123.8	123.9
1907-------	1946	83.2	92.6	100.2	106.2	110.9	114.3	116.5	117.8	118.4	118.7	118.8	118.9
1908-------	1947	80.3	89.1	96.1	102.0	106.3	109.7	111.8	113.0	113.7	114.0	114.1	114.2
1909-------	1948	78.3	86.8	93.9	99.5	103.9	107.2	109.2	110.4	111.0	111.3	111.5	111.6
1910-------	1949	76.9	85.5	92.3	97.9	102.1	105.2	107.2	108.3	108.9	109.2	109.4	109.5
1911-------	1950	76.4	84.6	91.3	96.7	100.8	104.0	105.9	107.1	107.7	108.0	108.1	108.2
1912-------	1951	74.3	82.3	88.7	94.0	98.1	101.1	103.1	104.2	104.8	105.1	105.2	105.3
1913-------	1952	72.5	80.3	86.6	91.7	95.6	98.7	100.6	101.7	102.2	102.5	102.6	102.7
1914-------	1953	71.5	79.0	85.2	90.2	94.2	97.2	99.1	100.1	100.7	101.0	101.1	101.2
1915-------	1954	70.4	77.8	83.9	89.0	92.9	95.7	97.5	98.5	99.0	99.2	99.3	99.3
1916-------	1955	69.6	76.9	83.0	88.0	91.8	94.5	96.3	97.3	97.8	98.0	98.1	98.1
1917-------	1956	69.2	76.6	82.8	87.7	91.4	94.2	96.0	97.0	97.5	97.7	97.8	97.8
1918-------	1957	69.6	77.1	83.1	88.1	91.9	94.7	96.4	97.3	97.8	98.0	98.1	98.1
1919-------	1958	72.7	80.1	86.5	91.6	95.5	98.4	100.2	101.1	101.6	101.8	101.9	101.9
1920-------	1959	74.0	81.8	88.2	93.4	97.3	100.1	101.8	102.7	103.2	103.4	103.5	103.5
1921-------	1960	75.5	83.2	89.7	94.9	98.8	101.6	103.2	104.1	104.5	104.7	104.8	104.8
1922-------	1961	75.7	83.4	89.7	94.7	98.5	100.9	102.4	103.2	103.5	103.7	103.7	103.7
1923-------	1962	78.2	86.0	92.2	97.2	100.6	102.9	104.3	105.0	105.3	105.4	105.4	105.4
1924-------	1963	81.8	89.6	96.0	100.6	103.8	106.0	107.2	107.9	108.2	108.3	108.3	108.3
1925-------	1964	86.0	93.8	99.7	104.0	107.0	108.9	110.0	110.6	110.9	111.0	111.0	
1926-------	1965	89.7	97.0	102.4	106.3	109.0	110.8	111.8	112.3	112.5	112.6		
1927-------	1966	92.4	99.0	103.8	107.3	109.8	111.4	112.3	112.8	113.0			
1928-------	1967	94.3	100.1	104.4	107.6	109.9	111.4	112.2	112.6				
1929-------	1968	96.2	101.5	105.6	108.7	110.8	112.1	112.9					
1930-------	1969	95.4	100.3	104.1	106.8	108.6	109.8						
1931-------	1970	93.7	98.3	101.7	104.0	105.7							
1932-------	1971	89.8	93.9	96.8	98.9								
1933-------	1972	85.3	88.7	91.2									
1934-------	1973	79.2	82.1										
1935-------	1974	71.3											

TABLE 6B. CUMULATIVE BIRTH RATES FOR WHITE WOMEN AS OF THE BEGINNING OF EACH YEAR 1917-74 BY AGE AND LIVE-BIRTH ORDER FOR EACH COHORT FROM 1867 TO 1959

LIVE-BIRTH ORDER AND COHORT	DIAGONAL LINE FOR JANUARY 1	EXACT AGE											
		15	16	17	18	19	20	21	22	23	24	25	26
TOTAL BIRTHS													
1891-------													1,249.9
1892-------												1,076.2	1,258.3
1893-------											901.8	1,085.3	1,265.5
1894-------										722.7	907.8	1,089.6	1,252.5
1895-------									554.4	728.8	912.2	1;074.8	1,250.2
1896-------								397.2	561.9	735.6	896.6	1,073.8	1,252.8
1897-------							261.1	404.9	569.5	719.8	897.6	1,078.2	1,247.9
1898-------						153.5	268.5	412.3	552.9	722.9	904.4	1,076.5	1,248.6
1899-------					76.8	154.7	268.4	390.5	550.9	722.0	891.8	1,064.2	1,234.7
1900-------				31.0	77.2	153.3	250.1	392.4	553.6	712.9	884.0	1,057.4	1,220.4
1901-------			9.7	31.0	75.7	141.3	256.8	402.8	552.0	711.4	884.8	1,051.8	1,208.7
1902-------	1917	2.0	9.8	30.8	69.6	151.5	274.9	412.7	563.6	728.3	895.2	1,056.4	1,210.8
1903-------	1918	2.0	9.9	28.0	77.3	167.3	282.8	421.1	575.0	734.8	897.8	1,056.7	1,204.7
1904-------	1919	2.1	8.5	31.5	84.9	168.1	282.7	423.0	571.2	727.4	886.1	1,037.8	1,180.0
1905-------	1920	1.6	9.8	34.4	82.8	165.4	282.3	416.3	560.2	711.8	862.3	1,007.0	1,148.9
1906-------	1921	2.0	10.8	32.8	80.6	166.3	278.3	408.3	549.7	693.5	837.5	981.6	1,115.6
1907-------	1922	2.2	10.1	31.7	81.8	164.6	274.0	402.7	537.6	676.1	820.1	956.9	1,085.7
1908-------	1923	2.0	9.8	32.8	81.9	162.9	271.2	393.8	523.5	662.0	797.5	928.0	1,048.3
1909-------	1924	2.0	10.3	33.3	81.5	161.5	264.9	382.0	512.4	643.6	773.7	896.1	1,020.6
1910-------	1925	2.1	10.4	32.7	81.1	157.3	255.5	373.7	496.7	622.2	744.0	870.3	991.8
1911-------	1926	2.1	10.2	33.6	79.8	152.9	253.3	365.4	483.8	602.5	729.4	854.8	977.3
1912-------	1927	2.1	11.0	32.9	78.1	153.1	247.3	355.0	466.5	589.7	715.7	841.3	966.0
1913-------	1928	2.4	10.5	32.4	78.9	148.7	239.2	340.0	456.8	580.2	706.3	835.4	965.4
1914-------	1929	2.1	10.4	32.9	75.5	142.3	226.3	332.3	449.4	573.3	703.4	837.6	965.5
1915-------	1930	2.2	10.8	31.6	72.3	134.1	222.5	329.2	446.5	574.1	709.1	840.7	974.1
1916-------	1931	2.3	10.2	29.7	67.1	131.7	220.5	326.9	446.6	577.9	708.9	844.7	986.5
1917-------	1932	2.0	9.3	27.2	66.4	131.3	218.9	326.9	450.1	577.0	711.2	855.9	1,017.5
1918-------	1933	1.8	8.5	27.4	66.9	130.8	220.3	331.2	449.4	579.7	722.7	890.6	1,055.4
1919-------	1934	1.8	9.0	28.4	67.3	133.8	227.0	335.1	459.6	601.5	771.8	940.8	1,091.1
1920-------	1935	1.9	9.4	28.5	69.6	138.4	228.4	341.1	475.2	638.3	807.0	960.6	1,100.2
1921-------	1936	2.1	9.5	29.9	72.8	139.4	233.2	354.4	503.9	663.2	816.5	958.0	1,140.6
1922-------	1937	1.9	9.5	30.1	70.3	137.1	234.9	367.2	513.3	659.4	798.1	985.4	1,186.1
1923-------	1938	2.0	9.5	28.8	69.2	139.0	247.1	377.7	512.1	644.8	831.6	1,040.4	1,226.8
1924-------	1939	2.0	9.3	28.9	71.5	148.6	256.3	374.9	497.3	677.9	889.6	1,084.4	1,272.2
1925-------	1940	1.9	9.3	30.3	75.3	152.4	247.7	356.9	521.8	730.1	927.7	1,123.4	1,310.1
1926-------	1941	1.9	9.9	31.4	76.6	143.6	231.4	373.4	569.3	764.0	962.0	1,155.8	1,353.7
1927-------	1942	2.1	10.3	32.1	71.5	133.7	243.7	419.7	604.6	799.2	993.9	1,199.2	1,401.8
1928-------	1943	2.1	10.4	29.2	65.6	140.3	283.1	451.5	635.8	827.0	1,034.9	1,245.2	1,449.8
1929-------	1944	2.1	9.3	26.9	69.1	170.8	310.7	479.3	660.7	867.7	1,082.4	1,298.0	1,509.8
1930-------	1945	1.9	8.7	28.0	88.1	190.8	330.8	496.1	693.8	907.3	1,127.2	1,351.3	1,567.0
1931-------	1946	1.9	9.1	37.9	101.0	204.7	342.6	524.7	729.3	950.0	1,181.6	1,411.8	1,636.3
1932-------	1947	1.9	12.5	43.5	106.9	208.5	359.5	545.6	757.0	988.8	1,226.6	1,466.4	1,697.5
1933-------	1948	2.8	14.8	46.6	109.5	221.1	374.6	568.0	789.5	1,027.6	1,275.7	1,522.4	1,752.0
1934-------	1949	3.2	15.5	47.1	115.2	226.6	386.2	587.2	814.2	1,063.1	1,318.3	1,563.3	1,794.0
1935-------	1950	3.0	15.3	48.8	116.0	231.1	394.4	598.3	835.4	1,090.5	1,343.3	1,588.2	1,818.5
1936-------	1951	3.1	15.8	48.8	118.5	236.4	401.2	615.2	858.2	1,110.3	1,362.5	1,607.3	1,834.5
1937-------	1952	3.2	15.7	49.8	120.7	238.8	412.6	631.8	872.3	1,125.2	1,379.1	1,621.4	1,840.1
1938-------	1953	3.1	15.9	50.9	121.7	246.6	425.1	642.7	886.1	1,140.1	1,390.4	1,622.9	1,833.0
1939-------	1954	3.2	16.8	52.0	127.5	257.1	434.7	656.3	899.1	1,149.7	1,390.6	1,614.2	1,816.0
1940-------	1955	3.5	17.1	54.6	132.7	260.3	439.5	657.3	895.7	1,137.2	1,367.8	1,581.2	1,762.9
1941-------	1956	3.5	18.1	56.9	132.7	258.4	431.9	644.5	873.7	1,103.2	1,321.9	1,513.4	1,683.1
1942-------	1957	3.6	18.4	55.3	128.6	249.8	418.3	621.3	838.4	1,054.7	1,250.0	1,430.1	1,594.5
1943-------	1958	3.6	17.6	52.9	123.1	240.6	401.6	594.6	798.2	990.3	1,174.2	1,348.1	1,510.7
1944-------	1959	3.5	17.2	51.6	120.6	233.2	387.7	569.6	750.8	932.1	1,108.9	1,278.5	1,442.6
1945-------	1960	3.6	17.2	51.3	117.6	226.2	371.5	533.9	704.8	876.8	1,046.1	1,214.8	1,378.6
1946-------	1961	3.6	17.0	49.2	112.6	214.9	346.7	501.1	663.2	828.6	998.8	1,168.9	1,320.7
1947-------	1962	3.2	15.3	45.8	105.3	199.2	324.7	470.0	625.3	790.0	959.9	1,116.0	1,249.3
1948-------	1963	3.0	14.5	43.3	98.9	188.9	307.6	447.7	601.8	765.4	920.1	1,055.7	1,180.8
1949-------	1964	2.9	13.9	41.1	94.4	179.5	293.6	430.9	583.1	731.2	863.9	989.4	
1950-------	1965	2.8	13.3	39.7	91.1	174.1	286.9	423.9	561.3	687.3	809.8		
1951-------	1966	2.7	13.2	39.0	89.7	172.5	286.5	410.2	527.4	643.5			
1952-------	1967	2.8	12.9	38.6	89.8	175.0	278.9	386.1	494.0				
1953-------	1968	2.7	13.2	39.7	94.0	173.5	266.7	365.8					
1954-------	1969	2.9	14.0	43.0	94.8	169.2	256.3						
1955-------	1970	3.2	15.8	44.4	95.6	166.5							
1956-------	1971	3.6	16.0	45.5	95.5								
1957-------	1972	3.7	16.9	46.4									
1958-------	1973	4.1	17.7										
1959-------	1974	4.3											

TABLE 6B. CUMULATIVE BIRTH RATES FOR WHITE WOMEN AS OF THE BEGINNING OF EACH YEAR 1917-74 BY AGE AND LIVE-BIRTH ORDER FOR EACH COHORT FROM 1867 TO 1959--CON.

LIVE-BIRTH ORDER AND COHORT	DIAGONAL LINE FOR JANUARY 1	EXACT AGE											
		27	28	29	30	31	32	33	34	35	36	37	38
TOTAL BIRTHS--CON.													
1879-------													3,059.9
1880-------												2,934.0	3,028.6
1881-------											2,802.5	2,902.6	2,996.0
1882-------										2,665.6	2,774.5	2,873.0	2,964.3
1883-------									2,526.4	2,641.2	2,748.6	2,845.3	2,936.1
1884-------								2,386.2	2,509.4	2,623.0	2,727.4	2,823.7	2,915.4
1885-------							2,241.4	2,366.8	2,489.2	2,598.8	2,703.3	2,801.0	2,886.3
1886-------						2,089.5	2,226.9	2,352.6	2,470.2	2,580.7	2,687.6	2,779.1	2,864.0
1887-------					1,932.2	2,081.4	2,219.3	2,340.1	2,459.3	2,572.7	2,673.2	2,764.7	2,849.2
1888-------				1,766.9	1,937.2	2,085.6	2,217.4	2,339.6	2,461.2	2,567.7	2,667.9	2,758.4	2,839.0
1889-------			1,553.7	1,769.5	1,938.1	2,078.1	2,211.5	2,335.6	2,449.9	2,555.9	2,655.1	2,742.3	2,819.8
1890-------	1917	1,420.1	1,598.9	1,773.3	1,931.1	2,074.5	2,210.4	2,327.8	2,442.1	2,547.4	2,642.0	2,724.6	2,800.0
1891-------	1918	1,423.8	1,601.8	1,763.0	1,925.5	2,070.7	2,199.1	2,316.0	2,429.2	2,530.4	2,620.9	2,702.0	2,772.3
1892-------	1919	1,431.5	1,594.6	1,761.7	1,925.2	2,060.6	2,187.8	2,303.3	2,411.1	2,506.5	2,593.9	2,668.5	2,733.0
1893-------	1920	1,423.1	1,593.2	1,760.8	1,912.3	2,045.7	2,171.7	2,282.3	2,384.1	2,476.8	2,557.7	2,627.0	2,690.2
1894-------	1921	1,420.1	1,592.3	1,748.1	1,898.6	2,031.1	2,151.9	2,257.5	2,357.1	2,443.9	2,520.1	2,588.7	2,648.7
1895-------	1922	1,421.3	1,583.1	1,738.5	1,887.6	2,015.4	2,132.0	2,235.6	2,329.6	2,411.6	2,487.6	2,553.0	2,610.2
1896-------	1923	1,414.6	1,576.2	1,729.0	1,871.9	1,995.4	2,109.0	2,206.5	2,295.1	2,376.4	2,447.5	2,509.5	2,562.3
1897-------	1924	1,409.3	1,568.9	1,715.4	1,853.0	1,972.6	2,079.9	2,172.4	2,260.2	2,336.2	2,404.5	2,462.2	2,514.6
1898-------	1925	1,409.9	1,562.8	1,703.6	1,836.7	1,950.2	2,052.8	2,145.2	2,227.8	2,300.8	2,364.4	2,421.9	2,472.4
1899-------	1926	1,391.2	1,539.5	1,677.7	1,805.5	1,915.2	2,018.4	2,107.2	2,189.1	2,259.0	2,324.1	2,380.7	2,429.6
1900-------	1927	1,369.9	1,514.7	1,645.4	1,766.9	1,876.4	1,974.5	2,060.5	2,137.0	2,207.9	2,271.3	2,325.6	2,373.3
1901-------	1928	1,356.8	1,493.8	1,618.2	1,738.8	1,843.2	1,937.5	2,017.5	2,094.9	2,163.2	2,223.6	2,276.2	2,323.2
1902-------	1929	1,350.8	1,481.3	1,605.3	1,719.7	1,818.5	1,905.8	1,986.2	2,060.1	2,125.3	2,183.9	2,236.0	2,280.8
1903-------	1930	1,339.8	1,470.8	1,589.9	1,699.6	1,792.4	1,881.5	1,959.3	2,031.1	2,094.9	2,153.4	2,203.7	2,247.8
1904-------	1931	1,315.5	1,441.1	1,555.9	1,659.3	1,755.1	1,842.4	1,918.8	1,989.9	2,054.4	2,111.8	2,162.4	2,207.0
1905-------	1932	1,278.1	1,398.6	1,506.1	1,612.4	1,705.7	1,790.4	1,866.5	1,938.1	2,001.4	2,059.1	2,110.0	2,156.7
1906-------	1933	1,238.9	1,351.9	1,462.2	1,565.8	1,656.7	1,741.6	1,818.8	1,889.5	1,953.7	2,011.9	2,064.5	2,115.8
1907-------	1934	1,202.1	1,318.7	1,426.8	1,528.2	1,620.3	1,707.0	1,783.6	1,855.7	1,921.0	1,983.2	2,041.6	2,094.5
1908-------	1935	1,167.5	1,281.0	1,386.5	1,488.0	1,581.8	1,667.5	1,745.9	1,819.1	1,890.3	1,958.5	2,018.9	2,073.4
1909-------	1936	1,137.8	1,249.7	1,357.0	1,461.9	1,555.4	1,644.2	1,725.3	1,806.6	1,884.3	1,953.7	2,016.9	2,073.4
1910-------	1937	1,107.9	1,221.4	1,332.3	1,435.9	1,533.2	1,624.9	1,713.0	1,801.6	1,879.7	1,952.0	2,018.0	2,075.3
1911-------	1938	1,096.7	1,215.4	1,325.3	1,433.4	1,535.1	1,633.0	1,729.4	1,817.1	1,898.3	1,974.9	2,041.9	2,095.2
1912-------	1939	1,089.6	1,205.9	1,320.1	1,432.6	1,542.9	1,649.4	1,744.2	1,834.3	1,920.8	1,998.3	2,060.0	2,112.0
1913-------	1940	1,087.2	1,208.8	1,329.4	1,453.5	1,571.8	1,676.1	1,773.7	1,870.9	1,958.8	2,030.2	2,090.6	2,141.9
1914-------	1941	1,093.6	1,223.1	1,358.3	1,490.0	1,603.4	1,710.9	1,818.3	1,918.0	1,999.2	2,069.7	2,130.2	2,182.9
1915-------	1942	1,110.9	1,256.5	1,398.7	1,523.0	1,638.6	1,758.5	1,869.2	1,960.7	2,040.9	2,111.5	2,173.7	2,228.7
1916-------	1943	1,139.4	1,291.0	1,422.2	1,546.3	1,676.7	1,800.6	1,901.3	1,991.3	2,071.0	2,143.1	2,207.3	2,262.3
1917-------	1944	1,174.9	1,313.6	1,443.0	1,586.2	1,723.0	1,836.6	1,936.4	2,026.5	2,108.6	2,183.0	2,247.8	2,304.3
1918-------	1945	1,198.7	1,331.9	1,482.8	1,633.7	1,757.9	1,869.7	1,969.0	2,061.3	2,145.7	2,220.3	2,286.1	2,341.8
1919-------	1946	1,228.1	1,391.3	1,555.8	1,695.2	1,820.5	1,934.0	2,038.6	2,136.1	2,222.4	2,299.9	2,366.4	2,423.6
1920-------	1947	1,272.8	1,451.1	1,602.5	1,742.7	1,869.1	1,987.4	2,096.9	2,195.6	2,284.3	2,361.7	2,428.6	2,485.7
1921-------	1948	1,331.4	1,496.2	1,649.0	1,790.7	1,922.9	2,047.1	2,157.4	2,258.8	2,347.8	2,425.7	2,493.3	2,549.4
1922-------	1949	1,361.2	1,526.1	1,679.1	1,826.0	1,963.1	2,087.1	2,199.4	2,299.9	2,388.6	2,466.8	2,531.8	2,586.9
1923-------	1950	1,402.9	1,568.0	1,728.4	1,881.1	2,018.7	2,145.5	2,257.4	2,358.3	2,448.0	2,524.1	2,589.0	2,643.1
1924-------	1951	1,449.0	1,624.3	1,791.2	1,944.5	2,085.8	2,212.2	2,325.4	2,427.9	2,515.4	2,590.7	2,654.7	2,708.4
1925-------	1952	1,496.9	1,677.5	1,844.5	2,001.2	2,141.4	2,268.6	2,382.5	2,481.8	2,568.0	2,642.6	2,705.9	2,756.7
1926-------	1953	1,545.9	1,726.7	1,897.1	2,053.2	2,193.9	2,321.6	2,432.1	2,529.6	2,614.6	2,688.0	2,747.7	2,796.8
1927-------	1954	1,595.8	1,779.8	1,949.9	2,107.2	2,249.3	2,374.2	2,483.7	2,580.3	2,664.4	2,733.9	2,791.7	2,839.3
1928-------	1955	1,647.4	1,831.9	2,003.1	2,161.7	2,301.3	2,425.7	2,534.1	2,629.3	2,708.8	2,776.2	2,832.7	2,876.4
1929-------	1956	1,709.9	1,898.5	2,074.7	2,232.3	2,373.1	2,497.2	2,606.1	2,697.9	2,776.2	2,842.3	2,894.3	2,933.9
1930-------	1957	1,772.6	1,966.3	2,140.8	2,299.7	2,439.8	2,563.5	2,668.0	2,758.2	2,834.8	2,895.6	2,942.4	2,979.0
1931-------	1958	1,849.4	2,042.5	2,218.5	2,377.4	2,517.8	2,637.2	2,739.5	2,828.0	2,898.2	2,952.9	2,996.1	3,029.8
1932-------	1959	1,909.4	2,104.0	2,280.4	2,437.9	2,572.0	2,688.2	2,787.6	2,868.0	2,931.2	2,981.6	3,021.6	3,052.9
1933-------	1960	1,964.7	2,159.3	2,333.8	2,484.5	2,614.5	2,727.0	2,817.2	2,889.0	2,947.1	2,994.0	3,031.8	3,061.6
1934-------	1961	2,006.7	2,198.6	2,365.9	2,511.9	2,638.3	2,740.5	2,821.1	2,887.0	2,940.6	2,985.4	3,021.2	3,048.0
1935-------	1962	2,028.2	2,212.9	2,374.4	2,516.4	2,630.3	2,721.7	2,796.0	2,857.4	2,909.4	2,952.0	2,984.3	3,007.5
1936-------	1963	2,037.1	2,215.2	2,372.6	2,500.2	2,603.1	2,687.5	2,757.0	2,816.9	2,866.7	2,905.1	2,933.0	2,953.3
1937-------	1964	2,035.0	2,207.6	2,348.8	2,464.9	2,561.1	2,641.6	2,710.9	2,769.3	2,814.4	2,847.7	2,872.3	
1938-------	1965	2,020.6	2,175.7	2,304.3	2,413.3	2,505.5	2,586.5	2,654.8	2,707.9	2,747.3	2,777.0		
1939-------	1966	1,985.4	2,127.9	2,250.4	2,356.8	2,450.6	2,531.8	2,594.8	2,641.9	2,677.9			
1940-------	1967	1,919.3	2,055.9	2,176.9	2,286.0	2,381.5	2,456.4	2,512.2	2,555.5				
1941-------	1968	1,834.2	1,970.4	2,094.9	2,206.5	2,294.9	2,361.5	2,413.4					
1942-------	1969	1,745.6	1,886.3	2,013.6	2,117.0	2,195.8	2,258.2						
1943-------	1970	1,664.5	1,806.2	1,924.0	2,015.8	2,089.7							
1944-------	1971	1,597.0	1,728.5	1,832.9	1,919.5								
1945-------	1972	1,521.5	1,637.8	1,737.2									
1946-------	1973	1,447.5	1,558.8										
1947-------	1974	1,369.3											

TABLE 6B. CUMULATIVE BIRTH RATES FOR WHITE WOMEN AS OF THE BEGINNING OF EACH YEAR 1917-74 BY AGE AND LIVE-BIRTH ORDER FOR EACH COHORT FROM 1867 TO 1959--CON.

LIVE-BIRTH ORDER AND COHORT	DIAGONAL LINE FOR JANUARY 1	EXACT AGE											
		39	40	41	42	43	44	45	46	47	48	49	50
TOTAL BIRTHS--CON.													
1867-------													3,938.6
1868-------												3,893.7	3,894.4
1869-------											3,846.6	3,848.2	3,848.9
1870-------										3,796.9	3,800.3	3,801.9	3,802.5
1871-------									3,743.6	3,750.1	3,753.7	3,755.2	3,755.9
1872-------								3,685.6	3,696.5	3,703.2	3,706.3	3,708.0	3,708.6
1873-------							3,623.6	3,640.7	3,651.6	3,657.8	3,661.2	3,662.8	3,663.4
1874-------						3,554.5	3,579.9	3,596.7	3,607.0	3,613.7	3,616.8	3,618.3	3,618.8
1875-------					3,476.0	3,508.3	3,533.4	3,549.6	3,560.3	3,566.6	3,569.7	3,571.1	3,571.6
1876-------				3,386.4	3,430.7	3,462.6	3,487.0	3,503.7	3,514.2	3,519.9	3,522.7	3,524.1	3,524.5
1877-------			3,286.0	3,341.7	3,385.6	3,416.8	3,441.7	3,458.2	3,467.9	3,473.4	3,476.2	3,477.5	3,477.8
1878-------	1917	3,178.9	3,253.3	3,308.9	3,352.2	3,384.1	3,409.2	3,424.8	3,434.3	3,439.8	3,442.4	3,443.5	3,443.9
1879-------	1918	3,143.7	3,217.6	3,272.4	3,316.1	3,348.2	3,371.8	3,387.1	3,396.5	3,401.9	3,404.3	3,405.5	3,405.8
1880-------	1919	3,111.6	3,184.6	3,239.4	3,283.4	3,313.4	3,336.7	3,352.1	3,361.2	3,366.3	3,368.7	3,369.7	3,370.0
1881-------	1920	3,077.5	3,150.0	3,205.0	3,245.9	3,275.3	3,298.5	3,313.1	3,321.6	3,326.4	3,328.6	3,329.5	3,329.8
1882-------	1921	3,045.0	3,117.8	3,168.8	3,208.8	3,238.1	3,260.1	3,273.6	3,281.6	3,286.1	3,288.3	3,289.1	3,289.4
1883-------	1922	3,017.4	3,084.8	3,134.7	3,174.6	3,202.8	3,223.3	3,236.3	3,243.9	3,248.1	3,250.1	3,251.0	3,251.3
1884-------	1923	2,990.8	3,057.2	3,107.0	3,145.1	3,171.6	3,191.4	3,203.6	3,210.7	3,214.6	3,216.6	3,217.4	3,217.7
1885-------	1924	2,960.9	3,026.9	3,074.5	3,110.6	3,136.7	3,155.4	3,166.6	3,173.5	3,177.3	3,179.0	3,179.9	3,180.2
1886-------	1925	2,938.3	3,001.1	3,046.1	3,081.3	3,105.4	3,122.3	3,133.3	3,139.7	3,143.3	3,144.9	3,145.7	3,145.9
1887-------	1926	2,920.8	2,981.0	3,025.7	3,059.0	3,081.4	3,098.5	3,109.0	3,115.1	3,118.5	3,120.0	3,120.6	3,120.8
1888-------	1927	2,906.6	2,964.9	3,006.3	3,037.0	3,059.2	3,075.0	3,084.7	3,090.4	3,093.5	3,094.9	3,095.5	3,095.7
1889-------	1928	2,886.6	2,941.7	2,980.7	3,011.1	3,032.1	3,047.6	3,057.0	3,062.5	3,065.6	3,066.9	3,067.5	3,067.7
1890-------	1929	2,862.2	2,913.4	2,951.8	2,980.2	3,000.5	3,015.1	3,024.4	3,029.5	3,032.1	3,033.3	3,033.9	3,034.1
1891-------	1930	2,830.0	2,880.3	2,916.1	2,943.4	2,962.5	2,976.8	2,985.5	2,990.4	2,992.8	2,994.0	2,994.6	2,994.7
1892-------	1931	2,789.7	2,836.1	2,870.0	2,895.3	2,914.0	2,927.4	2,935.4	2,939.9	2,942.4	2,943.4	2,943.7	2,943.8
1893-------	1932	2,743.0	2,787.0	2,818.8	2,843.5	2,860.7	2,872.9	2,880.2	2,884.6	2,886.9	2,887.8	2,888.1	2,888.2
1894-------	1933	2,698.8	2,739.9	2,771.2	2,794.5	2,810.5	2,821.7	2,829.0	2,833.0	2,835.1	2,836.0	2,836.2	2,836.3
1895-------	1934	2,657.1	2,697.7	2,727.3	2,749.0	2,764.3	2,775.6	2,782.2	2,786.0	2,788.1	2,788.7	2,788.9	2,789.0
1896-------	1935	2,608.7	2,647.0	2,674.6	2,695.4	2,710.4	2,720.9	2,727.0	2,730.4	2,732.3	2,733.0	2,733.2	2,733.3
1897-------	1936	2,558.7	2,594.6	2,621.3	2,641.8	2,656.0	2,665.7	2,671.5	2,675.1	2,676.9	2,677.6	2,677.8	2,677.9
1898-------	1937	2,514.2	2,548.8	2,575.4	2,595.0	2,608.8	2,618.1	2,624.6	2,628.4	2,630.3	2,631.2	2,631.4	2,631.5
1899-------	1938	2,471.0	2,505.9	2,531.6	2,550.6	2,564.1	2,573.8	2,580.2	2,583.9	2,585.9	2,586.8	2,587.0	2,587.1
1900-------	1939	2,414.4	2,447.9	2,472.9	2,491.6	2,504.6	2,514.7	2,521.3	2,525.0	2,527.0	2,527.8	2,528.0	2,528.1
1901-------	1940	2,362.1	2,394.2	2,418.4	2,436.4	2,450.4	2,460.8	2,467.3	2,470.8	2,472.6	2,473.1	2,473.3	2,473.4
1902-------	1941	2,318.9	2,350.3	2,374.9	2,394.7	2,409.5	2,420.0	2,426.3	2,429.7	2,431.2	2,431.7	2,431.9	2,432.0
1903-------	1942	2,285.4	2,318.2	2,344.7	2,365.4	2,380.6	2,390.9	2,397.2	2,400.3	2,401.8	2,402.2	2,402.3	2,402.4
1904-------	1943	2,246.7	2,282.3	2,309.6	2,331.0	2,345.8	2,356.3	2,362.0	2,365.0	2,366.5	2,366.8	2,366.9	2,367.0
1905-------	1944	2,200.0	2,236.4	2,264.8	2,285.8	2,300.7	2,310.1	2,315.6	2,318.5	2,319.8	2,320.1	2,320.2	2,320.3
1906-------	1945	2,160.3	2,198.0	2,226.7	2,248.1	2,262.0	2,270.9	2,276.1	2,279.0	2,280.3	2,280.9	2,281.0	2,281.1
1907-------	1946	2,140.6	2,179.0	2,207.8	2,227.8	2,241.0	2,249.9	2,255.3	2,258.1	2,259.5	2,260.0	2,260.1	2,260.1
1908-------	1947	2,120.4	2,158.7	2,185.4	2,204.5	2,217.5	2,226.2	2,231.5	2,234.2	2,235.6	2,235.9	2,236.0	2,236.1
1909-------	1948	2,120.8	2,156.7	2,182.9	2,201.9	2,215.0	2,224.2	2,229.6	2,232.3	2,233.6	2,234.1	2,234.2	2,234.2
1910-------	1949	2,119.5	2,154.9	2,180.9	2,200.0	2,213.6	2,222.7	2,228.1	2,230.7	2,232.2	2,232.5	2,232.6	2,232.7
1911-------	1950	2,138.7	2,173.5	2,199.9	2,219.5	2,233.1	2,242.4	2,247.9	2,250.9	2,252.2	2,252.6	2,252.7	2,252.8
1912-------	1951	2,154.9	2,190.0	2,217.0	2,236.9	2,251.0	2,260.2	2,265.6	2,268.4	2,269.7	2,270.2	2,270.3	2,270.4
1913-------	1952	2,185.4	2,221.8	2,249.0	2,269.7	2,283.7	2,293.1	2,298.5	2,301.3	2,302.7	2,303.1	2,303.2	2,303.2
1914-------	1953	2,228.6	2,265.3	2,293.7	2,314.4	2,328.5	2,337.8	2,343.1	2,345.9	2,347.2	2,347.5	2,347.6	2,347.6
1915-------	1954	2,274.4	2,312.1	2,340.6	2,361.4	2,375.7	2,384.6	2,389.9	2,392.5	2,393.8	2,394.3	2,394.4	2,394.4
1916-------	1955	2,308.9	2,346.8	2,374.4	2,395.2	2,408.9	2,417.9	2,423.1	2,425.9	2,427.2	2,427.5	2,427.6	2,427.6
1917-------	1956	2,351.5	2,389.3	2,417.9	2,438.1	2,452.0	2,460.7	2,465.9	2,468.5	2,469.6	2,469.9	2,469.9	2,469.9
1918-------	1957	2,388.2	2,425.8	2,453.0	2,472.9	2,486.6	2,495.4	2,500.2	2,502.5	2,503.3	2,503.5	2,503.6	2,503.6
1919-------	1958	2,471.2	2,508.3	2,536.3	2,556.3	2,570.1	2,578.9	2,583.8	2,586.1	2,587.0	2,587.2	2,587.2	2,587.2
1920-------	1959	2,531.9	2,569.0	2,596.5	2,616.7	2,629.9	2,638.1	2,642.7	2,644.8	2,645.6	2,645.7	2,645.7	2,645.7
1921-------	1960	2,595.6	2,631.9	2,659.3	2,678.5	2,691.3	2,699.3	2,703.6	2,705.7	2,706.5	2,706.6	2,706.6	2,706.6
1922-------	1961	2,631.6	2,667.5	2,693.5	2,712.1	2,724.2	2,731.6	2,735.7	2,737.7	2,738.5	2,738.6	2,738.6	2,738.6
1923-------	1962	2,687.5	2,721.4	2,746.4	2,764.3	2,775.8	2,782.6	2,786.4	2,788.1	2,788.7	2,788.8	2,788.8	2,788.8
1924-------	1963	2,750.5	2,783.5	2,808.0	2,824.7	2,835.1	2,841.4	2,844.9	2,846.4	2,847.1	2,847.2	2,847.2	2,847.2
1925-------	1964	2,797.5	2,829.8	2,852.4	2,867.3	2,876.7	2,882.4	2,885.5	2,886.9	2,887.4	2,887.5	2,887.5	
1926-------	1965	2,836.6	2,866.3	2,886.7	2,900.2	2,908.7	2,913.9	2,916.6	2,917.8	2,918.2	2,918.3		
1927-------	1966	2,875.7	2,902.4	2,920.6	2,933.0	2,940.8	2,945.3	2,947.5	2,948.5	2,948.8			
1928-------	1967	2,909.2	2,933.2	2,950.1	2,961.4	2,968.7	2,972.7	2,974.5	2,975.4				
1929-------	1968	2,964.2	2,986.4	3,002.1	3,012.7	3,018.9	3,022.5	3,024.3					
1930-------	1969	3,006.6	3,027.2	3,041.9	3,050.8	3,056.3	3,059.4						
1931-------	1970	3,055.7	3,075.3	3,088.0	3,096.1	3,100.8							
1932-------	1971	3,077.4	3,094.4	3,105.5	3,112.3								
1933-------	1972	3,083.1	3,097.8	3,107.3									
1934-------	1973	3,067.0	3,079.9										
1935-------	1974	3,023.9											

TABLE 6B. CUMULATIVE BIRTH RATES FOR WHITE WOMEN AS OF THE BEGINNING OF EACH YEAR 1917-74 BY AGE AND LIVE-BIRTH ORDER FOR EACH COHORT FROM 1867 TO 1959--CON.

LIVE-BIRTH ORDER AND COHORT	DIAGONAL LINE FOR JANUARY 1	EXACT AGE											
		15	16	17	18	19	20	21	22	23	24	25	26
FIRST BIRTHS													
1891-------													587.5
1892-------												545.4	595.7
1893-------											492.6	552.3	603.4
1894-------										428.0	498.2	558.4	598.0
1895-------									356.1	433.2	503.6	549.6	601.7
1896-------								278.1	362.4	440.0	492.9	554.2	608.7
1897-------							199.3	284.0	369.0	427.5	498.9	562.7	611.9
1898-------						127.1	205.2	290.3	354.7	434.1	508.2	565.5	613.7
1899-------					67.8	128.0	205.1	271.4	357.6	438.7	503.7	559.1	608.0
1900-------				28.8	68.1	126.7	188.8	276.8	364.7	435.7	498.8	555.9	602.7
1901-------			9.4	28.8	66.8	116.1	198.2	290.1	367.2	436.3	502.3	557.4	602.8
1902-------	1917	2.0	9.4	28.5	60.9	126.4	214.7	296.6	372.1	444.8	508.4	561.8	607.0
1903-------	1918	2.0	9.5	25.8	68.7	140.5	219.1	299.1	377.6	447.8	509.7	562.9	607.2
1904-------	1919	2.1	8.2	29.4	75.7	139.3	215.7	299.3	374.8	443.0	503.9	555.7	598.6
1905-------	1920	1.6	9.5	32.2	73.0	135.1	215.6	295.1	367.8	434.8	493.4	542.8	587.0
1906-------	1921	2.0	10.5	30.5	70.4	136.9	213.8	290.5	362.5	426.5	482.5	533.3	575.5
1907-------	1922	2.2	9.7	29.2	71.9	135.8	210.2	286.1	354.7	416.5	474.2	522.8	563.1
1908-------	1923	2.0	9.4	30.4	72.1	134.1	207.5	280.0	346.4	409.8	464.1	510.1	547.9
1909-------	1924	2.0	9.9	30.8	71.3	132.3	202.6	271.8	340.0	399.6	451.4	494.5	535.0
1910-------	1925	2.1	10.0	30.1	70.8	129.4	196.1	267.3	331.2	388.0	436.4	482.6	525.0
1911-------	1926	2.1	9.8	30.9	69.8	125.8	194.9	262.1	323.7	377.5	430.1	478.9	523.2
1912-------	1927	2.1	10.6	30.4	68.4	126.4	191.0	255.5	313.6	371.9	427.2	477.7	524.5
1913-------	1928	2.4	10.1	29.9	69.2	122.9	185.1	245.9	309.3	370.6	426.9	480.1	529.5
1914-------	1929	2.1	10.0	30.5	66.6	118.0	176.1	242.1	308.2	370.3	429.4	485.2	534.3
1915-------	1930	2.2	10.4	29.3	63.8	111.6	174.4	242.6	308.6	373.0	434.7	489.5	540.5
1916-------	1931	2.3	9.8	27.5	59.3	110.3	174.5	242.0	309.5	376.0	435.5	491.2	548.5
1917-------	1932	2.0	8.9	25.2	59.0	110.8	173.3	241.9	311.4	375.3	435.1	498.1	568.2
1918-------	1933	1.8	8.2	25.5	59.8	110.1	173.9	244.2	310.6	375.1	442.7	520.7	582.8
1919-------	1934	1.8	8.7	26.5	59.8	112.2	178.6	246.5	315.7	389.9	475.1	544.6	596.8
1920-------	1935	1.9	9.1	26.4	61.5	115.8	179.2	248.5	326.5	417.0	493.0	553.0	602.4
1921-------	1936	2.1	9.1	27.6	64.2	115.8	179.7	256.8	348.7	429.2	496.6	553.7	626.9
1922-------	1937	1.9	9.1	27.8	61.7	111.6	180.2	269.3	352.3	424.8	488.7	572.2	656.0
1923-------	1938	2.0	9.2	26.6	59.9	113.2	192.2	275.5	350.8	420.0	512.3	609.3	676.2
1924-------	1939	2.0	8.9	26.3	62.0	122.4	198.5	273.1	345.2	444.1	553.6	631.9	692.9
1925-------	1940	1.9	8.9	27.7	65.6	125.3	192.0	263.7	363.8	483.9	573.2	644.6	700.1
1926-------	1941	1.9	9.5	28.7	66.4	117.9	181.6	276.9	402.6	501.8	583.5	648.9	707.0
1927-------	1942	2.1	9.8	29.1	61.8	110.8	192.0	316.6	422.7	513.3	588.2	657.1	714.1
1928-------	1943	2.1	9.8	26.4	57.1	116.8	227.3	335.8	433.2	517.0	597.0	665.2	719.5
1929-------	1944	2.1	8.8	24.5	60.5	145.0	245.6	346.7	437.7	529.0	609.5	675.4	729.4
1930-------	1945	1.9	8.3	25.6	78.3	159.3	254.0	349.1	449.4	541.4	619.4	686.1	738.9
1931-------	1946	1.9	8.7	35.0	88.5	166.2	256.5	362.7	463.9	554.4	634.7	701.1	753.8
1932-------	1947	1.9	12.0	39.8	91.5	166.1	266.6	372.8	474.5	568.5	649.3	715.8	767.7
1933-------	1948	2.8	14.1	41.8	92.6	175.4	275.2	383.6	488.9	583.5	665.3	731.1	779.6
1934-------	1949	3.2	14.4	41.9	97.1	178.5	281.6	393.7	499.3	596.6	678.0	740.0	786.1
1935-------	1950	3.0	14.3	43.6	97.7	181.6	287.0	398.7	508.9	606.2	683.6	743.0	787.4
1936-------	1951	3.1	14.9	43.7	99.6	185.4	289.9	407.3	518.1	611.2	685.6	743.4	786.6
1937-------	1952	3.2	14.9	44.7	101.6	186.5	296.8	415.9	523.0	613.8	687.3	744.0	785.2
1938-------	1953	3.1	15.1	45.6	101.8	191.4	304.3	420.1	525.6	615.2	687.3	741.0	781.4
1939-------	1954	3.2	15.8	46.3	106.1	199.0	309.1	424.4	528.2	616.1	684.5	737.2	778.3
1940-------	1955	3.5	16.1	48.5	110.2	199.9	308.9	421.4	523.7	607.8	674.6	727.8	767.7
1941-------	1956	3.5	16.9	50.3	109.2	196.8	302.0	412.6	511.0	592.8	660.0	711.4	754.3
1942-------	1957	3.6	17.2	48.7	105.4	189.5	292.9	399.0	494.6	576.3	640.8	696.2	740.0
1943-------	1958	3.6	16.4	46.5	100.6	182.9	282.1	385.6	479.4	556.0	623.6	678.6	725.5
1944-------	1959	3.5	16.0	45.2	98.6	177.6	274.6	375.2	462.5	541.2	606.9	663.6	710.9
1945-------	1960	3.6	16.0	44.9	96.0	173.2	266.4	359.5	447.3	522.8	588.8	645.9	694.5
1946-------	1961	3.6	15.7	42.9	92.3	166.3	254.1	348.0	432.7	508.9	576.8	636.4	683.6
1947-------	1962	3.2	14.2	40.2	87.4	157.5	244.9	334.2	418.9	496.1	565.7	621.8	665.4
1948-------	1963	3.0	13.5	38.5	83.9	153.4	236.5	325.7	410.4	488.7	552.6	602.8	645.3
1949-------	1964	2.9	13.1	36.9	81.1	146.9	229.0	316.7	401.4	471.4	526.8	574.2	
1950-------	1965	2.8	12.6	36.0	78.8	144.3	225.7	314.0	389.4	449.5	501.3		
1951-------	1966	2.7	12.5	35.4	78.2	143.8	226.8	305.6	370.4	426.0			
1952-------	1967	2.8	12.3	35.4	78.8	147.0	222.2	291.0	350.6				
1953-------	1968	2.7	12.6	36.4	82.9	146.2	214.1	277.5					
1954-------	1969	2.9	13.4	39.6	84.0	143.8	207.1						
1955-------	1970	3.2	15.0	40.8	85.1	142.1							
1956-------	1971	3.6	15.3	42.2	85.4								
1957-------	1972	3.7	16.3	43.2									
1958-------	1973	4.1	17.0										
1959-------	1974	4.3											

TABLE 6B. CUMULATIVE BIRTH RATES FOR WHITE WOMEN AS OF THE BEGINNING OF EACH YEAR 1917-74 BY AGE AND LIVE-BIRTH ORDER FOR EACH COHORT FROM 1867 TO 1959--CON.

LIVE-BIRTH ORDER AND COHORT	DIAGONAL LINE FOR JANUARY 1	EXACT AGE											
		27	28	29	30	31	32	33	34	35	36	37	38
FIRST BIRTHS--CON.													
1879-------													769.3
1880-------												764.6	768.6
1881-------											760.5	765.4	769.5
1882-------										756.2	762.4	767.4	771.4
1883-------									749.4	756.8	763.2	768.2	772.4
1884-------								739.7	748.8	756.6	762.7	767.9	772.4
1885-------							728.5	739.2	748.9	756.1	762.7	768.3	772.4
1886-------						715.8	729.8	741.3	750.0	758.0	764.9	770.1	774.1
1887-------					700.5	718.7	733.7	744.0	753.9	762.1	768.7	773.8	777.9
1888-------				679.4	703.7	722.9	736.2	747.9	757.9	765.9	772.4	777.6	781.7
1889-------			653.1	682.7	708.1	724.3	739.4	751.1	760.9	768.6	775.1	780.2	784.1
1890-------	1917	622.6	657.9	688.7	709.4	728.8	744.1	755.7	765.2	773.0	779.3	784.1	788.1
1891-------	1918	628.0	664.7	689.0	714.6	734.3	749.3	760.5	770.1	777.8	783.8	788.7	792.5
1892-------	1919	637.6	666.5	697.4	723.6	742.1	756.5	767.7	777.0	784.2	790.2	794.9	798.4
1893-------	1920	636.4	673.2	705.2	729.1	746.8	761.2	772.2	780.9	788.0	793.7	798.1	801.8
1894-------	1921	640.6	679.1	707.9	730.9	748.7	762.9	773.4	782.3	789.2	794.7	799.3	802.9
1895-------	1922	646.6	681.5	709.3	732.5	750.1	763.9	774.5	783.1	789.9	795.8	800.3	803.6
1896-------	1923	649.6	683.3	711.3	734.0	751.0	764.7	775.0	783.5	790.7	796.3	800.5	803.6
1897-------	1924	651.5	685.6	712.7	734.6	751.4	764.8	775.0	783.9	790.7	796.0	799.9	803.1
1898-------	1925	653.9	686.7	712.7	734.1	750.5	763.8	774.5	782.9	789.2	794.1	798.2	801.5
1899-------	1926	647.0	679.0	704.9	726.1	742.5	756.5	767.0	775.2	781.5	786.8	791.2	794.7
1900-------	1927	640.2	671.7	696.9	717.8	735.0	748.6	758.6	766.5	773.2	778.8	783.4	787.1
1901-------	1928	640.5	671.2	696.1	717.9	734.7	747.9	757.4	765.8	772.7	778.5	783.3	787.3
1902-------	1929	643.5	673.7	699.6	720.9	736.9	749.1	759.3	768.1	775.3	781.5	786.7	790.8
1903-------	1930	643.3	674.8	700.3	720.6	735.7	748.9	759.8	769.1	776.9	783.6	789.2	793.6
1904-------	1931	636.1	666.9	691.1	710.4	727.0	741.4	753.0	763.0	771.5	778.7	784.7	789.6
1905-------	1932	623.2	652.3	675.2	696.2	713.8	728.9	741.3	752.1	761.2	768.9	775.5	781.5
1906-------	1933	609.7	637.4	662.4	684.6	703.1	719.2	732.7	744.2	753.8	762.2	769.7	776.1
1907-------	1934	595.6	625.6	652.0	675.1	695.2	712.8	727.2	739.3	749.9	760.2	768.3	774.6
1908-------	1935	582.6	614.1	641.3	666.0	687.7	706.2	721.2	734.4	747.6	758.1	766.0	772.4
1909-------	1936	571.6	604.1	633.6	660.5	683.2	702.7	719.4	736.2	749.1	758.8	766.8	774.4
1910-------	1937	563.0	597.8	629.5	657.1	681.1	702.5	722.3	738.3	749.8	759.5	769.1	777.5
1911-------	1938	563.9	601.5	633.7	662.9	689.5	713.5	732.4	746.1	757.6	769.5	780.2	787.2
1912-------	1939	567.6	605.3	639.3	671.6	701.6	724.4	740.5	754.1	768.4	781.4	790.0	796.3
1913-------	1940	572.9	612.8	651.0	688.2	715.8	735.2	751.0	768.3	784.1	794.6	802.4	808.2
1914-------	1941	580.4	625.4	670.2	703.6	726.6	745.5	766.4	785.6	798.2	807.8	815.0	820.6
1915-------	1942	592.3	645.7	685.2	712.7	735.0	760.5	783.8	798.9	810.2	819.0	825.9	831.4
1916-------	1943	610.8	657.7	689.7	716.0	746.6	775.1	793.1	806.5	816.7	825.1	831.8	837.0
1917-------	1944	622.7	660.7	691.4	728.5	762.9	785.0	801.0	813.1	823.1	831.3	837.6	842.5
1918-------	1945	627.1	663.0	706.7	748.1	774.5	794.0	808.3	820.2	829.9	837.4	843.3	847.8
1919-------	1946	639.0	691.6	741.2	773.6	797.4	815.2	829.5	841.2	850.2	857.4	863.0	867.3
1920-------	1947	664.8	724.6	763.3	792.4	813.9	831.6	845.7	856.4	864.9	871.6	876.8	880.9
1921-------	1948	698.3	745.3	780.1	806.4	827.9	845.1	857.9	868.3	876.3	882.6	887.5	891.3
1922-------	1949	712.1	754.2	785.8	812.3	833.0	848.7	861.0	870.5	877.9	883.9	888.5	891.9
1923-------	1950	726.8	765.3	797.4	822.9	842.3	857.6	868.9	877.9	885.1	890.6	894.8	898.0
1924-------	1951	739.4	779.1	810.4	834.2	852.6	866.6	877.4	886.1	892.7	897.9	901.9	904.9
1925-------	1952	748.3	786.9	816.0	838.6	855.8	869.1	879.5	887.5	893.7	898.6	902.3	905.0
1926-------	1953	753.8	789.8	817.4	838.6	854.8	867.6	877.2	884.7	890.5	895.0	898.4	901.0
1927-------	1954	758.7	793.1	819.4	839.6	855.4	867.3	876.4	883.5	888.9	893.1	896.2	899.1
1928-------	1955	762.6	795.6	820.7	840.5	855.2	866.4	874.9	881.4	886.4	890.3	893.9	896.6
1929-------	1956	771.1	803.1	828.1	846.7	860.5	871.2	879.2	885.3	890.0	894.4	897.8	900.3
1930-------	1957	779.9	811.5	834.9	852.3	865.4	875.4	882.8	888.6	893.9	898.0	901.1	903.3
1931-------	1958	794.5	824.2	846.0	862.6	875.0	884.2	891.3	897.6	902.5	906.2	908.9	911.3
1932-------	1959	805.6	833.5	854.2	869.7	880.9	889.8	897.3	903.1	907.6	911.0	914.0	916.0
1933-------	1960	815.3	841.7	861.1	875.2	886.2	895.5	902.5	908.0	912.1	915.8	918.4	920.4
1934-------	1961	820.1	845.0	863.2	877.0	888.8	897.6	904.4	909.4	913.8	917.0	919.5	921.2
1935-------	1962	820.1	843.9	861.5	876.3	887.2	895.8	901.8	907.3	911.2	914.4	916.7	918.4
1936-------	1963	818.1	841.2	860.2	874.1	885.0	892.9	899.7	904.6	908.6	911.5	913.7	915.3
1937-------	1964	815.8	840.1	858.2	872.3	882.7	891.5	897.9	903.0	906.7	909.5	911.6	
1938-------	1965	813.0	836.5	854.8	868.7	880.1	888.6	895.2	899.9	903.5	906.2		
1939-------	1966	809.0	833.3	851.6	866.9	878.2	887.1	893.5	898.2	901.8			
1940-------	1967	800.1	824.8	845.3	860.5	872.4	881.0	887.2	891.9				
1941-------	1968	787.6	815.4	836.1	852.5	864.2	872.6	879.0					
1942-------	1969	777.0	805.4	827.6	843.6	855.0	863.8						
1943-------	1970	763.0	792.6	814.4	829.9	841.9							
1944-------	1971	749.5	778.6	799.7	816.0								
1945-------	1972	732.2	760.1	781.9									
1946-------	1973	719.7	748.6										
1947-------	1974	701.4											

TABLE 6B. CUMULATIVE BIRTH RATES FOR WHITE WOMEN AS OF THE BEGINNING OF EACH YEAR 1917-74 BY AGE AND LIVE-BIRTH ORDER FOR EACH COHORT FROM 1867 TO 1959--CON.

LIVE-BIRTH ORDER AND COHORT	DIAGONAL LINE FOR JANUARY 1	EXACT AGE											
		39	40	41	42	43	44	45	46	47	48	49	50
FIRST BIRTHS--CON.													
1867-------													803.3
1868-------												801.3	801.3
1869-------											799.2	799.2	799.2
1870-------										797.0	797.0	797.0	797.0
1871-------									794.7	794.8	794.9	794.9	794.9
1872-------								792.3	792.5	792.6	792.6	792.6	792.6
1873-------							789.7	790.0	790.2	790.3	790.3	790.3	790.3
1874-------						786.8	787.3	787.6	787.8	787.9	787.9	787.9	787.9
1875-------					783.8	784.6	785.1	785.4	785.6	785.7	785.8	785.8	785.8
1876-------				781.0	782.2	783.0	783.6	783.9	784.1	784.2	784.2	784.2	784.2
1877-------			778.2	779.9	781.1	781.9	782.5	782.8	783.0	783.1	783.1	783.1	783.1
1878-------	1917	774.4	776.9	778.6	779.9	780.7	781.3	781.6	781.8	781.9	782.0	782.0	782.0
1879-------	1918	772.4	774.9	776.7	778.0	778.9	779.5	779.8	780.0	780.1	780.1	780.1	780.1
1880-------	1919	771.8	774.4	776.2	777.6	778.4	779.0	779.3	779.5	779.6	779.6	779.6	779.6
1881-------	1920	772.7	775.4	777.3	778.5	779.3	779.9	780.2	780.4	780.5	780.5	780.5	780.5
1882-------	1921	774.7	777.5	779.2	780.4	781.2	781.7	782.0	782.2	782.3	782.4	782.4	782.4
1883-------	1922	775.9	778.5	780.2	781.4	782.1	782.6	782.9	783.1	783.2	783.3	783.3	783.3
1884-------	1923	775.6	778.1	779.8	781.0	781.8	782.3	782.6	782.8	782.9	782.9	782.9	782.9
1885-------	1924	775.5	778.1	779.8	781.0	781.8	782.3	782.6	782.8	782.9	782.9	782.9	782.9
1886-------	1925	777.3	779.8	781.4	782.6	783.4	783.8	784.1	784.2	784.3	784.3	784.3	784.3
1887-------	1926	781.1	783.5	785.2	786.4	787.1	787.5	787.7	787.8	787.9	787.9	787.9	787.9
1888-------	1927	784.7	787.1	788.7	789.8	790.5	790.9	791.1	791.2	791.2	791.2	791.2	791.2
1889-------	1928	787.2	789.6	791.2	792.3	793.0	793.5	793.7	793.8	793.9	793.9	793.9	793.9
1890-------	1929	791.1	793.4	794.9	796.0	796.7	797.1	797.3	797.4	797.4	797.4	797.4	797.4
1891-------	1930	795.4	797.7	799.2	800.2	800.8	801.2	801.5	801.6	801.6	801.6	801.6	801.6
1892-------	1931	801.3	803.5	804.9	805.8	806.4	806.8	807.0	807.1	807.1	807.1	807.1	807.1
1893-------	1932	804.6	806.6	807.9	808.8	809.4	809.8	810.0	810.1	810.2	810.2	810.2	810.2
1894-------	1933	805.5	807.4	808.7	809.6	810.2	810.6	810.8	810.9	811.0	811.0	811.0	811.0
1895-------	1934	806.0	807.9	809.2	810.1	810.7	811.1	811.3	811.4	811.5	811.5	811.5	811.5
1896-------	1935	806.1	807.9	809.2	810.1	810.7	811.1	811.3	811.4	811.5	811.5	811.5	811.5
1897-------	1936	805.6	807.5	808.8	809.7	810.4	810.8	811.1	811.2	811.3	811.3	811.3	811.3
1898-------	1937	804.1	806.1	807.5	808.5	809.2	809.7	810.0	810.2	810.3	810.3	810.3	810.3
1899-------	1938	797.5	799.7	801.3	802.4	803.2	803.7	804.0	804.2	804.3	804.3	804.3	804.3
1900-------	1939	790.1	792.4	794.0	795.2	796.0	796.6	796.9	797.1	797.2	797.2	797.2	797.2
1901-------	1940	790.5	792.9	794.7	795.9	796.8	797.4	797.8	798.0	798.1	798.1	798.1	798.1
1902-------	1941	794.1	796.7	798.8	800.3	801.3	802.0	802.4	802.6	802.7	802.7	802.7	802.7
1903-------	1942	797.3	800.6	803.0	804.7	805.8	806.6	807.0	807.2	807.3	807.3	807.3	807.3
1904-------	1943	794.2	797.8	800.3	802.1	803.4	804.2	804.6	804.8	804.9	804.9	804.9	804.9
1905-------	1944	786.4	790.0	792.7	794.7	796.0	796.7	797.1	797.3	797.4	797.4	797.4	797.4
1906-------	1945	780.9	784.7	787.8	790.0	791.2	791.9	792.3	792.5	792.6	792.6	792.6	792.6
1907-------	1946	779.7	784.2	787.5	789.4	790.6	791.3	791.7	791.9	792.0	792.0	792.0	792.0
1908-------	1947	778.3	783.1	786.0	787.9	789.0	789.6	790.0	790.2	790.3	790.3	790.3	790.3
1909-------	1948	780.9	785.1	787.8	789.6	790.7	791.4	791.8	792.0	792.1	792.1	792.1	792.1
1910-------	1949	783.0	786.9	789.5	791.2	792.3	793.0	793.4	793.6	793.7	793.7	793.7	793.7
1911-------	1950	792.2	795.8	798.3	800.0	801.1	801.7	802.1	802.3	802.4	802.4	802.4	802.4
1912-------	1951	800.9	804.3	806.8	808.4	809.4	810.0	810.3	810.5	810.6	810.6	810.6	810.6
1913-------	1952	812.6	816.0	818.3	819.9	820.9	821.5	821.8	822.0	822.1	822.1	822.1	822.1
1914-------	1953	825.0	828.2	830.5	832.0	832.9	833.5	833.8	834.0	834.1	834.1	834.1	834.1
1915-------	1954	835.5	838.6	840.7	842.0	842.9	843.4	843.7	843.8	843.9	843.9	843.9	843.9
1916-------	1955	841.0	843.9	845.7	847.1	847.9	848.4	848.6	848.7	848.7	848.7	848.7	848.7
1917-------	1956	846.2	848.8	850.7	851.9	852.7	853.1	853.3	853.4	853.4	853.4	853.4	853.4
1918-------	1957	851.1	853.6	855.2	856.3	857.0	857.4	857.6	857.7	857.7	857.7	857.7	857.7
1919-------	1958	870.6	872.9	874.6	875.7	876.4	876.8	877.0	877.1	877.1	877.1	877.1	877.1
1920-------	1959	883.9	886.1	887.6	888.7	889.3	889.7	889.9	890.0	890.0	890.0	890.0	890.0
1921-------	1960	894.1	896.1	897.5	898.4	899.0	899.4	899.6	899.7	899.7	899.7	899.7	899.7
1922-------	1961	894.5	896.4	897.7	898.6	899.3	899.7	899.9	900.0	900.0	900.0	900.0	900.0
1923-------	1962	900.4	902.1	903.3	904.3	904.9	905.2	905.4	905.5	905.5	905.5	905.5	905.5
1924-------	1963	907.1	908.7	910.1	911.0	911.5	911.8	912.0	912.1	912.1	912.1	912.1	912.1
1925-------	1964	907.1	909.0	910.2	911.0	911.4	911.7	911.8	911.9	911.9	911.9	911.9	
1926-------	1965	903.3	905.0	906.1	906.8	907.3	907.5	907.6	907.7	907.7	907.7		
1927-------	1966	901.3	902.9	903.8	904.6	905.0	905.2	905.3	905.3	905.3			
1928-------	1967	898.6	899.9	901.0	901.6	902.0	902.2	902.3	902.3				
1929-------	1968	902.0	903.5	904.4	905.0	905.3	905.5	905.6					
1930-------	1969	905.2	906.4	907.3	907.8	908.1	908.3						
1931-------	1970	912.9	914.1	914.9	915.4	915.7							
1932-------	1971	917.6	918.6	919.3	919.7								
1933-------	1972	921.8	922.8	923.4									
1934-------	1973	922.5	923.4										
1935-------	1974	919.6											

TABLE 6B. CUMULATIVE BIRTH RATES FOR WHITE WOMEN AS OF THE BEGINNING OF EACH YEAR 1917-74 BY AGE AND LIVE-BIRTH ORDER FOR EACH COHORT FROM 1867 TO 1959--CON.

LIVE-BIRTH ORDER AND COHORT	DIAGONAL LINE FOR JANUARY 1	EXACT AGE											
		15	16	17	18	19	20	21	22	23	24	25	26
SECOND BIRTHS													
1891-------													358.4
1892-------												308.6	360.2
1893-------											255.2	310.7	361.5
1894-------										198.2	257.1	311.7	360.4
1895-------									143.3	199.8	257.6	309.8	358.1
1896-------								92.5	145.0	200.6	255.5	306.7	354.6
1897-------							51.5	94.2	146.1	199.0	252.3	303.1	352.9
1898-------						23.6	53.1	95.5	145.1	196.8	249.9	303.5	355.1
1899-------					8.4	23.7	52.9	93.2	141.0	191.7	247.2	301.9	351.7
1900-------				2.1	8.4	23.5	51.2	90.2	137.0	189.9	246.7	299.7	346.6
1901-------			0.3	2.1	8.2	22.3	49.0	88.0	136.7	190.8	245.9	296.3	341.3
1902-------	1917	*	0.4	2.2	8.1	22.3	50.4	92.2	142.7	195.9	248.0	296.6	340.3
1903-------	1918	*	0.4	2.1	8.0	23.8	54.2	97.4	146.5	197.6	248.6	295.7	337.8
1904-------	1919	*	0.3	2.0	8.5	25.7	56.8	97.9	144.7	194.8	243.8	288.8	329.7
1905-------	1920	*	0.3	2.1	9.1	26.9	56.1	95.3	141.2	189.4	235.7	279.1	319.7
1906-------	1921	*	0.3	2.2	9.4	25.9	54.0	92.7	137.6	183.2	228.1	270.9	309.8
1907-------	1922	*	0.4	2.4	9.1	25.3	53.4	91.7	134.5	178.8	223.1	264.4	302.1
1908-------	1923	*	0.4	2.3	9.1	25.5	53.4	89.7	131.0	174.6	216.9	256.6	292.3
1909-------	1924	*	0.4	2.4	9.4	25.7	52.1	87.0	127.6	169.4	210.3	247.9	284.4
1910-------	1925	*	0.4	2.5	9.4	24.5	49.7	83.9	122.6	162.9	201.5	239.6	274.3
1911-------	1926	*	0.4	2.5	9.1	23.8	48.9	81.8	119.5	157.6	196.9	233.6	268.8
1912-------	1927	*	0.4	2.4	8.9	23.5	47.4	79.3	114.5	153.1	190.6	227.8	264.2
1913-------	1928	*	0.4	2.4	8.9	22.9	45.9	75.3	110.8	147.8	186.1	224.7	263.3
1914-------	1929	*	0.4	2.3	8.3	21.7	42.7	72.2	106.2	144.0	183.7	224.4	263.0
1915-------	1930	*	0.4	2.2	7.9	20.0	40.8	69.2	104.2	143.5	185.1	225.5	266.1
1916-------	1931	*	0.4	2.1	7.3	19.1	39.1	68.3	104.2	144.8	185.5	227.1	269.5
1917-------	1932	*	0.4	1.9	6.9	18.3	39.0	68.7	105.8	145.3	186.8	230.0	278.4
1918-------	1933	*	0.3	1.8	6.6	18.5	39.6	70.2	106.1	146.6	189.1	239.3	293.7
1919-------	1934	*	0.3	1.8	7.0	19.3	41.2	71.5	109.3	151.4	201.9	257.4	307.0
1920-------	1935	*	0.3	2.0	7.5	20.2	42.0	74.3	113.0	159.2	214.0	263.8	309.3
1921-------	1936	*	0.4	2.2	7.9	20.9	44.9	77.9	117.5	167.5	216.0	260.7	321.4
1922-------	1937	*	0.4	2.2	7.9	22.1	45.7	78.0	121.4	166.3	208.6	269.9	336.9
1923-------	1938	*	0.3	2.1	8.4	22.3	45.7	80.9	120.2	159.2	218.8	286.8	354.1
1924-------	1939	*	0.4	2.4	8.5	22.7	48.0	79.8	113.6	168.9	234.9	304.7	375.3
1925-------	1940	*	0.4	2.4	8.7	23.5	46.0	73.4	120.2	180.9	250.2	323.7	394.9
1926-------	1941	*	0.4	2.5	9.2	22.2	41.4	77.2	128.7	194.4	267.7	341.6	415.0
1927-------	1942	*	0.5	2.8	8.7	19.9	43.4	83.4	141.6	211.7	285.0	361.1	434.7
1928-------	1943	*	0.6	2.6	7.7	20.6	47.4	94.6	157.5	227.7	303.6	380.4	454.7
1929-------	1944	*	0.5	2.2	7.8	22.8	55.8	107.8	171.2	244.5	322.2	401.5	476.4
1930-------	1945	*	0.4	2.2	8.9	28.0	65.2	117.9	184.3	260.2	341.2	422.0	496.3
1931-------	1946	*	0.4	2.7	11.4	33.8	72.1	127.8	197.6	278.0	362.1	443.5	519.3
1932-------	1947	*	0.5	3.5	14.0	37.0	77.1	135.3	209.1	292.9	378.4	462.6	539.5
1933-------	1948	*	0.7	4.5	15.3	39.6	81.8	143.7	220.7	306.8	395.8	482.0	557.4
1934-------	1949	*	1.0	4.8	16.3	41.4	85.9	149.7	229.5	319.2	410.9	496.0	570.1
1935-------	1950	*	0.9	4.8	16.5	42.7	87.8	153.9	236.6	329.3	420.5	504.5	576.9
1936-------	1951	*	0.9	4.8	17.0	43.7	90.7	159.6	245.1	337.2	428.1	510.9	580.5
1937-------	1952	*	0.8	4.8	17.2	44.9	94.3	165.4	251.2	344.3	434.4	514.4	580.4
1938-------	1953	*	0.8	5.0	17.9	47.3	97.9	169.9	257.9	350.2	437.7	513.8	577.7
1939-------	1954	*	1.0	5.4	19.3	49.8	102.1	176.3	263.1	353.2	436.6	510.3	572.5
1940-------	1955	*	1.0	5.7	20.1	51.5	105.0	177.4	261.7	348.1	428.7	499.7	557.7
1941-------	1956	*	1.1	6.1	20.9	52.0	103.5	173.2	254.0	336.6	413.2	478.9	535.4
1942-------	1957	*	1.1	6.1	20.5	50.7	99.7	166.2	242.6	319.7	389.6	452.9	510.3
1943-------	1958	*	1.1	5.9	19.9	48.5	95.3	157.5	227.8	297.0	363.4	427.2	485.4
1944-------	1959	*	1.1	5.9	19.4	46.9	90.6	147.6	209.6	274.1	340.3	403.7	463.7
1945-------	1960	*	1.1	5.9	19.0	44.6	84.4	134.0	190.9	253.6	317.2	380.6	441.0
1946-------	1961	*	1.2	5.8	17.9	40.9	75.0	119.6	174.2	234.2	298.3	362.6	419.6
1947-------	1962	*	1.0	5.1	15.7	35.4	65.7	108.2	159.4	219.1	283.3	343.2	395.7
1948-------	1963	*	0.9	4.4	13.4	30.7	59.6	99.0	149.8	209.1	268.5	322.6	373.7
1949-------	1964	*	0.8	3.9	11.9	28.4	54.6	93.1	143.3	198.1	250.5	301.9	
1950-------	1965	*	0.7	3.5	11.1	26.1	51.9	90.2	136.6	184.3	233.6		
1951-------	1966	*	0.7	3.4	10.4	25.2	51.0	86.6	126.7	171.3			
1952-------	1967	*	0.6	3.0	10.0	24.8	48.9	79.8	117.2				
1953-------	1968	*	0.6	3.1	10.1	24.3	45.7	74.7					
1954-------	1969	*	0.6	3.2	10.0	22.8	43.1						
1955-------	1970	*	0.7	3.3	9.6	21.9							
1956-------	1971	*	0.7	3.1	9.3								
1957-------	1972	*	0.6	3.0									
1958-------	1973	*	0.7										
1959-------	1974	*											

TABLE 6B. CUMULATIVE BIRTH RATES FOR WHITE WOMEN AS OF THE BEGINNING OF EACH YEAR 1917-74 BY AGE AND LIVE-BIRTH ORDER FOR EACH COHORT FROM 1867 TO 1959--CON.

LIVE-BIRTH ORDER AND COHORT	DIAGONAL LINE FOR JANUARY 1	EXACT AGE											
		27	28	29	30	31	32	33	34	35	36	37	38
SECOND BIRTHS--CON.													
1879-------													640.5
1880-------												631.3	637.7
1881-------											621.7	629.8	636.3
1882-------										611.0	621.0	629.1	635.5
1883-------									597.9	610.0	619.9	628.0	634.5
1884-------								582.6	597.4	609.3	619.2	627.3	634.0
1885-------							563.2	580.6	595.2	607.1	617.2	625.7	632.1
1886-------						538.4	560.0	577.3	591.9	604.1	614.6	622.7	629.2
1887-------					508.9	535.8	557.3	574.6	589.7	602.3	612.5	620.8	627.3
1888-------				478.9	512.9	539.6	561.0	578.8	594.1	606.6	616.9	625.1	631.4
1889-------			443.6	482.7	516.5	542.7	564.7	582.7	598.1	610.6	620.9	629.0	635.2
1890-------	1917	403.6	446.9	486.0	518.9	545.5	567.9	586.1	601.5	614.0	624.2	632.0	638.1
1891-------	1918	403.8	447.1	484.7	517.7	544.3	566.7	584.8	600.2	612.6	622.4	630.1	636.0
1892-------	1919	405.4	446.9	484.1	516.4	542.9	565.2	583.2	598.2	609.9	619.3	626.6	632.1
1893-------	1920	404.9	446.0	482.2	514.6	541.0	563.2	580.6	594.9	606.3	615.4	622.4	628.2
1894-------	1921	403.8	444.2	480.9	513.6	539.8	561.3	578.3	592.4	603.6	612.4	619.7	625.1
1895-------	1922	401.1	442.4	479.8	512.0	537.6	559.0	575.8	589.7	600.5	609.6	616.6	621.8
1896-------	1923	398.8	441.0	477.4	508.8	534.0	554.8	571.2	584.5	595.6	604.2	610.9	615.8
1897-------	1924	398.1	439.4	475.0	505.7	530.1	550.2	566.1	579.7	590.2	598.6	604.9	610.0
1898-------	1925	399.7	439.4	473.5	502.8	526.2	545.8	561.8	574.7	584.9	592.7	599.2	604.3
1899-------	1926	394.9	433.3	466.4	494.9	518.1	538.1	553.9	566.9	576.8	585.3	592.0	597.2
1900-------	1927	387.5	424.4	456.0	483.7	507.1	526.4	541.7	553.9	564.4	572.8	579.5	584.8
1901-------	1928	381.3	416.7	447.4	475.3	498.0	516.7	531.2	544.1	554.5	563.1	569.9	575.5
1902-------	1929	378.6	412.8	443.6	470.3	491.8	509.3	524.5	537.3	547.9	556.6	563.9	569.7
1903-------	1930	375.0	409.5	439.5	465.2	485.8	504.5	519.7	532.8	543.7	553.0	560.7	566.9
1904-------	1931	367.1	400.5	429.3	453.9	475.9	494.6	510.1	523.6	535.3	545.2	553.5	560.2
1905-------	1932	355.8	387.8	415.2	441.0	462.6	481.3	497.3	511.7	524.0	534.6	543.5	551.1
1906-------	1933	344.4	374.9	403.4	428.8	450.5	469.9	487.1	502.2	515.4	526.7	536.4	545.4
1907-------	1934	335.2	366.9	394.9	420.4	442.9	463.7	481.7	498.0	512.1	525.1	536.6	546.4
1908-------	1935	326.2	356.8	384.7	410.7	434.5	456.0	475.5	492.7	509.1	524.2	536.7	547.3
1909-------	1936	317.1	347.6	376.2	403.9	428.6	452.1	472.9	493.2	512.1	527.8	541.5	552.9
1910-------	1937	306.8	338.2	368.6	396.8	423.5	448.3	471.8	495.1	514.2	531.2	545.8	557.3
1911-------	1938	302.7	336.2	367.2	397.6	425.9	453.4	480.4	503.4	524.1	542.4	556.9	567.5
1912-------	1939	300.1	333.8	366.8	398.7	431.0	462.5	489.0	513.7	535.9	554.1	567.5	577.6
1913-------	1940	299.5	335.4	370.2	407.3	444.2	475.1	503.9	530.5	552.6	569.2	582.1	592.0
1914-------	1941	301.7	339.9	381.0	423.4	458.7	492.2	523.5	550.2	570.4	586.5	599.2	609.2
1915-------	1942	307.2	351.3	398.4	438.3	476.0	512.5	544.0	568.2	587.9	603.8	616.5	626.6
1916-------	1943	315.1	365.5	408.9	450.5	491.9	529.0	557.6	581.2	600.6	616.4	629.0	638.5
1917-------	1944	330.4	376.7	420.9	467.5	510.5	544.8	573.1	596.7	616.1	631.8	643.9	653.3
1918-------	1945	341.6	387.1	437.4	486.5	526.2	560.0	588.1	611.5	630.6	645.5	657.2	666.1
1919-------	1946	352.9	407.7	462.7	509.2	549.4	583.6	612.2	635.8	654.4	669.3	680.6	689.3
1920-------	1947	367.2	427.6	480.2	527.4	568.0	602.5	631.0	653.7	672.0	686.0	696.8	704.9
1921-------	1948	385.8	444.4	498.3	546.2	587.2	621.8	649.1	671.5	688.5	701.9	712.0	719.6
1922-------	1949	400.1	460.3	514.7	562.6	603.7	636.8	663.5	684.2	700.4	713.0	722.2	729.0
1923-------	1950	419.9	480.7	535.9	584.2	623.5	655.9	680.7	700.4	715.7	727.1	735.6	741.9
1924-------	1951	442.1	504.5	560.1	606.5	645.2	675.3	698.8	717.4	731.2	741.7	749.7	755.7
1925-------	1952	463.4	525.9	579.4	624.8	660.5	688.9	711.0	727.8	740.6	750.5	758.0	763.4
1926-------	1953	483.8	545.0	597.5	640.2	674.1	700.9	721.1	736.6	748.6	757.9	764.6	769.6
1927-------	1954	503.2	563.2	613.1	654.1	686.6	711.3	729.9	744.5	755.8	764.1	770.5	775.2
1928-------	1955	522.4	580.2	628.4	667.7	697.8	720.8	738.4	752.0	762.1	770.0	776.0	780.2
1929-------	1956	542.7	599.6	647.1	684.0	712.5	734.4	751.1	763.7	773.4	780.9	786.3	790.3
1930-------	1957	562.5	618.9	663.7	699.0	726.1	746.8	762.3	774.2	783.5	790.3	795.3	799.1
1931-------	1958	586.1	640.2	683.2	716.9	742.6	761.7	776.2	787.7	796.0	802.4	807.1	810.7
1932-------	1959	604.2	656.7	698.1	730.0	753.7	771.8	785.8	796.2	804.1	810.0	814.5	817.9
1933-------	1960	620.2	670.5	709.6	738.9	761.3	778.6	791.6	801.3	808.8	814.6	819.0	822.3
1934-------	1961	631.1	679.1	715.6	743.8	765.3	781.8	793.8	803.1	810.2	815.8	820.1	823.1
1935-------	1962	635.2	680.4	715.6	742.8	763.3	778.4	790.1	799.3	806.5	812.0	816.0	818.8
1936-------	1963	636.1	679.8	714.3	740.2	759.6	774.5	786.1	795.4	802.5	807.7	811.5	814.2
1937-------	1964	634.1	677.1	709.5	734.4	753.7	769.0	780.9	790.2	797.0	802.0	805.7	
1938-------	1965	630.2	670.5	702.1	726.9	746.7	762.6	774.9	783.9	790.5	795.6		
1939-------	1966	621.7	661.0	692.9	718.6	739.4	755.9	768.1	777.1	784.0			
1940-------	1967	605.6	645.4	678.4	706.2	728.4	744.9	757.2	766.5				
1941-------	1968	584.1	625.4	661.1	690.8	712.9	729.7	742.2					
1942-------	1969	560.9	605.9	644.3	673.8	696.5	713.6						
1943-------	1970	538.4	585.3	622.5	651.8	674.7							
1944-------	1971	518.2	563.2	599.4	629.0								
1945-------	1972	492.5	535.3	572.1									
1946-------	1973	468.2	511.7										
1947-------	1974	444.0											

TABLE 6B. CUMULATIVE BIRTH RATES FOR WHITE WOMEN AS OF THE BEGINNING OF EACH YEAR 1917-74 BY AGE AND LIVE-BIRTH ORDER FOR EACH COHORT FROM 1867 TO 1959--CON.

LIVE-BIRTH ORDER AND COHORT	DIAGONAL LINE FOR JANUARY 1	EXACT AGE											
		39	40	41	42	43	44	45	46	47	48	49	50
SECOND BIRTHS--CON.													
1867-------													701.6
1868-------												697.8	697.8
1869-------											694.0	694.0	694.0
1870-------										690.1	690.2	690.2	690.2
1871-------									686.2	686.4	686.5	686.5	686.5
1872-------								682.0	682.3	682.5	682.6	682.6	682.6
1873-------							677.4	677.9	678.2	678.3	678.4	678.4	678.4
1874-------						672.2	673.0	673.5	673.7	673.9	673.9	673.9	673.9
1875-------					666.9	668.0	668.8	669.2	669.5	669.6	669.7	669.7	669.7
1876-------				661.6	663.4	664.5	665.3	665.8	666.0	666.1	666.2	666.2	666.2
1877-------			656.0	658.6	660.4	661.5	662.3	662.7	662.9	663.0	663.1	663.1	663.1
1878-------	1917	649.1	652.9	655.5	657.3	658.5	659.3	659.7	659.9	660.0	660.0	660.0	660.0
1879-------	1918	645.4	649.2	651.8	653.6	654.8	655.6	656.0	656.2	656.3	656.3	656.3	656.3
1880-------	1919	642.7	646.6	649.3	651.2	652.3	653.1	653.5	653.7	653.8	653.8	653.8	653.8
1881-------	1920	641.3	645.2	647.9	649.7	650.8	651.6	652.0	652.3	652.4	652.4	652.4	652.4
1882-------	1921	640.5	644.5	647.1	648.8	649.9	650.7	651.1	651.3	651.4	651.4	651.4	651.4
1883-------	1922	639.7	643.5	646.0	647.8	649.0	649.7	650.1	650.3	650.4	650.4	650.4	650.4
1884-------	1923	638.9	642.7	645.3	647.0	648.0	648.7	649.1	649.3	649.4	649.4	649.4	649.4
1885-------	1924	637.1	640.9	643.4	645.1	646.2	646.9	647.2	647.4	647.5	647.5	647.5	647.5
1886-------	1925	634.2	637.9	640.4	642.0	643.0	643.6	643.9	644.1	644.2	644.2	644.2	644.2
1887-------	1926	632.2	635.9	638.3	639.9	640.8	641.4	641.8	642.0	642.1	642.1	642.1	642.1
1888-------	1927	636.1	639.6	641.9	643.4	644.3	644.9	645.2	645.4	645.5	645.5	645.5	645.5
1889-------	1928	639.9	643.4	645.7	647.2	648.1	648.7	649.0	649.1	649.2	649.2	649.2	649.2
1890-------	1929	642.7	646.1	648.3	649.8	650.7	651.3	651.6	651.7	651.8	651.8	651.8	651.8
1891-------	1930	640.4	643.8	645.9	647.4	648.3	648.8	649.0	649.1	649.1	649.1	649.1	649.1
1892-------	1931	636.6	639.7	641.8	643.2	644.0	644.5	644.7	644.8	644.8	644.8	644.8	644.8
1893-------	1932	632.3	635.3	637.3	638.5	639.2	639.7	639.9	640.0	640.0	640.0	640.0	640.0
1894-------	1933	629.0	631.9	633.8	635.0	635.8	636.2	636.5	636.6	636.6	636.6	636.6	636.6
1895-------	1934	625.6	628.6	630.5	631.7	632.4	632.9	633.1	633.2	633.3	633.3	633.3	633.3
1896-------	1935	619.7	622.5	624.4	625.6	626.4	626.9	627.1	627.3	627.4	627.4	627.4	627.4
1897-------	1936	613.9	616.7	618.6	620.0	620.8	621.3	621.6	621.8	621.9	621.9	621.9	621.9
1898-------	1937	608.1	610.9	613.0	614.3	615.1	615.6	615.9	616.1	616.2	616.2	616.2	616.2
1899-------	1938	601.2	604.3	606.5	607.9	608.8	609.4	609.8	610.0	610.1	610.1	610.1	610.1
1900-------	1939	589.0	592.3	594.6	596.1	597.0	597.7	598.1	598.3	598.4	598.4	598.4	598.4
1901-------	1940	579.9	583.3	585.7	587.3	588.4	589.1	589.5	589.7	589.8	589.8	589.8	589.8
1902-------	1941	574.4	578.0	580.7	582.6	583.9	584.7	585.2	585.4	585.5	585.5	585.5	585.5
1903-------	1942	571.9	576.0	579.1	581.3	582.8	583.7	584.2	584.4	584.5	584.5	584.5	584.5
1904-------	1943	565.9	570.7	574.2	576.7	578.3	579.3	579.8	580.0	580.1	580.1	580.1	580.1
1905-------	1944	557.8	563.1	566.9	569.6	571.3	572.2	572.7	572.9	573.0	573.0	573.0	573.0
1906-------	1945	552.7	558.4	562.6	565.4	567.0	567.9	568.4	568.6	568.7	568.7	568.7	568.7
1907-------	1946	554.4	560.7	565.0	567.7	569.2	570.1	570.6	570.8	570.9	570.9	570.9	570.9
1908-------	1947	555.9	562.3	566.4	569.0	570.5	571.4	571.9	572.1	572.2	572.2	572.2	572.2
1909-------	1948	561.6	567.6	571.6	574.1	575.6	576.6	577.1	577.3	577.4	577.4	577.4	577.4
1910-------	1949	565.4	571.2	575.1	577.7	579.4	580.4	580.9	581.1	581.2	581.2	581.2	581.2
1911-------	1950	575.3	581.0	585.0	587.6	589.2	590.2	590.7	591.0	591.1	591.1	591.1	591.1
1912-------	1951	585.3	591.1	595.0	597.7	599.3	600.2	600.7	600.9	601.0	601.0	601.0	601.0
1913-------	1952	599.6	605.3	609.3	611.9	613.5	614.5	615.0	615.2	615.3	615.3	615.3	615.3
1914-------	1953	617.0	622.7	626.6	629.1	630.7	631.6	632.0	632.2	632.3	632.3	632.3	632.3
1915-------	1954	634.0	639.5	643.3	645.8	647.3	648.1	648.5	648.7	648.8	648.8	648.8	648.8
1916-------	1955	645.8	651.1	654.6	656.9	658.2	659.0	659.4	659.6	659.7	659.7	659.7	659.7
1917-------	1956	660.3	665.4	668.8	671.0	672.3	673.0	673.4	673.6	673.7	673.7	673.7	673.7
1918-------	1957	672.7	677.5	680.6	682.6	683.8	684.5	684.9	685.1	685.1	685.1	685.1	685.1
1919-------	1958	695.7	700.2	703.1	705.0	706.2	706.9	707.3	707.4	707.4	707.4	707.4	707.4
1920-------	1959	710.8	714.9	717.6	719.4	720.5	721.1	721.4	721.5	721.5	721.5	721.5	721.5
1921-------	1960	725.0	728.7	731.4	733.1	734.1	734.6	734.9	735.0	735.0	735.0	735.0	735.0
1922-------	1961	733.9	737.6	740.0	741.6	742.4	742.9	743.1	743.2	743.2	743.2	743.2	743.2
1923-------	1962	746.6	749.8	752.0	753.4	754.3	754.8	755.0	755.1	755.1	755.1	755.1	755.1
1924-------	1963	759.9	762.9	764.9	766.3	767.1	767.5	767.7	767.8	767.8	767.8	767.8	767.8
1925-------	1964	767.3	770.2	772.1	773.3	774.0	774.4	774.6	774.7	774.7	774.7	774.7	
1926-------	1965	773.3	775.9	777.6	778.7	779.3	779.7	779.9	780.0	780.0	780.0		
1927-------	1966	778.5	780.8	782.3	783.3	783.9	784.2	784.3	784.4	784.4			
1928-------	1967	783.2	785.4	786.9	787.9	788.5	788.8	788.9	789.0				
1929-------	1968	793.2	795.3	796.8	797.7	798.2	798.5	798.6					
1930-------	1969	801.8	803.8	805.1	805.9	806.4	806.6						
1931-------	1970	813.3	815.1	816.3	817.0	817.4							
1932-------	1971	820.4	822.1	823.2	823.8								
1933-------	1972	824.5	826.0	827.0									
1934-------	1973	825.2	826.6										
1935-------	1974	820.8											

TABLE 6B. CUMULATIVE BIRTH RATES FOR WHITE WOMEN AS OF THE BEGINNING OF EACH YEAR 1917-74 BY AGE AND LIVE-BIRTH ORDER FOR EACH COHORT FROM 1867 TO 1959--CON.

LIVE-BIRTH ORDER AND COHORT	DIAGONAL LINE FOR JANUARY 1	EXACT AGE											
		15	16	17	18	19	20	21	22	23	24	25	26
THIRD BIRTHS													
1891-------													182.8
1892-------												143.8	182.8
1893-------											106.8	144.6	182.8
1894-------										71.7	106.7	143.8	179.8
1895-------									43.2	71.7	106.2	141.4	177.5
1896-------								22.1	43.3	71.5	104.3	139.4	175.8
1897-------							9.1	22.3	43.3	70.2	102.6	137.9	171.4
1898-------						2.8	9.2	22.3	42.4	69.1	101.7	134.3	168.9
1899-------					0.6	2.8	9.2	21.7	41.4	67.9	97.4	130.8	166.1
1900-------				0.1	0.7	2.9	9.0	21.2	40.8	64.7	95.5	130.5	164.6
1901-------			0.0	0.1	0.7	2.7	8.5	20.5	37.9	62.6	95.2	129.4	161.5
1902-------	1917	*	0.0	0.1	0.6	2.6	8.7	19.9	38.4	65.3	97.1	129.1	160.3
1903-------	1918	*	0.0	0.1	0.6	2.8	8.4	20.4	40.3	66.9	97.1	128.4	157.9
1904-------	1919	*	0.0	0.1	0.7	2.8	8.9	21.4	40.8	66.1	95.2	124.7	152.5
1905-------	1920	*	0.0	0.1	0.6	3.0	9.3	21.4	39.8	64.1	91.5	119.4	146.9
1906-------	1921	*	0.0	0.1	0.7	3.1	9.2	20.7	38.6	61.7	87.7	115.0	140.6
1907-------	1922	*	0.0	0.1	0.7	3.1	9.0	20.4	37.8	59.8	85.2	110.7	135.5
1908-------	1923	*	0.0	0.1	0.7	3.0	9.0	20.1	36.5	57.8	81.5	106.0	129.2
1909-------	1924	*	0.0	0.1	0.7	3.1	8.9	19.3	35.2	55.4	78.2	101.4	124.9
1910-------	1925	*	0.0	0.1	0.8	3.0	8.4	18.5	33.6	52.9	74.4	97.5	119.3
1911-------	1926	*	0.0	0.2	0.8	2.9	8.2	17.8	32.1	50.4	72.0	93.8	115.0
1912-------	1927	*	0.0	0.1	0.7	2.8	7.7	16.8	30.4	48.5	68.8	89.8	110.6
1913-------	1928	*	0.0	0.1	0.7	2.6	7.2	15.7	29.1	46.2	65.5	86.3	107.9
1914-------	1929	*	0.0	0.1	0.6	2.4	6.7	15.1	27.8	44.2	63.6	85.1	106.2
1915-------	1930	*	0.0	0.1	0.6	2.3	6.5	14.5	26.6	43.1	63.1	84.1	106.1
1916-------	1931	*	0.0	0.1	0.5	2.1	6.1	13.8	26.0	42.9	62.4	84.3	106.7
1917-------	1932	*	0.0	0.1	0.5	2.0	5.8	13.6	26.2	42.7	63.1	85.3	108.7
1918-------	1933	*	0.0	0.1	0.5	2.0	6.0	14.1	26.3	43.6	64.1	87.5	114.1
1919-------	1934	*	0.0	0.1	0.5	2.1	6.4	14.4	27.6	45.2	67.3	93.4	119.9
1920-------	1935	*	0.0	0.1	0.6	2.3	6.5	15.5	28.7	47.0	71.3	97.0	121.1
1921-------	1936	*	0.0	0.1	0.7	2.5	7.7	16.7	30.0	50.0	73.6	96.4	123.3
1922-------	1937	*	0.0	0.1	0.7	3.1	8.0	16.7	31.3	50.9	71.0	96.1	125.3
1923-------	1938	*	0.0	0.1	0.8	3.1	8.0	17.6	32.2	48.7	70.9	98.2	129.4
1924-------	1939	*	0.0	0.2	0.9	3.1	8.5	18.1	30.1	48.3	72.4	102.1	135.9
1925-------	1940	*	0.0	0.2	0.9	3.2	8.4	16.2	29.5	49.2	75.6	107.9	144.3
1926-------	1941	*	0.0	0.2	0.9	3.1	7.3	15.8	30.1	51.7	80.7	115.7	155.8
1927-------	1942	*	0.0	0.2	0.9	2.7	7.2	16.3	32.2	56.6	88.4	126.9	170.0
1928-------	1943	*	0.0	0.2	0.8	2.7	7.5	17.8	36.2	63.4	98.5	139.6	184.4
1929-------	1944	*	0.0	0.2	0.8	2.8	8.3	20.7	41.7	72.2	109.6	153.2	201.3
1930-------	1945	*	0.0	0.2	0.9	3.2	10.2	24.5	48.1	80.3	120.2	167.1	217.9
1931-------	1946	*	0.0	0.2	1.0	4.2	12.3	28.6	53.7	88.3	131.9	181.8	235.9
1932-------	1947	*	0.0	0.2	1.3	4.9	13.9	31.2	57.9	95.5	141.6	195.1	251.9
1933-------	1948	*	0.0	0.3	1.5	5.5	15.3	33.6	62.7	102.4	152.2	208.4	266.2
1934-------	1949	*	0.1	0.4	1.7	6.0	16.3	36.1	66.8	109.5	161.9	219.4	279.0
1935-------	1950	*	0.1	0.4	1.7	6.2	17.1	37.6	70.1	114.8	168.0	227.3	287.7
1936-------	1951	*	0.0	0.3	1.8	6.6	17.9	39.6	74.0	119.6	174.3	234.4	294.2
1937-------	1952	*	0.0	0.3	1.8	6.7	18.7	41.6	76.4	123.3	179.4	239.4	297.0
1938-------	1953	*	0.0	0.3	1.9	7.2	20.0	43.2	79.6	128.2	184.2	242.0	296.8
1939-------	1954	*	0.0	0.3	2.0	7.5	20.4	45.5	83.4	131.8	186.1	240.9	292.3
1940-------	1955	*	0.0	0.4	2.2	7.9	22.1	47.6	84.7	131.7	182.7	233.4	278.2
1941-------	1956	*	0.1	0.5	2.4	8.6	22.8	47.6	83.3	126.6	172.8	215.9	254.9
1942-------	1957	*	0.1	0.5	2.5	8.6	22.1	45.4	77.8	116.4	154.7	191.6	228.4
1943-------	1958	*	0.1	0.5	2.4	8.2	20.8	41.9	70.5	101.9	134.2	168.4	203.1
1944-------	1959	*	0.1	0.5	2.4	7.8	19.4	38.2	61.4	87.7	117.4	149.1	184.1
1945-------	1960	*	0.1	0.5	2.4	7.5	17.8	33.0	52.2	75.8	102.6	133.9	168.4
1946-------	1961	*	0.1	0.5	2.2	6.8	15.1	27.4	44.3	65.2	91.3	122.1	152.6
1947-------	1962	*	0.1	0.5	2.0	5.6	12.2	22.8	37.5	57.6	83.0	110.2	134.8
1948-------	1963	*	0.1	0.4	1.5	4.4	10.1	19.3	33.4	52.8	75.3	97.0	118.4
1949-------	1964	*	0.0	0.3	1.3	3.8	8.7	17.5	30.9	48.4	66.4	85.3	
1950-------	1965	*	0.0	0.2	1.1	3.3	8.1	16.5	28.8	42.6	58.4		
1951-------	1966	*	0.0	0.2	1.0	3.1	7.6	15.3	25.0	37.3			
1952-------	1967	*	0.0	0.2	0.9	2.9	7.0	13.2	21.9				
1953-------	1968	*	0.0	0.2	0.9	2.7	6.1	11.7					
1954-------	1969	*	0.0	0.2	0.8	2.4	5.5						
1955-------	1970	*	0.1	0.3	0.9	2.4							
1956-------	1971	*	0.0	0.2	0.8								
1957-------	1972	*	0.0	0.2									
1958-------	1973	*	0.0										
1959-------	1974	*											

TABLE 6B. CUMULATIVE BIRTH RATES FOR WHITE WOMEN AS OF THE BEGINNING OF EACH YEAR 1917-74 BY AGE AND LIVE-BIRTH ORDER FOR EACH COHORT FROM 1867 TO 1959--CON.

LIVE-BIRTH ORDER AND COHORT	DIAGONAL LINE FOR JANUARY 1	EXACT AGE											
		27	28	29	30	31	32	33	34	35	36	37	38
THIRD BIRTHS--CON.													
1879-------													495.8
1880-------												482.5	491.5
1881-------											467.5	478.4	487.4
1882-------										450.4	463.8	474.6	483.4
1883-------									431.7	447.5	460.6	471.2	480.1
1884-------								410.1	428.8	444.2	457.1	467.9	477.0
1885-------							386.2	406.7	424.9	440.0	453.0	464.1	472.7
1886-------						359.9	384.0	404.1	421.9	437.2	450.6	461.1	469.8
1887-------					330.6	359.0	382.7	402.4	420.5	436.2	449.0	459.7	468.5
1888-------				297.2	331.4	359.2	382.3	402.2	420.6	435.6	448.5	459.2	467.7
1889-------			259.5	296.6	330.1	356.7	380.0	400.2	417.8	432.8	445.9	456.3	464.6
1890-------	1917	220.8	259.2	295.8	327.6	354.5	378.2	397.6	415.3	430.7	443.2	453.4	461.5
1891-------	1918	220.6	258.5	292.8	324.7	351.8	374.5	393.9	412.0	426.7	438.9	448.7	456.5
1892-------	1919	220.0	255.4	289.6	321.4	346.6	369.2	389.0	406.3	420.5	432.2	441.5	448.7
1893-------	1920	217.5	252.7	286.6	315.7	340.6	363.6	382.6	399.1	412.7	423.8	432.5	439.6
1894-------	1921	214.7	250.0	280.8	309.8	335.2	357.4	375.8	391.7	404.8	415.3	424.1	431.0
1895-------	1922	212.9	245.3	276.0	305.5	330.0	351.4	369.2	384.5	397.0	407.7	416.2	422.8
1896-------	1923	208.4	240.8	271.8	300.1	323.9	344.7	361.7	376.3	388.8	399.0	407.1	413.3
1897-------	1924	204.0	236.8	266.7	294.0	316.8	336.4	352.6	367.1	379.0	388.8	396.4	402.7
1898-------	1925	202.4	234.1	262.6	288.6	310.2	329.1	345.3	359.0	370.5	379.7	387.4	393.5
1899-------	1926	198.9	229.2	256.7	281.5	302.3	321.1	336.7	350.3	361.2	370.7	378.4	384.5
1900-------	1927	195.3	224.5	250.4	273.9	294.4	312.3	327.2	339.9	351.1	360.4	367.9	373.9
1901-------	1928	191.6	218.9	243.3	266.3	286.0	303.0	317.1	330.0	340.8	349.8	357.1	363.1
1902-------	1929	188.3	214.0	237.9	259.6	278.1	294.2	308.3	320.5	330.9	339.7	347.0	353.0
1903-------	1930	184.5	210.0	232.8	253.7	271.2	287.4	300.9	312.9	323.1	331.9	339.3	345.4
1904-------	1931	178.8	202.8	225.0	244.8	262.6	278.1	291.3	303.2	313.6	322.6	330.2	336.6
1905-------	1932	171.7	195.2	215.9	235.9	252.8	267.7	280.8	292.8	303.2	312.4	320.3	327.3
1906-------	1933	164.6	186.6	207.7	226.5	242.8	257.6	270.8	282.8	293.5	303.0	311.6	320.0
1907-------	1934	158.2	180.5	200.3	218.6	234.8	249.8	263.1	275.5	286.6	297.1	307.4	316.5
1908-------	1935	151.9	172.6	191.6	209.4	225.7	240.6	254.3	267.1	279.4	291.8	303.0	313.0
1909-------	1936	146.1	166.0	184.7	202.8	219.1	234.6	248.9	263.1	277.7	291.1	303.4	313.9
1910-------	1937	139.8	159.3	178.3	196.2	213.2	229.3	244.9	261.8	277.5	292.3	305.4	316.2
1911-------	1938	135.4	155.6	174.4	193.1	210.7	228.0	246.6	264.6	281.7	297.4	310.7	320.9
1912-------	1939	131.4	151.0	170.5	189.6	208.9	229.5	249.3	268.6	286.8	302.7	315.3	325.4
1913-------	1940	128.2	148.7	168.7	189.9	212.6	234.5	255.6	276.3	294.8	310.1	322.6	332.9
1914-------	1941	127.4	148.5	170.8	195.6	219.2	242.3	265.1	286.4	304.3	319.4	332.3	343.2
1915-------	1942	127.9	150.8	176.8	202.2	226.7	251.9	275.6	296.2	314.0	329.7	343.3	355.1
1916-------	1943	129.4	156.0	182.1	207.7	234.1	260.1	282.9	303.4	321.8	338.3	352.9	364.8
1917-------	1944	135.0	161.7	187.5	215.3	243.1	268.5	291.6	313.0	332.5	350.2	365.1	377.5
1918-------	1945	140.6	166.1	193.7	223.0	250.1	275.9	299.9	322.5	343.4	361.5	376.9	389.0
1919-------	1946	145.0	173.1	203.4	232.8	261.2	288.7	315.0	339.7	361.4	380.2	395.5	407.9
1920-------	1947	148.5	179.2	209.8	240.7	271.0	300.8	329.0	354.7	377.0	395.6	410.9	422.9
1921-------	1948	153.8	185.4	217.9	251.2	284.3	316.8	346.3	372.5	394.8	413.3	428.3	439.7
1922-------	1949	156.8	190.5	225.4	261.4	297.3	330.9	360.9	387.1	409.1	427.2	441.3	452.1
1923-------	1950	163.4	199.5	237.6	277.0	314.3	348.6	378.6	404.5	426.4	443.7	457.2	467.5
1924-------	1951	172.6	212.6	254.4	295.2	333.7	368.2	398.2	424.3	445.1	461.6	474.4	484.3
1925-------	1952	184.7	228.2	271.6	313.9	352.5	387.1	417.1	441.6	461.3	477.0	489.3	498.4
1926-------	1953	199.7	244.5	289.8	332.6	371.3	405.7	434.1	457.4	476.1	491.2	502.4	510.9
1927-------	1954	215.4	262.6	308.7	352.1	391.1	424.3	451.6	473.9	491.9	505.6	516.1	524.1
1928-------	1955	232.4	280.8	327.6	371.4	409.4	441.6	467.8	489.2	505.6	518.6	528.5	535.7
1929-------	1956	251.5	301.9	350.3	393.4	430.9	462.1	487.7	507.5	523.3	535.6	544.6	551.1
1930-------	1957	270.4	322.6	370.3	413.5	450.1	480.6	504.5	523.6	538.6	549.8	558.0	564.1
1931-------	1958	291.1	343.3	391.7	434.3	470.5	499.2	522.1	540.5	554.3	564.4	572.0	577.4
1932-------	1959	307.8	360.9	409.4	451.5	485.5	512.9	534.8	551.6	564.0	573.5	580.4	585.5
1933-------	1960	323.3	377.0	424.7	464.2	496.4	522.9	542.9	558.0	569.5	578.2	584.8	589.7
1934-------	1961	337.0	389.9	434.9	472.6	503.9	528.0	546.0	560.0	570.8	579.2	585.6	590.0
1935-------	1962	344.7	395.0	438.0	474.7	503.1	524.8	541.8	555.1	565.7	573.9	579.6	583.5
1936-------	1963	349.0	397.2	438.8	471.9	497.7	518.2	534.2	547.5	557.9	565.2	570.3	573.8
1937-------	1964	349.4	395.5	432.9	463.1	487.7	507.3	523.9	537.1	546.5	553.1	557.7	
1938-------	1965	346.4	387.6	421.5	450.1	473.7	494.2	510.9	522.9	531.4	537.4		
1939-------	1966	336.3	373.3	405.7	433.8	458.6	479.7	494.9	505.7	513.6			
1940-------	1967	317.1	352.5	384.3	413.6	439.3	458.5	472.0	482.3				
1941-------	1968	291.9	326.4	359.6	390.0	413.5	430.4	443.4					
1942-------	1969	263.9	299.8	333.9	361.5	382.1	398.3						
1943-------	1970	239.7	275.9	306.7	330.4	349.6							
1944-------	1971	220.5	253.0	278.7	300.4								
1945-------	1972	200.8	227.4	250.6									
1946-------	1973	178.8	202.6										
1947-------	1974	157.9											

TABLE 6B. CUMULATIVE BIRTH RATES FOR WHITE WOMEN AS OF THE BEGINNING OF EACH YEAR 1917-74 BY AGE AND LIVE-BIRTH ORDER FOR EACH COHORT FROM 1867 TO 1959--CON.

LIVE-BIRTH ORDER AND COHORT	DIAGONAL LINE FOR JANUARY 1	EXACT AGE											
		39	40	41	42	43	44	45	46	47	48	49	50
THIRD BIRTHS--CON.													
1867-------													582.4
1868-------												577.2	577.2
1869-------											572.0	572.0	572.0
1870-------										566.7	566.8	566.8	566.8
1871-------									561.2	561.4	561.5	561.5	561.5
1872-------								555.5	555.9	556.1	556.2	556.2	556.2
1873-------							549.1	549.8	550.2	550.4	550.5	550.5	550.5
1874-------						542.1	543.2	543.9	544.3	544.5	544.6	544.6	544.6
1875-------					534.6	536.2	537.4	538.1	538.5	538.7	538.8	538.8	538.8
1876-------				526.5	529.1	530.8	531.9	532.6	533.0	533.2	533.3	533.3	533.3
1877-------			517.6	521.3	524.0	525.7	526.9	527.6	528.0	528.2	528.3	528.3	528.3
1878-------	1917	507.4	513.0	516.9	519.5	521.2	522.4	523.1	523.5	523.7	523.8	523.8	523.8
1879-------	1918	502.9	508.6	512.3	515.0	516.7	517.8	518.4	518.8	519.0	519.1	519.1	519.1
1880-------	1919	498.6	504.2	508.0	510.6	512.2	513.3	514.0	514.3	514.5	514.6	514.6	514.6
1881-------	1920	494.4	500.0	503.8	506.3	507.9	509.0	509.6	509.9	510.1	510.2	510.2	510.2
1882-------	1921	490.5	496.2	499.8	502.2	503.8	504.9	505.5	505.8	506.0	506.1	506.1	506.1
1883-------	1922	487.3	492.7	496.2	498.7	500.3	501.3	501.9	502.2	502.4	502.4	502.4	502.4
1884-------	1923	483.8	489.1	492.7	495.2	496.6	497.6	498.1	498.4	498.5	498.6	498.6	498.6
1885-------	1924	479.5	484.9	488.4	490.7	492.2	493.2	493.7	494.0	494.2	494.3	494.3	494.3
1886-------	1925	476.7	481.9	485.3	487.7	489.1	489.9	490.4	490.7	490.8	490.9	490.9	490.9
1887-------	1926	475.2	480.3	483.7	485.9	487.2	488.1	488.6	488.9	489.0	489.0	489.0	489.0
1888-------	1927	474.1	479.1	482.2	484.3	485.7	486.6	487.0	487.2	487.3	487.3	487.3	487.3
1889-------	1928	471.0	475.7	478.8	481.0	482.3	483.1	483.5	483.7	483.8	483.8	483.8	483.8
1890-------	1929	467.7	472.3	475.5	477.5	478.8	479.6	480.0	480.2	480.3	480.3	480.3	480.3
1891-------	1930	462.3	466.8	469.7	471.6	472.8	473.6	474.0	474.2	474.3	474.3	474.3	474.3
1892-------	1931	454.4	458.6	461.3	463.1	464.3	465.0	465.4	465.6	465.7	465.7	465.7	465.7
1893-------	1932	445.0	448.9	451.6	453.4	454.5	455.2	455.6	455.8	455.9	455.9	455.9	455.9
1894-------	1933	436.2	440.0	442.6	444.4	445.5	446.2	446.6	446.8	446.9	446.9	446.9	446.9
1895-------	1934	427.7	431.5	434.1	435.8	436.9	437.6	438.0	438.2	438.3	438.3	438.3	438.3
1896-------	1935	418.2	421.9	424.4	426.1	427.2	427.9	428.3	428.5	428.6	428.6	428.6	428.6
1897-------	1936	407.5	411.2	413.6	415.3	416.4	417.1	417.5	417.7	417.8	417.8	417.8	417.8
1898-------	1937	398.2	401.7	404.3	406.0	407.1	407.8	408.2	408.4	408.5	408.5	408.5	408.5
1899-------	1938	389.2	392.9	395.6	397.3	398.4	399.1	399.5	399.8	399.9	399.9	399.9	399.9
1900-------	1939	378.7	382.5	385.2	387.0	388.1	388.9	389.4	389.7	389.8	389.9	389.9	389.9
1901-------	1940	368.0	371.7	374.4	376.3	377.6	378.6	379.2	379.5	379.7	379.7	379.7	379.7
1902-------	1941	357.9	361.7	364.6	366.8	368.3	369.3	369.9	370.2	370.3	370.3	370.3	370.3
1903-------	1942	350.4	354.6	357.9	360.4	362.1	363.2	363.8	364.1	364.2	364.2	364.2	364.2
1904-------	1943	342.1	347.0	350.7	353.4	355.2	356.4	357.0	357.3	357.4	357.4	357.4	357.4
1905-------	1944	333.8	339.1	343.2	346.0	347.8	348.9	349.5	349.8	349.9	349.9	349.9	349.9
1906-------	1945	327.1	333.0	337.2	340.1	341.9	343.0	343.5	343.8	343.9	343.9	343.9	343.9
1907-------	1946	324.4	330.5	334.8	337.7	339.4	340.5	341.1	341.4	341.5	341.5	341.5	341.5
1908-------	1947	321.2	327.5	331.7	334.4	336.1	337.2	337.8	338.1	338.2	338.2	338.2	338.2
1909-------	1948	322.3	328.3	332.4	335.2	337.0	338.2	338.9	339.2	339.3	339.3	339.3	339.3
1910-------	1949	324.1	330.1	334.3	337.2	339.2	340.4	341.1	341.4	341.6	341.6	341.6	341.6
1911-------	1950	328.8	334.8	339.2	342.4	344.4	345.7	346.4	346.8	346.9	346.9	346.9	346.9
1912-------	1951	333.4	339.7	344.5	347.7	349.9	351.2	352.0	352.3	352.4	352.4	352.4	352.4
1913-------	1952	341.4	348.2	353.0	356.5	358.7	360.1	360.8	361.1	361.2	361.2	361.2	361.2
1914-------	1953	352.4	359.4	364.5	368.0	370.3	371.6	372.3	372.6	372.7	372.7	372.7	372.7
1915-------	1954	364.4	371.6	376.8	380.4	382.6	383.8	384.5	384.8	384.9	385.0	385.0	385.0
1916-------	1955	374.3	381.6	386.6	390.0	392.0	393.2	393.9	394.2	394.4	394.4	394.4	394.4
1917-------	1956	387.2	394.4	399.5	402.7	404.7	405.9	406.5	406.8	406.9	406.9	406.9	406.9
1918-------	1957	398.5	405.5	410.2	413.3	415.3	416.5	417.1	417.4	417.5	417.5	417.5	417.5
1919-------	1958	417.4	424.2	428.9	431.9	433.8	434.9	435.5	435.8	435.9	435.9	435.9	435.9
1920-------	1959	431.8	438.4	442.9	445.9	447.7	448.7	449.2	449.4	449.5	449.5	449.5	449.5
1921-------	1960	448.3	454.6	458.9	461.7	463.4	464.3	464.8	465.0	465.1	465.1	465.1	465.1
1922-------	1961	460.2	466.2	470.2	472.8	474.3	475.2	475.6	475.8	475.9	475.9	475.9	475.9
1923-------	1962	475.3	480.8	484.5	487.0	488.5	489.3	489.7	489.9	489.9	489.9	489.9	489.9
1924-------	1963	491.4	496.6	500.1	502.3	503.6	504.3	504.7	504.8	504.9	504.9	504.9	504.9
1925-------	1964	505.1	510.0	513.2	515.2	516.3	516.9	517.2	517.3	517.3	517.3	517.3	
1926-------	1965	517.2	521.6	524.5	526.3	527.3	527.9	528.2	528.3	528.4	528.4		
1927-------	1966	529.8	533.8	536.5	538.1	539.1	539.6	539.8	539.9	539.9			
1928-------	1967	540.8	544.5	546.8	548.3	549.2	549.6	549.8	549.9				
1929-------	1968	555.9	559.1	561.2	562.6	563.3	563.7	563.9					
1930-------	1969	568.4	571.4	573.4	574.5	575.1	575.4						
1931-------	1970	581.3	584.1	585.8	586.8	587.3							
1932-------	1971	589.2	591.6	593.1	593.9								
1933-------	1972	593.0	595.1	596.3									
1934-------	1973	593.0	594.9										
1935-------	1974	586.1											

TABLE 6B. CUMULATIVE BIRTH RATES FOR WHITE WOMEN AS OF THE BEGINNING OF EACH YEAR 1917-74 BY AGE AND LIVE-BIRTH ORDER FOR EACH COHORT FROM 1867 TO 1959--CON.

LIVE-BIRTH ORDER AND COHORT	DIAGONAL LINE FOR JANUARY 1	EXACT AGE											
		15	16	17	18	19	20	21	22	23	24	25	26
FOURTH BIRTHS													
1891-------													80.2
1892-------												55.3	79.2
1893-------											35.6	55.1	78.8
1894-------										19.6	34.2	53.7	76.4
1895-------									9.6	18.8	33.6	52.6	75.4
1896-------								3.9	9.1	18.4	32.9	52.0	75.2
1897-------							1.2	3.7	9.0	18.1	32.6	52.2	73.6
1898-------						0.0	1.0	3.6	8.8	18.0	33.1	51.2	72.6
1899-------					0.0	0.2	1.2	3.7	8.9	18.4	32.1	50.1	70.8
1900-------				0.0	0.0	0.2	1.1	3.6	9.0	17.5	31.4	49.1	69.3
1901-------			0.0	0.0	0.0	0.2	1.1	3.6	8.3	16.8	30.4	47.8	67.6
1902-------	1917	*	0.0	0.0	0.0	0.2	1.1	3.4	8.3	17.0	30.5	47.8	67.8
1903-------	1918	*	0.0	0.0	0.0	0.2	1.1	3.5	8.4	17.4	31.2	48.7	67.2
1904-------	1919	*	0.0	0.0	0.0	0.3	1.3	3.7	8.8	18.1	31.8	47.9	65.3
1905-------	1920	*	0.0	0.0	0.1	0.4	1.3	3.8	9.1	18.1	30.6	45.7	62.5
1906-------	1921	*	0.0	0.0	0.1	0.4	1.3	3.8	8.9	17.0	28.7	43.4	59.0
1907-------	1922	*	0.0	0.0	0.1	0.4	1.4	3.8	8.4	16.1	27.5	41.1	56.1
1908-------	1923	*	0.0	0.0	0.0	0.3	1.3	3.5	7.9	15.5	26.1	39.1	52.9
1909-------	1924	*	0.0	0.0	0.1	0.4	1.3	3.4	7.8	14.9	25.1	37.0	51.1
1910-------	1925	*	0.0	0.0	0.1	0.4	1.3	3.4	7.5	14.3	23.6	35.8	48.9
1911-------	1926	*	0.0	0.0	0.1	0.4	1.3	3.2	7.0	13.3	22.7	34.2	46.8
1912-------	1927	*	0.0	0.0	0.1	0.4	1.2	3.0	6.6	12.8	21.7	32.6	44.7
1913-------	1928	*	0.0	0.0	0.1	0.3	1.0	2.7	6.2	12.2	20.7	31.3	43.2
1914-------	1929	*	0.0	0.0	0.0	0.2	0.8	2.5	5.9	11.6	19.9	30.3	41.6
1915-------	1930	*	0.0	0.0	0.0	0.2	0.8	2.5	5.8	11.3	19.4	29.4	41.0
1916-------	1931	*	0.0	0.0	0.0	0.2	0.8	2.4	5.6	11.1	19.0	29.6	41.3
1917-------	1932	*	0.0	0.0	0.0	0.2	0.8	2.3	5.4	10.7	19.3	29.9	41.5
1918-------	1933	*	0.0	0.0	0.0	0.2	0.8	2.3	5.3	11.2	19.8	30.2	43.1
1919-------	1934	*	0.0	0.0	0.0	0.2	0.8	2.3	5.7	11.6	20.3	31.8	44.8
1920-------	1935	*	0.0	0.0	0.0	0.1	0.7	2.4	5.7	11.8	21.3	32.9	45.0
1921-------	1936	*	0.0	0.0	0.0	0.2	0.9	2.6	6.3	12.9	22.5	33.2	46.2
1922-------	1937	*	0.0	0.0	0.0	0.3	1.0	2.8	6.8	13.6	22.1	33.3	45.7
1923-------	1938	*	0.0	0.0	0.1	0.4	1.2	3.2	7.3	13.2	22.0	32.7	45.3
1924-------	1939	*	0.0	0.0	0.1	0.4	1.3	3.4	6.9	13.0	21.4	32.4	46.1
1925-------	1940	*	0.0	0.0	0.1	0.4	1.3	3.1	6.7	12.5	21.2	33.4	48.2
1926-------	1941	*	0.0	0.0	0.1	0.4	1.1	3.0	6.4	12.5	22.3	35.4	52.0
1927-------	1942	*	0.0	0.0	0.1	0.3	1.1	2.9	6.6	13.6	24.1	38.8	57.2
1928-------	1943	*	0.0	0.0	0.0	0.2	0.9	2.8	7.1	14.7	26.9	43.3	63.1
1929-------	1944	*	0.0	0.0	0.0	0.2	1.0	3.4	8.2	17.3	31.0	49.0	70.8
1930-------	1945	*	0.0	0.0	0.0	0.3	1.4	4.1	10.0	20.2	35.1	54.8	78.3
1931-------	1946	*	0.0	0.0	0.1	0.5	1.7	5.0	11.7	23.0	39.6	61.0	86.8
1932-------	1947	*	0.0	0.0	0.1	0.5	1.9	5.6	12.8	25.1	42.8	66.1	94.2
1933-------	1948	*	0.0	0.0	0.1	0.6	2.3	6.3	14.3	27.5	46.7	72.0	101.3
1934-------	1949	*	0.0	0.0	0.1	0.7	2.4	6.8	15.3	29.5	50.2	76.5	107.7
1935-------	1950	*	0.0	0.0	0.1	0.6	2.5	7.2	16.3	31.3	52.7	80.2	112.5
1936-------	1951	*	0.0	0.0	0.1	0.7	2.7	7.7	17.2	32.9	55.3	83.9	116.7
1937-------	1952	*	0.0	0.0	0.1	0.7	2.8	7.9	17.9	34.2	57.7	87.0	119.3
1938-------	1953	*	0.0	0.0	0.1	0.7	2.9	8.3	18.8	36.0	60.1	88.9	119.4
1939-------	1954	*	0.0	0.0	0.1	0.8	3.1	8.8	19.9	37.6	61.3	88.4	116.5
1940-------	1955	*	0.0	0.0	0.2	1.0	3.5	9.5	20.9	38.2	60.1	84.6	108.1
1941-------	1956	*	0.0	0.0	0.2	1.0	3.6	9.7	20.6	36.3	55.7	75.8	94.8
1942-------	1957	*	0.0	0.0	0.2	1.0	3.6	9.3	19.0	32.6	48.1	64.0	80.4
1943-------	1958	*	0.0	0.0	0.2	1.0	3.4	8.5	16.9	27.8	40.0	53.8	68.5
1944-------	1959	*	0.0	0.0	0.2	0.9	3.1	7.6	14.3	23.0	33.7	45.8	60.0
1945-------	1960	*	0.0	0.0	0.2	0.9	2.9	6.5	11.9	19.4	28.6	40.1	53.5
1946-------	1961	*	0.0	0.0	0.2	0.9	2.5	5.4	10.0	16.2	24.8	35.4	46.8
1947-------	1962	*	0.0	0.0	0.2	0.7	1.9	4.2	7.9	13.6	21.3	30.3	38.9
1948-------	1963	*	0.0	0.0	0.1	0.4	1.4	3.3	6.7	11.8	18.4	25.3	32.3
1949-------	1964	*	0.0	0.0	0.1	0.4	1.3	3.1	6.2	10.7	15.9	21.6	
1950-------	1965	*	0.0	0.0	0.1	0.4	1.2	2.8	5.4	8.9	13.1		
1951-------	1966	*	0.0	0.0	0.1	0.4	1.1	2.4	4.5	7.3			
1952-------	1967	*	0.0	0.0	0.1	0.3	0.8	1.9	3.6				
1953-------	1968	*	0.0	0.0	0.1	0.3	0.8	1.7					
1954-------	1969	*	0.0	0.0	0.0	0.2	0.6						
1955-------	1970	*	0.0	0.0	0.0	0.1							
1956-------	1971	*	0.0	0.0	0.0								
1957-------	1972	*	0.0	0.0									
1958-------	1973	*	0.0										
1959-------	1974	*											

TABLE 6B. CUMULATIVE BIRTH RATES FOR WHITE WOMEN AS OF THE BEGINNING OF EACH YEAR 1917-74 BY AGE AND LIVE-BIRTH ORDER FOR EACH COHORT FROM 1867 TO 1959--CON.

LIVE-BIRTH ORDER AND COHORT	DIAGONAL LINE FOR JANUARY 1	EXACT AGE											
		27	28	29	30	31	32	33	34	35	36	37	38
FOURTH BIRTHS--CON.													
1879-------													372.2
1880-------												357.0	367.8
1881-------											339.2	351.7	362.5
1882-------										319.2	334.1	346.6	357.0
1883-------									298.7	315.6	330.3	342.4	352.7
1884-------								276.1	295.3	311.9	326.0	338.0	348.5
1885-------							251.9	272.1	290.8	306.7	320.7	332.9	342.6
1886-------						226.2	249.0	268.9	286.9	302.8	317.3	328.7	338.5
1887-------					198.7	224.0	246.4	265.6	283.6	300.1	313.5	325.0	334.7
1888-------				169.2	198.2	223.1	244.6	263.7	282.3	297.3	310.7	322.1	331.7
1889-------			137.7	167.2	195.7	219.5	240.8	260.4	277.2	292.2	305.5	316.7	325.9
1890-------	1917	107.4	136.2	165.4	192.7	216.4	238.5	256.3	273.1	288.0	300.8	311.5	320.4
1891-------	1918	106.4	135.0	162.9	190.0	214.0	233.9	251.7	268.4	282.8	295.3	305.6	313.9
1892-------	1919	105.1	132.2	159.9	187.0	208.6	228.4	245.9	261.9	275.7	287.6	297.2	304.9
1893-------	1920	103.4	130.3	157.5	181.9	203.0	222.6	239.5	254.8	268.1	279.1	288.0	295.6
1894-------	1921	101.0	127.7	152.5	176.3	197.1	215.9	232.1	247.0	259.4	269.7	278.6	285.9
1895-------	1922	100.1	124.7	148.8	172.1	192.0	210.1	225.8	239.7	251.3	261.6	270.1	277.1
1896-------	1923	98.0	122.0	145.3	167.4	186.6	204.1	218.7	231.6	243.1	252.8	260.9	267.5
1897-------	1924	95.9	119.1	141.2	162.5	181.0	197.3	211.1	223.9	234.7	244.0	251.7	258.3
1898-------	1925	94.5	116.8	138.4	159.1	176.4	191.7	205.4	217.4	227.7	236.5	244.1	250.3
1899-------	1926	92.1	114.0	135.3	154.7	171.1	186.4	199.4	211.2	221.2	230.2	237.5	243.5
1900-------	1927	90.1	111.9	131.5	149.5	165.6	180.0	192.6	203.8	213.8	222.3	229.2	235.0
1901-------	1928	88.6	108.5	126.6	144.2	159.4	173.1	185.0	196.2	205.6	213.6	220.3	226.1
1902-------	1929	87.0	105.4	123.1	139.7	154.1	167.0	178.7	189.1	197.9	205.6	212.3	217.8
1903-------	1930	85.1	103.0	119.8	135.6	149.3	162.2	173.1	182.8	191.3	198.9	205.3	210.6
1904-------	1931	82.8	99.9	116.2	131.4	145.1	157.2	167.5	176.9	185.2	192.6	198.9	204.4
1905-------	1932	78.9	95.4	111.0	126.0	138.8	150.1	160.1	169.2	177.3	184.5	190.9	196.6
1906-------	1933	74.8	90.4	105.5	119.5	131.5	142.4	152.1	161.0	169.0	176.3	182.7	189.2
1907-------	1934	70.9	86.3	100.4	113.5	125.1	135.7	145.1	154.0	162.1	169.6	177.0	183.9
1908-------	1935	67.7	81.9	95.1	107.5	118.7	128.9	138.3	147.1	155.5	164.0	171.8	179.0
1909-------	1936	64.9	78.4	91.1	103.5	114.3	124.6	134.1	143.4	152.9	161.9	170.3	177.7
1910-------	1937	62.0	74.9	87.5	99.2	110.1	120.4	130.2	140.8	150.8	160.3	168.8	176.4
1911-------	1938	59.5	72.4	84.4	96.2	107.2	117.8	129.0	140.1	150.6	160.5	169.5	176.9
1912-------	1939	57.2	69.3	81.2	93.0	104.4	116.4	128.1	139.4	150.3	160.5	169.1	176.5
1913-------	1940	54.9	67.0	79.1	91.3	104.1	116.6	128.6	140.6	151.9	161.8	170.5	178.2
1914-------	1941	53.4	65.7	78.3	91.9	105.0	117.7	130.4	142.7	153.8	164.0	173.2	181.4
1915-------	1942	52.9	65.5	79.5	93.4	106.6	120.1	133.1	145.3	156.9	167.7	177.7	186.7
1916-------	1943	53.4	67.5	81.6	95.2	109.1	122.9	135.7	148.4	160.5	172.1	182.8	192.4
1917-------	1944	55.0	69.1	82.8	97.3	111.4	125.0	138.5	151.8	164.8	177.3	188.9	199.2
1918-------	1945	56.7	70.1	84.4	98.9	112.7	126.9	140.8	154.9	168.9	182.2	194.3	204.7
1919-------	1946	57.8	72.2	86.7	101.2	116.2	131.3	146.7	162.6	177.8	192.1	204.7	215.5
1920-------	1947	58.8	73.1	87.5	103.1	119.0	135.6	152.9	169.9	186.2	200.9	213.7	224.7
1921-------	1948	59.8	74.1	89.9	106.7	124.3	143.1	161.5	179.9	196.9	212.0	225.4	236.3
1922-------	1949	59.2	74.5	91.1	109.5	129.1	149.0	168.9	187.9	205.3	221.0	234.1	245.0
1923-------	1950	59.9	76.2	94.9	115.3	136.1	157.6	178.3	198.0	216.2	231.8	244.9	255.6
1924-------	1951	61.8	80.4	101.0	122.9	145.7	168.3	190.2	210.8	228.9	244.4	257.4	267.7
1925-------	1952	65.9	86.3	108.5	132.4	156.4	180.1	202.7	223.3	241.3	256.7	269.2	278.9
1926-------	1953	71.6	93.7	118.0	143.3	168.7	193.3	215.9	236.4	254.4	269.3	281.1	290.4
1927-------	1954	78.5	102.5	128.2	155.0	181.4	206.3	229.2	249.6	267.0	281.0	292.3	301.2
1928-------	1955	86.2	111.7	139.0	167.1	194.0	219.6	242.5	262.6	279.0	292.6	303.5	311.7
1929-------	1956	95.6	123.0	152.2	181.3	209.5	235.3	258.5	277.7	293.8	307.0	317.0	324.3
1930-------	1957	105.2	134.8	165.2	195.8	224.4	250.7	272.7	291.6	307.3	319.3	328.2	334.9
1931-------	1958	116.1	147.2	179.4	210.8	240.1	265.4	287.2	305.6	319.8	330.5	338.9	345.1
1932-------	1959	125.0	158.2	191.5	223.3	251.5	276.2	297.2	313.9	326.5	336.5	344.1	349.8
1933-------	1960	134.2	168.7	202.5	233.5	261.0	284.8	303.6	318.2	330.1	339.3	346.5	351.9
1934-------	1961	141.8	176.6	209.5	239.5	266.0	287.3	303.9	317.5	328.3	337.1	343.9	348.9
1935-------	1962	147.1	181.2	213.1	241.9	265.2	283.9	299.3	311.7	322.2	330.6	336.8	341.0
1936-------	1963	150.6	183.4	213.8	239.1	259.6	276.7	290.7	302.9	313.0	320.5	325.7	329.3
1937-------	1964	151.7	182.6	208.9	230.8	249.6	265.4	279.5	291.5	300.5	306.9	311.5	
1938-------	1965	149.6	176.0	198.5	218.6	236.0	251.9	265.7	276.5	284.2	289.8		
1939-------	1966	142.2	164.6	185.2	203.8	221.3	237.1	249.7	259.0	265.8			
1940-------	1967	129.4	149.5	168.5	187.3	204.8	219.1	229.7	237.7				
1941-------	1968	113.5	131.9	151.0	169.5	185.2	197.1	206.3					
1942-------	1969	97.3	115.6	134.1	150.6	163.2	173.4						
1943-------	1970	85.0	102.5	118.8	131.9	142.7							
1944-------	1971	75.8	91.1	103.8	114.8								
1945-------	1972	67.1	78.9	89.5									
1946-------	1973	57.1	66.7										
1947-------	1974	47.3											

TABLE 6B. CUMULATIVE BIRTH RATES FOR WHITE WOMEN AS OF THE BEGINNING OF EACH YEAR 1917-74 BY AGE AND LIVE-BIRTH ORDER FOR EACH COHORT FROM 1867 TO 1959--CON.

LIVE-BIRTH ORDER AND COHORT	DIAGONAL LINE FOR JANUARY 1	EXACT AGE											
		39	40	41	42	43	44	45	46	47	48	49	50
FOURTH BIRTHS--CON.													
1867-------													473.7
1868-------												467.8	467.9
1869-------											461.9	462.0	462.1
1870-------										455.9	456.1	456.2	456.3
1871-------									449.6	449.9	450.1	450.2	450.3
1872-------								442.8	443.4	443.7	443.8	443.9	444.0
1873-------							435.5	436.4	437.0	437.3	437.5	437.6	437.7
1874-------						427.4	429.0	429.9	430.4	430.7	430.8	430.9	430.9
1875-------					418.5	420.7	422.3	423.2	423.8	424.1	424.2	424.3	424.3
1876-------				408.6	412.0	414.2	415.8	416.8	417.3	417.6	417.7	417.8	417.8
1877-------			397.5	402.4	405.8	408.0	409.6	410.5	411.0	411.3	411.4	411.5	411.5
1878-------	1917	385.4	392.4	397.2	400.6	402.9	404.5	405.4	405.9	406.2	406.3	406.3	406.3
1879-------	1918	381.0	388.0	392.8	396.3	398.5	400.0	400.9	401.4	401.7	401.8	401.9	401.9
1880-------	1919	376.6	383.5	388.3	391.7	393.9	395.4	396.3	396.8	397.1	397.2	397.2	397.2
1881-------	1920	371.0	377.8	382.6	385.9	388.0	389.5	390.3	390.7	390.9	391.0	391.0	391.0
1882-------	1921	365.4	372.3	376.8	380.0	382.1	383.5	384.3	384.7	384.9	385.0	385.0	385.0
1883-------	1922	361.2	367.6	372.0	375.2	377.2	378.5	379.2	379.6	379.8	379.9	379.9	379.9
1884-------	1923	356.4	362.8	367.2	370.3	372.3	373.5	374.2	374.6	374.8	374.9	374.9	374.9
1885-------	1924	350.5	356.8	361.2	364.1	365.9	367.1	367.8	368.2	368.4	368.5	368.5	368.5
1886-------	1925	346.4	352.7	356.8	359.6	361.3	362.4	363.1	363.4	363.6	363.7	363.7	363.7
1887-------	1926	342.6	348.6	352.6	355.3	357.0	358.2	358.8	359.2	359.4	359.5	359.5	359.5
1888-------	1927	339.1	344.9	348.7	351.3	353.0	354.1	354.7	355.0	355.2	355.3	355.3	355.3
1889-------	1928	333.1	338.6	342.2	344.8	346.4	347.5	348.1	348.4	348.6	348.7	348.7	348.7
1890-------	1929	327.2	332.4	336.1	338.5	340.1	341.1	341.7	342.0	342.1	342.2	342.2	342.2
1891-------	1930	320.2	325.4	328.8	331.2	332.7	333.7	334.3	334.6	334.8	334.9	334.9	334.9
1892-------	1931	311.3	316.1	319.3	321.5	323.0	324.0	324.5	324.8	325.0	325.0	325.0	325.0
1893-------	1932	301.6	306.2	309.3	311.5	312.9	313.8	314.3	314.6	314.7	314.7	314.7	314.7
1894-------	1933	291.5	295.9	299.1	301.2	302.5	303.4	303.9	304.2	304.3	304.3	304.3	304.3
1895-------	1934	282.5	286.9	289.8	291.8	293.1	294.0	294.5	294.8	294.9	294.9	294.9	294.9
1896-------	1935	272.9	277.0	279.8	281.8	283.1	284.0	284.5	284.7	284.8	284.9	284.9	284.9
1897-------	1936	263.4	267.3	270.1	272.0	273.3	274.1	274.5	274.7	274.8	274.9	274.9	274.9
1898-------	1937	255.2	259.0	261.7	263.7	265.0	265.8	266.3	266.6	266.8	266.9	266.9	266.9
1899-------	1938	248.3	252.0	254.7	256.6	257.9	258.7	259.2	259.5	259.6	259.7	259.7	259.7
1900-------	1939	239.7	243.4	246.0	247.9	249.1	250.0	250.6	250.9	251.1	251.1	251.1	251.1
1901-------	1940	230.6	234.0	236.6	238.5	239.9	240.9	241.5	241.8	241.9	241.9	241.9	241.9
1902-------	1941	222.1	225.6	228.3	230.5	232.0	233.1	233.7	234.0	234.1	234.1	234.1	234.1
1903-------	1942	215.0	218.8	221.9	224.1	225.7	226.7	227.3	227.6	227.7	227.8	227.8	227.8
1904-------	1943	209.1	213.4	216.6	219.1	220.7	221.7	222.3	222.6	222.8	222.8	222.8	222.8
1905-------	1944	202.0	206.5	209.9	212.3	214.0	215.0	215.6	215.9	216.0	216.0	216.0	216.0
1906-------	1945	194.9	199.7	203.2	205.8	207.4	208.4	209.0	209.3	209.4	209.5	209.5	209.5
1907-------	1946	189.9	194.8	198.5	201.0	202.6	203.6	204.2	204.5	204.7	204.8	204.8	204.8
1908-------	1947	185.1	190.0	193.5	195.9	197.5	198.6	199.2	199.5	199.7	199.7	199.7	199.7
1909-------	1948	183.9	188.7	192.2	194.7	196.4	197.5	198.2	198.5	198.6	198.7	198.7	198.7
1910-------	1949	182.5	187.3	190.8	193.4	195.2	196.5	197.1	197.4	197.6	197.6	197.6	197.6
1911-------	1950	183.0	187.9	191.7	194.5	196.5	197.7	198.4	198.7	198.8	198.9	198.9	198.9
1912-------	1951	182.8	187.9	192.0	195.0	197.0	198.3	199.0	199.4	199.6	199.7	199.7	199.7
1913-------	1952	184.9	190.6	195.0	198.2	200.3	201.6	202.4	202.8	203.0	203.1	203.1	203.1
1914-------	1953	188.7	194.7	199.4	202.7	204.8	206.2	207.0	207.4	207.6	207.6	207.6	207.6
1915-------	1954	194.5	201.0	205.8	209.2	211.5	212.9	213.7	214.1	214.3	214.4	214.4	214.4
1916-------	1955	200.7	207.3	212.0	215.5	217.7	219.1	219.9	220.3	220.5	220.5	220.5	220.5
1917-------	1956	207.8	214.5	219.6	223.0	225.3	226.6	227.4	227.8	227.9	227.9	227.9	227.9
1918-------	1957	213.2	220.1	224.9	228.3	230.5	231.9	232.6	232.9	233.0	233.0	233.0	233.0
1919-------	1958	224.4	231.1	236.0	239.4	241.7	243.1	243.8	244.1	244.2	244.2	244.2	244.2
1920-------	1959	233.4	240.2	245.1	248.6	250.8	252.0	252.7	253.0	253.1	253.1	253.1	253.1
1921-------	1960	245.1	251.9	256.8	260.1	262.1	263.3	263.9	264.2	264.3	264.3	264.3	264.3
1922-------	1961	253.5	260.0	264.6	267.6	269.4	270.5	271.1	271.4	271.5	271.5	271.5	271.5
1923-------	1962	263.9	270.0	274.2	277.0	278.8	279.8	280.4	280.6	280.7	280.7	280.7	280.7
1924-------	1963	275.6	281.4	285.5	288.2	289.8	290.8	291.3	291.5	291.6	291.6	291.6	291.6
1925-------	1964	286.3	292.0	295.8	298.1	299.6	300.4	300.8	301.0	301.1	301.1	301.1	
1926-------	1965	297.7	302.8	306.2	308.5	309.8	310.5	310.9	311.0	311.0	311.0		
1927-------	1966	307.7	312.3	315.4	317.3	318.4	319.1	319.4	319.5	319.5			
1928-------	1967	317.6	321.8	324.5	326.2	327.3	327.8	328.0	328.1				
1929-------	1968	329.7	333.4	336.0	337.6	338.5	339.0	339.2					
1930-------	1969	339.8	343.3	345.7	347.0	347.8	348.2						
1931-------	1970	349.7	353.0	355.0	356.2	356.8							
1932-------	1971	354.1	356.9	358.6	359.6								
1933-------	1972	355.7	358.1	359.6									
1934-------	1973	352.2	354.3										
1935-------	1974	343.8											

TABLE 6B. CUMULATIVE BIRTH RATES FOR WHITE WOMEN AS OF THE BEGINNING OF EACH YEAR 1917-74 BY AGE AND LIVE-BIRTH ORDER FOR EACH COHORT FROM 1867 TO 1959--CON.

LIVE-BIRTH ORDER AND COHORT	DIAGONAL LINE FOR JANUARY 1	EXACT AGE											
		15	16	17	18	19	20	21	22	23	24	25	26
FIFTH BIRTHS													
1891-------													28.7
1892-------												16.9	28.3
1893-------											9.2	16.9	27.9
1894-------										4.1	8.8	16.2	26.8
1895-------									1.7	4.0	8.4	15.6	26.4
1896-------								0.5	1.6	3.8	8.1	15.5	26.7
1897-------							*	0.5	1.5	3.6	8.1	15.9	26.2
1898-------						*	*	0.4	1.4	3.6	8.4	15.6	26.2
1899-------					*	*	*	0.4	1.5	3.9	8.3	15.8	26.0
1900-------				*	*	*	*	0.5	1.6	3.8	8.5	15.7	25.4
1901-------			*	*	*	*	*	0.5	1.5	3.7	8.1	14.9	24.3
1902-------	1917	*	*	*	*	*	*	0.4	1.5	3.8	8.0	14.8	24.1
1903-------	1918	*	*	*	*	*	*	0.5	1.6	3.8	8.2	15.0	23.9
1904-------	1919	*	*	*	*	*	*	0.5	1.6	4.0	8.3	14.8	23.4
1905-------	1920	*	*	*	*	*	*	0.5	1.7	4.0	8.1	14.3	22.5
1906-------	1921	*	*	*	*	*	*	0.5	1.6	3.8	7.7	13.6	21.2
1907-------	1922	*	*	*	*	*	*	0.5	1.6	3.6	7.3	12.7	19.8
1908-------	1923	*	*	*	*	*	*	0.4	1.4	3.3	6.7	11.8	18.3
1909-------	1924	*	*	*	*	*	*	0.4	1.4	3.2	6.4	11.0	17.6
1910-------	1925	*	*	*	*	*	*	0.4	1.3	3.0	5.9	10.6	16.8
1911-------	1926	*	*	*	*	*	*	0.4	1.2	2.8	5.7	10.3	16.1
1912-------	1927	*	*	*	*	*	*	0.3	1.1	2.6	5.5	9.7	15.3
1913-------	1928	*	*	*	*	*	*	0.3	1.0	2.5	5.2	9.2	14.7
1914-------	1929	*	*	*	*	*	*	0.3	1.0	2.4	5.0	9.1	14.2
1915-------	1930	*	*	*	*	*	*	0.3	1.0	2.4	5.0	8.8	14.1
1916-------	1931	*	*	*	*	*	*	0.3	1.0	2.4	4.9	9.0	14.2
1917-------	1932	*	*	*	*	*	*	0.3	1.0	2.3	5.1	9.1	14.3
1918-------	1933	*	*	*	*	*	*	0.3	0.9	2.4	5.2	9.2	14.9
1919-------	1934	*	*	*	*	*	*	0.3	1.0	2.5	5.3	9.7	15.5
1920-------	1935	*	*	*	*	*	*	0.3	1.0	2.6	5.6	10.1	15.6
1921-------	1936	*	*	*	*	*	*	0.3	1.1	2.8	5.9	10.2	15.8
1922-------	1937	*	*	*	*	*	*	0.3	1.2	3.0	5.8	10.0	15.4
1923-------	1938	*	*	*	*	*	*	0.4	1.3	2.9	5.7	9.7	15.1
1924-------	1939	*	*	*	*	*	*	0.4	1.2	2.8	5.5	9.6	15.1
1925-------	1940	*	*	*	*	*	*	0.4	1.2	2.7	5.5	9.8	15.5
1926-------	1941	*	*	*	*	*	*	0.4	1.2	2.8	5.8	10.2	16.6
1927-------	1942	*	*	*	*	*	*	0.4	1.2	3.0	6.1	11.1	18.2
1928-------	1943	*	*	*	*	*	*	0.4	1.4	3.3	6.8	12.4	20.0
1929-------	1944	*	*	*	*	*	*	0.5	1.5	3.7	7.8	14.1	22.7
1930-------	1945	*	*	*	*	*	*	0.4	1.6	4.2	8.8	15.9	25.3
1931-------	1946	*	*	*	*	*	*	0.5	2.0	5.0	10.2	17.9	28.4
1932-------	1947	*	*	*	*	*	*	0.6	2.2	5.5	11.2	19.7	31.0
1933-------	1948	*	*	*	*	*	*	0.7	2.5	6.1	12.2	21.3	33.5
1934-------	1949	*	*	*	*	*	*	0.8	2.8	6.6	13.1	22.9	35.6
1935-------	1950	*	*	*	*	*	*	0.8	2.9	7.0	14.0	24.1	37.5
1936-------	1951	*	*	*	*	*	*	0.9	3.2	7.5	14.7	25.4	39.6
1937-------	1952	*	*	*	*	*	*	0.9	3.2	7.7	15.5	26.8	40.7
1938-------	1953	*	*	*	*	*	*	1.0	3.4	8.2	16.0	27.1	40.2
1939-------	1954	*	*	*	*	*	*	1.1	3.7	8.6	16.7	27.1	39.4
1940-------	1955	*	*	*	*	*	*	1.1	3.8	8.9	16.3	25.9	35.8
1941-------	1956	*	*	*	*	*	*	1.2	4.0	8.7	15.4	23.0	30.9
1942-------	1957	*	*	*	*	*	*	1.2	3.7	7.7	12.8	18.6	25.1
1943-------	1958	*	*	*	*	*	*	1.0	3.1	6.2	10.1	15.0	20.4
1944-------	1959	*	*	*	*	*	*	0.9	2.6	5.0	8.3	12.3	17.4
1945-------	1960	*	*	*	*	*	*	0.8	2.1	4.2	6.9	10.7	15.4
1946-------	1961	*	*	*	*	*	*	0.6	1.7	3.3	5.8	9.2	13.1
1947-------	1962	*	*	*	*	*	*	0.5	1.3	2.7	4.9	7.7	10.5
1948-------	1963	*	*	*	*	*	*	0.3	1.1	2.3	4.1	6.1	8.3
1949-------	1964	*	*	*	*	*	*	0.3	1.0	2.1	3.4	5.0	
1950-------	1965	*	*	*	*	*	*	0.3	0.9	1.6	2.7		
1951-------	1966	*	*	*	*	*	*	0.3	0.7	1.4			
1952-------	1967	*	*	*	*	*	*	0.2	0.6				
1953-------	1968	*	*	*	*	*	*	0.2					
1954-------	1969	*	*	*	*	*	*						
1955-------	1970	*	*	*	*	*							
1956-------	1971	*	*	*	*								
1957-------	1972	*	*	*									
1958-------	1973	*	*										
1959-------	1974	*											

TABLE 6B. CUMULATIVE BIRTH RATES FOR WHITE WOMEN AS OF THE BEGINNING OF EACH YEAR 1917-74 BY AGE AND LIVE-BIRTH ORDER FOR EACH COHORT FROM 1867 TO 1959--CON.

LIVE-BIRTH ORDER AND COHORT	DIAGONAL LINE FOR JANUARY 1	EXACT AGE											
		27	28	29	30	31	32	33	34	35	36	37	38
FIFTH BIRTHS--CON.													
1879-------													273.0
1880-------												257.3	269.1
1881-------											238.7	251.8	263.4
1882-------										218.0	233.1	246.0	257.3
1883-------									197.8	214.3	229.2	241.8	253.0
1884-------								176.6	194.8	211.1	225.4	237.8	248.9
1885-------							154.4	172.8	190.8	206.2	220.4	232.8	243.1
1886-------						131.3	151.3	169.7	186.7	202.1	216.3	227.9	238.1
1887-------					108.0	128.7	148.7	166.0	183.0	198.4	211.7	223.2	233.3
1888-------				85.2	107.4	127.8	146.6	163.9	180.7	195.1	208.2	219.5	229.0
1889-------			63.2	83.8	105.5	124.8	143.4	160.5	176.2	190.4	203.3	214.2	223.4
1890-------	1917	44.0	62.3	82.3	103.0	122.2	140.7	156.6	172.2	186.2	198.3	208.5	217.2
1891-------	1918	43.3	61.1	80.4	101.1	120.3	137.5	153.3	168.5	181.8	193.2	203.0	211.3
1892-------	1919	42.5	59.6	78.9	99.7	117.2	134.1	149.5	163.6	175.9	186.8	196.0	203.6
1893-------	1920	41.5	58.6	78.1	96.8	114.1	130.6	145.1	158.3	170.2	180.3	188.8	196.3
1894-------	1921	40.5	58.0	75.5	94.1	110.9	126.5	140.1	153.0	164.1	173.8	182.2	189.3
1895-------	1922	40.5	56.3	73.9	91.9	107.9	122.5	135.8	147.9	158.4	167.9	175.9	182.6
1896-------	1923	39.6	55.6	72.4	89.2	104.1	118.4	130.8	142.1	152.3	161.1	168.7	175.0
1897-------	1924	39.2	54.5	70.1	85.7	100.2	113.5	125.1	136.1	145.6	154.2	161.2	167.4
1898-------	1925	38.8	53.1	67.8	83.3	97.0	109.6	121.0	131.3	140.5	148.4	155.4	161.2
1899-------	1926	38.0	51.6	66.5	81.3	94.3	106.7	117.6	127.8	136.5	144.5	151.1	156.6
1900-------	1927	37.0	50.8	64.8	78.5	91.3	103.0	113.6	123.1	131.7	139.2	145.4	150.6
1901-------	1928	35.9	48.8	61.8	75.2	87.1	98.3	108.0	117.4	125.5	132.4	138.3	143.4
1902-------	1929	35.0	47.1	59.8	72.2	83.4	93.6	103.1	111.7	119.1	125.6	131.3	136.1
1903-------	1930	34.4	46.2	58.0	69.7	80.1	90.2	98.9	107.0	114.0	120.4	125.7	130.4
1904-------	1931	33.5	44.5	55.9	66.8	77.1	86.5	94.8	102.4	109.2	115.2	120.4	124.9
1905-------	1932	31.9	42.4	52.8	63.7	73.3	82.1	90.0	97.4	103.8	109.6	114.6	119.2
1906-------	1933	30.1	39.6	49.9	60.0	68.9	77.3	84.9	91.8	98.0	103.6	108.6	113.6
1907-------	1934	27.9	37.4	47.1	56.5	65.1	73.2	80.2	86.8	92.8	98.4	103.9	109.0
1908-------	1935	26.4	35.4	44.3	53.3	61.5	68.9	75.7	82.2	88.3	94.4	100.0	105.1
1909-------	1936	25.3	33.6	42.3	51.0	58.6	65.8	72.5	79.1	85.8	92.0	97.8	103.0
1910-------	1937	23.9	32.0	40.4	48.5	55.9	63.0	69.8	77.0	83.7	90.1	95.9	101.1
1911-------	1938	23.0	30.9	38.7	46.6	54.0	61.1	68.6	75.9	82.8	89.2	94.9	99.9
1912-------	1939	22.0	29.2	36.9	44.7	51.9	59.6	67.1	74.3	81.2	87.5	93.0	98.0
1913-------	1940	20.8	27.9	35.5	43.0	50.9	58.6	65.9	73.2	80.0	86.2	91.7	96.8
1914-------	1941	20.3	27.3	34.5	42.7	50.6	58.3	65.8	73.1	79.8	86.0	91.8	97.2
1915-------	1942	20.2	27.1	35.1	43.3	51.1	58.9	66.4	73.5	80.3	86.8	93.0	98.9
1916-------	1943	20.3	27.9	35.9	43.9	51.9	59.6	66.9	74.1	81.1	88.0	94.7	101.0
1917-------	1944	21.0	28.6	36.2	44.4	52.2	59.7	67.1	74.5	82.0	89.4	96.5	103.1
1918-------	1945	21.6	28.7	36.5	44.4	52.0	59.6	67.2	75.1	83.0	90.8	98.4	105.3
1919-------	1946	21.9	29.3	37.1	44.9	52.8	60.8	69.1	77.8	86.4	94.9	102.9	110.2
1920-------	1947	22.2	29.5	37.2	45.3	53.5	62.1	71.3	80.7	90.0	99.1	107.6	115.3
1921-------	1948	22.3	29.6	37.5	45.8	54.6	64.2	74.0	84.0	94.0	103.6	112.7	120.6
1922-------	1949	21.8	29.1	37.0	45.9	55.5	65.7	76.1	86.9	97.6	107.7	116.7	124.8
1923-------	1950	21.6	29.0	37.6	47.3	57.6	68.6	80.0	91.6	102.8	113.0	122.5	130.7
1924-------	1951	21.8	30.1	39.7	50.4	61.8	73.8	86.1	98.3	109.9	120.6	130.2	138.5
1925-------	1952	22.9	32.0	42.4	54.2	66.5	79.4	92.5	105.1	117.0	128.0	137.8	145.8
1926-------	1953	24.8	34.5	45.9	58.4	71.5	85.3	98.7	111.7	123.9	134.9	144.2	151.9
1927-------	1954	27.0	37.8	50.0	63.4	77.5	91.6	105.6	119.1	131.6	142.3	151.4	158.8
1928-------	1955	29.8	41.4	54.4	68.8	83.5	98.5	113.0	126.8	138.9	149.3	158.1	164.9
1929-------	1956	33.3	45.9	60.2	75.6	91.5	107.3	122.5	136.2	148.2	158.4	166.6	172.8
1930-------	1957	37.0	50.8	66.1	82.6	99.3	115.7	130.8	144.4	156.1	165.6	173.0	178.7
1931-------	1958	41.3	56.2	72.7	90.1	107.6	124.2	139.3	152.5	163.4	171.8	178.5	183.7
1932-------	1959	44.8	60.8	78.2	96.5	114.0	130.5	145.0	157.2	166.8	174.5	180.6	185.5
1933-------	1960	48.2	65.0	83.5	101.9	119.2	134.9	148.1	158.7	167.4	174.4	180.3	185.0
1934-------	1961	51.1	69.0	87.4	105.3	121.9	135.9	147.3	157.0	164.9	171.8	177.4	181.6
1935-------	1962	54.0	71.7	89.6	106.8	121.2	133.4	143.8	152.4	160.1	166.5	171.5	175.0
1936-------	1963	55.8	73.0	90.0	104.6	117.1	128.1	137.3	145.7	152.9	158.7	162.8	165.8
1937-------	1964	56.3	72.4	86.8	99.4	110.6	120.3	129.3	137.3	143.8	148.6	152.1	
1938-------	1965	54.6	68.0	80.0	91.1	101.0	110.6	119.4	126.6	132.0	136.0		
1939-------	1966	51.4	62.6	73.1	82.9	92.7	102.0	109.8	115.7	120.2			
1940-------	1967	45.5	55.1	64.4	74.1	83.6	91.8	98.1	103.0				
1941-------	1968	39.1	47.4	56.4	65.6	73.8	80.2	85.4					
1942-------	1969	32.0	39.9	48.2	56.1	62.4	67.7						
1943-------	1970	26.9	34.0	41.1	47.0	52.1							
1944-------	1971	23.3	29.4	34.7	39.5								
1945-------	1972	20.4	25.0	29.2									
1946-------	1973	16.8	20.3										
1947-------	1974	13.3											

TABLE 6B. CUMULATIVE BIRTH RATES FOR WHITE WOMEN AS OF THE BEGINNING OF EACH YEAR 1917-74 BY AGE AND LIVE-BIRTH ORDER FOR EACH COHORT FROM 1867 TO 1959--CON.

LIVE-BIRTH ORDER AND COHORT	DIAGONAL LINE FOR JANUARY 1	EXACT AGE											
		39	40	41	42	43	44	45	46	47	48	49	50
FIFTH BIRTHS--CON.													
1867-------													376.9
1868-------												371.1	371.1
1869-------											365.2	365.3	365.3
1870-------										359.3	359.5	359.6	359.6
1871-------									353.1	353.5	353.8	353.9	353.9
1872-------								346.4	347.1	347.6	347.8	347.9	347.9
1873-------							339.2	340.4	341.2	341.7	341.9	342.0	342.0
1874-------						331.4	333.3	334.6	335.3	335.8	336.0	336.1	336.1
1875-------					322.4	325.1	327.1	328.3	329.0	329.4	329.6	329.7	329.7
1876-------				311.7	315.7	318.4	320.3	321.5	322.2	322.5	322.7	322.8	322.8
1877-------			299.4	305.0	309.1	311.7	313.6	314.8	315.4	315.7	315.9	316.0	316.0
1878-------	1917	286.5	294.7	300.4	304.4	307.0	308.9	310.0	310.6	310.9	311.0	311.1	311.1
1879-------	1918	282.9	291.1	296.7	300.6	303.3	305.1	306.2	306.8	307.1	307.3	307.4	307.4
1880-------	1919	278.9	286.9	292.3	296.4	298.9	300.7	301.8	302.4	302.7	302.9	303.0	303.0
1881-------	1920	272.9	280.8	286.3	290.0	292.5	294.3	295.3	295.8	296.1	296.2	296.2	296.2
1882-------	1921	266.7	274.6	279.7	283.4	285.8	287.4	288.3	288.8	289.1	289.2	289.2	289.2
1883-------	1922	262.3	269.5	274.5	278.1	280.4	281.9	282.8	283.3	283.6	283.7	283.7	283.7
1884-------	1923	257.5	264.6	269.5	273.0	275.2	276.7	277.6	278.1	278.4	278.5	278.5	278.5
1885-------	1924	251.6	258.6	263.2	266.5	268.7	270.1	270.9	271.4	271.6	271.7	271.8	271.8
1886-------	1925	246.5	253.1	257.6	260.8	262.8	264.1	264.9	265.3	265.6	265.7	265.8	265.8
1887-------	1926	241.3	247.7	252.1	255.2	257.1	258.5	259.3	259.7	259.9	260.0	260.0	260.0
1888-------	1927	236.7	242.9	247.1	249.9	251.8	253.0	253.7	254.1	254.3	254.4	254.4	254.4
1889-------	1928	230.9	236.8	240.7	243.6	245.4	246.6	247.3	247.7	247.9	248.0	248.0	248.0
1890-------	1929	224.2	229.6	233.5	236.1	237.9	239.1	239.8	240.1	240.3	240.3	240.4	240.4
1891-------	1930	217.7	223.1	226.7	229.3	231.1	232.3	232.9	233.3	233.4	233.5	233.6	233.6
1892-------	1931	210.0	215.0	218.5	221.0	222.7	223.8	224.4	224.7	224.9	225.0	225.0	225.0
1893-------	1932	202.3	207.0	210.3	212.7	214.3	215.3	215.8	216.1	216.3	216.4	216.4	216.4
1894-------	1933	194.9	199.4	202.6	204.9	206.3	207.2	207.8	208.1	208.3	208.4	208.4	208.4
1895-------	1934	187.9	192.3	195.4	197.5	198.9	199.9	200.4	200.7	200.8	200.8	200.8	200.8
1896-------	1935	180.2	184.3	187.2	189.3	190.7	191.6	192.1	192.3	192.4	192.4	192.4	192.4
1897-------	1936	172.3	176.1	178.9	180.9	182.2	183.0	183.4	183.7	183.8	183.8	183.8	183.8
1898-------	1937	165.8	169.5	172.2	174.2	175.5	176.3	176.9	177.2	177.3	177.4	177.4	177.4
1899-------	1938	161.0	164.7	167.4	169.3	170.6	171.5	172.1	172.4	172.6	172.7	172.7	172.7
1900-------	1939	155.0	158.5	161.1	163.0	164.3	165.2	165.8	166.1	166.3	166.3	166.3	166.3
1901-------	1940	147.5	150.9	153.4	155.2	156.6	157.6	158.2	158.5	158.6	158.6	158.6	158.6
1902-------	1941	140.1	143.3	145.7	147.7	149.2	150.1	150.7	151.0	151.1	151.1	151.1	151.1
1903-------	1942	134.2	137.4	140.0	142.1	143.5	144.5	145.1	145.4	145.5	145.5	145.5	145.5
1904-------	1943	128.8	132.3	135.0	137.0	138.4	139.4	139.9	140.2	140.3	140.3	140.3	140.3
1905-------	1944	123.5	127.1	129.9	132.0	133.5	134.4	134.9	135.2	135.3	135.3	135.3	135.3
1906-------	1945	118.0	121.7	124.5	126.6	128.0	128.8	129.3	129.6	129.7	129.8	129.8	129.8
1907-------	1946	113.4	117.1	120.0	122.0	123.3	124.2	124.7	125.0	125.2	125.3	125.3	125.3
1908-------	1947	109.5	113.2	115.8	117.7	119.1	120.0	120.6	120.9	121.1	121.2	121.2	121.2
1909-------	1948	107.5	111.0	113.6	115.6	117.0	118.0	118.6	118.9	119.1	119.2	119.2	119.2
1910-------	1949	105.3	108.8	111.5	113.5	115.0	116.0	116.6	116.9	117.1	117.2	117.2	117.2
1911-------	1950	104.2	107.8	110.5	112.7	114.2	115.3	116.0	116.3	116.5	116.5	116.5	116.5
1912-------	1951	102.3	106.0	109.0	111.3	113.0	114.2	114.8	115.1	115.2	115.3	115.3	115.3
1913-------	1952	101.3	105.3	108.4	110.9	112.7	113.8	114.4	114.7	114.9	115.0	115.0	115.0
1914-------	1953	102.2	106.5	110.0	112.7	114.5	115.7	116.4	116.8	117.0	117.1	117.1	117.1
1915-------	1954	104.2	108.8	112.5	115.2	117.1	118.3	119.0	119.3	119.5	119.6	119.6	119.6
1916-------	1955	106.6	111.4	115.1	117.9	119.8	121.0	121.7	122.1	122.3	122.4	122.4	122.4
1917-------	1956	109.0	114.0	117.8	120.7	122.6	123.8	124.5	124.8	125.0	125.0	125.0	125.0
1918-------	1957	111.4	116.4	120.2	123.0	125.0	126.3	126.9	127.2	127.3	127.3	127.3	127.3
1919-------	1958	116.6	121.8	125.8	128.7	130.7	131.9	132.6	132.9	133.0	133.0	133.0	133.0
1920-------	1959	121.8	127.1	131.2	134.2	136.1	137.3	137.9	138.2	138.3	138.3	138.3	138.3
1921-------	1960	127.4	132.8	136.9	139.7	141.6	142.7	143.3	143.6	143.7	143.7	143.7	143.7
1922-------	1961	131.6	137.1	141.0	143.8	145.6	146.7	147.3	147.6	147.7	147.7	147.7	147.7
1923-------	1962	137.6	142.8	146.6	149.3	151.0	152.0	152.5	152.7	152.8	152.8	152.8	152.8
1924-------	1963	145.1	150.2	153.9	156.4	157.9	158.8	159.2	159.4	159.5	159.5	159.5	159.5
1925-------	1964	152.2	157.1	160.6	162.8	164.2	165.0	165.5	165.7	165.7	165.7	165.7	
1926-------	1965	158.0	162.6	165.6	167.6	168.8	169.6	170.0	170.1	170.2	170.2		
1927-------	1966	164.5	168.5	171.2	173.0	174.2	174.9	175.2	175.3	175.4			
1928-------	1967	170.0	173.5	176.0	177.7	178.7	179.3	179.5	179.6				
1929-------	1968	177.5	180.9	183.3	184.8	185.7	186.2	186.4					
1930-------	1969	182.9	186.1	188.3	189.6	190.3	190.7						
1931-------	1970	187.8	190.9	192.7	193.8	194.4							
1932-------	1971	189.4	192.0	193.6	194.6								
1933-------	1972	188.3	190.5	191.9									
1934-------	1973	184.4	186.3										
1935-------	1974	177.4											

TABLE 6B. CUMULATIVE BIRTH RATES FOR WHITE WOMEN AS OF THE BEGINNING OF EACH YEAR 1917-74 BY AGE AND LIVE-BIRTH ORDER FOR EACH COHORT FROM 1867 TO 1959--CON.

LIVE-BIRTH ORDER AND COHORT	DIAGONAL LINE FOR JANUARY 1	EXACT AGE											
		15	16	17	18	19	20	21	22	23	24	25	26
SIXTH BIRTHS													
1891-------													8.7
1892-------												4.5	8.6
1893-------											2.1	4.4	8.2
1894-------										0.9	2.1	4.2	7.9
1895-------									0.4	0.9	1.9	4.0	7.7
1896-------								0.1	0.4	0.9	2.0	4.2	8.3
1897-------							*	0.1	0.4	0.9	2.1	4.5	8.3
1898-------						*	*	0.1	0.3	0.8	2.1	4.4	8.3
1899-------					*	*	*	0.1	0.4	1.0	2.2	4.5	8.3
1900-------				*	*	*	*	0.1	0.4	0.9	2.2	4.5	8.1
1901-------			*	*	*	*	*	0.1	0.3	0.8	2.0	4.2	7.7
1902-------	1917	*	*	*	*	*	*	0.1	0.4	1.0	2.2	4.3	7.8
1903-------	1918	*	*	*	*	*	*	0.1	0.4	0.9	2.1	4.2	7.4
1904-------	1919	*	*	*	*	*	*	0.1	0.3	0.9	2.1	4.1	7.3
1905-------	1920	*	*	*	*	*	*	0.1	0.4	0.9	2.0	3.9	7.0
1906-------	1921	*	*	*	*	*	*	0.1	0.4	1.0	2.0	3.8	6.6
1907-------	1922	*	*	*	*	*	*	0.1	0.4	0.9	1.9	3.6	6.3
1908-------	1923	*	*	*	*	*	*	0.1	0.3	0.8	1.7	3.3	5.6
1909-------	1924	*	*	*	*	*	*	0.1	0.3	0.8	1.7	3.1	5.4
1910-------	1925	*	*	*	*	*	*	0.1	0.3	0.7	1.5	2.9	5.2
1911-------	1926	*	*	*	*	*	*	0.1	0.3	0.7	1.5	2.9	5.2
1912-------	1927	*	*	*	*	*	*	0.1	0.3	0.7	1.5	2.8	4.9
1913-------	1928	*	*	*	*	*	*	0.1	0.3	0.6	1.3	2.6	4.7
1914-------	1929	*	*	*	*	*	*	0.1	0.3	0.6	1.3	2.6	4.5
1915-------	1930	*	*	*	*	*	*	0.1	0.3	0.7	1.4	2.6	4.5
1916-------	1931	*	*	*	*	*	*	0.1	0.3	0.6	1.2	2.5	4.4
1917-------	1932	*	*	*	*	*	*	0.1	0.3	0.6	1.4	2.6	4.6
1918-------	1933	*	*	*	*	*	*	0.1	0.2	0.6	1.3	2.6	4.7
1919-------	1934	*	*	*	*	*	*	0.1	0.3	0.7	1.4	2.8	5.0
1920-------	1935	*	*	*	*	*	*	0.1	0.3	0.6	1.4	2.8	4.9
1921-------	1936	*	*	*	*	*	*	0.1	0.3	0.7	1.5	2.8	5.0
1922-------	1937	*	*	*	*	*	*	0.1	0.3	0.7	1.5	2.9	4.9
1923-------	1938	*	*	*	*	*	*	0.1	0.3	0.7	1.5	2.8	4.9
1924-------	1939	*	*	*	*	*	*	0.1	0.3	0.7	1.4	2.8	4.9
1925-------	1940	*	*	*	*	*	*	0.1	0.3	0.7	1.5	2.9	5.0
1926-------	1941	*	*	*	*	*	*	0.1	0.3	0.7	1.6	3.0	5.2
1927-------	1942	*	*	*	*	*	*	0.1	0.3	0.8	1.6	3.1	5.5
1928-------	1943	*	*	*	*	*	*	0.1	0.3	0.7	1.6	3.2	5.8
1929-------	1944	*	*	*	*	*	*	0.1	0.3	0.8	1.8	3.6	6.7
1930-------	1945	*	*	*	*	*	*	0.1	0.3	0.8	1.9	4.0	7.4
1931-------	1946	*	*	*	*	*	*	0.1	0.4	1.0	2.4	4.9	8.7
1932-------	1947	*	*	*	*	*	*	0.1	0.4	1.1	2.7	5.4	9.6
1933-------	1948	*	*	*	*	*	*	0.1	0.4	1.2	2.9	5.8	10.2
1934-------	1949	*	*	*	*	*	*	0.1	0.5	1.4	3.2	6.3	11.1
1935-------	1950	*	*	*	*	*	*	0.1	0.5	1.5	3.4	6.7	11.7
1936-------	1951	*	*	*	*	*	*	0.1	0.5	1.5	3.5	7.0	12.2
1937-------	1952	*	*	*	*	*	*	0.1	0.5	1.6	3.7	7.3	12.6
1938-------	1953	*	*	*	*	*	*	0.2	0.7	1.8	3.9	7.6	12.7
1939-------	1954	*	*	*	*	*	*	0.2	0.7	1.9	4.2	7.7	12.3
1940-------	1955	*	*	*	*	*	*	0.2	0.7	1.9	4.1	7.3	11.1
1941-------	1956	*	*	*	*	*	*	0.2	0.7	1.8	3.7	6.3	9.3
1942-------	1957	*	*	*	*	*	*	0.2	0.6	1.6	3.1	5.1	7.5
1943-------	1958	*	*	*	*	*	*	0.1	0.5	1.3	2.4	3.9	5.8
1944-------	1959	*	*	*	*	*	*	0.1	0.4	1.0	1.9	3.2	4.9
1945-------	1960	*	*	*	*	*	*	0.1	0.4	0.9	1.7	2.9	4.4
1946-------	1961	*	*	*	*	*	*	0.1	0.3	0.7	1.4	2.4	3.6
1947-------	1962	*	*	*	*	*	*	0.1	0.3	0.7	1.3	2.1	3.0
1948-------	1963	*	*	*	*	*	*	0.1	0.3	0.6	1.0	1.5	2.1
1949-------	1964	*	*	*	*	*	*	0.1	0.2	0.4	0.7	1.1	
1950-------	1965	*	*	*	*	*	*	0.1	0.2	0.4	0.6		
1951-------	1966	*	*	*	*	*	*	0.0	0.1	0.2			
1952-------	1967	*	*	*	*	*	*	0.0	0.1				
1953-------	1968	*	*	*	*	*	*	0.0					
1954-------	1969	*	*	*	*	*	*						
1955-------	1970	*	*	*	*	*							
1956-------	1971	*	*	*	*								
1957-------	1972	*	*	*									
1958-------	1973	*	*										
1959-------	1974	*											

TABLE 6B. CUMULATIVE BIRTH RATES FOR WHITE WOMEN AS OF THE BEGINNING OF EACH YEAR 1917-74 BY AGE AND LIVE-BIRTH ORDER FOR EACH COHORT FROM 1867 TO 1959--CON.

LIVE-BIRTH ORDER AND COHORT	DIAGONAL LINE FOR JANUARY 1	EXACT AGE											
		27	28	29	30	31	32	33	34	35	36	37	38
SIXTH BIRTHS--CON.													
1879-------													196.1
1880-------												180.0	192.4
1881-------											161.2	174.6	186.7
1882-------										140.9	155.5	168.5	180.2
1883-------									121.6	137.0	151.3	163.9	175.4
1884-------								103.4	119.5	134.6	148.3	160.7	172.0
1885-------							85.6	101.4	117.4	131.8	145.3	157.5	168.0
1886-------						68.1	84.0	99.8	115.0	129.2	142.7	154.2	164.4
1887-------					52.0	67.0	83.0	98.1	113.0	127.3	139.9	151.1	161.2
1888-------				37.0	51.5	66.3	81.5	96.1	111.2	124.5	136.9	147.9	157.4
1889-------			24.7	36.6	50.7	64.7	79.4	94.2	108.1	121.2	133.3	143.7	152.7
1890-------	1917	15.1	24.5	35.8	49.1	62.8	77.7	91.4	105.2	118.0	129.4	139.2	148.0
1891-------	1918	15.0	23.9	34.6	47.7	61.8	75.5	89.1	102.5	114.5	125.3	135.0	143.0
1892-------	1919	14.6	23.0	33.6	47.3	60.1	73.7	86.9	99.4	110.7	121.2	129.9	137.3
1893-------	1920	13.8	22.1	33.4	45.7	58.4	71.6	83.9	95.6	106.7	116.2	124.3	131.5
1894-------	1921	13.5	22.4	32.5	44.9	57.3	69.7	81.2	92.6	102.6	111.5	119.3	126.1
1895-------	1922	13.8	21.9	32.2	44.3	56.0	67.8	79.2	89.7	99.0	107.6	115.1	121.5
1896-------	1923	13.9	22.2	32.2	43.5	54.8	66.1	76.4	86.1	95.1	103.1	110.1	116.1
1897-------	1924	14.0	22.1	31.4	42.3	53.1	63.6	73.1	82.6	91.0	98.7	105.3	111.2
1898-------	1925	13.9	21.3	30.4	40.9	50.9	60.8	70.4	79.3	87.5	94.8	101.3	106.9
1899-------	1926	13.6	21.0	29.9	39.8	49.4	59.3	68.4	77.3	85.1	92.3	98.4	103.6
1900-------	1927	13.3	20.5	28.8	38.1	47.5	56.8	65.6	73.8	81.5	88.2	94.0	98.9
1901-------	1928	12.8	19.5	27.1	36.1	44.8	53.7	61.7	69.7	76.7	82.9	88.2	92.9
1902-------	1929	12.5	18.6	26.1	34.4	42.7	50.8	58.5	65.8	72.3	78.1	83.1	87.5
1903-------	1930	11.9	18.0	25.0	33.1	40.6	48.4	55.5	62.2	68.2	73.7	78.4	82.5
1904-------	1931	11.7	17.4	24.3	31.5	39.0	46.3	53.0	59.4	65.2	70.3	74.8	78.8
1905-------	1932	11.2	16.7	22.7	29.9	36.9	43.6	49.9	56.1	61.4	66.3	70.5	74.5
1906-------	1933	10.5	15.3	21.3	28.0	34.4	40.8	46.9	52.5	57.6	62.2	66.4	70.4
1907-------	1934	9.7	14.5	20.2	26.4	32.6	38.8	44.3	49.7	54.5	59.1	63.4	67.5
1908-------	1935	9.0	13.6	18.9	24.9	30.8	36.4	41.7	46.7	51.5	56.2	60.6	64.6
1909-------	1936	8.8	13.2	18.4	24.1	29.5	34.9	39.9	44.9	49.9	54.7	59.0	62.9
1910-------	1937	8.4	12.6	17.5	22.8	28.1	33.2	38.0	43.3	48.4	53.0	57.2	61.0
1911-------	1938	8.3	12.3	16.9	22.1	27.2	32.0	37.2	42.5	47.3	51.8	55.9	59.5
1912-------	1939	7.9	11.6	16.1	21.1	25.8	31.0	36.2	41.3	46.1	50.6	54.5	58.1
1913-------	1940	7.4	11.0	15.4	20.0	25.0	30.2	35.2	40.2	44.9	49.1	53.0	56.6
1914-------	1941	7.2	10.8	14.8	19.7	24.7	29.8	34.8	39.6	44.0	48.3	52.2	56.0
1915-------	1942	7.2	10.6	14.9	19.8	24.7	29.8	34.5	39.1	43.6	47.9	52.1	55.9
1916-------	1943	7.1	10.8	15.1	19.8	24.7	29.5	34.1	38.8	43.3	47.8	52.0	56.0
1917-------	1944	7.5	11.2	15.4	20.1	24.7	29.4	34.0	38.7	43.3	47.8	52.1	56.3
1918-------	1945	7.6	11.2	15.3	19.8	24.4	29.1	33.8	38.5	43.3	47.9	52.4	56.8
1919-------	1946	7.9	11.5	15.6	20.1	24.8	29.6	34.4	39.5	44.5	49.6	54.6	59.3
1920-------	1947	7.8	11.3	15.4	20.1	24.8	29.7	34.9	40.2	45.8	51.3	56.6	61.6
1921-------	1948	7.8	11.4	15.7	20.3	25.2	30.5	35.9	41.8	47.7	53.5	59.2	64.4
1922-------	1949	7.7	11.4	15.5	20.3	25.3	30.6	36.4	42.5	48.6	54.8	60.5	65.9
1923-------	1950	7.8	11.3	15.7	20.6	25.9	31.7	37.9	44.4	51.0	57.4	63.5	68.9
1924-------	1951	7.7	11.5	16.0	21.2	27.0	33.4	40.1	47.2	54.1	60.7	66.9	72.7
1925-------	1952	8.0	12.0	16.9	22.7	29.1	36.1	43.3	50.6	57.8	64.7	71.2	76.7
1926-------	1953	8.4	12.7	18.1	24.4	31.3	38.7	46.2	53.9	61.4	68.6	75.0	80.5
1927-------	1954	9.1	13.8	19.6	26.5	33.8	41.5	49.6	57.7	65.6	72.8	79.2	84.5
1928-------	1955	9.7	14.8	21.1	28.2	35.9	44.4	52.9	61.4	69.3	76.4	82.6	87.5
1929-------	1956	11.0	16.7	23.4	31.1	39.7	48.7	57.8	66.4	74.4	81.4	87.1	91.5
1930-------	1957	12.1	18.3	25.6	34.1	43.2	52.7	61.9	70.7	78.5	85.0	90.1	94.3
1931-------	1958	14.0	20.7	28.7	37.9	47.6	57.2	66.5	75.2	82.4	88.2	93.0	96.8
1932-------	1959	15.3	22.5	31.1	40.7	50.5	60.2	69.3	77.1	83.5	88.8	93.2	96.7
1933-------	1960	16.3	24.1	33.1	42.9	52.7	62.1	70.3	77.1	82.9	87.8	91.9	95.2
1934-------	1961	17.6	25.7	35.0	44.8	54.2	62.5	69.5	75.6	80.7	85.4	89.2	92.2
1935-------	1962	18.5	26.7	35.7	44.9	53.2	60.4	66.6	71.9	77.0	81.3	84.7	87.3
1936-------	1963	19.1	27.0	35.5	43.4	50.4	56.7	62.1	67.3	72.0	75.9	78.8	80.9
1937-------	1964	19.1	26.5	33.7	40.4	46.5	52.0	57.3	62.2	66.4	69.6	72.0	
1938-------	1965	18.7	24.9	30.8	36.5	41.7	47.0	51.9	56.2	59.6	62.2		
1939-------	1966	17.3	22.3	27.3	32.2	37.3	42.2	46.6	50.1	52.9			
1940-------	1967	15.1	19.4	23.7	28.4	33.1	37.4	40.8	43.7				
1941-------	1968	12.6	16.2	20.2	24.4	28.4	31.6	34.4					
1942-------	1969	10.2	13.4	16.9	20.3	23.2	25.8						
1943-------	1970	8.2	11.0	13.9	16.4	18.6							
1944-------	1971	7.0	9.3	11.4	13.3								
1945-------	1972	6.2	7.9	9.6									
1946-------	1973	4.9	6.2										
1947-------	1974	4.0											

TABLE 6B. CUMULATIVE BIRTH RATES FOR WHITE WOMEN AS OF THE BEGINNING OF EACH YEAR 1917-74 BY AGE AND LIVE-BIRTH ORDER FOR EACH COHORT FROM 1867 TO 1959--CON.

LIVE-BIRTH ORDER AND COHORT	DIAGONAL LINE FOR JANUARY 1	EXACT AGE											
		39	40	41	42	43	44	45	46	47	48	49	50
SIXTH BIRTHS--CON.													
1867-------													295.8
1868-------												290.6	290.6
1869-------											285.3	285.4	285.4
1870-------										279.9	280.1	280.2	280.2
1871-------									274.2	274.7	274.9	275.0	275.0
1872-------								268.0	268.9	269.5	269.7	269.8	269.8
1873-------							261.3	262.8	263.7	264.2	264.4	264.5	264.5
1874-------						254.2	256.6	258.1	259.0	259.6	259.8	259.9	259.9
1875-------					245.4	248.7	251.0	252.4	253.3	253.8	254.0	254.1	254.1
1876-------				234.4	239.2	242.4	244.6	246.1	247.0	247.4	247.6	247.7	247.7
1877-------			221.7	228.1	232.8	235.9	238.2	239.6	240.3	240.8	241.0	241.1	241.1
1878-------	1917	209.8	218.7	225.0	229.6	232.8	235.1	236.4	237.2	237.6	237.8	237.9	237.9
1879-------	1918	206.6	215.4	221.6	226.2	229.4	231.5	232.8	233.5	233.9	234.1	234.2	234.2
1880-------	1919	202.7	211.2	217.3	221.9	224.8	226.9	228.2	228.9	229.3	229.5	229.6	229.6
1881-------	1920	196.7	205.1	211.1	215.3	218.2	220.2	221.4	222.1	222.5	222.7	222.8	222.8
1882-------	1921	190.0	198.2	203.7	207.9	210.7	212.6	213.7	214.3	214.6	214.8	214.9	214.9
1883-------	1922	185.0	192.6	198.0	202.0	204.6	206.4	207.4	208.0	208.3	208.5	208.6	208.6
1884-------	1923	180.9	188.3	193.6	197.3	199.8	201.5	202.5	203.0	203.3	203.5	203.6	203.6
1885-------	1924	176.6	183.9	188.9	192.5	194.9	196.5	197.4	197.9	198.2	198.3	198.4	198.4
1886-------	1925	172.9	179.8	184.5	188.0	190.2	191.7	192.6	193.1	193.4	193.5	193.5	193.5
1887-------	1926	169.4	175.9	180.6	183.8	185.9	187.5	188.4	188.9	189.2	189.3	189.3	189.3
1888-------	1927	165.0	171.3	175.6	178.7	180.9	182.3	183.1	183.6	183.8	183.9	183.9	183.9
1889-------	1928	160.2	166.1	170.1	173.2	175.2	176.6	177.5	177.9	178.1	178.2	178.2	178.2
1890-------	1929	154.8	160.2	164.3	167.1	169.0	170.4	171.2	171.6	171.8	171.9	171.9	171.9
1891-------	1930	149.3	154.8	158.5	161.3	163.1	164.4	165.1	165.5	165.7	165.8	165.8	165.8
1892-------	1931	143.7	148.7	152.4	155.0	156.8	158.0	158.7	159.1	159.3	159.4	159.4	159.4
1893-------	1932	137.4	142.3	145.7	148.2	149.8	150.9	151.6	152.0	152.2	152.3	152.3	152.3
1894-------	1933	131.7	136.2	139.5	141.8	143.3	144.3	144.9	145.2	145.4	145.5	145.5	145.5
1895-------	1934	126.7	131.1	134.1	136.3	137.8	138.8	139.4	139.7	139.9	139.9	139.9	139.9
1896-------	1935	121.3	125.4	128.2	130.2	131.7	132.7	133.2	133.5	133.6	133.6	133.6	133.6
1897-------	1936	115.9	119.6	122.3	124.3	125.7	126.5	127.0	127.3	127.4	127.4	127.4	127.4
1898-------	1937	111.3	114.8	117.5	119.5	120.8	121.6	122.2	122.5	122.6	122.7	122.7	122.7
1899-------	1938	107.9	111.4	113.9	115.7	116.9	117.8	118.4	118.7	118.9	119.0	119.0	119.0
1900-------	1939	103.1	106.4	108.8	110.5	111.7	112.6	113.2	113.5	113.7	113.8	113.8	113.8
1901-------	1940	96.7	99.8	102.0	103.6	104.9	105.8	106.3	106.6	106.8	106.8	106.8	106.8
1902-------	1941	91.1	94.0	96.2	98.0	99.3	100.2	100.7	101.0	101.1	101.2	101.2	101.2
1903-------	1942	85.9	88.8	91.1	92.9	94.2	95.1	95.7	95.9	96.0	96.0	96.0	96.0
1904-------	1943	82.3	85.3	87.6	89.5	90.7	91.6	92.0	92.2	92.3	92.3	92.3	92.3
1905-------	1944	78.0	81.0	83.4	85.1	86.3	87.1	87.5	87.7	87.8	87.8	87.8	87.8
1906-------	1945	74.0	77.1	79.4	81.1	82.3	83.0	83.4	83.6	83.7	83.8	83.8	83.8
1907-------	1946	71.0	73.9	76.1	77.7	78.7	79.5	79.9	80.1	80.2	80.2	80.2	80.2
1908-------	1947	68.0	70.8	72.8	74.3	75.4	76.1	76.5	76.7	76.8	76.8	76.8	76.8
1909-------	1948	66.2	68.8	70.8	72.3	73.4	74.2	74.7	74.9	75.0	75.0	75.0	75.0
1910-------	1949	64.1	66.7	68.7	70.3	71.4	72.2	72.7	72.9	73.0	73.0	73.0	73.0
1911-------	1950	62.6	65.2	67.3	68.9	70.1	70.9	71.4	71.7	71.8	71.9	71.9	71.9
1912-------	1951	61.2	63.9	66.1	67.8	69.1	70.0	70.5	70.8	70.9	71.0	71.0	71.0
1913-------	1952	59.8	62.7	64.9	66.8	68.1	69.0	69.6	69.9	70.1	70.1	70.1	70.1
1914-------	1953	59.4	62.3	64.8	66.7	68.0	68.9	69.4	69.7	69.8	69.8	69.8	69.8
1915-------	1954	59.5	62.7	65.2	67.1	68.5	69.4	70.0	70.3	70.4	70.4	70.4	70.4
1916-------	1955	59.7	63.0	65.5	67.6	69.0	70.0	70.6	70.9	71.0	71.0	71.0	71.0
1917-------	1956	60.2	63.6	66.4	68.5	70.0	71.0	71.6	71.9	72.0	72.1	72.1	72.1
1918-------	1957	60.8	64.3	67.1	69.2	70.7	71.6	72.1	72.3	72.4	72.5	72.5	72.5
1919-------	1958	63.6	67.3	70.2	72.4	73.9	74.9	75.4	75.7	75.8	75.8	75.8	75.8
1920-------	1959	66.0	69.8	72.8	75.0	76.5	77.4	78.0	78.2	78.3	78.3	78.3	78.3
1921-------	1960	69.0	72.8	75.8	77.9	79.4	80.4	80.9	81.1	81.2	81.2	81.2	81.2
1922-------	1961	70.5	74.4	77.3	79.5	81.0	81.8	82.3	82.5	82.6	82.6	82.6	82.6
1923-------	1962	73.8	77.6	80.6	82.7	84.0	84.8	85.2	85.4	85.5	85.5	85.5	85.5
1924-------	1963	77.3	81.1	84.0	86.0	87.2	87.9	88.3	88.5	88.6	88.6	88.6	88.6
1925-------	1964	81.4	85.1	87.8	89.6	90.7	91.4	91.8	92.0	92.1	92.1	92.1	
1926-------	1965	85.0	88.5	90.9	92.4	93.4	94.0	94.3	94.5	94.5	94.5		
1927-------	1966	88.7	91.8	93.9	95.4	96.3	96.8	97.1	97.2	97.2			
1928-------	1967	91.2	94.0	96.0	97.3	98.1	98.6	98.8	98.9				
1929-------	1968	95.1	97.7	99.5	100.7	101.4	101.8	102.0					
1930-------	1969	97.4	99.8	101.5	102.6	103.3	103.7						
1931-------	1970	99.7	102.0	103.6	104.6	105.2							
1932-------	1971	99.5	101.6	102.9	103.7								
1933-------	1972	97.7	99.4	100.5									
1934-------	1973	94.4	95.9										
1935-------	1974	89.1											

TABLE 6B. CUMULATIVE BIRTH RATES FOR WHITE WOMEN AS OF THE BEGINNING OF EACH YEAR 1917-74 BY AGE AND LIVE-BIRTH ORDER FOR EACH COHORT FROM 1867 TO 1959--CON.

LIVE-BIRTH ORDER AND COHORT	DIAGONAL LINE FOR JANUARY 1	EXACT AGE											
		15	16	17	18	19	20	21	22	23	24	25	26
SEVENTH BIRTHS													
1891-------													2.5
1892-------												1.2	2.4
1893-------											0.3	1.0	2.1
1894-------										0.2	0.5	1.1	2.2
1895-------									0.1	0.3	0.6	1.2	2.3
1896-------								0.0	0.1	0.3	0.6	1.2	2.4
1897-------							*	0.1	0.2	0.4	0.7	1.3	2.4
1898-------						*	*	0.1	0.2	0.4	0.7	1.3	2.5
1899-------					*	*	*	0.0	0.1	0.3	0.6	1.3	2.5
1900-------				*	*	*	*	0.0	0.1	0.3	0.6	1.3	2.4
1901-------			*	*	*	*	*	0.0	0.1	0.3	0.6	1.2	2.3
1902-------	1917	*	*	*	*	*	*	0.1	0.2	0.4	0.7	1.3	2.3
1903-------	1918	*	*	*	*	*	*	0.1	0.2	0.3	0.6	1.2	2.2
1904-------	1919	*	*	*	*	*	*	0.1	0.2	0.4	0.7	1.2	2.1
1905-------	1920	*	*	*	*	*	*	0.1	0.2	0.4	0.7	1.2	2.2
1906-------	1921	*	*	*	*	*	*	0.0	0.1	0.2	0.5	1.0	1.9
1907-------	1922	*	*	*	*	*	*	0.1	0.2	0.3	0.6	1.1	1.9
1908-------	1923	*	*	*	*	*	*	0.0	0.0	0.1	0.3	0.7	1.4
1909-------	1924	*	*	*	*	*	*	0.0	0.1	0.2	0.4	0.8	1.5
1910-------	1925	*	*	*	*	*	*	0.1	0.2	0.3	0.5	0.9	1.6
1911-------	1926	*	*	*	*	*	*	0.0	0.0	0.1	0.3	0.7	1.4
1912-------	1927	*	*	*	*	*	*	0.0	0.0	0.1	0.3	0.6	1.2
1913-------	1928	*	*	*	*	*	*	0.0	0.1	0.2	0.4	0.8	1.4
1914-------	1929	*	*	*	*	*	*	0.0	0.0	0.1	0.3	0.6	1.2
1915-------	1930	*	*	*	*	*	*	0.0	0.0	0.1	0.3	0.6	1.3
1916-------	1931	*	*	*	*	*	*	0.0	0.0	0.1	0.3	0.7	1.3
1917-------	1932	*	*	*	*	*	*	0.0	0.0	0.1	0.3	0.6	1.2
1918-------	1933	*	*	*	*	*	*	0.0	0.0	0.1	0.3	0.7	1.4
1919-------	1934	*	*	*	*	*	*	0.0	0.0	0.1	0.3	0.7	1.4
1920-------	1935	*	*	*	*	*	*	0.0	0.0	0.1	0.3	0.7	1.3
1921-------	1936	*	*	*	*	*	*	0.0	0.0	0.1	0.3	0.7	1.4
1922-------	1937	*	*	*	*	*	*	0.0	0.0	0.1	0.3	0.7	1.3
1923-------	1938	*	*	*	*	*	*	0.0	0.0	0.1	0.3	0.7	1.4
1924-------	1939	*	*	*	*	*	*	0.0	0.0	0.1	0.3	0.7	1.4
1925-------	1940	*	*	*	*	*	*	0.0	0.1	0.2	0.4	0.8	1.5
1926-------	1941	*	*	*	*	*	*	0.0	0.0	0.1	0.3	0.7	1.5
1927-------	1942	*	*	*	*	*	*	0.0	0.0	0.1	0.3	0.7	1.4
1928-------	1943	*	*	*	*	*	*	0.0	0.1	0.2	0.4	0.8	1.6
1929-------	1944	*	*	*	*	*	*	0.1	0.1	0.2	0.4	0.9	1.8
1930-------	1945	*	*	*	*	*	*	0.0	0.1	0.2	0.5	1.1	2.2
1931-------	1946	*	*	*	*	*	*	0.0	0.0	0.2	0.5	1.2	2.5
1932-------	1947	*	*	*	*	*	*	0.0	0.1	0.2	0.5	1.3	2.7
1933-------	1948	*	*	*	*	*	*	0.0	0.0	0.1	0.5	1.4	2.8
1934-------	1949	*	*	*	*	*	*	0.0	0.0	0.2	0.7	1.6	3.2
1935-------	1950	*	*	*	*	*	*	0.0	0.1	0.3	0.8	1.8	3.5
1936-------	1951	*	*	*	*	*	*	0.0	0.1	0.3	0.8	1.8	3.5
1937-------	1952	*	*	*	*	*	*	0.0	0.1	0.3	0.9	1.9	3.6
1938-------	1953	*	*	*	*	*	*	0.0	0.1	0.4	0.9	1.9	3.6
1939-------	1954	*	*	*	*	*	*	0.0	0.1	0.4	0.9	1.9	3.4
1940-------	1955	*	*	*	*	*	*	0.1	0.2	0.5	1.0	1.9	3.2
1941-------	1956	*	*	*	*	*	*	0.0	0.1	0.3	0.8	1.5	2.5
1942-------	1957	*	*	*	*	*	*	0.0	0.1	0.3	0.7	1.3	2.1
1943-------	1958	*	*	*	*	*	*	0.0	0.0	0.1	0.4	0.9	1.5
1944-------	1959	*	*	*	*	*	*	0.0	0.0	0.1	0.3	0.6	1.2
1945-------	1960	*	*	*	*	*	*	0.0	0.0	0.1	0.3	0.6	1.1
1946-------	1961	*	*	*	*	*	*	0.0	0.0	0.1	0.3	0.6	1.0
1947-------	1962	*	*	*	*	*	*	0.0	0.0	0.1	0.2	0.4	0.6
1948-------	1963	*	*	*	*	*	*	0.0	0.0	0.0	0.1	0.2	0.4
1949-------	1964	*	*	*	*	*	*	0.0	0.0	0.0	0.1	0.2	
1950-------	1965	*	*	*	*	*	*	0.0	0.0	0.0	0.1		
1951-------	1966	*	*	*	*	*	*	0.0	0.0	0.0			
1952-------	1967	*	*	*	*	*	*	0.0	0.0				
1953-------	1968	*	*	*	*	*	*	0.0					
1954-------	1969	*	*	*	*	*	*						
1955-------	1970	*	*	*	*	*							
1956-------	1971	*	*	*	*								
1957-------	1972	*	*	*									
1958-------	1973	*	*										
1959-------	1974	*											

TABLE 6B. CUMULATIVE BIRTH RATES FOR WHITE WOMEN AS OF THE BEGINNING OF EACH YEAR 1917-74 BY AGE AND LIVE-BIRTH ORDER FOR EACH COHORT FROM 1867 TO 1959--CON.

LIVE-BIRTH ORDER AND COHORT	DIAGONAL LINE FOR JANUARY 1	EXACT AGE											
		27	28	29	30	31	32	33	34	35	36	37	38
SEVENTH BIRTHS--CON.													
1879-------													131.0
1880-------												116.7	128.5
1881-------											101.2	113.4	124.9
1882-------										85.1	97.7	109.5	120.8
1883-------									69.8	82.2	94.5	106.2	117.3
1884-------								55.4	67.7	79.9	91.9	103.4	114.3
1885-------							42.5	53.5	65.7	77.5	89.3	100.7	110.8
1886-------						30.8	41.0	52.1	63.7	75.3	87.2	97.7	107.5
1887-------					21.5	29.9	40.2	50.7	62.2	74.1	85.1	95.4	105.1
1888-------				13.4	20.7	29.0	38.7	49.1	60.9	71.8	82.6	92.7	101.6
1889-------			8.2	13.3	20.3	28.2	37.8	48.5	59.3	70.1	80.7	90.2	98.8
1890-------	1917	4.6	8.1	12.8	19.5	27.3	37.1	46.9	57.7	68.3	78.2	87.1	95.3
1891-------	1918	4.6	7.8	12.4	19.0	27.1	36.1	45.8	56.4	66.5	76.0	84.7	92.4
1892-------	1919	4.3	7.5	12.1	19.0	26.4	35.3	44.8	54.7	64.2	73.3	81.2	88.1
1893-------	1920	4.0	7.1	11.9	18.3	25.6	34.3	43.3	52.6	61.8	70.1	77.3	83.9
1894-------	1921	4.1	7.4	11.9	18.4	25.6	33.7	42.2	51.3	59.6	67.2	74.2	80.5
1895-------	1922	4.3	7.4	12.1	18.4	25.2	33.0	41.3	49.5	57.2	64.6	71.2	77.3
1896-------	1923	4.3	7.6	12.1	18.0	24.7	32.3	39.8	47.4	54.8	61.7	68.0	73.5
1897-------	1924	4.4	7.5	11.8	17.6	23.9	30.9	37.8	45.0	51.8	58.3	64.2	69.5
1898-------	1925	4.4	7.4	11.6	17.2	23.2	29.6	36.3	43.1	49.6	55.8	61.5	66.5
1899-------	1926	4.4	7.4	11.5	16.8	22.3	28.7	35.0	41.7	48.0	54.1	59.5	64.2
1900-------	1927	4.2	7.1	10.9	15.7	21.2	27.1	33.4	39.7	45.9	51.7	56.7	61.2
1901-------	1928	4.0	6.7	10.2	14.8	19.9	25.7	31.4	37.5	43.3	48.6	53.2	57.4
1902-------	1929	3.9	6.3	9.7	14.0	18.9	24.1	29.6	35.3	40.6	45.5	50.0	53.8
1903-------	1930	3.7	6.1	9.3	13.5	17.9	23.0	28.2	33.5	38.4	43.1	47.0	50.5
1904-------	1931	3.6	5.9	9.0	12.7	17.0	21.9	26.7	31.7	36.5	40.7	44.5	47.9
1905-------	1932	3.6	5.8	8.6	12.3	16.4	20.9	25.5	30.2	34.5	38.5	42.1	45.3
1906-------	1933	3.2	5.1	7.8	11.4	15.2	19.5	23.9	28.2	32.3	36.1	39.5	42.9
1907-------	1934	3.1	5.0	7.7	11.0	14.6	18.7	22.7	26.8	30.6	34.2	37.7	40.9
1908-------	1935	2.5	4.4	6.8	10.0	13.6	17.3	21.0	24.8	28.5	32.2	35.6	38.8
1909-------	1936	2.7	4.5	6.9	10.0	13.2	16.7	20.2	23.9	27.7	31.3	34.7	37.7
1910-------	1937	2.7	4.4	6.8	9.6	12.8	16.1	19.6	23.4	27.2	30.7	33.9	36.8
1911-------	1938	2.5	4.2	6.3	9.1	12.1	15.3	18.9	22.8	26.4	29.8	32.8	35.5
1912-------	1939	2.3	3.8	6.0	8.6	11.4	14.6	18.2	21.8	25.3	28.5	31.4	34.1
1913-------	1940	2.3	3.9	6.0	8.4	11.2	14.4	17.7	21.1	24.3	27.3	30.2	32.8
1914-------	1941	2.2	3.7	5.6	8.1	11.0	14.2	17.4	20.7	23.8	26.9	29.7	32.3
1915-------	1942	2.2	3.7	5.7	8.3	11.1	14.1	17.2	20.3	23.5	26.5	29.2	31.9
1916-------	1943	2.3	3.8	5.8	8.3	11.0	13.9	16.8	20.0	23.0	25.9	28.8	31.5
1917-------	1944	2.2	3.7	5.7	8.1	10.8	13.7	16.7	19.8	22.9	25.9	28.8	31.7
1918-------	1945	2.4	3.8	5.7	8.1	10.7	13.6	16.5	19.7	22.8	25.9	29.0	31.8
1919-------	1946	2.4	3.9	5.9	8.3	11.0	13.9	17.0	20.2	23.4	26.7	29.8	32.9
1920-------	1947	2.4	3.9	5.9	8.4	11.1	14.1	17.2	20.5	23.8	27.2	30.5	33.6
1921-------	1948	2.5	4.0	6.1	8.6	11.3	14.2	17.4	20.8	24.4	28.0	31.5	34.8
1922-------	1949	2.4	4.0	6.1	8.5	11.2	14.2	17.4	21.0	24.7	28.4	31.9	35.4
1923-------	1950	2.5	4.1	6.1	8.6	11.3	14.4	17.9	21.6	25.5	29.4	33.2	36.8
1924-------	1951	2.5	4.1	6.2	8.7	11.7	15.1	18.9	23.0	27.1	31.3	35.2	39.0
1925-------	1952	2.6	4.2	6.3	9.1	12.3	15.9	19.9	24.2	28.6	32.9	37.1	40.8
1926-------	1953	2.6	4.3	6.7	9.7	13.2	17.2	21.4	25.8	30.4	35.0	39.1	42.8
1927-------	1954	2.6	4.5	7.0	10.2	14.0	18.2	22.6	27.3	32.2	36.7	40.8	44.5
1928-------	1955	3.0	5.0	7.7	11.2	15.1	19.5	24.3	29.3	34.1	38.6	42.8	46.1
1929-------	1956	3.3	5.6	8.7	12.5	16.9	21.7	26.9	32.0	37.0	41.6	45.3	48.4
1930-------	1957	3.9	6.4	9.7	13.8	18.5	23.6	28.9	34.2	39.1	43.2	46.6	49.4
1931-------	1958	4.5	7.3	10.9	15.4	20.4	25.8	31.2	36.5	41.0	44.8	47.8	50.3
1932-------	1959	4.8	7.8	11.7	16.3	21.4	26.8	32.1	36.8	40.9	44.3	47.1	49.5
1933-------	1960	5.1	8.4	12.6	17.4	22.6	27.8	32.5	36.7	40.3	43.3	46.0	48.3
1934-------	1961	5.6	9.0	13.1	17.9	22.8	27.4	31.5	35.2	38.4	41.3	43.8	45.8
1935-------	1962	6.1	9.5	13.6	18.1	22.4	26.3	29.9	33.1	36.1	38.8	41.0	42.7
1936-------	1963	6.0	9.3	13.1	17.0	20.6	24.0	27.1	30.1	32.8	35.2	37.0	38.4
1937-------	1964	6.1	9.2	12.4	15.7	18.8	21.7	24.6	27.3	29.7	31.6	33.1	
1938-------	1965	5.8	8.4	11.1	13.8	16.4	19.2	21.8	24.2	26.1	27.7		
1939-------	1966	5.3	7.4	9.7	12.0	14.5	17.0	19.2	21.1	22.7			
1940-------	1967	4.7	6.4	8.3	10.4	12.6	14.6	16.4	18.0				
1941-------	1968	3.8	5.3	7.0	8.8	10.6	12.2	13.6					
1942-------	1969	3.1	4.4	5.8	7.3	8.6	9.8						
1943-------	1970	2.4	3.4	4.5	5.6	6.6							
1944-------	1971	1.9	2.7	3.6	4.4								
1945-------	1972	1.7	2.3	3.0									
1946-------	1973	1.4	1.9										
1947-------	1974	0.9											

TABLE 6B. CUMULATIVE BIRTH RATES FOR WHITE WOMEN AS OF THE BEGINNING OF EACH YEAR 1917-74 BY AGE AND LIVE-BIRTH ORDER FOR EACH COHORT FROM 1867 TO 1959--CON.

LIVE-BIRTH ORDER AND COHORT	DIAGONAL LINE FOR JANUARY 1	EXACT AGE											
		39	40	41	42	43	44	45	46	47	48	49	50
SEVENTH BIRTHS--CON.													
1867-------													225.0
1868-------												220.5	220.6
1869-------											215.9	216.0	216.1
1870-------										211.1	211.4	211.5	211.5
1871-------									205.9	206.5	206.8	206.9	207.0
1872-------								200.2	201.2	201.8	202.0	202.2	202.2
1873-------							194.1	195.8	196.8	197.3	197.6	197.7	197.7
1874-------						187.8	190.5	192.1	193.0	193.6	193.8	193.9	193.9
1875-------					179.6	183.1	185.8	187.3	188.3	188.8	189.0	189.1	189.1
1876-------				168.8	173.7	177.3	179.8	181.4	182.3	182.8	183.0	183.1	183.1
1877-------			156.1	162.4	167.3	170.7	173.3	174.8	175.7	176.2	176.4	176.5	176.5
1878-------	1917	144.0	152.8	159.2	163.9	167.4	170.0	171.5	172.4	172.9	173.1	173.2	173.2
1879-------	1918	141.4	150.1	156.3	161.1	164.5	167.0	168.5	169.3	169.8	170.0	170.1	170.1
1880-------	1919	138.7	147.3	153.5	158.2	161.5	163.9	165.3	166.1	166.5	166.7	166.8	166.8
1881-------	1920	134.9	143.4	149.5	154.0	157.1	159.4	160.8	161.5	161.9	162.1	162.2	162.2
1882-------	1921	130.6	138.9	144.6	148.9	152.0	154.2	155.4	156.1	156.5	156.7	156.8	156.8
1883-------	1922	126.9	134.6	140.1	144.3	147.2	149.2	150.3	150.9	151.2	151.4	151.5	151.5
1884-------	1923	123.2	130.6	136.0	140.0	142.7	144.5	145.6	146.2	146.5	146.7	146.8	146.8
1885-------	1924	119.4	126.7	131.8	135.6	138.1	139.9	140.9	141.5	141.8	141.9	142.0	142.0
1886-------	1925	116.0	122.8	127.6	131.2	133.6	135.3	136.3	136.9	137.2	137.3	137.4	137.4
1887-------	1926	113.0	119.6	124.4	127.8	130.1	131.7	132.6	133.1	133.4	133.5	133.6	133.6
1888-------	1927	109.0	115.3	119.6	122.7	124.8	126.3	127.2	127.7	128.0	128.1	128.2	128.2
1889-------	1928	106.1	112.0	116.0	119.0	121.1	122.6	123.4	123.9	124.2	124.3	124.4	124.4
1890-------	1929	102.1	107.5	111.5	114.4	116.4	117.8	118.7	119.2	119.4	119.5	119.5	119.5
1891-------	1930	98.6	103.9	107.6	110.4	112.3	113.7	114.5	114.9	115.1	115.2	115.3	115.3
1892-------	1931	94.1	98.9	102.5	105.1	106.9	108.2	109.0	109.4	109.6	109.7	109.7	109.7
1893-------	1932	89.4	94.1	97.4	99.9	101.6	102.8	103.5	103.9	104.1	104.2	104.2	104.2
1894-------	1933	85.9	90.2	93.4	95.7	97.3	98.3	99.0	99.4	99.6	99.7	99.7	99.7
1895-------	1934	82.3	86.5	89.5	91.6	93.0	94.1	94.7	95.0	95.2	95.3	95.3	95.3
1896-------	1935	78.3	82.2	84.9	86.9	88.3	89.3	89.8	90.1	90.3	90.4	90.4	90.4
1897-------	1936	74.0	77.5	80.1	82.1	83.4	84.3	84.8	85.1	85.3	85.4	85.4	85.4
1898-------	1937	70.6	74.0	76.5	78.3	79.5	80.3	80.9	81.2	81.4	81.5	81.5	81.5
1899-------	1938	68.2	71.5	73.8	75.5	76.7	77.6	78.2	78.5	78.7	78.8	78.8	78.8
1900-------	1939	65.1	68.1	70.3	71.9	73.0	73.9	74.5	74.8	75.0	75.1	75.1	75.1
1901-------	1940	60.8	63.6	65.6	67.1	68.3	69.2	69.7	70.0	70.1	70.2	70.2	70.2
1902-------	1941	57.0	59.6	61.6	63.2	64.4	65.3	65.8	66.0	66.1	66.1	66.1	66.1
1903-------	1942	53.5	56.0	58.1	59.7	61.0	61.8	62.2	62.4	62.5	62.5	62.5	62.5
1904-------	1943	50.8	53.5	55.5	57.2	58.3	59.1	59.5	59.7	59.8	59.8	59.8	59.8
1905-------	1944	48.4	51.0	53.1	54.6	55.7	56.4	56.8	57.0	57.1	57.1	57.1	57.1
1906-------	1945	45.8	48.4	50.3	51.8	52.8	53.4	53.8	54.0	54.1	54.1	54.1	54.1
1907-------	1946	43.9	46.3	48.1	49.5	50.4	51.0	51.4	51.6	51.7	51.7	51.7	51.7
1908-------	1947	41.5	43.8	45.5	46.7	47.6	48.2	48.6	48.8	48.9	48.9	48.9	48.9
1909-------	1948	40.3	42.4	44.0	45.3	46.2	46.8	47.2	47.4	47.5	47.5	47.5	47.5
1910-------	1949	39.3	41.4	43.1	44.3	45.3	45.9	46.3	46.5	46.6	46.6	46.6	46.6
1911-------	1950	37.9	40.0	41.7	43.0	43.9	44.6	45.0	45.2	45.3	45.3	45.3	45.3
1912-------	1951	36.5	38.6	40.2	41.5	42.5	43.1	43.5	43.7	43.8	43.8	43.8	43.8
1913-------	1952	35.2	37.2	38.8	40.1	41.0	41.7	42.1	42.3	42.4	42.4	42.4	42.4
1914-------	1953	34.7	36.8	38.5	39.9	40.9	41.6	42.0	42.2	42.3	42.3	42.3	42.3
1915-------	1954	34.3	36.5	38.3	39.8	40.8	41.5	41.9	42.1	42.2	42.2	42.2	42.2
1916-------	1955	34.0	36.3	38.1	39.6	40.7	41.4	41.8	42.1	42.2	42.2	42.2	42.2
1917-------	1956	34.3	36.7	38.6	40.1	41.2	41.9	42.4	42.6	42.7	42.7	42.7	42.7
1918-------	1957	34.5	36.9	38.9	40.5	41.6	42.3	42.7	42.9	43.0	43.0	43.0	43.0
1919-------	1958	35.7	38.3	40.4	42.0	43.2	44.0	44.4	44.6	44.7	44.7	44.7	44.7
1920-------	1959	36.6	39.2	41.3	43.0	44.1	44.8	45.2	45.4	45.5	45.5	45.5	45.5
1921-------	1960	37.9	40.6	42.8	44.4	45.5	46.3	46.7	46.9	47.0	47.0	47.0	47.0
1922-------	1961	38.6	41.4	43.5	45.1	46.2	46.9	47.3	47.5	47.6	47.6	47.6	47.6
1923-------	1962	40.0	42.7	44.8	46.4	47.4	48.0	48.4	48.6	48.7	48.7	48.7	48.7
1924-------	1963	42.2	44.9	47.0	48.4	49.4	50.0	50.4	50.5	50.6	50.6	50.6	50.6
1925-------	1964	44.0	46.6	48.5	49.8	50.7	51.3	51.6	51.7	51.8	51.8	51.8	
1926-------	1965	46.0	48.4	50.2	51.4	52.2	52.7	52.9	53.0	53.0	53.0		
1927-------	1966	47.4	49.7	51.3	52.4	53.1	53.5	53.7	53.8	53.8			
1928-------	1967	48.8	50.9	52.4	53.4	54.1	54.5	54.7	54.8				
1929-------	1968	50.8	52.6	53.9	54.9	55.5	55.8	56.0					
1930-------	1969	51.6	53.3	54.6	55.4	55.9	56.2						
1931-------	1970	52.4	54.1	55.2	56.0	56.4							
1932-------	1971	51.5	52.9	53.9	54.5								
1933-------	1972	50.0	51.3	52.1									
1934-------	1973	47.3	48.3										
1935-------	1974	44.0											

TABLE 68. CUMULATIVE BIRTH RATES FOR WHITE WOMEN AS OF THE BEGINNING OF EACH YEAR 1917-74 BY AGE AND LIVE-BIRTH ORDER FOR EACH COHORT FROM 1867 TO 1959--CON.

LIVE-BIRTH ORDER AND COHORT	DIAGONAL LINE FOR JANUARY 1	EXACT AGE											
		15	16	17	18	19	20	21	22	23	24	25	26
EIGHTH AND HIGHER BIRTHS													
1891-------													1.1
1892-------												0.5	1.1
1893-------											0.0	0.3	0.8
1894-------										0.0	0.2	0.5	1.0
1895-------									0.0	0.1	0.3	0.6	1.1
1896-------								0.0	0.0	0.1	0.3	0.6	1.1
1897-------							*	0.0	0.0	0.1	0.3	0.6	1.2
1898-------						*	*	0.0	0.0	0.1	0.3	0.7	1.3
1899-------					*	*	*	0.0	0.0	0.1	0.3	0.7	1.3
1900-------				*	*	*	*	0.0	0.0	0.1	0.3	0.7	1.3
1901-------			*	*	*	*	*	0.0	0.0	0.1	0.3	0.6	1.2
1902-------	1917	*	*	*	*	*	*	0.0	0.0	0.1	0.3	0.7	1.2
1903-------	1918	*	*	*	*	*	*	0.0	0.0	0.1	0.3	0.6	1.1
1904-------	1919	*	*	*	*	*	*	0.0	0.0	0.1	0.3	0.6	1.1
1905-------	1920	*	*	*	*	*	*	0.0	0.0	0.1	0.3	0.6	1.1
1906-------	1921	*	*	*	*	*	*	0.0	0.0	0.1	0.3	0.6	1.0
1907-------	1922	*	*	*	*	*	*	0.0	0.0	0.1	0.3	0.5	0.9
1908-------	1923	*	*	*	*	*	*	0.0	0.0	0.1	0.2	0.4	0.7
1909-------	1924	*	*	*	*	*	*	0.0	0.0	0.1	0.2	0.4	0.7
1910-------	1925	*	*	*	*	*	*	0.0	0.0	0.1	0.2	0.4	0.7
1911-------	1926	*	*	*	*	*	*	0.0	0.0	0.1	0.2	0.4	0.8
1912-------	1927	*	*	*	*	*	*	0.0	0.0	0.0	0.1	0.3	0.6
1913-------	1928	*	*	*	*	*	*	0.0	0.0	0.1	0.2	0.4	0.7
1914-------	1929	*	*	*	*	*	*	0.0	0.0	0.1	0.2	0.3	0.5
1915-------	1930	*	*	*	*	*	*	0.0	0.0	0.0	0.1	0.2	0.5
1916-------	1931	*	*	*	*	*	*	0.0	0.0	0.0	0.1	0.3	0.6
1917-------	1932	*	*	*	*	*	*	0.0	0.0	0.0	0.1	0.3	0.6
1918-------	1933	*	*	*	*	*	*	0.0	0.0	0.1	0.2	0.4	0.7
1919-------	1934	*	*	*	*	*	*	0.0	0.0	0.1	0.2	0.4	0.7
1920-------	1935	*	*	*	*	*	*	0.0	0.0	0.0	0.1	0.3	0.6
1921-------	1936	*	*	*	*	*	*	0.0	0.0	0.0	0.1	0.3	0.6
1922-------	1937	*	*	*	*	*	*	0.0	0.0	0.0	0.1	0.3	0.6
1923-------	1938	*	*	*	*	*	*	0.0	0.0	0.0	0.1	0.2	0.4
1924-------	1939	*	*	*	*	*	*	0.0	0.0	0.0	0.1	0.2	0.6
1925-------	1940	*	*	*	*	*	*	0.0	0.0	0.0	0.1	0.3	0.6
1926-------	1941	*	*	*	*	*	*	0.0	0.0	0.0	0.1	0.3	0.6
1927-------	1942	*	*	*	*	*	*	0.0	0.0	0.1	0.2	0.4	0.7
1928-------	1943	*	*	*	*	*	*	0.0	0.0	0.0	0.1	0.3	0.7
1929-------	1944	*	*	*	*	*	*	0.0	0.0	0.0	0.1	0.3	0.7
1930-------	1945	*	*	*	*	*	*	0.0	0.0	0.0	0.1	0.3	0.7
1931-------	1946	*	*	*	*	*	*	0.0	0.0	0.1	0.2	0.4	0.9
1932-------	1947	*	*	*	*	*	*	0.0	0.0	0.0	0.1	0.4	0.9
1933-------	1948	*	*	*	*	*	*	0.0	0.0	0.0	0.1	0.4	1.0
1934-------	1949	*	*	*	*	*	*	0.0	0.0	0.1	0.3	0.6	1.2
1935-------	1950	*	*	*	*	*	*	0.0	0.0	0.1	0.3	0.6	1.3
1936-------	1951	*	*	*	*	*	*	0.0	0.0	0.1	0.2	0.5	1.2
1937-------	1952	*	*	*	*	*	*	0.0	0.0	0.0	0.2	0.6	1.3
1938-------	1953	*	*	*	*	*	*	0.0	0.0	0.1	0.3	0.6	1.2
1939-------	1954	*	*	*	*	*	*	0.0	0.0	0.1	0.3	0.7	1.3
1940-------	1955	*	*	*	*	*	*	0.0	0.0	0.1	0.3	0.6	1.1
1941-------	1956	*	*	*	*	*	*	0.0	0.0	0.1	0.3	0.6	1.0
1942-------	1957	*	*	*	*	*	*	0.0	0.0	0.1	0.2	0.4	0.7
1943-------	1958	*	*	*	*	*	*	0.0	0.0	0.0	0.1	0.3	0.5
1944-------	1959	*	*	*	*	*	*	0.0	0.0	0.0	0.1	0.2	0.4
1945-------	1960	*	*	*	*	*	*	0.0	0.0	0.0	0.0	0.1	0.3
1946-------	1961	*	*	*	*	*	*	0.0	0.0	0.0	0.1	0.2	0.4
1947-------	1962	*	*	*	*	*	*	0.0	0.0	0.1	0.2	0.3	0.4
1948-------	1963	*	*	*	*	*	*	0.0	0.1	0.1	0.1	0.2	0.3
1949-------	1964	*	*	*	*	*	*	0.1	0.1	0.1	0.1	0.1	
1950-------	1965	*	*	*	*	*	*	0.0	0.0	0.0	0.0		
1951-------	1966	*	*	*	*	*	*	0.0	0.0	0.0			
1952-------	1967	*	*	*	*	*	*	0.0	0.0				
1953-------	1968	*	*	*	*	*	*	0.0					
1954-------	1969	*	*	*	*	*	*						
1955-------	1970	*	*	*	*	*							
1956-------	1971	*	*	*	*								
1957-------	1972	*	*	*									
1958-------	1973	*	*										
1959-------	1974	*											

TABLE 6B. CUMULATIVE BIRTH RATES FOR WHITE WOMEN AS OF THE BEGINNING OF EACH YEAR 1917-74 BY AGE AND LIVE-BIRTH ORDER FOR EACH COHORT FROM 1867 TO 1959--CON.

LIVE-BIRTH ORDER AND COHORT	DIAGONAL LINE FOR JANUARY 1	EXACT AGE											
		27	28	29	30	31	32	33	34	35	36	37	38
EIGHTH AND HIGHER BIRTHS--CON.													
1879-------													182.0
1880-------												144.6	173.0
1881-------											112.5	137.5	165.3
1882-------										84.8	106.9	131.3	158.7
1883-------									59.5	77.8	99.6	123.6	150.7
1884-------								42.3	57.1	75.4	96.8	120.7	148.3
1885-------							29.1	40.5	55.5	73.4	94.7	119.0	144.6
1886-------						19.0	27.8	39.4	54.1	72.0	94.0	116.7	142.4
1887-------					12.0	18.3	27.3	38.7	53.4	72.2	92.8	115.7	141.2
1888-------				6.6	11.4	17.7	26.5	37.9	53.5	70.9	91.7	114.3	138.5
1889-------			3.7	6.6	11.2	17.2	26.0	38.0	52.3	70.0	90.4	112.0	135.1
1890-------	1917	2.0	3.8	6.5	10.9	17.0	26.2	37.2	51.9	69.2	88.6	108.8	131.4
1891-------	1918	2.1	3.7	6.2	10.7	17.1	25.6	36.9	51.1	67.7	86.0	106.2	126.7
1892-------	1919	2.0	3.5	6.1	10.8	16.7	25.4	36.3	50.0	65.4	83.3	101.2	119.9
1893-------	1920	1.6	3.2	5.9	10.2	16.2	24.6	35.1	47.9	63.0	79.1	95.6	113.3
1894-------	1921	1.9	3.5	6.1	10.6	16.5	24.5	34.4	46.8	60.6	75.5	91.3	107.9
1895-------	1922	2.0	3.6	6.4	10.9	16.6	24.3	34.0	45.5	58.3	72.8	87.6	103.5
1896-------	1923	2.0	3.7	6.5	10.9	16.3	23.9	32.9	43.6	56.0	69.3	83.3	97.5
1897-------	1924	2.2	3.9	6.5	10.6	16.1	23.2	31.6	41.9	53.2	65.9	78.6	92.4
1898-------	1925	2.3	4.0	6.6	10.7	15.8	22.4	30.5	40.1	50.9	62.4	74.8	88.2
1899-------	1926	2.3	4.0	6.5	10.4	15.2	21.6	29.2	38.7	48.7	60.2	72.6	85.3
1900-------	1927	2.3	3.8	6.1	9.7	14.3	20.3	27.8	36.3	46.3	57.9	69.5	81.8
1901-------	1928	2.1	3.5	5.7	9.0	13.3	19.1	25.7	34.2	44.1	54.7	65.9	77.5
1902-------	1929	2.0	3.4	5.5	8.6	12.6	17.7	24.2	32.3	41.3	51.3	61.7	72.1
1903-------	1930	1.9	3.2	5.2	8.2	11.8	16.9	23.2	30.8	39.3	48.8	58.1	67.9
1904-------	1931	1.9	3.2	5.1	7.8	11.4	16.4	22.4	29.7	37.9	46.5	55.4	64.6
1905-------	1932	1.8	3.0	4.7	7.4	11.1	15.8	21.6	28.6	36.0	44.3	52.6	61.2
1906-------	1933	1.6	2.6	4.2	7.0	10.3	14.9	20.4	26.8	34.1	41.8	49.6	58.2
1907-------	1934	1.5	2.5	4.2	6.7	10.0	14.3	19.3	25.6	32.4	39.5	47.3	55.7
1908-------	1935	1.2	2.2	3.8	6.2	9.3	13.2	18.2	24.1	30.4	37.6	45.2	53.2
1909-------	1936	1.3	2.3	3.8	6.1	8.9	12.8	17.4	22.8	29.1	36.1	43.4	50.9
1910-------	1937	1.3	2.2	3.7	5.7	8.5	12.1	16.4	21.9	28.1	34.9	41.9	49.0
1911-------	1938	1.4	2.3	3.7	5.8	8.5	11.9	16.3	21.7	27.8	34.3	41.0	47.8
1912-------	1939	1.1	1.9	3.3	5.3	7.9	11.4	15.8	21.1	26.8	33.0	39.2	46.0
1913-------	1940	1.2	2.1	3.5	5.4	8.0	11.5	15.8	20.7	26.2	31.9	38.1	44.4
1914-------	1941	1.0	1.8	3.1	5.0	7.6	10.9	14.9	19.7	24.9	30.8	36.8	43.0
1915-------	1942	1.0	1.8	3.1	5.0	7.4	10.7	14.6	19.2	24.5	30.1	36.0	42.2
1916-------	1943	1.0	1.8	3.1	4.9	7.4	10.5	14.2	18.9	24.0	29.5	35.3	41.1
1917-------	1944	1.1	1.9	3.1	5.0	7.4	10.5	14.4	18.9	23.9	29.3	34.9	40.7
1918-------	1945	1.1	1.9	3.1	4.9	7.3	10.6	14.4	18.9	23.8	29.1	34.6	40.3
1919-------	1946	1.2	2.0	3.2	5.1	7.7	10.9	14.7	19.3	24.3	29.7	35.3	41.2
1920-------	1947	1.1	1.9	3.2	5.3	7.8	11.0	14.9	19.5	24.6	30.0	35.7	41.8
1921-------	1948	1.1	2.0	3.5	5.5	8.1	11.4	15.3	20.0	25.2	30.8	36.7	42.7
1922-------	1949	1.1	2.1	3.5	5.5	8.0	11.2	15.2	19.8	25.0	30.8	36.6	42.8
1923-------	1950	1.0	1.9	3.2	5.2	7.7	11.1	15.1	19.9	25.3	31.1	37.3	43.7
1924-------	1951	1.1	2.0	3.4	5.4	8.1	11.5	15.7	20.8	26.4	32.5	39.0	45.6
1925-------	1952	1.1	2.0	3.4	5.5	8.3	12.0	16.5	21.7	27.7	34.2	41.0	47.7
1926-------	1953	1.2	2.2	3.7	6.0	9.0	12.9	17.5	23.1	29.3	36.1	42.9	49.7
1927-------	1954	1.3	2.3	3.9	6.3	9.5	13.7	18.8	24.7	31.4	38.3	45.2	51.9
1928-------	1955	1.3	2.4	4.2	6.8	10.4	14.9	20.3	26.6	33.4	40.4	47.3	53.7
1929-------	1956	1.4	2.7	4.7	7.7	11.6	16.5	22.4	29.1	36.1	43.0	49.6	55.2
1930-------	1957	1.6	3.0	5.3	8.6	12.8	18.0	24.1	30.9	37.8	44.4	50.1	55.2
1931-------	1958	1.8	3.4	5.9	9.4	14.0	19.5	25.7	32.4	38.8	44.6	49.9	54.5
1932-------	1959	1.9	3.6	6.2	9.9	14.5	20.0	26.1	32.1	37.8	43.0	47.7	52.0
1933-------	1960	2.1	3.9	6.7	10.5	15.1	20.4	25.7	31.0	36.0	40.6	44.9	48.8
1934-------	1961	2.4	4.3	7.2	11.0	15.4	20.0	24.7	29.2	33.5	37.8	41.7	45.2
1935-------	1962	2.5	4.5	7.3	10.9	14.7	18.7	22.7	26.6	30.6	34.5	38.0	40.8
1936-------	1963	2.4	4.3	6.9	9.9	13.1	16.4	19.8	23.4	27.0	30.4	33.2	35.6
1937-------	1964	2.5	4.2	6.4	8.8	11.5	14.4	17.5	20.7	23.8	26.4	28.6	
1938-------	1965	2.3	3.8	5.5	7.6	9.9	12.4	15.0	17.7	20.0	22.1		
1939-------	1966	2.2	3.4	4.9	6.6	8.6	10.8	13.0	15.0	16.9			
1940-------	1967	1.8	2.8	4.0	5.5	7.3	9.1	10.8	12.4				
1941-------	1968	1.6	2.4	3.5	4.9	6.3	7.7	9.1					
1942-------	1969	1.2	1.9	2.8	3.8	4.8	5.8						
1943-------	1970	0.9	1.5	2.1	2.8	3.5							
1944-------	1971	0.8	1.2	1.6	2.1								
1945-------	1972	0.6	0.9	1.3									
1946-------	1973	0.6	0.8										
1947-------	1974	0.5											

TABLE 6B. CUMULATIVE BIRTH RATES FOR WHITE WOMEN AS OF THE BEGINNING OF EACH YEAR 1917-74 BY AGE AND LIVE-BIRTH ORDER FOR EACH COHORT FROM 1867 TO 1959--CON.

LIVE-BIRTH ORDER AND COHORT	DIAGONAL LINE FOR JANUARY 1	EXACT AGE											
		39	40	41	42	43	44	45	46	47	48	49	50
EIGHTH AND HIGHER BIRTHS--CON.													
1867-------													479.9
1868-------												467.4	467.9
1869-------											453.1	454.3	454.8
1870-------										436.9	439.2	440.4	440.9
1871-------									418.7	422.9	425.2	426.3	426.8
1872-------								398.4	405.2	409.4	411.6	412.8	413.3
1873-------							377.3	387.6	394.3	398.3	400.6	401.8	402.3
1874-------						352.6	367.0	377.0	383.5	387.7	390.0	391.1	391.6
1875-------					324.8	341.9	355.9	365.7	372.3	376.5	378.6	379.6	380.1
1876-------				293.8	315.4	332.0	345.7	355.6	362.3	366.1	368.0	369.0	369.4
1877-------			259.5	284.0	305.1	321.4	335.3	345.4	351.6	355.1	357.0	357.9	358.2
1878-------	1917	222.3	251.9	276.1	297.0	313.6	327.7	337.1	343.0	346.6	348.4	349.2	349.6
1879-------	1918	211.1	240.3	264.2	285.3	302.1	315.3	324.5	330.5	334.0	335.6	336.4	336.7
1880-------	1919	201.6	230.5	254.5	275.8	291.4	304.4	313.7	319.5	322.8	324.4	325.1	325.4
1881-------	1920	193.6	222.3	246.5	266.2	281.5	294.6	303.5	308.9	312.0	313.5	314.2	314.5
1882-------	1921	186.6	215.6	237.9	257.2	272.6	285.1	293.3	298.4	301.3	302.7	303.3	303.6
1883-------	1922	179.1	205.8	227.7	247.1	262.0	273.7	281.7	286.5	289.2	290.5	291.2	291.5
1884-------	1923	174.5	201.0	222.9	241.3	255.2	266.6	273.9	278.3	280.8	282.1	282.7	283.0
1885-------	1924	170.7	197.0	217.8	235.1	248.9	259.4	266.1	270.3	272.7	273.9	274.5	274.8
1886-------	1925	168.3	193.1	212.5	229.4	242.0	251.5	258.0	262.0	264.2	265.3	265.9	266.1
1887-------	1926	166.0	189.5	208.8	224.7	236.2	245.6	251.8	255.5	257.6	258.7	259.2	259.4
1888-------	1927	161.9	184.7	202.5	216.9	228.2	236.9	242.7	246.2	248.2	249.2	249.7	249.9
1889-------	1928	158.2	179.5	196.0	210.0	220.6	229.0	234.5	238.0	239.9	240.8	241.3	241.5
1890-------	1929	152.4	171.9	187.7	200.8	210.9	218.7	224.1	227.3	229.0	229.9	230.4	230.6
1891-------	1930	146.1	164.8	179.7	192.0	201.4	209.1	214.2	217.2	218.8	219.6	220.0	220.1
1892-------	1931	138.3	155.6	169.3	180.6	189.9	197.1	201.7	204.4	206.0	206.7	207.0	207.1
1893-------	1932	130.4	146.6	159.3	170.5	179.0	185.4	189.5	192.1	193.5	194.1	194.4	194.5
1894-------	1933	124.1	138.9	151.5	161.9	169.6	175.5	179.5	181.8	183.0	183.6	183.8	183.9
1895-------	1934	118.4	132.9	144.7	154.2	161.5	167.2	170.8	173.0	174.2	174.7	174.9	175.0
1896-------	1935	112.0	125.8	136.5	145.4	152.3	157.4	160.7	162.6	163.7	164.2	164.4	164.5
1897-------	1936	106.1	118.7	128.9	137.5	143.8	148.6	151.6	153.6	154.6	155.1	155.3	155.4
1898-------	1937	100.9	112.8	122.7	130.5	136.6	141.0	144.2	146.2	147.2	147.7	147.9	148.0
1899-------	1938	97.7	109.4	118.4	125.9	131.6	136.0	139.0	140.8	141.8	142.3	142.5	142.6
1900-------	1939	93.7	104.3	112.9	120.0	125.4	129.8	132.8	134.6	135.5	136.0	136.2	136.3
1901-------	1940	88.1	98.0	106.0	112.5	117.9	122.2	125.1	126.7	127.6	128.0	128.2	128.3
1902-------	1941	82.2	91.4	99.0	105.6	111.1	115.3	117.9	119.5	120.3	120.7	120.9	121.0
1903-------	1942	77.2	86.0	93.6	100.2	105.5	109.3	111.9	113.3	114.1	114.4	114.5	114.6
1904-------	1943	73.5	82.3	89.7	96.0	100.8	104.6	106.9	108.2	108.9	109.2	109.3	109.4
1905-------	1944	70.1	78.6	85.7	91.5	96.1	99.4	101.5	102.7	103.3	103.6	103.7	103.8
1906-------	1945	66.9	75.0	81.7	87.3	91.4	94.5	96.4	97.6	98.2	98.5	98.6	98.7
1907-------	1946	63.9	71.5	77.8	82.8	86.8	89.7	91.7	92.8	93.3	93.6	93.7	93.7
1908-------	1947	60.9	68.0	73.7	78.6	82.3	85.1	86.9	87.9	88.4	88.6	88.7	88.8
1909-------	1948	58.1	64.8	70.5	75.1	78.7	81.5	83.1	84.1	84.6	84.9	85.0	85.0
1910-------	1949	55.8	62.5	67.9	72.4	75.8	78.3	80.0	80.9	81.4	81.6	81.7	81.8
1911-------	1950	54.7	61.0	66.2	70.4	73.7	76.3	77.9	78.9	79.4	79.6	79.7	79.8
1912-------	1951	52.5	58.5	63.4	67.5	70.8	73.2	74.8	75.7	76.2	76.4	76.5	76.6
1913-------	1952	50.6	56.5	61.3	65.4	68.5	70.9	72.4	73.3	73.7	73.9	74.0	74.0
1914-------	1953	49.2	54.7	59.4	63.3	66.4	68.7	70.2	71.0	71.4	71.6	71.7	71.7
1915-------	1954	48.0	53.4	58.0	61.9	65.0	67.2	68.6	69.4	69.8	70.0	70.1	70.1
1916-------	1955	46.8	52.2	56.8	60.6	63.6	65.8	67.2	68.0	68.4	68.6	68.7	68.7
1917-------	1956	46.5	51.9	56.5	60.2	63.2	65.4	66.8	67.6	68.0	68.2	68.2	68.2
1918-------	1957	46.0	51.5	55.9	59.7	62.7	64.9	66.3	67.0	67.3	67.4	67.5	67.5
1919-------	1958	47.2	52.5	57.3	61.2	64.2	66.4	67.8	68.5	68.9	69.1	69.1	69.1
1920-------	1959	47.6	53.3	58.0	61.9	64.9	67.1	68.4	69.1	69.4	69.5	69.5	69.5
1921-------	1960	48.8	54.4	59.2	63.2	66.2	68.3	69.5	70.2	70.5	70.6	70.6	70.6
1922-------	1961	48.8	54.4	59.2	63.1	66.0	67.9	69.1	69.7	70.0	70.1	70.1	70.1
1923-------	1962	49.9	55.6	60.4	64.2	66.9	68.7	69.8	70.3	70.5	70.6	70.6	70.6
1924-------	1963	51.9	57.7	62.5	66.1	68.6	70.3	71.3	71.8	72.0	72.1	72.1	72.1
1925-------	1964	54.1	59.8	64.2	67.5	69.8	71.3	72.2	72.6	72.8	72.9	72.9	
1926-------	1965	56.1	61.5	65.6	68.5	70.6	72.0	72.8	73.2	73.4	73.5		
1927-------	1966	57.8	62.6	66.2	68.9	70.8	72.0	72.7	73.1	73.3			
1928-------	1967	59.0	63.2	66.5	69.0	70.8	71.9	72.5	72.8				
1929-------	1968	60.0	63.9	67.0	69.4	71.0	72.0	72.6					
1930-------	1969	59.5	63.1	66.0	68.0	69.4	70.3						
1931-------	1970	58.6	62.0	64.5	66.3	67.6							
1932-------	1971	55.7	58.7	60.9	62.5								
1933-------	1972	52.1	54.6	56.5									
1934-------	1973	48.0	50.2										
1935-------	1974	43.1											

TABLE 6C. CUMULATIVE BIRTH RATES FOR ALL OTHER WOMEN AS OF THE BEGINNING OF EACH YEAR 1917-74 BY AGE AND LIVE-BIRTH ORDER FOR EACH COHORT FROM 1867 TO 1959

LIVE-BIRTH ORDER AND COHORT	DIAGONAL LINE FOR JANUARY 1	EXACT AGE											
		15	16	17	18	19	20	21	22	23	24	25	26
TOTAL BIRTHS													
1891-------													1,693.5
1892-------												1,498.0	1,667.1
1893-------											1,336.7	1,517.1	1,683.4
1894-------										1,105.7	1,294.3	1,473.2	1,639.3
1895-------									896.7	1,078.4	1,267.0	1,441.2	1,619.4
1896-------								693.8	880.7	1,062.1	1,241.3	1,426.6	1,609.9
1897-------							509.4	689.0	875.3	1,047.5	1,237.1	1,428.0	1,598.0
1898-------						322.9	496.4	674.1	851.8	1,038.4	1,235.4	1,417.0	1,587.2
1899-------					194.1	334.0	502.8	670.1	863.4	1,051.8	1,237.9	1,416.9	1,592.8
1900-------				98.5	203.9	338.6	497.5	682.9	876.5	1,054.8	1,241.8	1,430.2	1,603.6
1901-------			42.0	104.9	205.6	330.9	507.9	695.8	875.9	1,051.1	1,246.1	1,426.9	1,591.9
1902-------	1917	11.3	45.8	106.7	201.4	344.6	530.1	705.9	885.1	1,072.5	1,258.0	1,428.8	1,576.7
1903-------	1918	12.8	45.7	102.5	211.4	364.0	533.8	710.0	899.0	1,079.6	1,256.2	1,412.7	1,546.1
1904-------	1919	12.1	42.7	108.4	222.4	360.1	533.3	718.7	902.7	1,080.2	1,244.9	1,389.7	1,517.9
1905-------	1920	11.2	46.7	114.6	216.2	360.5	542.9	723.6	903.8	1,068.3	1,220.3	1,358.4	1,485.4
1906-------	1921	13.0	49.7	109.8	216.4	368.8	546.6	724.9	894.1	1,046.6	1,191.5	1,330.7	1,454.2
1907-------	1922	13.6	46.3	109.8	223.1	375.8	551.1	718.1	876.0	1,022.0	1,168.9	1,301.7	1,424.5
1908-------	1923	12.3	47.2	114.9	231.7	381.8	546.9	703.0	856.6	1,004.5	1,145.8	1,279.1	1,396.4
1909-------	1924	13.2	50.5	122.8	239.0	381.6	538.2	692.1	848.7	994.7	1,139.6	1,269.8	1,393.1
1910-------	1925	14.3	54.3	126.3	238.3	373.3	527.3	684.2	837.6	987.6	1,127.8	1,264.0	1,385.0
1911-------	1926	15.6	57.2	128.9	236.0	367.9	525.8	679.3	838.1	981.0	1,128.6	1,263.9	1,384.1
1912-------	1927	16.4	57.0	124.2	227.2	361.4	513.3	670.6	818.0	966.9	1,111.8	1,243.0	1,365.6
1913-------	1928	16.1	54.3	118.8	223.8	354.7	509.7	657.0	812.1	961.3	1,103.4	1,239.8	1,364.2
1914-------	1929	14.7	50.9	116.6	218.3	350.5	496.2	651.1	807.1	954.5	1,103.5	1,241.9	1,367.7
1915-------	1930	14.2	51.3	115.4	217.7	342.1	495.6	651.8	805.5	959.2	1,108.9	1,248.9	1,378.4
1916-------	1931	14.5	50.1	115.2	210.9	342.0	497.2	650.2	810.4	964.0	1,115.3	1,260.4	1,394.0
1917-------	1932	13.9	50.1	110.6	212.1	346.7	498.4	658.6	818.4	972.6	1,130.6	1,281.2	1,419.3
1918-------	1933	14.2	48.4	111.9	217.7	349.5	509.1	670.4	827.9	985.8	1,147.9	1,302.3	1,446.1
1919-------	1934	13.6	49.0	117.2	223.2	364.8	528.5	690.5	853.5	1,016.9	1,184.3	1,342.6	1,485.1
1920-------	1935	13.9	53.1	121.6	235.2	380.7	545.2	713.3	879.3	1,046.7	1,216.3	1,370.6	1,507.8
1921-------	1936	15.5	55.1	129.4	246.4	394.0	564.2	738.2	908.5	1,077.3	1,240.7	1,387.3	1,541.0
1922-------	1937	14.8	56.1	131.1	245.6	394.0	567.5	739.8	911.6	1,073.8	1,224.4	1,387.9	1,551.3
1923-------	1938	15.7	58.0	130.5	243.9	398.1	570.8	745.8	911.1	1,063.5	1,235.5	1,413.0	1,584.1
1924-------	1939	16.4	57.8	130.4	248.7	405.2	581.2	747.7	904.9	1,082.5	1,275.6	1,466.3	1,646.5
1925-------	1940	16.8	59.5	136.5	262.5	422.5	587.4	747.0	928.4	1,131.4	1,338.1	1,536.9	1,725.6
1926-------	1941	17.0	62.2	145.7	274.3	421.4	579.7	761.2	973.1	1,190.0	1,404.8	1,611.3	1,809.3
1927-------	1942	17.9	66.1	151.0	268.6	410.8	582.9	795.8	1,020.5	1,243.9	1,462.4	1,675.7	1,878.5
1928-------	1943	18.2	67.2	144.4	258.9	408.1	611.3	836.2	1,065.8	1,290.4	1,514.3	1,728.6	1,936.4
1929-------	1944	18.5	63.4	140.2	257.0	436.0	651.2	881.2	1,112.2	1,343.4	1,571.0	1,794.2	2,010.8
1930-------	1945	17.1	61.7	137.9	277.3	465.9	683.6	912.4	1,147.7	1,379.5	1,610.9	1,841.3	2,061.3
1931-------	1946	17.5	61.9	154.6	303.5	495.9	713.8	947.7	1,183.9	1,422.5	1,666.3	1,903.9	2,135.0
1932-------	1947	16.4	69.4	168.2	319.0	510.9	732.6	964.2	1,203.6	1,452.9	1,703.6	1,951.4	2,185.2
1933-------	1948	20.4	78.0	179.6	332.2	528.5	747.8	986.9	1,241.8	1,502.8	1,767.7	2,023.5	2,259.7
1934-------	1949	22.1	81.9	184.9	340.9	534.9	760.9	1,014.3	1,281.0	1,557.9	1,830.6	2,088.8	2,332.3
1935-------	1950	22.6	82.6	187.9	341.5	540.3	776.2	1,038.4	1,319.6	1,603.9	1,879.1	2,142.7	2,383.3
1936-------	1951	23.2	84.7	187.2	343.1	548.4	787.9	1,061.6	1,347.7	1,630.3	1,906.2	2,164.3	2,402.9
1937-------	1952	24.3	83.0	185.9	344.3	549.5	797.8	1,075.1	1,356.3	1,636.5	1,905.5	2,160.0	2,393.2
1938-------	1953	22.1	80.1	184.9	340.7	550.9	797.8	1,066.7	1,344.3	1,616.7	1,880.0	2,125.2	2,347.4
1939-------	1954	22.0	82.7	186.3	346.8	556.4	797.9	1,066.6	1,340.2	1,612.5	1,868.0	2,106.2	2,319.2
1940-------	1955	23.8	82.6	187.9	348.0	553.9	794.4	1,059.1	1,331.9	1,596.2	1,844.4	2,072.6	2,266.8
1941-------	1956	22.7	83.3	189.6	344.3	547.8	783.1	1,043.8	1,309.1	1,565.0	1,804.2	2,012.6	2,189.9
1942-------	1957	22.7	83.3	184.1	337.2	534.6	764.0	1,018.5	1,276.7	1,524.2	1,743.3	1,934.0	2,096.5
1943-------	1958	23.0	79.4	179.6	327.1	519.3	742.1	991.1	1,241.3	1,472.1	1,674.4	1,849.4	1,999.9
1944-------	1959	21.5	79.0	176.2	322.5	511.3	733.3	979.1	1,217.2	1,432.5	1,620.0	1,784.0	1,935.1
1945-------	1960	22.3	77.7	173.9	316.2	503.4	724.6	959.9	1,184.5	1,385.7	1,563.2	1,727.2	1,884.8
1946-------	1961	21.3	76.3	170.0	311.4	500.7	714.9	940.6	1,152.7	1,344.2	1,522.4	1,692.1	1,841.2
1947-------	1962	21.2	74.1	167.4	310.2	493.9	702.6	919.6	1,122.3	1,312.4	1,493.0	1,654.7	1,788.0
1948-------	1963	20.1	72.4	165.4	304.9	485.2	687.2	894.0	1,094.4	1,286.2	1,458.0	1,600.4	1,724.8
1949-------	1964	19.9	72.2	164.6	303.0	479.2	675.3	879.8	1,080.8	1,262.5	1,413.1	1,545.7	
1950-------	1965	19.9	72.5	164.5	301.3	474.0	669.5	876.1	1,065.0	1,224.8	1,365.4		
1951-------	1966	20.4	73.1	166.4	301.8	474.7	672.4	867.3	1,036.6	1,185.9			
1952-------	1967	20.5	74.7	166.9	301.8	477.6	665.5	842.4	1,000.2				
1953-------	1968	21.3	75.6	167.4	306.7	475.8	650.8	816.4					
1954-------	1969	21.9	76.3	172.6	308.4	469.9	633.9						
1955-------	1970	22.4	80.4	175.7	309.4	461.7							
1956-------	1971	23.8	81.4	177.0	303.5								
1957-------	1972	23.6	81.8	173.7									
1958-------	1973	24.1	81.1										
1959-------	1974	24.5											

TABLE 6C. CUMULATIVE BIRTH RATES FOR ALL OTHER WOMEN AS OF THE BEGINNING OF EACH YEAR 1917-74 BY AGE AND LIVE-BIRTH ORDER FOR EACH COHORT FROM 1867 TO 1959--CON.

LIVE-BIRTH ORDER AND COHORT	DIAGONAL LINE FOR JANUARY 1	EXACT AGE											
		27	28	29	30	31	32	33	34	35	36	37	38
TOTAL BIRTHS--CON.													
1879-------													3,761.0
1880-------												3,575.5	3,676.2
1881-------											3,395.3	3,507.7	3,610.5
1882-------										3,219.8	3,335.9	3,449.7	3,558.5
1883-------									3,045.3	3,157.8	3,272.9	3,390.0	3,500.3
1884-------								2,864.7	2,965.8	3,075.0	3,190.3	3,306.4	3,408.9
1885-------							2,704.5	2,800.3	2,896.8	3,003.9	3,116.5	3,223.0	3,317.4
1886-------						2,557.5	2,669.0	2,761.0	2,854.2	2,957.9	3,064.6	3,162.8	3,250.6
1887-------					2,418.9	2,531.9	2,640.9	2,730.3	2,820.4	2,923.2	3,022.2	3,114.4	3,201.0
1888-------				2,261.6	2,395.5	2,505.7	2,613.1	2,700.7	2,796.1	2,892.6	2,987.4	3,079.3	3,166.5
1889-------			2,074.1	2,204.6	2,334.6	2,446.1	2,553.2	2,646.7	2,737.7	2,832.2	2,928.5	3,023.7	3,108.5
1890-------	1917	1,881.9	2,025.1	2,150.9	2,285.0	2,399.9	2,514.2	2,603.8	2,694.7	2,792.3	2,891.3	2,982.9	3,063.8
1891-------	1918	1,843.4	1,982.2	2,114.0	2,255.2	2,377.8	2,487.7	2,577.4	2,672.5	2,772.3	2,868.6	2,954.9	3,025.8
1892-------	1919	1,813.0	1,957.4	2,099.7	2,249.4	2,365.3	2,474.9	2,568.4	2,666.3	2,763.1	2,851.4	2,926.4	2,992.7
1893-------	1920	1,834.0	1,990.9	2,140.8	2,280.2	2,394.9	2,508.4	2,604.1	2,698.4	2,787.0	2,865.0	2,936.7	3,003.4
1894-------	1921	1,803.2	1,965.8	2,102.4	2,239.6	2,358.7	2,471.2	2,563.8	2,652.0	2,730.4	2,805.7	2,875.9	2,939.6
1895-------	1922	1,787.3	1,935.6	2,069.8	2,212.9	2,329.3	2,437.5	2,523.9	2,601.9	2,677.7	2,751.4	2,818.1	2,882.4
1896-------	1923	1,763.3	1,908.2	2,048.7	2,187.0	2,300.6	2,400.2	2,476.4	2,550.5	2,624.9	2,694.3	2,760.5	2,819.6
1897-------	1924	1,747.1	1,898.6	2,034.6	2,167.4	2,270.6	2,361.6	2,432.8	2,506.6	2,577.4	2,645.7	2,706.8	2,766.5
1898-------	1925	1,745.7	1,894.7	2,027.1	2,151.8	2,247.4	2,334.1	2,407.8	2,480.2	2,551.1	2,616.7	2,679.5	2,735.2
1899-------	1926	1,750.8	1,898.3	2,026.7	2,144.1	2,237.9	2,328.8	2,403.8	2,481.0	2,553.2	2,624.8	2,687.1	2,743.8
1900-------	1927	1,758.7	1,858.4	2,014.3	2,128.4	2,225.3	2,314.9	2,392.5	2,469.1	2,544.6	2,612.7	2,673.9	2,732.8
1901-------	1928	1,733.3	1,856.2	1,965.7	2,077.6	2,170.1	2,257.6	2,330.6	2,407.4	2,475.6	2,539.1	2,599.5	2,656.5
1902-------	1929	1,701.3	1,815.4	1,921.7	2,026.6	2,113.8	2,193.4	2,263.4	2,329.8	2,391.8	2,452.1	2,508.6	2,562.8
1903-------	1930	1,663.6	1,774.0	1,875.7	1,977.6	2,058.6	2,137.2	2,200.2	2,262.0	2,322.2	2,380.1	2,433.8	2,486.1
1904-------	1931	1,633.7	1,743.0	1,844.5	1,943.0	2,026.0	2,100.9	2,162.4	2,225.2	2,284.8	2,341.7	2,394.7	2,447.8
1905-------	1932	1,599.8	1,708.1	1,805.6	1,904.5	1,984.1	2,055.5	2,117.3	2,180.6	2,239.4	2,296.0	2,349.5	2,400.9
1906-------	1933	1,567.8	1,671.8	1,770.7	1,864.5	1,941.0	2,013.2	2,076.1	2,139.1	2,198.6	2,256.1	2,308.6	2,362.1
1907-------	1934	1,531.8	1,637.5	1,730.7	1,820.9	1,897.8	1,970.2	2,033.1	2,097.8	2,159.1	2,217.7	2,272.7	2,327.2
1908-------	1935	1,506.1	1,605.6	1,696.1	1,787.4	1,864.0	1,935.7	2,000.4	2,067.2	2,130.9	2,192.9	2,249.4	2,304.9
1909-------	1936	1,501.2	1,601.6	1,696.0	1,789.3	1,866.7	1,941.2	2,008.8	2,078.4	2,146.3	2,210.5	2,271.5	2,328.7
1910-------	1937	1,492.6	1,596.2	1,693.3	1,786.6	1,866.2	1,943.7	2,014.0	2,088.6	2,159.2	2,227.8	2,290.3	2,349.3
1911-------	1938	1,494.9	1,601.8	1,700.0	1,795.5	1,878.0	1,956.7	2,032.1	2,110.0	2,183.8	2,253.7	2,319.3	2,380.0
1912-------	1939	1,477.8	1,584.6	1,684.6	1,783.0	1,868.9	1,953.7	2,032.7	2,111.5	2,185.3	2,257.6	2,322.7	2,384.2
1913-------	1940	1,476.8	1,586.0	1,689.1	1,788.4	1,880.1	1,969.0	2,048.9	2,130.0	2,207.5	2,280.5	2,347.0	2,409.8
1914-------	1941	1,482.7	1,595.5	1,700.6	1,806.2	1,901.8	1,991.7	2,075.2	2,160.3	2,239.1	2,313.7	2,382.4	2,449.0
1915-------	1942	1,496.6	1,610.2	1,720.9	1,830.1	1,925.4	2,019.5	2,107.1	2,193.8	2,275.0	2,351.3	2,423.3	2,488.9
1916-------	1943	1,515.0	1,635.1	1,748.8	1,857.0	1,957.4	2,055.6	2,144.7	2,233.5	2,316.0	2,396.2	2,467.5	2,535.1
1917-------	1944	1,546.8	1,669.3	1,780.2	1,895.0	2,000.3	2,101.7	2,194.3	2,285.6	2,371.4	2,451.5	2,525.2	2,595.4
1918-------	1945	1,575.2	1,694.3	1,814.6	1,935.7	2,046.1	2,152.0	2,248.9	2,344.9	2,434.8	2,518.6	2,596.2	2,667.4
1919-------	1946	1,612.2	1,745.7	1,876.8	2,007.7	2,126.2	2,238.6	2,343.5	2,447.5	2,542.8	2,633.0	2,714.6	2,790.2
1920-------	1947	1,649.4	1,792.9	1,932.5	2,068.8	2,191.6	2,311.3	2,421.5	2,528.9	2,629.7	2,721.9	2,805.6	2,881.8
1921-------	1948	1,693.1	1,843.1	1,987.1	2,126.3	2,256.4	2,380.0	2,493.7	2,605.7	2,707.7	2,802.4	2,886.8	2,960.0
1922-------	1949	1,707.2	1,859.4	2,005.2	2,149.6	2,280.4	2,406.1	2,523.5	2,635.2	2,737.7	2,831.4	2,911.7	2,984.3
1923-------	1950	1,746.1	1,904.2	2,057.6	2,205.8	2,341.6	2,473.0	2,592.1	2,707.7	2,812.7	2,904.1	2,985.3	3,056.9
1924-------	1951	1,818.3	1,986.7	2,148.1	2,305.6	2,452.1	2,588.9	2,714.2	2,833.5	2,937.8	3,033.6	3,114.9	3,188.0
1925-------	1952	1,907.5	2,085.8	2,256.8	2,424.1	2,574.3	2,717.8	2,847.4	2,965.9	3,073.9	3,167.8	3,251.3	3,322.2
1926-------	1953	1,999.7	2,186.9	2,368.1	2,539.5	2,695.7	2,842.3	2,970.8	3,092.7	3,198.8	3,294.2	3,374.2	3,441.7
1927-------	1954	2,075.4	2,268.7	2,450.0	2,626.6	2,786.1	2,930.9	3,061.0	3,179.2	3,285.4	3,377.5	3,453.7	3,519.7
1928-------	1955	2,137.8	2,331.8	2,515.3	2,691.7	2,846.1	2,991.1	3,117.8	3,235.6	3,337.6	3,422.9	3,496.7	3,557.5
1929-------	1956	2,216.0	2,416.8	2,604.3	2,778.0	2,936.0	3,079.9	3,209.5	3,325.7	3,423.2	3,509.0	3,578.5	3,633.8
1930-------	1957	2,273.0	2,474.1	2,657.9	2,833.1	2,988.8	3,132.5	3,257.3	3,367.2	3,462.8	3,541.1	3,603.6	3,654.2
1931-------	1958	2,350.9	2,551.6	2,738.9	2,911.5	3,068.5	3,206.8	3,327.4	3,435.9	3,523.8	3,595.0	3,651.5	3,697.2
1932-------	1959	2,400.8	2,604.1	2,787.1	2,961.7	3,111.0	3,246.0	3,361.3	3,460.2	3,539.3	3,603.4	3,655.3	3,698.4
1933-------	1960	2,480.3	2,681.6	2,871.4	3,039.1	3,187.1	3,318.7	3,426.8	3,515.9	3,588.4	3,648.6	3,698.5	3,740.6
1934-------	1961	2,552.2	2,759.2	2,944.1	3,111.0	3,254.6	3,377.7	3,475.9	3,558.3	3,625.8	3,684.4	3,733.6	3,773.0
1935-------	1962	2,606.2	2,809.1	2,990.8	3,153.8	3,287.9	3,398.9	3,490.1	3,566.6	3,632.3	3,688.7	3,734.5	3,769.8
1936-------	1963	2,621.2	2,817.6	2,991.6	3,141.9	3,262.5	3,363.7	3,446.4	3,520.3	3,583.9	3,637.0	3,677.5	3,708.1
1937-------	1964	2,603.4	2,790.0	2,951.1	3,084.3	3,194.0	3,286.2	3,366.9	3,438.5	3,498.7	3,544.6	3,580.5	
1938-------	1965	2,545.0	2,716.2	2,856.6	2,975.8	3,074.9	3,165.0	3,245.0	3,312.6	3,363.7	3,404.7		
1939-------	1966	2,502.6	2,655.1	2,784.2	2,895.5	2,994.3	3,085.3	3,162.0	3,221.3	3,269.0			
1940-------	1967	2,431.1	2,572.4	2,693.0	2,803.6	2,903.6	2,990.9	3,058.0	3,112.3				
1941-------	1968	2,341.0	2,471.7	2,590.5	2,701.8	2,799.1	2,875.0	2,936.0					
1942-------	1969	2,236.1	2,364.7	2,485.6	2,593.0	2,677.4	2,746.9						
1943-------	1970	2,138.0	2,271.3	2,387.8	2,482.3	2,560.2							
1944-------	1971	2,079.9	2,206.7	2,310.2	2,398.3								
1945-------	1972	2,022.5	2,135.6	2,232.0									
1946-------	1973	1,964.1	2,070.4										
1947-------	1974	1,903.2											

TABLE 6C. CUMULATIVE BIRTH RATES FOR ALL OTHER WOMEN AS OF THE BEGINNING OF EACH YEAR 1917-74 BY AGE AND LIVE-BIRTH ORDER FOR EACH COHORT FROM 1867 TO 1959--CON.

LIVE-BIRTH ORDER AND COHORT	DIAGONAL LINE FOR JANUARY 1	EXACT AGE											
		39	40	41	42	43	44	45	46	47	48	49	50
TOTAL BIRTHS--CON.													
1867-------													5,349.1
1868-------												5,253.1	5,258.0
1869-------											5,151.8	5,160.0	5,169.2
1870-------										5,044.1	5,055.9	5,070.7	5,075.2
1871-------									4,930.7	4,948.9	4,970.6	4,978.0	4,983.3
1872-------								4,810.7	4,831.7	4,865.4	4,876.1	4,885.1	4,888.9
1873-------							4,679.9	4,703.9	4,738.3	4,755.1	4,768.3	4,774.6	4,778.2
1874-------						4,543.5	4,569.5	4,603.3	4,622.7	4,643.3	4,652.7	4,658.4	4,662.2
1875-------					4,404.1	4,434.5	4,463.1	4,485.0	4,507.7	4,522.5	4,531.3	4,537.6	4,541.0
1876-------				4,262.2	4,306.5	4,340.3	4,364.2	4,388.5	4,406.1	4,419.6	4,428.9	4,434.7	4,437.4
1877-------			4,112.9	4,169.0	4,219.1	4,247.6	4,272.0	4,293.3	4,309.4	4,324.4	4,333.1	4,337.8	4,340.7
1878-------	1917	3,945.3	4,027.0	4,087.9	4,131.2	4,160.7	4,186.4	4,205.9	4,223.5	4,238.0	4,244.9	4,250.1	4,252.6
1879-------	1918	3,849.6	3,935.2	3,993.3	4,039.1	4,070.7	4,094.1	4,114.7	4,131.7	4,145.0	4,153.1	4,157.6	4,160.7
1880-------	1919	3,766.2	3,853.5	3,914.9	3,964.4	3,993.3	4,017.2	4,037.7	4,053.8	4,068.1	4,074.7	4,079.4	4,082.5
1881-------	1920	3,707.3	3,799.0	3,862.5	3,907.9	3,937.3	3,961.2	3,981.7	3,998.6	4,010.6	4,017.6	4,022.5	4,025.2
1882-------	1921	3,658.5	3,749.4	3,808.5	3,853.7	3,882.7	3,907.3	3,927.7	3,942.9	3,954.6	3,961.8	3,966.1	3,968.8
1883-------	1922	3,595.1	3,679.3	3,736.4	3,780.1	3,810.3	3,834.5	3,853.1	3,867.1	3,878.2	3,884.5	3,888.7	3,891.3
1884-------	1923	3,496.7	3,576.5	3,631.7	3,674.5	3,702.9	3,724.1	3,740.8	3,753.6	3,764.4	3,769.9	3,774.2	3,776.7
1885-------	1924	3,399.2	3,476.3	3,530.6	3,571.5	3,595.9	3,614.4	3,629.0	3,641.6	3,651.2	3,656.6	3,660.3	3,663.1
1886-------	1925	3,330.5	3,405.1	3,455.4	3,491.9	3,513.0	3,529.6	3,544.1	3,555.5	3,565.1	3,569.5	3,573.6	3,576.3
1887-------	1926	3,281.7	3,352.3	3,399.1	3,430.4	3,450.5	3,466.9	3,480.6	3,492.4	3,500.5	3,505.2	3,508.9	3,511.5
1888-------	1927	3,242.3	3,308.3	3,348.1	3,378.0	3,397.7	3,413.2	3,427.7	3,437.7	3,445.3	3,449.5	3,453.1	3,455.2
1889-------	1928	3,181.3	3,240.0	3,280.0	3,311.1	3,330.0	3,346.7	3,359.3	3,368.9	3,376.1	3,380.4	3,383.8	3,386.0
1890-------	1929	3,127.2	3,183.6	3,224.7	3,253.7	3,273.9	3,289.2	3,302.2	3,311.4	3,318.2	3,322.2	3,325.5	3,327.5
1891-------	1930	3,086.7	3,145.5	3,183.8	3,214.2	3,233.3	3,249.7	3,261.7	3,270.5	3,277.3	3,281.1	3,284.1	3,285.8
1892-------	1931	3,055.2	3,109.9	3,149.8	3,178.4	3,197.9	3,213.4	3,224.7	3,233.5	3,239.7	3,243.3	3,246.2	3,247.6
1893-------	1932	3,062.2	3,118.0	3,155.0	3,183.4	3,202.1	3,216.7	3,227.7	3,235.4	3,241.0	3,244.3	3,246.6	3,247.9
1894-------	1933	2,999.4	3,051.1	3,087.6	3,115.4	3,133.0	3,147.2	3,157.4	3,164.4	3,170.1	3,173.0	3,174.8	3,175.7
1895-------	1934	2,937.4	2,989.0	3,024.0	3,049.5	3,066.8	3,079.8	3,088.9	3,096.1	3,100.8	3,103.6	3,105.0	3,105.9
1896-------	1935	2,874.6	2,922.1	2,954.2	2,979.2	2,995.6	3,007.4	3,017.0	3,023.1	3,027.6	3,030.0	3,031.4	3,032.5
1897-------	1936	2,816.8	2,860.8	2,892.7	2,916.7	2,931.7	2,944.1	2,952.6	2,959.7	2,963.9	2,965.9	2,967.6	2,968.8
1898-------	1937	2,783.7	2,828.3	2,861.4	2,884.3	2,900.7	2,912.9	2,923.1	2,930.4	2,934.4	2,937.2	2,938.9	2,939.8
1899-------	1938	2,795.9	2,843.3	2,874.3	2,898.7	2,914.9	2,928.3	2,938.1	2,944.4	2,948.7	2,951.1	2,952.7	2,953.7
1900-------	1939	2,786.5	2,832.0	2,864.1	2,888.9	2,905.3	2,919.2	2,928.8	2,935.4	2,939.5	2,941.7	2,943.2	2,944.0
1901-------	1940	2,706.4	2,750.0	2,781.5	2,803.7	2,820.2	2,833.8	2,843.2	2,849.1	2,852.7	2,854.7	2,856.1	2,856.7
1902-------	1941	2,610.7	2,654.1	2,684.4	2,707.9	2,724.7	2,738.3	2,747.1	2,752.4	2,755.5	2,757.2	2,758.4	2,758.9
1903-------	1942	2,533.8	2,575.8	2,607.1	2,630.4	2,647.6	2,660.6	2,668.7	2,673.3	2,676.1	2,677.6	2,678.8	2,679.2
1904-------	1943	2,495.1	2,538.6	2,569.9	2,594.3	2,611.4	2,623.9	2,631.4	2,636.1	2,639.0	2,640.6	2,641.6	2,642.2
1905-------	1944	2,450.2	2,493.9	2,526.2	2,550.2	2,566.9	2,578.5	2,586.4	2,591.1	2,593.7	2,594.9	2,595.8	2,596.4
1906-------	1945	2,411.9	2,456.4	2,487.6	2,511.3	2,527.1	2,539.4	2,546.8	2,551.2	2,553.7	2,555.1	2,556.1	2,556.5
1907-------	1946	2,377.0	2,419.3	2,450.8	2,473.2	2,489.3	2,501.1	2,508.1	2,512.3	2,514.8	2,515.9	2,516.9	2,517.2
1908-------	1947	2,352.9	2,395.3	2,425.2	2,448.3	2,463.5	2,475.1	2,481.9	2,486.1	2,488.4	2,489.6	2,490.1	2,490.5
1909-------	1948	2,379.7	2,423.0	2,455.4	2,479.2	2,496.5	2,508.9	2,517.1	2,521.6	2,523.9	2,525.0	2,525.8	2,526.2
1910-------	1949	2,401.1	2,447.0	2,480.2	2,506.8	2,524.1	2,537.4	2,545.3	2,549.9	2,552.3	2,553.7	2,554.7	2,555.1
1911-------	1950	2,434.4	2,481.1	2,517.1	2,542.9	2,561.5	2,575.0	2,583.3	2,587.8	2,590.4	2,591.7	2,592.4	2,592.8
1912-------	1951	2,438.8	2,487.4	2,522.2	2,549.1	2,568.0	2,581.7	2,590.0	2,594.9	2,597.3	2,598.6	2,599.4	2,599.8
1913-------	1952	2,466.7	2,514.7	2,550.8	2,577.8	2,596.6	2,610.8	2,619.2	2,624.0	2,626.6	2,627.8	2,628.4	2,628.6
1914-------	1953	2,506.6	2,556.4	2,593.7	2,620.5	2,640.2	2,654.8	2,663.0	2,667.7	2,670.2	2,671.1	2,671.7	2,671.9
1915-------	1954	2,547.4	2,598.2	2,634.9	2,663.2	2,682.9	2,696.2	2,704.3	2,708.7	2,710.9	2,712.0	2,712.5	2,712.6
1916-------	1955	2,596.2	2,646.6	2,684.9	2,712.9	2,731.6	2,744.8	2,752.8	2,756.9	2,759.2	2,760.3	2,760.8	2,760.9
1917-------	1956	2,656.6	2,709.1	2,746.6	2,774.2	2,793.4	2,806.3	2,814.2	2,818.4	2,820.7	2,821.8	2,822.1	2,822.3
1918-------	1957	2,730.6	2,782.4	2,819.9	2,847.5	2,866.9	2,880.3	2,887.8	2,892.1	2,894.2	2,895.1	2,895.5	2,895.6
1919-------	1958	2,854.9	2,907.9	2,947.5	2,976.2	2,996.4	3,010.0	3,018.0	3,022.3	3,024.5	3,025.5	3,025.8	3,026.0
1920-------	1959	2,945.9	2,999.7	3,038.9	3,067.8	3,087.4	3,100.9	3,109.2	3,113.5	3,115.5	3,116.3	3,116.6	3,116.7
1921-------	1960	3,023.7	3,075.7	3,114.8	3,142.6	3,161.9	3,175.1	3,182.6	3,186.4	3,188.1	3,188.8	3,189.2	3,189.3
1922-------	1961	3,046.1	3,097.4	3,133.9	3,160.5	3,179.0	3,191.0	3,197.9	3,201.5	3,203.2	3,204.1	3,204.3	3,204.4
1923-------	1962	3,118.6	3,167.6	3,203.0	3,229.3	3,246.4	3,257.6	3,263.9	3,267.0	3,268.5	3,269.2	3,269.5	3,269.6
1924-------	1963	3,247.4	3,294.7	3,331.0	3,355.9	3,372.4	3,382.9	3,388.8	3,391.7	3,393.2	3,393.7	3,393.9	3,393.9
1925-------	1964	3,380.8	3,428.8	3,462.7	3,486.6	3,502.0	3,511.5	3,517.2	3,520.3	3,521.7	3,522.2	3,522.3	
1926-------	1965	3,499.2	3,544.4	3,576.0	3,597.7	3,611.6	3,621.0	3,626.2	3,629.1	3,630.3	3,630.6		
1927-------	1966	3,573.1	3,613.8	3,642.8	3,662.0	3,675.1	3,683.5	3,688.4	3,690.8	3,692.0			
1928-------	1967	3,604.5	3,641.4	3,666.7	3,684.9	3,697.1	3,704.9	3,708.8	3,710.7				
1929-------	1968	3,677.9	3,711.1	3,735.2	3,752.1	3,763.5	3,769.9	3,773.4					
1930-------	1969	3,693.6	3,724.6	3,747.1	3,762.9	3,772.3	3,777.8						
1931-------	1970	3,733.8	3,763.2	3,784.3	3,797.9	3,806.4							
1932-------	1971	3,734.2	3,761.7	3,780.0	3,791.8								
1933-------	1972	3,773.8	3,797.3	3,813.1									
1934-------	1973	3,802.2	3,822.7										
1935-------	1974	3,795.8											

TABLE 6C. CUMULATIVE BIRTH RATES FOR ALL OTHER WOMEN AS OF THE BEGINNING OF EACH YEAR 1917-74 BY AGE AND LIVE-BIRTH ORDER FOR EACH COHORT FROM 1867 TO 1959--CON.

LIVE-BIRTH ORDER AND COHORT	DIAGONAL LINE FOR JANUARY 1	EXACT AGE											
		15	16	17	18	19	20	21	22	23	24	25	26
FIRST BIRTHS													
1891-------													656.7
1892-------												634.6	663.1
1893-------											603.9	639.8	669.5
1894-------										563.7	609.6	646.5	673.4
1895-------									513.8	569.8	616.5	650.1	682.4
1896-------								446.3	520.1	577.1	619.8	659.9	689.4
1897-------							364.0	453.6	528.8	580.9	631.6	668.7	694.0
1898-------						248.8	355.1	445.0	514.3	576.7	624.4	656.5	680.5
1899-------					163.0	264.1	368.1	450.6	532.6	590.6	631.6	662.0	686.8
1900-------				88.7	174.5	272.2	368.6	466.4	543.2	593.4	632.8	665.3	690.7
1901-------			39.8	95.6	178.0	268.5	382.1	476.6	542.9	591.0	633.9	666.6	689.6
1902-------	1917	11.3	43.7	97.9	175.0	282.2	395.4	477.8	541.7	594.3	636.5	666.0	686.1
1903-------	1918	12.8	43.8	94.2	185.0	293.9	392.6	475.0	544.5	596.9	635.3	661.5	679.1
1904-------	1919	12.1	40.9	100.1	192.2	287.5	389.0	477.6	545.9	596.2	631.0	654.3	671.4
1905-------	1920	11.2	44.8	104.7	185.1	285.8	394.3	481.2	546.6	590.6	622.3	645.1	663.0
1906-------	1921	13.0	47.4	99.8	184.9	292.1	399.1	482.0	541.5	582.0	612.6	636.6	653.6
1907-------	1922	13.6	44.1	99.7	190.5	298.9	400.3	476.4	531.6	571.3	603.3	625.7	643.1
1908-------	1923	12.3	44.9	104.5	198.3	301.5	396.2	466.0	520.2	561.4	592.3	615.7	631.5
1909-------	1924	13.2	48.2	111.5	203.2	300.3	389.2	458.8	515.0	555.8	587.9	609.4	627.1
1910-------	1925	14.3	51.7	114.7	201.7	293.3	380.4	452.2	507.0	548.6	577.9	601.7	618.6
1911-------	1926	15.6	54.5	116.1	199.9	289.1	379.5	449.4	505.3	543.3	575.1	598.3	615.0
1912-------	1927	16.4	54.0	112.2	192.2	284.4	370.9	441.8	492.5	533.4	564.6	587.1	604.1
1913-------	1928	16.1	51.7	107.3	190.1	279.5	367.3	433.0	487.8	528.9	559.3	582.2	599.7
1914-------	1929	14.7	48.4	105.6	185.1	275.4	356.8	427.7	482.2	521.4	552.6	575.7	593.8
1915-------	1930	14.2	48.8	104.3	184.7	268.8	356.5	426.5	478.5	519.0	549.5	573.0	591.1
1916-------	1931	14.5	47.5	104.1	178.7	268.8	356.2	422.0	476.1	515.8	546.3	569.5	588.7
1917-------	1932	13.9	47.7	100.3	179.8	270.8	353.7	422.8	476.1	515.7	545.8	570.4	592.0
1918-------	1933	14.2	46.0	101.0	183.6	270.4	357.6	426.9	478.9	517.6	548.8	577.2	599.2
1919-------	1934	13.6	46.4	105.2	186.6	280.2	369.7	438.1	490.6	531.3	567.9	595.9	617.1
1920-------	1935	13.9	50.2	108.8	196.2	292.3	380.0	447.4	501.5	545.4	580.8	607.2	627.8
1921-------	1936	15.5	51.9	115.2	205.0	298.9	383.9	453.6	508.0	550.5	583.5	609.1	635.1
1922-------	1937	14.8	52.9	117.0	202.8	290.8	376.7	445.8	498.8	538.5	569.5	601.4	633.6
1923-------	1938	15.7	54.8	116.0	197.6	287.9	374.7	442.9	492.9	531.1	570.3	610.7	640.4
1924-------	1939	16.4	54.5	114.2	198.8	292.9	379.5	442.8	491.6	540.2	591.2	628.9	657.7
1925-------	1940	16.8	55.3	118.4	206.2	300.7	380.0	442.5	502.4	565.7	613.0	648.7	676.4
1926-------	1941	17.0	57.8	123.0	211.3	296.5	373.6	447.2	524.7	583.2	627.4	661.4	689.0
1927-------	1942	17.9	59.2	124.8	204.5	287.6	373.7	467.3	539.3	593.3	634.7	667.6	694.6
1928-------	1943	18.2	59.9	119.1	196.8	285.0	392.5	480.8	547.2	597.0	636.5	668.4	694.9
1929-------	1944	18.5	56.6	115.6	195.2	305.6	410.4	492.8	554.4	603.1	642.2	674.8	702.6
1930-------	1945	17.1	55.1	113.0	210.4	320.4	418.2	494.6	555.5	603.8	643.7	677.5	704.4
1931-------	1946	17.5	54.8	125.8	226.3	330.6	423.3	500.6	561.4	611.8	655.0	689.1	716.9
1932-------	1947	16.4	60.7	135.4	232.5	333.7	428.8	505.1	569.3	623.4	667.1	702.3	730.0
1933-------	1948	20.4	68.4	142.9	239.6	344.2	436.8	518.3	587.6	643.9	689.8	725.7	752.0
1934-------	1949	22.1	71.3	146.9	246.3	348.1	445.8	533.2	604.5	663.3	709.8	744.1	770.9
1935-------	1950	22.6	72.5	150.3	247.8	353.1	457.6	546.3	620.8	679.9	724.7	759.1	785.8
1936-------	1951	23.2	74.6	150.5	249.6	360.1	463.0	554.8	629.3	686.1	729.8	763.6	790.0
1937-------	1952	24.3	73.6	150.2	252.1	360.5	467.3	559.3	630.1	685.8	729.2	761.9	787.2
1938-------	1953	22.1	71.2	149.3	248.2	358.9	464.6	552.0	621.7	676.9	719.0	750.4	776.1
1939-------	1954	22.0	73.4	149.8	251.3	361.1	462.2	549.1	619.0	674.1	715.0	747.8	772.8
1940-------	1955	23.8	72.9	150.2	251.5	357.3	457.7	544.3	614.9	669.4	711.6	744.5	770.4
1941-------	1956	22.7	73.0	151.2	246.6	351.4	450.2	536.7	607.1	662.0	704.8	738.1	764.8
1942-------	1957	22.7	73.8	146.6	241.8	343.7	441.4	528.2	599.2	656.0	699.3	733.8	760.9
1943-------	1958	23.0	69.8	143.1	234.9	335.1	431.9	519.2	591.5	648.5	692.7	727.2	756.9
1944-------	1959	21.5	69.4	139.7	230.7	329.2	427.3	517.0	590.0	648.2	692.8	729.3	759.5
1945-------	1960	22.3	68.3	138.3	226.4	325.8	426.8	516.4	591.0	649.3	695.5	732.7	765.6
1946-------	1961	21.3	67.0	134.8	223.7	326.3	426.5	519.3	594.4	654.7	702.9	743.6	775.6
1947-------	1962	21.2	64.9	132.8	223.4	325.1	429.3	522.7	600.4	662.8	713.4	753.0	785.2
1948-------	1963	20.1	63.6	131.6	222.0	326.7	431.5	527.4	607.1	671.1	719.7	758.3	789.2
1949-------	1964	19.9	63.4	132.5	224.6	329.9	437.0	534.0	613.5	673.9	719.2	755.1	
1950-------	1965	19.9	64.2	133.8	226.9	334.5	443.7	542.1	616.9	671.7	713.9		
1951-------	1966	20.4	65.1	136.5	231.8	341.7	452.8	546.2	614.6	665.6			
1952-------	1967	20.5	66.9	139.4	236.5	349.8	456.5	542.7	606.4				
1953-------	1968	21.3	68.6	142.0	243.0	353.0	454.7	535.4					
1954-------	1969	21.9	69.7	147.3	246.8	354.5	449.8						
1955-------	1970	22.4	73.6	150.8	251.5	353.6							
1956-------	1971	23.8	74.8	153.9	249.7								
1957-------	1972	23.6	76.0	152.6									
1958-------	1973	24.1	75.6										
1959-------	1974	24.5											

TABLE 6C. CUMULATIVE BIRTH RATES FOR ALL OTHER WOMEN AS OF THE BEGINNING OF EACH YEAR 1917-74 BY AGE AND LIVE-BIRTH ORDER FOR EACH COHORT FROM 1867 TO 1959--CON.

LIVE-BIRTH ORDER AND COHORT	DIAGONAL LINE FOR JANUARY 1	EXACT AGE											
		27	28	29	30	31	32	33	34	35	36	37	38
FIRST BIRTHS--CON.													
1879-------													778.0
1880-------												771.3	774.4
1881-------											764.9	768.6	772.6
1882-------										758.3	762.8	767.5	771.0
1883-------									750.3	755.1	760.4	764.5	768.4
1884-------								740.2	745.3	750.7	755.3	759.7	763.4
1885-------							731.3	736.8	742.4	747.1	752.1	756.2	759.5
1886-------						724.8	732.4	738.4	743.3	748.4	753.0	756.7	759.4
1887-------					718.5	727.9	736.3	741.6	747.0	751.7	755.8	758.9	761.7
1888-------				705.3	718.1	728.3	735.9	741.8	746.8	751.1	754.7	757.9	760.7
1889-------			690.6	705.1	718.9	728.2	736.8	742.3	746.9	750.8	754.5	758.2	760.7
1890-------	1917	674.4	692.3	707.7	720.3	731.2	739.2	744.3	748.7	752.7	756.9	760.0	762.8
1891-------	1918	678.4	697.4	711.4	726.4	736.4	743.8	748.7	753.0	757.4	760.6	764.0	766.0
1892-------	1919	686.1	703.4	720.5	734.2	743.3	750.4	755.2	759.9	763.3	766.8	769.2	771.0
1893-------	1920	690.4	711.5	726.9	739.0	747.6	754.6	759.6	763.1	766.9	769.6	771.9	773.9
1894-------	1921	698.7	717.6	730.8	742.1	750.6	757.7	762.0	765.9	768.9	771.6	773.9	775.7
1895-------	1922	705.1	721.3	733.5	744.7	752.8	758.8	762.9	766.2	769.1	771.7	773.9	775.7
1896-------	1923	708.8	723.7	735.9	746.7	753.8	759.1	762.6	765.7	768.6	771.1	773.1	774.6
1897-------	1924	711.9	726.9	738.7	747.9	754.3	759.4	762.6	766.0	768.8	771.1	773.0	774.7
1898-------	1925	698.7	713.8	724.3	733.1	739.0	743.7	747.5	750.6	753.1	755.3	757.1	758.5
1899-------	1926	706.1	720.1	730.9	739.2	745.0	750.4	754.1	757.4	760.2	762.5	764.5	766.2
1900-------	1927	708.6	721.9	731.0	739.1	745.5	750.6	754.3	757.5	760.3	762.8	764.9	766.6
1901-------	1928	705.7	717.1	726.1	734.4	740.6	745.8	749.3	752.7	755.4	757.8	759.9	761.6
1902-------	1929	699.7	710.5	719.7	727.7	733.6	738.0	741.4	744.3	746.8	749.0	750.9	752.7
1903-------	1930	692.1	703.3	712.1	719.8	724.8	729.2	732.2	734.9	737.3	739.5	741.5	743.3
1904-------	1931	685.2	696.0	704.8	711.5	716.8	721.0	724.0	726.8	729.4	731.8	733.8	735.8
1905-------	1932	676.1	686.8	694.6	701.6	706.7	710.9	714.0	717.0	719.7	722.1	724.3	726.4
1906-------	1933	667.0	676.8	685.0	692.0	697.2	701.4	704.8	708.0	710.8	713.5	716.0	718.2
1907-------	1934	655.1	665.5	673.7	680.8	685.8	690.4	694.0	697.3	700.4	703.4	706.1	708.6
1908-------	1935	644.5	654.7	662.9	669.7	675.2	680.0	683.8	687.6	691.2	694.5	697.6	700.2
1909-------	1936	640.0	650.2	658.4	665.8	671.7	676.8	681.1	685.4	689.5	693.2	696.5	699.5
1910-------	1937	631.2	641.7	650.3	658.0	664.1	669.9	674.7	679.7	684.2	688.2	691.9	695.2
1911-------	1938	627.9	638.9	647.9	655.8	662.5	668.5	674.1	679.5	684.2	688.8	693.2	696.7
1912-------	1939	617.7	629.1	638.3	646.9	654.4	661.4	667.4	672.9	678.1	683.5	687.7	691.5
1913-------	1940	613.9	625.6	635.5	645.2	653.5	661.0	667.1	673.2	679.7	684.8	689.1	692.8
1914-------	1941	608.3	620.9	632.5	643.1	651.9	659.4	666.2	673.8	679.7	685.1	689.6	693.5
1915-------	1942	606.6	620.4	632.6	643.5	652.2	660.9	669.5	676.5	682.8	688.2	692.9	696.5
1916-------	1943	605.0	619.6	631.9	642.6	652.7	663.1	670.8	678.3	684.4	689.9	694.3	698.3
1917-------	1944	609.2	623.8	635.9	648.7	660.9	670.8	679.3	686.3	692.7	698.0	702.5	706.0
1918-------	1945	616.3	630.5	645.1	660.2	672.1	682.5	690.7	698.0	704.2	709.4	713.7	717.3
1919-------	1946	633.9	651.9	670.1	685.5	697.9	708.1	716.8	724.1	730.3	735.8	740.3	743.9
1920-------	1947	649.1	671.2	689.3	704.4	716.6	727.0	735.2	742.8	749.0	754.2	758.3	761.4
1921-------	1948	661.5	682.7	700.1	714.7	726.7	736.9	745.5	752.7	758.7	763.6	767.4	770.6
1922-------	1949	658.2	678.3	694.9	709.1	720.9	730.8	739.1	746.0	751.4	755.7	759.3	762.2
1923-------	1950	663.9	683.2	699.6	713.9	725.1	735.2	743.0	749.6	754.8	759.1	762.7	765.3
1924-------	1951	680.4	700.0	717.0	730.9	743.1	752.6	760.3	766.5	771.5	775.9	779.1	781.7
1925-------	1952	699.7	719.7	736.5	751.0	762.1	771.5	778.6	784.7	789.8	793.8	796.8	799.2
1926-------	1953	712.4	732.1	748.9	762.2	772.9	781.5	788.4	794.2	798.8	802.5	805.3	807.8
1927-------	1954	717.4	737.0	752.4	765.1	775.1	783.3	789.9	795.3	799.6	803.0	805.9	808.2
1928-------	1955	717.6	735.8	750.4	762.8	772.3	780.3	786.4	791.4	795.4	798.7	801.4	803.5
1929-------	1956	724.4	742.6	756.9	768.6	778.2	785.8	791.9	796.7	800.5	803.6	806.2	808.3
1930-------	1957	726.5	743.9	757.9	769.5	778.7	786.1	791.7	796.4	800.2	803.3	806.0	807.9
1931-------	1958	738.2	755.0	768.7	780.0	788.9	795.9	801.5	806.1	809.8	813.0	815.3	817.5
1932-------	1959	750.8	767.7	781.3	792.3	800.8	807.8	813.3	817.8	821.8	824.5	827.2	829.3
1933-------	1960	772.9	789.7	803.1	813.5	822.0	828.8	834.3	839.0	842.4	845.7	848.3	850.4
1934-------	1961	791.8	808.7	821.7	832.5	840.8	847.8	853.4	857.7	861.7	865.0	867.6	869.7
1935-------	1962	806.7	823.1	836.3	846.9	855.5	862.6	867.9	872.9	876.9	880.1	882.6	884.4
1936-------	1963	810.4	826.7	839.5	850.5	859.0	865.6	871.6	876.7	880.7	883.8	886.2	888.1
1937-------	1964	807.5	823.1	836.8	847.8	856.0	863.6	870.0	875.1	878.8	882.0	884.5	
1938-------	1965	795.7	812.5	825.9	836.3	845.7	853.7	860.0	864.9	869.0	872.2		
1939-------	1966	793.6	810.6	824.0	836.4	846.6	854.9	861.3	866.6	870.6			
1940-------	1967	791.7	809.1	824.6	837.7	848.1	856.4	863.0	868.0				
1941-------	1968	786.7	806.1	822.4	835.9	846.6	855.2	861.6					
1942-------	1969	784.8	805.0	822.0	836.0	846.8	855.3						
1943-------	1970	781.5	803.2	820.8	834.9	846.2							
1944-------	1971	786.4	808.0	825.3	839.7								
1945-------	1972	791.6	812.9	830.9									
1946-------	1973	801.8	823.7										
1947-------	1974	811.4											

TABLE 6C. CUMULATIVE BIRTH RATES FOR ALL OTHER WOMEN AS OF THE BEGINNING OF EACH YEAR 1917-74 BY AGE AND LIVE-BIRTH ORDER FOR EACH COHORT FROM 1867 TO 1959--CON.

LIVE-BIRTH ORDER AND COHORT	DIAGONAL LINE FOR JANUARY 1	EXACT AGE											
		39	40	41	42	43	44	45	46	47	48	49	50
FIRST BIRTHS--CON.													
1867-------													837.3
1868-------												834.0	834.1
1869-------											830.4	830.7	831.0
1870-------										826.4	826.8	827.3	827.4
1871-------									822.1	822.6	823.2	823.4	823.5
1872-------								817.5	818.0	818.8	819.0	819.2	819.3
1873-------							812.5	812.9	813.6	813.9	814.2	814.4	814.5
1874-------						807.2	807.6	808.3	808.6	809.0	809.3	809.5	809.6
1875-------					801.8	802.2	802.8	803.1	803.5	803.9	804.2	804.4	804.5
1876-------				796.3	797.0	797.8	798.1	798.6	799.0	799.4	799.6	799.8	799.9
1877-------			790.7	791.9	793.3	793.7	794.2	794.6	795.0	795.3	795.6	795.8	795.9
1878-------	1917	784.6	786.6	788.6	789.3	789.9	790.3	790.7	791.0	791.4	791.7	791.9	792.0
1879-------	1918	780.4	783.3	784.7	785.9	786.4	786.8	787.2	787.6	787.9	788.2	788.3	788.4
1880-------	1919	777.5	779.8	781.6	782.6	783.2	783.7	784.1	784.4	784.9	785.2	785.3	785.4
1881-------	1920	775.4	778.2	779.9	781.0	781.6	782.0	782.4	782.9	783.3	783.5	783.6	783.6
1882-------	1921	774.2	776.8	778.5	779.7	780.2	780.6	781.1	781.5	781.8	781.9	782.0	782.1
1883-------	1922	771.4	773.9	775.5	776.4	776.9	777.3	777.7	778.1	778.2	778.3	778.4	778.5
1884-------	1923	766.1	768.3	769.7	770.6	771.1	771.5	771.9	772.1	772.3	772.4	772.5	772.6
1885-------	1924	761.7	763.8	765.0	765.9	766.4	766.7	766.9	767.1	767.3	767.4	767.5	767.6
1886-------	1925	761.7	763.5	764.7	765.6	766.0	766.3	766.5	766.8	766.9	767.0	767.1	767.2
1887-------	1926	763.9	765.7	766.9	767.6	768.0	768.3	768.6	768.8	769.0	769.1	769.2	769.3
1888-------	1927	762.8	764.7	765.7	766.3	766.6	766.9	767.1	767.3	767.5	767.6	767.7	767.9
1889-------	1928	763.0	764.5	765.4	766.0	766.3	766.6	766.8	767.0	767.1	767.2	767.4	767.4
1890-------	1929	764.5	765.8	766.8	767.4	767.8	768.0	768.2	768.4	768.5	768.6	768.7	768.7
1891-------	1930	767.5	769.1	769.9	770.5	770.8	771.1	771.3	771.5	771.7	771.8	771.8	771.8
1892-------	1931	772.8	774.1	774.9	775.4	775.7	775.9	776.1	776.3	776.5	776.6	776.7	776.7
1893-------	1932	775.4	776.6	777.3	777.8	778.1	778.3	778.5	778.7	778.8	778.9	778.9	779.0
1894-------	1933	777.2	778.3	778.9	779.4	779.7	779.9	780.1	780.2	780.4	780.5	780.6	780.6
1895-------	1934	777.0	778.1	778.8	779.3	779.6	779.8	779.9	780.1	780.2	780.3	780.3	780.3
1896-------	1935	776.0	777.0	777.6	778.0	778.3	778.5	778.7	778.8	778.9	778.9	778.9	778.9
1897-------	1936	775.8	776.8	777.4	777.8	778.1	778.3	778.4	778.5	778.6	778.6	778.6	778.7
1898-------	1937	759.8	760.7	761.3	761.7	762.0	762.2	762.3	762.4	762.5	762.5	762.6	762.7
1899-------	1938	767.5	768.6	769.3	769.9	770.2	770.4	770.5	770.6	770.7	770.8	770.9	771.0
1900-------	1939	768.0	769.2	770.0	770.5	770.9	771.1	771.3	771.4	771.5	771.6	771.7	771.7
1901-------	1940	763.0	764.2	765.0	765.5	765.9	766.2	766.4	766.5	766.6	766.7	766.7	766.7
1902-------	1941	754.1	755.3	756.1	756.6	757.1	757.4	757.6	757.7	757.8	757.8	757.8	757.8
1903-------	1942	744.8	746.0	746.9	747.5	748.0	748.3	748.5	748.6	748.7	748.7	748.7	748.7
1904-------	1943	737.5	738.8	739.8	740.6	741.1	741.4	741.5	741.6	741.7	741.7	741.7	741.8
1905-------	1944	728.2	729.6	730.7	731.5	732.0	732.3	732.6	732.8	732.8	732.8	732.9	732.9
1906-------	1945	720.2	721.8	723.0	723.8	724.4	724.8	725.0	725.1	725.2	725.3	725.3	725.3
1907-------	1946	710.7	712.5	713.8	714.7	715.4	715.8	716.0	716.2	716.3	716.3	716.3	716.3
1908-------	1947	702.4	704.3	705.6	706.7	707.2	707.6	707.9	708.0	708.1	708.1	708.1	708.1
1909-------	1948	702.1	704.0	705.6	706.6	707.3	707.8	708.1	708.3	708.3	708.3	708.3	708.3
1910-------	1949	697.9	700.3	701.9	703.1	703.7	704.2	704.4	704.5	704.6	704.6	704.7	704.7
1911-------	1950	699.6	702.0	703.7	704.7	705.5	705.9	706.2	706.3	706.3	706.4	706.4	706.4
1912-------	1951	694.4	696.8	698.3	699.3	700.0	700.5	700.7	700.8	700.9	701.0	701.1	701.1
1913-------	1952	695.8	698.1	699.7	700.7	701.5	701.9	702.2	702.4	702.5	702.6	702.6	702.6
1914-------	1953	696.4	698.8	700.4	701.4	702.1	702.6	702.8	703.0	703.1	703.1	703.1	703.1
1915-------	1954	699.8	702.1	703.5	704.6	705.2	705.6	705.9	706.0	706.1	706.1	706.1	706.1
1916-------	1955	701.1	703.2	704.8	705.8	706.3	706.8	707.0	707.1	707.1	707.2	707.2	707.2
1917-------	1956	708.9	711.1	712.5	713.4	714.1	714.5	714.7	714.8	714.9	714.9	714.9	714.9
1918-------	1957	720.1	722.1	723.4	724.3	724.9	725.3	725.5	725.6	725.6	725.6	725.6	725.6
1919-------	1958	746.5	748.5	749.8	750.7	751.3	751.7	751.9	752.0	752.1	752.1	752.1	752.1
1920-------	1959	763.9	765.6	767.0	767.8	768.4	768.7	768.9	769.0	769.0	769.0	769.0	769.0
1921-------	1960	772.9	774.7	775.8	776.5	777.0	777.4	777.6	777.7	777.7	777.7	777.8	777.8
1922-------	1961	764.4	766.1	767.1	767.8	768.3	768.6	768.7	768.7	768.7	768.8	768.8	768.8
1923-------	1962	767.4	768.9	769.9	770.7	771.2	771.4	771.5	771.5	771.6	771.6	771.6	771.6
1924-------	1963	783.6	785.0	786.0	786.7	787.1	787.4	787.5	787.6	787.6	787.6	787.6	787.6
1925-------	1964	801.3	802.8	803.9	804.6	805.0	805.2	805.4	805.5	805.5	805.5	805.5	
1926-------	1965	809.7	811.2	812.2	812.8	813.2	813.5	813.6	813.7	813.7	813.7		
1927-------	1966	810.1	811.4	812.4	813.0	813.4	813.6	813.7	813.8	813.9			
1928-------	1967	805.2	806.4	807.4	808.1	808.5	808.7	808.8	808.9				
1929-------	1968	810.0	811.4	812.4	812.9	813.2	813.4	813.6					
1930-------	1969	809.7	811.0	811.8	812.4	812.7	812.9						
1931-------	1970	819.1	820.3	821.1	821.5	821.9							
1932-------	1971	831.0	832.2	832.9	833.4								
1933-------	1972	851.9	852.9	853.6									
1934-------	1973	871.1	872.1										
1935-------	1974	885.8											

TABLE 6C. CUMULATIVE BIRTH RATES FCR ALL OTHER WOMEN AS OF THE BEGINNING OF EACH YEAR 1917-74 BY AGE AND LIVE-BIRTH ORDER FOR EACH COHORT FROM 1867 TO 1959--CON.

LIVE-BIRTH ORDER AND COHORT	DIAGONAL LINE FOR JANUARY 1	EXACT AGE											
		15	16	17	18	19	20	21	22	23	24	25	26
SECOND BIRTHS													
1891-------													436.9
1892-------												403.9	438.0
1893-------											358.6	401.3	433.1
1894-------										299.6	351.6	391.6	425.0
1895-------									237.4	293.5	342.3	383.0	419.2
1896-------								171.4	232.5	285.1	333.5	376.9	412.6
1897-------							110.6	168.3	225.6	277.9	328.9	372.1	407.8
1898-------						60.9	110.4	164.9	222.3	277.9	329.6	373.8	407.4
1899-------					26.9	58.6	105.2	158.4	218.6	274.1	326.5	367.7	399.6
1900-------				8.9	25.8	55.8	100.8	156.7	217.3	274.1	324.0	364.6	396.2
1901-------			2.1	8.5	24.2	52.1	98.5	157.7	219.4	273.1	323.0	361.4	392.0
1902-------	1917	*	2.0	8.1	23.1	52.2	105.1	165.2	224.3	278.7	325.1	362.1	388.0
1903-------	1918	*	1.8	7.5	23.0	58.9	111.3	169.1	228.4	280.9	326.2	359.0	382.0
1904-------	1919	*	1.7	7.6	26.6	61.2	112.1	170.7	228.2	279.7	320.7	350.4	372.4
1905-------	1920	*	1.8	9.0	27.3	61.5	113.6	169.8	227.2	274.8	311.8	340.5	363.0
1906-------	1921	*	2.2	9.1	27.2	62.8	112.3	169.7	223.3	266.2	302.3	331.6	354.3
1907-------	1922	*	2.1	9.1	28.0	62.9	115.2	168.9	217.8	259.9	296.5	325.6	348.1
1908-------	1923	*	2.2	9.4	28.9	65.6	114.7	164.7	213.2	255.5	292.1	321.5	342.6
1909-------	1924	*	2.2	10.2	30.9	66.5	112.9	162.8	212.1	254.8	292.7	321.0	342.9
1910-------	1925	*	2.4	10.4	31.5	65.0	111.8	162.5	211.3	255.9	291.8	320.9	343.1
1911-------	1926	*	2.6	11.7	31.1	64.7	112.1	161.6	213.1	255.0	292.2	321.0	343.4
1912-------	1927	*	2.8	10.8	30.3	63.5	109.1	161.1	209.2	252.2	288.8	317.8	340.5
1913-------	1928	*	2.4	10.3	29.2	61.9	109.1	158.3	208.0	250.6	287.6	317.6	340.5
1914-------	1929	*	2.3	9.9	28.7	61.8	107.1	157.4	207.1	250.8	289.5	319.4	342.3
1915-------	1930	*	2.4	10.1	28.7	60.4	106.5	157.7	207.9	253.2	291.4	321.6	344.5
1916-------	1931	*	2.4	10.0	27.8	59.9	107.3	159.1	211.3	256.1	294.8	324.5	348.7
1917-------	1932	*	2.3	9.4	27.9	62.3	110.5	164.5	216.3	261.5	299.4	330.6	356.0
1918-------	1933	*	2.2	9.8	29.6	64.7	115.4	169.7	221.0	264.9	303.9	336.4	363.4
1919-------	1934	*	2.4	10.9	31.7	69.4	120.9	176.4	227.5	273.1	313.6	347.3	373.1
1920-------	1935	*	2.7	11.6	33.8	72.4	125.8	183.0	235.2	281.3	322.7	354.1	378.9
1921-------	1936	*	3.0	12.8	35.6	77.1	133.9	193.7	246.0	293.1	331.0	360.9	392.3
1922-------	1937	*	3.0	12.8	36.7	81.2	140.1	196.4	250.1	293.5	328.6	366.4	400.0
1923-------	1938	*	3.0	13.1	38.7	86.0	141.7	200.2	250.1	290.4	335.0	376.1	413.9
1924-------	1939	*	3.1	14.4	41.7	87.1	145.5	200.0	247.1	298.5	348.8	396.1	435.6
1925-------	1940	*	3.8	16.0	46.5	94.5	148.9	200.5	257.5	315.8	373.2	421.9	461.8
1926-------	1941	*	3.9	19.7	52.0	96.5	148.7	208.1	272.8	339.6	398.6	446.6	485.9
1927-------	1942	*	6.4	23.1	53.0	95.9	151.9	218.8	293.5	361.5	418.6	465.6	503.6
1928-------	1943	*	6.7	22.2	51.4	95.8	158.7	236.5	313.1	378.7	433.9	478.3	515.7
1929-------	1944	*	6.2	21.6	51.1	101.5	175.2	256.6	331.4	395.6	448.6	493.3	531.5
1930-------	1945	*	6.1	21.7	55.1	113.6	191.8	271.6	344.3	404.9	457.4	503.0	541.6
1931-------	1946	*	6.4	25.0	63.9	127.9	206.4	285.1	354.6	416.7	471.7	519.0	558.8
1932-------	1947	*	7.8	28.5	71.2	135.8	213.0	288.1	358.5	423.7	481.7	531.3	572.2
1933-------	1948	*	8.6	31.9	75.9	140.3	216.2	293.5	368.3	437.6	499.7	551.4	592.2
1934-------	1949	*	9.4	32.7	76.6	139.9	217.0	297.7	377.8	452.6	516.0	567.4	609.1
1935-------	1950	*	9.1	32.4	75.6	140.1	218.3	304.3	389.7	465.2	528.3	579.6	619.7
1936-------	1951	*	9.0	31.4	75.3	140.1	222.7	313.1	397.6	472.2	534.0	583.4	622.3
1937-------	1952	*	8.5	30.7	74.2	141.1	227.0	316.6	399.7	472.2	531.5	579.6	617.8
1938-------	1953	*	7.9	30.6	74.5	143.1	227.4	314.2	396.2	465.7	523.8	569.9	607.4
1939-------	1954	*	8.4	31.4	76.7	145.1	227.8	314.9	394.3	464.3	520.6	566.8	603.4
1940-------	1955	*	8.8	32.4	77.4	145.3	227.9	312.5	391.8	459.6	516.0	560.9	596.1
1941-------	1956	*	9.2	32.8	78.1	144.5	224.6	306.9	383.1	449.7	504.9	548.5	583.1
1942-------	1957	*	8.6	32.1	75.9	140.2	217.0	296.5	371.9	437.8	490.7	533.0	568.0
1943-------	1958	*	8.5	31.0	73.3	134.6	208.4	286.5	360.3	423.1	474.3	516.7	550.4
1944-------	1959	*	8.6	31.1	72.4	132.8	206.2	282.9	353.1	413.4	463.8	504.6	542.0
1945-------	1960	*	8.4	30.1	70.8	130.2	202.2	275.5	342.7	401.3	449.6	493.4	534.2
1946-------	1961	*	8.3	29.9	69.7	128.5	197.4	266.7	331.8	388.4	439.6	487.3	527.7
1947-------	1962	*	8.2	29.2	68.8	124.7	189.9	257.0	318.6	376.5	430.9	478.3	516.3
1948-------	1963	*	7.8	28.7	66.0	118.9	181.1	244.5	307.1	367.9	422.3	465.3	503.6
1949-------	1964	*	7.9	27.4	63.5	113.9	172.6	235.9	300.8	361.1	409.3	452.1	
1950-------	1965	*	7.4	26.5	61.1	108.8	167.1	232.1	295.6	349.2	396.7		
1951-------	1966	*	7.3	26.0	58.0	104.7	164.3	227.4	284.9	337.2			
1952-------	1967	*	7.0	24.1	54.7	101.9	158.9	216.7	271.7				
1953-------	1968	*	6.5	22.4	53.8	98.9	151.3	206.3					
1954-------	1969	*	6.1	22.5	52.4	94.2	143.5						
1955-------	1970	*	6.3	22.2	49.7	89.0							
1956-------	1971	*	6.1	20.7	46.4								
1957-------	1972	*	5.4	19.1									
1958-------	1973	*	5.2										
1959-------	1974	*											

TABLE 6C. CUMULATIVE BIRTH RATES FOR ALL OTHER WOMEN AS OF THE BEGINNING OF EACH YEAR 1917-74 BY AGE AND LIVE-BIRTH ORDER FOR EACH COHORT FROM 1867 TO 1959--CON.

LIVE-BIRTH ORDER AND COHORT	DIAGONAL LINE FOR JANUARY 1	EXACT AGE											
		27	28	29	30	31	32	33	34	35	36	37	38
SECOND BIRTHS--CON.													
1879-------													637.7
1880-------												626.6	630.9
1881-------											615.6	620.9	625.7
1882-------										604.4	610.4	616.1	620.8
1883-------									591.4	598.1	604.4	609.9	615.0
1884-------								576.2	583.3	590.1	596.1	602.0	606.4
1885-------							561.2	569.0	576.2	582.8	589.1	594.1	598.6
1886-------						547.5	557.5	565.3	572.3	579.0	584.7	589.8	593.8
1887-------					533.2	545.2	555.3	563.1	570.1	576.6	582.3	586.9	590.4
1888-------				513.5	529.6	541.3	551.5	559.3	566.8	573.2	578.3	582.4	585.3
1889-------			489.6	507.8	523.2	535.5	545.9	554.3	561.6	567.4	572.1	576.0	578.9
1890-------	1917	464.1	486.0	503.0	519.6	532.7	543.9	552.1	558.6	564.2	569.1	572.7	575.5
1891-------	1918	462.5	482.9	501.6	519.8	533.4	544.5	551.9	558.4	563.8	568.2	571.6	573.7
1892-------	1919	461.8	484.3	505.2	523.5	537.0	546.9	554.2	560.6	565.7	569.7	572.4	575.0
1893-------	1920	459.3	484.3	504.8	522.9	535.1	544.9	551.8	557.9	562.3	565.6	568.8	571.1
1894-------	1921	454.0	478.4	498.6	515.0	526.6	535.9	542.6	547.8	551.6	555.2	558.0	560.3
1895-------	1922	447.5	471.6	490.1	505.5	516.2	525.2	530.8	535.2	539.0	542.2	544.9	546.9
1896-------	1923	440.5	462.5	479.5	493.9	504.4	511.7	516.5	520.8	524.4	527.6	530.0	532.0
1897-------	1924	433.3	453.6	469.9	483.7	492.1	498.5	503.2	507.4	510.9	513.7	516.2	518.0
1898-------	1925	431.3	451.6	466.9	478.4	485.9	492.2	496.8	500.8	504.0	506.9	509.2	511.0
1899-------	1926	424.6	444.5	458.8	469.4	477.2	484.1	488.7	492.9	496.5	499.7	502.3	504.3
1900-------	1927	420.4	438.3	450.7	461.4	469.9	476.4	481.2	485.5	489.3	492.5	495.0	497.1
1901-------	1928	413.3	428.6	440.8	452.0	459.7	466.2	470.9	475.3	479.2	482.1	484.7	487.0
1902-------	1929	406.2	420.7	432.9	442.8	450.1	455.9	460.4	464.6	467.8	470.7	473.2	475.5
1903-------	1930	399.3	413.7	424.9	434.7	441.6	447.5	451.9	455.6	458.8	461.7	464.3	466.5
1904-------	1931	390.1	404.1	415.4	424.9	432.2	437.9	442.1	445.8	449.1	452.1	454.6	457.1
1905-------	1932	380.6	394.7	405.7	415.4	422.3	427.8	432.1	436.1	439.5	442.5	445.3	447.8
1906-------	1933	371.7	385.0	396.2	405.3	412.1	418.0	422.5	426.6	430.2	433.6	436.5	439.3
1907-------	1934	364.5	377.9	388.5	397.7	404.8	410.5	415.2	419.6	423.6	427.3	430.6	433.6
1908-------	1935	359.0	372.1	382.8	392.4	399.4	405.3	410.3	415.2	419.8	423.9	427.5	430.6
1909-------	1936	359.6	373.3	384.6	394.2	401.4	407.7	413.3	418.9	424.0	428.4	432.2	436.0
1910-------	1937	360.0	374.1	386.0	395.5	403.0	410.0	416.3	422.5	428.0	432.9	437.3	441.4
1911-------	1938	360.7	375.3	387.0	396.8	405.0	412.7	419.7	426.4	432.1	437.5	442.6	447.1
1912-------	1939	358.3	372.6	384.5	395.1	404.3	412.8	420.4	427.3	433.7	439.9	445.3	449.8
1913-------	1940	357.9	372.6	385.3	397.1	407.3	416.5	424.1	432.0	439.3	445.9	451.5	456.0
1914-------	1941	360.2	375.9	389.7	402.7	413.5	422.9	431.8	440.7	448.5	455.5	461.0	465.7
1915-------	1942	363.5	379.9	395.1	408.5	419.5	430.4	440.5	449.8	458.1	464.6	470.3	475.3
1916-------	1943	368.0	386.1	401.5	414.7	427.4	439.4	449.9	459.7	467.6	474.7	480.8	485.9
1917-------	1944	377.1	395.3	410.2	425.8	439.9	453.0	463.8	473.3	481.7	489.1	495.3	500.7
1918-------	1945	384.4	401.5	419.3	436.7	452.4	465.6	476.8	486.7	495.7	503.4	509.9	515.2
1919-------	1946	393.6	415.3	436.4	456.1	472.4	486.2	498.3	509.3	518.7	526.6	533.4	538.6
1920-------	1947	404.6	429.4	452.3	472.9	489.4	504.4	517.2	528.3	537.4	545.6	551.9	557.0
1921-------	1948	420.9	447.5	471.8	492.0	509.6	525.2	538.0	549.0	558.6	566.4	572.6	577.7
1922-------	1949	430.9	458.6	482.1	502.7	520.4	535.5	548.3	559.3	568.6	576.1	582.2	586.4
1923-------	1950	446.0	473.8	497.3	518.0	535.7	551.3	563.9	575.2	584.3	591.6	596.8	601.1
1924-------	1951	468.5	496.4	520.6	542.1	560.8	576.2	589.0	599.8	608.7	615.4	620.8	625.3
1925-------	1952	494.5	523.3	548.5	570.3	588.4	603.4	616.0	626.4	634.6	641.3	646.7	651.0
1926-------	1953	519.0	548.6	573.9	595.6	612.8	628.0	639.8	649.8	658.1	664.4	669.7	673.6
1927-------	1954	536.6	565.0	589.7	610.5	628.1	642.0	653.4	663.2	670.7	677.2	682.2	685.8
1928-------	1955	548.2	576.4	600.2	620.7	636.5	650.0	661.3	670.3	677.8	683.6	688.0	691.6
1929-------	1956	564.0	592.4	616.1	635.0	650.7	664.2	674.9	683.8	691.0	696.5	701.0	704.3
1930-------	1957	574.5	602.7	624.8	643.7	659.5	672.6	683.0	691.7	698.1	703.5	707.6	710.9
1931-------	1958	592.2	619.0	641.4	660.5	675.9	688.2	698.6	706.4	713.0	718.1	722.4	725.7
1932-------	1959	605.1	632.3	654.5	673.4	688.0	700.5	709.8	717.9	724.0	729.3	733.3	736.7
1933-------	1960	625.4	652.2	674.6	692.5	707.1	719.1	728.8	736.4	742.8	748.0	752.4	755.7
1934-------	1961	641.5	668.5	690.5	708.4	722.7	734.7	744.0	751.6	758.1	763.4	767.7	770.9
1935-------	1962	652.1	678.7	700.1	717.9	732.3	744.0	753.3	761.5	768.1	773.5	777.6	781.2
1936-------	1963	653.9	679.4	700.3	717.9	732.1	743.7	753.5	761.8	768.6	773.9	778.3	781.4
1937-------	1964	648.5	673.8	694.7	712.2	726.2	738.1	748.3	757.0	763.8	769.4	773.5	
1938-------	1965	637.4	661.7	682.5	699.8	714.0	726.7	737.7	746.6	753.4	758.9		
1939-------	1966	632.7	657.2	678.0	695.7	711.5	725.5	736.9	745.9	753.1			
1940-------	1967	624.9	649.9	671.1	690.3	707.4	722.1	733.6	742.9				
1941-------	1968	612.1	637.1	659.8	680.6	698.6	713.2	725.1					
1942-------	1969	596.9	623.5	648.2	669.5	687.4	702.2						
1943-------	1970	581.9	611.2	636.3	657.9	676.1							
1944-------	1971	576.7	606.3	631.3	653.0								
1945-------	1972	568.8	597.4	622.4									
1946-------	1973	560.7	589.7										
1947-------	1974	549.5											

TABLE 6C. CUMULATIVE BIRTH RATES FOR ALL OTHER WOMEN AS OF THE BEGINNING OF EACH YEAR 1917-74 BY AGE AND LIVE-BIRTH ORDER FOR EACH COHORT FROM 1867 TO 1959--CON.

LIVE-BIRTH ORDER AND COHORT	DIAGONAL LINE FOR JANUARY 1	EXACT AGE											
		39	40	41	42	43	44	45	46	47	48	49	50
SECOND BIRTHS--CON.													
1867-------													735.3
1868-------												729.6	729.8
1869-------											723.5	723.8	723.9
1870-------										716.9	717.2	717.3	717.4
1871-------									710.0	710.6	710.7	710.8	711.0
1872-------								702.5	703.1	703.3	703.4	703.7	703.8
1873-------							694.7	695.4	695.7	696.0	696.3	696.4	696.5
1874-------						686.3	686.8	687.3	687.7	688.3	688.4	688.5	688.6
1875-------					677.6	678.3	679.0	679.5	680.2	680.4	680.5	680.6	680.7
1876-------				668.5	669.5	670.5	671.2	672.0	672.2	672.3	672.4	672.5	672.6
1877-------			659.0	660.6	661.9	662.9	663.6	664.1	664.3	664.6	664.7	664.9	665.0
1878-------	1917	648.7	651.5	653.4	654.8	655.8	656.6	657.0	657.4	657.7	657.9	658.1	658.2
1879-------	1918	641.3	644.4	646.3	647.6	648.8	649.5	650.0	650.3	650.7	650.8	651.0	651.0
1880-------	1919	634.8	637.9	639.9	641.5	642.5	643.1	643.5	643.9	644.2	644.4	644.5	644.6
1881-------	1920	629.6	633.1	635.2	636.6	637.6	638.1	638.6	638.8	639.1	639.3	639.4	639.4
1882-------	1921	625.2	628.5	630.5	631.8	632.5	633.1	633.5	633.8	634.1	634.3	634.4	634.5
1883-------	1922	618.9	622.1	623.9	624.9	625.6	625.9	626.2	626.5	626.8	626.9	627.0	627.0
1884-------	1923	610.3	613.2	614.7	615.7	616.2	616.6	616.9	617.2	617.4	617.5	617.6	617.6
1885-------	1924	602.1	604.5	605.9	606.9	607.3	607.7	607.9	608.1	608.2	608.3	608.4	608.4
1886-------	1925	596.8	598.9	600.3	601.1	601.6	601.8	602.0	602.1	602.2	602.3	602.3	602.4
1887-------	1926	592.8	594.9	596.0	596.8	597.2	597.4	597.6	597.8	598.0	598.0	598.1	598.2
1888-------	1927	587.6	589.4	590.5	591.2	591.5	591.8	592.0	592.2	592.3	592.4	592.6	592.7
1889-------	1928	581.1	582.8	583.8	584.4	584.7	585.0	585.2	585.4	585.5	585.6	585.7	585.8
1890-------	1929	577.3	578.9	579.9	580.4	580.8	581.1	581.3	581.4	581.5	581.6	581.7	581.8
1891-------	1930	575.7	577.2	578.1	578.7	579.0	579.2	579.4	579.5	579.6	579.7	579.8	579.8
1892-------	1931	576.9	578.5	579.4	579.9	580.2	580.5	580.7	580.9	581.0	581.1	581.1	581.1
1893-------	1932	573.0	574.4	575.2	575.8	576.2	576.4	576.6	576.7	576.8	576.8	576.9	576.9
1894-------	1933	561.9	563.2	564.0	564.6	564.9	565.1	565.2	565.3	565.3	565.3	565.3	565.3
1895-------	1934	548.5	549.7	550.4	550.9	551.2	551.4	551.5	551.5	551.6	551.7	551.7	551.7
1896-------	1935	533.4	534.4	535.2	535.7	536.0	536.2	536.3	536.4	536.5	536.6	536.6	536.6
1897-------	1936	519.3	520.4	521.3	521.8	522.1	522.3	522.4	522.6	522.7	522.7	522.7	522.7
1898-------	1937	512.4	513.7	514.5	515.0	515.3	515.5	515.7	515.9	516.0	516.0	516.0	516.0
1899-------	1938	506.0	507.4	508.1	508.7	509.0	509.3	509.5	509.6	509.7	509.7	509.7	509.8
1900-------	1939	498.9	500.3	501.1	501.7	502.1	502.4	502.6	502.7	502.8	502.8	502.9	502.9
1901-------	1940	488.8	490.2	491.1	491.8	492.2	492.5	492.7	492.9	492.9	493.0	493.1	493.1
1902-------	1941	477.2	478.7	479.8	480.5	480.9	481.3	481.6	481.7	481.8	481.9	482.0	482.0
1903-------	1942	468.4	470.0	471.1	471.8	472.3	472.7	472.9	473.0	473.1	473.1	473.2	473.2
1904-------	1943	459.2	461.0	462.2	463.0	463.5	463.9	464.1	464.3	464.4	464.5	464.5	464.5
1905-------	1944	450.1	452.0	453.2	454.1	454.7	455.1	455.4	455.5	455.6	455.6	455.6	455.6
1906-------	1945	441.7	443.5	444.9	445.9	446.5	447.0	447.2	447.3	447.4	447.4	447.5	447.5
1907-------	1946	436.0	438.3	439.8	440.8	441.5	442.0	442.2	442.3	442.4	442.4	442.4	442.4
1908-------	1947	433.5	435.8	437.3	438.4	439.1	439.5	439.8	440.0	440.1	440.1	440.1	440.1
1909-------	1948	439.1	441.5	443.2	444.5	445.4	446.0	446.3	446.5	446.5	446.5	446.5	446.5
1910-------	1949	444.7	447.4	449.3	450.8	451.7	452.2	452.5	452.6	452.7	452.7	452.8	452.8
1911-------	1950	450.7	453.5	455.8	457.2	458.1	458.7	459.0	459.2	459.3	459.4	459.4	459.4
1912-------	1951	453.4	456.6	458.7	460.2	461.1	461.8	462.1	462.3	462.4	462.4	462.4	462.4
1913-------	1952	459.9	462.9	465.1	466.6	467.6	468.2	468.6	468.8	468.9	468.9	468.9	468.9
1914-------	1953	469.8	473.0	475.2	476.8	477.7	478.3	478.6	478.7	478.8	478.8	478.8	478.8
1915-------	1954	479.3	482.5	484.7	486.1	487.0	487.6	487.9	488.0	488.1	488.1	488.1	488.1
1916-------	1955	490.2	493.3	495.4	496.8	497.8	498.4	498.7	498.8	498.9	498.9	498.9	498.9
1917-------	1956	504.7	507.8	509.9	511.3	512.3	512.8	513.1	513.2	513.3	513.3	513.3	513.3
1918-------	1957	519.3	522.4	524.4	525.7	526.5	527.0	527.2	527.4	527.4	527.4	527.4	527.4
1919-------	1958	542.7	545.7	547.7	548.9	549.7	550.2	550.5	550.6	550.6	550.6	550.6	550.6
1920-------	1959	561.2	564.0	565.7	566.9	567.7	568.2	568.5	568.6	568.7	568.7	568.7	568.7
1921-------	1960	581.2	583.8	585.6	586.9	587.7	588.2	588.5	588.6	588.7	588.7	588.7	588.7
1922-------	1961	589.9	592.6	594.5	595.7	596.4	596.9	597.1	597.2	597.3	597.3	597.3	597.3
1923-------	1962	604.7	607.4	609.1	610.2	610.9	611.4	611.6	611.7	611.7	611.7	611.7	611.7
1924-------	1963	628.7	631.1	632.8	633.9	634.6	634.9	635.2	635.3	635.3	635.3	635.3	635.3
1925-------	1964	654.3	656.6	658.2	659.3	660.0	660.5	660.8	660.9	660.9	660.9	660.9	
1926-------	1965	676.6	679.0	680.5	681.6	682.3	682.8	683.0	683.1	683.1	683.1		
1927-------	1966	688.7	690.8	692.5	693.4	694.2	694.6	694.8	694.9	694.9			
1928-------	1967	694.1	696.1	697.4	698.5	699.1	699.5	699.7	699.8				
1929-------	1968	707.0	708.9	710.3	711.2	711.9	712.3	712.5					
1930-------	1969	713.4	715.2	716.5	717.4	718.0	718.3						
1931-------	1970	728.3	730.2	731.5	732.5	733.0							
1932-------	1971	739.2	741.0	742.3	743.1								
1933-------	1972	758.2	760.0	761.2									
1934-------	1973	773.4	775.1										
1935-------	1974	783.5											

TABLE 6C. CUMULATIVE BIRTH RATES FOR ALL OTHER WOMEN AS OF THE BEGINNING OF EACH YEAR 1917-74 BY AGE AND LIVE-BIRTH ORDER FOR EACH COHORT FROM 1867 TO 1959--CON.

LIVE-BIRTH ORDER AND COHORT	DIAGONAL LINE FOR JANUARY 1	EXACT AGE											
		15	16	17	18	19	20	21	22	23	24	25	26
THIRD BIRTHS													
1891-------													284.0
1892-------												239.3	276.2
1893-------											212.5	253.9	292.1
1894-------										152.9	196.8	240.1	277.0
1895-------									101.0	140.6	187.0	227.9	266.8
1896-------								57.9	91.7	133.5	176.5	218.8	259.9
1897-------							28.8	52.2	87.9	126.7	170.3	215.5	252.8
1898-------						11.3	25.7	50.4	83.7	123.4	171.1	213.3	252.2
1899-------					3.7	9.9	24.9	47.9	81.6	124.4	168.5	212.0	253.0
1900-------				0.8	3.2	9.5	23.7	47.1	83.7	123.7	170.6	217.4	254.3
1901-------			0.1	0.7	3.1	9.0	23.1	48.2	81.9	123.8	173.6	215.4	248.4
1902-------	1917	*	0.1	0.7	3.0	9.2	25.0	49.1	85.5	131.2	175.3	212.9	243.5
1903-------	1918	*	0.1	0.7	3.1	9.9	25.0	51.1	90.2	130.9	171.8	208.2	236.6
1904-------	1919	*	0.1	0.7	3.3	10.0	26.8	54.6	90.1	129.4	169.3	203.0	229.5
1905-------	1920	*	0.1	0.8	3.4	11.4	29.0	54.5	88.7	127.6	164.3	195.8	222.3
1906-------	1921	*	0.1	0.8	3.8	11.9	28.7	54.3	88.2	124.2	159.0	190.3	215.8
1907-------	1922	*	0.1	0.9	4.0	11.7	28.8	54.3	86.5	120.5	155.1	185.1	211.1
1908-------	1923	*	0.1	0.9	3.9	12.4	29.5	54.1	85.1	119.0	152.0	182.5	207.8
1909-------	1924	*	0.1	1.0	4.2	12.6	29.4	52.9	84.4	117.6	152.3	183.1	209.0
1910-------	1925	*	0.2	1.1	4.5	12.7	28.7	52.7	83.3	118.0	152.7	184.6	209.5
1911-------	1926	*	0.1	1.0	4.4	12.1	28.1	51.7	83.8	117.9	154.0	184.7	209.1
1912-------	1927	*	0.2	1.1	4.2	11.5	27.3	51.4	81.5	116.7	151.1	180.7	206.1
1913-------	1928	*	0.2	1.1	3.9	11.2	27.3	49.8	81.1	115.6	149.3	180.8	207.0
1914-------	1929	*	0.2	1.0	3.9	11.3	26.4	49.9	81.3	115.3	150.8	183.3	209.4
1915-------	1930	*	0.1	0.9	3.8	11.0	26.8	50.9	82.0	118.1	154.9	187.3	213.8
1916-------	1931	*	0.2	1.0	3.8	11.4	27.7	51.9	84.8	122.0	158.7	192.0	219.1
1917-------	1932	*	0.1	0.8	3.9	11.7	28.2	54.0	87.8	124.7	163.1	197.3	224.4
1918-------	1933	*	0.2	1.0	4.0	12.4	29.9	56.2	89.2	127.6	166.4	199.9	227.8
1919-------	1934	*	0.2	1.0	4.3	13.1	31.3	57.9	92.9	132.0	170.5	204.6	232.7
1920-------	1935	*	0.2	1.1	4.6	13.7	32.6	62.2	97.3	136.1	175.0	208.6	234.8
1921-------	1936	*	0.2	1.2	5.0	15.4	37.9	68.3	104.9	144.2	182.2	213.1	241.9
1922-------	1937	*	0.2	1.2	5.4	18.6	41.4	72.5	109.7	148.2	182.3	215.5	246.4
1923-------	1938	*	0.2	1.3	6.6	20.4	44.0	75.7	112.4	147.6	184.2	219.5	254.1
1924-------	1939	*	0.2	1.6	7.1	21.2	45.3	76.8	110.6	148.9	188.4	229.4	266.7
1925-------	1940	*	0.3	1.8	8.5	22.9	46.9	75.8	112.4	153.7	199.8	243.9	284.7
1926-------	1941	*	0.4	2.7	9.6	23.8	45.7	77.2	117.4	165.3	215.4	263.9	307.1
1927-------	1942	*	0.5	2.9	9.7	22.8	46.0	80.3	126.2	179.0	233.4	283.9	326.6
1928-------	1943	*	0.6	2.9	9.3	23.0	48.4	87.4	138.3	195.6	251.7	300.7	343.5
1929-------	1944	*	0.6	2.8	9.4	24.4	52.9	97.0	153.0	212.4	268.1	317.2	359.8
1930-------	1945	*	0.5	2.9	10.2	26.9	59.8	108.3	166.4	224.9	278.9	328.6	371.4
1931-------	1946	*	0.6	3.4	11.6	31.7	68.1	118.8	176.3	233.3	289.3	339.9	384.6
1932-------	1947	*	0.8	3.9	13.5	35.0	73.1	123.3	179.2	238.5	295.9	348.8	394.8
1933-------	1948	*	0.9	4.3	14.5	36.9	75.2	125.4	184.2	245.7	306.1	361.1	407.8
1934-------	1949	*	1.1	4.8	15.7	39.0	77.3	129.9	190.9	256.4	319.2	375.3	423.0
1935-------	1950	*	0.9	4.7	15.7	39.0	79.0	132.5	197.0	265.5	330.4	387.3	433.9
1936-------	1951	*	1.0	4.8	15.7	39.9	80.4	136.4	203.8	272.0	335.6	390.9	436.7
1937-------	1952	*	0.9	4.5	15.6	39.7	81.4	139.9	206.4	273.5	335.9	390.0	433.6
1938-------	1953	*	0.9	4.5	15.6	40.3	83.0	140.1	204.6	270.4	331.0	382.7	424.4
1939-------	1954	*	0.8	4.5	16.2	41.4	84.3	141.0	205.3	269.3	328.0	378.0	418.7
1940-------	1955	*	0.8	4.7	16.5	42.2	84.7	140.8	203.1	266.2	321.8	369.3	406.4
1941-------	1956	*	1.0	4.9	16.8	42.6	84.2	138.2	198.8	257.7	310.6	353.7	388.3
1942-------	1957	*	0.8	4.8	16.8	41.5	81.9	134.0	190.7	246.5	294.2	333.5	365.7
1943-------	1958	*	1.0	4.9	16.2	40.5	79.0	128.4	182.2	232.9	276.3	312.3	342.2
1944-------	1959	*	0.9	4.8	16.6	40.3	77.3	124.6	174.1	220.2	259.4	293.5	324.4
1945-------	1960	*	0.9	4.9	16.4	39.0	74.8	118.5	163.3	204.3	241.7	276.3	309.1
1946-------	1961	*	0.9	4.7	15.5	37.9	71.2	110.6	150.4	188.5	225.7	261.8	294.3
1947-------	1962	*	0.9	4.8	15.5	36.2	65.6	101.0	137.4	174.6	212.2	247.6	275.8
1948-------	1963	*	0.9	4.5	14.5	32.8	59.4	90.2	124.4	162.1	198.2	228.2	254.7
1949-------	1964	*	0.8	4.2	12.9	29.5	52.9	82.1	116.9	152.5	183.4	211.5	
1950-------	1965	*	0.8	3.8	11.7	26.0	47.8	77.2	109.0	139.3	168.4		
1951-------	1966	*	0.7	3.6	10.6	24.1	45.4	72.0	100.0	128.5			
1952-------	1967	*	0.7	3.0	9.3	22.1	41.3	64.7	90.9				
1953-------	1968	*	0.5	2.7	8.8	20.6	37.5	59.1					
1954-------	1969	*	0.5	2.6	8.3	18.5	34.2						
1955-------	1970	*	0.5	2.5	7.4	16.8							
1956-------	1971	*	0.5	2.2	6.7								
1957-------	1972	*	0.4	1.9									
1958-------	1973	*	0.3										
1959-------	1974	*											

TABLE 6C. CUMULATIVE BIRTH RATES FOR ALL OTHER WOMEN AS OF THE BEGINNING OF EACH YEAR 1917-74 BY AGE AND LIVE-BIRTH ORDER FOR EACH COHORT FROM 1867 TO 1959--CON.

LIVE-BIRTH ORDER AND COHORT	DIAGONAL LINE FOR JANUARY 1	EXACT AGE											
		27	28	29	30	31	32	33	34	35	36	37	38
THIRD BIRTHS--CON.													
1879-------													534.5
1880-------												521.7	527.5
1881-------											508.6	515.9	522.7
1882-------										494.8	502.5	510.8	517.3
1883-------									478.5	486.6	495.1	502.8	510.4
1884-------								461.4	470.1	478.8	486.8	495.7	502.1
1885-------							443.7	453.2	462.1	470.3	479.2	486.7	492.9
1886-------						425.4	438.1	447.9	456.7	465.5	473.2	480.4	486.1
1887-------					405.5	420.0	433.2	442.9	452.1	460.2	467.6	474.3	480.0
1888-------				382.3	401.4	416.5	429.8	440.0	449.0	456.8	463.8	470.6	475.6
1889-------			355.4	377.1	396.8	412.0	426.2	436.3	445.0	452.6	459.9	465.9	470.6
1890-------	1917	322.2	348.5	370.7	390.5	406.9	421.0	430.9	439.5	447.6	454.7	460.5	464.7
1891-------	1918	314.3	341.3	363.4	384.9	401.6	415.4	425.2	434.6	442.5	449.4	454.5	457.9
1892-------	1919	307.2	334.0	358.3	380.5	396.3	409.9	420.6	429.5	437.4	443.1	447.4	450.6
1893-------	1920	322.9	352.2	377.5	397.9	413.5	428.3	438.0	446.8	453.2	458.3	462.6	465.8
1894-------	1921	310.4	340.9	363.5	383.8	400.6	413.5	422.7	430.1	435.8	440.7	444.7	447.9
1895-------	1922	301.5	328.6	351.3	373.1	388.2	399.6	407.9	414.3	419.9	424.4	428.1	431.2
1896-------	1923	290.8	318.0	342.1	361.5	374.7	385.4	392.3	398.3	403.5	407.8	411.4	414.2
1897-------	1924	283.8	312.8	334.4	352.0	364.1	373.0	379.3	384.9	389.7	393.7	397.0	399.7
1898-------	1925	286.0	312.0	332.4	348.1	358.5	366.9	373.2	378.9	383.6	387.4	390.7	393.3
1899-------	1926	283.9	309.0	327.7	342.2	352.7	361.4	367.8	373.8	378.6	383.0	386.6	389.5
1900-------	1927	282.9	305.8	322.2	336.3	347.0	355.5	362.2	368.1	373.3	377.6	381.1	384.2
1901-------	1928	275.0	295.1	310.7	324.7	334.5	342.9	349.3	355.4	360.2	364.1	367.7	370.5
1902-------	1929	266.9	285.0	300.0	312.7	321.9	329.9	336.1	341.2	345.6	349.6	353.0	355.7
1903-------	1930	258.1	276.0	290.4	302.7	312.0	319.8	325.4	330.3	334.7	338.7	341.9	344.5
1904-------	1931	250.8	268.8	283.0	295.6	304.6	312.3	317.9	323.1	327.6	331.5	334.7	337.5
1905-------	1932	243.6	261.5	275.7	287.8	296.9	304.0	309.5	314.7	319.2	323.1	326.5	329.5
1906-------	1933	237.1	254.4	268.4	280.3	288.9	296.2	302.0	307.3	311.8	316.0	319.4	322.8
1907-------	1934	231.7	249.0	262.3	273.6	282.2	289.7	295.6	300.9	305.8	310.1	314.0	317.7
1908-------	1935	228.3	244.5	257.4	268.9	277.8	285.3	291.2	296.9	302.1	307.0	311.2	315.0
1909-------	1936	229.0	245.0	258.5	270.6	279.5	287.1	293.6	299.9	305.7	310.9	315.5	319.9
1910-------	1937	228.9	245.6	259.9	271.9	280.9	289.2	296.2	303.2	309.3	314.8	319.9	324.6
1911-------	1938	229.6	247.3	261.4	273.3	282.9	291.5	299.2	306.6	313.1	319.3	324.9	329.7
1912-------	1939	227.2	244.6	258.6	271.1	281.3	290.8	298.9	306.7	313.6	320.1	325.9	330.9
1913-------	1940	227.8	245.2	259.7	272.8	283.8	293.9	302.4	310.8	318.3	325.3	331.4	336.8
1914-------	1941	230.2	248.2	263.5	277.4	289.0	299.1	308.6	317.5	325.8	333.3	339.7	345.7
1915-------	1942	235.2	253.5	269.5	284.1	295.5	307.0	317.0	326.8	335.8	343.5	350.8	356.7
1916-------	1943	240.5	259.7	276.5	290.5	303.5	315.6	326.4	336.8	345.9	354.6	361.1	367.5
1917-------	1944	246.7	266.7	282.5	298.4	312.4	325.4	337.0	347.8	357.6	365.9	373.4	379.9
1918-------	1945	250.9	269.5	287.6	304.6	319.6	333.8	346.3	357.8	368.1	377.1	385.2	391.6
1919-------	1946	254.7	276.5	296.3	315.3	332.3	347.8	361.2	374.2	385.2	394.9	403.0	409.7
1920-------	1947	259.5	282.9	304.9	325.7	343.8	360.2	374.7	388.3	399.9	409.8	417.8	424.6
1921-------	1948	269.0	294.8	318.5	340.2	359.3	376.3	391.7	405.0	416.6	426.4	434.8	441.3
1922-------	1949	275.3	302.2	326.8	349.6	368.8	386.9	401.9	415.5	427.0	436.9	444.9	451.4
1923-------	1950	285.1	314.0	340.5	363.6	383.6	401.3	416.6	430.4	442.2	451.8	459.5	465.7
1924-------	1951	301.0	332.8	360.0	384.6	405.6	424.0	440.0	454.0	465.7	475.2	482.8	489.0
1925-------	1952	321.8	354.1	382.2	407.4	428.4	447.4	463.4	477.1	488.2	497.3	504.9	511.1
1926-------	1953	344.2	377.2	406.0	431.4	452.9	471.9	487.1	500.5	511.2	520.4	527.8	533.3
1927-------	1954	363.7	396.3	425.2	450.7	472.5	490.2	505.0	517.6	528.2	537.1	543.6	549.0
1928-------	1955	379.9	412.7	440.9	466.4	486.1	503.6	517.9	530.1	540.3	548.3	554.8	559.9
1929-------	1956	397.0	429.9	458.9	482.6	502.5	519.6	534.1	545.9	555.5	563.5	569.7	574.5
1930-------	1957	409.0	442.2	469.3	492.8	512.6	529.8	543.2	554.7	564.1	571.5	577.4	582.2
1931-------	1958	423.6	455.8	483.2	506.3	526.4	542.4	555.7	567.0	575.9	583.2	588.6	592.9
1932-------	1959	432.8	465.5	492.6	516.3	535.2	551.0	563.9	574.5	583.3	589.9	595.4	599.7
1933-------	1960	447.2	479.2	506.7	529.5	548.4	564.1	576.5	587.0	594.9	601.8	607.2	611.7
1934-------	1961	461.8	494.3	521.4	544.1	562.1	577.3	589.4	599.0	607.2	614.2	619.8	624.0
1935-------	1962	472.0	503.7	530.3	552.3	569.7	583.9	595.4	605.1	613.4	620.4	625.8	629.9
1936-------	1963	473.9	504.3	529.6	550.4	566.7	580.5	591.6	601.7	610.3	617.0	622.2	626.0
1937-------	1964	469.3	499.0	523.1	542.4	558.4	571.6	583.3	593.6	602.0	608.3	613.3	
1938-------	1965	458.9	486.8	508.5	527.0	542.3	556.3	568.7	578.9	586.4	592.6		
1939-------	1966	451.1	476.7	497.9	515.7	532.0	546.9	559.4	568.8	576.5			
1940-------	1967	436.0	460.8	480.9	499.9	517.4	532.3	543.8	552.9				
1941-------	1968	416.5	439.1	460.3	480.8	498.6	512.3	523.2					
1942-------	1969	391.7	415.7	438.7	459.2	474.9	488.0						
1943-------	1970	369.2	395.3	418.4	436.3	451.5							
1944-------	1971	353.6	379.6	400.0	417.7								
1945-------	1972	338.4	361.3	381.1									
1946-------	1973	319.7	342.0										
1947-------	1974	300.1											

TABLE 6C. CUMULATIVE BIRTH RATES FOR ALL OTHER WOMEN AS OF THE BEGINNING OF EACH YEAR 1917-74 BY AGE AND LIVE-BIRTH ORDER FOR EACH COHORT FROM 1867 TO 1959--CON.

LIVE-BIRTH ORDER AND COHORT	DIAGONAL LINE FOR JANUARY 1	EXACT AGE											
		39	40	41	42	43	44	45	46	47	48	49	50
THIRD BIRTHS--CON.													
1867-------													650.0
1868-------												643.1	643.2
1869-------											635.6	635.8	636.0
1870-------										627.5	627.9	628.3	628.4
1871-------									618.9	619.6	620.3	620.5	620.6
1872-------								609.8	610.5	611.8	612.1	612.4	612.5
1873-------							600.1	600.7	602.0	602.5	603.0	603.1	603.2
1874-------						589.7	590.2	591.2	591.8	592.6	592.9	593.0	593.1
1875-------					579.2	579.9	580.7	581.2	582.1	582.6	582.9	583.0	583.1
1876-------				568.8	570.0	571.1	571.7	572.5	573.1	573.6	573.8	574.0	574.1
1877-------			558.3	560.1	562.0	562.7	563.5	564.1	564.7	565.1	565.4	565.6	565.8
1878-------	1917	546.9	550.1	552.7	554.0	555.0	555.8	556.4	556.9	557.5	557.7	558.0	558.0
1879-------	1918	539.0	543.0	545.1	547.0	548.1	548.8	549.3	550.0	550.5	550.9	551.0	551.1
1880-------	1919	532.8	536.4	539.2	541.3	542.3	543.1	543.7	544.3	544.8	544.9	545.0	545.1
1881-------	1920	527.8	532.3	535.1	537.0	538.1	538.8	539.5	540.1	540.5	540.7	540.8	540.8
1882-------	1921	523.3	527.5	530.2	532.2	533.2	533.9	534.5	534.9	535.1	535.2	535.2	535.3
1883-------	1922	515.6	519.6	522.2	523.9	524.9	525.5	526.0	526.2	526.5	526.6	526.8	526.9
1884-------	1923	507.2	511.0	513.4	514.9	515.7	516.3	516.6	516.9	517.2	517.4	517.6	517.7
1885-------	1924	497.5	501.1	503.6	504.9	505.7	506.1	506.4	506.8	507.1	507.2	507.3	507.4
1886-------	1925	490.7	494.3	496.3	497.5	498.0	498.4	498.7	498.9	499.1	499.2	499.4	499.5
1887-------	1926	484.3	487.3	489.0	489.9	490.5	490.8	491.1	491.3	491.5	491.7	491.8	491.9
1888-------	1927	479.4	482.0	483.4	484.4	484.9	485.2	485.5	485.7	485.9	486.0	486.1	486.1
1889-------	1928	474.0	476.3	477.8	478.8	479.2	479.6	479.9	480.1	480.2	480.3	480.4	480.5
1890-------	1929	467.4	469.6	471.1	471.8	472.3	472.7	473.0	473.2	473.4	473.5	473.6	473.7
1891-------	1930	460.6	462.8	463.9	464.8	465.3	465.7	465.9	466.1	466.2	466.3	466.4	466.5
1892-------	1931	453.2	455.1	456.4	457.3	457.8	458.2	458.5	458.7	458.8	458.9	459.0	459.1
1893-------	1932	468.2	470.2	471.4	472.2	472.7	473.0	473.2	473.3	473.4	473.5	473.6	473.6
1894-------	1933	450.4	452.3	453.5	454.3	454.7	455.1	455.3	455.4	455.5	455.6	455.7	455.7
1895-------	1934	433.4	435.2	436.4	437.1	437.5	437.7	437.9	438.0	438.1	438.2	438.2	438.2
1896-------	1935	416.4	418.2	419.3	420.0	420.4	420.6	420.8	420.9	421.0	421.0	421.1	421.1
1897-------	1936	401.8	403.6	404.6	405.3	405.7	405.9	406.1	406.3	406.4	406.5	406.6	406.6
1898-------	1937	395.5	397.2	398.4	399.1	399.5	399.7	400.0	400.2	400.3	400.4	400.5	400.6
1899-------	1938	391.9	393.8	395.0	395.7	396.1	396.4	396.6	396.8	396.9	397.0	397.1	397.2
1900-------	1939	386.6	388.5	389.7	390.5	390.9	391.2	391.5	391.7	391.9	392.0	392.1	392.2
1901-------	1940	372.8	374.6	375.8	376.6	377.0	377.4	377.7	377.9	378.0	378.1	378.2	378.2
1902-------	1941	357.9	359.7	360.9	361.7	362.2	362.6	362.8	362.9	363.0	363.1	363.1	363.2
1903-------	1942	346.8	348.8	350.1	351.0	351.6	352.0	352.3	352.5	352.6	352.6	352.7	352.7
1904-------	1943	339.9	342.1	343.5	344.5	345.1	345.6	345.9	346.1	346.2	346.3	346.3	346.3
1905-------	1944	332.3	334.7	336.3	337.2	338.0	338.5	338.8	339.0	339.1	339.1	339.2	339.2
1906-------	1945	325.8	328.2	329.6	330.8	331.6	332.1	332.4	332.6	332.7	332.8	332.8	332.8
1907-------	1946	320.7	323.1	324.9	326.1	326.9	327.4	327.7	327.9	328.1	328.1	328.2	328.2
1908-------	1947	318.2	320.9	322.7	323.9	324.6	325.2	325.5	325.7	325.8	325.9	326.0	326.0
1909-------	1948	323.6	326.5	328.4	329.7	330.7	331.4	331.8	331.9	332.0	332.1	332.1	332.1
1910-------	1949	328.4	331.4	333.5	335.1	336.2	336.9	337.2	337.5	337.6	337.7	337.8	337.8
1911-------	1950	333.8	337.2	339.5	341.2	342.3	343.0	343.5	343.7	343.8	343.9	343.9	343.9
1912-------	1951	335.3	338.7	341.1	342.8	344.0	344.8	345.1	345.3	345.4	345.4	345.4	345.4
1913-------	1952	341.4	345.3	347.8	349.7	350.8	351.5	351.9	352.1	352.2	352.2	352.2	352.2
1914-------	1953	350.6	354.4	357.1	358.9	360.1	361.0	361.4	361.6	361.8	361.8	361.8	361.8
1915-------	1954	361.8	365.5	368.2	370.1	371.3	371.9	372.3	372.6	372.7	372.7	372.7	372.7
1916-------	1955	372.6	376.5	379.3	381.1	382.1	382.8	383.3	383.5	383.6	383.6	383.6	383.6
1917-------	1956	385.0	389.1	391.7	393.3	394.6	395.3	395.7	395.9	396.0	396.0	396.0	396.0
1918-------	1957	396.9	400.7	403.2	405.1	406.2	407.0	407.3	407.5	407.6	407.6	407.6	407.6
1919-------	1958	415.0	418.8	421.7	423.5	424.8	425.4	425.8	426.0	426.1	426.2	426.2	426.2
1920-------	1959	430.0	434.0	436.7	438.7	439.7	440.4	440.8	441.0	441.1	441.1	441.1	441.1
1921-------	1960	446.6	450.5	453.4	455.2	456.3	457.1	457.5	457.7	457.8	457.8	457.8	457.8
1922-------	1961	456.4	460.3	462.9	464.5	465.7	466.3	466.7	467.0	467.1	467.2	467.2	467.2
1923-------	1962	470.7	474.5	476.9	478.6	479.6	480.3	480.8	481.0	481.1	481.1	481.1	481.1
1924-------	1963	493.9	497.3	499.9	501.4	502.4	503.1	503.4	503.6	503.7	503.8	503.8	503.8
1925-------	1964	515.7	519.3	521.6	523.2	524.2	524.8	525.2	525.4	525.5	525.5	525.5	
1926-------	1965	537.8	541.1	543.4	545.0	545.9	546.5	546.8	547.0	547.1	547.1		
1927-------	1966	553.2	556.2	558.5	559.7	560.5	561.0	561.2	561.3	561.4			
1928-------	1967	563.7	567.0	568.8	570.1	570.9	571.3	571.6	571.7				
1929-------	1968	578.5	581.0	582.9	584.1	584.7	585.1	585.3					
1930-------	1969	585.6	588.2	589.8	590.9	591.6	591.9						
1931-------	1970	596.2	598.7	600.5	601.6	602.3							
1932-------	1971	603.1	605.6	607.3	608.3								
1933-------	1972	615.0	617.3	618.8									
1934-------	1973	627.1	629.2										
1935-------	1974	632.8											

TABLE 6C. CUMULATIVE BIRTH RATES FOR ALL OTHER WOMEN AS OF THE BEGINNING OF EACH YEAR 1917-74 BY AGE AND LIVE-BIRTH ORDER FOR EACH COHORT FROM 1867 TO 1959--CON.

LIVE-BIRTH ORDER AND COHORT	DIAGONAL LINE FOR JANUARY 1	EXACT AGE											
		15	16	17	18	19	20	21	22	23	24	25	26
FOURTH BIRTHS													
1891-------													167.2
1892-------												126.8	157.0
1893-------											100.1	130.1	159.9
1894-------										60.4	87.2	117.2	147.0
1895-------									32.8	51.9	79.3	108.5	140.3
1896-------								15.0	27.7	47.2	73.0	103.2	136.8
1897-------							6.0	12.6	25.5	43.9	69.8	102.6	133.7
1898-------						1.9	5.2	11.8	24.1	42.8	71.9	103.0	134.6
1899-------					0.5	1.4	4.6	11.0	23.3	44.0	71.5	102.6	135.9
1900-------				0.1	0.4	1.1	4.4	10.7	24.4	44.1	72.5	105.8	140.0
1901-------			0.0	0.1	0.3	1.3	4.2	11.1	23.8	43.6	73.0	106.9	139.9
1902-------	1917	*	0.0	0.0	0.3	1.0	4.6	11.5	25.0	46.5	76.6	109.0	137.7
1903-------	1918	*	0.0	0.1	0.3	1.3	4.9	12.2	26.5	49.0	78.1	107.2	133.6
1904-------	1919	*	0.0	0.0	0.3	1.4	5.4	13.1	28.6	51.2	77.9	105.3	130.8
1905-------	1920	*	0.0	0.1	0.4	1.8	6.0	14.6	30.0	51.0	76.0	102.1	126.9
1906-------	1921	*	0.0	0.1	0.5	2.0	6.5	15.2	29.6	49.3	72.9	99.0	123.3
1907-------	1922	*	0.0	0.1	0.6	2.3	6.8	14.9	28.6	47.1	71.5	96.4	121.0
1908-------	1923	*	0.0	0.1	0.6	2.3	6.5	14.6	27.7	46.6	69.4	94.5	118.3
1909-------	1924	*	0.0	0.1	0.7	2.2	6.7	14.4	27.4	45.7	68.9	94.2	119.2
1910-------	1925	*	0.0	0.1	0.6	2.3	6.4	13.7	26.5	45.0	68.3	94.3	118.9
1911-------	1926	*	0.0	0.1	0.6	2.0	6.1	13.6	26.8	45.1	69.7	96.0	120.1
1912-------	1927	*	0.0	0.1	0.5	2.0	6.0	13.4	25.7	44.7	69.2	94.0	118.3
1913-------	1928	*	0.0	0.1	0.6	2.1	6.0	13.1	26.3	45.9	69.3	95.0	119.4
1914-------	1929	*	0.0	0.1	0.6	2.0	5.9	13.3	27.0	46.1	70.8	96.9	121.5
1915-------	1930	*	0.0	0.1	0.5	1.9	5.8	13.6	27.2	47.1	72.0	98.3	124.1
1916-------	1931	*	0.0	0.1	0.6	1.9	6.0	14.0	27.9	47.9	73.2	101.8	127.7
1917-------	1932	*	0.0	0.1	0.5	1.9	6.0	14.0	28.1	48.3	76.7	105.6	131.3
1918-------	1933	*	0.0	0.1	0.5	2.0	6.2	14.5	28.6	51.3	79.8	107.9	134.7
1919-------	1934	*	0.0	0.1	0.6	2.1	6.6	14.9	30.9	53.7	81.6	110.6	137.5
1920-------	1935	*	0.0	0.1	0.6	2.3	6.8	16.8	32.6	56.2	84.6	113.8	139.4
1921-------	1936	*	0.0	0.2	0.8	2.6	8.5	18.6	36.3	60.3	89.2	116.6	143.2
1922-------	1937	*	0.0	0.1	0.7	3.4	9.3	20.7	38.8	63.3	89.6	117.4	143.7
1923-------	1938	*	0.0	0.1	1.0	3.8	10.4	22.3	40.9	63.5	90.5	118.1	145.7
1924-------	1939	*	0.0	0.2	1.1	4.0	10.9	23.2	40.7	64.0	91.2	121.3	151.9
1925-------	1940	*	0.1	0.3	1.3	4.4	11.6	23.3	41.1	64.7	94.7	128.1	161.9
1926-------	1941	*	0.1	0.3	1.4	4.6	11.7	23.5	42.1	68.4	101.7	138.3	175.9
1927-------	1942	*	0.0	0.2	1.4	4.5	11.3	23.8	44.5	74.1	110.0	151.0	191.1
1928-------	1943	*	0.0	0.2	1.4	4.3	11.7	25.7	48.9	80.7	121.7	164.5	205.3
1929-------	1944	*	0.0	0.2	1.3	4.5	12.7	28.4	53.7	90.4	133.9	178.9	221.1
1930-------	1945	*	0.0	0.3	1.6	5.0	13.8	31.0	59.9	99.1	143.4	188.4	230.2
1931-------	1946	*	0.1	0.4	1.7	5.7	16.0	35.5	67.2	107.2	151.8	197.2	240.6
1932-------	1947	*	0.1	0.4	1.8	6.4	17.7	39.2	70.5	110.6	155.9	202.8	245.9
1933-------	1948	*	0.1	0.5	2.2	7.1	19.6	41.7	73.9	115.6	163.4	211.0	255.2
1934-------	1949	*	0.1	0.5	2.3	7.9	20.8	43.6	77.3	121.6	170.0	218.8	265.2
1935-------	1950	*	0.1	0.5	2.4	8.1	21.3	44.9	80.7	125.8	175.6	226.3	271.9
1936-------	1951	*	0.1	0.5	2.5	8.3	21.8	46.7	83.3	129.8	181.5	231.0	275.7
1937-------	1952	*	0.0	0.5	2.4	8.2	22.1	47.8	85.4	132.6	182.3	231.3	275.1
1938-------	1953	*	0.1	0.5	2.4	8.6	22.8	48.9	87.0	131.9	180.6	227.6	268.1
1939-------	1954	*	0.1	0.6	2.6	8.8	23.6	50.1	86.5	132.3	179.2	223.4	261.9
1940-------	1955	*	0.1	0.6	2.6	9.1	24.1	49.7	86.6	129.5	173.7	215.5	249.8
1941-------	1956	*	0.1	0.7	2.8	9.3	24.1	50.2	84.9	125.8	167.2	204.0	234.5
1942-------	1957	*	0.1	0.6	2.7	9.2	23.7	48.2	81.3	119.0	155.2	187.1	213.6
1943-------	1958	*	0.1	0.6	2.7	9.1	22.8	46.0	76.4	110.0	141.3	168.6	192.5
1944-------	1959	*	0.1	0.6	2.8	9.0	22.5	44.4	71.9	100.4	126.8	151.4	174.4
1945-------	1960	*	0.1	0.6	2.6	8.4	20.8	40.6	64.1	88.5	112.5	136.1	159.3
1946-------	1961	*	0.1	0.6	2.5	8.0	19.8	36.6	56.7	78.3	101.0	124.0	145.4
1947-------	1962	*	0.1	0.6	2.5	7.9	17.8	32.6	50.1	69.9	91.5	112.5	130.1
1948-------	1963	*	0.1	0.6	2.4	6.8	15.2	27.2	42.7	61.4	80.6	97.7	112.9
1949-------	1964	*	0.1	0.5	2.0	5.9	12.8	23.5	38.2	54.6	70.8	85.8	
1950-------	1965	*	0.1	0.4	1.6	4.7	10.9	21.1	33.9	48.0	61.8		
1951-------	1966	*	0.0	0.3	1.4	4.2	9.9	18.7	29.6	41.6			
1952-------	1967	*	0.1	0.4	1.3	3.8	8.8	16.0	25.4				
1953-------	1968	*	0.0	0.3	1.1	3.3	7.3	13.7					
1954-------	1969	*	0.0	0.2	0.9	2.7	6.4						
1955-------	1970	*	0.0	0.2	0.8	2.3							
1956-------	1971	*	0.0	0.2	0.7								
1957-------	1972	*	0.0	0.1									
1958-------	1973	*	0.0										
1959-------	1974	*											

TABLE 6C. CUMULATIVE BIRTH RATES FOR ALL OTHER WOMEN AS OF THE BEGINNING OF EACH YEAR 1917-74 BY AGE AND LIVE-BIRTH ORDER FOR EACH COHORT FROM 1867 TO 1959--CON.

LIVE-BIRTH ORDER AND COHORT	DIAGONAL LINE FOR JANUARY 1	EXACT AGE											
		27	28	29	30	31	32	33	34	35	36	37	38
FOURTH BIRTHS--CON.													
1879-------													441.9
1880-------												426.8	433.6
1881-------											410.7	419.5	426.7
1882-------										393.5	403.6	412.8	420.4
1883-------									369.9	380.4	390.7	400.3	408.4
1884-------								347.6	358.1	368.7	379.2	389.1	396.5
1885-------							328.9	339.5	349.8	360.4	371.1	380.1	386.8
1886-------						315.1	329.0	339.4	349.8	360.5	370.5	378.6	384.7
1887-------					300.9	316.8	330.6	341.1	351.5	361.8	370.9	378.4	384.5
1888-------				277.1	297.7	313.3	327.4	338.1	348.6	358.2	366.9	374.4	380.7
1889-------			242.8	264.6	284.7	300.9	315.4	326.4	336.5	346.0	354.9	362.3	368.4
1890-------	1917	205.5	230.4	251.5	272.4	289.6	304.6	315.2	325.4	335.2	343.4	350.7	356.0
1891-------	1918	193.9	217.9	239.9	262.7	280.6	295.1	305.8	316.5	325.4	334.1	340.6	345.5
1892-------	1919	182.8	207.8	232.2	255.8	272.7	287.3	298.5	308.8	318.4	325.8	331.3	335.8
1893-------	1920	186.6	214.4	239.7	261.7	278.5	293.7	305.1	315.9	324.2	330.5	335.8	340.1
1894-------	1921	176.6	205.2	228.3	249.9	267.6	282.8	294.2	303.5	310.7	317.2	322.2	326.4
1895-------	1922	170.7	196.8	219.3	242.3	259.6	274.3	284.2	292.3	299.6	305.5	310.5	314.4
1896-------	1923	164.6	190.1	214.4	237.1	253.8	266.7	275.2	283.1	289.5	295.3	299.8	303.7
1897-------	1924	160.8	188.2	213.0	234.3	249.0	260.2	268.2	275.2	281.6	286.9	291.2	294.9
1898-------	1925	164.5	193.1	216.7	236.3	249.6	260.3	268.1	275.3	281.5	286.6	291.0	294.5
1899-------	1926	167.0	195.1	217.0	235.0	247.7	258.6	266.7	274.3	280.5	286.1	290.5	294.3
1900-------	1927	170.8	196.2	216.0	232.7	245.9	256.7	265.2	272.6	279.2	284.6	289.3	293.1
1901-------	1928	166.8	189.3	207.3	223.9	236.4	247.2	255.1	262.5	268.7	274.2	278.6	282.5
1902-------	1929	162.0	182.4	200.0	216.0	228.0	237.9	245.4	252.3	258.0	262.7	266.9	270.6
1903-------	1930	156.6	176.4	193.8	209.3	220.7	230.1	237.5	243.6	248.8	253.5	257.6	261.1
1904-------	1931	152.8	172.9	190.3	205.5	216.9	226.5	233.1	239.1	244.4	249.1	253.1	256.5
1905-------	1932	149.0	169.1	185.7	200.8	211.8	220.5	227.1	233.3	238.7	243.2	247.1	250.7
1906-------	1933	146.0	165.2	182.2	196.5	207.1	216.0	222.9	229.3	234.5	239.0	243.2	247.0
1907-------	1934	142.2	162.0	177.8	191.6	202.1	211.1	218.2	224.4	229.8	235.0	239.4	243.5
1908-------	1935	140.2	158.7	174.0	187.7	198.3	207.4	214.3	220.8	227.0	232.5	237.2	241.5
1909-------	1936	140.6	159.2	174.7	189.0	199.9	208.9	216.2	223.4	230.1	236.0	241.2	245.8
1910-------	1937	140.1	158.8	175.2	189.5	200.3	209.8	217.5	225.4	232.5	238.7	244.1	248.8
1911-------	1938	141.4	160.7	177.1	191.4	202.5	211.7	220.1	228.4	235.5	242.0	247.9	252.8
1912-------	1939	139.6	158.8	175.3	189.7	201.0	211.0	219.9	228.1	235.6	242.6	248.3	253.4
1913-------	1940	140.7	160.1	176.6	190.6	202.7	213.3	222.3	231.4	239.4	246.4	252.4	258.0
1914-------	1941	143.1	162.5	178.9	193.9	206.5	217.6	227.7	236.8	244.9	252.1	258.9	265.1
1915-------	1942	145.6	164.6	181.9	197.2	209.8	221.6	231.4	240.8	249.2	257.3	264.3	270.5
1916-------	1943	149.6	169.7	187.2	202.5	215.7	227.5	237.6	247.4	256.7	265.1	272.6	279.1
1917-------	1944	154.5	174.8	191.7	207.6	221.3	233.7	244.6	255.3	264.9	273.5	281.1	288.0
1918-------	1945	157.9	177.5	195.4	212.3	226.8	240.1	252.0	263.6	273.9	283.1	291.3	298.4
1919-------	1946	160.1	181.3	200.7	219.3	234.9	249.4	262.7	275.5	286.7	296.9	305.7	312.9
1920-------	1947	163.2	185.2	205.8	225.0	241.8	258.1	272.7	285.9	297.9	308.3	317.1	325.1
1921-------	1948	167.2	190.3	211.6	232.0	250.7	267.7	282.5	296.6	309.0	319.7	328.9	336.1
1922-------	1949	168.2	192.2	215.1	237.2	256.4	273.8	289.4	303.6	315.9	326.6	335.0	341.9
1923-------	1950	172.5	198.9	224.1	247.3	267.7	286.5	302.5	317.1	329.6	339.8	348.1	355.5
1924-------	1951	182.1	211.4	238.4	263.6	285.7	305.0	321.5	336.5	348.5	358.7	367.4	374.9
1925-------	1952	195.3	226.7	255.7	282.5	305.0	324.8	341.8	356.2	368.2	378.7	387.7	394.8
1926-------	1953	211.5	244.6	275.0	302.1	324.8	344.7	361.2	375.1	387.2	397.8	405.9	412.1
1927-------	1954	227.7	262.3	292.5	319.8	342.3	362.0	377.8	391.8	404.1	413.7	421.1	427.6
1928-------	1955	243.1	277.0	307.1	333.1	355.1	373.9	389.5	403.6	415.0	423.8	431.2	436.8
1929-------	1956	258.8	293.4	323.1	348.9	371.2	389.9	406.3	420.0	430.6	439.7	446.7	452.2
1930-------	1957	268.3	302.0	330.8	357.0	378.0	396.8	412.0	424.8	435.0	443.4	449.8	455.0
1931-------	1958	278.9	312.7	342.3	366.8	388.7	406.3	421.2	433.7	443.6	451.1	457.2	461.6
1932-------	1959	284.6	319.0	347.0	372.5	392.6	410.3	424.2	436.0	444.7	451.9	457.4	462.1
1933-------	1960	295.0	328.9	359.0	383.6	404.0	420.9	434.5	445.1	453.9	460.8	466.5	471.4
1934-------	1961	304.8	339.6	368.5	392.5	412.1	428.2	440.7	451.3	459.4	466.4	472.3	476.7
1935-------	1962	312.0	346.1	374.0	397.6	416.0	431.1	443.7	453.3	461.6	468.8	474.4	478.7
1936-------	1963	314.4	346.5	373.3	395.1	412.3	426.1	437.0	446.7	455.2	462.1	467.2	470.9
1937-------	1964	312.0	342.4	367.4	386.7	402.1	414.7	425.8	435.7	443.8	449.6	454.2	
1938-------	1965	302.0	330.2	351.2	368.6	382.7	395.8	407.4	416.6	423.4	429.1		
1939-------	1966	293.6	317.7	337.6	354.1	368.9	382.3	393.2	401.2	407.9			
1940-------	1967	277.2	299.8	318.3	335.3	350.6	363.6	373.1	380.9				
1941-------	1968	259.2	280.1	298.6	315.7	330.7	341.6	350.4					
1942-------	1969	236.0	256.3	275.4	292.2	304.9	315.0						
1943-------	1970	214.1	235.1	253.2	267.5	278.9							
1944-------	1971	196.7	216.2	232.0	244.9								
1945-------	1972	180.1	197.0	211.0									
1946-------	1973	163.0	177.9										
1947-------	1974	145.5											

TABLE 6C. CUMULATIVE BIRTH RATES FOR ALL OTHER WOMEN AS OF THE BEGINNING OF EACH YEAR 1917-74 BY AGE AND LIVE-BIRTH ORDER FOR EACH COHORT FROM 1867 TO 1959--CON.

LIVE-BIRTH ORDER AND COHORT	DIAGONAL LINE FOR JANUARY 1	EXACT AGE											
		39	40	41	42	43	44	45	46	47	48	49	50
FOURTH BIRTHS--CON.													
1867-------													574.0
1868-------												566.1	566.3
1869-------											557.6	558.0	558.5
1870-------										548.4	548.8	549.7	549.8
1871-------									538.6	539.3	540.3	540.6	540.8
1872-------								528.3	529.0	530.8	531.1	531.5	531.7
1873-------							517.3	518.2	519.8	520.4	520.8	521.1	521.2
1874-------						505.5	506.5	508.1	508.7	509.5	509.8	510.0	510.1
1875-------					493.5	494.7	495.6	496.4	497.3	498.0	498.2	498.4	498.5
1876-------				481.5	483.6	484.7	485.5	486.5	487.3	487.8	488.0	488.3	488.4
1877-------			469.3	472.4	474.4	475.5	476.5	477.4	478.0	478.5	478.8	479.0	479.2
1878-------	1917	456.1	460.9	464.0	466.0	467.3	468.4	469.1	469.7	470.3	470.6	470.9	470.9
1879-------	1918	447.5	452.4	455.6	458.1	459.5	460.3	461.0	461.7	462.2	462.6	462.7	462.8
1880-------	1919	439.5	444.7	448.5	451.1	452.1	453.0	453.9	454.5	455.2	455.4	455.5	455.6
1881-------	1920	433.0	438.9	442.7	444.7	445.8	446.9	447.5	448.4	448.9	449.1	449.3	449.4
1882-------	1921	427.3	433.0	436.2	438.3	439.7	440.5	441.5	442.2	442.7	442.9	443.1	443.1
1883-------	1922	414.8	419.8	423.0	425.6	427.0	428.0	428.8	429.4	429.8	430.0	430.1	430.3
1884-------	1923	402.3	407.1	410.6	413.0	414.0	415.0	415.7	416.1	416.5	416.6	416.9	417.1
1885-------	1924	392.1	397.0	400.2	402.0	403.1	403.8	404.3	404.8	405.2	405.4	405.6	405.7
1886-------	1925	389.9	394.3	397.0	398.6	399.5	400.1	400.6	401.0	401.3	401.5	401.6	401.7
1887-------	1926	389.6	393.9	396.1	397.5	398.2	398.8	399.3	399.6	399.9	400.1	400.2	400.4
1888-------	1927	385.8	389.2	391.0	392.3	393.0	393.5	394.0	394.4	394.7	394.8	395.0	395.0
1889-------	1928	372.7	376.0	377.9	379.3	380.0	380.6	381.1	381.5	381.8	382.0	382.1	382.2
1890-------	1929	359.9	363.1	365.2	366.5	367.2	367.7	368.2	368.5	368.7	368.8	368.9	369.0
1891-------	1930	349.1	352.4	354.3	355.4	356.1	356.7	357.1	357.4	357.6	357.7	357.8	357.9
1892-------	1931	339.5	342.6	344.5	345.8	346.6	347.1	347.5	347.8	348.0	348.1	348.2	348.3
1893-------	1932	343.7	346.7	348.6	349.8	350.5	351.0	351.4	351.6	351.8	351.9	352.0	352.1
1894-------	1933	329.9	332.8	334.5	335.7	336.4	336.9	337.2	337.4	337.6	337.7	337.8	337.8
1895-------	1934	317.6	320.2	321.8	322.8	323.5	323.9	324.1	324.3	324.4	324.5	324.5	324.5
1896-------	1935	306.7	309.1	310.5	311.6	312.2	312.6	312.9	313.1	313.3	313.3	313.3	313.4
1897-------	1936	297.8	300.1	301.6	302.5	303.0	303.4	303.7	304.0	304.1	304.1	304.2	304.3
1898-------	1937	297.3	299.6	301.1	302.0	302.6	303.0	303.4	303.7	303.8	303.9	304.0	304.0
1899-------	1938	297.2	299.8	301.2	302.2	302.8	303.4	303.8	304.0	304.2	304.3	304.4	304.4
1900-------	1939	296.5	299.0	300.5	301.6	302.3	303.0	303.4	303.7	303.9	304.0	304.0	304.1
1901-------	1940	285.7	288.1	289.6	290.6	291.4	292.1	292.5	292.8	292.9	293.0	293.1	293.1
1902-------	1941	273.6	276.0	277.5	278.7	279.5	280.0	280.4	280.6	280.7	280.8	280.8	280.8
1903-------	1942	264.0	266.4	268.0	269.2	270.0	270.6	271.0	271.2	271.3	271.4	271.4	271.4
1904-------	1943	259.5	262.0	263.7	265.0	265.9	266.5	266.8	267.0	267.2	267.2	267.3	267.3
1905-------	1944	253.9	256.5	258.4	259.7	260.6	261.2	261.6	261.9	262.0	262.0	262.0	262.1
1906-------	1945	250.4	253.3	255.3	256.7	257.6	258.3	258.8	259.1	259.2	259.3	259.4	259.4
1907-------	1946	247.0	249.9	251.9	253.4	254.3	255.0	255.5	255.7	255.8	255.9	256.0	256.0
1908-------	1947	245.0	247.8	249.8	251.2	252.1	252.9	253.2	253.4	253.6	253.7	253.7	253.7
1909-------	1948	249.5	252.7	254.9	256.3	257.4	258.1	258.6	258.9	259.1	259.1	259.1	259.2
1910-------	1949	252.8	256.1	258.3	260.1	261.1	261.9	262.4	262.7	262.8	262.8	262.9	262.9
1911-------	1950	257.0	260.4	262.9	264.8	266.0	267.0	267.6	267.8	267.9	268.0	268.0	268.0
1912-------	1951	257.9	261.7	264.6	266.5	268.0	268.9	269.4	269.7	269.8	269.9	269.9	269.9
1913-------	1952	262.9	266.8	269.6	271.9	273.3	274.1	274.5	274.7	274.9	274.9	274.9	274.9
1914-------	1953	270.2	274.4	277.7	279.8	281.1	282.0	282.4	282.8	282.9	282.9	282.9	282.9
1915-------	1954	275.8	280.5	283.7	285.7	287.1	287.9	288.5	288.8	288.9	289.0	289.0	289.0
1916-------	1955	284.9	289.4	292.4	294.5	295.9	296.8	297.3	297.6	297.7	297.7	297.7	297.7
1917-------	1956	293.8	298.1	301.1	303.4	304.7	305.5	306.1	306.4	306.5	306.6	306.6	306.6
1918-------	1957	304.0	308.5	311.7	313.8	315.3	316.3	316.7	316.9	317.0	317.0	317.0	317.0
1919-------	1958	319.2	323.9	327.2	329.5	331.1	332.0	332.5	332.7	332.8	332.8	332.9	332.9
1920-------	1959	331.0	335.7	339.0	341.3	342.7	343.6	344.0	344.3	344.4	344.5	344.5	344.5
1921-------	1960	341.8	346.4	349.6	351.9	353.4	354.2	354.7	355.0	355.1	355.1	355.1	355.1
1922-------	1961	347.8	352.3	355.4	357.6	358.9	359.8	360.3	360.5	360.6	360.7	360.7	360.7
1923-------	1962	361.4	365.8	369.1	371.3	372.7	373.5	373.9	374.2	374.3	374.3	374.3	374.3
1924-------	1963	380.6	384.9	387.9	390.0	391.3	392.0	392.4	392.6	392.7	392.7	392.7	392.7
1925-------	1964	400.1	404.3	407.2	409.2	410.4	411.1	411.5	411.7	411.8	411.8	411.8	
1926-------	1965	417.1	421.0	423.6	425.2	426.3	427.0	427.4	427.6	427.7	427.7		
1927-------	1966	432.3	435.8	438.1	439.8	440.9	441.6	442.0	442.2	442.3			
1928-------	1967	441.1	444.3	446.6	448.3	449.4	449.9	450.2	450.3				
1929-------	1968	456.4	459.4	461.8	463.5	464.5	465.0	465.2					
1930-------	1969	458.6	461.9	464.1	465.5	466.3	466.7						
1931-------	1970	465.4	468.5	470.6	471.8	472.5							
1932-------	1971	465.9	468.6	470.4	471.5								
1933-------	1972	474.8	477.3	478.9									
1934-------	1973	480.1	482.3										
1935-------	1974	481.6											

TABLE 6C. CUMULATIVE BIRTH RATES FOR ALL OTHER WOMEN AS OF THE BEGINNING OF EACH YEAR 1917-74 BY AGE AND LIVE-BIRTH ORDER FOR EACH COHORT FROM 1867 TO 1959--CON.

LIVE-BIRTH ORDER AND COHORT	DIAGONAL LINE FOR JANUARY 1	EXACT AGE											
		15	16	17	18	19	20	21	22	23	24	25	26
FIFTH BIRTHS													
1891-------													82.6
1892-------												55.0	74.3
1893-------											39.4	55.7	73.8
1894-------										19.4	31.1	46.4	66.0
1895-------									8.2	15.0	26.1	42.4	62.2
1896-------								2.3	6.0	12.5	24.0	40.3	61.5
1897-------							*	1.5	5.0	11.7	22.9	40.5	60.5
1898-------						*	*	1.4	5.1	11.7	24.1	41.4	62.2
1899-------					*	*	*	1.5	5.1	12.3	24.8	42.6	64.6
1900-------				*	*	*	*	1.5	5.5	12.8	26.0	45.0	66.3
1901-------			*	*	*	*	*	1.6	5.5	12.9	26.5	44.4	66.0
1902-------	1917	*	*	*	*	*	*	1.6	5.9	14.1	27.0	45.0	66.4
1903-------	1918	*	*	*	*	*	*	1.8	6.3	13.9	26.9	44.8	63.5
1904-------	1919	*	*	*	*	*	*	1.8	6.4	14.9	28.2	44.8	63.7
1905-------	1920	*	*	*	*	*	*	2.3	7.4	15.6	28.2	44.6	62.4
1906-------	1921	*	*	*	*	*	*	2.4	7.5	15.7	28.0	43.8	60.9
1907-------	1922	*	*	*	*	*	*	2.4	7.6	15.2	26.9	41.7	58.7
1908-------	1923	*	*	*	*	*	*	2.4	7.0	14.6	25.6	40.0	56.5
1909-------	1924	*	*	*	*	*	*	2.1	6.7	13.8	24.4	38.6	56.0
1910-------	1925	*	*	*	*	*	*	2.2	6.5	13.5	24.2	39.1	56.1
1911-------	1926	*	*	*	*	*	*	2.0	6.3	13.3	24.6	39.7	56.6
1912-------	1927	*	*	*	*	*	*	2.1	6.4	13.5	24.9	39.3	56.5
1913-------	1928	*	*	*	*	*	*	2.0	6.2	13.7	24.6	39.6	57.3
1914-------	1929	*	*	*	*	*	*	2.0	6.7	14.3	26.0	41.4	59.4
1915-------	1930	*	*	*	*	*	*	2.2	7.0	14.8	26.8	42.8	61.6
1916-------	1931	*	*	*	*	*	*	2.3	7.2	14.9	27.5	44.7	64.2
1917-------	1932	*	*	*	*	*	*	2.3	6.9	15.0	29.3	47.5	66.8
1918-------	1933	*	*	*	*	*	*	2.1	7.0	16.1	31.4	49.4	69.5
1919-------	1934	*	*	*	*	*	*	2.2	7.9	17.7	32.4	51.0	71.3
1920-------	1935	*	*	*	*	*	*	2.7	8.7	18.8	34.0	52.9	72.5
1921-------	1936	*	*	*	*	*	*	2.8	9.5	19.9	35.5	53.6	73.8
1922-------	1937	*	*	*	*	*	*	3.4	10.3	21.0	35.6	53.6	73.2
1923-------	1938	*	*	*	*	*	*	3.6	10.8	21.3	36.1	54.0	74.4
1924-------	1939	*	*	*	*	*	*	3.8	10.8	21.2	36.1	54.8	76.4
1925-------	1940	*	*	*	*	*	*	3.6	10.7	21.4	36.9	57.1	80.6
1926-------	1941	*	*	*	*	*	*	3.7	11.2	22.3	39.4	61.5	87.4
1927-------	1942	*	*	*	*	*	*	4.0	11.9	24.4	42.7	67.0	95.3
1928-------	1943	*	*	*	*	*	*	4.2	13.2	26.7	46.9	73.2	103.9
1929-------	1944	*	*	*	*	*	*	4.8	14.4	29.5	52.1	81.6	114.7
1930-------	1945	*	*	*	*	*	*	5.1	15.9	32.9	58.5	89.7	123.7
1931-------	1946	*	*	*	*	*	*	5.9	18.0	37.9	65.0	97.6	132.7
1932-------	1947	*	*	*	*	*	*	6.5	19.3	39.3	67.0	99.8	135.1
1933-------	1948	*	*	*	*	*	*	6.1	20.2	41.1	69.5	104.0	140.2
1934-------	1949	*	*	*	*	*	*	7.3	22.0	43.9	74.1	109.4	146.3
1935-------	1950	*	*	*	*	*	*	7.8	23.0	46.2	77.2	113.5	149.9
1936-------	1951	*	*	*	*	*	*	8.1	24.6	48.3	80.0	115.8	152.7
1937-------	1952	*	*	*	*	*	*	8.7	25.7	49.9	80.9	116.6	153.1
1938-------	1953	*	*	*	*	*	*	8.8	25.3	48.8	79.4	114.3	147.9
1939-------	1954	*	*	*	*	*	*	8.7	25.1	48.8	79.0	111.8	143.5
1940-------	1955	*	*	*	*	*	*	8.7	25.4	48.3	76.7	107.4	135.2
1941-------	1956	*	*	*	*	*	*	8.9	25.5	47.5	73.8	100.1	123.5
1942-------	1957	*	*	*	*	*	*	8.7	24.2	43.8	66.4	88.6	107.7
1943-------	1958	*	*	*	*	*	*	8.3	22.3	39.6	58.3	76.6	92.5
1944-------	1959	*	*	*	*	*	*	7.6	20.3	34.5	50.1	65.3	80.3
1945-------	1960	*	*	*	*	*	*	6.8	17.2	29.6	42.7	56.7	71.3
1946-------	1961	*	*	*	*	*	*	5.8	14.5	24.5	36.2	49.0	61.6
1947-------	1962	*	*	*	*	*	*	4.8	11.8	20.4	30.6	41.6	51.4
1948-------	1963	*	*	*	*	*	*	3.7	9.7	16.8	25.5	34.1	42.1
1949-------	1964	*	*	*	*	*	*	3.2	8.3	14.6	21.4	28.3	
1950-------	1965	*	*	*	*	*	*	2.7	7.1	12.2	17.7		
1951-------	1966	*	*	*	*	*	*	2.3	5.7	9.7			
1952-------	1967	*	*	*	*	*	*	1.8	4.5				
1953-------	1968	*	*	*	*	*	*	1.4					
1954-------	1969	*	*	*	*	*	*						
1955-------	1970	*	*	*	*	*							
1956-------	1971	*	*	*	*								
1957-------	1972	*	*	*									
1958-------	1973	*	*										
1959-------	1974	*											

TABLE 6C. CUMULATIVE BIRTH RATES FOR ALL OTHER WOMEN AS OF THE BEGINNING OF EACH YEAR 1917-74 BY AGE AND LIVE-BIRTH ORDER FOR EACH COHORT FROM 1867 TO 1959--CON.

LIVE-BIRTH ORDER AND COHORT	DIAGONAL LINE FOR JANUARY 1	EXACT AGE											
		27	28	29	30	31	32	33	34	35	36	37	38
FIFTH BIRTHS--CON.													
1879-------													356.8
1880-------												339.6	347.7
1881-------											321.2	331.6	339.4
1882-------										301.6	313.2	323.2	331.6
1883-------									277.6	290.1	301.3	311.8	320.4
1884-------								254.3	266.1	278.2	289.6	300.0	308.2
1885-------							233.8	245.8	257.4	269.5	280.5	290.4	298.1
1886-------						217.3	231.7	243.5	254.8	266.2	277.0	286.3	293.0
1887-------					200.6	215.8	230.1	241.8	252.3	264.0	274.2	282.4	289.5
1888-------				176.6	195.0	209.9	224.3	235.2	246.6	257.7	267.1	275.8	282.8
1889-------			144.7	163.0	180.6	196.2	209.8	221.8	232.7	243.3	253.2	261.7	268.4
1890-------	1917	112.7	132.5	149.7	168.7	184.0	199.0	210.5	221.5	232.5	242.1	250.7	257.2
1891-------	1918	102.4	121.0	140.1	159.3	176.0	190.5	202.2	213.3	224.0	233.6	241.1	247.0
1892-------	1919	92.9	113.5	133.2	153.9	169.8	184.5	196.3	207.7	218.1	226.8	233.9	239.7
1893-------	1920	94.3	115.6	136.7	156.1	172.1	186.8	198.7	209.4	219.0	227.2	234.1	240.0
1894-------	1921	87.0	109.6	129.0	148.5	165.0	179.6	191.5	201.8	210.7	218.5	225.4	230.7
1895-------	1922	84.5	105.3	124.9	145.4	161.7	176.7	187.7	197.5	205.9	213.8	220.1	225.1
1896-------	1923	82.0	103.0	124.0	143.8	160.4	174.3	184.4	193.3	202.0	208.8	215.0	219.8
1897-------	1924	81.2	103.7	123.9	143.5	159.2	172.2	181.6	190.9	198.6	205.5	211.2	216.0
1898-------	1925	85.0	106.7	126.7	146.6	161.3	174.0	183.9	192.2	200.0	206.6	212.3	216.7
1899-------	1926	86.3	108.5	129.6	148.5	163.6	176.6	186.0	195.3	203.3	210.4	216.0	220.6
1900-------	1927	89.0	112.1	131.8	150.8	165.5	177.6	187.7	197.0	205.1	211.9	217.4	222.2
1901-------	1928	88.5	108.8	127.9	145.8	159.5	171.7	181.2	190.4	197.9	204.3	209.7	214.3
1902-------	1929	86.2	106.0	123.8	140.3	153.8	165.2	174.4	182.3	189.1	195.0	200.1	204.2
1903-------	1930	83.0	101.4	118.2	134.7	147.2	158.5	166.7	174.3	181.0	186.8	191.4	195.8
1904-------	1931	82.0	99.9	116.9	133.2	146.1	156.6	164.5	172.2	178.9	184.4	189.3	193.9
1905-------	1932	80.3	98.2	115.0	131.2	143.6	153.8	162.0	169.8	176.2	182.0	187.1	191.6
1906-------	1933	78.9	96.8	113.7	129.0	140.6	150.8	158.9	166.4	173.1	179.0	184.0	188.6
1907-------	1934	76.1	94.1	110.1	124.7	136.5	146.4	154.3	162.2	169.0	174.9	180.0	184.6
1908-------	1935	74.2	91.0	106.4	121.1	132.4	141.9	150.2	158.0	164.8	171.0	176.1	180.8
1909-------	1936	73.3	90.5	106.5	121.0	132.1	142.3	150.6	158.5	165.7	172.0	177.7	182.6
1910-------	1937	73.7	91.3	107.0	121.3	132.8	142.9	151.5	159.9	167.2	174.1	179.8	184.9
1911-------	1938	74.6	92.2	108.0	122.5	134.1	144.4	153.5	162.1	170.1	176.9	182.9	188.3
1912-------	1939	74.3	91.8	107.5	122.2	134.3	145.2	154.6	163.7	171.3	178.2	184.5	189.9
1913-------	1940	75.2	92.7	108.9	123.6	136.4	147.7	157.4	166.3	174.3	181.7	188.0	193.7
1914-------	1941	77.4	95.5	111.7	127.2	140.3	152.0	161.4	170.6	178.9	186.4	193.1	199.3
1915-------	1942	80.0	97.8	114.8	130.7	143.8	155.2	165.2	174.7	183.2	191.0	198.0	204.1
1916-------	1943	82.8	101.5	118.8	134.5	147.6	159.2	169.4	179.1	188.0	196.4	203.5	210.2
1917-------	1944	86.2	105.1	122.2	138.0	151.1	163.1	173.6	184.1	193.4	201.9	209.6	216.8
1918-------	1945	89.0	107.9	125.2	140.9	154.6	167.2	178.6	189.4	199.5	208.4	216.6	223.8
1919-------	1946	91.2	110.7	128.3	145.2	160.1	174.0	186.3	198.6	209.3	219.6	228.3	235.9
1920-------	1947	92.7	112.1	130.9	148.7	164.3	179.1	192.9	205.8	218.1	228.6	237.8	246.0
1921-------	1948	93.7	114.0	133.2	151.6	168.8	185.0	199.5	214.0	226.3	237.1	246.5	254.5
1922-------	1949	93.7	114.1	133.8	153.5	171.3	188.2	203.5	217.6	230.0	240.8	249.9	257.8
1923-------	1950	95.5	117.2	138.2	158.9	177.8	195.3	210.7	225.2	237.9	248.6	257.5	264.7
1924-------	1951	99.6	122.7	146.0	168.7	189.0	207.6	224.1	239.2	251.8	262.9	271.4	279.1
1925-------	1952	105.5	131.9	157.4	182.1	203.6	223.8	241.2	256.0	269.0	279.5	288.6	296.0
1926-------	1953	115.3	144.0	172.1	197.7	220.4	240.7	257.2	272.6	285.2	295.8	304.6	311.7
1927-------	1954	125.9	156.8	185.0	211.5	234.5	253.8	271.0	285.6	297.7	307.9	316.4	323.0
1928-------	1955	136.2	167.2	195.3	221.6	243.1	262.9	279.1	293.4	305.4	315.0	322.6	328.8
1929-------	1956	147.7	179.8	208.9	234.3	256.8	275.9	291.9	306.2	317.5	326.7	334.3	340.1
1930-------	1957	157.5	189.4	217.3	243.1	264.8	283.7	299.6	312.7	323.5	332.2	339.0	344.3
1931-------	1958	166.8	198.2	226.9	252.3	273.7	291.9	306.9	319.9	330.1	338.0	344.2	349.2
1932-------	1959	169.2	201.4	229.5	255.0	275.6	293.5	307.8	319.7	328.9	336.3	342.2	347.2
1933-------	1960	175.2	206.8	235.6	260.0	280.8	298.0	311.6	322.5	331.1	338.3	344.1	348.7
1934-------	1961	180.8	213.4	241.7	266.1	285.9	302.0	314.5	324.6	332.6	339.6	345.3	349.8
1935-------	1962	185.4	217.3	245.3	268.8	287.1	301.7	313.4	322.6	330.7	337.7	343.0	346.9
1936-------	1963	187.8	219.0	245.1	266.2	282.3	295.7	305.8	315.0	323.1	329.3	334.2	337.8
1937-------	1964	186.7	215.2	238.3	256.6	271.2	282.8	293.1	302.4	309.6	315.3	319.6	
1938-------	1965	178.4	203.6	223.2	239.1	251.8	263.3	273.7	282.1	288.8	293.8		
1939-------	1966	170.5	192.1	209.3	223.3	236.1	247.7	257.3	264.8	270.7			
1940-------	1967	158.2	176.9	192.0	206.1	219.0	230.1	238.5	245.2				
1941-------	1968	142.9	158.8	173.7	187.7	199.9	209.0	216.2					
1942-------	1969	124.0	139.2	154.0	166.9	176.7	184.6						
1943-------	1970	107.7	122.9	136.4	146.8	154.9							
1944-------	1971	95.3	109.0	119.7	128.5								
1945-------	1972	85.0	95.9	104.7									
1946-------	1973	72.3	81.3										
1947-------	1974	60.0											

TABLE 6C. CUMULATIVE BIRTH RATES FOR ALL OTHER WOMEN AS OF THE BEGINNING OF EACH YEAR 1917-74 BY AGE AND LIVE-BIRTH ORDER FOR EACH COHORT FROM 1867 TO 1959--CON.

LIVE-BIRTH ORDER AND COHORT	DIAGONAL LINE FOR JANUARY 1	EXACT AGE											
		39	40	41	42	43	44	45	46	47	48	49	50
FIFTH BIRTHS--CON.													
1867-------													499.5
1868-------												490.8	491.0
1869-------											481.8	482.2	482.4
1870-------										472.3	472.8	473.3	473.5
1871-------									462.3	463.2	463.9	464.2	464.4
1872-------								451.8	452.8	454.0	454.4	454.8	454.9
1873-------							440.6	441.7	442.8	443.6	444.2	444.5	444.6
1874-------						428.8	430.0	431.2	432.1	433.1	433.5	433.8	434.0
1875-------					416.2	417.7	418.9	419.9	420.9	421.5	421.9	422.3	422.5
1876-------				402.7	405.2	406.8	407.9	409.0	409.7	410.3	410.8	411.1	411.3
1877-------			388.2	391.8	394.6	396.0	397.2	398.0	398.7	399.6	400.1	400.3	400.4
1878-------	1917	372.9	378.7	382.5	385.1	386.7	387.8	388.6	389.5	390.4	390.6	390.9	391.0
1879-------	1918	363.5	369.3	373.1	376.1	377.6	378.6	379.6	380.5	381.2	381.6	381.8	382.0
1880-------	1919	354.2	360.3	364.5	367.3	368.6	369.7	370.8	371.6	372.2	372.6	372.8	373.0
1881-------	1920	346.5	353.1	357.1	359.6	361.0	362.2	363.3	363.9	364.5	364.9	365.2	365.4
1882-------	1921	339.0	345.4	349.2	351.7	353.2	354.5	355.3	356.0	356.5	356.9	357.1	357.2
1883-------	1922	327.6	333.6	337.2	339.9	341.7	342.8	343.6	344.2	344.7	345.0	345.3	345.5
1884-------	1923	315.0	320.4	324.2	326.4	327.8	328.8	329.5	330.1	330.6	330.9	331.1	331.2
1885-------	1924	304.0	309.7	312.7	315.0	316.3	317.2	317.9	318.5	319.2	319.4	319.5	319.6
1886-------	1925	299.2	303.8	306.9	308.8	309.9	310.6	311.4	312.1	312.5	312.7	312.9	313.1
1887-------	1926	295.5	300.2	303.0	304.9	305.8	306.7	307.4	307.9	308.2	308.4	308.6	308.7
1888-------	1927	288.2	292.7	295.4	297.0	298.1	298.8	299.4	299.8	300.1	300.3	300.4	300.6
1889-------	1928	273.9	278.1	280.5	282.4	283.3	284.1	284.6	285.0	285.3	285.5	285.7	285.8
1890-------	1929	262.0	265.9	268.7	270.4	271.5	272.2	272.8	273.2	273.5	273.6	273.7	273.8
1891-------	1930	251.7	256.3	258.9	260.7	261.6	262.3	262.9	263.3	263.6	263.7	263.9	264.0
1892-------	1931	244.9	248.8	251.2	252.8	253.7	254.4	254.9	255.2	255.3	255.5	255.7	255.8
1893-------	1932	244.6	248.0	250.3	251.8	252.8	253.5	254.0	254.2	254.4	254.6	254.7	254.8
1894-------	1933	234.8	238.3	240.5	242.1	243.0	243.6	243.9	244.2	244.4	244.6	244.7	244.7
1895-------	1934	229.2	232.6	234.9	236.3	237.0	237.4	237.7	238.0	238.2	238.3	238.3	238.4
1896-------	1935	223.7	227.0	229.0	230.1	230.8	231.2	231.5	231.7	231.9	232.0	232.1	232.1
1897-------	1936	219.7	222.7	224.5	225.7	226.4	226.9	227.2	227.5	227.7	227.8	227.9	228.0
1898-------	1937	220.2	223.2	225.3	226.6	227.4	227.9	228.4	228.7	228.9	229.1	229.2	229.2
1899-------	1938	224.6	227.8	229.8	231.2	232.0	232.7	233.2	233.6	233.8	233.9	234.0	234.0
1900-------	1939	226.2	229.2	231.3	232.7	233.5	234.1	234.6	234.9	235.1	235.2	235.3	235.3
1901-------	1940	217.8	220.9	223.0	224.2	224.9	225.6	226.0	226.3	226.5	226.6	226.7	226.8
1902-------	1941	207.8	210.9	212.8	214.0	214.8	215.5	216.0	216.2	216.3	216.4	216.5	216.5
1903-------	1942	199.6	202.6	204.5	205.8	206.8	207.5	207.8	208.0	208.2	208.3	208.4	208.4
1904-------	1943	197.6	200.6	202.6	204.1	205.0	205.6	206.0	206.2	206.3	206.4	206.5	206.5
1905-------	1944	195.5	198.6	200.9	202.3	203.3	203.9	204.3	204.5	204.6	204.7	204.7	204.7
1906-------	1945	192.4	195.7	197.6	199.1	200.0	200.6	201.0	201.2	201.3	201.4	201.4	201.5
1907-------	1946	188.6	191.7	193.9	195.3	196.2	196.9	197.3	197.5	197.6	197.6	197.7	197.7
1908-------	1947	184.7	187.9	190.0	191.6	192.6	193.3	193.6	193.8	193.9	194.0	194.0	194.0
1909-------	1948	186.8	190.2	192.6	194.3	195.4	196.1	196.7	196.9	197.1	197.2	197.2	197.2
1910-------	1949	189.2	192.8	195.2	197.1	198.2	199.2	199.7	200.0	200.2	200.3	200.3	200.3
1911-------	1950	192.7	196.2	199.0	200.8	202.3	203.2	203.7	204.0	204.2	204.2	204.2	204.3
1912-------	1951	194.4	198.4	201.1	203.2	204.6	205.5	206.0	206.4	206.5	206.6	206.7	206.7
1913-------	1952	198.6	202.7	205.7	207.7	209.1	210.2	210.8	211.1	211.3	211.4	211.4	211.4
1914-------	1953	204.4	208.8	211.9	214.1	215.6	216.7	217.2	217.5	217.7	217.7	217.8	217.8
1915-------	1954	209.7	214.2	217.4	219.9	221.5	222.4	223.0	223.3	223.4	223.5	223.6	223.6
1916-------	1955	216.1	220.7	224.2	226.6	228.0	229.1	229.6	229.9	230.1	230.2	230.3	230.3
1917-------	1956	222.6	227.5	230.8	233.1	234.8	235.8	236.3	236.6	236.7	236.8	236.8	236.8
1918-------	1957	229.9	234.7	238.1	240.5	242.2	243.2	243.7	244.0	244.2	244.3	244.3	244.3
1919-------	1958	242.3	247.4	250.9	253.5	255.0	256.1	256.7	257.0	257.2	257.3	257.3	257.3
1920-------	1959	252.6	257.7	261.2	263.4	265.2	266.3	266.9	267.2	267.4	267.5	267.5	267.5
1921-------	1960	260.9	265.7	269.1	271.6	273.2	274.1	274.7	275.0	275.1	275.1	275.2	275.2
1922-------	1961	263.7	268.4	271.6	274.1	275.6	276.6	277.1	277.4	277.5	277.6	277.6	277.6
1923-------	1962	271.0	275.5	278.8	281.2	282.7	283.5	283.9	284.2	284.3	284.4	284.4	284.4
1924-------	1963	285.0	289.4	292.7	295.0	296.4	297.2	297.7	297.9	298.0	298.0	298.0	298.0
1925-------	1964	301.7	306.1	309.2	311.3	312.5	313.2	313.7	313.9	314.0	314.1	314.1	
1926-------	1965	317.2	321.3	324.4	326.1	327.3	328.2	328.6	328.9	329.0	329.0		
1927-------	1966	328.2	332.2	334.6	336.2	337.4	338.1	338.6	338.8	338.9			
1928-------	1967	333.7	337.1	339.3	341.0	342.1	342.7	343.1	343.3				
1929-------	1968	344.3	347.3	349.5	351.2	352.1	352.7	353.0					
1930-------	1969	348.2	351.4	353.8	355.1	356.0	356.5						
1931-------	1970	353.1	356.1	358.0	359.2	360.0							
1932-------	1971	351.0	353.8	355.6	356.8								
1933-------	1972	352.4	354.8	356.5									
1934-------	1973	352.9	355.2										
1935-------	1974	349.8											

TABLE 6C. CUMULATIVE BIRTH RATES FOR ALL OTHER WOMEN AS OF THE BEGINNING OF EACH YEAR 1917-74 BY AGE AND LIVE-BIRTH ORDER FOR EACH COHORT FROM 1867 TO 1959--CON.

LIVE-BIRTH ORDER AND COHORT	DIAGONAL LINE FOR JANUARY 1	EXACT AGE											
		15	16	17	18	19	20	21	22	23	24	25	26
SIXTH BIRTHS													
1891-------													39.7
1892-------												24.0	35.5
1893-------											15.6	24.0	35.1
1894-------										6.8	12.0	20.2	31.2
1895-------									2.5	5.1	10.4	18.3	29.7
1896-------								0.6	1.8	4.4	9.2	17.3	29.7
1897-------							*	0.5	1.7	4.1	8.9	17.9	29.8
1898-------						*	*	0.4	1.5	3.9	9.5	18.4	30.4
1899-------					*	*	*	0.4	1.5	4.3	9.9	18.8	31.9
1900-------				*	*	*	*	0.4	1.7	4.5	10.4	20.2	33.1
1901-------			*	*	*	*	*	0.4	1.6	4.4	10.5	19.8	33.2
1902-------	1917	*	*	*	*	*	*	0.5	1.9	5.2	11.2	20.6	32.0
1903-------	1918	*	*	*	*	*	*	0.5	2.1	5.3	11.2	19.1	29.6
1904-------	1919	*	*	*	*	*	*	0.6	2.4	5.6	10.9	18.9	29.4
1905-------	1920	*	*	*	*	*	*	0.8	2.7	5.7	11.1	18.7	28.7
1906-------	1921	*	*	*	*	*	*	0.9	2.7	5.9	10.6	18.1	27.9
1907-------	1922	*	*	*	*	*	*	0.8	2.6	5.2	9.8	16.9	25.6
1908-------	1923	*	*	*	*	*	*	0.8	2.3	4.8	9.3	15.6	24.4
1909-------	1924	*	*	*	*	*	*	0.7	2.1	4.7	8.7	15.0	24.1
1910-------	1925	*	*	*	*	*	*	0.7	2.2	4.6	8.7	15.1	24.0
1911-------	1926	*	*	*	*	*	*	0.7	2.0	4.4	8.7	15.5	24.6
1912-------	1927	*	*	*	*	*	*	0.6	2.0	4.4	8.8	15.5	24.9
1913-------	1928	*	*	*	*	*	*	0.6	1.9	4.5	8.8	15.7	25.0
1914-------	1929	*	*	*	*	*	*	0.5	1.9	4.4	9.0	16.1	25.6
1915-------	1930	*	*	*	*	*	*	0.6	2.0	4.7	9.4	16.6	26.6
1916-------	1931	*	*	*	*	*	*	0.6	2.1	4.9	9.7	17.6	27.9
1917-------	1932	*	*	*	*	*	*	0.7	2.2	5.0	10.5	18.8	29.7
1918-------	1933	*	*	*	*	*	*	0.7	2.2	5.5	11.5	20.1	31.4
1919-------	1934	*	*	*	*	*	*	0.7	2.5	6.1	12.1	21.2	32.9
1920-------	1935	*	*	*	*	*	*	0.9	2.8	6.2	12.8	22.1	33.7
1921-------	1936	*	*	*	*	*	*	0.9	2.8	6.5	13.1	22.1	33.9
1922-------	1937	*	*	*	*	*	*	0.8	2.9	6.7	12.8	21.8	33.4
1923-------	1938	*	*	*	*	*	*	0.9	3.0	6.8	13.1	22.4	34.1
1924-------	1939	*	*	*	*	*	*	0.9	3.0	6.8	13.3	22.8	35.6
1925-------	1940	*	*	*	*	*	*	1.0	3.1	7.0	13.6	23.9	37.1
1926-------	1941	*	*	*	*	*	*	1.0	3.3	7.4	14.7	25.4	39.9
1927-------	1942	*	*	*	*	*	*	1.1	3.4	7.9	15.3	26.8	42.5
1928-------	1943	*	*	*	*	*	*	1.1	3.5	8.0	16.1	28.8	46.2
1929-------	1944	*	*	*	*	*	*	1.1	3.6	8.6	18.0	32.1	51.1
1930-------	1945	*	*	*	*	*	*	1.2	3.9	9.8	20.0	35.8	56.3
1931-------	1946	*	*	*	*	*	*	1.2	4.5	11.1	23.0	40.1	63.0
1932-------	1947	*	*	*	*	*	*	1.4	5.0	12.6	24.9	43.6	66.1
1933-------	1948	*	*	*	*	*	*	1.4	5.6	13.5	26.7	45.6	68.5
1934-------	1949	*	*	*	*	*	*	1.9	6.2	14.2	28.3	47.9	71.5
1935-------	1950	*	*	*	*	*	*	1.9	6.2	15.3	29.7	50.0	74.5
1936-------	1951	*	*	*	*	*	*	1.9	6.8	15.9	31.2	51.7	76.4
1937-------	1952	*	*	*	*	*	*	2.2	6.9	16.3	31.5	52.3	76.9
1938-------	1953	*	*	*	*	*	*	2.1	7.1	16.5	31.6	52.1	74.6
1939-------	1954	*	*	*	*	*	*	2.1	7.3	16.9	31.6	50.3	71.6
1940-------	1955	*	*	*	*	*	*	2.2	7.4	16.8	30.6	48.5	66.8
1941-------	1956	*	*	*	*	*	*	2.2	7.3	16.1	29.2	44.1	59.0
1942-------	1957	*	*	*	*	*	*	2.3	7.1	15.2	25.8	38.3	50.9
1943-------	1958	*	*	*	*	*	*	2.0	6.3	12.9	22.0	32.1	41.8
1944-------	1959	*	*	*	*	*	*	2.0	5.8	11.6	19.1	26.9	35.3
1945-------	1960	*	*	*	*	*	*	1.7	4.9	9.4	15.1	21.8	29.4
1946-------	1961	*	*	*	*	*	*	1.3	3.7	7.2	12.1	18.1	24.3
1947-------	1962	*	*	*	*	*	*	1.1	2.9	5.9	10.1	14.9	19.5
1948-------	1963	*	*	*	*	*	*	0.7	2.3	4.8	8.1	11.5	15.0
1949-------	1964	*	*	*	*	*	*	0.7	2.1	4.1	6.4	9.0	
1950-------	1965	*	*	*	*	*	*	0.6	1.7	3.1	4.9		
1951-------	1966	*	*	*	*	*	*	0.5	1.3	2.4			
1952-------	1967	*	*	*	*	*	*	0.3	0.9				
1953-------	1968	*	*	*	*	*	*	0.3					
1954-------	1969	*	*	*	*	*	*						
1955-------	1970	*	*	*	*	*							
1956-------	1971	*	*	*	*								
1957-------	1972	*	*	*									
1958-------	1973	*	*										
1959-------	1974	*											

TABLE 6C. CUMULATIVE BIRTH RATES FOR ALL OTHER WOMEN AS OF THE BEGINNING OF EACH YEAR 1917-74 BY AGE AND LIVE-BIRTH ORDER FOR EACH COHORT FROM 1867 TO 1959--CON.

LIVE-BIRTH ORDER AND COHORT	DIAGONAL LINE FOR JANUARY 1	EXACT AGE											
		27	28	29	30	31	32	33	34	35	36	37	38
SIXTH BIRTHS--CON.													
1879-------													293.2
1880-------												275.5	285.9
1881-------											258.0	271.0	283.3
1882-------										239.8	254.4	269.5	281.2
1883-------									218.9	234.1	250.2	264.2	275.4
1884-------								195.2	209.9	225.7	240.3	253.4	264.0
1885-------							172.6	186.8	201.2	215.3	228.9	241.2	250.5
1886-------						148.1	164.6	178.4	191.2	204.4	217.7	228.5	237.5
1887-------					124.9	140.8	157.1	169.5	181.5	195.1	207.0	217.5	225.8
1888-------				107.3	125.3	140.9	155.7	167.5	180.8	193.1	204.9	214.7	223.1
1889-------			82.4	98.4	115.9	130.6	144.9	158.1	170.5	183.0	194.5	204.5	213.3
1890-------	1917	59.0	74.8	90.1	107.3	122.1	138.2	150.5	163.3	176.0	187.5	198.2	206.1
1891-------	1918	53.3	68.5	84.2	101.9	118.3	133.3	146.1	159.6	172.4	184.4	193.5	200.7
1892-------	1919	48.5	64.0	80.6	99.9	115.3	130.9	144.3	157.6	169.9	180.0	188.4	195.1
1893-------	1920	48.3	64.7	82.6	100.8	116.4	132.7	145.8	158.4	169.1	178.5	186.5	193.7
1894-------	1921	45.1	62.6	79.4	97.5	114.2	129.8	142.4	154.1	164.1	173.3	181.1	187.6
1895-------	1922	44.5	61.0	77.4	97.1	113.2	127.9	140.0	150.6	160.5	169.4	177.1	184.3
1896-------	1923	43.7	59.8	78.2	96.5	112.3	126.3	137.2	147.5	156.9	165.3	173.2	179.1
1897-------	1924	43.4	61.4	78.2	96.5	111.0	124.4	134.5	144.9	154.0	162.7	169.4	175.2
1898-------	1925	45.9	62.6	80.4	97.8	111.9	124.7	135.5	145.4	155.0	162.9	169.8	175.3
1899-------	1926	47.0	64.9	82.1	98.9	112.6	126.2	137.0	148.1	157.4	166.0	172.8	178.4
1900-------	1927	49.0	66.1	81.8	98.6	113.1	126.6	138.1	148.8	158.5	166.5	173.1	178.7
1901-------	1928	47.3	62.4	77.3	93.7	107.7	120.9	131.6	142.1	150.7	158.0	164.3	169.9
1902-------	1929	44.7	59.1	73.6	89.0	102.2	114.4	124.4	133.5	141.4	148.3	154.3	159.6
1903-------	1930	41.8	55.2	69.4	84.6	96.9	108.4	117.4	125.9	133.2	139.8	145.5	150.6
1904-------	1931	41.2	54.8	69.0	83.7	95.9	106.9	115.7	124.0	131.3	137.8	143.3	148.4
1905-------	1932	40.7	54.1	67.7	82.1	94.0	104.5	113.4	121.8	128.9	135.2	140.8	145.6
1906-------	1933	38.9	52.0	65.7	79.4	90.8	101.4	110.3	118.6	125.6	131.9	137.2	142.1
1907-------	1934	36.4	49.7	62.4	75.6	87.2	97.8	106.6	114.8	121.9	128.3	133.8	138.8
1908-------	1935	35.5	47.5	60.0	73.4	84.5	94.9	103.6	111.9	119.3	126.1	131.7	136.9
1909-------	1936	34.7	46.9	59.9	73.3	84.5	94.9	103.8	112.3	120.2	127.2	133.3	138.4
1910-------	1937	34.9	47.5	60.8	74.2	85.4	96.0	105.1	114.1	122.3	129.5	135.6	141.0
1911-------	1938	35.7	49.0	62.5	76.1	87.5	98.0	107.7	117.1	125.2	132.4	138.7	144.2
1912-------	1939	36.2	49.6	63.4	77.2	88.9	100.2	110.3	119.4	127.5	134.9	141.2	147.0
1913-------	1940	36.4	50.2	64.2	77.5	89.8	101.5	111.2	120.4	128.6	135.8	142.3	148.1
1914-------	1941	37.4	51.4	65.0	78.8	91.7	103.3	113.1	122.6	130.7	138.2	144.6	150.8
1915-------	1942	38.5	52.0	65.9	80.4	93.0	104.2	114.0	123.5	132.0	139.4	146.4	152.6
1916-------	1943	40.3	54.1	68.8	83.2	95.3	106.6	116.9	126.6	134.9	142.9	150.0	156.5
1917-------	1944	42.3	56.8	71.0	84.8	96.9	108.8	119.1	128.9	138.0	146.4	153.9	160.8
1918-------	1945	44.6	59.0	73.2	87.2	99.9	111.8	122.4	133.0	142.8	151.9	160.0	167.1
1919-------	1946	46.2	60.9	75.4	90.3	103.9	116.8	128.8	140.5	150.9	160.6	169.1	176.8
1920-------	1947	47.3	61.9	77.2	92.6	106.9	120.9	133.3	145.1	156.4	166.5	175.3	183.3
1921-------	1948	47.4	62.6	78.2	94.5	109.6	123.8	136.5	149.5	161.1	171.5	180.8	188.3
1922-------	1949	46.9	62.2	78.4	95.3	110.5	125.2	139.2	152.1	163.8	174.5	183.1	191.1
1923-------	1950	48.3	64.3	81.5	98.6	115.1	130.7	144.8	158.5	170.7	180.9	190.0	197.6
1924-------	1951	50.5	68.1	86.1	105.1	122.6	139.4	154.8	169.2	181.1	192.3	201.1	208.5
1925-------	1952	53.6	72.3	92.1	112.4	131.4	149.7	165.9	180.2	193.0	203.6	212.4	219.8
1926-------	1953	57.7	78.2	100.2	122.4	143.0	161.8	178.0	193.0	205.1	215.7	224.4	231.2
1927-------	1954	62.0	84.5	107.4	130.8	151.7	170.7	186.9	200.8	213.2	223.7	231.7	238.3
1928-------	1955	67.3	90.9	114.8	138.6	159.5	178.2	193.5	207.6	219.4	228.6	236.4	242.8
1929-------	1956	73.6	98.5	123.7	147.6	168.6	186.8	202.7	216.7	227.6	237.1	244.6	250.3
1930-------	1957	80.6	106.5	131.7	155.6	176.3	194.6	210.2	222.8	234.0	242.6	249.1	254.3
1931-------	1958	87.8	113.8	139.1	162.6	183.3	201.4	215.8	229.1	238.7	246.2	252.3	257.3
1932-------	1959	91.0	116.6	141.2	164.9	184.8	201.7	216.1	227.3	235.8	242.9	248.6	252.6
1933-------	1960	93.5	119.3	145.1	167.3	186.3	202.9	215.6	225.7	233.8	240.3	245.2	249.4
1934-------	1961	97.3	124.6	148.9	170.5	189.1	204.4	216.2	225.6	233.1	239.3	244.3	248.5
1935-------	1962	101.5	127.6	151.1	172.7	189.8	203.5	214.0	222.6	229.8	235.8	240.9	244.6
1936-------	1963	102.9	127.9	151.3	170.5	185.7	197.7	206.9	215.1	222.0	227.9	232.2	235.4
1937-------	1964	101.7	125.6	145.6	161.9	175.0	185.2	193.8	201.5	208.3	213.1	216.9	
1938-------	1965	97.7	118.2	134.9	148.8	159.8	169.4	177.9	185.3	190.6	194.8		
1939-------	1966	91.8	108.5	122.7	134.9	144.9	154.6	162.7	168.8	173.6			
1940-------	1967	83.2	97.8	110.3	121.3	131.5	140.2	146.9	152.1				
1941-------	1968	72.7	84.9	95.9	106.4	115.3	122.4	128.0					
1942-------	1969	61.9	72.7	82.8	92.0	99.2	104.9						
1943-------	1970	51.5	61.2	69.9	77.1	82.7							
1944-------	1971	44.2	52.5	59.6	65.3								
1945-------	1972	36.7	43.4	48.9									
1946-------	1973	30.1	35.3										
1947-------	1974	23.9											

TABLE 6C. CUMULATIVE BIRTH RATES FOR ALL OTHER WOMEN AS OF THE BEGINNING OF EACH YEAR 1917-74 BY AGE AND LIVE-BIRTH ORDER FOR EACH COHORT FROM 1867 TO 1959--CON.

LIVE-BIRTH ORDER AND COHORT	DIAGONAL LINE FOR JANUARY 1	EXACT AGE											
		39	40	41	42	43	44	45	46	47	48	49	50
SIXTH BIRTHS--CON.													
1867-------													438.8
1868-------												430.5	430.9
1869-------											421.9	422.4	423.6
1870-------										412.8	413.4	414.8	415.1
1871-------									403.3	404.3	406.1	406.5	406.9
1872-------								393.1	394.3	397.4	397.9	398.4	398.6
1873-------							382.2	383.8	387.0	387.9	388.5	388.8	389.1
1874-------						370.8	372.5	375.8	376.9	378.0	378.3	378.6	378.9
1875-------					358.1	360.3	362.3	363.7	365.0	365.6	366.0	366.4	366.7
1876-------				343.9	347.4	350.0	351.5	353.1	353.9	354.5	355.0	355.4	355.6
1877-------			328.4	333.4	337.6	339.5	341.0	342.3	343.1	344.0	344.5	344.8	345.0
1878-------	1917	311.0	318.6	324.5	327.7	329.7	331.3	332.5	333.6	334.5	334.8	335.1	335.2
1879-------	1918	301.9	310.9	316.0	319.3	321.5	323.0	324.4	325.5	326.2	326.7	327.0	327.2
1880-------	1919	296.2	304.4	309.6	313.3	315.3	316.7	318.1	319.0	320.0	320.6	320.9	321.2
1881-------	1920	293.2	301.5	306.9	310.4	312.3	313.8	314.9	316.0	316.8	317.2	317.6	317.8
1882-------	1921	290.9	299.2	304.2	307.3	309.2	310.7	312.0	312.9	313.6	314.1	314.3	314.5
1883-------	1922	284.8	292.3	297.0	300.1	302.1	303.7	304.6	305.5	306.4	306.7	307.0	307.1
1884-------	1923	272.3	279.4	283.9	287.2	289.1	290.3	291.4	292.4	293.1	293.5	293.8	293.9
1885-------	1924	258.5	265.1	269.6	272.5	274.0	275.1	276.2	277.0	277.6	278.0	278.2	278.4
1886-------	1925	244.8	251.5	255.4	257.9	259.2	260.2	261.2	261.8	262.6	262.8	263.1	263.4
1887-------	1926	233.3	239.0	242.6	244.7	246.0	247.0	247.7	248.6	249.1	249.4	249.7	249.9
1888-------	1927	230.0	235.5	238.6	240.6	241.8	242.7	243.7	244.3	244.9	245.1	245.3	245.5
1889-------	1928	219.8	224.9	227.9	230.0	231.3	232.2	232.9	233.5	233.9	234.1	234.4	234.6
1890-------	1929	212.0	216.8	219.8	222.1	223.4	224.2	224.9	225.4	225.7	226.0	226.2	226.4
1891-------	1930	206.2	211.3	214.5	216.8	217.9	218.7	219.3	219.7	220.1	220.3	220.5	220.6
1892-------	1931	201.1	206.0	209.5	211.5	212.6	213.4	213.9	214.3	214.6	214.8	215.0	215.1
1893-------	1932	199.4	204.7	207.6	209.6	210.7	211.5	212.0	212.3	212.6	212.8	212.9	213.0
1894-------	1933	193.8	198.2	201.1	203.0	204.1	204.8	205.3	205.6	205.9	206.0	206.1	206.1
1895-------	1934	189.2	193.5	196.2	197.9	198.9	199.6	200.1	200.4	200.6	200.8	200.9	200.9
1896-------	1935	184.0	187.8	190.2	191.8	192.7	193.4	193.9	194.1	194.4	194.5	194.6	194.7
1897-------	1936	179.6	183.2	185.7	187.2	188.2	188.9	189.3	189.8	190.0	190.1	190.2	190.3
1898-------	1937	179.7	183.3	185.7	187.3	188.3	189.0	189.6	190.0	190.3	190.5	190.6	190.7
1899-------	1938	182.9	186.8	189.1	190.7	191.7	192.4	193.0	193.4	193.7	193.9	194.0	194.0
1900-------	1939	183.6	187.4	189.7	191.3	192.2	193.0	193.6	194.0	194.3	194.4	194.5	194.6
1901-------	1940	174.4	177.9	180.2	181.5	182.5	183.3	183.8	184.2	184.4	184.5	184.6	184.6
1902-------	1941	163.8	167.3	169.5	171.0	172.0	172.7	173.2	173.5	173.7	173.8	173.9	173.9
1903-------	1942	154.8	158.3	160.6	162.1	163.2	164.0	164.5	164.8	165.0	165.1	165.2	165.2
1904-------	1943	152.6	156.2	158.6	160.4	161.5	162.3	162.7	163.0	163.2	163.3	163.3	163.4
1905-------	1944	150.0	153.7	156.3	158.0	159.1	159.7	160.2	160.5	160.7	160.7	160.8	160.9
1906-------	1945	146.6	150.3	152.8	154.4	155.3	156.0	156.5	156.8	156.9	157.0	157.1	157.1
1907-------	1946	143.3	146.7	149.2	150.7	151.8	152.6	153.0	153.2	153.4	153.5	153.6	153.6
1908-------	1947	141.0	144.5	146.8	148.4	149.5	150.1	150.6	150.8	150.9	151.0	151.0	151.1
1909-------	1948	142.8	146.3	148.8	150.6	151.7	152.6	153.1	153.4	153.6	153.7	153.8	153.9
1910-------	1949	145.5	149.2	151.9	153.8	155.1	156.0	156.5	156.8	157.0	157.1	157.2	157.2
1911-------	1950	149.0	153.0	155.8	157.8	159.2	160.1	160.7	161.0	161.1	161.2	161.3	161.3
1912-------	1951	151.9	155.9	158.7	160.9	162.2	163.2	163.9	164.2	164.4	164.5	164.5	164.6
1913-------	1952	153.1	157.0	160.1	162.3	163.8	164.9	165.4	165.7	165.9	166.0	166.1	166.1
1914-------	1953	155.9	160.2	163.4	165.6	167.2	168.3	168.9	169.3	169.4	169.5	169.6	169.6
1915-------	1954	157.8	162.4	165.8	168.2	169.9	170.9	171.5	171.8	172.0	172.1	172.1	172.1
1916-------	1955	162.1	166.9	170.4	172.7	174.2	175.2	175.9	176.2	176.4	176.5	176.5	176.5
1917-------	1956	166.9	171.8	175.1	177.3	178.7	179.8	180.4	180.7	180.9	181.0	181.0	181.0
1918-------	1957	173.3	178.0	181.0	183.2	184.8	185.8	186.4	186.7	186.9	187.0	187.0	187.0
1919-------	1958	183.2	187.9	191.4	193.8	195.5	196.5	197.0	197.4	197.6	197.6	197.6	197.6
1920-------	1959	189.5	194.9	198.5	201.2	202.8	203.8	204.6	205.0	205.1	205.1	205.1	205.1
1921-------	1960	195.1	200.2	204.1	206.4	207.9	209.0	209.6	209.9	210.0	210.1	210.1	210.1
1922-------	1961	197.5	202.7	206.0	208.4	210.0	211.1	211.7	212.0	212.1	212.1	212.1	212.1
1923-------	1962	203.8	208.4	211.7	213.9	215.5	216.5	217.0	217.2	217.3	217.4	217.4	217.4
1924-------	1963	214.4	219.1	222.3	224.7	226.2	227.1	227.6	227.8	228.0	228.0	228.0	228.0
1925-------	1964	225.6	230.0	233.1	235.3	236.6	237.4	237.9	238.2	238.3	238.3	238.3	
1926-------	1965	236.7	240.9	243.9	246.0	247.2	248.0	248.5	248.7	248.8	248.8		
1927-------	1966	243.5	247.6	250.5	252.3	253.5	254.2	254.6	254.8	254.9			
1928-------	1967	247.5	251.2	253.6	255.3	256.4	257.1	257.4	257.5				
1929-------	1968	254.7	258.1	260.4	262.0	263.0	263.5	263.8					
1930-------	1969	258.6	261.5	263.8	265.3	266.2	266.8						
1931-------	1970	260.7	263.7	265.8	267.1	267.9							
1932-------	1971	256.2	258.9	260.7	261.9								
1933-------	1972	252.8	255.1	256.6									
1934-------	1973	251.6	253.6										
1935-------	1974	247.1											

TABLE 6C. CUMULATIVE BIRTH RATES FOR ALL OTHER WOMEN AS OF THE BEGINNING OF EACH YEAR 1917-74 BY AGE AND LIVE-BIRTH ORDER FOR EACH COHORT FROM 1867 TO 1959--CON.

LIVE-BIRTH ORDER AND COHORT	DIAGONAL LINE FOR JANUARY 1	EXACT AGE											
		15	16	17	18	19	20	21	22	23	24	25	26
SEVENTH BIRTHS													
1891-------													16.1
1892-------												9.0	14.1
1893-------											5.0	8.5	12.9
1894-------										2.2	4.2	7.1	12.2
1895-------									0.8	1.8	3.4	6.8	11.4
1896-------								0.2	0.6	1.4	3.3	6.2	11.9
1897-------							*	0.2	0.5	1.5	3.0	6.4	11.5
1898-------						*	*	0.1	0.5	1.3	2.9	6.3	11.7
1899-------					*	*	*	0.2	0.5	1.3	3.1	6.7	12.5
1900-------				*	*	*	*	0.1	0.5	1.4	3.5	7.3	13.6
1901-------			*	*	*	*	*	0.1	0.5	1.5	3.6	7.6	13.4
1902-------	1917	*	*	*	*	*	*	0.1	0.5	1.6	3.9	7.8	13.1
1903-------	1918	*	*	*	*	*	*	0.2	0.7	1.8	4.0	7.4	12.3
1904-------	1919	*	*	*	*	*	*	0.2	0.8	2.0	4.1	7.5	11.9
1905-------	1920	*	*	*	*	*	*	0.3	0.8	1.9	3.9	6.8	11.2
1906-------	1921	*	*	*	*	*	*	0.3	0.9	2.1	3.7	6.7	10.9
1907-------	1922	*	*	*	*	*	*	0.3	0.9	1.8	3.5	6.2	10.1
1908-------	1923	*	*	*	*	*	*	0.3	0.8	1.7	3.2	5.7	9.2
1909-------	1924	*	*	*	*	*	*	0.3	0.7	1.5	2.9	5.2	8.9
1910-------	1925	*	*	*	*	*	*	0.2	0.6	1.3	2.7	5.2	9.1
1911-------	1926	*	*	*	*	*	*	0.2	0.5	1.2	2.6	5.2	9.2
1912-------	1927	*	*	*	*	*	*	0.1	0.4	1.2	2.7	5.2	9.3
1913-------	1928	*	*	*	*	*	*	0.1	0.5	1.3	2.8	5.5	9.4
1914-------	1929	*	*	*	*	*	*	0.2	0.6	1.4	3.1	5.8	9.8
1915-------	1930	*	*	*	*	*	*	0.2	0.6	1.5	3.2	5.9	10.3
1916-------	1931	*	*	*	*	*	*	0.2	0.7	1.6	3.3	6.5	10.9
1917-------	1932	*	*	*	*	*	*	0.2	0.7	1.6	3.8	6.9	11.8
1918-------	1933	*	*	*	*	*	*	0.2	0.7	1.9	4.0	7.3	12.6
1919-------	1934	*	*	*	*	*	*	0.2	0.8	1.9	3.9	7.6	12.8
1920-------	1935	*	*	*	*	*	*	0.2	0.8	1.8	4.2	7.7	13.2
1921-------	1936	*	*	*	*	*	*	0.2	0.7	1.9	4.1	7.8	13.2
1922-------	1937	*	*	*	*	*	*	0.2	0.8	1.9	4.1	7.7	13.2
1923-------	1938	*	*	*	*	*	*	0.2	0.8	2.0	4.3	8.0	13.7
1924-------	1939	*	*	*	*	*	*	0.2	0.9	2.1	4.5	8.5	14.2
1925-------	1940	*	*	*	*	*	*	0.3	0.9	2.1	4.6	8.6	14.6
1926-------	1941	*	*	*	*	*	*	0.3	1.0	2.4	4.9	9.2	15.4
1927-------	1942	*	*	*	*	*	*	0.3	1.1	2.5	5.1	9.1	16.2
1928-------	1943	*	*	*	*	*	*	0.3	1.0	2.4	5.0	9.8	17.4
1929-------	1944	*	*	*	*	*	*	0.3	1.1	2.5	5.5	11.0	19.7
1930-------	1945	*	*	*	*	*	*	0.4	1.2	2.8	6.2	12.5	22.2
1931-------	1946	*	*	*	*	*	*	0.4	1.3	3.2	7.4	14.4	25.5
1932-------	1947	*	*	*	*	*	*	0.4	1.2	3.4	7.8	15.8	27.2
1933-------	1948	*	*	*	*	*	*	0.3	1.4	3.8	8.8	16.8	28.2
1934-------	1949	*	*	*	*	*	*	0.5	1.6	4.3	9.2	17.4	29.9
1935-------	1950	*	*	*	*	*	*	0.5	1.6	4.2	9.1	18.1	30.9
1936-------	1951	*	*	*	*	*	*	0.4	1.6	4.2	9.8	19.0	31.9
1937-------	1952	*	*	*	*	*	*	0.4	1.5	4.4	10.0	19.4	32.1
1938-------	1953	*	*	*	*	*	*	0.4	1.7	4.7	10.4	19.2	31.5
1939-------	1954	*	*	*	*	*	*	0.5	1.9	4.9	10.4	19.1	30.7
1940-------	1955	*	*	*	*	*	*	0.6	1.9	4.7	10.0	18.0	27.8
1941-------	1956	*	*	*	*	*	*	0.5	1.8	4.6	9.6	16.6	24.4
1942-------	1957	*	*	*	*	*	*	0.4	1.7	4.2	8.4	13.8	20.1
1943-------	1958	*	*	*	*	*	*	0.5	1.6	3.7	6.8	11.2	15.9
1944-------	1959	*	*	*	*	*	*	0.4	1.4	3.0	5.8	9.1	13.0
1945-------	1960	*	*	*	*	*	*	0.3	0.9	2.4	4.4	7.1	10.7
1946-------	1961	*	*	*	*	*	*	0.2	0.8	1.9	3.5	5.8	8.3
1947-------	1962	*	*	*	*	*	*	0.3	0.9	1.7	3.1	4.8	6.7
1948-------	1963	*	*	*	*	*	*	0.2	0.7	1.4	2.4	3.5	4.9
1949-------	1964	*	*	*	*	*	*	0.2	0.6	1.1	1.7	2.6	
1950-------	1965	*	*	*	*	*	*	0.2	0.5	0.8	1.3		
1951-------	1966	*	*	*	*	*	*	0.1	0.3	0.6			
1952-------	1967	*	*	*	*	*	*	0.1	0.2				
1953-------	1968	*	*	*	*	*	*	0.1					
1954-------	1969	*	*	*	*	*	*						
1955-------	1970	*	*	*	*	*							
1956-------	1971	*	*	*	*								
1957-------	1972	*	*	*									
1958-------	1973	*	*										
1959-------	1974	*											

TABLE 6C. CUMULATIVE BIRTH RATES FOR ALL OTHER WOMEN AS OF THE BEGINNING OF EACH YEAR 1917-74 BY AGE AND LIVE-BIRTH ORDER FOR EACH COHORT FROM 1867 TO 1959--CON.

LIVE-BIRTH ORDER AND COHORT	DIAGONAL LINE FOR JANUARY 1	EXACT AGE											
		27	28	29	30	31	32	33	34	35	36	37	38
SEVENTH BIRTHS--CON.													
1879-------													225.2
1880-------												207.3	220.0
1881-------											190.0	204.7	216.8
1882-------										172.3	187.4	201.2	214.2
1883-------									152.3	167.2	181.3	195.7	207.4
1884-------								130.0	143.8	157.6	171.8	184.6	195.2
1885-------							109.5	122.6	135.4	148.8	161.3	172.7	183.4
1886-------						88.5	103.0	115.2	127.2	139.1	150.8	162.3	172.4
1887-------					70.1	82.9	96.5	108.0	118.9	130.8	142.4	153.4	163.5
1888-------				55.7	68.8	80.7	93.8	104.4	116.2	127.9	139.3	150.4	160.6
1889-------			39.8	49.9	61.9	73.9	86.0	97.5	108.9	120.6	132.1	143.5	153.4
1890-------	1917	26.3	35.4	44.4	57.2	68.5	81.8	93.0	104.7	116.6	128.6	139.6	148.6
1891-------	1918	23.1	31.2	41.6	53.6	66.6	79.5	91.0	102.9	115.2	127.2	137.6	145.5
1892-------	1919	20.3	29.6	39.4	53.8	66.0	79.3	91.1	103.4	115.7	126.5	135.4	142.8
1893-------	1920	20.0	28.8	41.3	54.4	66.8	80.3	92.2	104.6	116.0	125.6	134.0	141.1
1894-------	1921	18.9	30.0	40.8	54.1	67.0	80.3	92.4	104.2	113.9	123.0	131.1	138.3
1895-------	1922	19.9	29.5	40.5	54.6	67.5	81.2	93.2	103.2	112.8	121.8	129.8	137.2
1896-------	1923	19.3	29.1	41.1	55.0	68.5	81.6	91.4	101.0	110.5	119.4	127.8	134.5
1897-------	1924	19.0	29.7	41.2	55.0	67.7	79.3	88.6	98.4	107.9	116.8	124.3	131.1
1898-------	1925	20.0	30.3	41.7	55.5	67.1	78.0	87.9	98.1	107.7	116.5	124.2	130.9
1899-------	1926	20.6	30.6	42.5	55.3	66.3	77.9	88.5	99.1	109.1	118.2	126.0	132.6
1900-------	1927	21.7	32.0	42.7	54.8	66.2	78.3	89.0	99.9	109.8	118.5	125.9	132.4
1901-------	1928	20.9	30.0	39.6	51.3	62.7	74.1	84.4	94.7	103.5	111.6	118.9	125.4
1902-------	1929	19.8	28.0	37.8	49.3	60.0	70.6	80.1	88.9	96.9	104.6	111.4	117.5
1903-------	1930	18.4	26.6	35.9	47.1	57.1	67.6	75.9	84.0	92.1	99.3	105.7	111.3
1904-------	1931	18.2	26.2	35.5	46.3	56.6	66.2	74.4	82.8	90.7	97.6	103.6	109.5
1905-------	1932	17.2	25.0	34.0	44.9	54.4	63.4	71.6	80.4	88.0	94.7	100.9	106.3
1906-------	1933	16.5	23.9	32.7	42.6	51.6	60.8	69.5	77.8	85.3	92.1	97.9	103.5
1907-------	1934	15.2	22.3	30.5	39.8	49.2	58.7	67.0	75.6	83.3	90.1	96.1	101.9
1908-------	1935	14.4	21.3	29.1	38.8	48.2	57.2	65.8	74.4	81.9	89.0	95.3	100.7
1909-------	1936	14.2	21.1	29.7	39.9	49.1	58.5	67.2	75.8	83.5	90.9	97.2	102.9
1910-------	1937	14.3	21.6	30.3	40.4	50.0	59.4	68.0	76.8	84.8	92.2	98.8	104.5
1911-------	1938	14.9	22.3	31.3	41.8	51.5	61.2	70.0	79.1	87.5	95.0	101.6	107.3
1912-------	1939	14.7	22.1	31.5	42.1	51.9	61.9	71.1	80.3	88.4	95.7	102.1	107.9
1913-------	1940	14.9	22.7	32.3	42.4	52.6	63.0	72.5	81.5	89.6	97.0	103.5	109.6
1914-------	1941	15.6	23.6	32.5	43.0	53.5	63.9	73.3	82.5	90.8	98.3	105.1	111.1
1915-------	1942	16.2	24.0	33.3	44.2	54.5	64.8	74.3	83.5	91.8	99.4	106.3	112.3
1916-------	1943	17.3	25.5	35.1	46.0	56.4	66.9	76.5	85.7	94.1	101.9	108.7	115.2
1917-------	1944	18.5	26.9	36.6	47.4	58.0	68.5	78.0	87.4	96.1	104.0	111.3	118.0
1918-------	1945	19.5	28.4	38.3	49.4	60.1	70.8	80.7	90.8	99.8	108.0	115.4	122.6
1919-------	1946	20.0	28.9	39.0	50.5	61.9	73.1	84.2	94.7	104.1	112.8	120.8	128.6
1920-------	1947	20.3	29.4	39.9	51.9	63.5	75.5	86.3	97.0	107.1	116.0	124.9	132.7
1921-------	1948	20.3	29.7	40.6	52.7	65.1	77.0	88.2	99.6	109.6	119.8	128.6	136.1
1922-------	1949	20.6	30.0	40.9	53.4	65.4	77.8	90.0	101.2	112.2	122.3	130.5	138.1
1923-------	1950	21.2	30.8	42.4	55.4	68.2	81.4	93.5	105.7	117.0	126.6	135.2	142.6
1924-------	1951	22.1	32.4	44.6	58.6	72.7	86.5	99.7	112.8	123.9	134.4	143.0	150.5
1925-------	1952	22.7	34.0	47.5	62.6	77.4	92.7	106.9	119.9	132.0	142.0	150.7	157.8
1926-------	1953	24.6	37.0	51.9	67.9	84.4	100.6	114.9	129.1	140.8	151.2	159.2	166.0
1927-------	1954	26.5	40.1	55.4	73.4	90.9	107.5	122.7	136.2	148.2	157.8	165.8	172.5
1928-------	1955	28.5	42.7	59.6	77.7	95.5	112.5	127.1	140.7	151.4	160.4	168.0	174.0
1929-------	1956	31.8	47.7	65.0	84.1	102.2	119.1	134.1	146.8	157.2	166.4	173.3	178.8
1930-------	1957	35.7	51.6	70.0	89.2	107.2	123.4	137.4	149.4	160.2	168.3	174.7	179.8
1931-------	1958	39.8	57.0	75.8	95.1	112.8	128.7	142.3	154.6	163.9	171.2	176.9	181.3
1932-------	1959	41.8	59.3	77.7	96.4	113.4	128.7	141.9	152.8	161.1	167.5	172.5	176.7
1933-------	1960	43.5	61.0	79.9	98.0	114.3	129.2	141.1	150.3	157.7	163.5	168.4	172.4
1934-------	1961	45.6	63.4	81.7	99.9	115.7	129.4	139.3	147.9	154.5	160.3	165.0	169.1
1935-------	1962	46.8	64.7	83.2	100.3	114.8	125.8	135.3	142.7	149.0	154.3	159.0	162.3
1936-------	1963	47.8	65.8	82.7	98.3	110.1	120.2	128.0	134.9	140.8	146.1	149.8	152.5
1937-------	1964	47.6	64.2	79.5	92.3	102.8	111.2	118.5	125.0	130.6	134.7	137.9	
1938-------	1965	45.9	60.1	72.5	83.0	91.4	99.2	105.9	111.9	116.1	119.7		
1939-------	1966	43.0	54.7	65.2	73.9	81.4	88.5	94.8	99.5	103.4			
1940-------	1967	37.9	47.5	55.9	63.3	70.1	76.7	81.4	85.4				
1941-------	1968	32.6	40.2	46.8	53.6	59.9	64.7	68.7					
1942-------	1969	26.4	32.4	38.5	44.5	49.1	53.0						
1943-------	1970	20.9	26.6	32.0	36.4	40.1							
1944-------	1971	17.6	22.1	25.9	29.2								
1945-------	1972	14.3	17.6	20.5									
1946-------	1973	10.9	13.3										
1947-------	1974	8.7											

TABLE 6C. CUMULATIVE BIRTH RATES FOR ALL OTHER WOMEN AS OF THE BEGINNING OF EACH YEAR 1917-74 BY AGE AND LIVE-BIRTH ORDER FOR EACH COHORT FROM 1867 TO 1959--CON.

LIVE-BIRTH ORDER AND COHORT	DIAGONAL LINE FOR JANUARY 1	EXACT AGE											
		39	40	41	42	43	44	45	46	47	48	49	50
SEVENTH BIRTHS--CON.													
1867-------													373.6
1868-------												365.2	365.7
1869-------											356.5	357.1	358.0
1870-------										347.3	348.2	349.1	349.6
1871-------									337.6	339.0	340.5	341.1	341.6
1872-------								327.3	329.0	331.4	332.3	332.9	333.2
1873-------							316.4	318.1	320.8	322.2	323.1	323.4	323.8
1874-------						304.9	306.4	308.8	310.5	311.9	312.4	312.8	313.2
1875-------					292.0	294.0	295.8	297.5	299.2	300.0	300.7	301.2	301.5
1876-------				277.2	280.7	283.0	284.6	286.3	287.4	288.5	289.3	289.7	289.8
1877-------			260.9	266.2	270.3	272.5	274.0	275.4	276.7	277.9	278.5	278.7	279.0
1878-------	1917	243.2	251.9	257.6	261.5	263.5	265.3	266.8	268.3	269.4	269.8	270.3	270.4
1879-------	1918	235.7	244.5	250.3	253.9	256.3	257.9	259.5	260.8	261.9	262.6	262.9	263.0
1880-------	1919	230.0	239.3	244.7	249.2	251.4	253.0	254.5	255.8	256.9	257.2	257.5	257.8
1881-------	1920	227.7	236.3	242.3	246.3	248.5	250.1	251.8	253.1	253.9	254.4	254.8	255.0
1882-------	1921	224.2	232.9	238.6	242.6	244.8	246.6	247.9	248.9	249.9	250.4	250.6	250.8
1883-------	1922	216.6	225.2	230.7	234.6	236.7	238.4	239.7	240.8	241.5	242.0	242.3	242.5
1884-------	1923	204.6	212.8	218.2	221.3	223.3	224.8	226.0	226.8	227.5	227.8	228.1	228.2
1885-------	1924	192.3	200.3	204.7	208.1	209.9	211.3	212.2	213.1	213.8	214.1	214.4	214.6
1886-------	1925	181.2	188.2	192.9	196.0	197.5	198.6	199.7	200.6	201.3	201.6	201.9	202.0
1887-------	1926	172.1	179.2	183.3	185.7	187.2	188.6	189.7	190.5	191.2	191.5	191.7	191.9
1888-------	1927	168.7	175.0	178.1	180.5	182.2	183.4	184.4	185.2	185.7	186.0	186.3	186.4
1889-------	1928	160.7	165.9	169.4	172.2	173.8	174.9	175.8	176.4	176.9	177.2	177.4	177.6
1890-------	1929	155.0	160.3	164.2	166.7	168.2	169.4	170.2	170.8	171.3	171.6	171.9	172.1
1891-------	1930	151.8	157.5	161.0	163.5	165.1	166.2	167.0	167.6	168.1	168.4	168.7	168.8
1892-------	1931	149.2	154.5	158.1	160.5	161.9	163.0	163.7	164.3	164.8	165.1	165.3	165.4
1893-------	1932	147.2	152.6	155.9	158.2	159.5	160.5	161.2	161.7	162.1	162.3	162.5	162.6
1894-------	1933	144.6	149.6	153.0	155.2	156.5	157.5	158.2	158.6	159.0	159.2	159.3	159.4
1895-------	1934	142.9	148.1	151.1	153.3	154.6	155.5	156.1	156.6	156.9	157.1	157.2	157.3
1896-------	1935	140.5	145.1	148.0	150.0	151.2	151.9	152.6	152.9	153.2	153.4	153.5	153.6
1897-------	1936	136.6	141.0	143.6	145.4	146.4	147.3	147.8	148.2	148.5	148.7	148.8	148.9
1898-------	1937	136.0	140.0	142.8	144.4	145.6	146.4	147.0	147.4	147.7	147.9	148.0	148.1
1899-------	1938	137.9	142.4	145.0	146.8	148.0	148.8	149.4	149.8	150.1	150.3	150.4	150.5
1900-------	1939	138.1	142.4	145.1	146.9	148.0	148.9	149.5	149.9	150.2	150.3	150.4	150.5
1901-------	1940	130.7	134.7	137.3	139.0	140.1	140.9	141.5	141.8	142.0	142.1	142.2	142.2
1902-------	1941	122.4	126.4	128.9	130.8	131.9	132.8	133.3	133.6	133.8	133.9	134.0	134.0
1903-------	1942	116.3	120.0	122.6	124.4	125.7	126.5	127.0	127.3	127.5	127.6	127.7	127.7
1904-------	1943	114.0	117.9	120.5	122.4	123.7	124.6	125.1	125.4	125.6	125.7	125.8	125.8
1905-------	1944	110.9	114.9	117.6	119.6	120.8	121.6	122.1	122.4	122.6	122.7	122.7	122.8
1906-------	1945	108.3	112.2	115.0	116.9	118.0	118.9	119.4	119.7	119.9	119.9	120.0	120.0
1907-------	1946	106.6	110.4	112.9	114.6	115.7	116.6	117.1	117.5	117.6	117.7	117.8	117.8
1908-------	1947	105.2	108.8	111.3	113.1	114.3	115.1	115.6	115.9	116.0	116.1	116.1	116.1
1909-------	1948	107.6	111.4	114.1	116.0	117.3	118.1	118.7	119.0	119.2	119.2	119.3	119.3
1910-------	1949	109.2	113.3	116.1	118.2	119.5	120.5	121.0	121.4	121.5	121.6	121.6	121.7
1911-------	1950	112.3	116.4	119.4	121.4	122.8	123.8	124.4	124.7	124.9	125.0	125.1	125.1
1912-------	1951	112.9	117.0	119.7	121.9	123.4	124.4	125.0	125.3	125.4	125.5	125.6	125.6
1913-------	1952	114.6	118.5	121.5	123.7	125.1	126.2	126.7	127.0	127.2	127.3	127.3	127.3
1914-------	1953	116.0	120.4	123.5	125.6	127.2	128.2	128.7	129.1	129.3	129.4	129.4	129.4
1915-------	1954	117.7	122.1	125.2	127.7	129.1	130.1	130.7	131.1	131.3	131.4	131.4	131.4
1916-------	1955	120.8	125.5	128.9	131.3	132.7	133.8	134.5	134.8	135.0	135.1	135.1	135.1
1917-------	1956	124.1	129.2	132.6	135.1	136.8	137.9	138.6	138.9	139.2	139.2	139.2	139.2
1918-------	1957	128.8	133.8	137.3	139.8	141.5	142.6	143.3	143.7	143.8	143.9	144.0	144.0
1919-------	1958	134.8	140.0	143.6	146.2	147.9	149.1	149.6	149.9	150.0	150.1	150.1	150.1
1920-------	1959	139.1	144.3	148.0	150.6	152.3	153.3	153.9	154.2	154.3	154.3	154.3	154.3
1921-------	1960	142.5	147.4	150.9	153.3	155.0	156.1	156.7	156.9	157.0	157.1	157.1	157.1
1922-------	1961	144.3	149.2	152.5	155.0	156.6	157.6	158.1	158.3	158.5	158.6	158.6	158.6
1923-------	1962	148.6	153.3	156.7	159.1	160.6	161.4	161.9	162.2	162.3	162.4	162.5	162.5
1924-------	1963	156.3	160.7	164.0	166.2	167.6	168.5	169.1	169.4	169.5	169.5	169.5	169.5
1925-------	1964	163.4	167.9	171.1	173.2	174.6	175.5	176.0	176.3	176.4	176.4	176.4	
1926-------	1965	171.7	176.0	178.8	180.8	182.1	182.9	183.3	183.5	183.6	183.6		
1927-------	1966	177.8	181.5	184.3	186.2	187.3	188.0	188.4	188.7	188.8			
1928-------	1967	178.5	182.1	184.7	186.3	187.3	187.9	188.3	188.4				
1929-------	1968	183.3	186.7	189.0	190.5	191.5	192.2	192.5					
1930-------	1969	183.8	186.8	188.9	190.4	191.3	191.7						
1931-------	1970	184.9	187.7	189.7	191.0	191.7							
1932-------	1971	180.2	182.9	184.5	185.5								
1933-------	1972	175.8	177.9	179.4									
1934-------	1973	171.7	173.6										
1935-------	1974	164.7											

TABLE 6C. CUMULATIVE BIRTH RATES FOR ALL OTHER WOMEN AS OF THE BEGINNING OF EACH YEAR 1917-74 BY AGE AND LIVE-BIRTH ORDER FOR EACH COHORT FROM 1867 TO 1959--CON.

LIVE-BIRTH ORDER AND COHORT	DIAGONAL LINE FOR JANUARY 1	EXACT AGE											
		15	16	17	18	19	20	21	22	23	24	25	26
EIGHTH AND HIGHER BIRTHS													
1891-------													10.3
1892-------												5.4	8.9
1893-------											1.6	3.8	7.0
1894-------										0.7	1.8	4.1	7.5
1895-------									0.2	0.7	2.0	4.2	7.4
1896-------								0.1	0.3	0.9	2.0	4.0	8.1
1897-------							*	0.1	0.3	0.8	1.7	4.3	7.9
1898-------						*	*	0.1	0.3	0.7	1.9	4.3	8.2
1899-------					*	*	*	0.1	0.2	0.8	2.0	4.5	8.5
1900-------				*	*	*	*	0.0	0.2	0.8	2.0	4.6	9.4
1901-------			*	*	*	*	*	0.1	0.3	0.8	2.0	4.8	9.4
1902-------	1917	*	*	*	*	*	*	0.1	0.3	0.9	2.4	5.4	9.9
1903-------	1918	*	*	*	*	*	*	0.1	0.3	0.9	2.7	5.5	9.4
1904-------	1919	*	*	*	*	*	*	0.1	0.3	1.2	2.8	5.5	8.8
1905-------	1920	*	*	*	*	*	*	0.1	0.4	1.1	2.7	4.8	7.9
1906-------	1921	*	*	*	*	*	*	0.1	0.4	1.2	2.4	4.6	7.5
1907-------	1922	*	*	*	*	*	*	0.1	0.4	1.0	2.3	4.1	6.8
1908-------	1923	*	*	*	*	*	*	0.1	0.3	0.9	1.9	3.6	6.1
1909-------	1924	*	*	*	*	*	*	0.1	0.3	0.8	1.8	3.3	5.9
1910-------	1925	*	*	*	*	*	*	0.0	0.2	0.7	1.5	3.1	5.7
1911-------	1926	*	*	*	*	*	*	0.1	0.3	0.8	1.7	3.5	6.1
1912-------	1927	*	*	*	*	*	*	0.1	0.3	0.8	1.7	3.4	5.9
1913-------	1928	*	*	*	*	*	*	0.1	0.3	0.8	1.7	3.4	5.9
1914-------	1929	*	*	*	*	*	*	0.1	0.3	0.8	1.7	3.3	5.9
1915-------	1930	*	*	*	*	*	*	0.1	0.3	0.8	1.7	3.4	6.4
1916-------	1931	*	*	*	*	*	*	0.1	0.3	0.8	1.8	3.8	6.8
1917-------	1932	*	*	*	*	*	*	0.1	0.3	0.8	2.0	4.1	7.3
1918-------	1933	*	*	*	*	*	*	0.1	0.3	0.9	2.1	4.1	7.5
1919-------	1934	*	*	*	*	*	*	0.1	0.4	1.1	2.3	4.4	7.7
1920-------	1935	*	*	*	*	*	*	0.1	0.4	0.9	2.2	4.2	7.5
1921-------	1936	*	*	*	*	*	*	0.1	0.3	0.9	2.1	4.1	7.6
1922-------	1937	*	*	*	*	*	*	0.0	0.2	0.7	1.9	4.1	7.8
1923-------	1938	*	*	*	*	*	*	0.0	0.2	0.8	2.0	4.2	7.8
1924-------	1939	*	*	*	*	*	*	0.0	0.2	0.8	2.1	4.5	8.4
1925-------	1940	*	*	*	*	*	*	0.0	0.3	1.0	2.3	4.7	8.5
1926-------	1941	*	*	*	*	*	*	0.2	0.6	1.4	2.7	5.0	8.7
1927-------	1942	*	*	*	*	*	*	0.2	0.6	1.2	2.6	4.7	8.6
1928-------	1943	*	*	*	*	*	*	0.2	0.6	1.3	2.5	4.9	9.5
1929-------	1944	*	*	*	*	*	*	0.2	0.6	1.3	2.6	5.3	10.3
1930-------	1945	*	*	*	*	*	*	0.2	0.6	1.3	2.8	5.8	11.5
1931-------	1946	*	*	*	*	*	*	0.2	0.6	1.3	3.1	6.6	12.9
1932-------	1947	*	*	*	*	*	*	0.2	0.6	1.4	3.3	7.0	13.9
1933-------	1948	*	*	*	*	*	*	0.2	0.6	1.6	3.7	7.9	15.6
1934-------	1949	*	*	*	*	*	*	0.2	0.7	1.6	4.0	8.5	16.4
1935-------	1950	*	*	*	*	*	*	0.2	0.6	1.8	4.1	8.8	16.7
1936-------	1951	*	*	*	*	*	*	0.2	0.7	1.8	4.3	8.9	17.2
1937-------	1952	*	*	*	*	*	*	0.2	0.6	1.8	4.2	8.9	17.4
1938-------	1953	*	*	*	*	*	*	0.2	0.7	1.8	4.2	9.0	17.4
1939-------	1954	*	*	*	*	*	*	0.2	0.8	1.9	4.2	9.0	16.6
1940-------	1955	*	*	*	*	*	*	0.3	0.8	1.7	4.0	8.5	14.3
1941-------	1956	*	*	*	*	*	*	0.2	0.6	1.6	4.1	7.5	12.3
1942-------	1957	*	*	*	*	*	*	0.2	0.6	1.7	3.3	5.9	9.6
1943-------	1958	*	*	*	*	*	*	0.2	0.7	1.4	2.7	4.7	7.7
1944-------	1959	*	*	*	*	*	*	0.2	0.6	1.2	2.2	3.9	6.2
1945-------	1960	*	*	*	*	*	*	0.1	0.4	0.9	1.7	3.1	5.2
1946-------	1961	*	*	*	*	*	*	0.1	0.4	0.7	1.4	2.5	4.0
1947-------	1962	*	*	*	*	*	*	0.1	0.2	0.6	1.2	2.0	3.0
1948-------	1963	*	*	*	*	*	*	0.1	0.4	0.7	1.2	1.8	2.4
1949-------	1964	*	*	*	*	*	*	0.2	0.4	0.6	0.9	1.3	
1950-------	1965	*	*	*	*	*	*	0.1	0.3	0.5	0.7		
1951-------	1966	*	*	*	*	*	*	0.1	0.2	0.3			
1952-------	1967	*	*	*	*	*	*	0.1	0.2				
1953-------	1968	*	*	*	*	*	*	0.1					
1954-------	1969	*	*	*	*	*	*						
1955-------	1970	*	*	*	*	*							
1956-------	1971	*	*	*	*								
1957-------	1972	*	*	*									
1958-------	1973	*	*										
1959-------	1974	*											

TABLE 6C. CUMULATIVE BIRTH RATES FOR ALL OTHER WOMEN AS OF THE BEGINNING OF EACH YEAR 1917-74 BY AGE AND LIVE-BIRTH ORDER FOR EACH COHORT FROM 1867 TO 1959--CON.

LIVE-BIRTH ORDER AND COHORT	DIAGONAL LINE FOR JANUARY 1	EXACT AGE											
		27	28	29	30	31	32	33	34	35	36	37	38
EIGHTH AND HIGHER BIRTHS--CON.													
1879-------													493.7
1880-------												406.7	456.2
1881-------											326.3	375.5	423.3
1882-------										255.1	301.6	348.6	402.0
1883-------									206.4	246.2	289.5	340.8	394.9
1884-------								159.8	189.2	225.2	271.2	321.9	373.1
1885-------							123.5	146.6	172.3	209.7	254.3	301.6	347.6
1886-------						90.8	112.7	132.9	158.9	194.8	237.7	280.2	323.7
1887-------					65.2	82.5	101.8	122.3	147.0	183.0	222.0	262.6	305.6
1888-------				43.8	59.6	74.8	94.7	114.4	141.3	174.6	212.4	253.1	297.7
1889-------			28.8	38.7	52.6	68.8	88.2	110.0	135.6	168.5	207.3	251.6	294.8
1890-------	1917	17.7	25.2	33.8	49.0	64.9	86.5	107.3	133.0	167.5	209.0	250.5	292.9
1891-------	1918	15.5	22.0	31.8	46.6	64.9	85.6	106.5	134.2	171.6	211.1	252.0	289.5
1892-------	1919	13.4	20.8	30.3	47.8	64.9	85.7	108.2	138.8	174.6	212.7	248.4	282.7
1893-------	1920	12.2	19.4	31.3	47.4	64.9	87.1	112.9	142.3	176.3	209.7	243.0	277.7
1894-------	1921	12.5	21.5	32.0	48.7	67.1	91.6	116.0	144.6	174.7	206.2	239.5	272.7
1895-------	1922	13.6	21.5	32.8	50.2	70.1	93.8	117.2	142.6	170.9	202.6	233.7	267.6
1896-------	1923	13.6	22.0	33.5	52.5	72.7	95.1	116.8	140.8	169.5	199.0	230.2	261.7
1897-------	1924	13.7	22.3	35.3	54.5	73.2	94.6	114.8	138.9	165.9	195.3	224.5	256.9
1898-------	1925	14.3	24.6	38.0	56.0	74.1	94.3	114.9	138.9	166.2	194.5	225.2	255.0
1899-------	1926	15.3	25.6	38.1	55.6	72.8	93.6	115.0	140.1	167.6	198.9	228.4	257.9
1900-------	1927	16.3	26.0	38.1	54.7	72.2	93.2	114.8	139.7	169.1	198.3	227.2	258.5
1901-------	1928	15.8	24.9	36.0	51.8	69.0	88.8	108.8	134.3	160.0	187.0	215.7	245.3
1902-------	1929	15.8	23.7	33.9	48.8	64.2	81.5	101.2	122.7	146.2	172.2	198.8	227.0
1903-------	1930	14.3	21.4	31.0	44.7	58.3	76.1	93.2	113.4	136.3	160.8	185.9	213.0
1904-------	1931	13.4	20.3	29.6	42.3	56.9	73.5	90.7	111.4	133.4	157.4	182.3	209.1
1905-------	1932	12.3	18.7	27.2	40.7	54.4	70.6	87.6	107.5	129.2	153.2	177.5	203.0
1906-------	1933	11.7	17.7	26.8	39.4	52.7	68.6	85.2	105.1	127.3	151.0	174.4	200.6
1907-------	1934	10.6	17.0	25.4	37.1	50.0	65.6	82.2	103.0	125.3	148.6	172.7	198.5
1908-------	1935	10.0	15.8	23.5	35.4	48.2	63.7	81.2	102.4	124.8	148.9	172.8	199.2
1909-------	1936	9.8	15.4	23.7	35.5	48.5	65.0	83.0	104.2	127.6	151.9	177.9	203.6
1910-------	1937	9.5	15.6	23.8	35.8	49.7	66.5	84.7	107.0	130.9	157.4	182.9	208.9
1911-------	1938	10.1	16.1	24.8	37.8	52.0	68.7	87.8	110.8	136.1	161.8	187.5	213.9
1912-------	1939	9.8	16.0	25.5	38.7	52.8	70.4	90.1	113.1	137.1	162.7	187.7	213.8
1913-------	1940	10.0	16.9	26.6	39.2	54.0	72.1	91.9	114.4	138.3	163.6	188.8	214.8
1914-------	1941	10.5	17.5	26.8	40.1	55.4	73.5	93.1	115.8	139.8	164.8	190.4	217.8
1915-------	1942	11.0	18.0	27.8	41.5	57.1	75.4	95.2	118.2	142.1	167.9	194.3	220.9
1916-------	1943	11.5	18.9	29.0	43.0	58.8	77.3	97.2	119.9	144.4	170.7	196.5	222.4
1917-------	1944	12.3	19.9	30.1	44.3	59.8	78.4	98.9	122.5	147.0	172.7	198.1	225.2
1918-------	1945	12.6	20.0	30.5	44.4	60.6	80.2	101.4	125.6	150.8	177.3	204.1	231.4
1919-------	1946	12.5	20.2	30.6	45.5	62.8	83.2	105.2	130.6	157.6	185.8	214.0	243.8
1920-------	1947	12.7	20.8	32.2	47.6	65.3	86.1	109.2	135.7	163.9	192.9	222.5	251.7
1921-------	1948	13.1	21.5	33.1	48.6	66.6	88.1	111.8	139.3	167.8	197.9	227.2	255.4
1922-------	1949	13.4	21.8	33.2	48.8	66.7	87.9	112.1	139.9	168.8	198.5	226.8	255.4
1923-------	1950	13.6	22.0	34.0	50.1	68.4	91.3	117.1	146.0	176.2	205.7	235.5	264.4
1924-------	1951	14.1	22.9	35.4	52.0	72.6	97.6	124.8	155.5	186.6	218.8	249.3	279.0
1925-------	1952	14.4	23.8	36.9	55.8	78.0	104.5	133.6	165.4	199.1	231.6	263.5	292.5
1926-------	1953	15.0	25.2	40.1	60.2	84.5	113.1	144.2	178.4	212.4	246.4	277.3	306.0
1927-------	1954	15.6	26.7	42.4	64.8	91.0	121.4	154.3	188.7	223.7	257.1	287.0	315.3
1928-------	1955	17.0	29.1	47.0	70.8	98.0	129.7	163.0	198.5	232.9	264.5	294.3	320.1
1929-------	1956	18.7	32.5	51.7	76.9	105.8	138.6	173.6	209.6	243.3	275.5	302.7	325.3
1930-------	1957	20.9	35.8	56.1	82.2	111.7	145.5	180.2	214.7	247.7	276.3	300.0	319.8
1931-------	1958	23.6	40.1	61.5	87.9	118.8	152.0	185.4	219.1	248.8	274.2	294.6	311.7
1932-------	1959	25.5	42.3	63.3	90.9	120.6	152.5	184.3	214.2	239.7	261.1	278.7	294.1
1933-------	1960	27.6	44.5	67.4	94.7	124.2	155.7	184.4	209.9	231.8	250.2	266.4	280.9
1934-------	1961	28.6	46.7	69.7	97.0	126.2	153.9	178.4	200.6	219.2	236.2	251.6	264.3
1935-------	1962	29.7	47.9	70.5	97.3	122.7	146.3	167.1	185.9	202.8	218.1	231.2	241.8
1936-------	1963	30.1	48.0	69.8	93.0	114.3	134.2	152.0	168.4	183.2	196.9	207.4	216.0
1937-------	1964	30.1	46.7	65.7	84.4	102.3	119.0	134.1	148.2	161.8	172.2	180.6	
1938-------	1965	29.0	43.1	57.9	73.2	87.2	100.6	113.7	126.3	136.0	143.6		
1939-------	1966	26.3	37.6	49.5	61.5	72.9	84.9	96.4	105.7	113.2			
1940-------	1967	22.0	30.6	39.9	49.7	59.5	69.5	77.7	84.9				
1941-------	1968	18.3	25.4	33.0	41.1	49.5	56.6	62.8					
1942-------	1969	14.4	19.9	26.0	32.7	38.4	43.9						
1943-------	1970	11.2	15.8	20.8	25.4	29.8							
1944-------	1971	9.4	13.0	16.4	20.0								
1945-------	1972	7.6	10.1	12.5									
1946-------	1973	5.6	7.2										
1947-------	1974	4.1											

TABLE 6C. CUMULATIVE BIRTH RATES FOR ALL OTHER WOMEN AS OF THE BEGINNING OF EACH YEAR 1917-74 BY AGE AND LIVE-BIRTH ORDER FOR EACH COHORT FROM 1867 TO 1959--CON.

LIVE-BIRTH ORDER AND COHORT	DIAGONAL LINE FOR JANUARY 1	EXACT AGE											
		39	40	41	42	43	44	45	46	47	48	49	50
EIGHTH AND HIGHER BIRTHS--CON.													
1867-------													1,240.6
1868-------												1,193.8	1,197.0
1869-------											1,144.5	1,150.0	1,155.8
1870-------										1,092.5	1,100.8	1,110.9	1,114.0
1871-------									1,037.9	1,050.3	1,065.6	1,070.9	1,074.5
1872-------								980.4	995.0	1,017.9	1,025.9	1,032.2	1,034.9
1873-------							916.1	933.1	956.6	968.6	978.2	982.9	985.3
1874-------						850.3	869.5	892.6	906.4	920.9	928.1	932.2	934.7
1875-------					785.7	807.4	828.0	843.7	859.5	870.5	876.9	881.3	883.5
1876-------				723.3	753.1	776.4	793.7	810.5	823.5	833.2	840.0	843.9	845.7
1877-------			658.1	692.6	725.0	744.8	762.0	777.4	788.9	799.4	805.5	808.7	810.4
1878-------	1917	581.9	628.7	664.6	692.8	712.8	730.9	744.8	757.1	766.8	771.8	774.9	776.9
1879-------	1918	540.3	587.4	622.2	651.2	672.5	689.2	703.7	715.3	724.4	729.7	732.9	735.2
1880-------	1919	501.2	550.7	586.9	618.1	637.9	654.9	669.1	680.3	689.9	694.4	697.9	699.8
1881-------	1920	474.1	525.6	563.3	592.3	612.4	629.3	643.7	655.4	663.6	668.5	671.8	673.8
1882-------	1921	454.4	506.1	541.1	570.1	589.9	607.4	621.9	632.7	640.9	646.1	649.4	651.3
1883-------	1922	445.4	492.8	526.9	554.7	575.4	592.9	606.5	616.4	624.3	629.0	631.8	633.5
1884-------	1923	418.9	464.3	497.0	525.4	545.7	560.8	572.8	582.0	589.8	593.8	596.6	598.4
1885-------	1924	391.0	434.8	468.9	496.2	513.2	526.5	537.2	546.2	552.8	556.8	559.4	561.4
1886-------	1925	366.2	410.6	441.9	466.4	481.3	493.6	504.0	512.2	519.2	522.4	525.3	527.0
1887-------	1926	350.2	392.1	422.2	443.3	457.6	469.3	479.2	487.9	493.6	497.0	499.6	501.2
1888-------	1927	339.8	379.8	405.4	425.7	439.6	450.9	461.6	468.8	474.2	477.3	479.7	481.0
1889-------	1928	336.1	371.5	397.3	418.0	431.4	443.7	453.0	460.0	465.4	468.5	470.7	472.1
1890-------	1929	329.1	363.2	389.0	408.4	422.7	433.9	443.6	450.5	455.6	458.5	460.8	462.0
1891-------	1930	324.1	358.9	383.2	403.8	417.5	429.8	438.8	445.4	450.4	453.2	455.2	456.4
1892-------	1931	317.6	350.3	375.8	395.2	409.4	420.9	429.4	436.0	440.7	443.2	445.2	446.1
1893-------	1932	310.7	344.8	368.7	388.2	401.6	412.5	420.8	426.9	431.1	433.5	435.1	435.9
1894-------	1933	306.8	338.4	362.1	381.1	393.7	404.3	412.2	417.7	422.0	424.1	425.3	426.1
1895-------	1934	299.6	331.6	354.4	371.9	384.5	394.5	401.6	407.2	410.8	412.7	413.9	414.6
1896-------	1935	293.9	323.5	344.4	362.0	374.0	383.0	390.3	395.2	398.4	400.3	401.3	402.1
1897-------	1936	286.2	313.0	334.0	351.0	361.8	371.1	377.7	382.8	385.9	387.4	388.6	389.3
1898-------	1937	282.8	310.6	332.3	348.2	360.0	369.2	376.7	382.1	384.9	386.9	388.0	388.5
1899-------	1938	287.9	316.7	336.8	353.5	365.1	374.9	382.1	386.6	389.6	391.2	392.2	392.8
1900-------	1939	288.6	316.0	336.7	353.7	365.4	375.5	382.3	387.1	389.8	391.4	392.3	392.7
1901-------	1940	273.2	299.4	319.5	334.5	346.2	355.8	362.6	366.7	369.4	370.7	371.5	372.0
1902-------	1941	253.9	279.8	298.9	314.6	326.3	336.0	342.2	346.2	348.4	349.5	350.3	350.7
1903-------	1942	239.1	263.7	283.3	298.6	310.0	319.0	324.7	327.9	329.7	330.8	331.5	331.9
1904-------	1943	234.8	260.0	279.0	294.3	305.6	314.0	319.3	322.5	324.4	325.5	326.2	326.6
1905-------	1944	229.3	253.9	272.8	287.8	298.4	306.2	311.4	314.5	316.3	317.3	317.9	318.2
1906-------	1945	226.5	251.4	269.4	283.7	293.7	301.7	306.5	309.4	311.1	312.0	312.6	312.9
1907-------	1946	224.1	246.7	264.4	277.6	287.5	294.8	299.3	302.0	303.6	304.4	304.9	305.2
1908-------	1947	222.9	245.3	261.7	275.0	284.1	291.4	295.7	298.5	300.0	300.7	301.1	301.4
1909-------	1948	228.2	250.4	267.8	281.2	291.3	298.8	303.8	306.7	308.1	308.9	309.5	309.7
1910-------	1949	233.4	256.5	274.0	288.6	298.6	306.5	311.6	314.4	315.9	316.9	317.4	317.7
1911-------	1950	239.3	262.4	281.0	295.0	305.3	313.3	318.2	321.1	322.9	323.6	324.1	324.4
1912-------	1951	238.6	262.3	280.0	294.3	304.7	312.6	317.8	320.9	322.5	323.3	323.8	324.1
1913-------	1952	240.4	263.4	281.3	295.2	305.4	313.8	319.1	322.2	323.7	324.5	325.0	325.2
1914-------	1953	243.3	266.4	284.5	298.3	309.2	317.7	323.0	325.7	327.2	327.9	328.3	328.5
1915-------	1954	245.5	268.9	286.4	300.9	311.8	319.8	324.5	327.1	328.4	329.1	329.5	329.6
1916-------	1955	248.4	271.1	289.5	304.1	314.6	321.9	326.5	329.0	330.4	331.1	331.5	331.6
1917-------	1956	250.6	274.5	292.9	307.3	317.4	324.7	329.3	331.9	333.2	334.0	334.3	334.5
1918-------	1957	258.3	282.2	300.8	315.1	325.5	333.1	337.7	340.3	341.7	342.3	342.6	342.7
1919-------	1958	271.2	295.7	315.2	330.1	341.1	349.0	354.0	356.7	358.1	358.8	359.0	359.2
1920-------	1959	278.6	303.5	322.8	337.9	348.6	356.6	361.6	364.2	365.5	366.1	366.4	366.5
1921-------	1960	282.7	307.0	326.3	340.8	351.4	359.0	363.3	365.6	366.7	367.2	367.4	367.5
1922-------	1961	282.1	305.8	323.9	337.4	347.5	354.1	358.2	360.4	361.4	361.8	362.0	362.1
1923-------	1962	291.0	313.8	330.8	344.3	353.2	359.6	363.3	365.0	365.9	366.3	366.5	366.6
1924-------	1963	304.9	327.2	345.4	358.0	366.8	372.7	375.9	377.5	378.4	378.8	379.0	379.0
1925-------	1964	318.7	341.8	358.4	370.5	378.7	383.8	386.7	388.4	389.3	389.7	389.8	
1926-------	1965	332.4	353.9	369.2	380.2	387.3	392.1	395.0	396.6	397.3	397.6		
1927-------	1966	339.3	358.3	371.9	381.4	387.9	392.4	395.1	396.3	396.9			
1928-------	1967	340.7	357.2	368.9	377.3	383.4	387.8	389.7	390.8				
1929-------	1968	343.7	358.3	368.9	376.7	382.6	385.7	387.5					
1930-------	1969	335.7	348.6	358.4	365.9	370.2	373.0						
1931-------	1970	326.1	338.0	347.1	353.2	357.1							
1932-------	1971	307.6	318.7	326.3	331.3								
1933-------	1972	292.9	302.0	308.1									
1934-------	1973	274.3	281.6										
1935-------	1974	250.5											

TABLE 7A. DISTRIBUTIONS OF ALL WOMEN BY PARITY AS OF THE BEGINNING OF EACH YEAR 1917-74 BY AGE FOR GROUPS OF COHORTS FROM 1867-71 TO 1955-59

(BASED ON CUMULATIVE BIRTH RATES FOR GROUPS OF COHORTS)

EXACT AGE AND COHORT	AS OF JANUARY 1	TOTAL	PARITY							
			0	1	2	3	4	5	6	7 AND HIGHER
15-19 YEARS										
1898-1902	1917	1,000.0	944.3	47.0	7.7	0.9	0.1	*	*	*
1899-1903	1918	1,000.0	942.8	48.7	7.5	0.9	0.1	*	*	*
1900-1904	1919	1,000.0	942.9	48.8	7.3	0.9	0.1	*	*	*
1901-1905	1920	1,000.0	946.9	45.2	7.0	0.8	0.1	*	*	*
1902-1906	1921	1,000.0	941.8	50.2	7.0	0.9	0.1	*	*	*
1903-1907	1922	1,000.0	936.8	54.5	7.7	0.9	0.1	*	*	*
1904-1908	1923	1,000.0	938.7	52.1	8.2	0.9	0.1	*	*	*
1905-1909	1924	1,000.0	940.3	50.2	8.4	1.0	0.1	*	*	*
1906-1910	1925	1,000.0	939.0	51.7	8.1	1.1	0.1	*	*	*
1907-1911	1926	1,000.0	938.5	52.3	8.1	1.0	0.1	*	*	*
1908-1912	1927	1,000.0	938.8	51.8	8.3	1.0	0.1	*	*	*
1909-1913	1928	1,000.0	939.2	51.3	8.4	1.0	0.1	*	*	*
1910-1914	1929	1,000.0	940.6	50.2	8.1	1.0	0.1	*	*	*
1911-1915	1930	1,000.0	942.2	48.9	7.8	1.0	0.1	*	*	*
1912-1916	1931	1,000.0	942.1	49.2	7.7	0.9	0.1	*	*	*
1913-1917	1932	1,000.0	944.0	47.6	7.4	0.9	0.1	*	*	*
1914-1918	1933	1,000.0	946.0	45.9	7.2	0.8	0.1	*	*	*
1915-1919	1934	1,000.0	949.1	43.3	6.7	0.8	0.1	*	*	*
1916-1920	1935	1,000.0	949.2	43.5	6.4	0.8	0.1	*	*	*
1917-1921	1936	1,000.0	948.4	44.4	6.3	0.8	0.1	*	*	*
1918-1922	1937	1,000.0	948.4	44.1	6.6	0.8	0.1	*	*	*
1919-1923	1938	1,000.0	946.7	45.3	7.1	0.8	0.1	*	*	*
1920-1924	1939	1,000.0	944.9	46.7	7.4	0.9	0.1	*	*	*
1921-1925	1940	1,000.0	945.5	45.9	7.5	1.0	0.1	*	*	*
1922-1926	1941	1,000.0	946.8	44.0	7.8	1.2	0.2	*	*	*
1923-1927	1942	1,000.0	945.5	44.9	8.1	1.3	0.2	*	*	*
1924-1928	1943	1,000.0	942.5	47.4	8.6	1.3	0.2	*	*	*
1925-1929	1944	1,000.0	941.4	47.9	9.0	1.5	0.2	*	*	*
1926-1930	1945	1,000.0	944.6	45.0	8.7	1.5	0.2	*	*	*
1927-1931	1946	1,000.0	947.6	42.7	8.2	1.3	0.2	*	*	*
1928-1932	1947	1,000.0	945.7	44.4	8.4	1.3	0.2	*	*	*
1929-1933	1948	1,000.0	933.6	55.4	9.4	1.4	0.2	*	*	*
1930-1934	1949	1,000.0	926.6	60.2	11.3	1.7	0.2	*	*	*
1931-1935	1950	1,000.0	923.6	60.7	13.3	2.1	0.3	*	*	*
1932-1936	1951	1,000.0	922.8	60.3	14.2	2.4	0.3	*	*	*
1933-1937	1952	1,000.0	919.4	62.9	14.8	2.5	0.4	*	*	*
1934-1938	1953	1,000.0	918.7	63.4	14.8	2.7	0.4	*	*	*
1935-1939	1954	1,000.0	917.5	64.3	15.0	2.8	0.4	*	*	*
1936-1940	1955	1,000.0	915.8	65.8	15.2	2.7	0.5	*	*	*
1937-1941	1956	1,000.0	915.5	65.6	15.7	2.7	0.5	*	*	*
1938-1942	1957	1,000.0	913.3	66.9	16.4	2.9	0.5	*	*	*
1939-1943	1958	1,000.0	910.9	68.6	16.9	3.1	0.5	*	*	*
1940-1944	1959	1,000.0	912.0	67.1	17.2	3.2	0.5	*	*	*
1941-1945	1960	1,000.0	914.2	65.1	16.9	3.3	0.5	*	*	*
1942-1946	1961	1,000.0	917.2	62.7	16.4	3.2	0.5	*	*	*
1943-1947	1962	1,000.0	919.3	61.3	15.8	3.1	0.5	*	*	*
1944-1948	1963	1,000.0	921.7	59.3	15.5	3.0	0.5	*	*	*
1945-1949	1964	1,000.0	924.1	57.8	14.7	2.9	0.5	*	*	*
1946-1950	1965	1,000.0	926.6	56.6	13.7	2.6	0.5	*	*	*
1947-1951	1966	1,000.0	929.0	55.8	12.4	2.4	0.4	*	*	*
1948-1952	1967	1,000.0	929.8	56.4	11.4	2.1	0.3	*	*	*
1949-1953	1968	1,000.0	930.8	55.9	11.2	1.8	0.3	*	*	*
1950-1954	1969	1,000.0	930.5	57.0	10.6	1.7	0.2	*	*	*
1951-1955	1970	1,000.0	929.6	58.4	10.2	1.6	0.2	*	*	*
1952-1956	1971	1,000.0	926.5	61.6	10.2	1.5	0.2	*	*	*
1953-1957	1972	1,000.0	925.7	62.6	10.1	1.4	0.2	*	*	*
1954-1958	1973	1,000.0	924.9	63.9	9.8	1.3	0.1	*	*	*
1955-1959	1974	1,000.0	924.7	64.6	9.4	1.2	0.1	*	*	*

TABLE 7A. DISTRIBUTIONS OF ALL WOMEN BY PARITY AS OF THE BEGINNING OF EACH YEAR 1917-74 BY AGE FOR GROUPS OF COHORTS FROM 1867-71 TO 1955-59--CON.

(BASED ON CUMULATIVE BIRTH RATES FOR GROUPS OF COHORTS)

EXACT AGE AND COHORT	AS OF JANUARY 1	TOTAL	PARITY							
			0	1	2	3	4	5	6	7 AND HIGHER
20-24 YEARS										
1893-1897	1917	1,000.0	631.2	208.7	101.7	40.6	13.4	3.1	1.0	0.3
1894-1898	1918	1,000.0	623.9	215.4	103.7	40.6	12.5	2.8	0.8	0.3
1895-1899	1919	1,000.0	618.6	221.0	104.1	40.5	12.3	2.4	0.8	0.3
1896-1900	1920	1,000.0	631.1	210.8	103.2	39.6	11.9	2.4	0.7	0.3
1897-1901	1921	1,000.0	624.3	220.4	101.5	38.7	11.7	2.4	0.7	0.3
1898-1902	1922	1,000.0	614.3	232.4	99.8	38.0	11.9	2.5	0.8	0.3
1899-1903	1923	1,000.0	612.8	233.0	102.7	36.5	11.4	2.5	0.8	0.3
1900-1904	1924	1,000.0	613.0	230.1	105.5	36.5	11.2	2.6	0.7	0.4
1901-1905	1925	1,000.0	609.5	231.9	105.7	37.9	11.3	2.6	0.7	0.4
1902-1906	1926	1,000.0	609.1	232.7	104.5	38.2	11.8	2.6	0.7	0.4
1903-1907	1927	1,000.0	612.6	230.9	103.5	37.1	12.0	2.7	0.8	0.4
1904-1908	1928	1,000.0	618.1	228.4	101.6	36.1	11.9	2.7	0.8	0.4
1905-1909	1929	1,000.0	626.1	224.8	98.8	35.2	11.3	2.6	0.8	0.4
1906-1910	1930	1,000.0	635.2	220.0	96.4	34.1	10.7	2.5	0.8	0.3
1907-1911	1931	1,000.0	641.0	217.5	94.6	33.1	10.4	2.4	0.7	0.3
1908-1912	1932	1,000.0	648.9	213.4	92.6	31.9	10.0	2.2	0.7	0.3
1909-1913	1933	1,000.0	657.6	208.3	90.5	30.9	9.7	2.1	0.6	0.3
1910-1914	1934	1,000.0	668.6	202.3	87.3	29.7	9.2	2.1	0.6	0.2
1911-1915	1935	1,000.0	673.2	201.1	85.1	28.8	9.0	2.0	0.6	0.2
1912-1916	1936	1,000.0	674.8	203.4	82.8	27.5	8.7	2.0	0.5	0.3
1913-1917	1937	1,000.0	675.9	204.4	82.0	26.5	8.5	2.0	0.4	0.3
1914-1918	1938	1,000.0	675.0	205.3	82.4	26.3	8.3	2.0	0.4	0.3
1915-1919	1939	1,000.0	671.9	206.7	83.7	26.8	8.2	2.0	0.4	0.3
1916-1920	1940	1,000.0	671.1	206.3	84.8	27.1	8.1	1.9	0.4	0.3
1917-1921	1941	1,000.0	669.2	205.4	86.2	27.9	8.4	2.1	0.5	0.3
1918-1922	1942	1,000.0	661.1	209.9	88.3	29.0	8.7	2.1	0.6	0.3
1919-1923	1943	1,000.0	641.4	224.3	92.0	30.0	9.2	2.2	0.6	0.3
1920-1924	1944	1,000.0	632.9	226.6	95.9	31.4	9.8	2.4	0.7	0.3
1921-1925	1945	1,000.0	635.1	224.6	94.4	32.0	10.4	2.5	0.7	0.3
1922-1926	1946	1,000.0	642.4	223.0	90.4	30.5	10.2	2.5	0.7	0.3
1923-1927	1947	1,000.0	626.0	232.7	97.1	30.5	10.2	2.5	0.7	0.3
1924-1928	1948	1,000.0	589.1	259.8	105.7	31.9	10.0	2.5	0.7	0.3
1925-1929	1949	1,000.0	570.2	265.3	116.3	34.4	10.2	2.6	0.7	0.3
1926-1930	1950	1,000.0	559.7	260.2	127.1	38.0	11.1	2.8	0.8	0.3
1927-1931	1951	1,000.0	555.8	250.5	134.3	42.8	12.5	3.0	0.7	0.4
1928-1932	1952	1,000.0	545.2	248.2	139.9	47.7	14.4	3.4	0.8	0.4
1929-1933	1953	1,000.0	534.3	247.3	145.2	51.6	16.2	4.0	1.0	0.4
1930-1934	1954	1,000.0	524.3	245.7	151.4	54.7	17.8	4.6	1.0	0.5
1931-1935	1955	1,000.0	512.2	247.1	156.4	58.3	19.2	5.0	1.3	0.5
1932-1936	1956	1,000.0	502.1	248.0	160.8	61.4	20.4	5.2	1.5	0.6
1933-1937	1957	1,000.0	490.9	249.7	165.3	64.5	21.8	5.5	1.7	0.6
1934-1938	1958	1,000.0	481.3	250.7	169.3	67.6	22.7	6.0	1.8	0.6
1935-1939	1959	1,000.0	476.6	249.3	172.1	69.6	23.7	6.2	1.9	0.6
1936-1940	1960	1,000.0	474.9	245.6	174.5	71.3	24.7	6.4	1.9	0.7
1937-1941	1961	1,000.0	476.4	241.6	174.1	73.2	25.4	6.6	2.0	0.7
1938-1942	1962	1,000.0	481.3	238.0	171.6	73.4	26.2	6.8	2.0	0.7
1939-1943	1963	1,000.0	490.7	234.0	167.3	72.5	25.8	6.9	2.1	0.7
1940-1944	1964	1,000.0	502.5	231.1	162.6	69.8	24.7	6.7	1.9	0.7
1941-1945	1965	1,000.0	514.4	231.4	157.2	65.6	22.8	6.2	1.7	0.7
1942-1946	1966	1,000.0	529.6	232.8	150.6	59.4	20.2	5.3	1.5	0.6
1943-1947	1967	1,000.0	541.5	238.3	143.9	52.7	17.5	4.4	1.2	0.5
1944-1948	1968	1,000.0	553.8	240.9	138.1	47.0	15.1	3.7	1.0	0.4
1945-1949	1969	1,000.0	563.7	244.9	132.3	41.8	13.1	3.1	0.8	0.3
1946-1950	1970	1,000.0	570.2	248.5	128.0	38.3	11.5	2.5	0.7	0.3
1947-1951	1971	1,000.0	573.6	251.6	125.3	36.2	10.3	2.2	0.5	0.3
1948-1952	1972	1,000.0	581.9	250.2	122.0	34.1	9.2	2.0	0.4	0.2
1949-1953	1973	1,000.0	597.1	245.0	116.7	31.0	8.0	1.7	0.4	0.1
1950-1954	1974	1,000.0	612.9	238.6	111.6	28.2	6.9	1.4	0.3	0.1

TABLE 7A. DISTRIBUTIONS OF ALL WOMEN BY PARITY AS OF THE BEGINNING OF EACH YEAR 1917-74 BY AGE FOR GROUPS OF COHORTS FROM 1867-71 TO 1955-59--CON.

(BASED ON CUMULATIVE BIRTH RATES FOR GROUPS OF COHORTS)

EXACT AGE AND COHORT	AS OF JANUARY 1	TOTAL	PARITY							
			0	1	2	3	4	5	6	7 AND HIGHER
25-29 YEARS										
1888-1892----------	1917	1,000.0	374.5	218.7	172.5	112.3	66.2	32.4	14.7	8.7
1889-1893----------	1918	1,000.0	369.0	222.1	176.3	113.8	65.3	30.9	14.4	8.2
1890-1894----------	1919	1,000.0	361.8	228.2	178.4	114.7	65.1	30.2	14.0	7.6
1891-1895----------	1920	1,000.0	363.4	227.8	180.3	114.3	64.1	29.5	13.2	7.4
1892-1896----------	1921	1,000.0	357.3	235.6	181.4	113.5	63.2	29.0	12.8	7.2
1893-1897----------	1922	1,000.0	350.0	246.0	180.5	112.5	62.1	28.7	12.8	7.4
1894-1898----------	1923	1,000.0	347.4	250.5	183.7	110.3	60.6	27.7	12.5	7.3
1895-1899----------	1924	1,000.0	347.2	252.0	186.6	108.4	58.8	27.2	12.4	7.4
1896-1900----------	1925	1,000.0	347.5	254.0	186.6	107.8	57.4	26.7	12.5	7.5
1897-1901----------	1926	1,000.0	348.9	255.9	185.9	106.9	56.5	26.1	12.3	7.5
1898-1902----------	1927	1,000.0	350.8	257.8	185.2	105.0	56.2	25.3	12.2	7.5
1899-1903----------	1928	1,000.0	352.3	261.3	183.6	102.7	55.4	25.3	12.0	7.4
1900-1904----------	1929	1,000.0	355.1	264.9	181.8	100.3	54.2	25.0	11.5	7.2
1901-1905----------	1930	1,000.0	359.6	267.4	180.5	97.7	52.3	24.7	11.1	6.7
1902-1906----------	1931	1,000.0	364.8	269.1	179.0	95.2	50.7	24.1	10.7	6.4
1903-1907----------	1932	1,000.0	373.4	268.8	176.9	92.4	49.0	23.0	10.3	6.2
1904-1908----------	1933	1,000.0	385.6	266.4	173.6	89.4	47.1	22.1	9.9	5.9
1905-1909----------	1934	1,000.0	400.3	262.2	169.8	86.6	45.4	20.9	9.3	5.5
1906-1910----------	1935	1,000.0	412.5	258.5	166.8	84.2	43.9	20.0	8.9	5.2
1907-1911----------	1936	1,000.0	421.9	257.2	164.4	81.5	42.3	19.2	8.5	5.0
1908-1912----------	1937	1,000.0	428.7	257.8	162.6	78.8	40.8	18.3	8.2	4.8
1909-1913----------	1938	1,000.0	431.3	260.5	161.9	76.7	39.2	17.8	7.8	4.8
1910-1914----------	1939	1,000.0	429.9	264.3	162.8	75.3	38.1	17.3	7.6	4.7
1911-1915----------	1940	1,000.0	426.7	268.1	164.7	74.7	37.0	16.8	7.4	4.6
1912-1916----------	1941	1,000.0	422.4	271.0	167.2	74.7	36.5	16.4	7.1	4.7
1913-1917----------	1942	1,000.0	413.6	276.0	170.6	75.5	36.2	16.4	7.0	4.7
1914-1918----------	1943	1,000.0	395.8	284.7	177.4	77.5	36.4	16.5	7.0	4.7
1915-1919----------	1944	1,000.0	381.5	283.9	186.9	81.3	37.4	17.0	7.2	4.8
1916-1920----------	1945	1,000.0	374.6	280.6	191.9	84.6	38.4	17.4	7.6	4.9
1917-1921----------	1946	1,000.0	369.7	278.7	195.6	86.7	39.0	17.5	7.8	5.0
1918-1922----------	1947	1,000.0	348.8	285.5	205.8	89.0	40.2	17.7	7.9	5.1
1919-1923----------	1948	1,000.0	317.8	298.0	218.9	93.4	41.0	17.8	7.9	5.2
1920-1924----------	1949	1,000.0	299.2	299.9	230.2	98.2	41.4	17.9	7.9	5.3
1921-1925----------	1950	1,000.0	285.8	294.5	241.9	103.7	42.8	17.9	8.0	5.4
1922-1926----------	1951	1,000.0	277.6	283.3	251.9	110.4	44.9	18.4	8.0	5.5
1923-1927----------	1952	1,000.0	267.6	272.1	260.2	118.4	48.2	19.4	8.5	5.6
1924-1928----------	1953	1,000.0	259.0	259.7	265.6	127.3	52.3	21.2	9.0	5.9
1925-1929----------	1954	1,000.0	252.8	246.1	269.4	135.3	57.1	23.3	9.7	6.3
1926-1930----------	1955	1,000.0	247.2	232.6	271.4	143.3	62.2	25.8	10.7	6.8
1927-1931----------	1956	1,000.0	240.2	221.3	272.2	151.4	67.3	28.3	11.8	7.5
1928-1932----------	1957	1,000.0	231.1	211.8	273.0	159.6	72.6	30.5	13.0	8.4
1929-1933----------	1958	1,000.0	219.4	203.8	274.4	167.8	78.0	33.0	14.3	9.3
1930-1934----------	1959	1,000.0	208.9	197.2	275.3	174.6	83.1	35.4	15.3	10.2
1931-1935----------	1960	1,000.0	199.9	191.4	275.1	180.5	88.2	37.5	16.3	11.1
1932-1936----------	1961	1,000.0	194.0	186.7	273.4	185.1	92.5	39.3	17.2	11.8
1933-1937----------	1962	1,000.0	190.7	183.4	270.8	187.9	95.6	41.2	18.1	12.3
1934-1938----------	1963	1,000.0	191.0	181.4	267.8	188.9	97.4	42.2	18.7	12.6
1935-1939----------	1964	1,000.0	193.4	180.7	265.6	188.4	97.8	42.8	18.7	12.6
1936-1940----------	1965	1,000.0	197.0	181.9	264.4	187.1	96.8	42.1	18.4	12.3
1937-1941----------	1966	1,000.0	204.1	185.5	264.8	183.6	93.3	40.0	17.3	11.4
1938-1942----------	1967	1,000.0	212.5	192.7	267.4	177.8	87.3	36.6	15.5	10.2
1939-1943----------	1968	1,000.0	222.8	200.9	270.7	170.5	80.1	32.6	13.6	8.8
1940-1944----------	1969	1,000.0	232.6	211.3	274.4	161.7	72.6	28.4	11.7	7.3
1941-1945----------	1970	1,000.0	244.1	219.4	276.6	153.1	65.9	24.9	10.0	6.0
1942-1946----------	1971	1,000.0	254.2	227.6	277.4	145.2	60.1	22.0	8.6	4.9
1943-1947----------	1972	1,000.0	265.7	236.5	276.2	136.5	54.4	19.4	7.3	4.0
1944-1948----------	1973	1,000.0	279.2	244.9	275.3	126.5	48.2	16.7	6.0	3.2
1945-1949----------	1974	1,000.0	295.2	250.6	273.5	116.8	42.4	14.1	4.9	2.5

TABLE 7A. DISTRIBUTIONS OF ALL WOMEN BY PARITY AS OF THE BEGINNING OF EACH YEAR 1917-74 BY AGE FOR GROUPS OF COHORTS FROM 1867-71 TO 1955-59--CON.

(BASED ON CUMULATIVE BIRTH RATES FOR GROUPS OF COHORTS)

EXACT AGE AND COHORT	AS OF JANUARY 1	TOTAL	PARITY							
			0	1	2	3	4	5	6	7 AND HIGHER
30-34 YEARS										
1883-1887----------	1917	1,000.0	271.6	169.3	168.2	130.9	96.9	66.5	45.8	50.8
1884-1888----------	1918	1,000.0	270.5	171.7	168.8	131.9	97.0	66.6	44.0	49.5
1885-1889----------	1919	1,000.0	267.7	175.1	170.2	133.0	96.8	65.2	44.2	47.8
1886-1890----------	1920	1,000.0	265.8	176.9	172.4	134.4	97.0	63.7	43.7	46.1
1887-1891----------	1921	1,000.0	261.7	179.8	175.6	135.8	97.0	62.7	42.9	44.5
1888-1892----------	1922	1,000.0	256.5	183.3	179.5	136.7	97.0	61.2	42.2	43.6
1889-1893----------	1923	1,000.0	251.3	187.6	184.0	137.9	96.2	59.9	40.9	42.2
1890-1894----------	1924	1,000.0	246.6	192.6	188.2	138.6	94.5	58.6	39.6	41.3
1891-1895----------	1925	1,000.0	242.3	198.4	191.2	139.3	92.6	57.0	38.4	40.8
1892-1896----------	1926	1,000.0	238.8	204.7	194.2	139.2	90.6	55.2	37.3	40.0
1893-1897----------	1927	1,000.0	237.0	210.4	196.8	138.5	88.8	53.2	36.1	39.2
1894-1898----------	1928	1,000.0	236.8	214.9	199.8	137.0	86.7	51.4	34.8	38.6
1895-1899----------	1929	1,000.0	238.4	219.1	201.8	135.1	84.4	49.8	34.0	37.4
1896-1900----------	1930	1,000.0	241.7	223.2	202.6	132.9	82.0	48.6	32.9	36.1
1897-1901----------	1931	1,000.0	244.7	227.7	203.1	130.5	79.7	47.4	32.1	34.8
1898-1902----------	1932	1,000.0	247.7	232.6	203.3	127.9	77.8	46.1	31.1	33.5
1899-1903----------	1933	1,000.0	250.4	238.2	203.4	125.2	75.5	44.8	30.1	32.4
1900-1904----------	1934	1,000.0	254.8	243.5	202.8	122.2	73.5	43.6	28.7	30.9
1901-1905----------	1935	1,000.0	259.6	247.6	202.7	119.3	71.6	42.3	27.5	29.4
1902-1906----------	1936	1,000.0	266.0	250.8	202.2	116.4	69.7	40.8	26.2	27.9
1903-1907----------	1937	1,000.0	274.1	252.4	201.6	113.8	67.4	39.3	24.9	26.5
1904-1908----------	1938	1,000.0	283.2	253.4	200.8	111.0	65.1	37.5	23.7	25.3
1905-1909----------	1939	1,000.0	291.2	253.8	200.8	108.9	62.8	35.8	22.5	24.2
1906-1910----------	1940	1,000.0	297.2	254.6	201.5	107.2	60.9	34.2	21.3	23.1
1907-1911----------	1941	1,000.0	300.1	255.1	203.8	106.2	59.4	32.8	20.4	22.2
1908-1912----------	1942	1,000.0	299.2	257.4	206.9	105.5	58.3	31.7	19.4	21.6
1909-1913----------	1943	1,000.0	292.0	261.0	212.3	106.3	57.7	31.0	18.7	21.0
1910-1914----------	1944	1,000.0	283.1	260.8	219.2	109.3	57.7	30.9	18.3	20.7
1911-1915----------	1945	1,000.0	275.2	257.9	225.4	113.4	58.5	30.9	18.1	20.6
1912-1916----------	1946	1,000.0	268.2	251.7	232.7	118.2	59.7	31.1	17.9	20.5
1913-1917----------	1947	1,000.0	255.8	247.2	241.5	124.2	61.4	31.6	18.0	20.3
1914-1918----------	1948	1,000.0	240.1	245.1	250.3	130.6	63.4	32.3	17.9	20.3
1915-1919----------	1949	1,000.0	226.7	241.8	258.5	136.6	65.3	32.8	18.0	20.3
1916-1920----------	1950	1,000.0	213.5	238.3	266.5	142.1	67.6	33.4	18.1	20.5
1917-1921----------	1951	1,000.0	200.3	233.4	274.2	148.6	70.4	34.0	18.4	20.7
1918-1922----------	1952	1,000.0	187.7	227.6	280.5	155.7	73.9	34.8	18.7	21.1
1919-1923----------	1953	1,000.0	174.9	220.8	285.0	164.0	78.1	36.4	19.3	21.5
1920-1924----------	1954	1,000.0	165.1	212.1	287.2	172.4	82.9	38.4	20.0	21.9
1921-1925----------	1955	1,000.0	157.3	201.5	287.9	180.5	88.4	40.7	21.1	22.6
1922-1926----------	1956	1,000.0	152.5	190.0	286.1	188.0	93.9	43.5	22.4	23.6
1923-1927----------	1957	1,000.0	148.2	178.5	282.7	194.7	100.1	46.7	24.1	25.0
1924-1928----------	1958	1,000.0	145.4	167.1	277.4	200.7	106.4	50.3	25.7	27.0
1925-1929----------	1959	1,000.0	143.7	156.5	270.9	205.7	112.8	53.9	27.5	29.0
1926-1930----------	1960	1,000.0	142.4	146.3	264.2	209.7	119.0	57.7	29.6	31.1
1927-1931----------	1961	1,000.0	139.3	137.2	258.2	213.5	124.9	61.6	31.8	33.5
1928-1932----------	1962	1,000.0	134.7	129.6	252.8	216.8	130.8	65.4	33.9	36.0
1929-1933----------	1963	1,000.0	128.9	123.8	248.6	219.8	135.8	68.9	36.0	38.2
1930-1934----------	1964	1,000.0	123.3	119.5	245.3	222.2	140.1	71.9	37.8	39.9
1931-1935----------	1965	1,000.0	117.3	118.0	242.8	224.2	143.5	74.1	39.0	41.1
1932-1936----------	1966	1,000.0	113.8	118.0	241.7	225.8	145.2	75.2	39.5	40.8
1933-1937----------	1967	1,000.0	112.2	119.6	242.5	227.0	145.4	74.9	39.1	39.3
1934-1938----------	1968	1,000.0	113.3	121.6	245.3	227.8	144.0	73.3	37.7	37.0
1935-1939----------	1969	1,000.0	114.8	125.4	250.2	228.2	141.3	70.6	35.7	33.8
1936-1940----------	1970	1,000.0	117.7	129.2	256.4	228.4	137.4	67.1	33.4	30.4
1937-1941----------	1971	1,000.0	121.5	133.9	263.8	227.6	132.2	63.3	30.7	27.0
1938-1942----------	1972	1,000.0	126.6	139.5	273.5	224.9	125.7	58.4	27.8	23.6
1939-1943----------	1973	1,000.0	133.4	146.1	285.3	220.2	117.4	53.0	24.6	20.0
1940-1944----------	1974	1,000.0	142.0	153.5	297.6	213.6	108.3	47.2	21.3	16.5

TABLE 7A. DISTRIBUTIONS OF ALL WOMEN BY PARITY AS OF THE BEGINNING OF EACH YEAR 1917-74 BY AGE FOR GROUPS OF COHORTS FROM 1867-71 TO 1955-59--CON.

(BASED ON CUMULATIVE BIRTH RATES FOR GROUPS OF COHORTS)

EXACT AGE AND COHORT	AS OF JANUARY 1	TOTAL	PARITY							
			0	1	2	3	4	5	6	7 AND HIGHER
35-39 YEARS										
1878-1882----------	1917	1,000.0	233.8	135.7	144.9	122.9	98.4	75.8	62.7	125.8
1879-1883----------	1918	1,000.0	233.9	137.9	146.8	123.5	98.5	75.8	60.9	122.7
1880-1884----------	1919	1,000.0	233.6	140.0	149.0	124.3	98.8	75.5	59.6	119.2
1881-1885----------	1920	1,000.0	233.4	141.9	151.4	125.5	98.9	75.1	58.2	115.6
1882-1886----------	1921	1,000.0	232.7	144.6	153.1	126.8	99.1	74.4	57.3	112.0
1883-1887----------	1922	1,000.0	231.4	147.7	154.4	128.0	99.4	73.6	56.9	108.6
1884-1888----------	1923	1,000.0	229.9	150.4	156.0	129.8	99.8	72.2	56.8	105.1
1885-1889----------	1924	1,000.0	227.8	152.8	158.2	131.9	100.5	70.8	56.2	101.8
1886-1890----------	1925	1,000.0	224.7	155.2	160.9	134.3	101.2	69.5	55.3	98.9
1887-1891----------	1926	1,000.0	220.9	157.9	164.7	136.4	101.7	68.1	54.3	96.0
1888-1892----------	1927	1,000.0	216.8	160.9	169.5	138.4	101.8	66.6	52.8	93.2
1889-1893----------	1928	1,000.0	212.3	165.5	174.0	140.2	101.6	65.1	51.0	90.3
1890-1894----------	1929	1,000.0	208.3	171.2	178.5	141.5	100.6	63.6	49.2	87.1
1891-1895----------	1930	1,000.0	205.1	177.7	182.8	142.3	98.8	61.9	47.5	83.9
1892-1896----------	1931	1,000.0	202.5	184.5	186.9	142.6	96.6	60.3	46.0	80.6
1893-1897----------	1932	1,000.0	201.2	191.1	190.7	142.3	94.3	58.6	44.4	77.4
1894-1898----------	1933	1,000.0	201.8	196.3	194.5	141.6	91.8	56.5	43.0	74.5
1895-1899----------	1934	1,000.0	203.7	201.2	197.5	139.9	89.5	54.7	41.8	71.7
1896-1900----------	1935	1,000.0	207.2	205.8	199.0	137.7	87.4	53.1	40.6	69.2
1897-1901----------	1936	1,000.0	210.8	210.7	200.3	135.4	85.2	51.7	39.2	66.7
1898-1902----------	1937	1,000.0	213.8	216.2	201.6	133.1	83.2	50.3	37.9	63.9
1899-1903----------	1938	1,000.0	215.7	222.4	203.2	131.0	81.1	49.3	36.3	61.0
1900-1904----------	1939	1,000.0	217.9	228.5	204.8	128.7	79.4	48.1	34.6	58.0
1901-1905----------	1940	1,000.0	220.4	233.8	206.8	126.7	77.8	46.8	32.9	54.8
1902-1906----------	1941	1,000.0	224.3	237.2	208.9	125.0	76.1	45.4	31.3	51.8
1903-1907----------	1942	1,000.0	229.2	238.9	210.7	123.9	74.3	43.9	29.9	49.2
1904-1908----------	1943	1,000.0	234.1	239.7	212.8	122.9	72.6	42.3	28.8	46.8
1905-1909----------	1944	1,000.0	237.7	238.7	215.4	123.1	71.6	41.1	27.5	44.9
1906-1910----------	1945	1,000.0	240.0	236.3	218.4	124.2	71.2	39.9	26.6	43.4
1907-1911----------	1946	1,000.0	239.7	232.8	222.3	126.5	71.2	39.4	25.8	42.3
1908-1912----------	1947	1,000.0	236.0	230.0	226.9	129.5	71.8	39.3	25.1	41.4
1909-1913----------	1948	1,000.0	228.5	228.0	232.1	133.6	73.1	39.4	24.8	40.5
1910-1914----------	1949	1,000.0	220.1	225.4	237.7	138.3	74.7	39.6	24.5	39.7
1911-1915----------	1950	1,000.0	210.2	222.3	243.7	143.8	76.5	40.1	24.4	39.0
1912-1916----------	1951	1,000.0	201.2	217.8	249.4	149.1	78.9	40.9	24.2	38.5
1913-1917----------	1952	1,000.0	192.2	211.9	254.5	154.9	81.9	42.0	24.6	38.0
1914-1918----------	1953	1,000.0	184.2	204.8	258.5	161.0	85.3	43.4	24.8	38.0
1915-1919----------	1954	1,000.0	174.6	198.4	262.0	166.9	89.2	45.3	25.3	38.3
1916-1920----------	1955	1,000.0	164.1	192.7	264.4	172.9	93.5	47.4	26.0	39.0
1917-1921----------	1956	1,000.0	152.7	187.0	266.3	179.2	98.3	49.6	27.2	39.7
1918-1922----------	1957	1,000.0	142.6	181.2	266.9	185.2	103.0	51.9	28.4	40.8
1919-1923----------	1958	1,000.0	132.5	175.4	266.5	190.8	108.2	54.6	29.9	42.1
1920-1924----------	1959	1,000.0	124.9	168.7	264.8	195.9	113.2	57.4	31.6	43.5
1921-1925----------	1960	1,000.0	119.7	161.1	261.6	200.4	117.9	60.6	33.3	45.4
1922-1926----------	1961	1,000.0	117.0	152.4	257.6	203.9	122.7	63.7	35.1	47.6
1923-1927----------	1962	1,000.0	114.6	143.8	252.7	207.0	127.4	67.2	37.0	50.3
1924-1928----------	1963	1,000.0	114.0	135.3	247.0	209.3	131.8	70.5	39.0	53.1
1925-1929----------	1964	1,000.0	114.4	126.6	240.8	211.3	136.1	73.9	41.0	55.9
1926-1930----------	1965	1,000.0	114.4	118.6	234.7	213.0	140.5	77.2	43.0	58.6
1927-1931----------	1966	1,000.0	112.4	112.0	229.5	215.0	144.9	80.2	45.2	60.8
1928-1932----------	1967	1,000.0	108.9	106.7	225.8	217.3	148.9	83.2	46.9	62.3
1929-1933----------	1968	1,000.0	103.8	102.9	223.4	220.0	152.9	85.5	48.4	63.1
1930-1934----------	1969	1,000.0	98.4	100.9	222.5	222.9	156.1	87.1	49.3	62.8
1931-1935----------	1970	1,000.0	93.7	100.3	222.8	225.6	158.3	88.2	49.5	61.6
1932-1936----------	1971	1,000.0	90.9	100.9	224.1	228.2	159.2	88.4	49.1	59.2
1933-1937----------	1972	1,000.0	89.9	102.4	226.9	230.3	159.0	87.5	48.0	56.0
1934-1938----------	1973	1,000.0	91.0	104.4	231.7	232.4	157.4	85.2	46.1	51.8
1935-1939----------	1974	1,000.0	93.1	107.2	238.5	234.2	154.6	81.9	43.5	47.0

TABLE 7A. DISTRIBUTIONS OF ALL WOMEN BY PARITY AS OF THE BEGINNING OF EACH YEAR 1917-74 BY AGE FOR GROUPS OF COHORTS FROM 1867-71 TO 1955-59--CON.

(BASED ON CUMULATIVE BIRTH RATES FOR GROUPS OF COHORTS)

EXACT AGE AND COHORT	AS OF JANUARY 1	TOTAL	PARITY							
			0	1	2	3	4	5	6	7 AND HIGHER
40-44 YEARS										
1873-1877----------	1917	1,000.0	214.1	118.0	129.0	113.5	94.7	75.7	66.1	188.9
1874-1878----------	1918	1,000.0	216.1	120.0	130.7	114.2	94.7	74.7	65.9	183.7
1875-1879----------	1919	1,000.0	217.9	122.1	132.1	114.9	94.5	74.0	65.7	178.8
1876-1880----------	1920	1,000.0	219.3	124.2	133.6	115.5	94.4	73.4	65.5	174.1
1877-1881----------	1921	1,000.0	220.2	126.4	135.1	116.2	94.5	72.9	64.7	170.0
1878-1882----------	1922	1,000.0	220.5	128.7	136.9	116.9	94.6	72.7	63.3	166.4
1879-1883----------	1923	1,000.0	220.3	131.2	138.8	118.0	94.9	72.9	61.5	162.4
1880-1884----------	1924	1,000.0	220.0	133.3	141.2	119.3	95.3	73.1	59.9	157.9
1881-1885----------	1925	1,000.0	219.7	135.3	143.8	120.7	95.9	73.1	58.5	153.0
1882-1886----------	1926	1,000.0	219.2	137.9	145.8	122.2	96.6	72.7	57.6	148.0
1883-1887----------	1927	1,000.0	218.4	140.9	147.3	123.9	97.3	72.1	57.1	143.0
1884-1888----------	1928	1,000.0	217.0	143.8	148.9	125.9	98.2	70.9	57.1	138.2
1885-1889----------	1929	1,000.0	215.1	146.4	151.3	128.1	99.2	69.9	56.5	133.5
1886-1890----------	1930	1,000.0	212.2	149.1	154.4	130.8	100.2	68.8	55.7	128.8
1887-1891----------	1931	1,000.0	208.8	152.0	158.3	133.4	100.8	67.5	54.8	124.4
1888-1892----------	1932	1,000.0	204.9	155.3	163.6	135.7	101.0	66.1	53.5	119.9
1889-1893----------	1933	1,000.0	200.9	160.0	168.6	137.7	100.9	64.7	51.9	115.3
1890-1894----------	1934	1,000.0	197.3	165.7	173.6	139.2	99.9	63.4	50.1	110.8
1891-1895----------	1935	1,000.0	194.3	172.4	178.1	140.1	98.4	61.7	48.5	106.5
1892-1896----------	1936	1,000.0	192.2	179.3	182.5	140.6	96.4	60.1	46.9	102.0
1893-1897----------	1937	1,000.0	191.3	186.0	186.4	140.6	94.2	58.5	45.4	97.6
1894-1898----------	1938	1,000.0	192.0	191.4	190.5	140.0	92.1	56.6	43.9	93.5
1895-1899----------	1939	1,000.0	193.5	196.4	193.8	138.8	89.9	55.0	42.7	89.9
1896-1900----------	1940	1,000.0	196.5	201.3	195.8	137.0	87.9	53.6	41.5	86.4
1897-1901----------	1941	1,000.0	199.6	206.1	197.8	135.2	85.9	52.3	40.2	82.9
1898-1902----------	1942	1,000.0	202.0	211.6	199.6	133.4	84.2	51.1	38.9	79.2
1899-1903----------	1943	1,000.0	202.9	217.8	201.9	131.8	82.5	50.2	37.4	75.5
1900-1904----------	1944	1,000.0	203.8	223.7	204.2	130.3	81.1	49.2	36.0	71.7
1901-1905----------	1945	1,000.0	204.9	228.6	206.7	129.1	80.0	48.2	34.4	68.1
1902-1906----------	1946	1,000.0	207.2	231.4	209.1	128.2	79.1	47.1	33.0	64.9
1903-1907----------	1947	1,000.0	210.4	231.9	211.4	128.3	78.0	46.1	31.8	62.1
1904-1908----------	1948	1,000.0	214.3	230.9	213.7	128.5	77.2	45.1	30.8	59.5
1905-1909----------	1949	1,000.0	217.3	228.9	216.2	129.5	76.9	44.3	29.7	57.2
1906-1910----------	1950	1,000.0	218.6	226.2	219.4	131.3	76.8	43.7	28.8	55.2
1907-1911----------	1951	1,000.0	217.4	223.2	223.1	133.8	77.2	43.4	28.2	53.7
1908-1912----------	1952	1,000.0	214.5	220.3	226.9	136.6	78.2	43.3	27.6	52.6
1909-1913----------	1953	1,000.0	209.0	217.3	231.0	140.3	79.8	43.6	27.4	51.6
1910-1914----------	1954	1,000.0	201.7	213.9	235.4	144.8	81.8	44.2	27.4	50.8
1911-1915----------	1955	1,000.0	192.7	210.0	239.8	149.9	84.4	45.3	27.7	50.2
1912-1916----------	1956	1,000.0	184.2	205.2	243.8	154.9	87.3	46.6	28.2	49.8
1913-1917----------	1957	1,000.0	176.1	198.9	247.1	160.4	90.7	48.5	28.6	49.7
1914-1918----------	1958	1,000.0	169.0	192.0	249.6	165.4	94.5	50.3	29.1	50.1
1915-1919----------	1959	1,000.0	160.2	185.7	252.0	170.5	98.3	52.6	29.9	50.8
1916-1920----------	1960	1,000.0	150.7	180.3	253.7	175.4	102.3	54.8	30.9	51.9
1917-1921----------	1961	1,000.0	140.1	175.3	254.8	180.5	106.6	57.2	32.4	53.1
1918-1922----------	1962	1,000.0	130.8	170.3	255.0	185.2	110.8	59.4	33.9	54.6
1919-1923----------	1963	1,000.0	121.4	165.4	254.5	189.9	115.1	62.0	35.5	56.2
1920-1924----------	1964	1,000.0	114.7	159.4	252.9	194.1	119.2	64.6	37.1	58.0
1921-1925----------	1965	1,000.0	110.0	152.6	250.1	197.9	123.3	67.4	38.8	59.9
1922-1926----------	1966	1,000.0	107.7	144.8	246.6	201.1	127.2	70.2	40.4	62.0
1923-1927----------	1967	1,000.0	105.7	137.2	242.5	203.9	131.2	73.1	42.1	64.3
1924-1928----------	1968	1,000.0	105.5	129.3	237.6	206.1	135.4	75.9	43.7	66.5
1925-1929----------	1969	1,000.0	105.8	121.7	232.3	208.1	139.4	78.8	45.4	68.5
1926-1930----------	1970	1,000.0	106.4	114.1	227.1	210.2	143.3	81.7	47.2	70.0
1927-1931----------	1971	1,000.0	104.9	107.7	223.0	212.3	147.5	84.3	49.0	71.3
1928-1932----------	1972	1,000.0	101.9	102.6	220.0	215.0	151.3	86.8	50.5	71.9
1929-1933----------	1973	1,000.0	97.1	99.1	218.4	217.9	154.9	89.0	51.7	71.9
1930-1934----------	1974	1,000.0	92.3	97.0	218.0	221.2	157.9	90.4	52.4	70.8

TABLE 7A. DISTRIBUTIONS OF ALL WOMEN BY PARITY AS OF THE BEGINNING OF EACH YEAR 1917-74 BY AGE FOR GROUPS OF COHORTS FROM 1867-71 TO 1955-59--CON.

(BASED ON CUMULATIVE BIRTH RATES FOR GROUPS OF COHORTS)

EXACT AGE AND COHORT	AS OF JANUARY 1	TOTAL	PARITY							
			0	1	2	3	4	5	6	7 AND HIGHER
45-49 YEARS										
1868-1872----------	1917	1,000.0	200.2	107.3	119.9	108.0	94.5	77.5	68.5	224.1
1869-1873----------	1918	1,000.0	202.5	109.1	121.4	108.7	94.3	76.8	67.9	219.3
1870-1874----------	1919	1,000.0	204.9	111.0	122.7	109.5	94.0	76.0	67.3	214.6
1871-1875----------	1920	1,000.0	207.4	112.8	124.3	110.3	93.6	75.3	66.5	209.8
1872-1876----------	1921	1,000.0	209.7	114.8	125.8	111.2	93.4	74.6	65.9	204.6
1873-1877----------	1922	1,000.0	211.8	117.0	127.5	111.9	93.3	74.1	65.4	199.0
1874-1878----------	1923	1,000.0	213.7	119.2	129.1	112.7	93.2	73.4	65.0	193.7
1875-1879----------	1924	1,000.0	215.5	121.1	130.7	113.4	93.2	72.6	64.9	188.6
1876-1880----------	1925	1,000.0	216.9	123.3	132.1	114.0	93.2	72.0	64.7	183.8
1877-1881----------	1926	1,000.0	217.8	125.5	133.7	114.8	93.1	71.8	63.9	179.4
1878-1882----------	1927	1,000.0	218.2	127.7	135.5	115.7	93.4	71.6	62.5	175.4
1879-1883----------	1928	1,000.0	218.1	130.2	137.5	116.6	93.9	71.8	60.8	171.1
1880-1884----------	1929	1,000.0	217.8	132.4	140.0	117.8	94.5	72.0	59.3	166.2
1881-1885----------	1930	1,000.0	217.5	134.6	142.6	119.4	95.1	72.1	57.9	160.8
1882-1886----------	1931	1,000.0	217.0	137.2	144.7	121.1	95.7	71.9	57.1	155.3
1883-1887----------	1932	1,000.0	216.3	140.3	146.1	122.9	96.5	71.4	56.6	149.9
1884-1888----------	1933	1,000.0	215.1	143.1	147.8	124.9	97.4	70.4	56.6	144.7
1885-1889----------	1934	1,000.0	213.2	145.8	150.1	127.3	98.5	69.3	56.1	139.7
1886-1890----------	1935	1,000.0	210.4	148.5	153.3	129.9	99.5	68.1	55.5	134.8
1887-1891----------	1936	1,000.0	207.1	151.4	157.3	132.4	100.2	66.9	54.6	130.1
1888-1892----------	1937	1,000.0	203.2	154.8	162.6	134.8	100.4	65.5	53.4	125.3
1889-1893----------	1938	1,000.0	199.3	159.5	167.7	136.8	100.2	64.4	51.7	120.4
1890-1894----------	1939	1,000.0	195.8	165.3	172.5	138.4	99.4	63.0	50.1	115.5
1891-1895----------	1940	1,000.0	192.8	171.9	177.3	139.3	97.9	61.5	48.4	110.9
1892-1896----------	1941	1,000.0	190.6	179.0	181.6	139.9	96.0	59.9	46.8	106.2
1893-1897----------	1942	1,000.0	189.7	185.6	185.6	140.0	94.0	58.3	45.3	101.5
1894-1898----------	1943	1,000.0	190.3	191.0	189.8	139.5	91.8	56.5	43.8	97.3
1895-1899----------	1944	1,000.0	191.8	195.9	193.2	138.3	89.8	54.8	42.7	93.5
1896-1900----------	1945	1,000.0	194.6	200.7	195.3	136.6	87.9	53.5	41.5	89.9
1897-1901----------	1946	1,000.0	197.5	205.6	197.2	134.9	85.9	52.3	40.3	86.3
1898-1902----------	1947	1,000.0	199.6	211.1	199.1	133.0	84.3	51.2	39.1	82.6
1899-1903----------	1948	1,000.0	200.3	217.2	201.3	131.6	82.7	50.4	37.6	78.9
1900-1904----------	1949	1,000.0	201.0	222.9	203.7	130.3	81.4	49.5	36.1	75.1
1901-1905----------	1950	1,000.0	202.0	227.6	206.2	129.4	80.3	48.6	34.7	71.2
1902-1906----------	1951	1,000.0	204.1	230.4	208.7	128.5	79.6	47.6	33.3	67.8
1903-1907----------	1952	1,000.0	207.2	230.9	211.0	128.6	78.6	46.7	32.2	64.8
1904-1908----------	1953	1,000.0	211.3	229.9	213.2	128.8	77.8	45.8	31.1	62.1
1905-1909----------	1954	1,000.0	214.3	227.9	215.7	129.7	77.6	44.9	30.1	59.8
1906-1910----------	1955	1,000.0	215.6	225.2	218.7	131.5	77.5	44.4	29.2	57.9
1907-1911----------	1956	1,000.0	214.5	222.0	222.2	134.0	78.1	44.2	28.6	56.4
1908-1912----------	1957	1,000.0	211.7	219.0	225.8	136.8	79.0	44.2	28.2	55.3
1909-1913----------	1958	1,000.0	206.3	215.9	229.7	140.5	80.6	44.6	28.1	54.3
1910-1914----------	1959	1,000.0	199.1	212.5	233.7	145.1	82.5	45.3	28.2	53.6
1911-1915----------	1960	1,000.0	190.2	208.6	238.1	149.9	85.2	46.2	28.8	53.0
1912-1916----------	1961	1,000.0	181.9	203.7	242.1	154.7	88.1	47.7	29.1	52.7
1913-1917----------	1962	1,000.0	173.9	197.6	245.3	159.8	91.6	49.5	29.6	52.7
1914-1918----------	1963	1,000.0	167.0	190.6	247.8	164.9	95.1	51.4	30.1	53.1
1915-1919----------	1964	1,000.0	158.4	184.3	250.1	169.9	98.9	53.6	30.9	53.9
1916-1920----------	1965	1,000.0	149.0	179.0	251.8	174.6	102.8	55.8	32.0	55.0
1917-1921----------	1966	1,000.0	138.5	174.1	253.0	179.6	107.1	58.1	33.3	56.3
1918-1922----------	1967	1,000.0	129.3	169.3	253.2	184.4	111.1	60.3	34.7	57.7
1919-1923----------	1968	1,000.0	119.9	164.7	252.7	189.1	115.3	62.7	36.4	59.2
1920-1924----------	1969	1,000.0	113.1	159.0	251.2	193.2	119.5	65.2	38.0	60.8
1921-1925----------	1970	1,000.0	108.6	152.0	248.8	197.0	123.5	68.0	39.5	62.6
1922-1926----------	1971	1,000.0	106.4	144.3	245.4	200.3	127.4	70.7	41.0	64.5
1923-1927----------	1972	1,000.0	104.5	136.7	241.4	203.2	131.5	73.5	42.6	66.6
1924-1928----------	1973	1,000.0	104.3	128.9	236.8	205.5	135.4	76.3	44.3	68.5
1925-1929----------	1974	1,000.0	104.9	121.1	231.6	207.6	139.4	79.2	45.9	70.3

TABLE 7A. DISTRIBUTIONS OF ALL WOMEN BY PARITY AS OF THE BEGINNING OF EACH YEAR 1917-74 BY AGE FOR GROUPS OF COHORTS FROM 1867-71 TO 1955-59--CON.

(BASED ON CUMULATIVE BIRTH RATES FOR GROUPS OF COHORTS)

EXACT AGE AND COHORT	AS OF JANUARY 1	TOTAL	PARITY							
			0	1	2	3	4	5	6	7 AND HIGHER
50-54 YEARS										
1863-1867----------	1917	---	---	---	---	---	---	---	---	---
1864-1868----------	1918	---	---	---	---	---	---	---	---	---
1865-1869----------	1919	---	---	---	---	---	---	---	---	---
1866-1870----------	1920	---	---	---	---	---	---	---	---	---
1867-1871----------	1921	1,000.0	197.8	105.5	118.4	107.0	94.5	77.9	69.1	229.8
1868-1872----------	1922	1,000.0	200.0	107.2	119.9	107.7	94.5	77.2	68.4	225.1
1869-1873----------	1923	1,000.0	202.3	109.0	121.3	108.5	94.2	76.6	67.9	220.2
1870-1874----------	1924	1,000.0	204.7	110.9	122.7	109.2	94.0	75.8	67.2	215.5
1871-1875----------	1925	1,000.0	207.2	112.8	124.2	110.0	93.6	75.1	66.4	210.7
1872-1876----------	1926	1,000.0	209.5	114.9	125.7	110.9	93.4	74.4	65.8	205.4
1873-1877----------	1927	1,000.0	211.7	116.9	127.4	111.8	93.2	73.9	65.2	199.9
1874-1878----------	1928	1,000.0	213.6	119.1	129.0	112.6	93.1	73.2	64.9	194.5
1875-1879----------	1929	1,000.0	215.4	121.0	130.7	113.3	93.0	72.5	64.8	189.3
1876-1880----------	1930	1,000.0	216.8	123.2	132.0	114.0	93.0	72.0	64.5	184.5
1877-1881----------	1931	1,000.0	217.7	125.4	133.6	114.7	93.1	71.6	63.8	180.1
1878-1882----------	1932	1,000.0	218.0	127.8	135.4	115.5	93.4	71.4	62.5	176.0
1879-1883----------	1933	1,000.0	218.0	130.2	137.4	116.6	93.8	71.6	60.8	171.6
1880-1884----------	1934	1,000.0	217.7	132.4	139.9	117.8	94.3	71.9	59.3	166.7
1881-1885----------	1935	1,000.0	217.4	134.6	142.5	119.3	95.0	72.0	57.9	161.3
1882-1886----------	1936	1,000.0	217.0	137.1	144.6	121.0	95.7	71.8	57.0	155.8
1883-1887----------	1937	1,000.0	216.2	140.3	146.0	122.8	96.5	71.3	56.5	150.4
1884-1888----------	1938	1,000.0	215.0	143.2	147.7	124.7	97.4	70.3	56.5	145.2
1885-1889----------	1939	1,000.0	213.1	145.9	150.0	127.2	98.4	69.2	56.0	140.2
1886-1890----------	1940	1,000.0	210.4	148.5	153.2	129.7	99.5	68.0	55.4	135.3
1887-1891----------	1941	1,000.0	207.0	151.4	157.3	132.3	100.2	66.8	54.5	130.5
1888-1892----------	1942	1,000.0	203.2	154.7	162.7	134.6	100.4	65.4	53.3	125.7
1889-1893----------	1943	1,000.0	199.2	159.6	167.6	136.7	100.2	64.4	51.6	120.7
1890-1894----------	1944	1,000.0	195.7	165.3	172.6	138.3	99.3	63.0	50.0	115.8
1891-1895----------	1945	1,000.0	192.7	172.0	177.2	139.3	97.8	61.5	48.3	111.2
1892-1896----------	1946	1,000.0	190.5	179.0	181.6	139.9	96.0	59.9	46.7	106.4
1893-1897----------	1947	1,000.0	189.6	185.6	185.6	140.0	94.0	58.2	45.3	101.7
1894-1898----------	1948	1,000.0	190.2	191.0	189.8	139.4	91.9	56.4	43.8	97.5
1895-1899----------	1949	1,000.0	191.7	195.9	193.2	138.2	89.8	54.9	42.6	93.7
1896-1900----------	1950	1,000.0	194.6	200.7	195.2	136.6	87.8	53.5	41.5	90.1
1897-1901----------	1951	1,000.0	197.4	205.6	197.2	134.8	85.9	52.3	40.3	86.5
1898-1902----------	1952	1,000.0	199.5	211.1	199.1	133.0	84.2	51.3	39.0	82.8
1899-1903----------	1953	1,000.0	200.2	217.2	201.3	131.6	82.6	50.4	37.7	79.0
1900-1904----------	1954	1,000.0	200.9	222.9	203.7	130.3	81.4	49.4	36.2	75.2
1901-1905----------	1955	1,000.0	201.9	227.6	206.2	129.3	80.4	48.6	34.7	71.3
1902-1906----------	1956	1,000.0	204.0	230.4	208.7	128.5	79.5	47.7	33.3	67.9
1903-1907----------	1957	1,000.0	207.1	230.9	211.0	128.5	78.7	46.7	32.2	64.9
1904-1908----------	1958	1,000.0	211.2	230.0	213.1	128.7	77.9	45.8	31.1	62.2
1905-1909----------	1959	1,000.0	214.2	227.9	215.7	129.6	77.6	45.0	30.1	59.9
1906-1910----------	1960	1,000.0	215.6	225.1	218.7	131.4	77.5	44.6	29.2	57.9
1907-1911----------	1961	1,000.0	214.4	222.1	222.0	134.1	78.0	44.3	28.6	56.5
1908-1912----------	1962	1,000.0	211.6	219.0	225.7	136.8	79.0	44.3	28.3	55.3
1909-1913----------	1963	1,000.0	206.2	215.9	229.6	140.5	80.6	44.6	28.2	54.4
1910-1914----------	1964	1,000.0	199.0	212.5	233.7	145.0	82.5	45.3	28.3	53.7
1911-1915----------	1965	1,000.0	190.1	208.6	238.1	149.8	85.2	46.3	28.8	53.1
1912-1916----------	1966	1,000.0	181.9	203.7	241.9	154.7	88.1	47.7	29.2	52.8
1913-1917----------	1967	1,000.0	173.9	197.5	245.2	159.9	91.5	49.5	29.7	52.8
1914-1918----------	1968	1,000.0	167.0	190.5	247.8	164.9	95.0	51.4	30.2	53.2
1915-1919----------	1969	1,000.0	158.4	184.3	250.0	169.9	98.8	53.7	30.9	54.0
1916-1920----------	1970	1,000.0	149.0	179.0	251.7	174.6	102.8	55.8	32.0	55.1
1917-1921----------	1971	1,000.0	138.5	174.0	253.0	179.6	107.1	58.1	33.3	56.4
1918-1922----------	1972	1,000.0	129.3	169.2	253.2	184.4	111.1	60.3	34.7	57.8
1919-1923----------	1973	1,000.0	119.9	164.6	252.7	189.1	115.3	62.8	36.3	59.3
1920-1924----------	1974	1,000.0	113.1	158.9	251.2	193.2	119.5	65.3	37.9	60.9

TABLE 7B. DISTRIBUTIONS OF WHITE WOMEN BY PARITY AS OF THE BEGINNING OF EACH YEAR 1917-74 BY AGE FOR GROUPS OF COHORTS FROM 1867-71 TO 1955-59

(BASED ON CUMULATIVE BIRTH RATES FOR GROUPS OF COHORTS)

EXACT AGE AND COHORT	AS OF JANUARY 1	TOTAL	PARITY							
			0	1	2	3	4	5	6	7 AND HIGHER
15-19 YEARS										
1898-1902----------	1917	1,000.0	953.0	40.1	6.2	0.7	0.0	*	*	*
1899-1903----------	1918	1,000.0	952.7	40.4	6.2	0.7	*	*	*	*
1900-1904----------	1919	1,000.0	953.3	39.8	6.2	0.7	*	*	*	*
1901-1905----------	1920	1,000.0	957.5	35.9	5.9	0.7	*	*	*	*
1902-1906----------	1921	1,000.0	952.8	40.7	5.8	0.7	*	*	*	*
1903-1907----------	1922	1,000.0	947.8	45.3	6.2	0.7	*	*	*	*
1904-1908----------	1923	1,000.0	949.1	43.4	6.8	0.6	0.1	*	*	*
1905-1909----------	1924	1,000.0	950.8	41.4	7.0	0.7	0.1	*	*	*
1906-1910----------	1925	1,000.0	949.8	42.7	6.7	0.7	0.1	*	*	*
1907-1911----------	1926	1,000.0	949.8	42.8	6.6	0.7	0.1	*	*	*
1908-1912----------	1927	1,000.0	950.5	41.9	6.8	0.7	0.1	*	*	*
1909-1913----------	1928	1,000.0	950.6	41.8	6.8	0.7	0.1	*	*	*
1910-1914----------	1929	1,000.0	951.6	41.1	6.5	0.7	0.1	*	*	*
1911-1915----------	1930	1,000.0	952.7	40.2	6.4	0.6	0.1	*	*	*
1912-1916----------	1931	1,000.0	952.2	40.8	6.3	0.6	0.1	*	*	*
1913-1917----------	1932	1,000.0	953.9	39.3	6.1	0.6	0.1	*	*	*
1914-1918----------	1933	1,000.0	956.0	37.6	5.8	0.6	*	*	*	*
1915-1919----------	1934	1,000.0	958.8	35.3	5.3	0.6	*	*	*	*
1916-1920----------	1935	1,000.0	958.9	35.5	5.1	0.5	*	*	*	*
1917-1921----------	1936	1,000.0	958.3	36.3	4.9	0.5	*	*	*	*
1918-1922----------	1937	1,000.0	958.5	35.9	5.1	0.5	*	*	*	*
1919-1923----------	1938	1,000.0	957.5	36.6	5.3	0.6	*	*	*	*
1920-1924----------	1939	1,000.0	956.2	37.7	5.5	0.6	*	*	*	*
1921-1925----------	1940	1,000.0	957.0	36.7	5.6	0.7	*	*	*	*
1922-1926----------	1941	1,000.0	958.3	35.0	5.9	0.7	0.1	*	*	*
1923-1927----------	1942	1,000.0	957.1	36.2	5.9	0.7	0.1	*	*	*
1924-1928----------	1943	1,000.0	954.3	38.8	6.1	0.7	0.1	*	*	*
1925-1929----------	1944	1,000.0	953.5	39.3	6.3	0.8	0.1	*	*	*
1926-1930----------	1945	1,000.0	956.6	36.6	6.0	0.7	0.1	*	*	*
1927-1931----------	1946	1,000.0	959.5	34.5	5.3	0.6	0.1	*	*	*
1928-1932----------	1947	1,000.0	957.3	36.5	5.5	0.7	*	*	*	*
1929-1933----------	1948	1,000.0	945.4	47.6	6.2	0.8	*	*	*	*
1930-1934----------	1949	1,000.0	939.0	52.3	7.8	0.8	0.1	*	*	*
1931-1935----------	1950	1,000.0	936.6	52.7	9.5	1.1	0.1	*	*	*
1932-1936----------	1951	1,000.0	936.4	52.0	10.2	1.3	0.1	*	*	*
1933-1937----------	1952	1,000.0	933.2	54.5	10.8	1.4	0.1	*	*	*
1934-1938----------	1953	1,000.0	932.4	54.9	11.1	1.4	0.2	*	*	*
1935-1939----------	1954	1,000.0	931.2	55.7	11.4	1.6	0.1	*	*	*
1936-1940----------	1955	1,000.0	929.6	57.0	11.7	1.5	0.2	*	*	*
1937-1941----------	1956	1,000.0	929.2	57.0	12.0	1.6	0.2	*	*	*
1938-1942----------	1957	1,000.0	926.7	58.6	12.8	1.7	0.2	*	*	*
1939-1943----------	1958	1,000.0	923.9	60.7	13.3	1.9	0.2	*	*	*
1940-1944----------	1959	1,000.0	924.5	59.6	13.7	2.0	0.2	*	*	*
1941-1945----------	1960	1,000.0	926.3	57.8	13.6	2.1	0.2	*	*	*
1942-1946----------	1961	1,000.0	929.0	55.5	13.2	2.1	0.2	*	*	*
1943-1947----------	1962	1,000.0	930.9	54.1	12.8	2.0	0.2	*	*	*
1944-1948----------	1963	1,000.0	933.3	52.2	12.3	2.0	0.2	*	*	*
1945-1949----------	1964	1,000.0	935.6	50.7	11.6	1.9	0.2	*	*	*
1946-1950----------	1965	1,000.0	938.4	49.2	10.6	1.6	0.2	*	*	*
1947-1951----------	1966	1,000.0	941.3	48.0	9.2	1.3	0.2	*	*	*
1948-1952----------	1967	1,000.0	942.8	47.8	8.2	1.1	0.1	*	*	*
1949-1953----------	1968	1,000.0	944.8	46.5	7.7	0.9	0.1	*	*	*
1950-1954----------	1969	1,000.0	945.3	46.7	7.1	0.8	0.1	*	*	*
1951-1955----------	1970	1,000.0	944.9	47.3	7.0	0.7	0.1	*	*	*
1952-1956----------	1971	1,000.0	942.4	49.8	7.0	0.7	0.1	*	*	*
1953-1957----------	1972	1,000.0	942.0	50.3	6.9	0.7	0.1	*	*	*
1954-1958----------	1973	1,000.0	941.7	51.1	6.5	0.7	*	*	*	*
1955-1959----------	1974	1,000.0	941.6	51.4	6.3	0.7	*	*	*	*

TABLE 7B. DISTRIBUTIONS OF WHITE WOMEN BY PARITY AS OF THE BEGINNING OF EACH YEAR 1917-74 BY AGE FOR GROUPS OF COHORTS FROM 1867-71 TO 1955-59--CON.

(BASED ON CUMULATIVE BIRTH RATES FOR GROUPS OF COHORTS)

EXACT AGE AND COHORT	AS OF JANUARY 1	TOTAL	PARITY							
			0	1	2	3	4	5	6	7 AND HIGHER
20-24 YEARS										
1893-1897----------	1917	1,000.0	650.7	201.1	97.5	36.7	10.9	2.4	0.6	0.1
1894-1898----------	1918	1,000.0	643.4	206.8	99.2	37.2	10.4	2.3	0.5	0.2
1895-1899----------	1919	1,000.0	638.4	211.1	100.0	37.3	10.4	2.1	0.5	0.2
1896-1900----------	1920	1,000.0	652.9	198.3	99.3	36.6	10.2	2.0	0.5	0.2
1897-1901----------	1921	1,000.0	646.9	207.2	97.3	35.8	10.1	2.0	0.5	0.2
1898-1902----------	1922	1,000.0	636.7	219.9	95.5	34.9	10.1	2.2	0.5	0.2
1899-1903----------	1923	1,000.0	635.5	220.5	98.3	33.2	9.7	2.1	0.5	0.2
1900-1904----------	1924	1,000.0	635.6	217.5	101.7	32.9	9.5	2.1	0.5	0.2
1901-1905----------	1925	1,000.0	632.1	219.4	102.2	34.1	9.4	2.1	0.4	0.3
1902-1906----------	1926	1,000.0	632.0	220.1	100.8	34.7	9.6	2.1	0.4	0.3
1903-1907----------	1927	1,000.0	635.8	218.1	99.6	33.8	9.8	2.2	0.5	0.2
1904-1908----------	1928	1,000.0	641.0	215.8	97.7	32.7	9.9	2.2	0.4	0.3
1905-1909----------	1929	1,000.0	648.6	212.4	95.0	31.8	9.4	2.1	0.5	0.2
1906-1910----------	1930	1,000.0	657.3	207.8	92.6	30.8	8.9	1.9	0.5	0.2
1907-1911----------	1931	1,000.0	662.8	205.6	90.6	29.9	8.6	1.9	0.4	0.2
1908-1912----------	1932	1,000.0	670.4	202.0	88.4	28.6	8.3	1.7	0.5	0.1
1909-1913----------	1933	1,000.0	679.3	197.1	86.2	27.3	7.9	1.6	0.5	0.1
1910-1914----------	1934	1,000.0	690.1	191.6	82.8	26.1	7.4	1.5	0.4	0.1
1911-1915----------	1935	1,000.0	694.4	190.8	80.6	25.2	7.1	1.4	0.4	0.1
1912-1916----------	1936	1,000.0	695.4	194.0	77.9	24.1	6.7	1.4	0.4	0.1
1913-1917----------	1937	1,000.0	695.8	195.9	77.1	22.9	6.5	1.3	0.4	0.1
1914-1918----------	1938	1,000.0	694.5	197.6	77.4	22.5	6.3	1.2	0.4	0.1
1915-1919----------	1939	1,000.0	691.0	199.6	78.9	22.7	6.1	1.2	0.4	0.1
1916-1920----------	1940	1,000.0	690.6	199.3	79.6	22.9	5.9	1.3	0.3	0.1
1917-1921----------	1941	1,000.0	689.2	198.4	80.9	23.6	6.1	1.3	0.4	0.1
1918-1922----------	1942	1,000.0	680.8	203.8	82.9	24.4	6.3	1.3	0.4	0.1
1919-1923----------	1943	1,000.0	659.5	220.0	86.7	25.3	6.6	1.4	0.4	0.1
1920-1924----------	1944	1,000.0	650.3	223.3	90.7	26.6	7.1	1.5	0.4	0.1
1921-1925----------	1945	1,000.0	652.5	221.8	89.1	27.0	7.5	1.6	0.4	0.1
1922-1926----------	1946	1,000.0	660.2	220.6	84.5	25.4	7.2	1.6	0.4	0.1
1923-1927----------	1947	1,000.0	642.2	232.1	91.4	25.1	7.2	1.5	0.4	0.1
1924-1928----------	1948	1,000.0	603.2	261.7	100.0	26.3	6.8	1.5	0.4	0.1
1925-1929----------	1949	1,000.0	584.2	268.5	110.2	28.3	6.8	1.5	0.4	0.1
1926-1930----------	1950	1,000.0	573.9	264.1	121.1	31.3	7.5	1.5	0.5	0.1
1927-1931----------	1951	1,000.0	570.3	254.9	128.7	35.5	8.3	1.8	0.4	0.1
1928-1932----------	1952	1,000.0	559.1	253.4	135.2	40.1	9.7	1.9	0.5	0.1
1929-1933----------	1953	1,000.0	547.4	253.2	141.4	43.8	11.3	2.3	0.5	0.1
1930-1934----------	1954	1,000.0	537.3	251.1	148.3	47.4	12.6	2.6	0.5	0.2
1931-1935----------	1955	1,000.0	525.4	252.0	153.9	51.0	13.9	3.0	0.7	0.1
1932-1936----------	1956	1,000.0	515.9	252.2	158.6	54.2	14.9	3.3	0.8	0.1
1933-1937----------	1957	1,000.0	505.0	253.9	163.1	57.4	16.1	3.5	0.8	0.2
1934-1938----------	1958	1,000.0	495.5	254.8	167.2	60.6	17.1	3.7	0.9	0.2
1935-1939----------	1959	1,000.0	490.6	253.2	170.7	62.5	17.9	4.0	0.9	0.2
1936-1940----------	1960	1,000.0	488.3	249.4	173.3	64.9	18.7	4.2	1.0	0.2
1937-1941----------	1961	1,000.0	489.2	245.1	173.4	67.0	19.6	4.4	1.0	0.3
1938-1942----------	1962	1,000.0	493.5	241.4	171.0	67.7	20.5	4.6	1.0	0.3
1939-1943----------	1963	1,000.0	503.1	236.9	166.5	66.9	20.4	4.8	1.1	0.3
1940-1944----------	1964	1,000.0	515.6	233.2	161.5	64.3	19.5	4.6	1.0	0.3
1941-1945----------	1965	1,000.0	528.5	233.0	155.4	60.0	17.7	4.2	1.0	0.2
1942-1946----------	1966	1,000.0	545.4	233.6	147.8	53.4	15.3	3.5	0.8	0.2
1943-1947----------	1967	1,000.0	559.0	238.3	140.0	46.3	12.8	2.8	0.7	0.1
1944-1948----------	1968	1,000.0	573.4	239.4	133.1	40.4	10.8	2.3	0.5	0.1
1945-1949----------	1969	1,000.0	585.7	241.4	126.2	35.2	9.1	1.8	0.5	0.1
1946-1950----------	1970	1,000.0	594.9	242.7	120.8	31.7	7.9	1.5	0.4	0.1
1947-1951----------	1971	1,000.0	600.7	243.9	117.2	29.6	6.9	1.3	0.4	0.0
1948-1952----------	1972	1,000.0	611.8	240.5	112.7	27.5	6.0	1.2	0.3	0.0
1949-1953----------	1973	1,000.0	629.6	233.0	106.7	24.3	5.2	1.0	0.2	0.0
1950-1954----------	1974	1,000.0	647.5	224.5	101.0	21.7	4.3	0.8	0.2	0.0

TABLE 7B. DISTRIBUTIONS OF WHITE WOMEN BY PARITY AS OF THE BEGINNING OF EACH YEAR 1917-74 BY AGE FOR GROUPS OF COHORTS FROM 1867-71 TO 1955-59--CON.

(BASED ON CUMULATIVE BIRTH RATES FOR GROUPS OF COHORTS)

EXACT AGE AND COHORT	AS OF JANUARY 1	TOTAL	PARITY							
			0	1	2	3	4	5	6	7 AND HIGHER
25-29 YEARS										
1888-1892----------	1917	1,000.0	382.4	219.0	176.7	111.1	62.8	29.9	12.1	6.0
1889-1893----------	1918	1,000.0	376.7	222.4	180.1	112.0	61.9	29.1	11.9	5.9
1890-1894----------	1919	1,000.0	369.4	228.3	182.1	112.6	61.6	28.7	11.7	5.6
1891-1895----------	1920	1,000.0	372.1	226.6	183.9	111.9	60.7	28.1	11.2	5.5
1892-1896----------	1921	1,000.0	366.6	233.7	184.9	111.1	59.7	27.8	10.8	5.4
1893-1897----------	1922	1,000.0	359.5	243.5	184.4	110.1	58.7	27.3	11.0	5.5
1894-1898----------	1923	1,000.0	356.7	247.6	187.7	108.0	57.4	26.4	10.7	5.5
1895-1899----------	1924	1,000.0	356.6	248.2	191.1	106.2	55.8	25.9	10.6	5.6
1896-1900----------	1925	1,000.0	357.1	249.3	192.1	105.7	54.3	25.3	10.6	5.6
1897-1901----------	1926	1,000.0	358.7	250.9	191.7	105.3	53.1	24.6	10.3	5.4
1898-1902----------	1927	1,000.0	360.7	252.9	190.9	103.9	52.5	23.8	9.9	5.4
1899-1903----------	1928	1,000.0	362.6	255.8	189.3	101.8	52.0	23.5	9.8	5.2
1900-1904----------	1929	1,000.0	365.1	259.3	187.6	99.6	50.9	23.0	9.5	5.0
1901-1905----------	1930	1,000.0	369.1	262.1	186.1	97.1	49.4	22.4	9.1	4.7
1902-1906----------	1931	1,000.0	373.8	264.0	184.5	94.7	47.9	21.8	8.8	4.5
1903-1907----------	1932	1,000.0	382.3	263.7	182.3	92.0	46.0	20.9	8.4	4.4
1904-1908----------	1933	1,000.0	394.7	261.3	178.7	89.0	44.3	19.8	8.1	4.1
1905-1909----------	1934	1,000.0	409.9	257.0	174.8	85.9	42.5	18.6	7.5	3.8
1906-1910----------	1935	1,000.0	422.4	253.5	171.6	83.2	40.9	17.8	7.1	3.5
1907-1911----------	1936	1,000.0	431.7	253.0	168.9	80.3	39.1	16.9	6.7	3.4
1908-1912----------	1937	1,000.0	438.1	254.8	166.7	77.4	37.5	15.8	6.5	3.2
1909-1913----------	1938	1,000.0	440.0	258.8	165.9	75.0	35.9	15.0	6.2	3.2
1910-1914----------	1939	1,000.0	437.3	264.2	166.8	73.6	34.7	14.4	5.9	3.1
1911-1915----------	1940	1,000.0	432.9	269.3	169.0	72.9	33.6	13.7	5.8	2.8
1912-1916----------	1941	1,000.0	427.2	273.4	172.0	73.0	32.8	13.3	5.5	2.8
1913-1917----------	1942	1,000.0	416.9	279.7	176.0	73.6	32.5	13.2	5.3	2.8
1914-1918----------	1943	1,000.0	396.9	290.1	183.6	75.6	32.7	13.2	5.2	2.7
1915-1919----------	1944	1,000.0	381.4	289.5	194.0	79.7	33.7	13.6	5.3	2.8
1916-1920----------	1945	1,000.0	374.5	285.9	199.3	83.3	34.7	14.0	5.5	2.8
1917-1921----------	1946	1,000.0	370.1	283.7	203.0	85.4	35.3	14.1	5.6	2.8
1918-1922----------	1947	1,000.0	347.6	291.7	213.8	87.9	36.2	14.3	5.7	2.8
1919-1923----------	1948	1,000.0	314.1	305.9	228.0	92.4	36.8	14.3	5.6	2.9
1920-1924----------	1949	1,000.0	294.2	309.1	240.0	97.0	37.0	14.3	5.5	2.9
1921-1925----------	1950	1,000.0	280.3	304.2	252.4	102.3	38.2	14.1	5.5	3.0
1922-1926----------	1951	1,000.0	272.1	293.1	263.3	109.0	39.8	14.2	5.5	3.0
1923-1927----------	1952	1,000.0	262.2	281.8	272.5	117.1	42.7	15.0	5.7	3.0
1924-1928----------	1953	1,000.0	253.9	269.1	278.6	126.5	46.5	16.4	6.0	3.0
1925-1929----------	1954	1,000.0	248.1	255.1	283.0	135.2	51.0	18.0	6.5	3.1
1926-1930----------	1955	1,000.0	242.3	241.4	285.7	144.1	56.1	19.9	7.1	3.4
1927-1931----------	1956	1,000.0	234.8	230.0	287.1	153.1	61.4	22.1	7.8	3.7
1928-1932----------	1957	1,000.0	225.3	220.2	288.3	162.2	66.9	24.3	8.6	4.2
1929-1933----------	1958	1,000.0	213.4	211.9	289.8	171.0	73.0	26.7	9.5	4.7
1930-1934----------	1959	1,000.0	203.1	204.6	290.9	178.4	78.3	29.1	10.4	5.2
1931-1935----------	1960	1,000.0	195.2	197.9	290.5	184.5	83.6	31.2	11.3	5.8
1932-1936----------	1961	1,000.0	190.6	191.9	288.4	189.4	88.3	33.1	12.1	6.2
1933-1937----------	1962	1,000.0	188.6	187.6	285.2	192.6	91.4	35.2	12.8	6.6
1934-1938----------	1963	1,000.0	189.7	185.0	281.7	193.7	93.4	36.3	13.4	6.8
1935-1939----------	1964	1,000.0	192.6	183.9	279.0	193.3	94.0	36.8	13.5	6.9
1936-1940----------	1965	1,000.0	196.1	185.1	277.5	191.9	92.9	36.4	13.4	6.7
1937-1941----------	1966	1,000.0	203.4	188.9	277.5	188.0	89.2	34.3	12.5	6.2
1938-1942----------	1967	1,000.0	212.3	196.3	279.7	181.4	82.8	31.0	11.1	5.4
1939-1943----------	1968	1,000.0	223.5	204.5	282.6	172.9	75.0	27.4	9.5	4.6
1940-1944----------	1969	1,000.0	234.6	214.6	285.4	163.0	67.1	23.5	8.0	3.8
1941-1945----------	1970	1,000.0	247.7	222.4	286.5	153.1	60.0	20.4	6.8	3.1
1942-1946----------	1971	1,000.0	259.9	229.8	286.1	143.9	54.3	17.7	5.7	2.6
1943-1947----------	1972	1,000.0	273.9	237.9	283.5	133.9	48.5	15.3	4.9	2.1
1944-1948----------	1973	1,000.0	290.5	245.3	280.9	122.5	42.2	12.9	4.1	1.6
1945-1949----------	1974	1,000.0	309.7	249.6	277.7	111.5	36.3	10.6	3.3	1.3

TABLE 7B. DISTRIBUTIONS OF WHITE WOMEN BY PARITY AS OF THE BEGINNING OF EACH YEAR 1917-74 BY AGE FOR GROUPS OF COHORTS FROM 1867-71 TO 1955-59--CON.

(BASED ON CUMULATIVE BIRTH RATES FOR GROUPS OF COHORTS)

EXACT AGE AND COHORT	AS OF JANUARY 1	TOTAL	PARITY							
			0	1	2	3	4	5	6	7 AND HIGHER
30-34 YEARS										
1883-1887----------	1917	1,000.0	273.2	168.6	174.5	133.4	96.7	66.2	43.7	43.7
1884-1888----------	1918	1,C00.0	272.0	170.7	175.3	134.3	96.7	66.3	42.1	42.6
1885-1889----------	1919	1,000.0	269.0	173.8	177.0	135.2	96.5	65.1	41.9	41.5
1886-1890----------	1920	1,000.0	267.2	175.0	179.6	136.3	96.5	63.7	41.5	40.2
1887-1891----------	1921	1,000.0	263.1	177.6	182.9	137.5	96.2	62.9	40.7	39.1
1888-1892----------	1922	1,000.0	257.8	181.1	186.7	138.0	96.0	62.0	39.9	38.5
1889-1893----------	1923	1,000.0	252.6	185.7	191.3	138.8	94.7	60.7	38.8	37.4
1890-1894----------	1924	1,000.0	248.0	190.8	195.4	139.3	92.9	59.3	37.7	36.6
1891-1895----------	1925	1,000.0	244.0	196.3	198.6	139.9	90.9	57.8	36.6	35.9
1892-1896----------	1926	1,000.0	240.8	201.9	202.0	140.0	88.8	56.0	35.5	35.0
1893-1897----------	1927	1,000.0	239.2	206.4	205.6	139.6	87.1	53.8	34.3	34.0
1894-1898----------	1928	1,000.0	238.6	210.2	209.0	138.8	85.3	51.7	33.2	33.2
1895-1899----------	1929	1,000.0	240.1	213.5	211.5	137.5	83.3	50.0	32.1	32.0
1896-1900----------	1930	1,000.0	243.5	216.9	212.8	135.8	81.1	48.4	30.9	30.6
1897-1901----------	1931	1,000.0	246.4	221.2	213.6	133.7	79.0	46.9	30.0	29.2
1898-1902----------	1932	1,000.0	249.2	226.1	214.0	131.5	77.0	45.5	28.9	27.8
1899-1903----------	1933	1,000.0	252.2	231.3	214.0	129.2	74.7	44.1	27.9	26.6
1900-1904----------	1934	1,000.0	256.2	237.0	213.4	126.1	73.0	42.6	26.5	25.2
1901-1905----------	1935	1,000.0	260.6	241.4	213.2	123.2	71.3	41.2	25.2	23.9
1902-1906----------	1936	1,000.0	266.5	244.9	212.8	120.3	69.4	39.6	23.9	22.6
1903-1907----------	1937	1,000.0	274.2	246.8	212.3	117.6	67.2	38.0	22.4	21.5
1904-1908----------	1938	1,000.0	283.1	248.0	211.7	114.8	64.8	36.1	21.2	20.3
1905-1909----------	1939	1,000.0	290.8	249.0	211.8	112.6	62.2	34.3	20.0	19.3
1906-1910----------	1940	1,000.0	296.4	250.5	212.7	110.7	60.1	32.5	18.9	18.2
1907-1911----------	1941	1,000.0	298.6	252.1	215.2	109.5	58.4	30.9	18.0	17.3
1908-1912----------	1942	1,000.0	296.5	255.8	218.6	108.7	57.1	29.7	17.2	16.4
1909-1913----------	1943	1,000.0	287.6	261.1	224.3	109.6	56.4	28.9	16.4	15.7
1910-1914----------	1944	1,000.0	277.1	261.8	231.9	112.8	56.6	28.6	16.0	15.2
1911-1915----------	1945	1,000.0	267.8	259.3	238.9	117.4	57.5	28.4	15.8	14.9
1912-1916----------	1946	1,000.0	259.7	253.0	247.1	122.7	58.8	28.5	15.6	14.6
1913-1917----------	1947	1,000.0	245.9	248.9	256.7	129.0	60.7	28.9	15.6	14.3
1914-1918----------	1948	1,000.0	228.9	247.1	266.4	135.8	62.7	29.5	15.5	14.1
1915-1919----------	1949	1,000.0	215.0	243.8	275.1	142.1	64.6	30.0	15.4	14.0
1916-1920----------	1950	1,000.0	201.7	240.1	283.6	148.0	66.8	30.4	15.5	13.9
1917-1921----------	1951	1,000.0	188.6	234.9	291.7	154.9	69.5	31.0	15.4	14.0
1918-1922----------	1952	1,000.0	175.7	229.1	298.4	162.6	72.8	31.8	15.5	14.1
1919-1923----------	1953	1,000.0	162.4	222.3	303.3	171.4	77.4	33.0	15.9	14.3
1920-1924----------	1954	1,000.0	152.1	214.0	305.6	180.4	82.2	34.9	16.4	14.4
1921-1925----------	1955	1,000.0	144.4	203.4	306.3	189.0	88.0	37.0	17.2	14.7
1922-1926----------	1956	1,000.0	139.9	191.9	304.4	197.0	93.7	39.6	18.3	15.2
1923-1927----------	1957	1,000.0	136.2	180.5	300.7	204.2	100.0	42.7	19.7	16.0
1924-1928----------	1958	1,000.0	134.2	169.1	294.8	210.8	106.6	46.3	21.1	17.1
1925-1929----------	1959	1,000.0	133.2	158.4	287.8	216.4	113.3	49.8	22.8	18.3
1926-1930----------	1960	1,000.0	131.9	148.3	280.8	220.9	120.1	53.7	24.6	19.7
1927-1931----------	1961	1,000.0	128.5	139.4	274.5	225.1	126.7	57.7	26.7	21.4
1928-1932----------	1962	1,000.0	123.9	131.6	268.6	228.9	133.2	61.8	28.7	23.3
1929-1933----------	1963	1,000.0	118.3	125.6	263.9	232.0	138.8	65.6	30.7	25.1
1930-1934----------	1964	1,000.0	113.4	121.1	260.0	234.4	143.4	68.7	32.5	26.5
1931-1935----------	1965	1,000.0	108.9	119.1	256.6	236.3	146.9	71.1	33.6	27.5
1932-1936----------	1966	1,000.0	107.1	118.3	255.1	237.7	148.4	72.1	34.1	27.2
1933-1937----------	1967	1,000.0	106.9	119.6	255.6	238.6	148.1	71.6	33.4	26.2
1934-1938----------	1968	1,000.0	108.9	121.4	258.1	239.3	146.2	69.7	32.1	24.3
1935-1939----------	1969	1,000.0	110.9	125.2	263.1	239.3	142.7	66.8	29.9	22.1
1936-1940----------	1970	1,000.0	114.0	129.1	269.3	239.0	138.1	63.0	27.7	19.8
1937-1941----------	1971	1,C00.0	118.0	134.0	276.6	237.7	132.1	58.8	25.3	17.5
1938-1942----------	1972	1,000.0	123.6	139.7	286.4	234.1	124.6	53.8	22.6	15.2
1939-1943----------	1973	1,000.0	131.4	146.1	298.4	227.9	115.5	48.3	19.6	12.8
1940-1944----------	1974	1,C00.0	141.5	153.3	310.4	219.8	105.5	42.3	16.7	10.5

TABLE 7B. DISTRIBUTIONS OF WHITE WOMEN BY PARITY AS OF THE BEGINNING OF EACH YEAR 1917-74 BY AGE FOR GROUPS OF COHORTS FROM 1867-71 TO 1955-59--CON.

(BASED ON CUMULATIVE BIRTH RATES FOR GROUPS OF COHORTS)

EXACT AGE AND COHORT	AS OF JANUARY 1	TOTAL	PARITY							
			0	1	2	3	4	5	6	7 AND HIGHER
35-39 YEARS										
1878-1882----------	1917	1,000.0	235.0	134.3	150.0	126.1	99.9	77.1	62.0	115.6
1879-1883----------	1918	1,000.0	234.9	136.3	152.0	126.8	99.8	77.0	60.6	112.6
1880-1884----------	1919	1,000.0	234.3	138.2	154.4	127.5	99.9	76.9	59.3	109.5
1881-1885----------	1920	1,000.0	233.8	140.0	157.0	128.6	99.9	76.5	57.9	106.3
1882-1886----------	1921	1,000.0	232.9	142.4	159.0	129.8	99.9	75.9	56.9	103.2
1883-1887----------	1922	1,000.0	231.3	145.4	160.3	131.0	100.3	74.8	56.3	100.6
1884-1888----------	1923	1,000.0	229.5	147.9	162.2	132.7	100.6	73.6	55.8	97.7
1885-1889----------	1924	1,000.0	227.1	150.0	164.8	134.7	101.1	72.3	55.0	95.0
1886-1890----------	1925	1,000.0	223.8	151.9	168.1	136.9	101.5	71.1	54.1	92.6
1887-1891----------	1926	1,000.0	220.0	154.1	172.1	138.9	102.0	70.0	53.0	89.9
1888-1892----------	1927	1,000.0	215.8	157.1	176.8	140.8	102.0	68.9	51.6	87.0
1889-1893----------	1928	1,000.0	211.6	161.7	181.5	142.2	101.4	67.4	50.0	84.2
1890-1894----------	1929	1,000.0	207.7	167.4	186.0	143.5	100.2	65.9	48.2	81.1
1891-1895----------	1930	1,000.0	204.7	173.7	190.4	144.4	98.3	64.2	46.6	77.7
1892-1896----------	1931	1,000.0	202.2	179.9	195.0	144.9	96.3	62.3	45.1	74.3
1893-1897----------	1932	1,000.0	201.0	185.3	199.7	145.0	94.2	60.3	43.6	70.9
1894-1898----------	1933	1,000.0	201.0	190.0	203.9	144.9	92.0	58.3	42.1	67.8
1895-1899----------	1934	1,000.0	203.0	193.8	207.5	143.8	90.1	56.2	40.8	64.8
1896-1900----------	1935	1,000.0	206.5	197.8	209.7	142.1	88.1	54.3	39.6	61.9
1897-1901----------	1936	1,000.0	210.0	202.5	211.4	140.3	85.9	52.7	38.2	59.0
1898-1902----------	1937	1,000.0	212.8	208.0	212.9	138.4	84.0	51.1	36.7	56.1
1899-1903----------	1938	1,000.0	214.7	214.1	214.6	136.5	82.2	49.6	35.0	53.3
1900-1904----------	1939	1,000.0	216.2	220.5	216.4	134.5	80.5	48.3	33.2	50.4
1901-1905----------	1940	1,000.0	217.9	226.2	218.7	132.5	79.0	46.8	31.5	47.4
1902-1906----------	1941	1,000.0	221.0	230.0	221.1	130.9	77.3	45.2	29.9	44.6
1903-1907----------	1942	1,000.0	225.1	232.0	223.5	129.7	75.7	43.6	28.4	42.0
1904-1908----------	1943	1,000.0	229.4	233.1	226.0	128.8	74.0	41.9	27.1	39.7
1905-1909----------	1944	1,000.0	232.4	232.4	229.1	129.1	72.8	40.6	25.8	37.8
1906-1910----------	1945	1,000.0	234.0	230.4	232.6	130.3	72.2	39.5	24.8	36.2
1907-1911----------	1946	1,000.0	232.8	227.5	236.7	133.0	72.2	38.8	24.1	34.9
1908-1912----------	1947	1,000.0	228.1	225.3	241.7	136.4	72.7	38.6	23.6	33.6
1909-1913----------	1948	1,000.0	219.2	224.3	247.2	140.9	74.2	38.5	23.2	32.5
1910-1914----------	1949	1,000.0	209.4	222.6	253.1	146.1	76.0	38.6	22.7	31.5
1911-1915----------	1950	1,000.0	198.2	219.9	259.9	151.8	78.2	38.9	22.6	30.5
1912-1916----------	1951	1,000.0	188.0	215.8	266.2	157.5	80.7	39.6	22.5	29.7
1913-1917----------	1952	1,000.0	178.5	209.9	271.9	163.5	83.9	40.5	22.7	29.1
1914-1918----------	1953	1,000.0	170.1	202.9	276.2	169.9	87.3	41.9	22.9	28.8
1915-1919----------	1954	1,000.0	160.5	196.2	279.9	176.2	91.4	43.8	23.2	28.8
1916-1920----------	1955	1,000.0	150.2	190.3	282.3	182.7	95.9	45.8	23.8	29.0
1917-1921----------	1956	1,000.0	139.0	184.7	283.9	189.4	100.9	48.0	24.6	29.5
1918-1922----------	1957	1,000.0	128.9	178.9	284.3	196.0	105.8	50.3	25.7	30.1
1919-1923----------	1958	1,000.0	118.4	173.3	283.9	202.1	111.3	53.0	27.1	30.9
1920-1924----------	1959	1,000.0	110.6	167.2	281.9	207.4	116.5	55.9	28.5	32.0
1921-1925----------	1960	1,000.0	105.5	160.1	278.3	212.0	121.6	59.1	30.1	33.3
1922-1926----------	1961	1,000.0	103.3	151.8	273.9	215.5	126.6	62.4	31.7	34.8
1923-1927----------	1962	1,000.0	101.7	143.5	268.4	219.0	131.3	65.7	33.7	36.7
1924-1928----------	1963	1,000.0	102.0	135.2	262.1	221.6	135.8	69.1	35.6	38.6
1925-1929----------	1964	1,000.0	103.1	126.7	255.4	223.7	140.5	72.2	37.8	40.6
1926-1930----------	1965	1,000.0	103.1	119.1	249.0	225.5	145.4	75.5	39.6	42.8
1927-1931----------	1966	1,000.0	100.8	112.9	243.5	227.7	150.1	78.9	41.5	44.6
1928-1932----------	1967	1,000.0	97.2	107.7	239.4	230.3	154.5	82.0	43.0	45.9
1929-1933----------	1968	1,000.0	92.5	103.9	236.6	233.0	158.7	84.5	44.3	46.5
1930-1934----------	1969	1,000.0	88.0	101.6	235.4	235.7	162.0	86.1	45.1	46.1
1931-1935----------	1970	1,000.0	84.9	100.6	235.2	238.2	164.0	87.0	45.0	45.1
1932-1936----------	1971	1,000.0	83.9	100.6	236.2	240.6	164.5	86.8	44.4	43.0
1933-1937----------	1972	1,000.0	84.4	101.9	238.8	242.4	163.7	85.4	43.1	40.3
1934-1938----------	1973	1,000.0	86.5	103.9	243.3	244.3	161.4	82.7	41.0	36.9
1935-1939----------	1974	1,000.0	89.1	106.8	250.4	245.7	157.7	78.9	38.2	33.2

TABLE 7B. DISTRIBUTIONS OF WHITE WOMEN BY PARITY AS OF THE BEGINNING OF EACH YEAR 1917-74 BY AGE FOR GROUPS OF COHORTS FROM 1867-71 TO 1955-59--CON.

(BASED ON CUMULATIVE BIRTH RATES FOR GROUPS OF COHORTS)

EXACT AGE AND COHORT	AS OF JANUARY 1	TOTAL	PARITY							
			0	1	2	3	4	5	6	7 AND HIGHER
40-44 YEARS										
1873-1877----------	1917	1,000.0	216.1	117.1	132.8	116.5	96.7	77.4	66.1	177.3
1874-1878----------	1918	1,000.0	217.8	119.0	134.6	117.3	96.5	76.5	65.8	172.5
1875-1879----------	1919	1,000.0	219.5	120.8	136.2	118.0	96.3	75.9	65.4	167.9
1876-1880----------	1920	1,000.0	220.7	122.8	137.8	118.6	96.1	75.4	65.0	163.6
1877-1881----------	1921	1,000.0	221.4	124.8	139.6	119.2	96.1	75.0	64.2	159.7
1878-1882----------	1922	1,000.0	221.5	127.0	141.6	120.0	96.0	74.8	62.9	156.2
1879-1883----------	1923	1,000.0	221.2	129.2	143.8	121.0	96.2	75.0	61.3	152.3
1880-1884----------	1924	1,000.0	220.6	131.1	146.6	122.1	96.5	75.2	59.8	148.1
1881-1885----------	1925	1,000.0	219.9	133.0	149.3	123.6	96.9	75.2	58.4	143.7
1882-1886----------	1926	1,000.0	219.1	135.3	151.5	125.1	97.6	74.8	57.4	139.2
1883-1887----------	1927	1,000.0	217.9	138.3	153.0	126.7	98.3	74.0	56.9	134.9
1884-1888----------	1928	1,000.0	216.2	140.8	154.9	128.8	99.1	72.9	56.6	130.7
1885-1889----------	1929	1,000.0	213.9	143.1	157.8	131.0	99.8	72.0	55.8	126.6
1886-1890----------	1930	1,000.0	210.9	145.2	161.4	133.4	100.8	71.0	55.0	122.3
1887-1891----------	1931	1,000.0	207.4	147.6	165.6	135.9	101.4	70.0	53.9	118.2
1888-1892----------	1932	1,000.0	203.5	150.8	170.8	138.1	101.6	68.8	52.7	113.7
1889-1893----------	1933	1,000.0	199.6	155.6	176.1	139.8	101.0	67.6	51.1	109.2
1890-1894----------	1934	1,000.0	196.2	161.4	181.0	141.3	99.9	66.1	49.5	104.6
1891-1895----------	1935	1,000.0	193.4	167.9	185.6	142.3	98.3	64.5	47.9	100.1
1892-1896----------	1936	1,000.0	191.4	174.3	190.3	143.0	96.5	62.7	46.4	95.4
1893-1897----------	1937	1,000.0	190.6	179.7	195.3	143.4	94.5	60.8	44.9	90.8
1894-1898----------	1938	1,000.0	190.7	184.6	199.8	143.4	92.7	58.9	43.4	86.5
1895-1899----------	1939	1,000.0	192.3	188.4	203.8	142.9	90.9	57.0	42.2	82.5
1896-1900----------	1940	1,000.0	195.3	192.5	206.5	141.9	89.0	55.2	41.0	78.6
1897-1901----------	1941	1,000.0	198.1	197.5	208.7	140.6	87.1	53.7	39.7	74.6
1898-1902----------	1942	1,000.0	200.1	203.1	210.9	139.1	85.5	52.3	38.2	70.8
1899-1903----------	1943	1,000.0	201.0	208.9	213.6	137.8	83.9	51.2	36.5	67.1
1900-1904----------	1944	1,000.0	201.1	215.2	216.1	136.5	82.7	50.0	35.0	63.4
1901-1905----------	1945	1,000.0	201.3	220.4	218.9	135.4	81.8	48.9	33.3	60.0
1902-1906----------	1946	1,000.0	202.5	223.6	221.7	134.7	81.1	47.5	31.9	57.0
1903-1907----------	1947	1,000.0	204.7	224.3	224.6	134.9	80.2	46.5	30.5	54.3
1904-1908----------	1948	1,000.0	207.8	223.5	227.4	135.3	79.5	45.3	29.5	51.7
1905-1909----------	1949	1,000.0	210.3	221.5	230.5	136.6	78.9	44.5	28.4	49.3
1906-1910----------	1950	1,000.0	211.0	219.2	233.9	138.6	78.9	43.7	27.5	47.2
1907-1911----------	1951	1,000.0	209.0	216.8	238.0	141.3	79.3	43.4	26.8	45.4
1908-1912----------	1952	1,000.0	205.2	214.6	242.1	144.5	80.2	43.2	26.4	43.8
1909-1913----------	1953	1,000.0	198.7	212.5	246.3	148.5	82.0	43.3	26.2	42.5
1910-1914----------	1954	1,000.0	190.2	209.9	250.9	153.5	84.2	43.8	26.1	41.5
1911-1915----------	1955	1,000.0	180.0	206.5	255.9	158.9	87.1	44.7	26.5	40.4
1912-1916----------	1956	1,000.0	170.5	202.1	260.1	164.4	90.2	46.1	26.9	39.7
1913-1917----------	1957	1,000.0	161.8	196.0	263.8	170.0	93.9	47.9	27.2	39.4
1914-1918----------	1958	1,000.0	154.4	189.2	266.6	175.2	97.6	49.9	27.6	39.5
1915-1919----------	1959	1,000.0	145.7	182.7	269.0	180.7	101.7	51.9	28.4	39.9
1916-1920----------	1960	1,000.0	136.4	177.2	270.7	185.9	105.9	54.1	29.3	40.5
1917-1921----------	1961	1,000.0	126.1	172.3	271.5	191.4	110.4	56.4	30.4	41.5
1918-1922----------	1962	1,000.0	116.7	167.5	271.5	196.5	114.8	58.9	31.6	42.5
1919-1923----------	1963	1,000.0	107.1	162.8	271.0	201.4	119.4	61.5	33.1	43.7
1920-1924----------	1964	1,000.0	100.1	157.6	269.1	205.7	123.6	64.3	34.6	45.0
1921-1925----------	1965	1,000.0	95.6	151.3	266.0	209.7	127.7	67.1	36.1	46.5
1922-1926----------	1966	1,000.0	93.8	143.9	262.1	213.0	131.7	69.9	37.7	47.9
1923-1927----------	1967	1,000.0	92.7	136.6	257.4	216.1	135.8	72.5	39.5	49.4
1924-1928----------	1968	1,000.0	93.3	129.1	252.0	218.4	140.1	75.3	40.9	50.9
1925-1929----------	1969	1,000.0	94.4	121.8	246.2	220.5	144.4	77.9	42.6	52.2
1926-1930----------	1970	1,000.0	95.0	114.6	240.8	222.7	148.7	80.8	44.1	53.3
1927-1931----------	1971	1,000.0	93.3	108.6	236.3	225.3	153.0	83.7	45.6	54.2
1928-1932----------	1972	1,000.0	90.2	103.5	233.3	228.0	157.1	86.3	46.9	54.7
1929-1933----------	1973	1,000.0	85.8	100.0	231.4	230.9	161.0	88.5	47.8	54.6
1930-1934----------	1974	1,000.0	81.9	97.8	230.7	233.9	164.1	89.8	48.3	53.5

TABLE 7B. DISTRIBUTIONS OF WHITE WOMEN BY PARITY AS OF THE BEGINNING OF EACH YEAR 1917-74 BY AGE FOR GROUPS OF COHORTS FROM 1867-71 TO 1955-59--CON.

(BASED ON CUMULATIVE BIRTH RATES FOR GROUPS OF COHORTS)

EXACT AGE AND COHORT	AS OF JANUARY 1	TOTAL	PARITY							
			0	1	2	3	4	5	6	7 AND HIGHER
45-49 YEARS										
1868-1872----------	1917	1,000.0	203.1	106.9	123.5	110.9	96.6	79.4	68.9	210.7
1869-1873----------	1918	1,000.0	205.3	108.5	125.0	111.6	96.4	78.8	68.2	206.2
1870-1874----------	1919	1,000.0	207.5	110.3	126.5	112.3	96.0	78.1	67.5	201.8
1871-1875----------	1920	1,000.0	209.8	112.1	128.0	113.1	95.6	77.3	66.8	197.3
1872-1876----------	1921	1,000.0	211.9	114.1	129.5	114.0	95.3	76.6	66.0	192.6
1873-1877----------	1922	1,000.0	213.8	116.1	131.2	114.8	95.2	76.0	65.4	187.5
1874-1878----------	1923	1,000.0	215.5	118.0	133.0	115.7	95.1	75.1	65.0	182.6
1875-1879----------	1924	1,000.0	217.1	119.9	134.6	116.4	95.0	74.5	64.7	177.8
1876-1880----------	1925	1,000.0	218.3	121.9	136.2	117.0	95.0	74.0	64.2	173.4
1877-1881----------	1926	1,000.0	219.0	124.0	138.0	117.7	94.9	73.8	63.3	169.3
1878-1882----------	1927	1,000.0	219.2	126.1	140.1	118.6	95.0	73.6	62.1	165.3
1879-1883----------	1928	1,000.0	218.9	128.3	142.5	119.5	95.2	74.0	60.6	161.0
1880-1884----------	1929	1,000.0	218.4	130.2	145.2	120.8	95.6	74.3	59.1	156.4
1881-1885----------	1930	1,000.0	217.7	132.2	147.9	122.6	96.0	74.3	57.9	151.4
1882-1886----------	1931	1,000.0	216.9	134.6	150.2	124.1	96.7	74.1	56.9	146.5
1883-1887----------	1932	1,000.0	215.8	137.6	151.7	125.8	97.4	73.3	56.5	141.9
1884-1888----------	1933	1,000.0	214.2	140.1	153.8	127.7	98.4	72.3	56.3	137.2
1885-1889----------	1934	1,000.0	212.0	142.4	156.6	130.1	99.1	71.4	55.6	132.8
1886-1890----------	1935	1,000.0	209.1	144.4	160.3	132.5	100.2	70.4	54.8	128.3
1887-1891----------	1936	1,000.0	205.6	146.9	164.6	135.0	100.8	69.5	53.7	123.9
1888-1892----------	1937	1,000.0	201.8	150.1	169.9	137.2	100.9	68.5	52.4	119.2
1889-1893----------	1938	1,000.0	198.0	155.0	175.1	138.9	100.6	67.1	50.9	114.4
1890-1894----------	1939	1,000.0	194.6	161.0	179.9	140.4	99.6	65.7	49.4	109.4
1891-1895----------	1940	1,000.0	191.8	167.5	184.6	141.4	98.0	64.3	47.8	104.6
1892-1896----------	1941	1,000.0	189.8	173.9	189.3	142.3	96.2	62.5	46.3	99.7
1893-1897----------	1942	1,000.0	189.0	179.2	194.4	142.8	94.3	60.7	44.8	94.8
1894-1898----------	1943	1,000.0	189.0	184.0	199.1	142.9	92.6	58.7	43.4	90.3
1895-1899----------	1944	1,000.0	190.3	188.0	203.2	142.4	90.8	56.9	42.3	86.1
1896-1900----------	1945	1,000.0	193.2	192.1	205.9	141.5	89.0	55.2	41.1	82.0
1897-1901----------	1946	1,000.0	195.8	197.0	208.2	140.2	87.2	53.8	39.8	78.0
1898-1902----------	1947	1,000.0	197.6	202.5	210.4	138.9	85.5	52.6	38.3	74.2
1899-1903----------	1948	1,000.0	198.2	208.2	212.9	137.9	84.1	51.4	36.9	70.4
1900-1904----------	1949	1,000.0	198.0	214.4	215.4	136.8	83.1	50.4	35.2	66.7
1901-1905----------	1950	1,000.0	198.0	219.5	218.3	135.8	82.3	49.4	33.6	63.1
1902-1906----------	1951	1,000.0	199.1	222.6	221.3	135.1	81.6	48.2	32.3	59.8
1903-1907----------	1952	1,000.0	201.2	223.4	224.1	135.3	80.9	47.2	30.9	57.0
1904-1908----------	1953	1,000.0	204.6	222.5	226.8	135.7	80.2	46.1	29.9	54.2
1905-1909----------	1954	1,000.0	207.2	220.4	229.9	136.9	79.6	45.4	28.8	51.8
1906-1910----------	1955	1,000.0	207.9	218.1	233.2	138.9	79.6	44.6	28.0	49.7
1907-1911----------	1956	1,000.0	206.0	215.5	237.1	141.6	80.1	44.4	27.4	47.9
1908-1912----------	1957	1,000.0	202.3	213.2	240.9	144.9	81.0	44.3	27.1	46.3
1909-1913----------	1958	1,000.0	195.9	211.0	244.9	148.8	82.9	44.5	27.0	45.0
1910-1914----------	1959	1,000.0	187.5	208.4	249.2	153.7	85.2	45.0	27.0	44.0
1911-1915----------	1960	1,000.0	177.4	205.0	254.1	159.0	88.0	46.0	27.4	43.1
1912-1916----------	1961	1,000.0	168.2	200.5	258.3	164.1	91.2	47.3	27.9	42.5
1913-1917----------	1962	1,000.0	159.6	194.5	262.0	169.4	94.9	49.0	28.3	42.3
1914-1918----------	1963	1,000.0	152.5	187.6	264.7	174.6	98.5	51.1	28.6	42.4
1915-1919----------	1964	1,000.0	143.9	181.2	267.1	179.9	102.5	53.2	29.3	42.9
1916-1920----------	1965	1,000.0	134.6	175.9	268.7	185.2	106.5	55.3	30.3	43.5
1917-1921----------	1966	1,000.0	124.4	171.1	269.6	190.5	111.0	57.5	31.4	44.5
1918-1922----------	1967	1,000.0	115.1	166.5	269.7	195.6	115.2	59.9	32.5	45.5
1919-1923----------	1968	1,000.0	105.6	162.0	269.2	200.5	119.7	62.4	34.0	46.6
1920-1924----------	1969	1,000.0	98.6	156.9	267.5	204.8	123.9	65.1	35.4	47.8
1921-1925----------	1970	1,000.0	94.2	150.7	264.5	208.8	128.0	67.9	36.8	49.1
1922-1926----------	1971	1,000.0	92.6	143.3	260.9	212.1	132.0	70.5	38.3	50.3
1923-1927----------	1972	1,000.0	91.5	136.1	256.4	215.2	136.1	73.1	40.0	51.6
1924-1928----------	1973	1,000.0	92.1	128.7	251.1	217.9	140.2	75.8	41.4	52.8
1925-1929----------	1974	1,000.0	93.4	121.3	245.4	220.1	144.3	78.6	43.0	53.9

TABLE 7B. DISTRIBUTIONS OF WHITE WOMEN BY PARITY AS OF THE BEGINNING OF EACH YEAR 1917-74 BY AGE FOR GROUPS OF COHORTS FROM 1867-71 TO 1955-59--CON.

(BASED ON CUMULATIVE BIRTH RATES FOR GROUPS OF COHORTS)

EXACT AGE AND COHORT	AS OF JANUARY 1	TOTAL	PARITY							
			0	1	2	3	4	5	6	7 AND HIGHER
50-54 YEARS										
1863-1867----------	1917	---	---	---	---	---	---	---	---	---
1864-1868----------	1918	---	---	---	---	---	---	---	---	---
1865-1869----------	1919	---	---	---	---	---	---	---	---	---
1866-1870----------	1920	---	---	---	---	---	---	---	---	---
1867-1871----------	1921	1,000.0	200.9	105.1	122.0	109.9	96.7	80.0	69.4	216.0
1868-1872----------	1922	1,000.0	203.0	106.8	123.5	110.6	96.5	79.4	68.7	211.5
1869-1873----------	1923	1,000.0	205.2	108.5	124.9	111.3	96.4	78.7	68.1	206.9
1870-1874----------	1924	1,000.0	207.5	110.2	126.4	112.1	95.9	78.0	67.4	202.5
1871-1875----------	1925	1,000.0	209.7	112.1	127.9	112.9	95.5	77.2	66.7	198.0
1872-1876----------	1926	1,000.0	211.8	114.0	129.5	113.8	95.2	76.5	66.0	193.2
1873-1877----------	1927	1,000.0	213.7	116.0	131.2	114.7	95.1	75.8	65.4	188.1
1874-1878----------	1928	1,000.0	215.4	118.0	132.8	115.6	95.1	75.0	64.9	183.2
1875-1879----------	1929	1,000.0	217.0	119.9	134.4	116.3	95.0	74.4	64.6	178.4
1876-1880----------	1930	1,000.0	218.2	121.9	136.1	116.9	94.8	74.0	64.2	173.9
1877-1881----------	1931	1,000.0	218.9	124.0	137.9	117.6	94.9	73.6	63.3	169.8
1878-1882----------	1932	1,000.0	219.1	126.1	140.0	118.5	94.9	73.5	62.1	165.8
1879-1883----------	1933	1,000.0	218.8	128.3	142.4	119.5	95.1	73.9	60.5	161.5
1880-1884----------	1934	1,000.0	218.3	130.2	145.1	120.8	95.5	74.2	59.1	156.8
1881-1885----------	1935	1,000.0	217.6	132.2	147.9	122.4	96.0	74.2	57.8	151.9
1882-1886----------	1936	1,000.0	216.8	134.6	150.1	124.1	96.6	74.0	56.9	146.9
1883-1887----------	1937	1,000.0	215.7	137.6	151.7	125.7	97.3	73.3	56.4	142.3
1884-1888----------	1938	1,000.0	214.2	140.1	153.7	127.6	98.3	72.4	56.1	137.6
1885-1889----------	1939	1,000.0	212.0	142.3	156.6	130.0	99.1	71.3	55.6	133.1
1886-1890----------	1940	1,000.0	209.1	144.3	160.3	132.4	100.2	70.3	54.8	128.6
1887-1891----------	1941	1,000.0	205.6	146.9	164.6	134.8	100.8	69.5	53.6	124.2
1888-1892----------	1942	1,000.0	201.8	150.1	169.8	137.1	100.9	68.5	52.4	119.4
1889-1893----------	1943	1,000.0	198.0	155.0	175.0	138.9	100.4	67.2	50.9	114.6
1890-1894----------	1944	1,000.0	194.5	161.0	179.9	140.4	99.4	65.8	49.3	109.7
1891-1895----------	1945	1,000.0	191.7	167.5	184.6	141.4	98.0	64.2	47.8	104.8
1892-1896----------	1946	1,000.0	189.7	173.9	189.3	142.3	96.2	62.5	46.2	99.9
1893-1897----------	1947	1,000.0	188.9	179.3	194.3	142.8	94.3	60.7	44.7	95.0
1894-1898----------	1948	1,000.0	188.9	184.0	199.1	142.8	92.6	58.8	43.3	90.5
1895-1899----------	1949	1,000.0	190.2	188.0	203.2	142.3	90.9	56.9	42.2	86.3
1896-1900----------	1950	1,000.0	193.1	192.1	205.9	141.4	89.0	55.2	41.1	82.2
1897-1901----------	1951	1,000.0	195.8	196.9	208.1	140.3	87.1	53.9	39.7	78.2
1898-1902----------	1952	1,000.0	197.5	202.5	210.3	139.0	85.5	52.5	38.4	74.3
1899-1903----------	1953	1,000.0	198.1	208.2	212.9	137.9	84.1	51.4	36.9	70.5
1900-1904----------	1954	1,000.0	198.0	214.3	215.4	136.8	83.1	50.4	35.3	66.7
1901-1905----------	1955	1,000.0	197.9	219.5	218.3	135.8	82.3	49.4	33.7	63.1
1902-1906----------	1956	1,000.0	199.0	222.6	221.3	135.1	81.6	48.2	32.3	59.9
1903-1907----------	1957	1,000.0	201.2	223.4	224.0	135.2	81.0	47.2	31.0	57.0
1904-1908----------	1958	1,000.0	204.6	222.4	226.8	135.6	80.2	46.2	29.9	54.3
1905-1909----------	1959	1,000.0	207.1	220.5	229.8	136.9	79.5	45.5	28.8	51.9
1906-1910----------	1960	1,000.0	207.9	218.0	233.2	138.8	79.6	44.7	28.0	49.8
1907-1911----------	1961	1,000.0	205.9	215.5	237.1	141.6	80.0	44.5	27.4	48.0
1908-1912----------	1962	1,000.0	202.2	213.2	240.9	144.8	81.0	44.4	27.1	46.4
1909-1913----------	1963	1,000.0	195.8	211.0	244.9	148.7	83.0	44.4	27.1	45.1
1910-1914----------	1964	1,000.0	187.4	208.4	249.2	153.6	85.2	45.0	27.1	44.1
1911-1915----------	1965	1,000.0	177.4	204.9	254.1	158.9	88.0	46.1	27.4	43.2
1912-1916----------	1966	1,000.0	168.1	200.5	258.3	164.0	91.2	47.4	27.9	42.6
1913-1917----------	1967	1,000.0	159.6	194.4	262.0	169.3	94.9	49.1	28.3	42.4
1914-1918----------	1968	1,000.0	152.4	187.7	264.6	174.6	98.4	51.1	28.7	42.5
1915-1919----------	1969	1,000.0	143.8	181.3	267.0	179.9	102.5	53.1	29.4	43.0
1916-1920----------	1970	1,000.0	134.6	175.9	268.7	185.1	106.5	55.3	30.3	43.6
1917-1921----------	1971	1,000.0	124.4	171.1	269.5	190.5	111.0	57.5	31.4	44.6
1918-1922----------	1972	1,000.0	115.1	166.5	269.6	195.6	115.2	59.9	32.5	45.6
1919-1923----------	1973	1,000.0	105.5	162.1	269.1	200.5	119.7	62.4	34.0	46.7
1920-1924----------	1974	1,000.0	98.5	157.0	267.4	204.9	123.8	65.2	35.3	47.9

TABLE 7C. DISTRIBUTIONS OF ALL OTHER WOMEN BY PARITY AS OF THE BEGINNING OF EACH YEAR 1917-74 BY AGE FOR GROUPS OF COHORTS FROM 1867-71 TO 1955-59

(BASED ON CUMULATIVE BIRTH RATES FOR GROUPS OF COHORTS)

EXACT AGE AND COHORT	AS OF JANUARY 1	TOTAL	PARITY							
			0	1	2	3	4	5	6	7 AND HIGHER
15-19 YEARS										
1898-1902----------	1917	1,000.0	890.2	90.0	16.6	2.7	0.5	*	*	*
1899-1903----------	1918	1,000.0	881.9	99.1	16.2	2.4	0.4	*	*	*
1900-1904----------	1919	1,000.0	879.2	102.8	15.3	2.4	0.3	*	*	*
1901-1905----------	1920	1,000.0	882.0	101.1	14.3	2.3	0.3	*	*	*
1902-1906----------	1921	1,000.0	875.0	108.1	14.3	2.3	0.3	*	*	*
1903-1907----------	1922	1,000.0	869.6	111.1	16.5	2.5	0.3	*	*	*
1904-1908----------	1923	1,000.0	874.2	105.9	17.0	2.5	0.4	*	*	*
1905-1909----------	1924	1,000.0	874.3	105.7	16.8	2.7	0.5	*	*	*
1906-1910----------	1925	1,000.0	870.1	109.4	17.1	2.9	0.5	*	*	*
1907-1911----------	1926	1,000.0	864.8	114.3	17.5	2.8	0.6	*	*	*
1908-1912----------	1927	1,000.0	861.9	116.2	18.3	3.0	0.6	*	*	*
1909-1913----------	1928	1,000.0	862.4	115.1	18.8	3.1	0.6	*	*	*
1910-1914----------	1929	1,000.0	865.6	112.5	18.2	3.1	0.6	*	*	*
1911-1915----------	1930	1,000.0	869.8	108.7	18.0	3.0	0.5	*	*	*
1912-1916----------	1931	1,000.0	871.3	107.7	17.7	2.8	0.5	*	*	*
1913-1917----------	1932	1,000.0	873.9	105.5	17.4	2.6	0.6	*	*	*
1914-1918----------	1933	1,C00.0	874.8	104.6	17.4	2.7	0.5	*	*	*
1915-1919----------	1934	1,000.0	878.5	101.5	16.8	2.7	0.5	*	*	*
1916-1920----------	1935	1,000.0	878.0	102.0	16.7	2.8	0.5	*	*	*
1917-1921----------	1936	1,000.0	874.9	104.0	17.7	2.9	0.5	*	*	*
1918-1922----------	1937	1,000.0	873.5	104.3	18.6	3.1	0.5	*	*	*
1919-1923----------	1938	1,000.0	868.0	108.2	20.0	3.2	0.6	*	*	*
1920-1924----------	1939	1,000.0	862.9	112.3	20.8	3.4	0.6	*	*	*
1921-1925----------	1940	1,000.0	862.2	111.8	21.5	3.8	0.7	*	*	*
1922-1926----------	1941	1,000.0	865.0	107.4	22.2	4.5	0.9	*	*	*
1923-1927----------	1942	1,000.0	863.8	106.7	23.6	4.8	1.1	*	*	*
1924-1928----------	1943	1,000.0	860.1	108.0	25.3	5.5	1.1	*	*	*
1925-1929----------	1944	1,000.0	857.0	107.7	28.1	6.0	1.2	*	*	*
1926-1930----------	1945	1,000.0	861.2	103.2	28.2	6.2	1.2	*	*	*
1927-1931----------	1946	1,000.0	865.5	99.5	27.9	5.9	1.2	*	*	*
1928-1932----------	1947	1,000.0	867.1	97.9	27.8	6.0	1.2	*	*	*
1929-1933----------	1948	1,000.0	855.4	106.7	30.1	6.5	1.3	*	*	*
1930-1934----------	1949	1,000.0	845.5	111.6	34.2	7.3	1.4	*	*	*
1931-1935----------	1950	1,000.0	840.0	111.9	38.0	8.5	1.6	*	*	*
1932-1936----------	1951	1,000.0	836.8	112.5	39.7	9.2	1.8	*	*	*
1933-1937----------	1952	1,000.0	832.1	116.2	40.0	9.7	2.0	*	*	*
1934-1938----------	1953	1,000.0	831.6	117.3	39.0	9.9	2.2	*	*	*
1935-1939----------	1954	1,000.0	830.8	118.4	38.8	9.8	2.2	*	*	*
1936-1940----------	1955	1,000.0	828.3	121.0	38.5	9.9	2.3	*	*	*
1937-1941----------	1956	1,000.0	829.2	119.6	39.1	9.8	2.3	*	*	*
1938-1942----------	1957	1,000.0	828.8	118.9	39.9	10.0	2.4	*	*	*
1939-1943----------	1958	1,000.0	827.9	119.3	40.1	10.3	2.4	*	*	*
1940-1944----------	1959	1,000.0	831.6	115.6	39.8	10.5	2.5	*	*	*
1941-1945----------	1960	1,000.0	834.4	113.6	39.0	10.5	2.5	*	*	*
1942-1946----------	1961	1,000.0	838.4	111.0	37.9	10.2	2.5	*	*	*
1943-1947----------	1962	1,000.0	841.5	109.4	36.5	10.1	2.5	*	*	*
1944-1948----------	1963	1,000.0	844.9	106.8	35.8	10.0	2.5	*	*	*
1945-1949----------	1964	1,000.0	846.8	105.8	35.4	9.7	2.3	*	*	*
1946-1950----------	1965	1,000.0	847.1	106.1	35.1	9.5	2.2	*	*	*
1947-1951----------	1966	1,000.0	847.2	107.7	34.0	8.9	2.2	*	*	*
1948-1952----------	1967	1,000.0	845.9	110.9	33.2	8.2	1.8	*	*	*
1949-1953----------	1968	1,000.0	843.7	114.7	32.5	7.5	1.6	*	*	*
1950-1954----------	1969	1,000.0	840.8	119.7	31.5	6.7	1.3	*	*	*
1951-1955----------	1970	1,000.0	837.5	124.9	30.3	6.1	1.2	*	*	*
1952-1956----------	1971	1,000.0	832.5	130.6	30.1	5.8	1.0	*	*	*
1953-1957----------	1972	1,000.0	830.2	133.9	29.5	5.5	0.9	*	*	*
1954-1958----------	1973	1,000.0	828.0	138.0	28.3	5.0	0.7	*	*	*
1955-1959----------	1974	1,000.0	828.8	139.3	26.8	4.5	0.6	*	*	*

TABLE 7C. DISTRIBUTIONS OF ALL OTHER WOMEN BY PARITY AS OF THE BEGINNING OF EACH YEAR 1917-74 BY AGE FOR GROUPS OF COHORTS FROM 1867-71 TO 1955-59--CON.

(BASED ON CUMULATIVE BIRTH RATES FOR GROUPS OF COHORTS)

EXACT AGE AND COHORT	AS OF JANUARY 1	TOTAL	PARITY							
			0	1	2	3	4	5	6	7 AND HIGHER
20-24 YEARS										
1893-1897----------	1917	1,000.0	505.5	255.8	128.8	67.3	28.8	8.7	3.5	1.6
1894-1898----------	1918	1,000.0	498.4	270.3	129.9	64.5	26.2	6.8	2.5	1.4
1895-1899----------	1919	1,000.0	492.9	282.5	127.9	63.0	24.7	5.6	2.3	1.1
1896-1900----------	1920	1,000.0	493.2	288.2	126.9	60.4	22.8	5.5	1.9	1.1
1897-1901----------	1921	1,000.0	482.1	301.8	127.0	58.9	22.0	5.3	1.9	1.0
1898-1902----------	1922	1,000.0	474.0	309.2	126.3	59.3	22.5	5.5	2.2	1.0
1899-1903----------	1923	1,000.0	472.3	308.4	129.7	58.4	22.3	5.6	2.3	1.0
1900-1904----------	1924	1,000.0	474.1	305.4	128.9	59.9	22.4	5.9	2.3	1.1
1901-1905----------	1925	1,000.0	471.1	306.0	127.2	62.7	23.3	6.0	2.5	1.2
1902-1906----------	1926	1,000.0	468.1	308.6	127.4	60.8	25.2	6.0	2.5	1.4
1903-1907----------	1927	1,000.0	467.9	308.5	129.0	58.3	26.0	6.2	2.7	1.4
1904-1908----------	1928	1,000.0	472.9	306.6	126.7	57.8	25.3	6.7	2.6	1.4
1905-1909----------	1929	1,000.0	481.8	303.5	123.0	56.7	24.2	6.7	2.7	1.4
1906-1910----------	1930	1,000.0	491.3	298.7	120.8	55.5	23.2	6.7	2.5	1.3
1907-1911----------	1931	1,000.0	497.7	294.6	119.8	54.8	23.0	6.6	2.3	1.2
1908-1912----------	1932	1,000.0	504.9	289.3	119.4	54.2	22.6	6.2	2.3	1.1
1909-1913----------	1933	1,000.0	509.8	283.8	119.8	54.6	22.7	6.1	2.2	1.0
1910-1914----------	1934	1,000.0	519.3	276.4	118.6	54.1	22.4	6.1	2.2	0.9
1911-1915----------	1935	1,000.0	523.9	272.8	117.6	53.7	22.7	6.2	2.2	0.9
1912-1916----------	1936	1,000.0	528.3	269.4	117.0	53.0	22.8	6.3	2.2	1.0
1913-1917----------	1937	1,000.0	533.0	263.8	117.9	52.8	22.9	6.4	2.2	1.0
1914-1918----------	1938	1,000.0	534.4	258.8	119.3	54.3	23.1	6.8	2.2	1.1
1915-1919----------	1939	1,000.0	532.4	256.7	120.5	56.6	23.7	6.7	2.3	1.1
1916-1920----------	1940	1,000.0	528.2	255.9	123.3	58.2	24.1	6.8	2.3	1.2
1917-1921----------	1941	1,000.0	522.9	255.4	125.0	59.9	25.6	7.3	2.6	1.3
1918-1922----------	1942	1,000.0	517.6	253.2	128.1	62.3	26.7	7.8	2.9	1.4
1919-1923----------	1943	1,000.0	511.6	252.6	130.2	64.6	28.2	8.4	3.1	1.3
1920-1924----------	1944	1,000.0	509.5	248.2	132.3	66.6	29.8	9.0	3.2	1.4
1921-1925----------	1945	1,000.0	512.5	242.8	131.4	67.7	31.4	9.5	3.3	1.4
1922-1926----------	1946	1,000.0	518.3	238.6	130.7	66.6	31.5	9.6	3.2	1.5
1923-1927----------	1947	1,000.0	513.2	236.6	136.5	67.6	31.8	9.5	3.3	1.5
1924-1928----------	1948	1,000.0	491.7	245.3	145.4	70.9	32.2	9.6	3.3	1.6
1925-1929----------	1949	1,000.0	474.7	241.7	157.3	77.1	34.1	10.0	3.4	1.7
1926-1930----------	1950	1,000.0	464.2	231.5	166.4	84.5	37.0	11.0	3.7	1.7
1927-1931----------	1951	1,000.0	459.2	219.5	169.6	93.4	40.5	12.2	3.8	1.8
1928-1932----------	1952	1,000.0	455.1	210.5	169.9	99.5	45.4	13.6	4.2	1.8
1929-1933----------	1953	1,000.0	450.1	207.4	168.9	101.8	49.9	15.2	4.7	2.0
1930-1934----------	1954	1,000.0	442.2	209.2	169.8	102.1	52.3	16.9	5.3	2.2
1931-1935----------	1955	1,000.0	428.6	215.5	171.7	104.0	53.8	17.8	6.1	2.5
1932-1936----------	1956	1,000.0	415.0	220.2	175.7	106.0	55.5	18.3	6.6	2.7
1933-1937----------	1957	1,000.0	400.8	222.8	180.9	108.6	58.0	19.1	6.8	3.0
1934-1938----------	1958	1,000.0	391.4	224.0	182.3	112.4	59.2	20.2	7.4	3.1
1935-1939----------	1959	1,000.0	389.0	222.6	181.8	113.9	60.7	21.1	7.9	3.0
1936-1940----------	1960	1,000.0	391.2	219.8	181.1	112.8	62.3	21.5	8.0	3.3
1937-1941----------	1961	1,000.0	396.1	218.2	178.4	112.4	62.2	21.2	8.1	3.4
1938-1942----------	1962	1,000.0	402.8	216.4	176.1	110.0	62.2	20.9	8.1	3.5
1939-1943----------	1963	1,000.0	409.7	216.7	172.4	108.3	60.6	20.7	8.1	3.5
1940-1944----------	1964	1,000.0	416.1	217.8	170.9	105.3	58.6	20.1	7.8	3.4
1941-1945----------	1965	1,000.0	420.8	221.6	169.9	102.1	56.1	19.0	7.3	3.2
1942-1946----------	1966	1,000.0	423.9	228.1	169.8	98.7	52.9	17.4	6.4	2.8
1943-1947----------	1967	1,000.0	423.9	238.7	170.2	95.2	48.8	15.2	5.8	2.2
1944-1948----------	1968	1,000.0	421.9	251.1	172.1	90.9	44.2	13.1	4.8	1.9
1945-1949----------	1969	1,000.0	417.0	268.3	172.6	85.9	39.7	11.3	3.7	1.5
1946-1950----------	1970	1,000.0	409.9	284.9	174.3	81.3	35.7	9.7	3.0	1.2
1947-1951----------	1971	1,000.0	401.4	299.4	176.4	78.4	32.7	8.2	2.4	1.1
1948-1952----------	1972	1,000.0	397.4	309.5	178.5	75.3	29.4	7.0	2.1	0.8
1949-1953----------	1973	1,000.0	399.4	318.3	177.3	70.7	26.1	6.0	1.6	0.6
1950-1954----------	1974	1,000.0	405.8	323.1	174.9	66.4	23.1	5.0	1.3	0.4

TABLE 7C. DISTRIBUTIONS OF ALL OTHER WOMEN BY PARITY AS OF THE BEGINNING OF EACH YEAR 1917-74 BY AGE FOR GROUPS OF COHORTS FROM 1867-71 TO 1955-59--CON.

(BASED ON CUMULATIVE BIRTH RATES FOR GROUPS OF COHORTS)

EXACT AGE AND COHORT	AS OF JANUARY 1	TOTAL	PARITY							
			0	1	2	3	4	5	6	7 AND HIGHER
25-29 YEARS										
1888-1892----------	1917	1,000.0	327.7	210.7	140.7	119.8	89.1	50.5	32.6	28.9
1889-1893----------	1918	1,000.0	324.3	216.6	145.1	118.8	89.6	48.4	31.0	26.2
1890-1894----------	1919	1,000.0	318.6	226.9	144.2	124.4	89.1	44.3	29.3	23.2
1891-1895----------	1920	1,000.0	314.3	235.1	145.6	127.0	86.7	42.1	27.2	22.0
1892-1896----------	1921	1,000.0	305.4	246.7	146.6	128.0	85.6	40.2	26.6	20.9
1893-1897----------	1922	1,000.0	298.5	258.4	144.0	128.1	84.4	39.1	25.6	21.9
1894-1898----------	1923	1,000.0	297.7	263.8	148.7	124.5	81.7	37.1	25.0	21.5
1895-1899----------	1924	1,000.0	297.7	270.1	148.7	122.0	78.7	36.8	24.6	21.4
1896-1900----------	1925	1,000.0	297.3	277.0	143.4	120.5	77.3	37.0	25.4	22.1
1897-1901----------	1926	1,000.0	296.8	282.5	140.7	116.0	78.5	37.4	25.4	22.7
1898-1902----------	1927	1,000.0	298.3	284.5	140.1	110.8	79.3	37.4	26.6	23.0
1899-1903----------	1928	1,000.0	298.8	289.7	139.5	107.0	76.7	39.0	26.1	23.2
1900-1904----------	1929	1,000.0	303.8	292.6	138.8	103.6	74.2	39.5	25.0	22.5
1901-1905----------	1930	1,000.0	311.0	294.3	138.9	100.0	70.8	39.7	24.4	20.9
1902-1906----------	1931	1,000.0	318.4	295.3	138.4	96.9	68.3	39.3	23.3	20.1
1903-1907----------	1932	1,000.0	327.3	294.8	137.2	93.6	66.9	38.3	22.6	19.3
1904-1908----------	1933	1,000.0	336.5	293.2	135.3	90.8	65.7	37.9	22.0	18.6
1905-1909----------	1934	1,000.0	346.5	289.7	133.3	89.4	64.5	37.5	21.6	17.5
1906-1910----------	1935	1,000.0	355.2	285.4	131.5	88.3	64.2	37.4	21.3	16.7
1907-1911----------	1936	1,000.0	362.9	280.2	130.9	87.6	64.4	37.2	20.7	16.1
1908-1912----------	1937	1,000.0	370.7	273.8	131.3	86.7	64.2	36.9	20.6	15.8
1909-1913----------	1938	1,000.0	377.1	267.4	131.4	86.5	63.9	37.0	20.5	16.2
1910-1914----------	1939	1,000.0	383.5	260.6	131.0	86.5	64.0	37.0	20.9	16.5
1911-1915----------	1940	1,000.0	388.5	255.2	130.2	86.8	63.9	37.3	21.3	16.8
1912-1916----------	1941	1,000.0	393.4	249.3	129.3	87.1	64.1	37.8	21.7	17.3
1913-1917----------	1942	1,000.0	395.6	243.6	128.9	88.3	64.4	39.0	22.2	18.0
1914-1918----------	1943	1,000.0	394.6	239.4	129.6	89.9	64.8	40.3	22.8	18.6
1915-1919----------	1944	1,000.0	388.7	237.5	132.1	91.4	65.7	41.6	23.5	19.5
1916-1920----------	1945	1,000.0	380.7	237.6	134.6	92.9	66.8	42.4	24.6	20.4
1917-1921----------	1946	1,000.0	372.6	238.4	138.1	93.8	67.6	43.1	25.2	21.2
1918-1922----------	1947	1,000.0	363.5	236.9	143.4	96.1	68.9	43.8	25.7	21.7
1919-1923----------	1948	1,000.0	350.6	236.8	149.8	99.8	70.7	44.2	26.1	22.0
1920-1924----------	1949	1,000.0	340.1	231.8	156.4	105.4	72.7	44.9	26.2	22.5
1921-1925----------	1950	1,000.0	330.3	222.9	163.5	112.0	76.0	45.7	26.7	22.9
1922-1926----------	1951	1,000.0	320.7	212.7	168.5	118.8	80.8	47.4	27.6	23.5
1923-1927----------	1952	1,000.0	308.8	203.3	170.7	125.7	87.3	50.2	29.6	24.4
1924-1928----------	1953	1,000.0	297.6	193.4	171.9	130.7	94.1	54.8	31.7	25.8
1925-1929----------	1954	1,000.0	288.9	182.6	171.7	134.4	99.8	60.5	34.2	27.9
1926-1930----------	1955	1,000.0	283.3	172.4	170.2	136.1	104.1	66.1	37.3	30.5
1927-1931----------	1956	1,000.0	278.8	163.1	168.9	138.1	106.9	70.5	40.4	33.3
1928-1932----------	1957	1,000.0	272.3	156.3	168.8	140.2	109.4	72.9	43.2	36.9
1929-1933----------	1958	1,000.0	261.1	152.0	170.8	143.9	111.4	74.9	45.8	40.1
1930-1934----------	1959	1,000.0	248.0	150.3	173.5	147.8	113.5	76.3	47.7	42.9
1931-1935----------	1960	1,000.0	232.1	150.3	176.4	151.6	116.9	78.6	48.8	45.3
1932-1936----------	1961	1,000.0	217.6	152.1	178.6	155.0	120.1	79.8	50.0	46.8
1933-1937----------	1962	1,000.0	205.9	154.7	179.5	156.4	122.8	80.7	51.7	48.3
1934-1938----------	1963	1,000.0	201.4	156.4	179.1	156.8	123.5	81.1	52.6	49.1
1935-1939----------	1964	1,000.0	201.1	158.5	179.1	156.5	122.7	81.0	51.7	49.4
1936-1940----------	1965	1,000.0	204.9	159.9	180.1	156.1	121.1	79.0	50.6	48.3
1937-1941----------	1966	1,000.0	209.7	163.6	182.5	155.2	119.5	76.2	47.9	45.4
1938-1942----------	1967	1,000.0	214.6	169.3	187.5	155.1	116.4	72.3	44.1	40.7
1939-1943----------	1968	1,000.0	218.4	176.7	194.3	154.8	113.1	67.5	39.9	35.3
1940-1944----------	1969	1,000.0	219.7	188.3	202.5	153.8	109.2	61.3	35.7	29.5
1941-1945----------	1970	1,000.0	219.8	200.1	210.9	153.3	104.4	56.1	31.4	24.0
1942-1946----------	1971	1,000.0	215.8	212.7	219.8	153.6	99.6	51.4	27.3	19.8
1943-1947----------	1972	1,000.0	210.2	226.3	227.8	154.2	94.8	47.0	23.4	16.3
1944-1948----------	1973	1,000.0	203.3	242.5	237.2	153.0	89.3	41.9	19.9	12.9
1945-1949----------	1974	1,000.0	197.9	258.6	245.6	151.3	83.3	36.9	16.4	10.0

TABLE 7C. DISTRIBUTIONS OF ALL OTHER WOMEN BY PARITY AS OF THE BEGINNING OF EACH YEAR 1917-74 BY AGE FOR GROUPS OF COHORTS FROM 1867-71 TO 1955-59--CON.

(BASED ON CUMULATIVE BIRTH RATES FOR GROUPS OF COHORTS)

EXACT AGE AND COHORT	AS OF JANUARY 1	TOTAL	PARITY							
			0	1	2	3	4	5	6	7 AND HIGHER
30-34 YEARS										
1883-1887----------	1917	1,000.0	267.0	171.1	119.0	110.4	95.8	67.8	61.3	107.6
1884-1888----------	1918	1,000.0	267.9	175.2	120.3	108.4	97.3	65.4	61.3	104.2
1885-1889----------	1919	1,000.0	267.1	180.6	121.0	107.7	99.3	65.6	60.8	97.9
1886-1890----------	1920	1,000.0	266.1	185.5	122.0	108.1	101.1	66.3	58.9	92.0
1887-1891----------	1921	1,000.0	263.4	191.0	123.6	110.5	103.4	64.5	57.3	86.3
1888-1892----------	1922	1,000.0	260.2	195.4	126.7	114.5	103.7	60.4	55.9	83.2
1889-1893----------	1923	1,000.0	256.5	199.9	126.5	120.9	104.3	57.8	53.7	80.4
1890-1894----------	1924	1,000.0	252.5	206.0	127.1	125.0	103.6	55.0	51.6	79.2
1891-1895----------	1925	1,000.0	248.4	213.7	126.5	127.7	102.3	51.8	50.4	79.2
1892-1896----------	1926	1,000.0	244.7	223.6	125.6	127.4	100.4	49.7	48.9	79.7
1893-1897----------	1927	1,000.0	242.9	234.3	123.6	124.7	98.2	48.8	47.2	80.3
1894-1898----------	1928	1,000.0	244.9	242.9	125.1	119.2	94.0	48.1	45.4	80.4
1895-1899----------	1929	1,000.0	246.7	252.2	125.0	113.6	89.7	48.2	45.3	79.3
1896-1900----------	1930	1,000.0	248.8	260.2	124.3	108.3	85.7	49.1	45.9	77.7
1897-1901----------	1931	1,000.0	251.2	266.8	123.8	103.9	81.8	49.8	46.4	76.3
1898-1902----------	1932	1,000.0	255.3	271.0	123.8	99.7	79.1	50.0	45.7	75.4
1899-1903----------	1933	1,000.0	257.8	277.2	124.3	95.9	76.2	49.8	44.9	73.9
1900-1904----------	1934	1,000.0	263.8	280.4	124.8	92.6	73.6	49.7	43.4	71.7
1901-1905----------	1935	1,000.0	271.7	282.1	125.5	89.6	71.0	49.5	41.8	68.8
1902-1906----------	1936	1,000.0	280.8	282.8	125.2	86.3	69.3	49.4	40.6	65.6
1903-1907----------	1937	1,000.0	290.4	282.5	124.2	83.7	67.6	49.1	39.9	62.6
1904-1908----------	1938	1,000.0	300.5	280.9	122.6	81.6	65.9	48.6	39.3	60.6
1905-1909----------	1939	1,000.0	309.4	278.1	121.5	80.1	65.2	48.2	38.2	59.3
1906-1910----------	1940	1,000.0	317.7	273.5	120.9	79.0	65.7	47.4	37.5	58.3
1907-1911----------	1941	1,000.0	324.4	268.1	120.8	78.8	65.9	47.0	36.7	58.3
1908-1912----------	1942	1,000.0	330.4	261.9	121.0	78.9	66.2	46.3	36.4	58.9
1909-1913----------	1943	1,000.0	334.4	255.7	121.6	79.5	66.3	46.1	36.5	59.9
1910-1914----------	1944	1,000.0	337.6	249.4	122.1	80.3	66.2	46.3	37.2	60.9
1911-1915----------	1945	1,000.0	339.3	243.6	122.6	81.4	66.0	46.9	38.0	62.2
1912-1916----------	1946	1,000.0	341.2	237.1	122.9	82.7	65.8	48.3	38.6	63.4
1913-1917----------	1947	1,000.0	339.7	230.8	123.8	84.9	67.1	50.1	38.9	64.7
1914-1918----------	1948	1,000.0	334.5	226.1	126.0	87.5	68.5	51.9	39.3	66.2
1915-1919----------	1949	1,000.0	324.9	222.9	129.5	91.1	70.2	53.5	40.1	67.8
1916-1920----------	1950	1,000.0	311.5	221.6	133.8	94.7	72.7	54.9	41.1	69.7
1917-1921----------	1951	1,000.0	296.7	219.8	138.3	99.1	75.6	56.6	42.4	71.5
1918-1922----------	1952	1,000.0	284.5	215.2	142.7	103.1	79.1	57.9	43.7	73.8
1919-1923----------	1953	1,000.0	273.8	208.2	146.5	107.6	82.6	60.0	45.5	75.8
1920-1924----------	1954	1,000.0	265.0	199.1	148.9	112.3	86.7	62.6	47.4	78.0
1921-1925----------	1955	1,000.0	255.8	188.3	151.7	116.1	91.3	65.9	49.6	81.3
1922-1926----------	1956	1,000.0	246.8	176.5	153.5	119.6	96.2	69.4	52.7	85.3
1923-1927----------	1957	1,000.0	236.1	165.7	153.9	122.7	100.6	73.6	56.2	91.2
1924-1928----------	1958	1,000.0	227.1	154.4	152.9	125.9	104.3	78.0	59.6	97.8
1925-1929----------	1959	1,000.0	220.5	143.6	151.3	127.9	107.8	81.7	62.8	104.4
1926-1930----------	1960	1,000.0	217.6	132.9	148.6	129.9	109.7	84.8	65.4	111.1
1927-1931----------	1961	1,000.0	214.8	123.5	146.9	131.6	111.7	87.5	67.1	116.9
1928-1932----------	1962	1,000.0	209.9	116.7	146.1	133.7	114.1	88.9	69.1	121.5
1929-1933----------	1963	1,000.0	200.3	112.6	147.9	136.3	116.2	90.6	71.2	124.9
1930-1934----------	1964	1,000.0	188.0	110.7	150.5	140.2	118.6	92.6	72.5	126.9
1931-1935----------	1965	1,000.0	172.8	112.0	153.3	144.2	121.6	94.1	73.7	128.3
1932-1936----------	1966	1,000.0	158.8	114.9	156.6	147.7	124.7	95.8	74.2	127.3
1933-1937----------	1967	1,000.0	147.6	118.7	159.8	150.7	127.7	96.9	75.0	123.6
1934-1938----------	1968	1,000.0	143.3	121.8	162.8	153.7	129.6	96.6	74.4	117.8
1935-1939----------	1969	1,000.0	142.0	125.4	167.3	156.9	131.1	95.4	72.5	109.4
1936-1940----------	1970	1,000.0	143.1	129.2	173.1	160.1	131.8	93.8	69.4	99.5
1937-1941----------	1971	1,000.0	145.2	133.2	180.1	163.2	132.2	91.7	65.8	88.6
1938-1942----------	1972	1,000.0	147.0	138.3	189.0	166.4	132.0	88.2	61.5	77.6
1939-1943----------	1973	1,000.0	146.7	145.7	200.4	169.5	130.5	84.3	56.7	66.2
1940-1944----------	1974	1,000.0	145.8	154.3	213.2	172.7	128.1	79.3	51.3	55.3

TABLE 7C. DISTRIBUTIONS OF ALL OTHER WOMEN BY PARITY AS OF THE BEGINNING OF EACH YEAR 1917-74 BY AGE FOR GROUPS OF COHORTS FROM 1867-71 TO 1955-59--CON.

(BASED ON CUMULATIVE BIRTH RATES FOR GROUPS OF COHORTS)

EXACT AGE AND COHORT	AS OF JANUARY 1	TOTAL	PARITY							
			0	1	2	3	4	5	6	7 AND HIGHER
35-39 YEARS										
1878-1882----------	1917	1,000.0	228.6	144.8	105.3	95.5	87.4	62.9	67.9	207.6
1879-1883----------	1918	1,000.0	231.7	148.0	106.0	97.4	87.7	59.7	66.5	203.0
1880-1884----------	1919	1,000.0	234.3	151.5	106.2	100.3	88.4	54.3	67.6	197.4
1881-1885----------	1920	1,000.0	237.3	154.9	106.8	102.3	88.9	51.0	67.2	191.6
1882-1886----------	1921	1,000.0	239.4	158.5	107.3	103.5	90.1	50.6	67.3	183.3
1883-1887----------	1922	1,000.0	240.9	163.0	108.5	102.9	91.3	52.8	67.4	173.2
1884-1888----------	1923	1,000.0	242.2	167.0	109.8	101.6	93.1	56.0	66.2	164.1
1885-1889----------	1924	1,000.0	242.9	171.4	110.8	101.3	95.6	57.7	64.7	155.6
1886-1890----------	1925	1,000.0	242.3	176.5	111.4	102.0	97.8	58.8	62.4	148.8
1887-1891----------	1926	1,000.0	240.6	182.0	112.8	104.3	99.1	57.0	60.2	144.0
1888-1892----------	1927	1,000.0	238.5	186.9	115.1	108.0	99.7	52.6	58.3	140.9
1889-1893----------	1928	1,000.0	235.3	192.7	114.1	114.0	100.3	49.9	55.8	137.9
1890-1894----------	1929	1,000.0	232.4	199.5	114.7	117.8	99.4	47.5	53.6	135.1
1891-1895----------	1930	1,000.0	229.8	207.5	115.8	119.4	97.5	45.7	51.4	132.9
1892-1896----------	1931	1,000.0	227.8	217.7	116.2	118.9	94.2	44.8	49.7	130.7
1893-1897----------	1932	1,000.0	227.0	229.7	115.0	116.8	90.9	43.9	48.2	128.5
1894-1898----------	1933	1,000.0	230.0	238.7	117.2	111.6	86.4	42.3	47.0	126.8
1895-1899----------	1934	1,000.0	232.0	248.0	117.9	106.2	81.9	42.4	46.1	125.5
1896-1900----------	1935	1,000.0	233.9	256.2	117.3	101.0	78.1	42.8	45.9	124.8
1897-1901----------	1936	1,000.0	236.6	262.5	117.0	96.7	74.8	43.4	45.9	123.1
1898-1902----------	1937	1,000.0	240.9	266.8	117.1	92.6	72.3	44.2	45.5	120.6
1899-1903----------	1938	1,000.0	243.9	272.6	117.9	89.5	69.6	45.0	44.3	117.2
1900-1904----------	1939	1,000.0	250.1	275.9	118.7	86.5	67.5	45.5	42.8	113.0
1901-1905----------	1940	1,000.0	258.3	277.7	119.8	83.9	65.5	45.6	41.3	107.9
1902-1906----------	1941	1,000.0	267.2	278.6	119.8	81.3	63.5	45.9	40.2	103.5
1903-1907----------	1942	1,000.0	276.2	278.2	119.1	79.2	61.6	46.1	39.2	100.4
1904-1908----------	1943	1,000.0	285.1	276.8	117.9	77.1	60.5	46.0	38.6	98.0
1905-1909----------	1944	1,000.0	292.7	273.7	117.2	75.8	60.4	45.8	37.8	96.6
1906-1910----------	1945	1,000.0	299.2	269.0	116.8	75.1	61.4	45.2	37.1	96.2
1907-1911----------	1946	1,000.0	304.0	263.2	117.0	75.0	62.5	44.7	36.8	96.8
1908-1912----------	1947	1,000.0	307.9	256.5	117.4	75.7	63.4	44.1	36.9	98.1
1909-1913----------	1948	1,000.0	309.3	250.2	118.2	76.7	64.2	44.2	37.4	99.8
1910-1914----------	1949	1,000.0	310.6	243.1	119.3	78.0	64.5	45.0	38.2	101.3
1911-1915----------	1950	1,000.0	310.4	236.5	120.1	80.2	64.8	46.3	38.9	102.8
1912-1916----------	1951	1,000.0	310.1	229.4	120.3	82.4	65.8	48.2	39.6	104.2
1913-1917----------	1952	1,000.0	307.0	222.5	120.5	85.5	67.4	50.9	40.2	106.0
1914-1918----------	1953	1,000.0	302.1	215.8	121.6	88.4	69.4	53.2	41.3	108.2
1915-1919----------	1954	1,000.0	291.9	211.6	123.5	91.8	71.8	55.2	42.9	111.3
1916-1920----------	1955	1,000.0	278.9	208.1	126.5	94.7	74.4	57.4	45.2	114.8
1917-1921----------	1956	1,000.0	264.1	204.4	130.3	98.2	77.1	59.8	47.5	118.6
1918-1922----------	1957	1,000.0	252.5	198.5	133.4	101.7	79.8	62.0	49.2	122.9
1919-1923----------	1958	1,000.0	242.8	190.7	135.8	104.8	83.2	64.2	51.4	127.1
1920-1924----------	1959	1,000.0	235.1	180.6	137.6	108.6	86.6	66.9	53.4	131.2
1921-1925----------	1960	1,000.0	227.3	169.8	138.7	112.5	90.1	69.3	55.9	136.4
1922-1926----------	1961	1,000.0	219.7	158.1	139.5	115.4	94.4	71.9	58.5	142.5
1923-1927----------	1962	1,000.0	210.4	147.2	139.8	117.4	98.8	75.7	60.9	149.8
1924-1928----------	1963	1,000.0	202.7	136.4	138.9	120.0	102.2	79.5	63.8	156.5
1925-1929----------	1964	1,000.0	197.2	125.9	137.6	121.8	105.0	83.6	66.3	162.6
1926-1930----------	1965	1,000.0	195.4	115.6	135.2	123.7	107.5	86.1	68.7	167.8
1927-1931----------	1966	1,000.0	193.4	107.0	133.6	125.4	109.9	88.3	70.9	171.5
1928-1932----------	1967	1,000.0	189.1	101.3	133.2	128.6	111.9	90.1	72.9	172.9
1929-1933----------	1968	1,000.0	180.0	97.5	135.7	131.9	114.9	92.4	74.6	173.0
1930-1934----------	1969	1,000.0	167.6	96.7	139.1	137.0	117.5	94.5	76.5	171.1
1931-1935----------	1970	1,000.0	152.3	97.9	143.7	141.7	121.5	97.4	77.6	167.9
1932-1936----------	1971	1,000.0	138.0	101.1	147.8	146.4	125.5	99.7	79.0	162.5
1933-1937----------	1972	1,000.0	126.6	104.5	152.1	150.4	129.6	101.1	79.6	156.1
1934-1938----------	1973	1,000.0	121.5	107.4	156.3	155.0	132.2	101.2	79.5	146.9
1935-1939----------	1974	1,000.0	119.8	110.1	161.9	159.5	134.4	100.7	78.0	135.6

TABLE 7C. DISTRIBUTIONS OF ALL OTHER WOMEN BY PARITY AS OF THE BEGINNING OF EACH YEAR 1917-74 BY AGE FOR GROUPS OF COHORTS FROM 1867-71 TO 1955-59--CON.

(BASED ON CUMULATIVE BIRTH RATES FOR GROUPS OF COHORTS)

EXACT AGE AND COHORT	AS OF JANUARY 1	TOTAL	PARITY							
			0	1	2	3	4	5	6	7 AND HIGHER
40-44 YEARS										
1873-1877----------	1917	1,000.0	198.3	124.5	98.0	85.8	78.1	58.6	66.4	290.3
1874-1878----------	1918	1,000.0	202.9	127.8	99.2	86.5	78.9	58.3	66.6	279.8
1875-1879----------	1919	1,000.0	206.8	131.4	99.9	87.7	79.8	57.3	66.9	270.2
1876-1880----------	1920	1,000.0	210.9	134.5	100.6	88.5	81.0	56.7	66.2	261.6
1877-1881----------	1921	1,000.0	214.0	138.0	100.6	89.5	82.4	55.3	65.7	254.5
1878-1882----------	1922	1,000.0	216.8	141.1	100.5	90.7	83.9	52.6	65.2	249.2
1879-1883----------	1923	1,000.0	219.3	144.5	100.6	93.0	84.7	48.9	65.1	243.9
1880-1884----------	1924	1,000.0	222.2	147.9	100.6	95.9	85.4	45.5	65.0	237.5
1881-1885----------	1925	1,000.0	225.6	151.5	100.8	98.1	86.2	43.4	64.8	229.6
1882-1886----------	1926	1,000.0	228.7	155.5	101.5	99.3	87.2	43.6	64.7	219.5
1883-1887----------	1927	1,000.0	231.1	160.1	102.9	98.9	88.5	46.6	63.5	208.4
1884-1888----------	1928	1,000.0	233.0	164.9	104.0	97.7	90.5	49.8	62.3	197.8
1885-1889----------	1929	1,000.0	233.9	170.2	105.2	97.1	92.5	52.6	60.8	187.7
1886-1890----------	1930	1,000.0	233.6	175.8	106.5	97.8	94.3	53.7	59.1	179.2
1887-1891----------	1931	1,000.0	232.6	181.3	108.4	100.0	95.3	52.4	57.1	172.9
1888-1892----------	1932	1,000.0	231.1	186.2	111.7	103.6	95.4	48.7	55.4	167.9
1889-1893----------	1933	1,000.0	228.7	191.6	111.0	109.8	95.8	45.8	53.8	163.5
1890-1894----------	1934	1,000.0	226.0	198.3	111.9	113.6	95.2	43.1	51.8	160.1
1891-1895----------	1935	1,000.0	223.7	206.5	112.9	115.3	93.4	41.1	49.6	157.5
1892-1896----------	1936	1,000.0	222.2	216.6	113.2	115.2	90.6	40.0	47.4	154.8
1893-1897----------	1937	1,000.0	221.7	228.7	112.1	113.3	87.3	39.5	45.5	151.9
1894-1898----------	1938	1,000.0	224.9	237.7	114.5	108.3	82.9	38.8	43.8	149.1
1895-1899----------	1939	1,000.0	226.8	247.0	115.1	103.2	78.5	39.0	42.9	147.5
1896-1900----------	1940	1,000.0	228.6	255.1	114.5	98.2	75.0	39.5	43.1	146.0
1897-1901----------	1941	1,000.0	231.1	261.4	114.4	93.7	71.9	40.4	43.2	143.9
1898-1902----------	1942	1,000.0	235.4	265.4	114.8	89.8	69.3	41.4	42.9	141.0
1899-1903----------	1943	1,000.0	238.2	271.2	115.9	86.7	66.8	42.4	41.9	136.9
1900-1904----------	1944	1,000.0	244.1	274.5	117.0	83.8	65.0	42.9	40.6	132.1
1901-1905----------	1945	1,000.0	252.0	276.1	118.1	81.6	62.7	43.6	39.4	126.5
1902-1906----------	1946	1,000.0	260.3	277.0	118.1	79.3	60.7	44.0	38.5	122.1
1903-1907----------	1947	1,000.0	268.7	276.6	117.3	77.1	59.5	44.2	37.6	119.0
1904-1908----------	1948	1,000.0	276.9	275.1	116.0	75.3	58.7	44.1	37.1	116.8
1905-1909----------	1949	1,000.0	283.8	272.0	115.1	74.2	59.0	44.1	36.4	115.4
1906-1910----------	1950	1,000.0	289.4	267.1	115.0	73.5	60.2	44.0	35.8	115.0
1907-1911----------	1951	1,000.0	293.3	261.0	115.2	74.1	61.4	43.5	35.6	115.9
1908-1912----------	1952	1,000.0	296.3	254.1	115.8	74.8	62.4	43.1	36.1	117.4
1909-1913----------	1953	1,000.0	297.5	247.2	116.3	75.9	63.3	43.6	36.8	119.4
1910-1914----------	1954	1,000.0	298.5	239.8	116.9	77.1	63.9	44.5	37.9	121.4
1911-1915----------	1955	1,000.0	298.2	233.0	116.9	78.9	64.7	46.2	38.8	123.3
1912-1916----------	1956	1,000.0	298.0	225.2	117.0	80.8	65.6	48.3	39.9	125.2
1913-1917----------	1957	1,000.0	295.1	217.9	117.0	83.7	66.8	51.0	40.7	127.8
1914-1918----------	1958	1,000.0	290.4	210.7	117.7	86.6	68.5	53.3	41.8	131.0
1915-1919----------	1959	1,000.0	280.6	206.0	119.5	89.3	70.8	55.5	43.3	135.0
1916-1920----------	1960	1,000.0	267.9	202.5	122.0	92.0	73.0	57.9	45.0	139.7
1917-1921----------	1961	1,000.0	253.6	198.9	125.1	95.3	75.4	60.3	47.2	144.2
1918-1922----------	1962	1,000.0	242.7	192.9	127.6	98.7	78.3	61.9	49.7	148.2
1919-1923----------	1963	1,000.0	233.5	185.2	129.8	101.9	81.6	64.0	51.9	152.1
1920-1924----------	1964	1,000.0	226.3	175.3	131.3	105.4	85.3	66.2	54.1	156.1
1921-1925----------	1965	1,000.0	219.0	164.2	132.7	108.8	89.4	68.9	56.3	160.7
1922-1926----------	1966	1,000.0	211.7	152.5	133.8	111.9	93.1	71.9	58.8	166.3
1923-1927----------	1967	1,000.0	202.7	142.0	134.2	114.4	97.1	75.7	61.4	172.5
1924-1928----------	1968	1,000.0	195.2	131.8	133.4	117.6	100.5	79.2	64.2	178.1
1925-1929----------	1969	1,000.0	190.0	121.5	132.5	119.4	103.9	83.0	66.7	183.0
1926-1930----------	1970	1,000.0	188.3	111.5	130.6	121.6	106.5	85.8	69.2	186.5
1927-1931----------	1971	1,000.0	186.6	103.1	129.4	123.5	109.1	88.3	71.5	188.5
1928-1932----------	1972	1,000.0	182.5	97.2	129.7	126.8	111.5	90.3	73.5	188.5
1929-1933----------	1973	1,000.0	173.3	93.7	132.4	130.4	114.5	93.2	75.1	187.4
1930-1934----------	1974	1,000.0	161.2	92.7	136.0	135.7	117.4	95.6	77.0	184.4

TABLE 7C. DISTRIBUTIONS OF ALL OTHER WOMEN BY PARITY AS OF THE BEGINNING OF EACH YEAR 1917-74 BY AGE FOR GROUPS OF COHORTS FROM 1867-71 TO 1955-59--CON.

(BASED ON CUMULATIVE BIRTH RATES FOR GROUPS OF COHORTS)

EXACT AGE AND COHORT	AS OF JANUARY 1	TOTAL	PARITY							
			0	1	2	3	4	5	6	7 AND HIGHER
45-49 YEARS										
1868-1872----------	1917	1,000.0	173.9	109.6	89.5	79.2	76.0	59.5	65.5	346.8
1869-1873----------	1918	1,000.0	177.8	112.2	91.1	80.2	76.2	58.9	65.3	338.3
1870-1874----------	1919	1,000.0	181.8	115.3	92.2	81.0	76.7	56.8	66.1	330.1
1871-1875----------	1920	1,000.0	186.4	118.1	93.9	82.2	76.6	56.2	65.9	320.7
1872-1876----------	1921	1,000.0	191.1	120.8	95.6	83.4	76.7	55.8	65.9	310.7
1873-1877----------	1922	1,000.0	195.8	123.9	97.1	84.5	77.3	55.6	66.1	299.7
1874-1878----------	1923	1,000.0	200.2	127.3	98.4	85.5	77.9	55.8	65.8	289.1
1875-1879----------	1924	1,000.0	204.5	130.5	99.4	86.5	78.7	55.7	65.5	279.2
1876-1880----------	1925	1,000.0	208.3	134.0	99.6	87.5	80.0	55.0	65.0	270.6
1877-1881----------	1926	1,000.0	211.6	137.2	99.7	88.7	81.4	53.5	64.3	263.6
1878-1882----------	1927	1,000.0	214.2	140.7	99.4	90.0	82.9	50.8	63.8	258.2
1879-1883----------	1928	1,000.0	216.8	144.3	99.4	91.9	83.9	47.3	63.9	252.5
1880-1884----------	1929	1,000.0	219.9	147.8	99.6	94.2	84.9	43.9	64.0	245.7
1881-1885----------	1930	1,000.0	223.5	151.4	99.9	96.7	85.5	41.7	64.2	237.1
1882-1886----------	1931	1,000.0	226.8	155.4	100.9	97.9	86.5	42.0	63.9	226.6
1883-1887----------	1932	1,000.0	229.3	160.2	102.2	97.9	87.4	45.5	62.7	214.8
1884-1888----------	1933	1,000.0	231.5	164.9	103.5	96.7	89.3	48.8	61.6	203.7
1885-1889----------	1934	1,000.0	232.5	170.3	104.5	96.2	91.5	51.5	59.9	193.6
1886-1890----------	1935	1,000.0	232.2	175.9	105.9	96.8	93.4	52.6	58.1	185.1
1887-1891----------	1936	1,000.0	231.3	181.3	108.0	98.9	94.4	51.4	56.2	178.5
1888-1892----------	1937	1,000.0	229.8	186.2	111.1	102.8	94.6	47.8	54.5	173.2
1889-1893----------	1938	1,000.0	227.5	191.6	110.5	108.9	95.1	45.0	52.9	168.5
1890-1894----------	1939	1,000.0	224.8	198.3	111.4	112.8	94.5	42.5	50.7	165.0
1891-1895----------	1940	1,000.0	222.5	206.6	112.5	114.6	92.7	40.4	48.6	162.1
1892-1896----------	1941	1,000.0	221.0	216.8	112.8	114.4	90.2	39.2	46.4	159.2
1893-1897----------	1942	1,000.0	220.6	228.9	111.6	112.7	86.9	38.7	44.7	155.9
1894-1898----------	1943	1,000.0	223.9	237.7	114.2	107.6	82.4	38.1	43.1	153.0
1895-1899----------	1944	1,000.0	225.9	246.8	114.8	102.6	77.9	38.3	42.5	151.2
1896-1900----------	1945	1,000.0	227.6	254.9	114.3	97.5	74.3	39.0	42.6	149.8
1897-1901----------	1946	1,000.0	230.1	261.1	114.1	93.0	71.4	39.9	42.8	147.6
1898-1902----------	1947	1,000.0	234.2	265.2	114.6	88.9	69.0	40.9	42.5	144.7
1899-1903----------	1948	1,000.0	236.9	271.1	115.5	85.9	66.7	41.7	41.5	140.7
1900-1904----------	1949	1,000.0	242.7	274.3	116.7	83.2	64.7	42.4	40.3	135.7
1901-1905----------	1950	1,000.0	250.5	275.9	117.8	81.0	62.4	43.1	39.1	130.2
1902-1906----------	1951	1,000.0	258.8	276.8	117.7	78.7	60.7	43.5	38.0	125.8
1903-1907----------	1952	1,000.0	267.1	276.3	116.9	76.7	59.4	43.8	37.2	122.6
1904-1908----------	1953	1,000.0	275.2	274.9	115.6	74.8	58.8	43.8	36.6	120.3
1905-1909----------	1954	1,000.0	281.9	271.8	114.8	73.7	59.0	43.8	36.0	119.0
1906-1910----------	1955	1,000.0	287.5	266.7	114.6	73.2	60.1	43.6	35.6	118.7
1907-1911----------	1956	1,000.0	291.3	260.6	114.7	73.6	61.3	43.4	35.3	119.8
1908-1912----------	1957	1,000.0	294.4	253.5	115.2	74.3	62.3	43.0	36.0	121.3
1909-1913----------	1958	1,000.0	295.6	246.5	115.7	75.4	63.0	43.5	36.7	123.6
1910-1914----------	1959	1,000.0	296.6	239.0	116.3	76.5	63.7	44.4	38.0	125.5
1911-1915----------	1960	1,000.0	296.2	232.3	116.4	78.3	64.3	46.0	39.0	127.5
1912-1916----------	1961	1,000.0	296.0	224.6	116.3	80.3	65.1	48.2	39.9	129.6
1913-1917----------	1962	1,000.0	293.3	217.2	116.3	83.1	66.4	50.9	40.5	132.3
1914-1918----------	1963	1,000.0	288.7	210.1	116.9	85.8	68.2	53.3	41.4	135.6
1915-1919----------	1964	1,000.0	278.9	205.5	118.5	88.6	70.3	55.6	42.8	139.8
1916-1920----------	1965	1,000.0	266.3	202.0	120.9	91.2	72.6	57.7	44.9	144.4
1917-1921----------	1966	1,000.0	252.2	198.1	124.1	94.5	75.1	60.0	47.2	148.8
1918-1922----------	1967	1,000.0	241.4	192.1	126.6	98.0	77.7	61.9	49.6	152.7
1919-1923----------	1968	1,000.0	232.2	184.4	128.8	101.2	81.2	63.9	52.0	156.3
1920-1924----------	1969	1,000.0	225.1	174.6	130.2	104.7	85.0	66.0	54.2	160.2
1921-1925----------	1970	1,000.0	217.8	163.4	131.8	108.2	89.1	68.7	56.3	164.7
1922-1926----------	1971	1,000.0	210.6	151.8	132.8	111.4	92.9	71.7	58.8	170.0
1923-1927----------	1972	1,000.0	201.6	141.2	133.5	114.0	96.9	75.4	61.3	176.1
1924-1928----------	1973	1,000.0	194.1	131.1	132.9	117.0	100.3	79.1	64.2	181.3
1925-1929----------	1974	1,000.0	188.9	120.9	132.0	118.7	103.8	83.0	66.8	185.9

TABLE 7C. DISTRIBUTIONS OF ALL OTHER WOMEN BY PARITY AS OF THE BEGINNING OF EACH YEAR 1917-74 BY AGE FOR GROUPS OF COHORTS FROM 1867-71 TO 1955-59--CON.

(BASED ON CUMULATIVE BIRTH RATES FOR GROUPS OF COHORTS)

EXACT AGE AND COHORT	AS OF JANUARY 1	TOTAL	PARITY							
			0	1	2	3	4	5	6	7 AND HIGHER
50-54 YEARS										
1863-1867----------	1917	---	---	---	---	---	---	---	---	---
1864-1868----------	1918	---	---	---	---	---	---	---	---	---
1865-1869----------	1919	---	---	---	---	---	---	---	---	---
1866-1870----------	1920	---	---	---	---	---	---	---	---	---
1867-1871----------	1921	1,000.0	169.3	107.2	87.9	77.7	75.7	59.1	65.4	357.7
1868-1872----------	1922	1,000.0	172.9	109.9	89.1	78.7	76.2	58.2	65.4	349.6
1869-1873----------	1923	1,000.0	176.9	112.6	90.4	79.7	76.4	57.3	65.5	341.2
1870-1874----------	1924	1,000.0	181.1	115.4	91.9	80.9	76.4	56.6	65.4	332.3
1871-1875----------	1925	1,000.0	185.7	118.2	93.6	82.0	76.4	56.1	65.3	322.7
1872-1876----------	1926	1,000.0	190.4	121.2	95.2	83.2	76.5	55.7	65.5	312.3
1873-1877----------	1927	1,000.0	195.1	124.2	96.8	84.4	76.9	55.5	65.6	301.5
1874-1878----------	1928	1,000.0	199.6	127.4	98.2	85.4	77.6	55.5	65.5	290.8
1875-1879----------	1929	1,000.0	203.9	130.6	99.1	86.4	78.6	55.5	65.2	280.7
1876-1880----------	1930	1,000.0	207.7	134.0	99.5	87.4	79.9	54.7	64.8	272.0
1877-1881----------	1931	1,000.0	210.9	137.5	99.4	88.6	81.2	53.1	64.3	265.0
1878-1882----------	1932	1,000.0	213.7	140.8	99.4	89.7	82.7	50.5	63.8	259.4
1879-1883----------	1933	1,000.0	216.4	144.3	99.5	91.6	83.6	47.0	63.8	253.8
1880-1884----------	1934	1,000.0	219.6	147.8	99.4	94.1	84.6	43.6	64.0	246.9
1881-1885----------	1935	1,000.0	223.1	151.5	99.8	96.5	85.3	41.5	64.1	238.2
1882-1886----------	1936	1,000.0	226.4	155.6	100.6	97.8	86.3	41.8	63.9	227.6
1883-1887----------	1937	1,000.0	229.0	160.3	102.0	97.7	87.4	45.1	62.7	215.8
1884-1888----------	1938	1,000.0	231.1	165.0	103.4	96.5	89.4	48.4	61.6	204.6
1885-1889----------	1939	1,000.0	232.1	170.4	104.4	96.1	91.4	51.2	59.9	194.5
1886-1890----------	1940	1,000.0	231.9	175.9	105.9	96.6	93.3	52.4	58.0	186.0
1887-1891----------	1941	1,000.0	231.0	181.3	108.0	98.8	94.3	51.2	56.0	179.4
1888-1892----------	1942	1,000.0	229.5	186.3	111.0	102.7	94.5	47.6	54.3	174.1
1889-1893----------	1943	1,000.0	227.3	191.6	110.4	108.8	95.1	44.9	52.6	169.3
1890-1894----------	1944	1,000.0	224.6	198.4	111.3	112.7	94.4	42.4	50.5	165.7
1891-1895----------	1945	1,000.0	222.3	206.7	112.4	114.5	92.6	40.4	48.4	162.7
1892-1896----------	1946	1,000.0	220.9	216.8	112.8	114.3	90.0	39.2	46.3	159.7
1893-1897----------	1947	1,000.0	220.5	228.9	111.6	112.6	86.8	38.6	44.6	156.4
1894-1898----------	1948	1,000.0	223.8	237.7	114.1	107.6	82.3	38.0	43.0	153.5
1895-1899----------	1949	1,000.0	225.7	246.9	114.7	102.6	77.8	38.2	42.4	151.7
1896-1900----------	1950	1,000.0	227.4	255.0	114.1	97.5	74.3	38.8	42.6	150.3
1897-1901----------	1951	1,000.0	229.8	261.3	113.9	93.0	71.3	39.9	42.8	148.0
1898-1902----------	1952	1,000.0	234.0	265.2	114.5	89.0	68.9	40.8	42.5	145.1
1899-1903----------	1953	1,000.0	236.8	271.0	115.5	85.9	66.6	41.7	41.5	141.0
1900-1904----------	1954	1,000.0	242.7	274.2	116.6	83.2	64.6	42.4	40.3	136.0
1901-1905----------	1955	1,000.0	250.4	275.9	117.8	81.0	62.3	43.0	39.1	130.5
1902-1906----------	1956	1,000.0	258.7	276.7	117.8	78.6	60.7	43.4	38.0	126.1
1903-1907----------	1957	1,000.0	267.0	276.4	116.8	76.6	59.4	43.8	37.2	122.8
1904-1908----------	1958	1,000.0	275.1	274.9	115.5	74.8	58.8	43.7	36.7	120.5
1905-1909----------	1959	1,000.0	281.8	271.8	114.7	73.6	59.1	43.7	36.1	119.2
1906-1910----------	1960	1,000.0	287.5	266.6	114.5	73.2	60.1	43.5	35.6	119.0
1907-1911----------	1961	1,000.0	291.2	260.6	114.6	73.6	61.3	43.3	35.4	120.0
1908-1912----------	1962	1,000.0	294.3	253.5	115.2	74.3	62.2	42.9	36.0	121.6
1909-1913----------	1963	1,000.0	295.4	246.6	115.7	75.3	63.0	43.4	36.8	123.8
1910-1914----------	1964	1,000.0	296.4	239.1	116.3	76.5	63.6	44.3	38.0	125.8
1911-1915----------	1965	1,000.0	296.1	232.4	116.3	78.3	64.1	46.1	38.9	127.8
1912-1916----------	1966	1,000.0	296.0	224.6	116.3	80.2	64.9	48.2	40.0	129.8
1913-1917----------	1967	1,000.0	293.2	217.2	116.3	83.1	66.2	50.9	40.6	132.5
1914-1918----------	1968	1,000.0	288.6	210.1	117.0	85.7	68.0	53.4	41.4	135.8
1915-1919----------	1969	1,000.0	278.8	205.5	118.5	88.6	70.1	55.7	42.8	140.0
1916-1920----------	1970	1,000.0	266.2	202.0	120.9	91.2	72.5	57.8	44.9	144.5
1917-1921----------	1971	1,000.0	252.1	198.2	124.0	94.5	75.0	60.0	47.3	148.9
1918-1922----------	1972	1,000.0	241.3	192.2	126.5	98.0	77.6	62.0	49.6	152.8
1919-1923----------	1973	1,000.0	232.1	184.5	128.7	101.2	81.1	63.9	52.0	156.5
1920-1924----------	1974	1,000.0	225.0	174.7	130.1	104.7	85.0	66.0	54.1	160.4

TABLE 8A. DISTRIBUTIONS OF ALL WOMEN BY PARITY AS OF THE BEGINNING OF EACH YEAR 1917-74 BY AGE FOR EACH COHORT FROM 1867 TO 1959

(BASED ON CUMULATIVE BIRTH RATES)

EXACT AGE AND COHORT	AS OF JANUARY 1	TOTAL	PARITY							
			0	1	2	3	4	5	6	7 AND HIGHER
15 YEARS										
1902---------------	1917	1,000.0	996.6	3.4	*	*	*	*	*	*
1903---------------	1918	1,000.0	996.5	3.5	*	*	*	*	*	*
1904---------------	1919	1,000.0	996.4	3.6	*	*	*	*	*	*
1905---------------	1920	1,000.0	997.0	3.0	*	*	*	*	*	*
1906---------------	1921	1,000.0	996.4	3.6	*	*	*	*	*	*
1907---------------	1922	1,000.0	996.2	3.8	*	*	*	*	*	*
1908---------------	1923	1,000.0	996.6	3.4	*	*	*	*	*	*
1909---------------	1924	1,000.0	996.5	3.5	*	*	*	*	*	*
1910---------------	1925	1,000.0	996.3	3.7	*	*	*	*	*	*
1911---------------	1926	1,000.0	996.1	3.9	*	*	*	*	*	*
1912---------------	1927	1,000.0	996.1	3.9	*	*	*	*	*	*
1913---------------	1928	1,000.0	995.9	4.1	*	*	*	*	*	*
1914---------------	1929	1,000.0	996.3	3.7	*	*	*	*	*	*
1915---------------	1930	1,000.0	996.3	3.7	*	*	*	*	*	*
1916---------------	1931	1,000.0	996.2	3.8	*	*	*	*	*	*
1917---------------	1932	1,000.0	996.5	3.5	*	*	*	*	*	*
1918---------------	1933	1,000.0	996.7	3.3	*	*	*	*	*	*
1919---------------	1934	1,000.0	996.8	3.2	*	*	*	*	*	*
1920---------------	1935	1,000.0	996.6	3.4	*	*	*	*	*	*
1921---------------	1936	1,000.0	996.3	3.7	*	*	*	*	*	*
1922---------------	1937	1,000.0	996.5	3.5	*	*	*	*	*	*
1923---------------	1938	1,000.0	996.3	3.7	*	*	*	*	*	*
1924---------------	1939	1,000.0	996.2	3.8	*	*	*	*	*	*
1925---------------	1940	1,000.0	996.3	3.7	*	*	*	*	*	*
1926---------------	1941	1,000.0	996.2	3.8	*	*	*	*	*	*
1927---------------	1942	1,000.0	995.9	4.1	*	*	*	*	*	*
1928---------------	1943	1,000.0	995.9	4.1	*	*	*	*	*	*
1929---------------	1944	1,000.0	995.8	4.2	*	*	*	*	*	*
1930---------------	1945	1,000.0	996.2	3.8	*	*	*	*	*	*
1931---------------	1946	1,000.0	996.1	3.9	*	*	*	*	*	*
1932---------------	1947	1,000.0	996.2	3.8	*	*	*	*	*	*
1933---------------	1948	1,000.0	994.8	5.2	*	*	*	*	*	*
1934---------------	1949	1,000.0	994.2	5.8	*	*	*	*	*	*
1935---------------	1950	1,000.0	994.3	5.7	*	*	*	*	*	*
1936---------------	1951	1,000.0	994.2	5.8	*	*	*	*	*	*
1937---------------	1952	1,000.0	994.0	6.0	*	*	*	*	*	*
1938---------------	1953	1,000.0	994.3	5.7	*	*	*	*	*	*
1939---------------	1954	1,000.0	994.2	5.8	*	*	*	*	*	*
1940---------------	1955	1,000.0	993.7	6.3	*	*	*	*	*	*
1941---------------	1956	1,000.0	993.9	6.1	*	*	*	*	*	*
1942---------------	1957	1,000.0	993.8	6.2	*	*	*	*	*	*
1943---------------	1958	1,000.0	993.9	6.1	*	*	*	*	*	*
1944---------------	1959	1,000.0	994.2	5.8	*	*	*	*	*	*
1945---------------	1960	1,000.0	994.0	6.0	*	*	*	*	*	*
1946---------------	1961	1,000.0	994.0	6.0	*	*	*	*	*	*
1947---------------	1962	1,000.0	994.5	5.5	*	*	*	*	*	*
1948---------------	1963	1,000.0	994.9	5.1	*	*	*	*	*	*
1949---------------	1964	1,000.0	994.9	5.1	*	*	*	*	*	*
1950---------------	1965	1,000.0	994.8	5.2	*	*	*	*	*	*
1951---------------	1966	1,000.0	994.8	5.2	*	*	*	*	*	*
1952---------------	1967	1,000.0	994.7	5.3	*	*	*	*	*	*
1953---------------	1968	1,000.0	994.7	5.3	*	*	*	*	*	*
1954---------------	1969	1,000.0	994.3	5.7	*	*	*	*	*	*
1955---------------	1970	1,000.0	994.0	6.0	*	*	*	*	*	*
1956---------------	1971	1,000.0	993.4	6.6	*	*	*	*	*	*
1957---------------	1972	1,000.0	993.3	6.7	*	*	*	*	*	*
1958---------------	1973	1,000.0	992.9	7.1	*	*	*	*	*	*
1959---------------	1974	1,000.0	992.6	7.4	*	*	*	*	*	*

TABLE 8A. DISTRIBUTIONS OF ALL WOMEN BY PARITY AS OF THE BEGINNING OF EACH YEAR 1917-74 BY AGE FOR EACH COHORT FROM 1867 TO 1959--CON.

(BASED ON CUMULATIVE BIRTH RATES)

EXACT AGE AND COHORT	AS OF JANUARY 1	TOTAL	PARITY							
			0	1	2	3	4	5	6	7 AND HIGHER
16 YEARS										
1901	1917	1,000.0	986.1	13.4	0.5	0.0	0.0	*	*	*
1902	1918	1,000.0	985.7	13.7	0.6	0.0	0.0	*	*	*
1903	1919	1,000.0	985.6	13.9	0.5	0.0	0.0	*	*	*
1904	1920	1,000.0	987.1	12.4	0.5	0.0	0.0	*	*	*
1905	1921	1,000.0	985.5	14.0	0.5	0.0	0.0	*	*	*
1906	1922	1,000.0	984.3	15.1	0.6	0.0	0.0	*	*	*
1907	1923	1,000.0	985.6	13.8	0.6	0.0	0.0	*	*	*
1908	1924	1,000.0	985.8	13.6	0.6	0.0	0.0	*	*	*
1909	1925	1,000.0	985.0	14.4	0.6	0.0	0.0	*	*	*
1910	1926	1,000.0	984.5	14.9	0.6	0.0	0.0	*	*	*
1911	1927	1,000.0	984.3	15.0	0.7	0.0	0.0	*	*	*
1912	1928	1,000.0	983.9	15.4	0.7	0.0	0.0	*	*	*
1913	1929	1,000.0	984.6	14.7	0.7	0.0	0.0	*	*	*
1914	1930	1,000.0	985.2	14.2	0.6	0.0	0.0	*	*	*
1915	1931	1,000.0	984.9	14.5	0.6	0.0	0.0	*	*	*
1916	1932	1,000.0	985.6	13.8	0.6	0.0	0.0	*	*	*
1917	1933	1,000.0	986.3	13.1	0.6	0.0	0.0	*	*	*
1918	1934	1,000.0	987.3	12.2	0.5	0.0	0.0	*	*	*
1919	1935	1,000.0	986.9	12.6	0.5	0.0	0.0	*	*	*
1920	1936	1,000.0	985.9	13.5	0.6	0.0	0.0	*	*	*
1921	1937	1,000.0	985.7	13.6	0.7	0.0	0.0	*	*	*
1922	1938	1,000.0	985.5	13.8	0.7	0.0	0.0	*	*	*
1923	1939	1,000.0	985.1	14.2	0.7	0.0	0.0	*	*	*
1924	1940	1,000.0	985.5	13.8	0.7	0.0	0.0	*	*	*
1925	1941	1,000.0	985.4	13.7	0.8	0.1	0.0	*	*	*
1926	1942	1,000.0	984.5	14.6	0.8	0.1	0.0	*	*	*
1927	1943	1,000.0	984.0	14.7	1.2	0.1	0.0	*	*	*
1928	1944	1,000.0	983.9	14.8	1.2	0.1	0.0	*	*	*
1929	1945	1,000.0	985.1	13.7	1.1	0.1	0.0	*	*	*
1930	1946	1,000.0	985.7	13.1	1.1	0.1	0.0	*	*	*
1931	1947	1,000.0	985.3	13.4	1.2	0.1	0.0	*	*	*
1932	1948	1,000.0	981.5	17.0	1.4	0.1	0.0	*	*	*
1933	1949	1,000.0	978.5	19.7	1.6	0.2	0.0	*	*	*
1934	1950	1,000.0	977.7	20.2	1.9	0.2	0.0	*	*	*
1935	1951	1,000.0	977.7	20.3	1.8	0.2	0.0	*	*	*
1936	1952	1,000.0	977.0	21.0	1.8	0.2	0.0	*	*	*
1937	1953	1,000.0	977.2	20.9	1.7	0.2	0.0	*	*	*
1938	1954	1,000.0	977.2	21.0	1.6	0.2	0.0	*	*	*
1939	1955	1,000.0	976.3	21.7	1.8	0.2	0.0	*	*	*
1940	1956	1,000.0	976.1	21.8	1.9	0.2	0.0	*	*	*
1941	1957	1,000.0	975.4	22.4	2.0	0.2	0.0	*	*	*
1942	1958	1,000.0	975.3	22.6	1.9	0.2	0.0	*	*	*
1943	1959	1,000.0	976.7	21.2	1.9	0.2	0.0	*	*	*
1944	1960	1,000.0	977.1	20.9	1.8	0.2	0.0	*	*	*
1945	1961	1,000.0	977.1	20.8	1.9	0.2	0.0	*	*	*
1946	1962	1,000.0	977.5	20.4	1.9	0.2	0.0	*	*	*
1947	1963	1,000.0	979.3	18.7	1.8	0.2	0.0	*	*	*
1948	1964	1,000.0	980.2	18.0	1.6	0.2	0.0	*	*	*
1949	1965	1,000.0	980.2	18.0	1.6	0.2	0.0	*	*	*
1950	1966	1,000.0	980.2	18.1	1.5	0.2	0.0	*	*	*
1951	1967	1,000.0	980.1	18.3	1.5	0.1	0.0	*	*	*
1952	1968	1,000.0	979.9	18.5	1.5	0.1	0.0	*	*	*
1953	1969	1,000.0	979.5	19.1	1.3	0.1	0.0	*	*	*
1954	1970	1,000.0	978.4	20.2	1.3	0.1	0.0	*	*	*
1955	1971	1,000.0	976.4	22.1	1.4	0.1	0.0	*	*	*
1956	1972	1,000.0	975.8	22.7	1.4	0.1	0.0	*	*	*
1957	1973	1,000.0	974.7	23.9	1.3	0.1	0.0	*	*	*
1958	1974	1,000.0	974.1	24.6	1.2	0.1	0.0	*	*	*

TABLE 8A. DISTRIBUTIONS OF ALL WOMEN BY PARITY AS OF THE BEGINNING OF EACH YEAR 1917-74 BY AGE FOR EACH COHORT FROM 1867 TO 1959--CON.

(BASED ON CUMULATIVE BIRTH RATES)

EXACT AGE AND COHORT	AS OF JANUARY 1	TOTAL	PARITY							
			0	1	2	3	4	5	6	7 AND HIGHER
17 YEARS										
1900---------------	1917	1,000.0	962.6	34.4	2.8	0.2	0.0	*	*	*
1901---------------	1918	1,000.0	961.7	35.4	2.7	0.2	0.0	*	*	*
1902---------------	1919	1,000.0	961.7	35.4	2.7	0.2	0.0	*	*	*
1903---------------	1920	1,000.0	964.5	32.7	2.6	0.2	0.0	*	*	*
1904---------------	1921	1,000.0	960.6	36.6	2.6	0.2	0.0	*	*	*
1905---------------	1922	1,000.0	957.7	39.3	2.8	0.2	0.0	*	*	*
1906---------------	1923	1,000.0	959.9	36.9	3.0	0.2	0.0	*	*	*
1907---------------	1924	1,000.0	961.2	35.5	3.1	0.2	0.0	*	*	*
1908---------------	1925	1,000.0	959.7	37.1	3.0	0.2	0.0	*	*	*
1909---------------	1926	1,000.0	958.5	38.1	3.2	0.2	0.0	*	*	*
1910---------------	1927	1,000.0	958.9	37.6	3.3	0.2	0.0	*	*	*
1911---------------	1928	1,000.0	958.0	38.3	3.5	0.2	0.0	*	*	*
1912---------------	1929	1,000.0	959.2	37.3	3.3	0.2	0.0	*	*	*
1913---------------	1930	1,000.0	960.3	36.3	3.2	0.2	0.0	*	*	*
1914---------------	1931	1,000.0	960.2	36.6	3.0	0.2	0.0	*	*	*
1915---------------	1932	1,000.0	961.5	35.4	2.9	0.2	0.0	*	*	*
1916---------------	1933	1,000.0	963.2	33.8	2.8	0.2	0.0	*	*	*
1917---------------	1934	1,000.0	965.7	31.5	2.6	0.2	0.0	*	*	*
1918---------------	1935	1,000.0	965.5	31.8	2.5	0.2	0.0	*	*	*
1919---------------	1936	1,000.0	964.2	33.0	2.6	0.2	0.0	*	*	*
1920---------------	1937	1,000.0	963.6	33.3	2.9	0.2	0.0	*	*	*
1921---------------	1938	1,000.0	961.8	34.7	3.3	0.2	0.0	*	*	*
1922---------------	1939	1,000.0	961.3	35.2	3.3	0.2	0.0	*	*	*
1923---------------	1940	1,000.0	962.3	34.2	3.3	0.2	0.0	*	*	*
1924---------------	1941	1,000.0	962.8	33.3	3.6	0.3	0.0	*	*	*
1925---------------	1942	1,000.0	961.0	34.8	3.8	0.4	0.0	*	*	*
1926---------------	1943	1,000.0	959.5	35.8	4.2	0.5	0.0	*	*	*
1927---------------	1944	1,000.0	958.9	35.7	4.8	0.6	0.0	*	*	*
1928---------------	1945	1,000.0	961.9	33.1	4.5	0.5	0.0	*	*	*
1929---------------	1946	1,000.0	963.8	31.5	4.2	0.5	0.0	*	*	*
1930---------------	1947	1,000.0	963.1	32.1	4.3	0.5	0.0	*	*	*
1931---------------	1948	1,000.0	953.0	41.3	5.1	0.6	0.0	*	*	*
1932---------------	1949	1,000.0	947.3	45.8	6.2	0.7	0.0	*	*	*
1933---------------	1950	1,000.0	944.4	47.4	7.3	0.8	0.1	*	*	*
1934---------------	1951	1,000.0	943.6	47.8	7.7	0.8	0.1	*	*	*
1935---------------	1952	1,000.0	941.8	49.6	7.6	0.9	0.1	*	*	*
1936---------------	1953	1,000.0	941.8	49.8	7.4	0.9	0.1	*	*	*
1937---------------	1954	1,000.0	941.0	50.7	7.3	0.9	0.1	*	*	*
1938---------------	1955	1,000.0	940.2	51.3	7.5	0.9	0.1	*	*	*
1939---------------	1956	1,000.0	939.5	51.5	8.0	0.9	0.1	*	*	*
1940---------------	1957	1,000.0	937.6	53.0	8.3	1.0	0.1	*	*	*
1941---------------	1958	1,000.0	936.0	54.3	8.6	1.0	0.1	*	*	*
1942---------------	1959	1,000.0	938.4	52.0	8.5	1.0	0.1	*	*	*
1943---------------	1960	1,000.0	941.0	49.8	8.1	1.0	0.1	*	*	*
1944---------------	1961	1,000.0	942.5	48.5	7.9	1.0	0.1	*	*	*
1945---------------	1962	1,000.0	942.8	48.1	8.0	1.0	0.1	*	*	*
1946---------------	1963	1,000.0	945.1	45.9	7.9	1.0	0.1	*	*	*
1947---------------	1964	1,000.0	947.9	43.8	7.3	0.9	0.1	*	*	*
1948---------------	1965	1,000.0	949.7	42.8	6.6	0.8	0.1	*	*	*
1949---------------	1966	1,000.0	950.3	42.6	6.2	0.8	0.1	*	*	*
1950---------------	1967	1,000.0	950.3	43.0	5.9	0.8	0.0	*	*	*
1951---------------	1968	1,000.0	950.4	43.0	5.9	0.7	0.0	*	*	*
1952---------------	1969	1,000.0	949.7	44.2	5.5	0.6	0.0	*	*	*
1953---------------	1970	1,000.0	948.6	45.6	5.2	0.6	0.0	*	*	*
1954---------------	1971	1,000.0	944.7	49.3	5.4	0.6	0.0	*	*	*
1955---------------	1972	1,000.0	943.0	51.0	5.5	0.5	0.0	*	*	*
1956---------------	1973	1,000.0	941.1	53.2	5.2	0.5	0.0	*	*	*
1957---------------	1974	1,000.0	940.3	54.2	5.1	0.4	0.0	*	*	*

TABLE 8A. DISTRIBUTIONS OF ALL WOMEN BY PARITY AS OF THE BEGINNING OF EACH YEAR 1917-74 BY AGE FOR EACH COHORT FROM 1867 TO 1959--CON.

(BASED ON CUMULATIVE BIRTH RATES)

EXACT AGE AND COHORT	AS OF JANUARY 1	TOTAL	PARITY							
			0	1	2	3	4	5	6	7 AND HIGHER
18 YEARS										
1899----------------	1917	1,000.0	919.0	70.0	10.0	0.9	0.1	*	*	*
1900----------------	1918	1,000.0	917.0	72.3	9.7	0.9	0.1	*	*	*
1901----------------	1919	1,000.0	917.6	72.1	9.3	0.9	0.1	*	*	*
1902----------------	1920	1,000.0	923.1	66.8	9.1	0.9	0.1	*	*	*
1903----------------	1921	1,000.0	914.9	75.0	9.1	0.9	0.1	*	*	*
1904----------------	1922	1,000.0	908.0	81.0	9.9	1.0	0.1	*	*	*
1905----------------	1923	1,000.0	911.5	77.0	10.5	0.9	0.1	*	*	*
1906----------------	1924	1,000.0	913.8	74.3	10.7	1.1	0.1	*	*	*
1907----------------	1925	1,000.0	912.1	76.3	10.4	1.1	0.1	*	*	*
1908----------------	1926	1,000.0	911.0	77.3	10.6	1.0	0.1	*	*	*
1909----------------	1927	1,000.0	911.3	76.5	11.0	1.1	0.1	*	*	*
1910----------------	1928	1,000.0	912.3	75.4	11.1	1.1	0.1	*	*	*
1911----------------	1929	1,000.0	913.4	74.6	10.8	1.1	0.1	*	*	*
1912----------------	1930	1,000.0	915.9	72.5	10.5	1.0	0.1	*	*	*
1913----------------	1931	1,000.0	915.6	73.0	10.3	1.0	0.1	*	*	*
1914----------------	1932	1,000.0	918.8	70.4	9.8	0.9	0.1	*	*	*
1915----------------	1933	1,000.0	921.4	68.2	9.4	0.9	0.1	*	*	*
1916----------------	1934	1,000.0	926.3	64.0	8.8	0.8	0.1	*	*	*
1917----------------	1935	1,000.0	926.5	64.1	8.5	0.8	0.1	*	*	*
1918----------------	1936	1,000.0	925.5	65.2	8.4	0.8	0.1	*	*	*
1919----------------	1937	1,000.0	925.1	65.0	8.9	0.9	0.1	*	*	*
1920----------------	1938	1,000.0	922.2	67.2	9.6	0.9	0.1	*	*	*
1921----------------	1939	1,000.0	918.8	69.9	10.2	1.0	0.1	*	*	*
1922----------------	1940	1,000.0	921.1	67.6	10.1	1.1	0.1	*	*	*
1923----------------	1941	1,000.0	923.1	64.8	10.6	1.3	0.2	*	*	*
1924----------------	1942	1,000.0	921.0	66.3	11.1	1.4	0.2	*	*	*
1925----------------	1943	1,000.0	916.9	69.6	11.7	1.6	0.2	*	*	*
1926----------------	1944	1,000.0	915.4	70.1	12.5	1.8	0.2	*	*	*
1927----------------	1945	1,000.0	920.3	65.4	12.2	1.9	0.2	*	*	*
1928----------------	1946	1,000.0	925.2	61.6	11.4	1.6	0.2	*	*	*
1929----------------	1947	1,000.0	922.2	64.4	11.6	1.6	0.2	*	*	*
1930----------------	1948	1,000.0	904.6	80.5	12.9	1.8	0.2	*	*	*
1931----------------	1949	1,000.0	893.2	88.4	16.0	2.2	0.2	*	*	*
1932----------------	1950	1,000.0	889.4	88.9	18.7	2.7	0.3	*	*	*
1933----------------	1951	1,000.0	887.4	89.1	20.2	2.9	0.4	*	*	*
1934----------------	1952	1,000.0	882.4	93.1	20.9	3.1	0.5	*	*	*
1935----------------	1953	1,000.0	881.8	93.6	20.9	3.3	0.4	*	*	*
1936----------------	1954	1,000.0	880.0	95.1	21.1	3.3	0.5	*	*	*
1937----------------	1955	1,000.0	878.1	97.0	21.1	3.3	0.5	*	*	*
1938----------------	1956	1,000.0	878.2	96.2	21.8	3.3	0.5	*	*	*
1939----------------	1957	1,000.0	874.0	98.8	23.1	3.6	0.5	*	*	*
1940----------------	1958	1,000.0	870.5	101.5	23.7	3.8	0.5	*	*	*
1941----------------	1959	1,000.0	872.2	99.2	24.3	3.8	0.5	*	*	*
1942----------------	1960	1,000.0	876.7	95.4	23.5	3.9	0.5	*	*	*
1943----------------	1961	1,000.0	882.0	91.1	22.7	3.7	0.5	*	*	*
1944----------------	1962	1,000.0	884.1	89.8	21.8	3.8	0.5	*	*	*
1945----------------	1963	1,000.0	886.9	87.2	21.6	3.8	0.5	*	*	*
1946----------------	1964	1,000.0	890.6	84.7	20.8	3.4	0.5	*	*	*
1947----------------	1965	1,000.0	895.2	82.2	18.9	3.2	0.5	*	*	*
1948----------------	1966	1,000.0	898.5	81.4	16.9	2.8	0.4	*	*	*
1949----------------	1967	1,000.0	899.6	81.5	16.0	2.5	0.4	*	*	*
1950----------------	1968	1,000.0	900.5	81.4	15.5	2.4	0.2	*	*	*
1951----------------	1969	1,000.0	900.2	82.7	14.7	2.2	0.2	*	*	*
1952----------------	1970	1,000.0	898.6	85.0	14.3	1.9	0.2	*	*	*
1953----------------	1971	1,000.0	894.2	89.5	14.2	1.9	0.2	*	*	*
1954----------------	1972	1,000.0	892.2	91.6	14.2	1.9	0.1	*	*	*
1955----------------	1973	1,000.0	890.3	94.2	13.8	1.6	0.1	*	*	*
1956----------------	1974	1,000.0	889.9	95.3	13.2	1.5	0.1	*	*	*

TABLE 8A. DISTRIBUTIONS OF ALL WOMEN BY PARITY AS OF THE BEGINNING OF EACH YEAR 1917-74 BY AGE FOR EACH COHORT FROM 1867 TO 1959--CON.

(BASED ON CUMULATIVE BIRTH RATES)

EXACT AGE AND COHORT	AS OF JANUARY 1	TOTAL	PARITY 0	1	2	3	4	5	6	7 AND HIGHER
19 YEARS										
1898---------------	1917	1,000.0	856.9	114.2	25.1	3.4	0.4	*	*	*
1899---------------	1918	1,000.0	853.3	118.2	24.8	3.3	0.4	*	*	*
1900---------------	1919	1,000.0	853.1	119.1	24.1	3.3	0.4	*	*	*
1901---------------	1920	1,000.0	862.7	111.0	22.8	3.1	0.4	*	*	*
1902---------------	1921	1,000.0	851.8	121.8	22.8	3.2	0.4	*	*	*
1903---------------	1922	1,000.0	838.0	133.3	24.8	3.5	0.4	*	*	*
1904---------------	1923	1,000.0	840.1	129.3	26.8	3.3	0.5	*	*	*
1905---------------	1924	1,000.0	844.1	124.4	27.3	3.6	0.6	*	*	*
1906---------------	1925	1,000.0	841.8	127.3	26.5	3.8	0.6	*	*	*
1907---------------	1926	1,000.0	842.3	127.4	26.0	3.7	0.6	*	*	*
1908---------------	1927	1,000.0	843.6	125.7	26.5	3.6	0.6	*	*	*
1909---------------	1928	1,000.0	845.7	123.3	26.7	3.8	0.5	*	*	*
1910---------------	1929	1,000.0	849.4	120.8	25.6	3.7	0.5	*	*	*
1911---------------	1930	1,000.0	853.2	117.7	25.1	3.5	0.5	*	*	*
1912---------------	1931	1,000.0	853.6	117.9	24.7	3.3	0.5	*	*	*
1913---------------	1932	1,000.0	857.5	114.8	24.0	3.2	0.5	*	*	*
1914---------------	1933	1,000.0	862.6	110.8	23.1	3.1	0.4	*	*	*
1915---------------	1934	1,000.0	869.2	105.9	21.6	2.9	0.4	*	*	*
1916---------------	1935	1,000.0	870.6	105.5	20.7	2.8	0.4	*	*	*
1917---------------	1936	1,000.0	870.0	106.5	20.3	2.8	0.4	*	*	*
1918---------------	1937	1,000.0	870.9	105.2	20.7	2.8	0.4	*	*	*
1919---------------	1938	1,000.0	867.8	107.0	21.8	3.0	0.4	*	*	*
1920---------------	1939	1,000.0	862.9	110.7	22.8	3.1	0.5	*	*	*
1921---------------	1940	1,000.0	862.1	110.2	23.7	3.5	0.5	*	*	*
1922---------------	1941	1,000.0	866.5	104.3	24.3	4.2	0.7	*	*	*
1923---------------	1942	1,000.0	865.2	104.7	24.9	4.4	0.8	*	*	*
1924---------------	1943	1,000.0	856.4	112.8	25.5	4.5	0.8	*	*	*
1925---------------	1944	1,000.0	852.8	114.8	26.8	4.8	0.8	*	*	*
1926---------------	1945	1,000.0	859.6	109.0	25.7	4.9	0.8	*	*	*
1927---------------	1946	1,000.0	867.1	103.3	24.3	4.5	0.8	*	*	*
1928---------------	1947	1,000.0	861.9	108.1	24.9	4.3	0.8	*	*	*
1929---------------	1948	1,000.0	834.3	132.8	27.5	4.6	0.8	*	*	*
1930---------------	1949	1,000.0	819.8	141.1	32.9	5.4	0.8	*	*	*
1931---------------	1950	1,000.0	812.0	141.7	38.4	6.8	1.1	*	*	*
1932---------------	1951	1,000.0	811.2	138.5	41.3	7.8	1.2	*	*	*
1933---------------	1952	1,000.0	801.6	145.2	43.3	8.4	1.5	*	*	*
1934---------------	1953	1,000.0	798.2	147.0	44.3	8.8	1.7	*	*	*
1935---------------	1954	1,000.0	795.0	149.0	45.2	9.2	1.6	*	*	*
1936---------------	1955	1,000.0	790.9	152.4	45.5	9.4	1.8	*	*	*
1937---------------	1956	1,000.0	790.0	152.1	46.7	9.4	1.8	*	*	*
1938---------------	1957	1,000.0	785.7	154.0	48.6	9.8	1.9	*	*	*
1939---------------	1958	1,000.0	778.8	158.4	50.5	10.3	2.0	*	*	*
1940---------------	1959	1,000.0	778.6	157.1	51.6	10.7	2.0	*	*	*
1941---------------	1960	1,000.0	782.4	153.1	51.3	11.2	2.0	*	*	*
1942---------------	1961	1,000.0	790.3	147.1	49.7	10.8	2.1	*	*	*
1943---------------	1962	1,000.0	797.4	142.9	47.3	10.4	2.0	*	*	*
1944---------------	1963	1,000.0	802.5	139.6	45.8	10.2	1.9	*	*	*
1945---------------	1964	1,000.0	806.7	137.4	44.2	9.8	1.9	*	*	*
1946---------------	1965	1,000.0	813.0	134.7	41.5	9.0	1.8	*	*	*
1947---------------	1966	1,000.0	821.1	132.0	37.4	7.8	1.7	*	*	*
1948---------------	1967	1,000.0	824.3	133.7	34.0	6.7	1.3	*	*	*
1949---------------	1968	1,000.0	828.4	131.6	32.7	6.1	1.2	*	*	*
1950---------------	1969	1,000.0	829.0	133.3	31.2	5.6	0.9	*	*	*
1951---------------	1970	1,000.0	828.3	135.2	30.3	5.4	0.8	*	*	*
1952---------------	1971	1,000.0	823.9	140.3	30.1	4.9	0.8	*	*	*
1953---------------	1972	1,000.0	824.1	141.0	29.6	4.6	0.7	*	*	*
1954---------------	1973	1,000.0	825.4	141.3	28.5	4.3	0.5	*	*	*
1955---------------	1974	1,000.0	826.6	141.5	27.6	3.8	0.5	*	*	*

TABLE 8A. DISTRIBUTIONS OF ALL WOMEN BY PARITY AS OF THE BEGINNING OF EACH YEAR 1917-74 BY AGE FOR EACH COHORT FROM 1867 TO 1959--CON.

(BASED ON CUMULATIVE BIRTH RATES)

EXACT AGE AND COHORT	AS OF JANUARY 1	TOTAL	PARITY							
			0	1	2	3	4	5	6	7 AND HIGHER
20 YEARS										
1897----------------	1917	1,000.0	778.3	162.4	47.7	9.7	1.9	*	*	*
1898----------------	1918	1,000.0	775.1	163.9	49.7	9.7	1.6	*	*	*
1899----------------	1919	1,000.0	772.6	167.4	48.7	9.6	1.7	*	*	*
1900----------------	1920	1,000.0	786.4	155.8	46.9	9.2	1.7	*	*	*
1901----------------	1921	1,000.0	776.4	167.9	45.3	8.8	1.6	*	*	*
1902----------------	1922	1,000.0	760.1	182.0	46.9	9.3	1.7	*	*	*
1903----------------	1923	1,000.0	756.7	181.2	51.3	9.1	1.7	*	*	*
1904----------------	1924	1,000.0	760.3	175.3	53.0	9.5	1.9	*	*	*
1905----------------	1925	1,000.0	759.8	176.4	51.8	10.0	2.0	*	*	*
1906----------------	1926	1,000.0	760.9	177.2	50.0	9.9	2.0	*	*	*
1907----------------	1927	1,000.0	764.3	174.2	49.8	9.7	2.0	*	*	*
1908----------------	1928	1,000.0	767.5	171.1	49.8	9.6	2.0	*	*	*
1909----------------	1929	1,000.0	773.0	167.0	48.5	9.7	1.8	*	*	*
1910----------------	1930	1,000.0	780.1	162.1	46.9	9.1	1.8	*	*	*
1911----------------	1931	1,000.0	781.4	161.6	46.4	8.8	1.8	*	*	*
1912----------------	1932	1,000.0	786.3	158.6	45.0	8.4	1.7	*	*	*
1913----------------	1933	1,000.0	792.2	154.1	43.9	8.2	1.6	*	*	*
1914----------------	1934	1,000.0	801.7	147.8	41.4	7.7	1.4	*	*	*
1915----------------	1935	1,000.0	803.4	147.9	39.8	7.5	1.4	*	*	*
1916----------------	1936	1,000.0	803.7	149.2	38.4	7.3	1.4	*	*	*
1917----------------	1937	1,000.0	805.2	147.3	39.0	7.1	1.4	*	*	*
1918----------------	1938	1,000.0	804.3	147.3	39.6	7.4	1.4	*	*	*
1919----------------	1939	1,000.0	798.6	150.8	41.3	7.9	1.4	*	*	*
1920----------------	1940	1,000.0	796.7	151.3	42.4	8.1	1.5	*	*	*
1921----------------	1941	1,C00.0	795.7	148.7	44.4	9.4	1.8	*	*	*
1922----------------	1942	1,000.0	795.7	147.3	45.0	10.0	2.0	*	*	*
1923----------------	1943	1,000.0	785.2	157.3	45.1	10.1	2.3	*	*	*
1924----------------	1944	1,000.0	779.0	160.8	47.2	10.6	2.4	*	*	*
1925----------------	1945	1,000.0	784.5	156.6	45.7	10.7	2.5	*	*	*
1926----------------	1946	1,000.0	794.3	150.9	42.7	9.8	2.3	*	*	*
1927----------------	1947	1,000.0	785.2	157.6	45.1	9.8	2.3	*	*	*
1928----------------	1948	1,000.0	751.7	186.9	48.9	10.1	2.4	*	*	*
1929----------------	1949	1,000.0	733.1	195.8	57.2	11.4	2.5	*	*	*
1930----------------	1950	1,000.0	724.7	193.6	65.1	13.7	2.9	*	*	*
1931----------------	1951	1,C00.0	721.4	188.7	70.2	16.2	3.5	*	*	*
1932----------------	1952	1,000.0	711.3	193.3	73.5	17.9	4.0	*	*	*
1933----------------	1953	1,000.0	702.8	197.3	76.3	19.0	4.6	*	*	*
1934----------------	1954	1,000.0	695.9	200.3	79.2	19.7	4.9	*	*	*
1935----------------	1955	1,000.0	689.8	204.6	79.9	20.6	5.1	*	*	*
1936----------------	1956	1,000.0	686.6	204.9	82.1	21.1	5.3	*	*	*
1937----------------	1957	1,000.0	680.2	207.6	85.0	21.8	5.4	*	*	*
1938----------------	1958	1,000.0	673.7	210.8	87.0	22.8	5.7	*	*	*
1939----------------	1959	1,000.0	669.9	210.9	89.9	23.3	6.0	*	*	*
1940----------------	1960	1,000.0	670.7	207.5	91.1	24.5	6.2	*	*	*
1941----------------	1961	1,000.0	678.1	202.0	88.8	24.8	6.3	*	*	*
1942----------------	1962	1,000.0	687.8	197.0	85.2	23.7	6.3	*	*	*
1943----------------	1963	1,000.0	698.5	191.5	81.6	22.5	5.9	*	*	*
1944----------------	1964	1,000.0	705.2	189.3	78.6	21.4	5.5	*	*	*
1945----------------	1965	1,000.0	712.5	187.5	74.6	20.2	5.2	*	*	*
1946----------------	1966	1,000.0	723.7	185.4	68.5	17.7	4.7	*	*	*
1947----------------	1967	1,000.0	731.6	186.8	62.6	14.9	4.1	*	*	*
1948----------------	1968	1,000.0	738.3	186.5	58.8	13.2	3.2	*	*	*
1949----------------	1969	1,000.0	742.8	186.6	55.9	11.9	2.8	*	*	*
1950----------------	1970	1,000.0	743.6	188.3	54.4	11.3	2.4	*	*	*
1951----------------	1971	1,000.0	741.3	191.5	54.1	10.9	2.2	*	*	*
1952----------------	1972	1,000.0	744.2	191.1	52.7	10.0	2.0	*	*	*
1953----------------	1973	1,000.0	751.4	187.8	50.1	9.0	1.7	*	*	*
1954----------------	1974	1,000.0	757.4	184.7	48.1	8.4	1.4	*	*	*

TABLE 8A. DISTRIBUTIONS OF ALL WOMEN BY PARITY AS OF THE BEGINNING OF EACH YEAR 1917-74 BY AGE FOR EACH COHORT FROM 1867 TO 1959--CON.

(BASED ON CUMULATIVE BIRTH RATES)

EXACT AGE AND COHORT	AS OF JANUARY 1	TOTAL	PARITY							
			0	1	2	3	4	5	6	7 AND HIGHER
21 YEARS										
1896	1917	1,000.0	699.2	197.9	76.3	21.2	4.7	0.5	0.1	0.1
1897	1918	1,000.0	692.9	203.1	77.9	21.2	4.3	0.4	0.1	0.1
1898	1919	1,000.0	689.4	205.6	79.1	21.2	4.2	0.3	0.1	0.1
1899	1920	1,000.0	704.2	193.8	76.8	20.5	4.2	0.3	0.1	0.1
1900	1921	1,000.0	697.1	203.8	74.5	19.9	4.1	0.4	0.1	0.1
1901	1922	1,000.0	684.0	218.6	73.2	19.5	4.1	0.4	0.1	0.1
1902	1923	1,000.0	678.1	219.7	78.3	19.2	4.1	0.4	0.1	0.1
1903	1924	1,000.0	676.3	216.4	82.6	19.9	4.1	0.5	0.1	0.1
1904	1925	1,000.0	676.0	216.2	81.9	20.9	4.3	0.5	0.1	0.1
1905	1926	1,000.0	679.3	215.5	79.3	20.6	4.6	0.5	0.1	0.1
1906	1927	1,000.0	683.4	213.6	77.7	20.0	4.6	0.5	0.1	0.1
1907	1928	1,000.0	688.4	209.8	76.8	19.9	4.4	0.5	0.1	0.1
1908	1929	1,000.0	695.3	205.2	75.1	19.4	4.3	0.5	0.1	0.1
1909	1930	1,000.0	703.8	199.4	73.2	19.0	4.0	0.4	0.1	0.1
1910	1931	1,000.0	708.8	197.1	71.4	18.1	4.0	0.4	0.1	0.1
1911	1932	1,000.0	713.9	194.1	70.0	17.6	3.8	0.4	0.1	0.1
1912	1933	1,000.0	721.1	189.3	68.5	16.9	3.6	0.4	0.2	0.0
1913	1934	1,000.0	730.8	183.7	65.5	16.1	3.4	0.4	0.1	0.0
1914	1935	1,000.0	735.1	182.4	63.2	15.5	3.3	0.4	0.0	0.1
1915	1936	1,000.0	734.9	185.3	61.0	15.0	3.3	0.4	0.0	0.1
1916	1937	1,000.0	736.4	184.6	60.7	14.5	3.3	0.4	0.0	0.1
1917	1938	1,000.0	736.5	183.5	61.6	14.7	3.2	0.4	0.1	0.0
1918	1939	1,000.0	734.1	184.1	62.7	15.4	3.2	0.4	0.0	0.1
1919	1940	1,000.0	730.7	185.4	64.4	15.8	3.2	0.4	0.0	0.1
1920	1941	1,000.0	727.6	185.1	66.2	16.9	3.6	0.4	0.1	0.1
1921	1942	1,000.0	719.5	188.7	69.0	18.3	3.9	0.4	0.1	0.1
1922	1943	1,000.0	709.0	198.8	68.8	18.4	4.3	0.5	0.1	0.1
1923	1944	1,000.0	703.7	200.7	70.9	19.2	4.8	0.5	0.1	0.1
1924	1945	1,000.0	705.8	199.4	69.5	19.5	5.0	0.6	0.1	0.1
1925	1946	1,000.0	714.0	196.7	65.7	18.0	4.8	0.6	0.1	0.1
1926	1947	1,000.0	701.7	204.7	70.1	18.1	4.6	0.6	0.1	0.1
1927	1948	1,000.0	664.4	235.1	76.2	18.9	4.6	0.6	0.1	0.1
1928	1949	1,000.0	645.7	241.9	86.0	20.6	5.0	0.6	0.1	0.1
1929	1950	1,000.0	634.3	238.8	96.5	23.8	5.6	0.8	0.1	0.1
1930	1951	1,000.0	632.0	230.1	102.6	27.8	6.5	0.8	0.1	0.1
1931	1952	1,000.0	619.0	232.3	108.2	31.6	7.7	1.0	0.1	0.1
1932	1953	1,000.0	609.1	235.0	112.3	33.5	8.7	1.1	0.2	0.1
1933	1954	1,000.0	598.1	238.0	117.7	35.1	9.7	1.1	0.2	0.1
1934	1955	1,000.0	587.2	242.9	121.0	37.1	10.1	1.3	0.3	0.1
1935	1956	1,000.0	581.2	244.4	123.7	38.4	10.5	1.4	0.3	0.1
1936	1957	1,000.0	572.7	247.1	127.5	39.8	11.0	1.5	0.3	0.1
1937	1958	1,000.0	564.7	249.6	130.8	41.6	11.3	1.6	0.3	0.1
1938	1959	1,000.0	561.7	248.8	133.2	42.4	11.9	1.6	0.3	0.1
1939	1960	1,000.0	558.4	246.4	136.6	44.1	12.4	1.6	0.4	0.1
1940	1961	1,000.0	561.7	242.4	135.5	45.5	12.8	1.7	0.3	0.1
1941	1962	1,000.0	570.9	237.8	131.4	44.7	13.0	1.7	0.4	0.1
1942	1963	1,000.0	584.2	232.4	126.3	42.6	12.3	1.7	0.4	0.1
1943	1964	1,000.0	597.0	228.8	121.0	39.8	11.5	1.5	0.3	0.1
1944	1965	1,000.0	606.0	228.9	115.7	37.2	10.4	1.5	0.2	0.1
1945	1966	1,000.0	619.9	227.4	108.4	33.3	9.5	1.2	0.2	0.1
1946	1967	1,000.0	630.1	231.3	100.4	28.8	8.1	1.0	0.2	0.1
1947	1968	1,000.0	641.8	231.0	94.4	24.8	7.0	0.8	0.2	0.0
1948	1969	1,000.0	648.1	234.1	89.4	22.0	5.7	0.6	0.0	0.1
1949	1970	1,000.0	653.7	233.8	86.2	20.5	5.1	0.5	0.1	0.1
1950	1971	1,000.0	653.8	236.0	85.1	19.9	4.5	0.6	0.0	0.1
1951	1972	1,000.0	660.4	232.9	83.2	18.9	4.0	0.5	0.1	0.0
1952	1973	1,000.0	672.9	227.6	78.8	16.8	3.5	0.3	0.1	0.0
1953	1974	1,000.0	685.4	221.0	75.0	15.2	3.1	0.2	0.1	0.0

TABLE 8A. DISTRIBUTIONS OF ALL WOMEN BY PARITY AS OF THE BEGINNING OF EACH YEAR 1917-74 BY AGE FOR EACH COHORT FROM 1867 TO 1959--CON.

(BASED ON CUMULATIVE BIRTH RATES)

EXACT AGE AND COHORT	AS OF JANUARY 1	TOTAL	PARITY							
			0	1	2	3	4	5	6	7 AND HIGHER
22 YEARS										
1895---------------	1917	1,000.0	622.9	221.4	105.2	37.9	10.2	1.7	0.5	0.2
1896---------------	1918	1,000.0	616.2	227.3	107.2	37.8	9.4	1.5	0.4	0.2
1897---------------	1919	1,000.0	609.1	234.4	107.6	37.8	9.2	1.3	0.4	0.2
1898---------------	1920	1,000.0	624.3	220.1	107.9	36.9	9.0	1.2	0.4	0.2
1899---------------	1921	1,000.0	618.6	229.9	104.7	35.9	9.0	1.3	0.4	0.2
1900---------------	1922	1,000.0	610.6	241.7	101.3	35.2	9.1	1.5	0.4	0.2
1901---------------	1923	1,000.0	608.3	243.8	104.2	33.3	8.4	1.4	0.4	0.2
1902---------------	1924	1,000.0	604.1	242.0	109.1	34.1	8.6	1.5	0.4	0.2
1903---------------	1925	1,000.0	598.9	243.4	110.6	36.1	8.7	1.7	0.4	0.2
1904---------------	1926	1,000.0	601.4	242.6	108.6	35.9	9.2	1.6	0.5	0.2
1905---------------	1927	1,000.0	607.6	239.8	106.2	34.5	9.5	1.7	0.5	0.2
1906---------------	1928	1,000.0	613.1	237.8	103.8	33.7	9.3	1.6	0.5	0.2
1907---------------	1929	1,000.0	621.5	233.1	101.1	33.4	8.6	1.6	0.5	0.2
1908---------------	1930	1,000.0	630.5	227.8	99.1	32.1	8.3	1.6	0.4	0.2
1909---------------	1931	1,000.0	637.1	224.4	97.0	31.4	8.1	1.4	0.4	0.2
1910---------------	1932	1,000.0	646.0	220.0	94.3	30.0	7.8	1.3	0.4	0.2
1911---------------	1933	1,000.0	653.1	215.5	92.8	29.2	7.5	1.4	0.3	0.2
1912---------------	1934	1,000.0	664.0	209.6	89.7	27.8	7.1	1.3	0.4	0.1
1913---------------	1935	1,000.0	668.5	208.7	87.3	26.9	7.0	1.2	0.3	0.1
1914---------------	1936	1,000.0	670.4	211.2	84.2	25.7	6.8	1.3	0.2	0.2
1915---------------	1937	1,000.0	670.5	212.9	83.4	24.9	6.6	1.3	0.2	0.2
1916---------------	1938	1,000.0	670.4	212.8	83.8	24.7	6.6	1.3	0.2	0.2
1917---------------	1939	1,000.0	668.8	212.3	85.4	25.4	6.5	1.2	0.3	0.1
1918---------------	1940	1,000.0	669.4	211.0	85.8	25.8	6.4	1.2	0.2	0.2
1919---------------	1941	1,000.0	663.5	213.2	88.1	26.7	6.7	1.3	0.3	0.2
1920---------------	1942	1,000.0	652.4	220.0	90.7	27.9	7.1	1.3	0.4	0.2
1921---------------	1943	1,000.0	632.0	235.0	94.1	29.1	7.7	1.5	0.4	0.2
1922---------------	1944	1,000.0	629.6	233.5	96.2	30.0	8.4	1.7	0.4	0.2
1923---------------	1945	1,000.0	631.4	232.4	94.2	30.6	9.0	1.8	0.4	0.2
1924---------------	1946	1,000.0	636.6	233.1	90.2	29.0	8.7	1.8	0.4	0.2
1925---------------	1947	1,000.0	618.9	243.8	97.5	28.9	8.5	1.8	0.4	0.2
1926---------------	1948	1,000.0	581.9	271.4	105.7	30.3	8.3	1.8	0.4	0.2
1927---------------	1949	1,000.0	562.6	276.6	116.9	32.7	8.7	1.9	0.4	0.2
1928---------------	1950	1,000.0	552.2	270.8	128.1	36.4	9.7	2.1	0.5	0.2
1929---------------	1951	1,000.0	547.0	261.2	136.0	41.7	11.0	2.4	0.5	0.2
1930---------------	1952	1,000.0	536.8	258.0	141.8	47.0	13.0	2.7	0.5	0.2
1931---------------	1953	1,000.0	523.1	258.4	148.6	51.0	14.8	3.3	0.5	0.3
1932---------------	1954	1,000.0	512.4	258.3	155.1	53.7	16.0	3.5	0.7	0.3
1933---------------	1955	1,000.0	497.7	261.7	161.2	57.0	17.5	3.7	0.9	0.3
1934---------------	1956	1,000.0	486.3	263.9	166.0	60.1	18.3	4.1	1.0	0.3
1935---------------	1957	1,000.0	475.8	266.7	170.0	62.6	19.2	4.3	1.1	0.3
1936---------------	1958	1,000.0	466.7	267.8	174.0	65.5	19.9	4.7	1.1	0.3
1937---------------	1959	1,000.0	462.4	266.4	177.3	66.9	20.8	4.8	1.1	0.3
1938---------------	1960	1,000.0	461.0	262.3	180.3	68.3	21.8	4.8	1.1	0.4
1939---------------	1961	1,000.0	459.2	259.8	180.9	71.1	22.4	5.0	1.2	0.4
1940---------------	1962	1,000.0	463.7	256.8	178.6	71.1	23.1	5.1	1.2	0.4
1941---------------	1963	1,000.0	476.3	252.2	172.5	69.7	22.4	5.3	1.2	0.4
1942---------------	1964	1,000.0	491.9	248.5	166.9	65.4	20.9	4.9	1.1	0.4
1943---------------	1965	1,000.0	506.0	249.0	160.0	60.3	19.1	4.3	1.0	0.3
1944---------------	1966	1,000.0	520.5	251.3	152.1	54.5	16.7	3.8	0.8	0.3
1945---------------	1967	1,000.0	533.9	255.2	144.1	48.0	14.8	3.0	0.7	0.3
1946---------------	1968	1,000.0	546.7	258.8	136.5	42.1	12.5	2.6	0.6	0.2
1947---------------	1969	1,000.0	557.9	262.3	129.5	36.9	10.8	2.0	0.5	0.1
1948---------------	1970	1,000.0	564.0	265.8	125.1	33.8	9.2	1.6	0.3	0.2
1949---------------	1971	1,000.0	569.7	265.5	122.1	32.2	8.5	1.5	0.3	0.2
1950---------------	1972	1,000.0	578.5	262.5	118.9	30.9	7.4	1.5	0.2	0.1
1951---------------	1973	1,000.0	595.1	255.6	113.5	27.8	6.6	1.1	0.3	0.0
1952---------------	1974	1,000.0	612.7	247.8	107.6	25.2	5.6	0.9	0.2	0.0

TABLE 8A. DISTRIBUTIONS OF ALL WOMEN BY PARITY AS OF THE BEGINNING OF EACH YEAR 1917-74 BY AGE FOR EACH COHORT FROM 1867 TO 1959--CON.

(BASED ON CUMULATIVE BIRTH RATES)

EXACT AGE AND COHORT	AS OF JANUARY 1	TOTAL	PARITY							
			0	1	2	3	4	5	6	7 AND HIGHER
23 YEARS										
1894	1917	1,000.0	554.1	234.2	129.7	57.2	18.9	4.2	1.3	0.4
1895	1918	1,000.0	548.3	239.5	131.9	57.3	17.8	3.7	1.0	0.5
1896	1919	1,000.0	541.1	247.2	132.5	57.2	17.2	3.4	1.0	0.4
1897	1920	1,000.0	551.4	239.2	132.1	55.9	16.8	3.3	0.9	0.4
1898	1921	1,000.0	547.1	245.0	131.8	54.9	16.6	3.2	1.0	0.4
1899	1922	1,000.0	540.4	256.8	127.4	53.6	16.9	3.4	1.1	0.4
1900	1923	1,000.0	542.3	256.6	128.7	51.2	16.3	3.5	0.9	0.5
1901	1924	1,000.0	541.9	256.1	131.4	50.3	15.4	3.5	0.9	0.5
1902	1925	1,000.0	534.0	258.7	133.2	53.0	16.0	3.6	1.0	0.5
1903	1926	1,000.0	531.0	260.0	133.4	53.8	16.6	3.7	1.0	0.5
1904	1927	1,000.0	535.5	258.2	131.8	52.0	17.0	3.9	1.1	0.5
1905	1928	1,000.0	543.6	255.6	128.2	50.1	17.0	3.9	1.1	0.5
1906	1929	1,000.0	552.1	253.5	124.4	48.8	16.0	3.6	1.1	0.5
1907	1930	1,000.0	562.5	248.1	121.6	47.8	15.0	3.5	1.1	0.4
1908	1931	1,000.0	569.9	245.0	119.6	45.9	14.8	3.5	0.9	0.4
1909	1932	1,000.0	579.8	239.7	117.1	44.8	14.2	3.1	0.9	0.4
1910	1933	1,000.0	591.1	234.1	113.9	43.0	13.7	3.0	0.8	0.4
1911	1934	1,000.0	601.3	228.7	111.1	41.7	13.1	3.0	0.7	0.4
1912	1935	1,000.0	607.8	226.6	108.8	40.1	12.7	2.9	0.8	0.3
1913	1936	1,000.0	609.7	229.8	105.8	38.5	12.3	2.9	0.7	0.3
1914	1937	1,000.0	611.0	232.1	104.2	36.9	11.9	2.9	0.6	0.4
1915	1938	1,000.0	608.9	234.5	104.5	36.5	11.7	2.9	0.6	0.4
1916	1939	1,000.0	607.1	235.0	105.6	36.8	11.7	2.8	0.6	0.4
1917	1940	1,000.0	607.7	233.2	106.7	37.3	11.4	2.7	0.7	0.3
1918	1941	1,000.0	607.9	231.6	106.9	37.8	11.8	2.9	0.7	0.4
1919	1942	1,000.0	593.2	241.0	110.5	38.9	12.2	3.0	0.8	0.4
1920	1943	1,000.0	567.4	258.8	116.2	40.4	12.7	3.2	0.9	0.4
1921	1944	1,000.0	556.0	261.3	121.6	42.6	13.7	3.4	1.0	0.4
1922	1945	1,000.0	561.0	257.4	119.0	43.0	14.5	3.7	1.0	0.4
1923	1946	1,000.0	566.0	258.7	114.5	41.4	14.3	3.7	1.0	0.4
1924	1947	1,000.0	543.9	271.0	124.3	41.5	14.2	3.7	1.0	0.4
1925	1948	1,000.0	505.8	296.5	135.5	43.3	13.8	3.7	1.0	0.4
1926	1949	1,000.0	487.8	299.6	146.7	46.6	14.2	3.7	1.0	0.4
1927	1950	1,000.0	476.6	292.7	158.9	50.8	15.4	4.1	1.0	0.5
1928	1951	1,000.0	472.7	280.6	166.9	56.6	17.1	4.5	1.1	0.5
1929	1952	1,000.0	461.1	275.0	174.0	63.2	19.8	5.2	1.2	0.5
1930	1953	1,000.0	450.5	270.3	180.2	68.7	22.4	6.0	1.4	0.5
1931	1954	1,000.0	437.9	265.5	189.1	73.5	24.7	7.1	1.5	0.7
1932	1955	1,000.0	423.8	265.6	195.8	78.3	26.5	7.4	1.9	0.7
1933	1956	1,000.0	408.3	267.2	202.4	82.6	28.7	7.8	2.2	0.8
1934	1957	1,000.0	394.3	268.2	207.9	87.6	30.4	8.4	2.4	0.8
1935	1958	1,000.0	383.6	268.6	212.4	91.5	31.5	8.9	2.7	0.8
1936	1959	1,000.0	378.4	266.3	215.2	94.3	32.9	9.4	2.7	0.8
1937	1960	1,000.0	376.3	262.2	218.0	96.1	34.1	9.7	2.7	0.9
1938	1961	1,000.0	376.1	258.0	218.6	98.2	35.5	9.8	2.8	1.0
1939	1962	1,000.0	375.8	255.9	217.7	100.1	36.4	10.2	2.9	1.0
1940	1963	1,000.0	383.6	253.0	213.3	99.6	36.3	10.3	2.9	1.0
1941	1964	1,000.0	398.2	249.9	207.5	96.0	34.5	10.2	2.7	1.0
1942	1965	1,000.0	413.5	251.3	201.7	89.4	31.6	9.1	2.5	0.9
1943	1966	1,000.0	432.0	254.6	194.5	80.4	28.0	7.7	2.1	0.7
1944	1967	1,000.0	444.5	263.3	187.3	72.1	24.0	6.4	1.8	0.6
1945	1968	1,000.0	460.7	266.2	180.3	64.3	21.1	5.4	1.4	0.6
1946	1969	1,000.0	472.5	273.5	172.9	57.0	18.0	4.5	1.2	0.4
1947	1970	1,000.0	482.6	278.1	166.7	51.8	15.9	3.6	1.0	0.3
1948	1971	1,000.0	487.6	282.6	162.9	48.8	14.0	3.1	0.6	0.4
1949	1972	1,000.0	500.9	278.7	157.7	46.1	12.8	2.8	0.7	0.3
1950	1973	1,000.0	519.1	273.4	151.2	42.1	11.0	2.6	0.4	0.2
1951	1974	1,000.0	540.2	264.8	144.6	38.2	9.7	2.0	0.4	0.1

TABLE 8A. DISTRIBUTIONS OF ALL WOMEN BY PARITY AS OF THE BEGINNING OF EACH YEAR 1917-74 BY AGE FOR EACH COHORT FROM 1867 TO 1959--CON.

(BASED ON CUMULATIVE BIRTH RATES)

EXACT AGE AND COHORT	AS OF JANUARY 1	TOTAL	PARITY							
			0	1	2	3	4	5	6	7 AND HIGHER
24 YEARS										
1893	1917	1,000.0	492.7	238.0	149.1	76.4	30.9	9.1	2.9	0.9
1894	1918	1,000.0	486.8	243.4	151.8	77.1	29.5	8.0	2.5	0.9
1895	1919	1,000.0	480.7	250.4	152.6	77.0	28.9	7.3	2.1	1.0
1896	1920	1,000.0	489.4	244.8	152.5	75.4	27.9	7.1	2.0	0.9
1897	1921	1,000.0	482.5	255.0	151.4	73.8	27.4	7.0	2.0	0.9
1898	1922	1,000.0	476.3	262.9	150.1	72.7	27.7	7.1	2.3	0.9
1899	1923	1,000.0	478.5	263.6	151.2	69.5	26.9	7.0	2.4	0.9
1900	1924	1,000.0	482.2	260.8	151.7	68.4	26.2	7.4	2.2	1.1
1901	1925	1,000.0	478.9	264.6	151.1	69.5	25.4	7.3	2.2	1.0
1902	1926	1,000.0	473.1	268.2	151.2	70.8	26.3	7.1	2.2	1.1
1903	1927	1,000.0	472.1	268.6	152.1	69.6	26.9	7.4	2.3	1.0
1904	1928	1,000.0	477.9	267.8	149.3	67.1	26.9	7.7	2.3	1.0
1905	1929	1,000.0	488.4	265.6	144.8	64.6	25.9	7.4	2.3	1.0
1906	1930	1,000.0	499.3	262.5	141.1	62.7	24.2	7.1	2.2	0.9
1907	1931	1,000.0	508.0	259.3	138.4	61.3	23.3	6.8	2.1	0.8
1908	1932	1,000.0	518.5	254.8	136.3	58.7	22.6	6.4	1.9	0.8
1909	1933	1,000.0	530.4	248.6	133.3	57.3	21.9	6.0	1.7	0.8
1910	1934	1,000.0	545.1	241.9	128.9	55.1	21.0	5.6	1.7	0.7
1911	1935	1,000.0	551.3	239.6	126.8	53.8	20.4	5.8	1.6	0.7
1912	1936	1,000.0	555.5	241.5	124.2	51.3	19.6	5.6	1.6	0.7
1913	1937	1,000.0	556.5	244.9	122.9	49.2	18.9	5.4	1.6	0.6
1914	1938	1,000.0	555.1	248.4	122.5	48.0	18.4	5.5	1.3	0.8
1915	1939	1,000.0	550.9	251.3	123.7	48.4	18.1	5.5	1.3	0.8
1916	1940	1,000.0	551.0	250.6	124.6	48.4	18.0	5.3	1.3	0.8
1917	1941	1,000.0	551.3	248.5	125.3	48.9	18.1	5.6	1.6	0.7
1918	1942	1,000.0	544.5	252.9	126.3	49.6	18.5	5.8	1.6	0.8
1919	1943	1,000.0	513.6	271.3	135.8	52.0	18.9	5.9	1.7	0.8
1920	1944	1,000.0	496.2	276.8	143.4	54.7	19.9	6.2	1.9	0.9
1921	1945	1,000.0	492.7	277.3	143.6	56.0	21.0	6.5	2.1	0.8
1922	1946	1,000.0	501.1	275.8	138.7	54.2	20.8	6.6	2.0	0.8
1923	1947	1,000.0	480.1	286.8	148.3	54.4	21.1	6.5	2.0	0.8
1924	1948	1,000.0	441.6	309.2	162.4	56.8	20.7	6.4	2.0	0.9
1925	1949	1,000.0	421.6	312.8	174.6	60.8	20.8	6.5	2.0	0.9
1926	1950	1,000.0	410.8	305.1	186.6	65.5	22.1	6.9	2.1	0.9
1927	1951	1,000.0	405.9	292.1	195.6	71.7	24.2	7.4	2.1	1.0
1928	1952	1,000.0	397.7	282.3	202.4	78.6	27.3	8.3	2.4	1.0
1929	1953	1,000.0	385.9	275.6	208.8	85.5	30.8	9.6	2.7	1.1
1930	1954	1,000.0	377.4	266.1	215.8	91.7	33.7	11.1	3.0	1.2
1931	1955	1,000.0	362.5	260.6	224.1	98.5	36.9	12.4	3.5	1.5
1932	1956	1,000.0	348.0	259.5	230.1	104.5	39.3	13.0	4.0	1.6
1933	1957	1,000.0	331.4	258.8	236.4	110.8	42.7	13.6	4.5	1.8
1934	1958	1,000.0	317.6	257.1	241.9	116.9	45.1	14.7	4.8	1.9
1935	1959	1,000.0	310.6	254.2	245.0	121.1	46.5	15.5	5.2	1.9
1936	1960	1,000.0	308.0	249.7	246.3	123.9	48.8	16.0	5.3	2.0
1937	1961	1,000.0	306.9	245.7	246.9	126.1	50.2	16.7	5.4	2.1
1938	1962	1,000.0	308.1	242.5	245.5	127.4	52.0	16.8	5.5	2.2
1939	1963	1,000.0	311.1	240.8	242.6	128.2	52.1	17.4	5.6	2.2
1940	1964	1,000.0	320.2	239.1	239.0	126.3	50.9	16.9	5.4	2.2
1941	1965	1,000.0	334.2	240.2	234.1	120.8	47.5	16.1	5.0	2.1
1942	1966	1,000.0	351.8	245.3	229.8	110.8	42.4	13.8	4.3	1.8
1943	1967	1,000.0	367.4	254.9	225.1	99.5	36.8	11.3	3.6	1.4
1944	1968	1,000.0	381.5	262.2	220.4	90.4	31.8	9.5	3.1	1.1
1945	1969	1,000.0	397.3	268.0	213.7	81.3	28.2	8.1	2.4	1.0
1946	1970	1,000.0	407.2	276.4	207.8	74.1	24.7	6.9	2.1	0.8
1947	1971	1,000.0	415.5	282.3	202.6	69.3	22.2	5.8	1.7	0.6
1948	1972	1,000.0	425.7	285.7	197.4	64.8	19.6	5.0	1.2	0.6
1949	1973	1,000.0	446.9	280.8	189.8	59.2	17.4	4.3	1.2	0.4
1950	1974	1,000.0	468.7	274.7	182.6	54.2	14.8	4.0	0.7	0.3

TABLE 8A. DISTRIBUTIONS OF ALL WOMEN BY PARITY AS OF THE BEGINNING OF EACH YEAR 1917-74 BY AGE FOR EACH COHORT FROM 1867 TO 1959--CON.

(BASED ON CUMULATIVE BIRTH RATES)

EXACT AGE AND COHORT	AS OF JANUARY 1	TOTAL	PARITY							
			0	1	2	3	4	5	6	7 AND HIGHER
25 YEARS										
1892	1917	1,000.0	442.6	235.8	165.9	92.1	42.5	14.2	4.8	2.1
1893	1918	1,000.0	435.8	240.8	165.0	93.9	42.9	14.8	4.9	1.9
1894	1919	1,000.0	429.3	248.0	166.8	94.3	41.9	13.5	4.4	1.8
1895	1920	1,000.0	436.2	244.1	167.5	92.7	40.8	12.8	4.0	1.9
1896	1921	1,000.0	430.6	253.3	166.9	90.9	39.8	12.7	4.0	1.8
1897	1922	1,000.0	422.0	265.7	164.7	89.2	39.5	12.8	4.2	1.9
1898	1923	1,000.0	422.1	264.6	168.8	86.8	39.0	12.5	4.3	1.9
1899	1924	1,000.0	426.2	262.9	169.5	84.5	37.8	12.7	4.5	1.9
1900	1925	1,000.0	428.2	263.3	166.8	85.1	37.3	12.8	4.4	2.1
1901	1926	1,000.0	426.6	268.0	164.9	85.1	36.7	12.4	4.3	2.0
1902	1927	1,000.0	422.8	271.3	165.6	84.3	37.4	12.3	4.2	2.1
1903	1928	1,000.0	422.3	273.1	165.5	82.5	37.7	12.7	4.3	1.9
1904	1929	1,000.0	429.8	272.8	162.4	79.6	36.6	12.7	4.2	1.9
1905	1930	1,000.0	442.4	270.0	158.1	76.4	34.9	12.3	4.1	1.8
1906	1931	1,000.0	451.9	268.8	154.4	74.4	33.2	11.7	3.9	1.7
1907	1932	1,000.0	462.7	264.8	152.1	72.4	31.8	10.9	3.7	1.6
1908	1933	1,000.0	475.3	259.6	149.4	69.5	30.8	10.5	3.4	1.5
1909	1934	1,000.0	489.9	252.7	145.6	67.8	29.7	9.8	3.1	1.4
1910	1935	1,000.0	501.6	248.4	141.7	65.4	28.9	9.6	3.1	1.3
1911	1936	1,000.0	505.6	249.6	139.6	63.5	27.8	9.5	3.0	1.4
1912	1937	1,000.0	508.4	252.4	138.4	60.7	26.8	9.0	3.0	1.3
1913	1938	1,000.0	506.9	257.0	138.3	58.9	25.9	8.9	2.9	1.2
1914	1939	1,000.0	503.1	261.0	139.2	58.5	25.2	9.0	2.6	1.4
1915	1940	1,000.0	499.8	263.2	140.6	58.8	24.8	8.8	2.6	1.4
1916	1941	1,000.0	499.1	262.3	141.6	58.9	25.1	8.9	2.6	1.5
1917	1942	1,000.0	492.7	265.3	143.5	59.9	25.0	9.3	2.9	1.4
1918	1943	1,000.0	472.2	277.1	149.9	61.6	25.3	9.4	3.0	1.5
1919	1944	1,000.0	448.9	283.0	161.7	65.6	26.3	9.7	3.2	1.6
1920	1945	1,000.0	440.2	285.2	164.4	67.6	27.4	10.0	3.6	1.6
1921	1946	1,000.0	439.3	287.7	162.8	67.1	27.8	10.2	3.5	1.6
1922	1947	1,000.0	423.7	294.7	171.1	67.1	28.2	10.1	3.5	1.6
1923	1948	1,000.0	390.0	312.2	184.7	70.0	28.1	9.9	3.5	1.6
1924	1949	1,000.0	368.2	315.5	198.4	74.6	28.1	10.0	3.5	1.7
1925	1950	1,000.0	354.6	309.3	211.3	79.8	29.3	10.3	3.6	1.8
1926	1951	1,000.0	349.3	295.9	220.6	86.2	31.5	11.0	3.7	1.8
1927	1952	1,000.0	341.5	284.0	228.1	93.7	34.8	12.1	3.9	1.9
1928	1953	1,000.0	334.0	273.2	233.1	101.0	38.8	13.5	4.4	2.0
1929	1954	1,000.0	324.3	262.2	239.5	108.4	42.9	15.5	5.0	2.2
1930	1955	1,000.0	315.0	252.2	244.8	116.0	46.5	17.4	5.6	2.5
1931	1956	1,000.0	300.4	245.8	251.0	124.0	50.4	19.0	6.4	3.0
1932	1957	1,000.0	285.6	242.3	256.2	131.5	54.1	19.8	7.2	3.3
1933	1958	1,000.0	269.6	239.1	261.9	138.5	58.4	21.1	7.8	3.6
1934	1959	1,000.0	259.3	234.9	265.1	144.9	61.2	22.5	8.3	3.8
1935	1960	1,000.0	254.5	230.7	265.6	149.5	63.5	23.5	8.7	4.0
1936	1961	1,000.0	253.4	226.0	265.1	151.9	66.2	24.3	9.0	4.1
1937	1962	1,000.0	253.4	223.5	263.4	153.3	67.7	25.3	9.2	4.2
1938	1963	1,000.0	257.4	221.1	260.6	153.2	68.9	25.2	9.3	4.3
1939	1964	1,000.0	261.1	220.8	258.5	152.9	68.0	25.3	9.2	4.2
1940	1965	1,000.0	269.7	222.1	256.3	149.7	65.3	24.1	8.8	4.0
1941	1966	1,000.0	285.2	226.5	253.7	141.5	59.8	22.0	7.7	3.6
1942	1967	1,000.0	299.1	237.5	253.2	130.0	52.3	18.4	6.5	3.0
1943	1968	1,000.0	315.0	246.3	251.6	118.5	45.7	15.2	5.3	2.4
1944	1969	1,000.0	327.5	255.8	248.8	108.7	40.0	12.9	4.5	1.8
1945	1970	1,000.0	342.9	261.6	242.8	99.9	36.2	11.2	3.8	1.6
1946	1971	1,000.0	350.0	271.5	238.4	93.4	32.3	9.9	3.1	1.4
1947	1972	1,000.0	361.5	278.0	232.7	86.9	29.0	8.3	2.6	1.0
1948	1973	1,000.0	377.0	281.7	227.3	79.4	25.0	6.9	1.9	0.8
1949	1974	1,000.0	401.1	276.4	219.8	72.4	22.0	6.0	1.7	0.6

TABLE 8A. DISTRIBUTIONS OF ALL WOMEN BY PARITY AS OF THE BEGINNING OF EACH YEAR 1917-74 BY AGE FOR EACH COHORT FROM 1867 TO 1959--CON.

(BASED ON CUMULATIVE BIRTH RATES)

EXACT AGE AND COHORT	AS OF JANUARY 1	TOTAL	PARITY 0	1	2	3	4	5	6	7 AND HIGHER
26 YEARS										
1891	1917	1,000.0	402.8	228.5	173.3	105.2	55.5	22.3	8.4	4.0
1892	1918	1,000.0	394.8	234.0	176.7	106.3	54.7	21.6	8.1	3.8
1893	1919	1,000.0	387.2	240.8	175.4	107.7	55.5	21.9	8.1	3.4
1894	1920	1,000.0	391.2	239.2	177.6	106.8	53.9	20.6	7.3	3.4
1895	1921	1,000.0	386.4	247.0	178.0	105.2	52.9	20.0	7.1	3.4
1896	1922	1,000.0	379.1	258.4	176.3	103.5	51.8	20.0	7.4	3.5
1897	1923	1,000.0	375.7	263.9	178.8	100.6	50.6	19.6	7.3	3.5
1898	1924	1,000.0	376.9	260.4	183.1	99.2	49.8	19.5	7.5	3.6
1899	1925	1,000.0	380.2	261.3	181.1	98.2	48.5	19.3	7.8	3.6
1900	1926	1,000.0	384.1	262.4	177.4	97.6	48.1	19.1	7.4	3.9
1901	1927	1,000.0	384.0	267.3	176.0	95.9	47.2	18.5	7.4	3.7
1902	1928	1,000.0	380.8	271.9	175.9	94.4	47.6	18.6	7.1	3.7
1903	1929	1,000.0	381.4	274.3	175.8	92.4	47.0	18.8	6.9	3.4
1904	1930	1,000.0	390.2	273.9	173.2	88.9	45.0	18.6	6.9	3.3
1905	1931	1,000.0	401.5	272.6	169.1	85.9	43.3	17.8	6.6	3.2
1906	1932	1,000.0	412.8	271.0	165.7	83.3	41.1	16.8	6.3	3.0
1907	1933	1,000.0	425.3	266.3	163.0	81.2	39.6	15.9	5.9	2.8
1908	1934	1,000.0	440.2	260.9	159.7	77.9	38.2	15.1	5.5	2.5
1909	1935	1,000.0	452.2	255.7	156.5	76.1	37.3	14.5	5.2	2.5
1910	1936	1,000.0	462.3	254.5	152.7	73.2	35.8	14.0	5.1	2.4
1911	1937	1,000.0	464.7	256.9	151.6	71.2	34.5	13.6	5.0	2.5
1912	1938	1,000.0	465.2	260.9	151.7	68.6	33.2	13.1	4.9	2.4
1913	1939	1,000.0	461.3	265.9	152.9	67.7	32.3	12.9	4.8	2.2
1914	1940	1,000.0	457.6	269.7	154.4	67.3	31.4	12.8	4.4	2.4
1915	1941	1,000.0	452.6	271.9	156.6	68.0	31.2	12.8	4.4	2.5
1916	1942	1,000.0	446.2	274.9	158.9	68.7	31.4	12.9	4.4	2.6
1917	1943	1,000.0	428.1	284.1	165.5	70.5	31.3	13.1	4.9	2.5
1918	1944	1,000.0	414.7	283.3	174.4	73.9	32.4	13.6	5.0	2.7
1919	1945	1,000.0	400.3	284.8	181.8	77.7	33.4	13.9	5.3	2.8
1920	1946	1,000.0	394.2	288.1	183.1	78.3	34.0	13.9	5.6	2.8
1921	1947	1,000.0	371.6	298.1	192.9	79.7	35.1	14.2	5.6	2.8
1922	1948	1,000.0	346.1	309.2	204.8	82.4	35.2	14.0	5.5	2.8
1923	1949	1,000.0	327.6	310.9	216.8	87.2	35.3	13.9	5.4	2.9
1924	1950	1,000.0	311.2	305.7	231.0	93.0	36.4	14.1	5.6	3.0
1925	1951	1,000.0	302.5	294.0	241.7	99.7	38.6	14.6	5.7	3.2
1926	1952	1,000.0	295.0	281.0	249.3	107.6	41.8	16.1	6.0	3.2
1927	1953	1,000.0	288.2	268.1	254.2	115.7	46.2	17.7	6.5	3.4
1928	1954	1,000.0	283.2	254.3	258.2	123.2	50.7	19.5	7.2	3.7
1929	1955	1,000.0	273.7	242.6	262.3	131.4	55.5	22.2	8.2	4.1
1930	1956	1,000.0	265.5	232.0	264.7	139.9	59.9	24.3	9.0	4.7
1931	1957	1,000.0	251.0	224.1	269.1	148.8	64.9	26.4	10.2	5.5
1932	1958	1,000.0	236.9	218.8	273.0	156.8	69.7	27.7	11.1	6.0
1933	1959	1,000.0	224.1	213.9	276.3	163.5	74.3	29.6	11.9	6.4
1934	1960	1,000.0	215.8	208.7	276.8	169.7	78.4	31.2	12.5	6.9
1935	1961	1,000.0	212.5	204.7	275.1	173.9	81.0	32.4	13.2	7.2
1936	1962	1,000.0	212.4	201.5	272.6	175.5	83.4	33.7	13.6	7.3
1937	1963	1,000.0	214.4	200.2	270.0	175.2	84.5	34.4	13.9	7.4
1938	1964	1,000.0	219.0	199.1	268.0	174.4	84.8	33.7	13.6	7.4
1939	1965	1,000.0	222.2	201.0	267.3	173.2	82.7	33.4	13.1	7.1
1940	1966	1,000.0	231.7	205.2	267.4	168.5	77.9	30.7	12.2	6.4
1941	1967	1,000.0	244.4	213.8	268.8	159.4	70.3	27.4	10.4	5.5
1942	1968	1,000.0	257.4	224.7	271.5	148.4	61.9	22.8	8.7	4.6
1943	1969	1,000.0	270.3	236.0	272.6	136.6	54.8	19.0	7.1	3.6
1944	1970	1,000.0	282.4	243.8	271.5	127.7	49.0	16.7	6.1	2.8
1945	1971	1,000.0	296.4	250.3	266.3	119.5	44.9	14.9	5.2	2.5
1946	1972	1,000.0	304.8	261.9	262.5	111.4	40.0	13.1	4.3	2.0
1947	1973	1,000.0	319.4	269.4	258.4	102.1	35.1	10.7	3.5	1.4
1948	1974	1,000.0	336.1	273.2	254.6	93.3	30.2	8.9	2.6	1.1

TABLE 8A. DISTRIBUTIONS OF ALL WOMEN BY PARITY AS OF THE BEGINNING OF EACH YEAR 1917-74 BY AGE FOR EACH COHORT FROM 1867 TO 1959--CON.

(BASED ON CUMULATIVE BIRTH RATES)

EXACT AGE AND COHORT	AS OF JANUARY 1	TOTAL	PARITY							
			0	1	2	3	4	5	6	7 AND HIGHER
27 YEARS										
1890	1917	1,000.0	369.8	219.0	177.6	115.0	67.1	31.1	13.3	7.1
1891	1918	1,000.0	364.5	223.7	179.4	116.0	66.5	30.3	13.0	6.6
1892	1919	1,000.0	355.0	231.0	183.0	116.9	65.9	29.5	12.5	6.2
1893	1920	1,000.0	355.6	231.0	182.5	117.2	65.9	29.8	12.1	5.9
1894	1921	1,000.0	350.6	238.0	184.6	116.5	64.5	28.5	11.5	5.8
1895	1922	1,000.0	344.1	248.0	184.0	115.1	63.2	28.0	11.5	6.1
1896	1923	1,000.0	340.7	254.5	186.2	112.5	61.4	27.3	11.4	6.0
1897	1924	1,000.0	338.7	258.0	189.2	110.2	59.6	26.8	11.4	6.1
1898	1925	1,000.0	339.3	255.9	191.6	109.9	58.9	26.5	11.6	6.3
1899	1926	1,000.0	343.6	256.9	189.5	108.3	57.8	26.0	11.6	6.3
1900	1927	1,000.0	349.0	258.6	185.9	106.0	57.1	25.6	11.3	6.5
1901	1928	1,000.0	349.0	264.6	184.0	103.9	55.9	25.3	11.2	6.1
1902	1929	1,000.0	347.2	269.8	184.1	102.0	55.5	24.9	10.5	6.0
1903	1930	1,000.0	348.2	272.8	184.5	99.9	53.9	24.9	10.3	5.5
1904	1931	1,000.0	355.7	273.5	182.4	96.5	52.0	24.4	10.1	5.4
1905	1932	1,000.0	368.2	272.1	178.5	93.1	50.1	23.1	9.7	5.2
1906	1933	1,000.0	381.1	270.3	174.4	90.3	47.8	22.0	9.2	4.9
1907	1934	1,000.0	395.3	265.3	171.6	88.0	46.0	20.7	8.6	4.5
1908	1935	1,000.0	408.2	261.2	168.9	84.8	44.5	20.0	8.3	4.1
1909	1936	1,000.0	418.5	258.7	166.1	82.5	43.2	19.0	7.8	4.2
1910	1937	1,000.0	427.3	258.9	163.0	79.5	41.4	18.3	7.6	4.0
1911	1938	1,000.0	427.4	262.3	163.1	77.9	39.9	17.8	7.5	4.1
1912	1939	1,000.0	425.6	266.8	164.6	75.9	38.7	17.2	7.2	4.0
1913	1940	1,000.0	421.4	271.8	166.6	75.1	37.7	16.6	7.1	3.7
1914	1941	1,000.0	415.3	275.7	169.5	75.6	36.8	16.5	6.6	4.0
1915	1942	1,000.0	405.1	280.9	173.3	76.8	36.7	16.6	6.5	4.1
1916	1943	1,000.0	389.2	289.3	178.9	78.0	37.2	16.6	6.6	4.2
1917	1944	1,000.0	377.8	285.9	188.2	81.7	37.8	17.2	7.2	4.2
1918	1945	1,000.0	373.5	279.6	193.2	85.3	39.0	17.6	7.4	4.4
1919	1946	1,000.0	361.0	281.1	200.0	88.4	39.6	17.7	7.7	4.5
1920	1947	1,000.0	336.5	291.7	210.1	90.4	40.9	17.9	7.9	4.6
1921	1948	1,000.0	305.5	304.0	223.0	95.0	41.8	18.3	7.8	4.6
1922	1949	1,000.0	293.8	302.1	233.0	98.8	42.0	17.9	7.8	4.6
1923	1950	1,000.0	280.3	296.5	244.8	104.8	43.2	17.9	7.7	4.8
1924	1951	1,000.0	267.6	286.6	257.3	111.9	45.2	18.5	8.0	4.9
1925	1952	1,000.0	257.3	275.1	265.8	120.1	48.7	19.5	8.3	5.2
1926	1953	1,000.0	251.0	260.6	270.6	129.2	52.7	21.7	8.9	5.3
1927	1954	1,000.0	246.3	245.9	273.9	136.9	57.9	23.7	9.7	5.7
1928	1955	1,000.0	242.7	231.5	274.9	144.8	63.1	26.1	10.6	6.3
1929	1956	1,000.0	234.5	219.7	275.8	153.6	68.5	29.0	11.9	7.0
1930	1957	1,000.0	226.9	208.7	275.9	162.3	73.7	31.6	13.0	7.9
1931	1958	1,000.0	212.8	199.8	278.5	171.4	79.7	34.2	14.5	9.1
1932	1959	1,000.0	201.3	194.0	279.9	178.4	85.1	36.0	15.6	9.7
1933	1960	1,000.0	190.4	188.8	280.3	184.5	90.7	38.3	16.5	10.5
1934	1961	1,000.0	183.6	183.8	278.5	190.3	95.1	40.2	17.3	11.2
1935	1962	1,000.0	181.4	181.0	275.5	193.0	97.2	42.0	18.3	11.6
1936	1963	1,000.0	182.4	179.1	272.5	193.5	99.2	42.9	18.8	11.6
1937	1964	1,000.0	185.2	178.8	270.4	192.4	99.5	43.4	18.7	11.6
1938	1965	1,000.0	189.0	179.6	270.0	191.1	99.0	42.0	18.0	11.3
1939	1966	1,000.0	192.8	183.9	271.4	189.1	95.2	40.3	16.9	10.4
1940	1967	1,000.0	200.8	190.8	275.1	184.0	88.5	36.5	15.2	9.1
1941	1968	1,000.0	212.6	199.5	279.1	175.7	80.1	32.4	12.9	7.7
1942	1969	1,000.0	222.1	212.3	284.9	165.1	71.4	27.1	10.8	6.3
1943	1970	1,000.0	234.5	221.6	287.5	154.7	64.4	23.2	9.1	5.0
1944	1971	1,000.0	245.3	229.0	287.9	146.6	58.5	20.8	7.9	4.0
1945	1972	1,000.0	260.3	237.1	283.6	137.0	53.3	18.5	6.7	3.5
1946	1973	1,000.0	270.0	250.1	283.0	126.3	46.6	15.9	5.4	2.7
1947	1974	1,000.0	284.7	257.8	281.4	116.1	40.9	12.8	4.4	1.9

TABLE 8A. DISTRIBUTIONS OF ALL WOMEN BY PARITY AS OF THE BEGINNING OF EACH YEAR 1917-74 BY AGE FOR EACH COHORT FROM 1867 TO 1959--CON.

(BASED ON CUMULATIVE BIRTH RATES)

EXACT AGE AND COHORT	AS OF JANUARY 1	TOTAL	PARITY							
			0	1	2	3	4	5	6	7 AND HIGHER
28 YEARS										
1889	1917	1,000.0	341.0	209.7	177.6	122.2	77.2	40.5	19.9	11.9
1890	1918	1,000.0	336.5	211.5	181.4	123.7	76.9	39.5	19.3	11.2
1891	1919	1,000.0	329.8	217.7	183.5	124.5	76.7	38.6	18.8	10.4
1892	1920	1,000.0	327.5	219.2	187.9	124.4	75.3	37.8	17.8	10.1
1893	1921	1,000.0	320.6	226.7	187.2	124.8	75.4	38.1	17.5	9.7
1894	1922	1,000.0	314.3	235.7	188.4	124.3	73.4	36.7	17.2	10.0
1895	1923	1,000.0	311.3	241.4	191.6	122.1	71.6	35.4	16.6	10.0
1896	1924	1,000.0	309.1	246.3	194.2	120.2	69.0	34.6	16.6	10.0
1897	1925	1,000.0	306.8	251.1	195.6	118.9	67.1	33.7	16.7	10.1
1898	1926	1,000.0	308.6	249.2	197.9	117.9	66.8	33.2	16.2	10.2
1899	1927	1,000.0	313.8	250.5	196.1	115.2	65.8	32.0	16.5	10.1
1900	1928	1,000.0	319.8	253.2	192.0	112.3	64.4	32.1	15.9	10.3
1901	1929	1,000.0	320.6	260.1	190.5	110.0	62.4	31.3	15.5	9.6
1902	1930	1,000.0	319.4	265.9	191.0	108.1	61.1	30.9	14.5	9.1
1903	1931	1,000.0	319.2	269.7	192.1	106.2	59.5	30.5	14.2	8.6
1904	1932	1,000.0	327.4	270.8	190.1	102.3	57.7	29.5	13.8	8.4
1905	1933	1,000.0	341.4	269.1	185.5	99.0	55.6	28.0	13.3	8.1
1906	1934	1,000.0	355.6	267.4	181.4	95.7	53.3	26.6	12.5	7.5
1907	1935	1,000.0	367.8	263.4	179.3	93.8	51.3	25.4	12.0	7.0
1908	1936	1,000.0	379.3	261.7	177.2	90.2	49.3	24.4	11.3	6.6
1909	1937	1,000.0	388.7	260.1	175.1	87.8	47.9	23.1	10.7	6.6
1910	1938	1,000.0	395.4	261.5	173.1	85.1	45.8	22.3	10.4	6.4
1911	1939	1,000.0	393.0	265.4	174.5	84.1	44.6	21.7	10.2	6.5
1912	1940	1,000.0	391.1	269.9	176.7	82.3	43.2	20.7	9.9	6.2
1913	1941	1,000.0	384.9	274.9	179.9	82.3	42.3	20.1	9.6	6.0
1914	1942	1,000.0	374.1	281.3	184.3	83.3	41.6	20.0	9.1	6.3
1915	1943	1,000.0	356.2	288.9	191.8	85.9	41.9	20.1	8.9	6.3
1916	1944	1,000.0	346.0	285.9	199.8	89.0	43.1	20.6	9.1	6.5
1917	1945	1,000.0	342.5	278.1	205.4	92.8	43.7	21.2	9.8	6.5
1918	1946	1,000.0	340.1	270.7	210.8	95.9	44.7	21.2	9.9	6.7
1919	1947	1,000.0	312.3	278.8	223.7	100.5	46.0	21.6	10.2	6.9
1920	1948	1,000.0	281.0	291.0	236.4	105.1	47.4	21.8	10.3	7.0
1921	1949	1,000.0	261.5	293.1	247.0	110.5	48.4	22.1	10.3	7.1
1922	1950	1,000.0	254.3	285.3	256.4	115.4	49.5	21.7	10.3	7.1
1923	1951	1,000.0	244.1	275.8	266.5	122.4	51.6	22.1	10.2	7.3
1924	1952	1,000.0	230.3	265.7	276.6	131.0	54.9	23.1	10.9	7.5
1925	1953	1,000.0	221.0	253.0	282.1	140.5	59.1	25.0	11.4	7.9
1926	1954	1,000.0	217.0	237.3	284.6	149.1	64.0	27.5	12.2	8.3
1927	1955	1,000.0	213.7	222.5	284.5	157.0	70.0	30.0	13.3	9.0
1928	1956	1,000.0	211.6	208.5	282.5	164.7	75.7	32.7	14.4	9.9
1929	1957	1,000.0	204.2	196.7	280.8	173.6	81.8	35.9	16.0	11.0
1930	1958	1,000.0	197.1	185.7	278.9	182.0	87.6	39.1	17.5	12.1
1931	1959	1,000.0	184.8	177.2	279.5	189.5	94.2	42.0	19.1	13.7
1932	1960	1,000.0	174.9	171.2	278.7	195.4	100.4	44.4	20.3	14.7
1933	1961	1,000.0	165.3	166.8	276.6	200.9	106.3	46.9	21.5	15.7
1934	1962	1,000.0	159.8	162.4	273.6	205.6	110.0	49.4	22.6	16.6
1935	1963	1,000.0	158.6	161.1	270.4	206.7	111.6	51.1	23.6	16.9
1936	1964	1,000.0	160.3	159.9	268.0	206.5	112.9	51.8	23.7	16.9
1937	1965	1,000.0	162.1	161.3	267.1	205.4	112.6	51.6	23.4	16.5
1938	1966	1,000.0	166.4	164.0	268.8	203.9	110.6	48.9	22.0	15.4
1939	1967	1,000.0	169.6	169.8	273.2	201.9	105.4	46.2	20.1	13.8
1940	1968	1,000.0	177.1	176.7	279.0	197.5	98.1	41.6	18.1	11.9
1941	1969	1,000.0	185.9	187.1	285.4	189.8	89.5	37.0	15.3	10.0
1942	1970	1,000.0	194.8	197.0	293.2	180.8	81.1	31.8	13.1	8.2
1943	1971	1,000.0	206.0	205.5	297.2	171.7	74.1	27.7	11.2	6.6
1944	1972	1,000.0	217.2	214.1	299.3	162.4	67.2	24.8	9.7	5.3
1945	1973	1,000.0	233.2	223.3	298.4	150.6	60.3	21.6	8.1	4.5
1946	1974	1,000.0	242.0	236.5	301.0	139.6	52.6	18.3	6.6	3.4

TABLE 8A. DISTRIBUTIONS OF ALL WOMEN BY PARITY AS OF THE BEGINNING OF EACH YEAR 1917-74 BY AGE FOR EACH COHORT FROM 1867 TO 1959--CON.

(BASED ON CUMULATIVE BIRTH RATES)

EXACT AGE AND COHORT	AS OF JANUARY 1	TOTAL	PARITY							
			0	1	2	3	4	5	6	7 AND HIGHER
29 YEARS										
1888---------------	1917	1,000.0	316.3	200.4	175.0	127.1	85.7	49.5	27.5	18.5
1889---------------	1918	1,000.0	313.2	200.8	179.0	128.9	85.4	48.5	26.6	17.6
1890---------------	1919	1,000.0	307.5	203.9	183.0	130.4	85.5	47.5	25.8	16.4
1891---------------	1920	1,000.0	306.7	205.3	186.1	130.2	84.6	46.6	24.8	15.7
1892---------------	1921	1,000.0	298.1	213.2	190.3	130.1	83.3	45.8	23.9	15.3
1893---------------	1922	1,000.0	290.4	222.5	188.7	130.7	82.7	45.8	23.9	15.3
1894---------------	1923	1,000.0	287.2	227.9	193.4	129.6	80.3	43.6	22.8	15.2
1895---------------	1924	1,000.0	285.3	232.2	197.0	128.0	77.7	42.2	22.2	15.4
1896---------------	1925	1,000.0	282.9	238.3	198.2	127.0	75.1	40.9	22.3	15.3
1897---------------	1926	1,000.0	281.5	243.0	200.0	125.5	73.3	39.7	21.7	15.3
1898---------------	1927	1,000.0	284.4	241.5	202.2	123.7	73.3	38.4	21.3	15.2
1899---------------	1928	1,000.0	289.7	243.7	200.5	120.4	71.5	37.8	21.3	15.1
1900---------------	1929	1,000.0	296.5	247.3	196.5	117.3	69.4	37.6	20.5	14.9
1901---------------	1930	1,000.0	297.7	254.5	195.7	115.2	66.7	36.6	19.8	13.8
1902---------------	1931	1,000.0	295.6	261.1	196.8	113.2	65.5	35.8	18.8	13.2
1903---------------	1932	1,000.0	295.7	265.5	198.0	111.1	64.0	35.0	18.1	12.6
1904---------------	1933	1,000.0	305.1	266.5	195.5	107.1	62.0	33.7	17.8	12.3
1905---------------	1934	1,000.0	320.4	264.7	191.0	103.2	60.1	32.2	16.7	11.7
1906---------------	1935	1,000.0	332.7	263.9	187.6	100.6	57.5	30.7	16.1	10.9
1907---------------	1936	1,000.0	343.6	261.8	186.1	98.5	55.2	29.2	15.2	10.4
1908---------------	1937	1,000.0	354.4	260.8	184.8	95.0	53.0	27.9	14.4	9.7
1909---------------	1938	1,000.0	361.8	260.5	183.5	92.8	51.4	26.6	13.7	9.7
1910---------------	1939	1,000.0	366.5	262.2	182.8	90.5	49.6	25.7	13.2	9.5
1911---------------	1940	1,000.0	363.6	266.1	185.0	89.8	48.3	24.9	12.9	9.4
1912---------------	1941	1,000.0	360.1	270.4	188.3	88.7	47.1	23.7	12.4	9.3
1913---------------	1942	1,000.0	350.1	277.4	192.8	89.1	46.3	23.2	12.1	9.0
1914---------------	1943	1,000.0	333.1	284.3	200.7	91.9	46.3	23.1	11.6	9.0
1915---------------	1944	1,000.0	319.9	281.8	210.4	96.3	47.3	23.7	11.5	9.1
1916---------------	1945	1,000.0	316.3	275.5	214.8	99.6	48.5	24.2	11.7	9.4
1917---------------	1946	1,000.0	313.9	265.8	221.6	103.5	48.9	24.7	12.3	9.3
1918---------------	1947	1,000.0	299.7	264.5	230.9	107.7	50.5	24.8	12.3	9.6
1919---------------	1948	1,000.0	266.3	273.7	245.7	114.5	52.2	25.3	12.5	9.8
1920---------------	1949	1,000.0	244.7	278.2	255.9	119.5	53.6	25.4	12.7	10.0
1921---------------	1950	1,000.0	228.7	275.4	266.0	125.6	55.6	25.7	12.8	10.2
1922---------------	1951	1,000.0	224.5	264.4	273.4	131.7	57.6	25.5	12.7	10.2
1923---------------	1952	1,000.0	213.9	254.6	281.2	139.6	61.0	26.3	13.0	10.4
1924---------------	1953	1,000.0	200.8	243.4	288.4	149.7	64.9	28.3	13.7	10.8
1925---------------	1954	1,000.0	193.4	230.5	290.7	159.0	69.9	30.5	14.6	11.4
1926---------------	1955	1,000.0	190.7	214.4	290.5	167.3	75.7	33.5	15.7	12.2
1927---------------	1956	1,000.0	188.8	200.6	287.3	174.8	82.0	36.3	17.1	13.1
1928---------------	1957	1,000.0	187.8	187.1	283.2	181.5	88.5	39.1	18.4	14.4
1929---------------	1958	1,000.0	180.6	175.8	279.4	190.2	94.9	43.0	20.2	15.9
1930---------------	1959	1,000.0	175.0	166.0	275.6	196.9	100.8	46.5	21.9	17.3
1931---------------	1960	1,000.0	164.1	157.6	274.1	203.3	108.0	49.8	23.8	19.3
1932---------------	1961	1,000.0	155.2	152.1	271.9	208.4	114.1	52.5	25.2	20.6
1933---------------	1962	1,000.0	146.7	148.6	268.5	212.5	119.7	55.5	26.6	21.9
1934---------------	1963	1,000.0	142.3	145.3	265.6	215.8	122.7	57.8	27.8	22.7
1935---------------	1964	1,000.0	141.6	144.8	262.9	216.1	123.7	59.5	28.4	23.0
1936---------------	1965	1,000.0	142.1	145.4	261.3	215.9	124.7	59.5	28.6	22.5
1937---------------	1966	1,000.0	144.6	147.9	262.4	214.9	123.2	58.2	27.5	21.3
1938---------------	1967	1,000.0	148.8	151.5	266.6	213.9	119.9	54.6	25.3	19.4
1939---------------	1968	1,000.0	152.0	157.0	272.7	212.2	114.6	51.3	23.0	17.2
1940---------------	1969	1,000.0	157.2	165.2	280.2	208.7	107.0	46.3	20.7	14.7
1941---------------	1970	1,000.0	165.8	173.2	287.8	202.4	98.7	41.9	17.9	12.3
1942---------------	1971	1,000.0	173.3	181.9	297.2	194.8	90.6	36.5	15.5	10.2
1943---------------	1972	1,000.0	184.7	191.2	303.0	185.0	82.6	32.0	13.2	8.3
1944---------------	1973	1,000.0	196.6	199.9	309.1	174.2	74.3	28.1	11.2	6.6
1945---------------	1974	1,000.0	211.9	209.4	310.8	162.3	66.5	24.3	9.3	5.5

TABLE 8A. DISTRIBUTIONS OF ALL WOMEN BY PARITY AS OF THE BEGINNING OF EACH YEAR 1917-74 BY AGE FOR EACH COHORT FROM 1867 TO 1959--CON.

(BASED ON CUMULATIVE BIRTH RATES)

EXACT AGE AND COHORT	AS OF JANUARY 1	TOTAL	PARITY							
			0	1	2	3	4	5	6	7 AND HIGHER
30 YEARS										
1887	1917	1,000.0	296.3	191.3	172.1	130.1	91.7	58.5	33.1	26.9
1888	1918	1,000.0	293.4	191.4	174.4	131.6	91.9	56.3	34.5	26.5
1889	1919	1,000.0	289.2	193.1	178.7	133.3	91.8	55.3	33.5	25.1
1890	1920	1,000.0	287.7	192.7	183.5	134.3	91.6	54.2	32.2	23.8
1891	1921	1,000.0	282.2	198.5	186.6	134.4	90.7	53.4	31.3	22.9
1892	1922	1,000.0	273.3	207.2	190.3	134.2	89.2	52.3	30.5	23.0
1893	1923	1,000.0	267.8	214.2	191.4	134.8	88.0	51.6	29.8	22.4
1894	1924	1,000.0	265.5	218.7	196.3	134.1	85.1	49.3	28.6	22.4
1895	1925	1,000.0	263.4	223.8	198.7	133.4	82.6	47.6	28.0	22.5
1896	1926	1,000.0	261.6	230.1	200.3	132.2	80.1	45.9	27.7	22.1
1897	1927	1,000.0	261.1	234.6	202.6	130.3	78.7	43.9	26.8	22.0
1898	1928	1,000.0	264.5	234.2	204.6	127.9	77.9	43.1	26.1	21.7
1899	1929	1,000.0	270.0	237.1	203.2	124.7	75.5	42.4	25.9	21.2
1900	1930	1,000.0	277.2	241.0	199.7	121.8	72.9	41.8	25.1	20.5
1901	1931	1,000.0	277.6	248.7	199.7	119.6	70.3	40.6	24.2	19.3
1902	1932	1,000.0	276.0	256.0	200.9	117.3	69.1	39.5	22.8	18.4
1903	1933	1,000.0	277.0	260.4	201.9	115.3	67.4	38.3	22.0	17.7
1904	1934	1,000.0	287.4	261.4	199.4	110.8	65.6	37.2	21.3	16.9
1905	1935	1,000.0	301.1	260.2	195.7	107.2	63.6	35.7	20.3	16.2
1906	1936	1,000.0	312.4	260.8	193.0	104.6	60.7	33.9	19.3	15.3
1907	1937	1,000.0	322.4	259.5	192.2	102.8	58.2	32.2	18.3	14.4
1908	1938	1,000.0	331.8	259.4	191.8	99.4	55.9	30.7	17.3	13.7
1909	1939	1,000.0	337.2	259.6	191.6	97.6	54.6	29.3	16.4	13.7
1910	1940	1,000.0	341.3	261.4	191.6	95.7	52.8	28.3	15.7	13.2
1911	1941	1,000.0	336.9	264.9	195.0	95.6	51.7	27.4	15.3	13.2
1912	1942	1,000.0	330.5	270.6	199.4	94.9	50.6	26.3	14.8	12.9
1913	1943	1,000.0	316.1	277.2	206.7	97.0	50.4	25.9	14.4	12.3
1914	1944	1,000.0	302.4	276.0	216.2	101.6	51.0	26.3	14.1	12.4
1915	1945	1,000.0	294.3	270.5	223.1	106.4	52.3	26.8	14.0	12.6
1916	1946	1,000.0	291.8	261.6	228.9	110.1	53.4	27.3	14.0	12.9
1917	1947	1,000.0	279.5	257.1	238.3	115.2	54.6	28.0	14.6	12.7
1918	1948	1,000.0	261.3	257.4	248.5	120.8	56.5	28.0	14.5	13.0
1919	1949	1,000.0	235.9	260.7	260.9	127.7	58.3	28.5	14.8	13.2
1920	1950	1,000.0	217.2	261.5	270.4	133.1	60.5	28.7	15.0	13.6
1921	1951	1,000.0	203.8	255.6	278.7	140.4	63.3	29.2	15.2	13.8
1922	1952	1,000.0	199.5	244.7	283.7	147.3	66.2	29.5	15.3	13.8
1923	1953	1,000.0	189.7	233.8	288.7	156.4	70.6	31.0	15.7	14.1
1924	1954	1,000.0	178.3	222.5	292.9	166.3	75.0	33.6	16.7	14.7
1925	1955	1,000.0	171.8	209.6	293.0	174.9	80.9	36.2	17.9	15.7
1926	1956	1,000.0	170.4	194.6	289.9	182.4	87.2	39.4	19.3	16.8
1927	1957	1,000.0	169.5	181.4	284.5	189.2	93.9	42.4	21.0	18.1
1928	1958	1,000.0	168.9	169.0	278.6	195.2	100.5	45.8	22.3	19.7
1929	1959	1,000.0	162.9	158.9	273.3	202.2	106.9	50.0	24.2	21.6
1930	1960	1,000.0	158.4	149.4	268.1	207.5	113.2	53.7	26.4	23.3
1931	1961	1,000.0	148.3	141.6	265.8	212.9	120.0	57.2	28.5	25.7
1932	1962	1,000.0	140.4	136.8	262.4	217.0	125.8	60.3	30.2	27.1
1933	1963	1,000.0	133.1	134.5	258.9	219.7	130.6	63.2	31.5	28.5
1934	1964	1,000.0	128.9	131.9	256.8	222.2	133.1	65.3	32.5	29.3
1935	1965	1,000.0	127.3	133.1	254.2	222.6	133.9	66.6	33.1	29.2
1936	1966	1,000.0	128.6	134.1	254.6	222.6	134.0	65.6	32.6	27.9
1937	1967	1,000.0	130.9	137.7	257.6	222.0	131.5	63.5	31.0	25.8
1938	1968	1,000.0	135.4	141.1	263.2	221.4	127.8	59.6	28.3	23.2
1939	1969	1,000.0	137.1	147.3	270.6	220.6	122.5	55.8	25.7	20.4
1940	1970	1,000.0	142.3	153.4	279.0	218.1	115.2	51.0	23.5	17.5
1941	1971	1,000.0	149.8	160.7	287.3	213.1	107.2	46.7	20.5	14.7
1942	1972	1,000.0	157.6	169.2	298.9	205.0	98.5	40.9	17.6	12.3
1943	1973	1,000.0	169.4	178.2	308.4	194.6	89.4	35.4	14.8	9.8
1944	1974	1,000.0	180.5	187.4	316.5	184.1	80.2	31.0	12.5	7.8

TABLE 8A. DISTRIBUTIONS OF ALL WOMEN BY PARITY AS OF THE BEGINNING OF EACH YEAR 1917-74 BY AGE FOR EACH COHORT FROM 1867 TO 1959--CON.

(BASED ON CUMULATIVE BIRTH RATES)

EXACT AGE AND COHORT	AS OF JANUARY 1	TOTAL	PARITY							
			0	1	2	3	4	5	6	7 AND HIGHER
31 YEARS										
1886---------------	1917	1,000.0	282.1	177.9	171.9	131.6	95.4	64.4	39.5	37.2
1887---------------	1918	1,000.0	279.2	183.2	170.5	132.7	95.8	63.5	39.3	35.8
1888---------------	1919	1,000.0	275.3	184.5	173.0	134.1	96.0	61.2	40.7	35.2
1889---------------	1920	1,000.0	273.8	183.9	177.9	135.8	95.9	60.0	39.2	33.5
1890---------------	1921	1,000.0	269.3	186.0	182.9	137.1	95.7	59.2	37.9	31.9
1891---------------	1922	1,000.0	263.5	192.1	185.8	137.0	95.1	57.9	37.1	31.5
1892---------------	1923	1,000.0	255.9	199.5	191.3	137.2	93.0	56.5	35.7	30.9
1893---------------	1924	1,000.0	251.1	206.0	192.4	138.0	91.6	55.7	34.9	30.3
1894---------------	1925	1,000.0	248.7	210.9	196.4	138.2	88.7	53.3	33.6	30.2
1895---------------	1926	1,000.0	246.9	216.3	199.2	137.3	86.2	51.3	32.8	30.0
1896---------------	1927	1,000.0	245.7	222.5	201.2	135.9	83.9	49.2	32.1	29.5
1897---------------	1928	1,000.0	245.5	227.6	203.6	133.8	82.1	47.4	30.9	29.1
1898---------------	1929	1,000.0	249.4	227.8	205.8	131.4	80.8	46.5	30.0	28.3
1899---------------	1930	1,000.0	254.8	230.9	205.0	128.3	78.2	45.7	29.7	27.4
1900---------------	1931	1,000.0	261.3	235.3	202.0	125.3	75.7	44.8	28.9	26.7
1901---------------	1932	1,000.0	262.1	243.3	202.1	123.2	73.1	43.4	27.6	25.2
1902---------------	1933	1,000.0	261.2	251.0	203.3	120.6	71.7	42.1	26.1	24.0
1903---------------	1934	1,000.0	263.2	255.3	204.3	118.4	70.1	40.9	25.0	22.8
1904---------------	1935	1,000.0	272.2	256.4	202.8	114.2	68.3	39.8	24.4	21.9
1905---------------	1936	1,000.0	285.0	256.5	199.6	110.5	66.3	38.0	23.1	21.0
1906---------------	1937	1,000.0	295.5	257.8	197.5	108.2	63.2	36.2	21.8	19.8
1907---------------	1938	1,000.0	304.1	257.2	197.5	106.6	60.7	34.3	20.9	18.7
1908---------------	1939	1,000.0	312.1	257.4	198.1	103.6	58.5	32.7	19.6	18.0
1909---------------	1940	1,000.0	316.5	257.7	198.7	102.3	57.3	31.3	18.6	17.6
1910---------------	1941	1,000.0	319.4	258.9	199.9	100.9	55.8	30.2	17.8	17.1
1911---------------	1942	1,000.0	312.7	263.2	204.3	101.2	54.8	29.5	17.3	17.0
1912---------------	1943	1,000.0	303.1	268.4	210.8	101.7	54.2	28.6	16.7	16.5
1913---------------	1944	1,000.0	290.8	268.8	219.1	105.6	54.6	28.6	16.5	16.0
1914---------------	1945	1,000.0	281.0	264.9	226.4	110.8	55.6	28.8	16.4	16.1
1915---------------	1946	1,000.0	273.6	256.5	234.8	116.2	57.1	29.4	16.1	16.3
1916---------------	1947	1,000.0	263.5	251.7	242.3	121.1	58.6	30.2	16.1	16.5
1917---------------	1948	1,000.0	247.6	249.3	251.7	127.4	60.3	30.9	16.5	16.3
1918---------------	1949	1,000.0	236.5	245.2	259.8	132.6	62.1	30.8	16.5	16.5
1919---------------	1950	1,000.0	213.4	245.7	271.3	139.7	64.7	31.5	16.8	16.9
1920---------------	1951	1,000.0	196.8	244.1	279.3	146.0	67.4	32.0	17.1	17.3
1921---------------	1952	1,000.0	183.4	237.7	285.5	154.1	71.3	32.9	17.5	17.6
1922---------------	1953	1,000.0	179.8	226.0	288.1	161.7	75.2	33.8	17.8	17.6
1923---------------	1954	1,000.0	171.3	215.5	290.2	170.9	79.9	35.8	18.4	18.0
1924---------------	1955	1,000.0	160.6	204.0	292.7	180.0	85.2	38.9	19.6	19.0
1925---------------	1956	1,000.0	155.4	192.4	290.1	187.6	91.3	41.7	21.2	20.3
1926---------------	1957	1,000.0	154.9	178.2	285.2	193.9	98.0	45.1	22.8	21.9
1927---------------	1958	1,000.0	154.4	165.9	278.2	200.2	104.6	48.6	24.5	23.6
1928---------------	1959	1,000.0	154.8	154.8	271.2	204.6	111.2	52.1	25.9	25.4
1929---------------	1960	1,000.0	149.6	145.3	264.9	210.1	117.6	56.5	28.3	27.7
1930---------------	1961	1,000.0	145.8	136.3	259.4	214.3	123.4	60.4	30.7	29.7
1931---------------	1962	1,000.0	136.4	129.2	256.1	218.6	130.3	64.0	33.0	32.4
1932---------------	1963	1,000.0	129.5	125.2	252.9	221.9	135.0	67.0	34.7	33.8
1933---------------	1964	1,000.0	122.5	123.8	249.8	223.6	139.3	70.0	35.8	35.2
1934---------------	1965	1,000.0	117.6	122.6	247.9	226.1	141.7	71.7	36.7	35.7
1935---------------	1966	1,000.0	116.7	124.1	246.9	226.9	141.6	72.0	36.9	34.9
1936---------------	1967	1,000.0	118.1	125.9	248.8	227.1	141.0	70.5	36.0	32.6
1937---------------	1968	1,000.0	120.8	129.2	252.8	227.1	138.1	68.2	33.9	29.9
1938---------------	1969	1,000.0	124.3	133.2	259.7	226.9	134.6	63.8	30.9	26.6
1939---------------	1970	1,000.0	125.9	138.3	267.1	227.2	129.4	60.2	28.4	23.5
1940---------------	1971	1,000.0	130.6	143.6	275.9	225.5	122.5	55.5	26.1	20.3
1941---------------	1972	1,000.0	138.2	150.7	286.2	220.2	114.0	50.9	22.7	17.1
1942---------------	1973	1,000.0	146.2	158.5	301.1	212.3	104.4	44.1	19.3	14.1
1943---------------	1974	1,000.0	157.5	167.8	312.0	202.4	94.8	38.2	16.1	11.2

TABLE 8A. DISTRIBUTIONS OF ALL WOMEN BY PARITY AS OF THE BEGINNING OF EACH YEAR 1917-74 BY AGE FOR EACH COHORT FROM 1867 TO 1959--CON.

(BASED ON CUMULATIVE BIRTH RATES)

EXACT AGE AND COHORT	AS OF JANUARY 1	TOTAL	PARITY							
			0	1	2	3	4	5	6	7 AND HIGHER
32 YEARS										
1885	1917	1,000.0	270.3	166.3	170.4	131.8	97.8	68.7	44.9	49.8
1886	1918	1,000.0	268.9	170.8	169.3	132.7	97.8	67.8	44.8	47.9
1887	1919	1,000.0	265.0	177.1	168.3	133.8	97.8	66.9	44.7	46.4
1888	1920	1,000.0	262.6	177.1	171.1	135.4	98.4	64.4	45.7	45.3
1889	1921	1,000.0	259.4	177.6	176.3	137.5	98.4	63.5	44.0	43.3
1890	1922	1,000.0	254.9	179.3	181.4	138.4	98.9	62.2	42.8	42.1
1891	1923	1,000.0	249.4	185.0	185.3	139.4	97.5	60.9	41.6	40.9
1892	1924	1,000.0	242.3	192.2	190.6	139.6	95.5	59.4	40.1	40.3
1893	1925	1,000.0	237.5	198.7	191.2	141.0	94.4	58.5	39.2	39.5
1894	1926	1,000.0	235.3	204.1	195.4	141.0	91.6	56.0	37.7	38.9
1895	1927	1,000.0	234.0	209.2	198.9	139.9	89.3	53.8	36.4	38.5
1896	1928	1,000.0	232.9	216.0	200.9	138.5	86.6	51.8	35.6	37.7
1897	1929	1,000.0	233.1	221.4	203.8	136.4	84.6	49.8	34.3	36.6
1898	1930	1,000.0	237.1	222.0	206.2	134.3	83.0	48.9	33.2	35.3
1899	1931	1,000.0	241.8	225.4	205.9	131.1	80.5	47.9	33.0	34.4
1900	1932	1,000.0	248.8	230.0	203.0	128.1	78.0	46.7	32.1	33.3
1901	1933	1,000.0	249.9	238.2	203.4	125.8	75.2	45.3	30.5	31.7
1902	1934	1,000.0	250.0	246.1	204.3	123.2	73.8	44.0	28.8	29.8
1903	1935	1,000.0	251.0	250.3	206.4	121.0	72.3	42.9	27.6	28.5
1904	1936	1,000.0	259.1	252.4	205.4	116.9	70.6	41.5	26.8	27.3
1905	1937	1,000.0	271.3	253.1	202.7	113.5	68.3	39.8	25.2	26.1
1906	1938	1,000.0	280.9	254.7	201.3	111.4	65.2	37.9	23.9	24.7
1907	1939	1,000.0	288.1	254.2	202.4	110.3	62.8	35.8	23.0	23.4
1908	1940	1,000.0	295.3	254.6	203.7	107.5	60.9	34.2	21.5	22.3
1909	1941	1,000.0	298.7	254.1	205.5	106.8	59.9	32.8	20.4	21.8
1910	1942	1,000.0	299.8	255.8	207.4	105.9	58.6	31.9	19.5	21.1
1911	1943	1,000.0	290.8	260.0	213.1	107.1	57.8	31.4	18.9	20.9
1912	1944	1,000.0	282.1	260.6	220.3	109.2	57.9	30.8	18.6	20.5
1913	1945	1,000.0	272.7	258.5	227.0	113.8	58.7	30.9	18.4	20.0
1914	1946	1,000.0	263.4	251.8	235.4	119.9	60.1	31.1	18.2	20.1
1915	1947	1,000.0	250.0	246.5	244.8	126.5	62.2	31.8	18.0	20.2
1916	1948	1,000.0	237.1	243.9	252.1	132.0	64.0	32.8	17.8	20.3
1917	1949	1,000.0	226.8	238.2	259.6	138.0	65.7	33.4	18.3	20.0
1918	1950	1,000.0	218.0	232.2	266.8	142.9	68.2	33.4	18.2	20.3
1919	1951	1,000.0	196.5	230.8	277.0	150.8	71.0	34.5	18.7	20.7
1920	1952	1,000.0	179.9	228.7	283.4	157.6	74.7	35.3	19.1	21.3
1921	1953	1,000.0	167.0	221.7	287.2	166.2	79.5	37.0	19.8	21.6
1922	1954	1,000.0	164.8	210.0	287.3	173.9	83.8	38.4	20.1	21.7
1923	1955	1,000.0	156.6	199.9	288.1	182.2	89.2	40.6	21.1	22.3
1924	1956	1,000.0	147.2	189.0	288.5	190.4	94.6	44.1	22.6	23.6
1925	1957	1,000.0	142.6	178.4	284.1	197.1	100.9	47.1	24.5	25.3
1926	1958	1,000.0	142.6	165.1	278.0	202.5	107.4	50.9	26.2	27.3
1927	1959	1,000.0	142.9	154.0	270.3	207.2	114.2	54.3	27.8	29.3
1928	1960	1,000.0	143.9	143.9	262.6	210.3	120.3	57.9	29.7	31.4
1929	1961	1,000.0	139.3	134.8	256.3	214.6	126.2	62.6	32.1	34.1
1930	1962	1,000.0	136.1	126.3	250.3	217.8	131.9	66.6	34.7	36.3
1931	1963	1,000.0	127.5	119.9	247.3	221.4	137.7	70.0	37.0	39.2
1932	1964	1,000.0	120.9	116.5	244.4	223.9	142.1	73.0	38.7	40.5
1933	1965	1,000.0	113.5	116.2	241.4	225.8	146.2	75.5	39.7	41.7
1934	1966	1,000.0	109.0	115.3	240.9	228.4	148.0	76.7	40.2	41.5
1935	1967	1,000.0	108.3	117.8	240.9	229.4	147.3	76.5	40.1	39.7
1936	1968	1,000.0	110.4	119.2	243.6	230.0	146.4	74.8	38.7	36.9
1937	1969	1,000.0	112.2	122.9	248.9	230.5	143.5	72.1	36.3	33.6
1938	1970	1,000.0	115.9	126.2	255.5	231.0	140.3	67.8	33.3	30.0
1939	1971	1,000.0	117.1	130.9	263.1	231.9	135.3	64.2	30.9	26.6
1940	1972	1,000.0	122.1	135.9	273.5	230.0	128.0	59.2	28.3	23.0
1941	1973	1,000.0	129.8	142.6	286.2	225.0	118.9	53.9	24.5	19.1
1942	1974	1,000.0	137.4	150.5	302.1	217.9	109.0	46.7	20.7	15.7

TABLE 8A. DISTRIBUTIONS OF ALL WOMEN BY PARITY AS OF THE BEGINNING OF EACH YEAR 1917-74 BY AGE FOR EACH COHORT FROM 1867 TO 1959--CON.

(BASED ON CUMULATIVE BIRTH RATES)

EXACT AGE AND COHORT	AS OF JANUARY 1	TOTAL	PARITY							
			0	1	2	3	4	5	6	7 AND HIGHER
33 YEARS										
1884---------------	1917	1,000.0	259.4	158.3	166.3	131.2	99.3	72.9	49.0	63.6
1885---------------	1918	1,000.0	260.2	160.0	167.5	131.9	99.2	70.9	49.2	61.1
1886---------------	1919	1,000.0	258.0	165.4	166.7	132.8	98.9	69.9	49.2	59.1
1887---------------	1920	1,000.0	255.3	170.6	165.9	134.2	99.3	68.8	48.8	57.1
1888---------------	1921	1,000.0	251.6	171.4	169.0	136.1	99.9	66.7	49.6	55.7
1889---------------	1922	1,000.0	248.4	171.7	174.1	137.9	100.6	65.4	47.8	54.1
1890---------------	1923	1,000.0	244.1	173.0	180.2	139.7	100.5	64.1	46.4	52.0
1891---------------	1924	1,000.0	238.9	178.6	183.8	140.8	99.1	62.8	45.2	50.8
1892---------------	1925	1,000.0	231.8	185.8	188.7	141.6	97.3	61.2	43.5	50.1
1893---------------	1926	1,000.0	227.1	192.8	189.5	142.7	96.4	60.5	42.2	48.8
1894---------------	1927	1,000.0	225.4	198.1	193.9	142.7	93.9	57.8	40.4	47.8
1895---------------	1928	1,000.0	224.1	203.5	197.7	141.6	91.3	55.4	39.2	47.2
1896---------------	1929	1,000.0	223.4	210.4	200.2	140.3	88.4	53.6	38.2	45.5
1897---------------	1930	1,000.0	223.7	216.2	203.3	138.4	86.3	51.7	36.6	43.8
1898---------------	1931	1,000.0	227.2	217.2	205.9	136.3	84.8	50.4	35.8	42.4
1899---------------	1932	1,000.0	232.2	220.5	205.8	133.2	82.3	49.4	35.4	41.2
1900---------------	1933	1,000.0	239.5	225.2	203.2	129.9	79.6	48.1	34.4	40.1
1901---------------	1934	1,000.0	241.1	233.7	203.5	127.6	76.9	46.7	32.5	38.0
1902---------------	1935	1,000.0	240.6	241.5	205.1	125.2	75.5	45.5	30.8	35.8
1903---------------	1936	1,000.0	241.1	246.3	207.7	123.1	74.1	44.3	29.3	34.1
1904---------------	1937	1,000.0	248.5	248.9	207.2	119.4	72.2	42.8	28.4	32.6
1905---------------	1938	1,000.0	260.0	249.8	205.1	116.1	69.9	41.1	26.8	31.2
1906---------------	1939	1,000.0	268.6	251.3	204.7	114.4	66.9	39.1	25.4	29.6
1907---------------	1940	1,000.0	275.0	250.9	206.4	113.6	64.7	37.1	24.4	27.9
1908---------------	1941	1,000.0	281.6	250.6	208.6	111.2	63.1	35.4	22.9	26.6
1909---------------	1942	1,000.0	283.5	250.3	211.1	111.0	62.2	34.2	21.8	25.9
1910---------------	1943	1,000.0	281.8	252.3	214.3	110.9	61.2	33.6	20.7	25.2
1911---------------	1944	1,000.0	273.4	252.8	220.4	113.5	61.1	33.3	20.4	25.1
1912---------------	1945	1,000.0	267.2	251.2	226.1	116.3	61.6	32.7	20.2	24.7
1913---------------	1946	1,000.0	257.9	247.0	233.7	121.8	62.6	33.1	19.8	24.1
1914---------------	1947	1,000.0	244.2	242.2	242.9	128.8	64.8	33.2	19.9	24.0
1915---------------	1948	1,000.0	228.3	239.2	251.7	136.0	67.0	34.3	19.5	24.0
1916---------------	1949	1,000.0	220.2	234.3	257.1	141.0	68.9	35.1	19.4	24.0
1917---------------	1950	1,000.0	211.6	227.1	264.1	146.6	71.2	35.8	19.9	23.7
1918---------------	1951	1,000.0	204.4	219.6	270.3	151.9	73.9	36.0	19.9	24.0
1919---------------	1952	1,000.0	182.8	217.7	279.0	160.4	77.4	37.7	20.3	24.7
1920---------------	1953	1,000.0	166.5	215.4	283.4	167.3	81.9	39.1	21.1	25.3
1921---------------	1954	1,000.0	154.7	208.3	285.0	176.0	87.2	41.2	21.9	25.7
1922---------------	1955	1,000.0	152.9	196.9	284.0	182.9	92.1	42.6	22.6	26.0
1923---------------	1956	1,000.0	145.7	187.4	283.2	190.3	97.5	45.4	23.8	26.7
1924---------------	1957	1,000.0	136.8	177.2	282.4	197.5	103.1	49.1	25.4	28.5
1925---------------	1958	1,000.0	132.6	167.5	276.7	203.5	109.2	52.3	27.6	30.6
1926---------------	1959	1,000.0	133.3	155.2	270.4	207.4	115.5	56.2	29.3	32.7
1927---------------	1960	1,000.0	134.1	145.1	262.2	211.0	121.8	59.6	31.2	35.0
1928---------------	1961	1,000.0	135.7	135.3	254.7	213.0	127.5	63.3	33.1	37.4
1929---------------	1962	1,000.0	131.5	126.7	248.0	216.5	133.1	68.0	35.6	40.6
1930---------------	1963	1,000.0	128.9	118.7	242.6	219.2	137.8	71.8	38.3	42.7
1931---------------	1964	1,000.0	120.7	112.7	239.7	222.1	143.5	75.1	40.5	45.7
1932---------------	1965	1,000.0	113.6	110.4	237.1	224.6	147.6	77.7	42.1	46.9
1933---------------	1966	1,000.0	106.6	110.6	234.9	226.7	151.0	80.0	42.8	47.4
1934---------------	1967	1,000.0	102.4	110.2	235.4	229.5	152.5	80.6	43.1	46.3
1935---------------	1968	1,000.0	102.3	112.5	236.0	230.5	151.9	80.2	42.5	44.1
1936---------------	1969	1,000.0	103.7	114.5	239.7	231.7	150.7	78.2	40.9	40.6
1937---------------	1970	1,000.0	105.8	117.6	244.7	232.7	148.0	75.6	38.5	37.1
1938---------------	1971	1,000.0	109.3	120.7	251.5	233.6	144.8	71.4	35.5	33.2
1939---------------	1972	1,000.0	110.7	125.2	260.3	234.4	139.7	67.3	33.0	29.4
1940---------------	1973	1,000.0	115.9	129.9	272.4	232.9	131.8	61.9	30.0	25.2
1941---------------	1974	1,000.0	123.4	136.6	285.9	228.5	122.6	56.2	25.9	20.9

TABLE 8A. DISTRIBUTIONS OF ALL WOMEN BY PARITY AS OF THE BEGINNING OF EACH YEAR 1917-74 BY AGE FOR EACH COHORT FROM 1867 TO 1959--CON.

(BASED ON CUMULATIVE BIRTH RATES)

EXACT AGE AND COHORT	AS OF JANUARY 1	TOTAL	PARITY							
			0	1	2	3	4	5	6	7 AND HIGHER
34 YEARS										
1883	1917	1,000.0	249.8	152.7	160.3	129.9	100.3	76.0	52.1	78.9
1884	1918	1,000.0	250.7	153.0	162.7	130.5	100.0	74.5	52.5	76.1
1885	1919	1,000.0	250.9	155.5	164.1	131.3	99.6	72.5	52.7	73.4
1886	1920	1,000.0	249.7	159.9	163.7	132.4	99.7	71.3	52.5	70.8
1887	1921	1,000.0	245.9	165.8	163.0	134.1	100.2	70.6	51.9	68.5
1888	1922	1,000.0	242.2	166.4	166.1	135.7	101.4	68.0	52.7	67.5
1889	1923	1,000.0	239.2	166.4	172.0	138.4	101.6	66.8	50.7	64.9
1890	1924	1,000.0	235.2	167.5	177.9	140.3	101.5	65.5	49.2	62.9
1891	1925	1,000.0	229.9	173.2	181.0	142.0	100.3	64.1	47.9	61.6
1892	1926	1,000.0	223.0	180.5	186.4	142.6	98.8	62.5	45.9	60.3
1893	1927	1,000.0	218.9	187.6	187.3	143.5	98.3	61.6	44.4	58.4
1894	1928	1,000.0	217.0	193.3	192.1	143.4	95.6	58.9	42.5	57.2
1895	1929	1,000.0	216.1	198.6	196.3	142.6	92.7	56.7	41.4	55.6
1896	1930	1,000.0	215.5	205.9	198.9	141.7	89.7	54.9	40.1	53.3
1897	1931	1,000.0	215.4	212.0	202.3	139.8	87.6	52.9	38.7	51.3
1898	1932	1,000.0	219.4	213.1	205.0	137.6	86.2	51.5	37.6	49.6
1899	1933	1,000.0	224.5	216.2	205.1	134.6	83.5	50.3	37.4	48.4
1900	1934	1,000.0	232.2	221.2	202.6	131.0	80.9	49.1	36.1	46.9
1901	1935	1,000.0	233.3	229.6	203.3	129.0	78.2	47.8	34.2	44.6
1902	1936	1,000.0	232.5	237.8	205.5	126.6	77.0	46.5	32.2	41.9
1903	1937	1,000.0	232.6	242.9	208.5	124.9	75.4	45.4	30.6	39.7
1904	1938	1,000.0	239.4	245.7	208.4	121.5	73.5	43.8	29.6	38.1
1905	1939	1,000.0	250.1	246.5	207.2	118.4	71.2	42.2	28.0	36.4
1906	1940	1,000.0	258.1	248.0	207.3	117.0	68.5	40.2	26.5	34.4
1907	1941	1,000.0	264.0	247.0	209.7	116.7	66.5	38.1	25.5	32.5
1908	1942	1,000.0	269.6	246.9	212.3	114.6	65.1	36.6	24.0	30.9
1909	1943	1,000.0	268.1	247.1	216.5	115.1	64.6	35.5	22.9	30.2
1910	1944	1,000.0	267.0	245.8	219.9	116.3	64.2	35.2	22.0	29.6
1911	1945	1,000.0	260.7	244.4	224.7	119.6	64.4	34.9	21.8	29.5
1912	1946	1,000.0	254.5	241.3	230.8	123.2	65.1	34.7	21.4	29.0
1913	1947	1,000.0	241.9	238.5	239.0	129.3	66.8	35.1	21.3	28.1
1914	1948	1,000.0	226.3	235.4	247.7	136.8	69.2	35.4	21.3	27.9
1915	1949	1,000.0	214.1	230.8	254.9	143.5	71.5	36.5	20.9	27.8
1916	1950	1,000.0	207.4	225.1	259.8	148.0	73.7	37.3	20.9	27.8
1917	1951	1,000.0	200.1	216.6	265.8	153.9	76.4	38.3	21.4	27.5
1918	1952	1,000.0	193.0	209.1	270.8	159.4	79.6	38.8	21.4	27.9
1919	1953	1,000.0	171.6	206.8	277.7	168.3	83.7	41.1	22.1	28.7
1920	1954	1,000.0	156.2	204.3	280.5	175.0	88.7	42.8	23.1	29.4
1921	1955	1,000.0	144.7	197.2	281.3	182.9	94.5	45.1	24.3	30.0
1922	1956	1,000.0	143.8	186.4	278.9	189.2	99.3	46.9	25.1	30.4
1923	1957	1,000.0	137.0	177.4	277.4	195.7	104.7	50.0	26.4	31.4
1924	1958	1,000.0	128.4	168.0	275.4	202.2	110.4	53.7	28.2	33.7
1925	1959	1,000.0	124.8	159.3	269.5	206.8	116.2	57.1	30.4	35.9
1926	1960	1,000.0	126.0	147.6	263.2	209.8	121.9	60.9	32.3	38.3
1927	1961	1,000.0	127.3	137.9	255.1	212.5	127.7	64.4	34.3	40.8
1928	1962	1,000.0	129.3	128.7	247.4	213.9	133.0	68.0	36.2	43.5
1929	1963	1,000.0	125.6	120.4	241.4	216.8	137.8	72.5	38.8	46.7
1930	1964	1,000.0	123.3	112.8	236.0	219.2	142.3	76.1	41.4	48.9
1931	1965	1,000.0	114.6	107.8	233.3	221.9	148.0	78.9	43.6	51.9
1932	1966	1,000.0	107.9	105.9	231.4	224.5	151.4	81.6	44.9	52.4
1933	1967	1,000.0	101.2	106.6	229.9	227.0	154.5	83.3	45.3	52.2
1934	1968	1,000.0	97.5	106.0	231.1	229.7	156.0	83.8	45.2	50.7
1935	1969	1,000.0	96.9	108.9	232.2	231.3	155.2	83.2	44.4	47.9
1936	1970	1,000.0	98.8	110.2	236.0	232.7	154.1	81.1	43.0	44.1
1937	1971	1,000.0	100.7	113.4	241.2	233.9	151.4	78.5	40.6	40.3
1938	1972	1,000.0	104.6	116.4	248.7	234.9	148.0	74.0	37.3	36.1
1939	1973	1,000.0	105.9	121.0	258.7	235.9	142.7	69.5	34.6	31.7
1940	1974	1,000.0	111.2	125.4	271.5	235.0	134.7	63.8	31.3	27.1

TABLE 8A. DISTRIBUTIONS OF ALL WOMEN BY PARITY AS OF THE BEGINNING OF EACH YEAR 1917-74 BY AGE FOR EACH COHORT FROM 1867 TO 1959--CON.

(BASED ON CUMULATIVE BIRTH RATES)

EXACT AGE AND COHORT	AS OF JANUARY 1	TOTAL	PARITY 0	1	2	3	4	5	6	7 AND HIGHER
35 YEARS										
1882	1917	1,000.0	242.9	146.5	154.8	127.9	100.3	76.8	56.0	94.8
1883	1918	1,000.0	242.6	148.4	156.8	128.6	100.5	76.7	54.8	91.6
1884	1919	1,000.0	243.2	149.1	159.4	129.3	100.0	75.2	55.3	88.5
1885	1920	1,000.0	244.0	151.1	161.1	130.2	99.9	73.2	55.2	85.3
1886	1921	1,000.0	242.0	156.0	160.7	131.7	100.0	72.3	54.9	82.4
1887	1922	1,000.0	238.1	161.7	160.0	133.2	101.0	71.4	54.2	80.4
1888	1923	1,000.0	234.7	162.1	163.7	135.5	101.8	68.8	54.9	78.5
1889	1924	1,000.0	231.9	162.0	169.5	138.2	102.2	67.6	52.8	75.8
1890	1925	1,000.0	227.8	163.2	175.0	140.5	102.2	66.4	51.2	73.7
1891	1926	1,000.0	222.5	169.0	178.6	142.2	101.1	65.0	49.7	71.9
1892	1927	1,000.0	216.2	176.3	183.9	142.7	100.1	63.2	47.5	70.1
1893	1928	1,000.0	212.1	183.7	185.1	143.6	99.4	62.3	45.9	67.9
1894	1929	1,000.0	210.5	189.4	190.2	143.8	96.6	59.8	44.0	65.7
1895	1930	1,000.0	209.7	194.9	194.7	143.2	93.5	57.6	42.9	63.5
1896	1931	1,000.0	208.8	202.3	197.5	142.5	90.6	55.8	41.6	60.9
1897	1932	1,000.0	209.0	208.6	201.0	140.6	88.6	53.8	40.0	58.4
1898	1933	1,000.0	213.5	209.6	203.7	138.5	86.9	52.2	39.1	56.5
1899	1934	1,000.0	218.6	212.9	204.1	135.2	84.5	50.9	38.7	55.1
1900	1935	1,000.0	226.0	217.7	201.8	131.8	82.0	49.8	37.3	53.6
1901	1936	1,000.0	226.8	226.4	202.9	130.1	79.2	48.6	35.2	50.8
1902	1937	1,000.0	225.8	234.8	205.6	127.7	78.2	47.2	33.2	47.5
1903	1938	1,000.0	225.5	240.0	208.9	126.4	76.5	46.2	31.5	45.0
1904	1939	1,000.0	231.5	242.9	209.5	123.1	74.7	44.6	30.5	43.2
1905	1940	1,000.0	241.7	243.7	208.7	120.4	72.5	43.1	28.8	41.1
1906	1941	1,000.0	249.3	244.7	209.4	119.3	70.0	41.1	27.3	38.9
1907	1942	1,000.0	254.3	243.8	212.2	119.3	68.2	39.1	26.3	36.8
1908	1943	1,000.0	257.5	244.0	215.9	117.9	67.0	37.7	25.0	35.0
1909	1944	1,000.0	256.2	241.7	220.2	119.5	67.1	36.8	24.0	34.5
1910	1945	1,000.0	256.3	238.9	222.9	121.2	67.1	36.5	23.2	33.9
1911	1946	1,000.0	249.9	236.3	227.8	125.3	67.4	36.8	22.8	33.7
1912	1947	1,000.0	241.2	234.2	234.4	129.5	68.6	36.5	22.6	33.0
1913	1948	1,000.0	227.2	232.8	242.1	135.7	70.8	36.9	22.6	31.9
1914	1949	1,000.0	214.4	228.5	249.7	142.8	73.1	37.5	22.4	31.6
1915	1950	1,000.0	203.3	223.3	256.4	149.1	75.7	38.5	22.2	31.5
1916	1951	1,000.0	197.6	216.8	260.5	153.6	78.3	39.5	22.2	31.5
1917	1952	1,000.0	190.5	208.0	265.5	159.8	81.3	40.9	22.8	31.2
1918	1953	1,000.0	183.7	200.4	269.1	165.5	85.0	41.7	23.0	31.6
1919	1954	1,000.0	162.9	198.0	274.7	174.0	89.6	44.3	23.9	32.6
1920	1955	1,000.0	147.9	195.3	276.7	180.3	94.8	46.3	25.2	33.5
1921	1956	1,000.0	137.0	188.7	276.4	187.5	100.7	48.8	26.6	34.3
1922	1957	1,000.0	136.6	178.2	273.5	193.2	105.3	50.9	27.4	34.9
1923	1958	1,000.0	130.0	169.8	271.3	198.9	110.8	54.1	28.9	36.2
1924	1959	1,000.0	122.0	161.2	268.9	204.5	116.1	57.9	30.8	38.6
1925	1960	1,000.0	118.7	153.1	263.2	208.1	121.4	61.3	33.0	41.2
1926	1961	1,000.0	120.3	141.7	257.0	210.4	126.8	65.1	34.9	43.8
1927	1962	1,000.0	122.0	132.4	248.8	212.8	132.0	68.5	36.9	46.6
1928	1963	1,000.0	124.4	123.8	241.6	213.8	136.6	71.7	39.0	49.1
1929	1964	1,000.0	121.0	115.7	235.7	216.4	141.2	76.2	41.4	52.4
1930	1965	1,000.0	118.2	108.9	230.7	218.5	145.7	79.4	44.0	54.6
1931	1966	1,000.0	109.9	104.4	228.2	221.5	150.8	82.2	46.0	57.0
1932	1967	1,000.0	103.5	102.7	227.1	224.3	154.0	84.4	47.0	57.0
1933	1968	1,000.0	97.2	103.3	226.1	226.7	157.2	85.9	47.3	56.3
1934	1969	1,000.0	93.1	103.4	227.6	229.8	158.5	86.3	47.0	54.3
1935	1970	1,000.0	93.0	105.7	229.0	231.4	157.6	85.6	46.4	51.3
1936	1971	1,000.0	94.8	107.1	232.9	233.0	156.6	83.6	44.7	47.3
1937	1972	1,000.0	97.0	110.3	238.7	234.3	153.7	80.6	42.2	43.2
1938	1973	1,000.0	100.9	113.4	247.1	235.6	150.1	75.8	38.7	38.4
1939	1974	1,000.0	102.3	117.7	257.7	237.0	144.8	71.1	35.8	33.6

TABLE 8A. DISTRIBUTIONS OF ALL WOMEN BY PARITY AS OF THE BEGINNING OF EACH YEAR 1917-74 BY AGE FOR EACH COHORT FROM 1867 TO 1959--CON.

(BASED ON CUMULATIVE BIRTH RATES)

EXACT AGE AND COHORT	AS OF JANUARY 1	TOTAL	PARITY							
			0	1	2	3	4	5	6	7 AND HIGHER
36 YEARS										
1881	1917	1,000.0	238.4	140.2	148.9	125.0	99.2	76.6	60.6	111.1
1882	1918	1,000.0	236.8	143.0	151.6	126.3	99.9	77.0	57.8	107.6
1883	1919	1,000.0	236.3	145.1	153.7	127.1	100.2	76.7	56.8	104.1
1884	1920	1,000.0	237.2	145.6	156.5	127.9	99.8	75.4	56.9	100.7
1885	1921	1,000.0	237.6	147.8	158.2	129.1	99.7	73.6	56.9	97.1
1886	1922	1,000.0	235.3	152.7	157.9	130.5	100.1	72.8	56.4	94.3
1887	1923	1,000.0	231.8	158.3	157.4	132.6	101.0	71.7	55.8	91.4
1888	1924	1,000.0	228.6	158.4	161.2	134.9	102.0	69.2	56.3	89.4
1889	1925	1,000.0	225.7	158.5	166.7	137.9	102.5	68.1	54.1	86.5
1890	1926	1,000.0	221.7	159.7	172.7	140.1	102.7	66.8	52.5	83.8
1891	1927	1,000.0	216.8	165.5	176.2	141.8	101.9	65.3	50.8	81.7
1892	1928	1,000.0	210.4	173.2	181.8	142.3	100.9	63.4	48.6	79.4
1893	1929	1,000.0	206.6	180.7	183.2	143.4	100.1	62.6	47.1	76.3
1894	1930	1,000.0	205.3	186.4	188.5	143.8	97.0	60.4	45.2	73.4
1895	1931	1,000.0	204.2	191.9	193.2	143.4	94.0	58.3	43.9	71.1
1896	1932	1,000.0	203.5	199.6	196.0	142.7	91.3	56.4	42.5	68.0
1897	1933	1,000.0	204.0	205.8	199.6	140.9	89.1	54.4	41.0	65.2
1898	1934	1,000.0	208.9	206.9	202.4	138.7	87.6	52.5	40.0	63.0
1899	1935	1,000.0	213.6	210.1	202.9	135.6	85.2	51.4	39.6	61.6
1900	1936	1,000.0	220.7	215.1	201.0	132.3	82.8	50.4	37.9	59.8
1901	1937	1,000.0	221.3	224.0	202.4	130.8	80.0	49.1	36.0	56.4
1902	1938	1,000.0	220.1	232.5	205.4	128.6	79.0	47.8	33.9	52.7
1903	1939	1,000.0	219.3	237.6	209.3	127.3	77.5	46.9	32.1	50.0
1904	1940	1,000.0	224.8	240.5	210.2	124.4	75.9	45.2	31.3	47.7
1905	1941	1,000.0	234.7	241.0	209.8	122.1	73.7	43.8	29.5	45.4
1906	1942	1,000.0	241.6	242.1	210.8	121.2	71.4	41.9	28.0	43.0
1907	1943	1,000.0	244.8	241.4	214.3	121.9	69.8	39.9	27.1	40.8
1908	1944	1,000.0	247.9	239.8	218.1	121.3	69.1	38.8	25.9	39.1
1909	1945	1,000.0	247.2	236.3	222.1	123.4	69.5	37.9	25.0	38.6
1910	1946	1,000.0	247.2	232.4	224.8	125.8	69.7	38.1	24.1	37.9
1911	1947	1,000.0	238.8	230.6	230.0	130.4	70.4	38.5	23.8	37.5
1912	1948	1,000.0	229.1	229.5	236.4	134.5	72.0	38.1	23.8	36.6
1913	1949	1,000.0	217.3	227.2	243.3	140.4	74.1	38.7	23.6	35.4
1914	1950	1,000.0	205.3	222.6	250.5	147.2	76.5	39.2	23.5	35.2
1915	1951	1,000.0	194.9	216.9	256.4	153.4	79.5	40.5	23.4	35.0
1916	1952	1,000.0	189.5	210.1	259.7	158.0	82.4	41.7	23.6	35.0
1917	1953	1,000.0	182.6	201.1	263.6	164.5	85.8	43.5	24.2	34.7
1918	1954	1,000.0	176.5	193.5	266.1	169.7	90.0	44.5	24.4	35.3
1919	1955	1,000.0	155.9	190.9	271.0	178.0	94.6	47.5	25.5	36.6
1920	1956	1,000.0	141.4	188.5	272.4	183.7	99.8	49.5	27.2	37.5
1921	1957	1,000.0	130.9	182.1	271.6	190.4	105.5	52.3	28.6	38.6
1922	1958	1,000.0	130.8	172.0	268.3	195.3	110.2	54.4	29.6	39.4
1923	1959	1,000.0	124.6	164.3	265.8	200.4	115.4	57.5	31.3	40.7
1924	1960	1,000.0	116.9	156.2	263.3	205.3	120.2	61.5	33.1	43.5
1925	1961	1,000.0	113.9	148.3	257.9	208.2	125.2	64.9	35.4	46.2
1926	1962	1,000.0	115.9	137.2	251.6	210.3	130.2	68.5	37.2	49.1
1927	1963	1,000.0	117.9	128.5	243.7	212.4	134.8	71.6	39.3	51.8
1928	1964	1,000.0	120.6	120.0	236.9	213.1	139.2	74.7	41.3	54.2
1929	1965	1,000.0	116.8	112.6	231.2	215.5	143.8	78.9	43.6	57.6
1930	1966	1,000.0	114.2	106.3	226.6	217.6	147.9	82.1	46.1	59.2
1931	1967	1,000.0	106.2	101.9	224.7	220.9	152.7	84.5	47.8	61.3
1932	1968	1,000.0	100.2	100.2	223.8	223.8	156.0	86.5	48.7	60.8
1933	1969	1,000.0	93.6	101.2	223.3	226.3	159.0	87.9	49.0	59.7
1934	1970	1,000.0	89.9	101.0	224.9	229.6	160.1	88.3	48.6	57.6
1935	1971	1,000.0	89.9	103.2	226.6	231.2	159.3	87.6	47.8	54.4
1936	1972	1,000.0	91.9	104.8	230.8	232.9	158.1	85.3	46.1	50.1
1937	1973	1,000.0	94.2	108.0	237.3	234.5	155.1	82.1	43.4	45.4
1938	1974	1,000.0	98.2	111.0	246.1	236.1	151.6	77.1	39.6	40.3

TABLE 8A. DISTRIBUTIONS OF ALL WOMEN BY PARITY AS OF THE BEGINNING OF EACH YEAR 1917-74 BY AGE FOR EACH COHORT FROM 1867 TO 1959--CON.

(BASED ON CUMULATIVE BIRTH RATES)

EXACT AGE AND COHORT	AS OF JANUARY 1	TOTAL	PARITY							
			0	1	2	3	4	5	6	7 AND HIGHER
37 YEARS										
1880	1917	1,000.0	234.2	134.8	143.7	122.3	98.1	75.7	64.3	126.9
1881	1918	1,000.0	233.6	137.2	146.1	123.4	98.6	76.1	61.5	123.5
1882	1919	1,000.0	231.8	140.1	148.9	124.7	99.5	76.4	59.0	119.6
1883	1920	1,000.0	231.4	142.2	151.1	125.7	99.6	76.4	57.6	116.0
1884	1921	1,000.0	232.1	142.8	153.8	126.8	99.2	75.2	57.8	112.3
1885	1922	1,000.0	232.2	145.0	155.7	127.9	99.4	73.6	57.7	108.5
1886	1923	1,000.0	230.3	149.9	155.5	129.6	99.8	72.8	57.2	104.9
1887	1924	1,000.0	226.9	155.3	155.0	131.8	100.9	71.8	56.5	101.8
1888	1925	1,000.0	223.6	155.6	158.7	134.2	102.0	69.3	57.0	99.6
1889	1926	1,000.0	220.7	155.9	164.4	137.0	102.7	68.3	54.8	96.2
1890	1927	1,000.0	217.1	156.9	170.4	139.4	103.0	67.0	53.2	93.0
1891	1928	1,000.0	212.0	163.0	174.2	141.2	102.2	65.2	51.6	90.6
1892	1929	1,000.0	205.9	170.9	179.8	141.9	101.2	63.6	49.3	87.4
1893	1930	1,000.0	202.4	178.3	181.5	143.2	100.3	62.8	47.9	83.6
1894	1931	1,000.0	201.0	183.9	187.0	143.6	97.2	60.9	45.9	80.5
1895	1932	1,000.0	199.9	189.7	191.8	143.2	94.3	58.6	44.7	77.8
1896	1933	1,000.0	199.5	197.4	194.5	142.7	91.6	56.7	43.1	74.5
1897	1934	1,000.0	200.3	203.7	198.2	140.8	89.5	54.7	41.6	71.2
1898	1935	1,000.0	205.1	204.7	201.1	138.7	88.1	52.7	40.7	68.9
1899	1936	1,000.0	209.4	208.1	201.8	135.9	85.7	51.8	40.0	67.3
1900	1937	1,000.0	216.4	213.2	200.2	132.6	83.3	50.7	38.5	65.1
1901	1938	1,000.0	216.8	222.1	201.9	131.3	80.6	49.5	36.5	61.3
1902	1939	1,000.0	215.3	230.6	205.3	129.0	79.8	48.3	34.3	57.4
1903	1940	1,000.0	214.1	235.8	209.4	128.0	78.5	47.3	32.7	54.2
1904	1941	1,000.0	219.3	238.3	210.8	125.5	76.8	45.7	31.8	51.8
1905	1942	1,000.0	228.6	238.9	210.6	123.4	74.8	44.4	30.0	49.3
1906	1943	1,000.0	234.7	240.1	211.7	123.0	72.6	42.6	28.6	46.7
1907	1944	1,000.0	237.4	238.2	215.4	124.4	71.4	40.9	27.7	44.6
1908	1945	1,000.0	240.6	235.6	219.2	124.2	71.1	39.8	26.7	42.8
1909	1946	1,000.0	239.8	231.2	223.2	126.8	71.7	39.2	25.8	42.3
1910	1947	1,000.0	238.3	227.9	226.1	129.7	72.1	39.5	24.9	41.5
1911	1948	1,000.0	228.9	227.1	231.0	134.2	73.2	39.9	24.7	41.0
1912	1949	1,000.0	221.0	225.1	237.1	138.0	74.7	39.5	24.7	39.9
1913	1950	1,000.0	209.9	222.6	243.5	143.8	76.9	40.1	24.5	38.7
1914	1951	1,000.0	198.4	217.7	250.2	150.4	79.5	40.9	24.5	38.4
1915	1952	1,000.0	188.2	211.7	255.4	156.7	82.8	42.3	24.7	38.2
1916	1953	1,000.0	183.0	204.7	257.9	161.4	86.0	43.9	24.8	38.3
1917	1954	1,000.0	176.5	195.8	261.0	167.3	89.8	46.0	25.5	38.1
1918	1955	1,000.0	170.8	188.1	262.6	172.7	93.9	47.3	25.7	38.9
1919	1956	1,000.0	150.5	185.5	267.4	180.2	98.7	50.2	27.2	40.3
1920	1957	1,000.0	136.3	183.3	268.3	185.8	103.6	52.3	29.0	41.4
1921	1958	1,000.0	126.1	177.2	267.1	191.6	109.4	55.3	30.6	42.7
1922	1959	1,000.0	126.3	167.6	263.8	196.2	113.7	57.3	31.6	43.5
1923	1960	1,000.0	120.4	160.4	261.1	200.7	118.5	60.5	33.3	45.1
1924	1961	1,000.0	113.0	152.4	258.8	205.0	123.2	64.4	35.2	48.0
1925	1962	1,000.0	110.2	144.7	253.4	207.9	127.6	67.8	37.5	50.9
1926	1963	1,000.0	112.6	134.0	247.4	209.6	132.3	71.1	39.3	53.7
1927	1964	1,000.0	114.8	125.4	239.9	211.5	136.6	74.1	41.3	56.4
1928	1965	1,000.0	117.2	117.6	233.2	212.2	140.9	77.0	43.1	58.8
1929	1966	1,000.0	113.5	110.6	227.8	214.6	145.3	81.1	45.4	61.7
1930	1967	1,000.0	111.1	104.5	223.6	216.9	149.2	84.1	47.6	63.0
1931	1968	1,000.0	103.5	99.9	222.0	220.2	154.2	86.1	49.4	64.7
1932	1969	1,000.0	97.2	98.8	221.4	223.3	157.2	88.0	50.2	63.9
1933	1970	1,000.0	91.0	99.5	221.2	225.7	160.1	89.5	50.3	62.7
1934	1971	1,000.0	87.4	99.2	222.9	229.2	161.2	89.9	49.8	60.4
1935	1972	1,000.0	87.6	101.5	224.9	230.8	160.3	89.0	49.0	56.9
1936	1973	1,000.0	89.7	103.1	229.6	232.8	159.1	86.4	47.1	52.2
1937	1974	1,000.0	92.1	106.3	236.4	234.6	156.1	83.2	44.1	47.2

TABLE 8A. DISTRIBUTIONS OF ALL WOMEN BY PARITY AS OF THE BEGINNING OF EACH YEAR 1917-74 BY AGE FOR EACH COHORT FROM 1867 TO 1959--CON.

(BASED ON CUMULATIVE BIRTH RATES)

EXACT AGE AND COHORT	AS OF JANUARY 1	TOTAL	PARITY							
			0	1	2	3	4	5	6	7 AND HIGHER
38 YEARS										
1879----------------	1917	1,000.0	229.3	130.3	140.0	120.3	97.5	75.1	66.1	141.4
1880----------------	1918	1,000.0	230.3	132.5	141.2	120.6	97.1	74.9	64.6	138.8
1881----------------	1919	1,000.0	229.5	135.0	143.6	121.8	97.8	75.2	62.1	135.0
1882----------------	1920	1,000.0	227.8	137.8	146.6	123.2	98.6	75.7	59.2	131.1
1883----------------	1921	1,000.0	227.2	140.1	148.6	124.5	98.7	75.8	57.9	127.2
1884----------------	1922	1,000.0	227.7	140.7	151.4	125.6	98.5	74.8	58.1	123.2
1885----------------	1923	1,000.0	228.1	142.9	153.5	126.9	98.8	73.2	58.0	118.6
1886----------------	1924	1,000.0	226.4	147.5	153.4	128.6	99.3	72.6	57.5	114.7
1887----------------	1925	1,000.0	222.9	153.1	152.7	130.9	100.6	71.5	56.8	111.5
1888----------------	1926	1,000.0	219.6	153.6	156.6	133.0	102.0	69.2	57.3	108.7
1889----------------	1927	1,000.0	217.0	153.8	162.2	136.1	102.6	68.3	55.1	104.9
1890----------------	1928	1,000.0	213.2	155.0	168.5	138.6	103.0	66.8	53.6	101.3
1891----------------	1929	1,000.0	208.3	161.2	172.4	140.5	102.2	65.2	51.9	98.3
1892----------------	1930	1,000.0	202.5	169.1	178.2	141.4	101.1	63.7	49.7	94.3
1893----------------	1931	1,000.0	198.9	176.4	180.2	142.6	100.3	62.9	48.4	90.3
1894----------------	1932	1,000.0	197.6	182.2	185.6	143.1	97.3	61.0	46.3	86.9
1895----------------	1933	1,000.0	196.7	188.0	190.4	142.9	94.4	58.6	45.0	84.0
1896----------------	1934	1,000.0	196.5	195.8	193.2	142.3	91.8	56.8	43.5	80.1
1897----------------	1935	1,000.0	197.3	202.0	197.0	140.4	89.7	54.9	42.0	76.7
1898----------------	1936	1,000.0	202.0	203.1	200.1	138.5	88.4	52.7	41.1	74.1
1899----------------	1937	1,000.0	206.0	206.7	200.9	135.9	86.0	52.0	40.3	72.2
1900----------------	1938	1,000.0	212.9	211.8	199.4	132.8	83.6	50.9	38.8	69.8
1901----------------	1939	1,000.0	213.1	220.7	201.4	131.3	81.1	49.8	36.8	65.8
1902----------------	1940	1,000.0	211.4	229.1	205.1	129.3	80.4	48.5	34.8	61.4
1903----------------	1941	1,000.0	210.0	234.2	209.4	128.6	79.0	47.7	33.1	58.0
1904----------------	1942	1,000.0	214.8	236.6	211.0	126.3	77.5	46.1	32.2	55.5
1905----------------	1943	1,000.0	223.0	237.5	211.0	124.6	75.7	44.9	30.5	52.8
1906----------------	1944	1,000.0	228.8	237.7	212.2	124.6	73.9	43.4	29.1	50.3
1907----------------	1945	1,000.0	231.6	235.0	215.9	126.4	72.9	41.7	28.4	48.1
1908----------------	1946	1,000.0	234.6	231.9	219.7	126.6	72.8	40.8	27.3	46.3
1909----------------	1947	1,000.0	232.7	227.8	223.9	129.5	73.6	40.4	26.5	45.6
1910----------------	1948	1,000.0	230.5	225.1	226.6	132.5	74.3	40.6	25.7	44.7
1911----------------	1949	1,000.0	222.4	223.7	231.3	136.7	75.3	41.1	25.4	44.1
1912----------------	1950	1,000.0	215.0	221.7	237.0	140.4	76.8	40.7	25.4	43.0
1913----------------	1951	1,000.0	204.3	218.9	243.1	146.1	79.1	41.5	25.3	41.7
1914----------------	1952	1,000.0	193.0	213.7	249.3	152.7	82.0	42.3	25.6	41.4
1915----------------	1953	1,000.0	182.9	207.5	253.8	159.1	85.6	44.1	25.7	41.3
1916----------------	1954	1,000.0	178.0	200.7	255.7	163.3	88.9	46.0	25.9	41.5
1917----------------	1955	1,000.0	171.7	191.6	258.2	169.2	93.0	48.2	26.7	41.4
1918----------------	1956	1,000.0	166.4	184.0	259.6	174.2	97.0	49.5	27.1	42.2
1919----------------	1957	1,000.0	146.3	181.4	264.0	181.5	101.8	52.5	28.6	43.9
1920----------------	1958	1,000.0	132.3	179.5	264.7	186.5	106.5	54.7	30.7	45.1
1921----------------	1959	1,000.0	122.4	173.6	263.5	192.0	112.0	57.7	32.3	46.5
1922----------------	1960	1,000.0	122.9	164.5	260.0	196.1	116.0	59.7	33.4	47.4
1923----------------	1961	1,000.0	117.2	157.5	257.4	200.2	120.7	62.9	35.0	49.1
1924----------------	1962	1,000.0	110.0	149.6	255.1	204.5	125.0	66.6	37.0	52.2
1925----------------	1963	1,000.0	107.5	142.1	250.0	207.2	129.1	70.0	39.1	55.0
1926----------------	1964	1,000.0	110.1	131.6	244.2	208.8	133.6	73.0	40.9	57.8
1927----------------	1965	1,000.0	112.0	123.6	236.8	210.6	137.9	75.9	42.7	60.5
1928----------------	1966	1,000.0	114.5	116.1	230.5	211.3	142.0	78.6	44.6	62.4
1929----------------	1967	1,000.0	111.0	109.2	225.4	213.8	146.2	82.7	46.6	65.1
1930----------------	1968	1,000.0	108.9	103.0	221.4	216.3	150.1	85.4	48.8	66.1
1931----------------	1969	1,000.0	101.1	98.8	220.2	219.5	155.0	87.3	50.7	67.4
1932----------------	1970	1,000.0	95.2	97.4	219.8	222.7	157.9	89.3	51.2	66.5
1933----------------	1971	1,000.0	89.0	98.2	219.7	225.2	160.8	90.7	51.2	65.2
1934----------------	1972	1,000.0	85.6	98.0	221.5	228.7	161.8	91.0	50.8	62.6
1935----------------	1973	1,000.0	85.9	100.2	224.0	230.5	160.9	89.9	49.8	58.8
1936----------------	1974	1,000.0	88.1	101.9	228.8	232.8	159.6	87.2	47.8	53.8

TABLE 8A. DISTRIBUTIONS OF ALL WOMEN BY PARITY AS OF THE BEGINNING OF EACH YEAR 1917-74 BY AGE FOR EACH COHORT FROM 1867 TO 1959--CON.

(BASED ON CUMULATIVE BIRTH RATES)

EXACT AGE AND COHORT	AS OF JANUARY 1	TOTAL	PARITY							
			0	1	2	3	4	5	6	7 AND HIGHER
39 YEARS										
1878---------------	1917	1,000.0	224.2	126.6	137.2	118.8	97.0	74.9	66.5	154.8
1879---------------	1918	1,000.0	226.3	128.5	137.9	118.8	96.3	74.4	66.0	151.8
1880---------------	1919	1,000.0	227.1	130.8	139.2	119.0	96.2	74.0	64.8	148.9
1881---------------	1920	1,000.0	226.4	133.2	141.7	120.3	96.8	74.6	61.9	145.1
1882---------------	1921	1,000.0	224.5	136.2	144.5	122.0	97.6	75.1	59.2	140.9
1883---------------	1922	1,000.0	223.8	138.4	146.7	123.2	97.9	75.3	57.9	136.8
1884---------------	1923	1,000.0	224.5	139.1	149.6	124.5	97.8	74.4	58.0	132.1
1885---------------	1924	1,000.0	225.1	141.1	151.7	125.9	98.2	72.9	57.9	127.2
1886---------------	1925	1,000.0	223.3	145.8	151.5	127.7	98.8	72.3	57.4	123.2
1887---------------	1926	1,000.0	219.8	151.6	150.9	129.7	100.4	71.2	56.9	119.5
1888---------------	1927	1,000.0	216.7	152.1	154.8	132.0	101.7	69.2	57.3	116.2
1889---------------	1928	1,000.0	214.0	152.3	160.6	135.3	102.2	68.2	55.1	112.3
1890---------------	1929	1,000.0	210.3	153.6	167.0	137.9	102.7	66.8	53.7	108.0
1891---------------	1930	1,000.0	205.6	159.8	171.0	140.0	102.0	65.2	51.9	104.5
1892---------------	1931	1,000.0	199.7	167.7	177.0	140.7	100.9	63.7	49.9	100.4
1893---------------	1932	1,000.0	196.2	175.2	179.0	141.9	100.2	62.9	48.7	95.9
1894---------------	1933	1,000.0	195.1	181.0	184.4	142.6	97.3	60.7	46.5	92.4
1895---------------	1934	1,000.0	194.4	186.7	189.3	142.4	94.4	58.6	45.2	89.0
1896---------------	1935	1,000.0	194.2	194.4	192.3	141.7	91.9	56.7	43.8	85.0
1897---------------	1936	1,000.0	194.9	200.8	196.1	140.0	89.8	55.0	42.1	81.3
1898---------------	1937	1,000.0	199.5	202.1	199.2	138.3	88.5	52.8	41.3	78.3
1899---------------	1938	1,000.0	203.4	205.6	200.1	135.9	86.1	52.1	40.5	76.3
1900---------------	1939	1,000.0	210.1	210.7	198.7	132.8	83.9	51.0	39.0	73.8
1901---------------	1940	1,000.0	210.1	219.6	200.9	131.5	81.4	50.0	37.1	69.4
1902---------------	1941	1,000.0	208.3	227.9	204.8	129.7	80.7	48.7	35.1	64.8
1903---------------	1942	1,000.0	206.6	233.0	209.3	129.1	79.4	48.0	33.3	61.3
1904---------------	1943	1,000.0	210.5	235.6	211.1	127.0	78.1	46.4	32.7	58.6
1905---------------	1944	1,000.0	218.4	235.9	211.1	125.6	76.6	45.4	31.0	56.0
1906---------------	1945	1,000.0	224.3	235.5	212.3	125.8	75.0	44.0	29.7	53.4
1907---------------	1946	1,000.0	226.9	232.4	215.9	128.0	74.2	42.5	28.9	51.2
1908---------------	1947	1,000.0	229.1	229.5	220.0	128.5	74.1	41.7	27.9	49.2
1909---------------	1948	1,000.0	226.7	225.8	224.0	131.4	75.2	41.3	27.1	48.5
1910---------------	1949	1,000.0	225.3	222.7	226.8	134.0	76.0	41.5	26.3	47.4
1911---------------	1950	1,000.0	217.7	221.1	231.1	138.3	76.9	42.1	26.0	46.8
1912---------------	1951	1,000.0	210.6	218.9	236.6	142.0	78.4	41.8	26.0	45.7
1913---------------	1952	1,000.0	200.0	216.0	242.3	147.6	81.0	42.7	26.0	44.4
1914---------------	1953	1,000.0	188.8	210.5	248.0	154.3	84.1	43.8	26.4	44.1
1915---------------	1954	1,000.0	178.9	204.4	252.1	160.3	87.8	45.7	26.7	44.1
1916---------------	1955	1,000.0	174.2	197.5	253.7	164.3	91.3	47.7	26.9	44.4
1917---------------	1956	1,000.0	168.1	188.5	255.8	170.1	95.3	50.0	27.8	44.4
1918---------------	1957	1,000.0	163.1	181.0	256.9	175.0	99.1	51.4	28.3	45.2
1919---------------	1958	1,000.0	143.1	178.5	261.1	181.9	104.0	54.4	29.9	47.1
1920---------------	1959	1,000.0	129.4	176.7	261.8	186.7	108.4	56.6	32.0	48.4
1921---------------	1960	1,000.0	119.7	171.1	260.5	191.8	113.6	59.6	33.8	49.9
1922---------------	1961	1,000.0	120.4	162.2	257.0	195.6	117.6	61.5	34.8	50.9
1923---------------	1962	1,000.0	114.8	155.3	254.5	199.7	121.9	64.6	36.5	52.7
1924---------------	1963	1,000.0	107.8	147.7	252.3	203.8	126.1	68.3	38.3	55.7
1925---------------	1964	1,000.0	105.5	140.3	247.4	206.4	130.0	71.5	40.4	58.5
1926---------------	1965	1,000.0	107.8	130.3	241.7	207.9	134.6	74.4	42.0	61.3
1927---------------	1966	1,000.0	109.8	122.5	234.6	209.8	138.6	77.1	43.9	63.7
1928---------------	1967	1,000.0	112.5	115.2	228.4	210.6	142.6	79.9	45.5	65.3
1929---------------	1968	1,000.0	109.3	108.0	223.6	213.3	146.8	83.6	47.6	67.8
1930---------------	1969	1,000.0	107.0	102.2	219.9	215.7	150.7	86.3	49.7	68.5
1931---------------	1970	1,000.0	99.5	97.8	219.0	218.8	155.5	88.3	51.4	69.7
1932---------------	1971	1,000.0	93.6	96.5	218.6	222.2	158.3	90.2	52.0	68.6
1933---------------	1972	1,000.0	87.6	97.4	218.6	224.8	161.1	91.5	51.9	67.1
1934---------------	1973	1,000.0	84.3	97.1	220.7	228.4	162.2	91.6	51.5	64.2
1935---------------	1974	1,000.0	84.7	99.3	223.4	230.4	161.2	90.5	50.3	60.2

TABLE 8A. DISTRIBUTIONS OF ALL WOMEN BY PARITY AS OF THE BEGINNING OF EACH YEAR 1917-74 BY AGE FOR EACH COHORT FROM 1867 TO 1959--CON.

(BASED ON CUMULATIVE BIRTH RATES)

EXACT AGE AND COHORT	AS OF JANUARY 1	TOTAL	PARITY							
			0	1	2	3	4	5	6	7 AND HIGHER
40 YEARS										
1877---------------	1917	1,000.0	220.2	123.4	134.2	116.9	96.2	76.1	65.8	167.2
1878---------------	1918	1,000.0	221.8	125.3	135.6	117.3	95.9	74.0	66.5	163.6
1879---------------	1919	1,C00.0	223.7	127.3	136.2	117.5	95.2	73.5	66.1	160.5
1880---------------	1920	1,000.0	224.5	129.6	137.6	117.7	95.1	73.3	64.7	157.5
1881---------------	1921	1,000.0	223.7	132.1	140.0	119.0	95.9	73.9	61.8	153.6
1882---------------	1922	1,000.0	221.7	135.1	142.8	120.8	96.7	74.5	59.2	149.2
1883---------------	1923	1,000.0	221.2	137.3	145.2	122.1	97.1	74.8	57.7	144.6
1884---------------	1924	1,000.0	222.0	137.9	148.1	123.5	97.0	74.0	57.9	139.6
1885---------------	1925	1,000.0	222.6	139.9	150.2	124.9	97.6	72.5	57.8	134.5
1886---------------	1926	1,000.0	220.8	144.8	150.0	126.6	98.5	71.8	57.4	130.1
1887---------------	1927	1,000.0	217.5	150.4	149.5	128.8	100.0	71.0	56.7	126.1
1888---------------	1928	1,000.0	214.3	151.1	153.4	131.3	101.2	68.9	57.3	122.5
1889---------------	1929	1,C00.0	211.7	151.3	159.4	134.5	101.8	68.1	55.0	118.2
1890---------------	1930	1,000.0	208.1	152.6	165.9	137.3	102.3	66.8	53.6	113.4
1891---------------	1931	1,000.0	203.4	158.8	169.9	139.3	101.7	65.0	52.1	109.8
1892---------------	1932	1,000.0	197.6	166.8	176.0	140.0	100.7	63.6	50.1	105.2
1893---------------	1933	1,000.0	194.2	174.3	178.1	141.3	100.1	62.5	48.8	100.7
1894---------------	1934	1,000.0	193.3	180.1	183.4	142.1	97.2	60.5	46.7	96.7
1895---------------	1935	1,000.0	192.6	185.7	188.5	141.8	94.3	58.5	45.3	93.3
1896---------------	1936	1,000.0	192.4	193.6	191.4	141.3	91.8	56.6	43.9	89.0
1897---------------	1937	1,000.0	193.0	200.1	195.2	139.7	89.9	55.0	42.2	84.9
1898---------------	1938	1,000.0	197.6	201.3	198.5	138.1	88.5	52.9	41.3	81.8
1899---------------	1939	1,000.0	201.4	204.7	199.5	135.8	86.1	52.1	40.7	79.7
1900---------------	1940	1,000.0	207.9	209.9	198.2	132.8	83.9	51.1	39.3	76.9
1901---------------	1941	1,000.0	207.9	218.6	200.6	131.7	81.4	50.2	37.3	72.3
1902---------------	1942	1,000.0	205.8	227.1	204.5	129.9	80.9	48.9	35.3	67.6
1903---------------	1943	1,000.0	203.5	232.3	209.2	129.4	79.8	48.2	33.6	64.0
1904---------------	1944	1,000.0	207.2	234.4	211.0	127.5	78.8	46.7	33.0	61.4
1905---------------	1945	1,000.0	215.1	234.4	210.9	126.3	77.4	45.8	31.4	58.7
1906---------------	1946	1,000.0	220.8	233.8	212.1	126.6	75.9	44.6	30.1	56.1
1907---------------	1947	1,000.0	222.8	230.7	216.0	129.1	75.1	43.2	29.3	53.8
1908---------------	1948	1,000.0	224.7	228.0	220.0	129.7	75.2	42.4	28.4	51.6
1909---------------	1949	1,000.0	222.8	224.2	223.9	132.4	76.3	42.1	27.5	50.8
1910---------------	1950	1,000.0	221.6	221.0	226.5	135.1	77.1	42.3	26.7	49.7
1911---------------	1951	1,000.0	214.3	219.1	230.8	139.3	78.0	42.9	26.5	49.1
1912---------------	1952	1,000.0	207.3	216.7	236.1	143.0	79.7	42.6	26.6	48.0
1913---------------	1953	1,000.0	196.7	213.9	241.3	148.5	82.4	43.8	26.8	46.6
1914---------------	1954	1,C00.0	185.7	208.2	246.8	155.1	85.6	45.0	27.1	46.5
1915---------------	1955	1,000.0	175.9	202.1	250.6	160.8	89.5	46.9	27.7	46.5
1916---------------	1956	1,000.0	171.4	195.2	251.9	164.9	92.8	49.0	27.9	46.9
1917---------------	1957	1,000.0	165.6	186.1	253.8	170.5	96.9	51.4	28.6	47.1
1918---------------	1958	1,000.0	160.6	178.8	255.0	175.0	100.7	52.8	29.2	47.9
1919---------------	1959	1,000.0	140.8	176.4	259.0	181.9	105.3	55.8	30.9	49.9
1920---------------	1960	1,000.0	127.3	174.8	259.5	186.4	109.7	57.9	33.1	51.3
1921---------------	1961	1,000.0	117.7	169.5	258.1	191.3	114.8	60.9	34.8	52.9
1922---------------	1962	1,000.0	118.5	160.5	254.9	195.0	118.5	62.8	35.9	53.9
1923---------------	1963	1,000.0	113.1	153.9	252.3	199.1	122.7	65.8	37.5	55.6
1924---------------	1964	1,000.0	106.2	146.4	250.3	203.1	126.7	69.4	39.3	58.6
1925---------------	1965	1,000.0	103.7	139.3	245.5	205.6	130.7	72.5	41.3	61.4
1926---------------	1966	1,000.0	106.1	129.4	240.0	207.2	135.1	75.3	42.9	64.0
1927---------------	1967	1,000.0	108.3	121.7	233.1	209.1	139.1	77.9	44.7	66.1
1928---------------	1968	1,000.0	111.2	114.4	226.9	210.1	143.2	80.5	46.1	67.6
1929---------------	1969	1,000.0	107.8	107.4	222.6	212.7	147.2	84.2	48.3	69.8
1930---------------	1970	1,000.0	105.8	101.4	219.0	215.1	151.0	87.0	50.4	70.3
1931---------------	1971	1,000.0	98.3	97.1	218.1	218.3	155.8	88.9	52.0	71.5
1932---------------	1972	1,000.0	92.6	95.8	217.9	221.8	158.5	90.6	52.6	70.2
1933---------------	1973	1,000.0	86.6	96.9	218.0	224.5	161.2	92.0	52.3	68.5
1934---------------	1974	1,000.0	83.4	96.5	220.3	228.2	162.3	92.0	51.9	65.4

TABLE 8A. DISTRIBUTIONS OF ALL WOMEN BY PARITY AS OF THE BEGINNING OF EACH YEAR 1917-74 BY AGE FOR EACH COHORT FROM 1867 TO 1959--CON.

(BASED ON CUMULATIVE BIRTH RATES)

EXACT AGE AND COHORT	AS OF JANUARY 1	TOTAL	PARITY							
			0	1	2	3	4	5	6	7 AND HIGHER
41 YEARS										
1876----------------	1917	1,000.0	217.2	120.4	131.2	114.9	95.0	75.5	65.7	180.1
1877----------------	1918	1,000.0	218.6	122.5	133.2	115.7	95.5	75.2	65.9	173.4
1878----------------	1919	1,000.0	220.1	124.5	134.4	116.3	95.1	73.3	66.4	169.9
1879----------------	1920	1,000.0	222.0	126.4	135.3	116.4	94.4	72.9	66.0	166.6
1880----------------	1921	1,000.0	222.7	128.8	136.5	116.7	94.5	72.6	64.6	163.6
1881----------------	1922	1,000.0	221.8	131.3	139.0	118.0	95.2	73.3	61.8	159.6
1882----------------	1923	1,000.0	220.0	134.3	141.8	119.9	96.1	74.0	59.0	154.9
1883----------------	1924	1,000.0	219.5	136.5	144.2	121.3	96.5	74.3	57.6	150.1
1884----------------	1925	1,000.0	220.3	137.1	147.1	122.7	96.5	73.6	57.8	144.9
1885----------------	1926	1,000.0	220.9	139.2	149.2	124.0	97.4	72.1	57.6	139.6
1886----------------	1927	1,000.0	219.2	144.0	149.2	125.9	98.1	71.5	57.2	134.9
1887----------------	1928	1,000.0	215.9	149.7	148.6	128.2	99.6	70.6	56.6	130.8
1888----------------	1929	1,000.0	212.8	150.4	152.6	130.7	100.8	68.7	57.3	126.7
1889----------------	1930	1,000.0	210.2	150.7	158.5	134.1	101.5	67.9	54.9	122.2
1890----------------	1931	1,000.0	206.6	152.0	164.9	136.9	102.0	66.6	53.6	117.4
1891----------------	1932	1,000.0	202.0	158.2	169.2	138.7	101.5	64.8	52.2	113.4
1892----------------	1933	1,000.0	196.2	166.3	175.3	139.5	100.5	63.3	50.1	108.8
1893----------------	1934	1,000.0	193.0	173.6	177.5	140.8	99.9	62.4	48.8	104.0
1894----------------	1935	1,000.0	192.1	179.5	182.7	141.6	97.0	60.4	46.8	99.9
1895----------------	1936	1,000.0	191.4	185.1	187.8	141.5	94.1	58.5	45.3	96.3
1896----------------	1937	1,000.0	191.1	193.2	190.7	141.0	91.7	56.6	44.0	91.7
1897----------------	1938	1,000.0	191.7	199.6	194.7	139.3	89.9	55.1	42.2	87.5
1898----------------	1939	1,000.0	196.3	200.7	198.0	138.0	88.4	52.9	41.3	84.4
1899----------------	1940	1,000.0	199.9	204.2	199.0	135.7	86.1	52.2	40.8	82.1
1900----------------	1941	1,000.0	206.4	209.2	197.9	132.8	83.9	51.2	39.4	79.2
1901----------------	1942	1,000.0	206.2	218.1	200.2	131.8	81.5	50.3	37.5	74.4
1902----------------	1943	1,000.0	203.8	226.6	204.3	130.0	81.1	49.1	35.5	69.6
1903----------------	1944	1,000.0	201.3	231.6	209.0	129.6	80.2	48.4	33.8	66.1
1904----------------	1945	1,000.0	204.9	233.5	210.8	127.9	79.2	47.0	33.2	63.5
1905----------------	1946	1,000.0	212.7	233.3	210.6	126.8	78.0	46.1	31.7	60.8
1906----------------	1947	1,000.0	218.0	232.8	212.1	127.1	76.5	45.0	30.4	58.1
1907----------------	1948	1,000.0	219.7	229.8	215.9	129.7	75.8	43.8	29.6	55.7
1908----------------	1949	1,000.0	221.9	227.1	219.8	130.3	75.9	43.0	28.6	53.4
1909----------------	1950	1,000.0	220.2	223.1	223.7	133.0	77.0	42.6	27.9	52.5
1910----------------	1951	1,000.0	219.1	219.8	226.2	135.7	77.8	42.9	27.0	51.5
1911----------------	1952	1,000.0	211.9	217.7	230.4	139.8	78.9	43.5	26.9	50.9
1912----------------	1953	1,000.0	204.9	215.4	235.3	143.5	80.7	43.3	27.1	49.8
1913----------------	1954	1,000.0	194.5	212.3	240.5	148.9	83.5	44.5	27.4	48.4
1914----------------	1955	1,000.0	183.5	206.7	245.7	155.4	86.7	45.8	27.8	48.4
1915----------------	1956	1,000.0	173.9	200.5	249.3	161.1	90.5	47.8	28.5	48.4
1916----------------	1957	1,000.0	169.6	193.6	250.6	165.1	93.6	50.0	28.6	48.9
1917----------------	1958	1,000.0	163.8	184.6	252.3	170.4	98.1	52.3	29.3	49.2
1918----------------	1959	1,000.0	159.0	177.4	253.5	174.8	101.6	53.8	29.9	50.0
1919----------------	1960	1,000.0	139.2	175.2	257.3	181.7	106.1	56.7	31.7	52.1
1920----------------	1961	1,000.0	125.8	173.7	257.8	186.0	110.4	58.9	33.8	53.6
1921----------------	1962	1,000.0	116.3	168.3	256.5	190.8	115.5	61.8	35.5	55.3
1922----------------	1963	1,000.0	117.3	159.4	253.4	194.4	119.1	63.6	36.6	56.2
1923----------------	1964	1,000.0	111.9	153.0	250.9	198.5	123.1	66.5	38.3	57.8
1924----------------	1965	1,000.0	104.9	145.7	248.9	202.5	127.1	70.1	40.0	60.8
1925----------------	1966	1,000.0	102.5	138.6	244.4	204.9	131.0	73.1	42.0	63.5
1926----------------	1967	1,000.0	105.0	128.9	238.8	206.7	135.4	75.8	43.5	65.9
1927----------------	1968	1,000.0	107.3	121.1	232.1	208.7	139.4	78.4	45.1	67.9
1928----------------	1969	1,000.0	110.1	114.0	226.2	209.6	143.5	80.9	46.5	69.2
1929----------------	1970	1,000.0	106.9	106.9	221.9	212.2	147.4	84.7	48.8	71.2
1930----------------	1971	1,000.0	104.9	101.0	218.4	214.6	151.1	87.5	50.8	71.7
1931----------------	1972	1,000.0	97.5	96.7	217.6	218.0	156.0	89.1	52.4	72.7
1932----------------	1973	1,000.0	91.9	95.4	217.5	221.6	158.6	90.8	52.9	71.3
1933----------------	1974	1,000.0	85.9	96.6	217.7	224.3	161.2	92.3	52.6	69.4

TABLE 8A. DISTRIBUTIONS OF ALL WOMEN BY PARITY AS OF THE BEGINNING OF EACH YEAR 1917-74 BY AGE FOR EACH COHORT FROM 1867 TO 1959--CON.

(BASED ON CUMULATIVE BIRTH RATES)

EXACT AGE AND COHORT	AS OF JANUARY 1	TOTAL	PARITY							
			0	1	2	3	4	5	6	7 AND HIGHER
42 YEARS										
1875	1917	1,000.0	214.2	117.8	128.6	113.1	94.2	75.2	65.8	191.1
1876	1918	1,000.0	216.1	119.8	130.5	114.0	94.5	74.6	65.7	184.8
1877	1919	1,000.0	217.4	121.9	132.3	115.2	94.7	74.6	65.7	178.2
1878	1920	1,000.0	218.9	123.9	133.7	115.5	94.6	72.7	66.2	174.5
1879	1921	1,000.0	220.7	125.9	134.5	115.6	94.0	72.2	65.8	171.3
1880	1922	1,000.0	221.4	128.3	135.7	116.0	93.9	72.0	64.4	168.3
1881	1923	1,000.0	220.6	130.7	138.4	117.3	94.6	72.9	61.5	164.0
1882	1924	1,000.0	218.8	133.8	141.1	119.2	95.6	73.5	58.8	159.2
1883	1925	1,000.0	218.3	136.0	143.5	120.6	96.1	73.8	57.4	154.3
1884	1926	1,000.0	219.1	136.6	146.4	122.0	96.3	73.2	57.5	148.9
1885	1927	1,000.0	219.8	138.6	148.7	123.4	97.0	71.7	57.4	143.4
1886	1928	1,000.0	218.1	143.6	148.4	125.5	97.8	71.1	57.0	138.5
1887	1929	1,000.0	214.8	149.3	148.0	127.7	99.3	70.4	56.4	134.1
1888	1930	1,000.0	211.8	150.0	152.0	130.3	100.5	68.5	57.2	129.7
1889	1931	1,000.0	209.2	150.3	157.8	133.7	101.2	67.7	54.9	125.2
1890	1932	1,000.0	205.6	151.6	164.4	136.5	101.7	66.4	53.6	120.2
1891	1933	1,000.0	201.0	157.9	168.7	138.2	101.3	64.6	52.1	116.2
1892	1934	1,000.0	195.3	165.9	174.8	139.2	100.2	63.2	50.0	111.4
1893	1935	1,000.0	192.1	173.3	177.0	140.4	99.6	62.4	48.7	106.5
1894	1936	1,000.0	191.3	179.1	182.2	141.3	96.8	60.3	46.8	102.2
1895	1937	1,000.0	190.5	184.8	187.4	141.2	93.9	58.5	45.2	98.5
1896	1938	1,000.0	190.2	192.9	190.4	140.6	91.6	56.7	43.9	93.7
1897	1939	1,000.0	190.8	199.2	194.4	139.1	89.8	55.0	42.3	89.4
1898	1940	1,000.0	195.4	200.4	197.6	137.7	88.4	52.9	41.4	86.2
1899	1941	1,000.0	198.9	203.8	198.8	135.5	86.1	52.2	40.9	83.8
1900	1942	1,000.0	205.3	208.9	197.6	132.7	83.9	51.2	39.5	80.9
1901	1943	1,000.0	205.0	217.8	200.0	131.7	81.6	50.4	37.6	75.9
1902	1944	1,000.0	202.4	226.2	204.1	130.0	81.2	49.2	35.7	71.2
1903	1945	1,000.0	199.7	231.2	208.7	129.8	80.4	48.5	34.0	67.7
1904	1946	1,000.0	203.3	232.8	210.6	128.1	79.5	47.1	33.4	65.2
1905	1947	1,000.0	210.9	232.7	210.4	127.1	78.3	46.3	31.9	62.4
1906	1948	1,000.0	216.0	232.2	212.0	127.4	76.9	45.4	30.5	59.6
1907	1949	1,000.0	217.9	229.1	215.7	130.0	76.3	44.1	29.8	57.1
1908	1950	1,000.0	220.1	226.5	219.6	130.6	76.3	43.4	28.8	54.7
1909	1951	1,000.0	218.5	222.4	223.5	133.3	77.3	43.0	28.2	53.8
1910	1952	1,000.0	217.5	218.9	225.9	136.0	78.3	43.3	27.2	52.9
1911	1953	1,000.0	210.3	216.8	229.9	140.1	79.4	44.0	27.2	52.3
1912	1954	1,000.0	203.3	214.5	234.7	143.8	81.3	43.7	27.5	51.2
1913	1955	1,000.0	193.0	211.3	239.7	149.1	84.1	45.1	27.9	49.8
1914	1956	1,000.0	182.1	205.7	244.8	155.6	87.2	46.4	28.4	49.8
1915	1957	1,000.0	172.6	199.4	248.3	161.3	91.0	48.5	28.9	50.0
1916	1958	1,000.0	168.3	192.7	249.5	165.0	94.3	50.6	29.1	50.5
1917	1959	1,000.0	162.6	183.7	251.3	170.2	98.6	53.1	29.7	50.8
1918	1960	1,000.0	157.9	176.6	252.4	174.5	102.1	54.5	30.4	51.6
1919	1961	1,000.0	138.2	174.4	256.2	181.3	106.5	57.4	32.2	53.8
1920	1962	1,000.0	124.8	172.9	256.7	185.6	110.8	59.5	34.3	55.4
1921	1963	1,000.0	115.4	167.6	255.5	190.2	115.9	62.4	36.0	57.0
1922	1964	1,000.0	116.5	158.7	252.4	194.0	119.3	64.1	37.1	57.9
1923	1965	1,000.0	110.9	152.7	249.8	198.1	123.3	67.0	38.8	59.4
1924	1966	1,000.0	104.0	145.3	248.1	202.0	127.2	70.6	40.5	62.3
1925	1967	1,000.0	101.7	138.2	243.7	204.5	131.1	73.4	42.5	64.9
1926	1968	1,000.0	104.3	128.5	238.1	206.3	135.6	76.2	43.8	67.2
1927	1969	1,000.0	106.5	120.9	231.6	208.3	139.5	78.7	45.4	69.1
1928	1970	1,000.0	109.5	113.6	225.8	209.3	143.5	81.2	46.9	70.2
1929	1971	1,000.0	106.3	106.6	221.5	211.9	147.4	85.0	49.1	72.2
1930	1972	1,000.0	104.4	100.7	218.0	214.5	151.1	87.7	51.0	72.6
1931	1973	1,000.0	97.0	96.5	217.3	217.8	156.0	89.3	52.6	73.5
1932	1974	1,000.0	91.4	95.2	217.3	221.5	158.6	90.9	53.2	71.9

TABLE 8A. DISTRIBUTIONS OF ALL WOMEN BY PARITY AS OF THE BEGINNING OF EACH YEAR 1917-74 BY AGE FOR EACH COHORT FROM 1867 TO 1959--CON.

(BASED ON CUMULATIVE BIRTH RATES)

EXACT AGE AND COHORT	AS OF JANUARY 1	TOTAL	PARITY							
			0	1	2	3	4	5	6	7 AND HIGHER
43 YEARS										
1874----------------	1917	1,000.0	211.0	115.4	126.4	111.8	94.0	75.5	66.2	199.7
1875----------------	1918	1,000.0	213.5	117.4	128.1	112.5	93.9	74.5	65.6	194.5
1876----------------	1919	1,000.0	215.3	119.5	129.9	113.6	94.0	74.1	65.4	188.2
1877----------------	1920	1,000.0	216.6	121.6	131.8	114.7	94.3	74.1	65.5	181.4
1878----------------	1921	1,000.0	218.1	123.6	133.2	115.0	94.2	72.2	65.9	177.8
1879----------------	1922	1,000.0	219.9	125.5	134.1	115.1	93.5	71.7	65.6	174.6
1880----------------	1923	1,000.0	220.6	128.0	135.2	115.6	93.5	71.6	64.1	171.4
1881----------------	1924	1,000.0	219.8	130.4	137.9	116.9	94.2	72.5	61.2	167.1
1882----------------	1925	1,000.0	218.0	133.5	140.6	118.8	95.2	73.2	58.5	162.2
1883----------------	1926	1,000.0	217.6	135.6	143.1	120.1	95.9	73.5	57.1	157.1
1884----------------	1927	1,000.0	218.3	136.4	146.0	121.5	96.0	72.9	57.4	151.5
1885----------------	1928	1,000.0	219.1	138.3	148.3	123.0	96.7	71.5	57.3	145.8
1886----------------	1929	1,000.0	217.4	143.3	148.0	125.2	97.6	70.9	56.8	140.8
1887----------------	1930	1,000.0	214.1	149.1	147.6	127.4	99.1	70.2	56.2	136.3
1888----------------	1931	1,000.0	211.1	149.8	151.6	130.0	100.3	68.3	57.1	131.8
1889----------------	1932	1,000.0	208.5	150.1	157.4	133.5	101.0	67.4	54.9	127.2
1890----------------	1933	1,000.0	205.0	151.4	164.0	136.2	101.5	66.2	53.5	122.2
1891----------------	1934	1,000.0	200.4	157.7	168.4	137.9	101.0	64.6	51.9	118.1
1892----------------	1935	1,000.0	194.7	165.8	174.4	138.9	100.0	63.1	49.9	113.2
1893----------------	1936	1,000.0	191.6	173.1	176.6	140.2	99.4	62.3	48.7	108.1
1894----------------	1937	1,000.0	190.8	178.9	181.9	141.1	96.6	60.2	46.7	103.8
1895----------------	1938	1,000.0	189.9	184.7	187.2	140.8	93.9	58.4	45.2	99.9
1896----------------	1939	1,000.0	189.6	192.7	190.2	140.4	91.5	56.6	43.9	95.1
1897----------------	1940	1,000.0	190.2	199.1	194.1	138.9	89.7	55.0	42.3	90.7
1898----------------	1941	1,000.0	194.8	200.2	197.4	137.5	88.4	52.9	41.4	87.4
1899----------------	1942	1,000.0	198.2	203.7	198.5	135.4	86.1	52.2	40.9	85.0
1900----------------	1943	1,000.0	204.6	208.7	197.4	132.6	83.9	51.2	39.6	82.0
1901----------------	1944	1,000.0	204.2	217.6	199.8	131.6	81.6	50.4	37.7	77.1
1902----------------	1945	1,000.0	201.4	226.0	203.9	130.0	81.2	49.3	35.8	72.4
1903----------------	1946	1,000.0	198.7	230.9	208.4	129.9	80.5	48.6	34.0	69.0
1904----------------	1947	1,000.0	202.2	232.5	210.4	128.2	79.6	47.3	33.5	66.3
1905----------------	1948	1,000.0	209.7	232.3	210.3	127.2	78.5	46.5	32.0	63.5
1906----------------	1949	1,000.0	214.9	231.8	211.8	127.6	77.1	45.6	30.6	60.6
1907----------------	1950	1,000.0	216.8	228.7	215.6	130.1	76.5	44.3	30.0	58.0
1908----------------	1951	1,000.0	219.1	226.1	219.4	130.7	76.5	43.6	29.0	55.6
1909----------------	1952	1,000.0	217.5	222.0	223.2	133.3	77.7	43.2	28.3	54.8
1910----------------	1953	1,000.0	216.4	218.4	225.6	136.2	78.6	43.6	27.3	53.9
1911----------------	1954	1,000.0	209.2	216.4	229.5	140.2	79.7	44.2	27.5	53.3
1912----------------	1955	1,000.0	202.3	213.9	234.2	143.9	81.6	44.1	27.8	52.2
1913----------------	1956	1,000.0	192.0	210.8	239.1	149.2	84.3	45.6	28.2	50.8
1914----------------	1957	1,000.0	181.2	205.1	244.2	155.6	87.5	46.8	28.7	50.9
1915----------------	1958	1,000.0	171.7	198.9	247.6	161.2	91.4	48.8	29.3	51.1
1916----------------	1959	1,000.0	167.5	192.2	248.9	164.8	94.6	51.0	29.4	51.6
1917----------------	1960	1,000.0	161.9	183.1	250.7	169.9	98.9	53.5	30.0	52.0
1918----------------	1961	1,000.0	157.2	176.1	251.8	174.2	102.3	54.9	30.8	52.7
1919----------------	1962	1,000.0	137.6	173.9	255.4	181.0	106.7	57.8	32.6	55.0
1920----------------	1963	1,000.0	124.2	172.4	256.1	185.2	111.0	59.9	34.6	56.6
1921----------------	1964	1,000.0	114.8	167.2	254.9	189.9	115.9	62.8	36.3	58.2
1922----------------	1965	1,000.0	115.9	158.5	251.7	193.7	119.4	64.3	37.5	59.0
1923----------------	1966	1,000.0	110.3	152.5	249.2	197.8	123.3	67.3	39.1	60.5
1924----------------	1967	1,000.0	103.5	145.1	247.6	201.6	127.3	70.8	40.8	63.3
1925----------------	1968	1,000.0	101.3	137.9	243.3	204.1	131.3	73.6	42.7	65.8
1926----------------	1969	1,000.0	103.8	128.3	237.8	206.1	135.6	76.3	44.0	68.1
1927----------------	1970	1,000.0	106.1	120.7	231.2	208.2	139.4	79.0	45.6	69.8
1928----------------	1971	1,000.0	109.1	113.4	225.6	209.0	143.6	81.3	47.1	70.9
1929----------------	1972	1,000.0	106.0	106.4	221.3	211.7	147.4	85.2	49.2	72.8
1930----------------	1973	1,000.0	104.1	100.5	217.9	214.3	151.2	87.7	51.2	73.1
1931----------------	1974	1,000.0	96.7	96.4	217.1	217.7	156.0	89.4	52.8	73.9

TABLE 8A. DISTRIBUTIONS OF ALL WOMEN BY PARITY AS OF THE BEGINNING OF EACH YEAR 1917-74 BY AGE FOR EACH COHORT FROM 1867 TO 1959--CON.

(BASED ON CUMULATIVE BIRTH RATES)

EXACT AGE AND COHORT	AS OF JANUARY 1	TOTAL	PARITY 0	1	2	3	4	5	6	7 AND HIGHER
44 YEARS										
1873	1917	1,000.0	207.9	113.0	124.6	110.8	94.2	76.1	67.0	206.4
1874	1918	1,000.0	210.5	115.2	126.0	111.4	93.7	75.0	65.9	202.3
1875	1919	1,000.0	213.0	117.1	127.8	112.2	93.4	74.2	65.2	197.1
1876	1920	1,000.0	214.7	119.3	129.6	113.2	93.7	73.8	65.1	190.6
1877	1921	1,000.0	216.0	121.4	131.5	114.3	94.0	73.8	65.1	183.9
1878	1922	1,000.0	217.5	123.4	132.9	114.6	93.8	71.9	65.6	180.3
1879	1923	1,000.0	219.3	125.3	133.8	114.8	93.2	71.4	65.3	176.9
1880	1924	1,000.0	220.0	127.9	134.8	115.3	93.2	71.3	63.8	173.7
1881	1925	1,C00.0	219.2	130.3	137.5	116.6	93.9	72.2	61.0	169.3
1882	1926	1,000.0	217.5	133.2	140.4	118.5	94.9	72.9	58.3	164.3
1883	1927	1,000.0	217.1	135.4	142.8	119.8	95.7	73.2	56.9	159.1
1884	1928	1,000.0	217.8	136.3	145.7	121.2	95.7	72.7	57.3	153.3
1885	1929	1,000.0	218.6	138.1	148.1	122.8	96.4	71.4	57.0	147.6
1886	1930	1,000.0	217.0	143.1	147.8	124.9	97.4	70.8	56.6	142.4
1887	1931	1,000.0	213.7	148.9	147.4	127.1	98.9	70.0	56.1	137.9
1888	1932	1,000.0	210.7	149.7	151.3	129.8	100.1	68.1	57.0	133.3
1889	1933	1,000.0	208.1	149.9	157.2	133.3	100.8	67.2	54.8	128.7
1890	1934	1,000.0	204.6	151.3	163.7	136.0	101.3	66.1	53.4	123.6
1891	1935	1,000.0	200.0	157.6	168.1	137.7	100.9	64.4	51.9	119.4
1892	1936	1,000.0	194.3	165.7	174.2	138.7	99.9	63.0	49.8	114.4
1893	1937	1,000.0	191.2	173.0	176.5	140.0	99.2	62.2	48.7	109.2
1894	1938	1,000.0	190.4	178.9	181.7	140.9	96.5	60.1	46.7	104.8
1895	1939	1,000.0	189.5	184.6	187.1	140.6	93.8	58.3	45.2	100.9
1896	1940	1,000.0	189.2	192.7	190.0	140.2	91.4	56.6	43.9	96.0
1897	1941	1,000.0	189.8	199.0	194.0	138.7	89.7	55.0	42.2	91.6
1898	1942	1,000.0	194.4	200.1	197.3	137.3	88.4	52.9	41.4	88.2
1899	1943	1,000.0	197.8	203.6	198.3	135.3	86.1	52.1	40.9	85.9
1900	1944	1,000.0	204.1	208.6	197.2	132.5	83.9	51.2	39.6	82.9
1901	1945	1,C00.0	203.6	217.5	199.6	131.5	81.7	50.4	37.7	78.0
1902	1946	1,000.0	200.7	226.0	203.6	130.0	81.3	49.3	35.8	73.3
1903	1947	1,000.0	198.0	230.7	208.3	129.9	80.5	48.7	34.1	69.8
1904	1948	1,000.0	201.5	232.3	210.2	128.3	79.7	47.3	33.6	67.1
1905	1949	1,000.0	209.0	232.1	210.1	127.3	78.7	46.5	32.1	64.2
1906	1950	1,000.0	214.2	231.6	211.7	127.6	77.3	45.7	30.6	61.3
1907	1951	1,000.0	216.1	228.5	215.5	130.1	76.6	44.4	30.2	58.6
1908	1952	1,000.0	218.5	225.9	219.1	130.8	76.6	43.8	29.1	56.2
1909	1953	1,000.0	216.8	221.8	223.0	133.3	77.9	43.3	28.4	55.5
1910	1954	1,000.0	215.7	218.2	225.3	136.2	78.8	43.8	27.4	54.6
1911	1955	1,000.0	208.6	216.1	229.1	140.3	79.8	44.5	27.6	54.0
1912	1956	1,000.0	201.7	213.6	233.9	143.8	81.7	44.4	28.0	52.9
1913	1957	1,000.0	191.4	210.5	238.7	149.2	84.5	45.8	28.4	51.5
1914	1958	1,000.0	180.6	204.9	243.7	155.6	87.7	46.9	28.9	51.7
1915	1959	1,000.0	171.2	198.6	247.2	161.1	91.5	49.1	29.4	51.9
1916	1960	1,000.0	167.0	191.9	248.5	164.6	94.8	51.2	29.6	52.4
1917	1961	1,000.0	161.5	182.8	250.2	169.8	99.0	53.7	30.3	52.7
1918	1962	1,000.0	156.8	175.8	251.4	174.0	102.3	55.2	31.0	53.5
1919	1963	1,000.0	137.2	173.7	255.0	180.7	106.8	58.0	32.8	55.8
1920	1964	1,000.0	123.9	172.1	255.7	185.0	111.0	60.2	34.7	57.4
1921	1965	1,000.0	114.4	167.1	254.5	189.6	116.0	62.9	36.5	59.0
1922	1966	1,000.0	115.5	158.4	251.3	193.6	119.4	64.4	37.7	59.7
1923	1967	1,000.0	110.0	152.3	248.9	197.6	123.4	67.4	39.3	61.1
1924	1968	1,000.0	103.2	145.0	247.3	201.3	127.5	70.9	40.9	63.9
1925	1969	1,000.0	101.0	137.8	243.1	203.9	131.3	73.7	42.8	66.4
1926	1970	1,000.0	103.6	128.1	237.6	206.0	135.5	76.5	44.1	68.6
1927	1971	1,000.0	105.9	120.6	231.0	208.0	139.5	79.0	45.7	70.3
1928	1972	1,000.0	108.9	113.3	225.5	208.9	143.5	81.4	47.2	71.3
1929	1973	1,000.0	105.8	106.3	221.2	211.6	147.4	85.3	49.2	73.2
1930	1974	1,000.0	103.9	100.5	217.8	214.2	151.2	87.7	51.3	73.4

TABLE 8A. DISTRIBUTIONS OF ALL WOMEN BY PARITY AS OF THE BEGINNING OF EACH YEAR 1917-74 BY AGE FOR EACH COHORT FROM 1867 TO 1959--CON.

(BASED ON CUMULATIVE BIRTH RATES)

EXACT AGE AND COHORT	AS OF JANUARY 1	TOTAL	PARITY							
			0	1	2	3	4	5	6	7 AND HIGHER
45 YEARS										
1872---------------	1917	1,000.0	205.1	110.9	122.9	109.8	94.3	76.6	67.5	212.9
1873---------------	1918	1,000.0	207.6	112.8	124.4	110.5	94.0	75.8	66.8	208.1
1874---------------	1919	1,000.0	210.1	115.1	125.8	111.1	93.5	74.6	65.8	204.0
1875---------------	1920	1,000.0	212.7	116.9	127.6	112.0	93.1	74.0	65.0	198.7
1876---------------	1921	1,000.0	214.4	119.1	129.4	112.9	93.5	73.6	64.9	192.2
1877---------------	1922	1,000.0	215.7	121.3	131.2	114.1	93.7	73.6	65.0	185.4
1878---------------	1923	1,000.0	217.2	123.3	132.6	114.4	93.6	71.7	65.4	181.8
1879---------------	1924	1,000.0	219.0	125.1	133.6	114.6	93.0	71.2	65.1	178.4
1880---------------	1925	1,000.0	219.7	127.7	134.6	115.1	93.0	71.1	63.7	175.1
1881---------------	1926	1,000.0	218.9	130.2	137.3	116.4	93.7	72.0	60.8	170.7
1882---------------	1927	1,000.0	217.2	133.1	140.2	118.3	94.8	72.6	58.3	165.5
1883---------------	1928	1,000.0	216.8	135.3	142.7	119.6	95.5	73.1	56.8	160.2
1884---------------	1929	1,000.0	217.5	136.2	145.6	121.0	95.5	72.6	57.2	154.4
1885---------------	1930	1,000.0	218.3	138.1	147.9	122.6	96.3	71.3	56.9	148.6
1886---------------	1931	1,000.0	216.7	143.1	147.6	124.7	97.3	70.7	56.5	143.4
1887---------------	1932	1,000.0	213.4	148.9	147.2	127.0	98.8	69.8	56.1	138.8
1888---------------	1933	1,000.0	210.5	149.6	151.2	129.6	100.0	67.9	57.0	134.2
1889---------------	1934	1,000.0	207.9	149.8	157.1	133.1	100.7	67.1	54.7	129.6
1890---------------	1935	1,000.0	204.4	151.3	163.5	135.8	101.2	66.0	53.4	124.4
1891---------------	1936	1,000.0	199.8	157.6	167.9	137.6	100.8	64.3	51.8	120.2
1892---------------	1937	1,000.0	194.1	165.7	174.0	138.6	99.8	62.9	49.8	115.1
1893---------------	1938	1,000.0	191.0	173.0	176.4	139.8	99.2	62.1	48.6	109.9
1894---------------	1939	1,000.0	190.2	178.8	181.6	140.8	96.5	60.0	46.6	105.5
1895---------------	1940	1,000.0	189.3	184.6	186.9	140.5	93.8	58.2	45.2	101.5
1896---------------	1941	1,000.0	189.0	192.7	189.8	140.2	91.3	56.6	43.9	96.5
1897---------------	1942	1,000.0	189.6	198.9	193.9	138.7	89.7	54.9	42.2	92.1
1898---------------	1943	1,000.0	194.2	200.0	197.2	137.2	88.3	52.9	41.4	88.8
1899---------------	1944	1,000.0	197.5	203.6	198.2	135.2	86.0	52.1	40.9	86.5
1900---------------	1945	1,000.0	203.8	208.5	197.1	132.4	83.9	51.3	39.5	83.5
1901---------------	1946	1,000.0	203.2	217.5	199.5	131.4	81.7	50.5	37.7	78.5
1902---------------	1947	1,000.0	200.3	225.9	203.6	129.9	81.3	49.4	35.8	73.8
1903---------------	1948	1,000.0	197.6	230.6	208.3	129.8	80.6	48.6	34.2	70.3
1904---------------	1949	1,000.0	201.2	232.1	210.1	128.4	79.7	47.4	33.6	67.5
1905---------------	1950	1,000.0	208.6	232.0	210.0	127.3	78.8	46.6	32.1	64.6
1906---------------	1951	1,000.0	213.8	231.5	211.7	127.6	77.3	45.8	30.6	61.7
1907---------------	1952	1,000.0	215.7	228.5	215.3	130.1	76.7	44.5	30.2	59.0
1908---------------	1953	1,000.0	218.1	225.8	219.0	130.8	76.7	43.9	29.1	56.6
1909---------------	1954	1,000.0	216.4	221.7	222.9	133.2	78.0	43.4	28.5	55.9
1910---------------	1955	1,000.0	215.3	218.1	225.1	136.3	78.8	43.9	27.5	55.0
1911---------------	1956	1,000.0	208.2	216.0	228.9	140.3	79.8	44.7	27.7	54.4
1912---------------	1957	1,000.0	201.4	213.4	233.7	143.8	81.8	44.5	28.1	53.3
1913---------------	1958	1,000.0	191.1	210.4	238.4	149.2	84.6	45.8	28.6	51.9
1914---------------	1959	1,000.0	180.3	204.8	243.4	155.6	87.7	47.1	29.0	52.1
1915---------------	1960	1,000.0	170.9	198.5	246.9	161.0	91.6	49.2	29.6	52.3
1916---------------	1961	1,000.0	166.8	191.7	248.2	164.6	94.8	51.3	29.8	52.8
1917---------------	1962	1,000.0	161.3	182.6	250.0	169.6	99.1	53.8	30.4	53.2
1918---------------	1963	1,000.0	156.6	175.6	251.2	173.9	102.4	55.2	31.2	53.9
1919---------------	1964	1,000.0	137.0	173.5	254.8	180.6	106.8	58.2	32.9	56.2
1920---------------	1965	1,000.0	123.7	172.0	255.5	184.8	111.1	60.2	34.9	57.8
1921---------------	1966	1,000.0	114.2	167.0	254.3	189.5	116.0	63.0	36.6	59.4
1922---------------	1967	1,000.0	115.3	158.4	251.1	193.4	119.4	64.5	37.8	60.1
1923---------------	1968	1,000.0	109.8	152.3	248.7	197.4	123.5	67.5	39.3	61.5
1924---------------	1969	1,000.0	103.0	145.0	247.1	201.2	127.6	70.9	40.9	64.3
1925---------------	1970	1,000.0	100.9	137.7	243.0	203.8	131.2	73.8	42.9	66.7
1926---------------	1971	1,000.0	103.5	128.0	237.5	205.9	135.5	76.5	44.2	68.9
1927---------------	1972	1,000.0	105.8	120.6	230.9	207.9	139.5	79.0	45.8	70.5
1928---------------	1973	1,000.0	108.8	113.2	225.5	208.9	143.5	81.4	47.2	71.5
1929---------------	1974	1,000.0	105.7	106.3	221.1	211.6	147.4	85.3	49.2	73.4

TABLE 8A. DISTRIBUTIONS OF ALL WOMEN BY PARITY AS OF THE BEGINNING OF EACH YEAR 1917-74 BY AGE FOR EACH COHORT FROM 1867 TO 1959--CON.

(BASED ON CUMULATIVE BIRTH RATES)

EXACT AGE AND COHORT	AS OF JANUARY 1	TOTAL	PARITY 0	1	2	3	4	5	6	7 AND HIGHER
46 YEARS										
1871---------------	1917	1,000.0	202.5	109.1	121.3	108.7	94.5	76.9	68.0	219.0
1872---------------	1918	1,000.0	204.9	110.8	122.8	109.6	94.2	76.4	67.3	214.0
1873---------------	1919	1,000.0	207.4	112.7	124.2	110.4	93.8	75.5	66.8	209.2
1874---------------	1920	1,000.0	209.9	115.0	125.7	111.0	93.3	74.4	65.7	205.0
1875---------------	1921	1,000.0	212.5	116.8	127.4	111.9	92.9	73.9	64.8	199.8
1876---------------	1922	1,000.0	214.2	119.1	129.2	112.7	93.4	73.5	64.8	193.1
1877---------------	1923	1,000.0	215.5	121.3	131.0	114.0	93.6	73.4	64.9	186.3
1878---------------	1924	1,000.0	217.0	123.2	132.5	114.3	93.4	71.6	65.3	182.7
1879---------------	1925	1,000.0	218.8	125.0	133.5	114.5	92.8	71.2	64.9	179.3
1880---------------	1926	1,000.0	219.5	127.7	134.4	115.0	92.9	70.9	63.6	176.0
1881---------------	1927	1,000.0	218.7	130.2	137.2	116.2	93.7	71.8	60.7	171.5
1882---------------	1928	1,000.0	217.0	133.1	140.1	118.1	94.8	72.4	58.3	166.2
1883---------------	1929	1,000.0	216.6	135.3	142.6	119.5	95.4	73.0	56.7	160.9
1884---------------	1930	1,000.0	217.3	136.2	145.5	120.9	95.4	72.5	57.2	155.0
1885---------------	1931	1,000.0	218.1	138.1	147.8	122.5	96.2	71.3	56.8	149.2
1886---------------	1932	1,000.0	216.5	143.1	147.5	124.6	97.3	70.6	56.4	144.0
1887---------------	1933	1,000.0	213.3	148.8	147.1	127.0	98.7	69.7	56.0	139.4
1888---------------	1934	1,000.0	210.4	149.5	151.2	129.5	99.9	67.8	57.0	134.7
1889---------------	1935	1,000.0	207.8	149.8	157.0	133.0	100.6	67.0	54.7	130.1
1890---------------	1936	1,000.0	204.2	151.4	163.4	135.7	101.1	66.0	53.3	124.9
1891---------------	1937	1,000.0	199.7	157.6	167.8	137.5	100.7	64.3	51.8	120.6
1892---------------	1938	1,000.0	194.0	165.7	173.9	138.5	99.8	62.8	49.8	115.5
1893---------------	1939	1,000.0	190.9	173.0	176.3	139.7	99.2	62.0	48.6	110.3
1894---------------	1940	1,000.0	190.1	178.8	181.5	140.7	96.5	60.0	46.5	105.9
1895---------------	1941	1,000.0	189.2	184.6	186.8	140.5	93.7	58.2	45.2	101.8
1896---------------	1942	1,000.0	188.9	192.6	189.8	140.2	91.3	56.5	43.9	96.8
1897---------------	1943	1,000.0	189.5	198.8	193.9	138.7	89.6	54.9	42.2	92.4
1898---------------	1944	1,000.0	194.0	200.0	197.2	137.1	88.3	52.9	41.4	89.1
1899---------------	1945	1,000.0	197.3	203.6	198.2	135.1	86.0	52.1	40.9	86.8
1900---------------	1946	1,000.0	203.6	208.5	197.0	132.4	83.9	51.3	39.5	83.8
1901---------------	1947	1,000.0	203.0	217.5	199.4	131.4	81.7	50.5	37.7	78.8
1902---------------	1948	1,000.0	200.1	225.9	203.6	129.8	81.3	49.4	35.8	74.1
1903---------------	1949	1,000.0	197.4	230.6	208.2	129.8	80.6	48.7	34.2	70.5
1904---------------	1950	1,000.0	201.0	232.1	210.0	128.4	79.7	47.5	33.6	67.7
1905---------------	1951	1,000.0	208.4	232.0	210.0	127.2	78.8	46.7	32.1	64.8
1906---------------	1952	1,000.0	213.6	231.5	211.6	127.6	77.3	45.9	30.6	61.9
1907---------------	1953	1,000.0	215.5	228.5	215.2	130.1	76.7	44.6	30.2	59.2
1908---------------	1954	1,000.0	217.9	225.8	218.9	130.8	76.7	44.0	29.1	56.8
1909---------------	1955	1,000.0	216.2	221.7	222.8	133.2	78.0	43.5	28.5	56.1
1910---------------	1956	1,000.0	215.1	218.1	225.0	136.3	78.8	44.0	27.5	55.2
1911---------------	1957	1,000.0	208.0	216.0	228.8	140.3	79.8	44.7	27.8	54.6
1912---------------	1958	1,000.0	201.2	213.4	233.6	143.7	81.9	44.5	28.2	53.5
1913---------------	1959	1,000.0	191.0	210.3	238.3	149.2	84.6	45.8	28.7	52.1
1914---------------	1960	1,000.0	180.1	204.8	243.3	155.5	87.7	47.2	29.1	52.3
1915---------------	1961	1,000.0	170.8	198.4	246.8	160.9	91.7	49.2	29.7	52.5
1916---------------	1962	1,000.0	166.7	191.6	248.1	164.5	94.8	51.4	29.8	53.1
1917---------------	1963	1,000.0	161.2	182.5	249.9	169.5	99.2	53.8	30.5	53.4
1918---------------	1964	1,000.0	156.5	175.5	251.1	173.9	102.4	55.3	31.2	54.1
1919---------------	1965	1,000.0	136.9	173.5	254.6	180.6	106.8	58.2	33.0	56.4
1920---------------	1966	1,000.0	123.6	172.0	255.4	184.7	111.1	60.2	35.0	58.0
1921---------------	1967	1,000.0	114.1	167.0	254.2	189.4	116.0	63.1	36.6	59.6
1922---------------	1968	1,000.0	115.2	158.4	251.0	193.3	119.4	64.6	37.8	60.3
1923---------------	1969	1,000.0	109.7	152.3	248.6	197.4	123.5	67.5	39.3	61.7
1924---------------	1970	1,000.0	102.9	145.0	247.1	201.1	127.6	70.9	40.9	64.5
1925---------------	1971	1,000.0	100.8	137.7	243.0	203.7	131.2	73.8	42.9	66.9
1926---------------	1972	1,000.0	103.4	128.0	237.5	205.8	135.6	76.4	44.3	69.0
1927---------------	1973	1,000.0	105.8	120.5	230.9	207.9	139.5	79.0	45.8	70.6
1928---------------	1974	1,000.0	108.8	113.1	225.5	208.9	143.5	81.4	47.2	71.6

TABLE 8A. DISTRIBUTIONS OF ALL WOMEN BY PARITY AS OF THE BEGINNING OF EACH YEAR 1917-74 BY AGE FOR EACH COHORT FROM 1867 TO 1959--CON.

(BASED ON CUMULATIVE BIRTH RATES)

EXACT AGE AND COHORT	AS OF JANUARY 1	TOTAL	PARITY							
			0	1	2	3	4	5	6	7 AND HIGHER
47 YEARS										
1870---------------	1917	1,000.0	200.1	107.2	119.9	107.9	94.5	77.4	68.5	224.5
1871---------------	1918	1,000.0	202.4	109.0	121.3	108.6	94.3	76.8	67.9	219.7
1872---------------	1919	1,000.0	204.7	110.8	122.6	109.6	94.1	76.1	67.4	214.7
1873---------------	1920	1,000.0	207.3	112.6	124.2	110.3	93.6	75.4	66.8	209.8
1874---------------	1921	1,000.0	209.8	114.9	125.6	110.9	93.2	74.3	65.6	205.7
1875---------------	1922	1,000.0	212.4	116.8	127.3	111.8	92.8	73.8	64.7	200.4
1876---------------	1923	1,000.0	214.1	119.1	129.1	112.6	93.3	73.4	64.7	193.7
1877---------------	1924	1,000.0	215.4	121.2	131.0	113.9	93.5	73.3	64.8	186.9
1878---------------	1925	1,000.0	216.9	123.1	132.5	114.2	93.3	71.5	65.3	183.2
1879---------------	1926	1,000.0	218.7	125.0	133.3	114.5	92.7	71.2	64.8	179.8
1880---------------	1927	1,000.0	219.4	127.6	134.4	114.9	92.9	70.7	63.6	176.5
1881---------------	1928	1,000.0	218.6	130.2	137.1	116.1	93.7	71.7	60.6	172.0
1882---------------	1929	1,000.0	216.9	133.1	140.0	118.0	94.8	72.3	58.3	166.6
1883---------------	1930	1,000.0	216.5	135.3	142.5	119.5	95.3	72.9	56.7	161.3
1884---------------	1931	1,000.0	217.2	136.2	145.5	120.8	95.3	72.5	57.1	155.4
1885---------------	1932	1,000.0	218.0	138.1	147.7	122.5	96.1	71.3	56.8	149.5
1886---------------	1933	1,000.0	216.4	143.1	147.5	124.5	97.2	70.6	56.3	144.4
1887---------------	1934	1,000.0	213.2	148.8	147.1	126.9	98.7	69.6	56.0	139.7
1888---------------	1935	1,000.0	210.4	149.4	151.2	129.4	99.9	67.7	57.0	135.0
1889---------------	1936	1,000.0	207.7	149.8	157.0	132.9	100.6	66.9	54.7	130.4
1890---------------	1937	1,000.0	204.1	151.4	163.4	135.6	101.1	65.9	53.4	125.1
1891---------------	1938	1,000.0	199.7	157.6	167.7	137.4	100.7	64.3	51.8	120.8
1892---------------	1939	1,000.0	193.9	165.7	173.9	138.4	99.8	62.8	49.8	115.7
1893---------------	1940	1,000.0	190.8	173.1	176.2	139.7	99.1	62.0	48.6	110.5
1894---------------	1941	1,000.0	190.0	178.9	181.4	140.7	96.4	60.0	46.5	106.1
1895---------------	1942	1,000.0	189.1	184.6	186.8	140.5	93.7	58.1	45.2	102.0
1896---------------	1943	1,000.0	188.8	192.6	189.8	140.2	91.3	56.4	43.9	97.0
1897---------------	1944	1,000.0	189.4	198.8	193.9	138.7	89.6	54.9	42.1	92.6
1898---------------	1945	1,000.0	193.9	200.0	197.2	137.0	88.4	52.9	41.3	89.3
1899---------------	1946	1,000.0	197.2	203.6	198.2	135.0	86.0	52.1	40.9	87.0
1900---------------	1947	1,000.0	203.5	208.5	197.0	132.3	83.9	51.3	39.5	84.0
1901---------------	1948	1,000.0	202.9	217.5	199.4	131.4	81.6	50.5	37.7	79.0
1902---------------	1949	1,000.0	200.0	225.9	203.6	129.8	81.3	49.4	35.8	74.2
1903---------------	1950	1,000.0	197.3	230.6	208.2	129.8	80.5	48.8	34.2	70.6
1904---------------	1951	1,000.0	200.9	232.1	210.0	128.3	79.8	47.5	33.6	67.8
1905---------------	1952	1,000.0	208.3	232.0	210.0	127.2	78.8	46.7	32.1	64.9
1906---------------	1953	1,000.0	213.5	231.5	211.6	127.6	77.3	45.9	30.6	62.0
1907---------------	1954	1,000.0	215.4	228.5	215.2	130.0	76.8	44.6	30.2	59.3
1908---------------	1955	1,000.0	217.8	225.8	218.9	130.7	76.7	44.1	29.1	56.9
1909---------------	1956	1,000.0	216.1	221.7	222.8	133.1	78.0	43.6	28.5	56.2
1910---------------	1957	1,000.0	215.0	218.1	225.0	136.2	78.8	44.1	27.5	55.3
1911---------------	1958	1,000.0	207.9	216.0	228.7	140.4	79.7	44.8	27.8	54.7
1912---------------	1959	1,000.0	201.2	213.3	233.5	143.7	82.0	44.5	28.2	53.6
1913---------------	1960	1,000.0	190.9	210.3	238.3	149.1	84.6	45.8	28.8	52.2
1914---------------	1961	1,000.0	180.0	204.8	243.3	155.4	87.7	47.3	29.1	52.4
1915---------------	1962	1,000.0	170.7	198.4	246.8	160.9	91.6	49.2	29.8	52.6
1916---------------	1963	1,000.0	166.7	191.5	248.0	164.5	94.8	51.4	29.9	53.2
1917---------------	1964	1,000.0	161.2	182.4	249.9	169.5	99.1	53.9	30.5	53.5
1918---------------	1965	1,000.0	156.5	175.5	251.0	173.9	102.3	55.3	31.3	54.2
1919---------------	1966	1,000.0	136.9	173.5	254.5	180.6	106.8	58.2	33.0	56.5
1920---------------	1967	1,000.0	123.6	172.0	255.3	184.7	111.1	60.2	35.0	58.1
1921---------------	1968	1,000.0	114.1	167.0	254.1	189.4	116.0	63.1	36.6	59.7
1922---------------	1969	1,000.0	115.2	158.4	250.9	193.3	119.4	64.6	37.8	60.4
1923---------------	1970	1,000.0	109.7	152.3	248.6	197.3	123.5	67.5	39.3	61.8
1924---------------	1971	1,000.0	102.9	145.0	247.0	201.1	127.6	70.9	40.9	64.6
1925---------------	1972	1,000.0	100.8	137.7	242.9	203.7	131.3	73.7	42.9	67.0
1926---------------	1973	1,000.0	103.4	128.0	237.4	205.9	135.5	76.4	44.4	69.0
1927---------------	1974	1,000.0	105.8	120.5	230.9	207.9	139.4	79.1	45.7	70.7

TABLE 8A. DISTRIBUTIONS OF ALL WOMEN BY PARITY AS OF THE BEGINNING OF EACH YEAR 1917-74 BY AGE FOR EACH COHORT FROM 1867 TO 1959--CON.

(BASED ON CUMULATIVE BIRTH RATES)

EXACT AGE AND COHORT	AS OF JANUARY 1	TOTAL	PARITY 0	1	2	3	4	5	6	7 AND HIGHER
48 YEARS										
1869	1917	1,000.0	197.8	105.5	118.4	107.1	94.6	78.0	69.0	229.6
1870	1918	1,000.0	200.0	107.2	119.9	107.8	94.5	77.3	68.5	224.8
1871	1919	1,000.0	202.3	109.0	121.2	108.6	94.2	76.7	67.9	220.1
1872	1920	1,000.0	204.6	110.8	122.6	109.6	94.0	76.0	67.4	215.0
1873	1921	1,000.0	207.2	112.6	124.1	110.3	93.5	75.4	66.8	210.1
1874	1922	1,000.0	209.7	115.0	125.5	110.8	93.2	74.3	65.5	206.0
1875	1923	1,000.0	212.3	116.8	127.3	111.8	92.7	73.8	64.6	200.7
1876	1924	1,000.0	214.0	119.1	129.1	112.6	93.2	73.3	64.7	194.0
1877	1925	1,000.0	215.3	121.2	131.0	113.9	93.4	73.3	64.7	187.2
1878	1926	1,000.0	216.8	123.2	132.4	114.2	93.2	71.5	65.3	183.4
1879	1927	1,000.0	218.7	124.9	133.3	114.5	92.6	71.2	64.7	180.1
1880	1928	1,000.0	219.4	127.5	134.4	114.8	92.9	70.7	63.6	176.7
1881	1929	1,000.0	218.6	130.1	137.1	116.1	93.7	71.6	60.6	172.2
1882	1930	1,000.0	216.8	133.1	140.0	118.0	94.8	72.2	58.3	166.8
1883	1931	1,000.0	216.4	135.3	142.6	119.4	95.2	72.9	56.7	161.5
1884	1932	1,000.0	217.2	136.2	145.4	120.8	95.3	72.4	57.1	155.6
1885	1933	1,000.0	218.0	138.1	147.6	122.5	96.1	71.3	56.7	149.7
1886	1934	1,000.0	216.4	143.1	147.4	124.5	97.2	70.6	56.2	144.6
1887	1935	1,000.0	213.2	148.8	147.1	126.8	98.7	69.6	55.9	139.9
1888	1936	1,000.0	210.4	149.4	151.1	129.4	99.9	67.7	57.0	135.1
1889	1937	1,000.0	207.7	149.8	157.0	132.8	100.6	66.8	54.8	130.5
1890	1938	1,000.0	204.1	151.4	163.4	135.5	101.1	65.9	53.4	125.2
1891	1939	1,000.0	199.7	157.6	167.7	137.3	100.7	64.3	51.8	120.9
1892	1940	1,000.0	193.9	165.7	173.9	138.4	99.7	62.8	49.8	115.8
1893	1941	1,000.0	190.8	173.1	176.2	139.7	99.0	62.0	48.6	110.6
1894	1942	1,000.0	190.0	178.9	181.4	140.7	96.3	60.0	46.5	106.2
1895	1943	1,000.0	189.1	184.6	186.8	140.5	93.7	58.0	45.2	102.1
1896	1944	1,000.0	188.8	192.6	189.8	140.2	91.3	56.4	43.8	97.1
1897	1945	1,000.0	189.4	198.8	193.9	138.6	89.7	54.9	42.0	92.7
1898	1946	1,000.0	193.9	200.0	197.2	136.9	88.4	52.9	41.3	89.4
1899	1947	1,000.0	197.2	203.6	198.2	134.9	86.0	52.1	40.9	87.1
1900	1948	1,000.0	203.5	208.5	196.9	132.4	83.8	51.3	39.5	84.1
1901	1949	1,000.0	202.9	217.4	199.5	131.4	81.6	50.4	37.7	79.1
1902	1950	1,000.0	200.0	225.9	203.6	129.8	81.2	49.4	35.9	74.2
1903	1951	1,000.0	197.3	230.6	208.2	129.7	80.6	48.7	34.3	70.6
1904	1952	1,000.0	200.9	232.1	210.0	128.3	79.7	47.6	33.6	67.8
1905	1953	1,000.0	208.3	232.0	210.0	127.1	78.9	46.7	32.1	64.9
1906	1954	1,000.0	213.5	231.5	211.6	127.5	77.4	45.8	30.7	62.0
1907	1955	1,000.0	215.4	228.5	215.2	129.9	76.8	44.7	30.2	59.3
1908	1956	1,000.0	217.8	225.8	218.9	130.6	76.7	44.2	29.1	56.9
1909	1957	1,000.0	216.1	221.7	222.8	133.0	78.0	43.7	28.5	56.2
1910	1958	1,000.0	215.0	218.1	224.9	136.3	78.7	44.2	27.5	55.3
1911	1959	1,000.0	207.9	216.0	228.6	140.4	79.8	44.7	27.9	54.7
1912	1960	1,000.0	201.2	213.3	233.5	143.6	82.0	44.5	28.3	53.6
1913	1961	1,000.0	190.9	210.3	238.3	149.0	84.6	45.9	28.7	52.3
1914	1962	1,000.0	180.0	204.8	243.3	155.4	87.6	47.3	29.2	52.4
1915	1963	1,000.0	170.7	198.4	246.7	160.9	91.6	49.2	29.9	52.6
1916	1964	1,000.0	166.7	191.5	248.0	164.5	94.7	51.5	29.9	53.2
1917	1965	1,000.0	161.2	182.4	249.9	169.5	99.0	53.9	30.6	53.5
1918	1966	1,000.0	156.5	175.5	251.0	173.9	102.3	55.3	31.3	54.2
1919	1967	1,000.0	136.9	173.5	254.5	180.6	106.8	58.2	33.0	56.5
1920	1968	1,000.0	123.6	172.0	255.3	184.7	111.1	60.2	35.0	58.1
1921	1969	1,000.0	114.1	167.0	254.1	189.4	116.0	63.1	36.6	59.7
1922	1970	1,000.0	115.2	158.4	250.9	193.3	119.4	64.6	37.8	60.4
1923	1971	1,000.0	109.7	152.3	248.6	197.3	123.5	67.5	39.3	61.8
1924	1972	1,000.0	102.9	145.0	247.0	201.1	127.6	70.9	40.9	64.6
1925	1973	1,000.0	100.8	137.7	242.9	203.7	131.3	73.7	42.9	67.0
1926	1974	1,000.0	103.4	128.0	237.4	205.9	135.5	76.4	44.4	69.0

TABLE 8A. DISTRIBUTIONS OF ALL WOMEN BY PARITY AS OF THE BEGINNING OF EACH YEAR 1917-74 BY AGE FOR EACH COHORT FROM 1867 TO 1959--CON.

(BASED ON CUMULATIVE BIRTH RATES)

EXACT AGE AND COHORT	AS OF JANUARY 1	TOTAL	PARITY							
			0	1	2	3	4	5	6	7 AND HIGHER
49 YEARS										
1868----------------	1917	1,000.0	195.6	103.7	117.1	106.4	94.6	78.5	69.6	234.5
1869----------------	1918	1,000.0	197.7	105.5	118.5	107.0	94.6	77.9	69.0	229.8
1870----------------	1919	1,000.0	199.9	107.3	119.8	107.7	94.6	77.2	68.5	225.0
1871----------------	1920	1,000.0	202.3	109.0	121.2	108.5	94.2	76.6	67.9	220.3
1872----------------	1921	1,000.0	204.6	110.7	122.6	109.6	94.0	75.9	67.4	215.2
1873----------------	1922	1,000.0	207.2	112.6	124.1	110.2	93.5	75.4	66.7	210.3
1874----------------	1923	1,000.0	209.6	115.1	125.5	110.7	93.2	74.3	65.4	206.2
1875----------------	1924	1,000.0	212.3	116.8	127.3	111.7	92.7	73.7	64.6	200.9
1876----------------	1925	1,000.0	214.0	119.1	129.1	112.5	93.2	73.2	64.7	194.2
1877----------------	1926	1,000.0	215.2	121.3	131.0	113.8	93.4	73.3	64.7	187.3
1878----------------	1927	1,000.0	216.8	123.1	132.4	114.2	93.2	71.5	65.2	183.6
1879----------------	1928	1,000.0	218.7	124.9	133.3	114.4	92.6	71.2	64.7	180.2
1880----------------	1929	1,000.0	219.4	127.5	134.3	114.8	92.9	70.7	63.6	176.8
1881----------------	1930	1,000.0	218.5	130.2	137.1	116.1	93.6	71.6	60.6	172.3
1882----------------	1931	1,000.0	216.8	133.1	140.0	118.0	94.7	72.2	58.3	166.9
1883----------------	1932	1,000.0	216.4	135.3	142.5	119.5	95.2	72.8	56.7	161.6
1884----------------	1933	1,000.0	217.2	136.2	145.4	120.7	95.3	72.4	57.1	155.7
1885----------------	1934	1,000.0	218.0	138.1	147.6	122.4	96.1	71.3	56.7	149.8
1886----------------	1935	1,000.0	216.4	143.1	147.4	124.5	97.1	70.6	56.2	144.7
1887----------------	1936	1,000.0	213.2	148.8	147.1	126.8	98.6	69.6	55.9	140.0
1888----------------	1937	1,000.0	210.4	149.4	151.1	129.3	100.0	67.6	57.0	135.2
1889----------------	1938	1,000.0	207.7	149.8	157.0	132.8	100.5	66.8	54.8	130.6
1890----------------	1939	1,000.0	204.1	151.4	163.4	135.4	101.1	65.9	53.4	125.3
1891----------------	1940	1,000.0	199.7	157.6	167.7	137.3	100.6	64.3	51.8	121.0
1892----------------	1941	1,000.0	193.9	165.7	173.9	138.4	99.6	62.9	49.7	115.9
1893----------------	1942	1,000.0	190.8	173.1	176.2	139.7	99.0	62.0	48.6	110.6
1894----------------	1943	1,000.0	190.0	178.9	181.4	140.7	96.3	60.0	46.5	106.2
1895----------------	1944	1,000.0	189.1	184.6	186.8	140.5	93.7	58.0	45.2	102.1
1896----------------	1945	1,000.0	188.8	192.6	189.8	140.2	91.3	56.4	43.8	97.1
1897----------------	1946	1,000.0	189.4	198.8	193.9	138.6	89.7	54.9	42.0	92.7
1898----------------	1947	1,000.0	193.9	200.0	197.2	136.9	88.4	52.9	41.3	89.4
1899----------------	1948	1,000.0	197.2	203.6	198.2	134.9	86.0	52.1	40.9	87.1
1900----------------	1949	1,000.0	203.5	208.5	196.9	132.4	83.8	51.3	39.5	84.1
1901----------------	1950	1,000.0	202.9	217.4	199.5	131.4	81.6	50.4	37.7	79.1
1902----------------	1951	1,000.0	200.0	225.9	203.6	129.8	81.2	49.4	35.9	74.2
1903----------------	1952	1,000.0	197.3	230.6	208.2	129.7	80.6	48.7	34.3	70.6
1904----------------	1953	1,000.0	200.9	232.1	210.0	128.3	79.7	47.6	33.6	67.8
1905----------------	1954	1,000.0	208.3	232.0	210.0	127.1	78.9	46.7	32.1	64.9
1906----------------	1955	1,000.0	213.5	231.5	211.6	127.5	77.4	45.8	30.7	62.0
1907----------------	1956	1,000.0	215.4	228.5	215.2	129.9	76.8	44.7	30.2	59.3
1908----------------	1957	1,000.0	217.8	225.8	218.9	130.6	76.7	44.2	29.1	56.9
1909----------------	1958	1,000.0	216.1	221.7	222.8	133.0	78.0	43.7	28.5	56.2
1910----------------	1959	1,000.0	215.0	218.1	224.9	136.3	78.7	44.2	27.5	55.3
1911----------------	1960	1,000.0	207.9	216.0	228.6	140.4	79.8	44.7	27.9	54.7
1912----------------	1961	1,000.0	201.2	213.3	233.5	143.6	82.0	44.5	28.3	53.6
1913----------------	1962	1,000.0	190.9	210.3	238.3	149.0	84.6	45.9	28.7	52.3
1914----------------	1963	1,000.0	180.0	204.8	243.3	155.4	87.6	47.3	29.2	52.4
1915----------------	1964	1,000.0	170.7	198.4	246.7	160.9	91.6	49.2	29.9	52.6
1916----------------	1965	1,000.0	166.7	191.5	248.0	164.5	94.7	51.5	29.9	53.2
1917----------------	1966	1,000.0	161.2	182.4	249.9	169.5	99.0	53.9	30.6	53.5
1918----------------	1967	1,000.0	156.5	175.5	251.0	173.9	102.3	55.3	31.3	54.2
1919----------------	1968	1,000.0	136.9	173.5	254.5	180.6	106.8	58.2	33.0	56.5
1920----------------	1969	1,000.0	123.6	172.0	255.3	184.7	111.1	60.2	35.0	58.1
1921----------------	1970	1,000.0	114.1	167.0	254.1	189.4	116.0	63.1	36.6	59.7
1922----------------	1971	1,000.0	115.2	158.4	250.9	193.3	119.4	64.6	37.8	60.4
1923----------------	1972	1,000.0	109.7	152.3	248.6	197.3	123.5	67.5	39.3	61.8
1924----------------	1973	1,000.0	102.9	145.0	247.0	201.1	127.6	70.9	40.9	64.6
1925----------------	1974	1,000.0	100.8	137.7	242.9	203.7	131.3	73.7	42.9	67.0

TABLE 8A. DISTRIBUTIONS OF ALL WOMEN BY PARITY AS OF THE BEGINNING OF EACH YEAR 1917-74 BY AGE FOR EACH COHORT FROM 1867 TO 1959--CON.

(BASED ON CUMULATIVE BIRTH RATES)

EXACT AGE AND COHORT	AS OF JANUARY 1	TOTAL	PARITY							
			0	1	2	3	4	5	6	7 AND HIGHER
50 YEARS										
1867	1917	1,000.0	193.4	102.0	115.6	105.8	94.6	79.1	70.3	239.2
1868	1918	1,000.0	195.6	103.7	117.1	106.3	94.6	78.5	69.6	234.6
1869	1919	1,000.0	197.7	105.5	118.5	106.9	94.6	77.9	69.0	229.9
1870	1920	1,000.0	199.9	107.3	119.8	107.6	94.6	77.2	68.5	225.1
1871	1921	1,000.0	202.3	108.9	121.3	108.4	94.2	76.6	67.9	220.4
1872	1922	1,000.0	204.6	110.7	122.6	109.5	94.1	75.8	67.4	215.3
1873	1923	1,000.0	207.2	112.6	124.1	110.1	93.6	75.4	66.6	210.4
1874	1924	1,000.0	209.6	115.1	125.5	110.6	93.3	74.2	65.4	206.3
1875	1925	1,000.0	212.3	116.8	127.3	111.6	92.8	73.6	64.6	201.0
1876	1926	1,000.0	214.0	119.1	129.1	112.5	93.1	73.3	64.7	194.2
1877	1927	1,000.0	215.2	121.3	131.0	113.8	93.4	73.2	64.7	187.4
1878	1928	1,000.0	216.8	123.1	132.4	114.2	93.2	71.5	65.1	183.7
1879	1929	1,000.0	218.7	124.9	133.3	114.4	92.6	71.2	64.7	180.2
1880	1930	1,000.0	219.4	127.5	134.3	114.8	92.9	70.6	63.6	176.9
1881	1931	1,000.0	218.5	130.2	137.1	116.1	93.6	71.5	60.6	172.4
1882	1932	1,000.0	216.8	133.1	140.0	118.0	94.7	72.2	58.3	166.9
1883	1933	1,000.0	216.4	135.3	142.5	119.5	95.2	72.8	56.7	161.6
1884	1934	1,000.0	217.2	136.2	145.4	120.7	95.3	72.4	57.0	155.8
1885	1935	1,000.0	218.0	138.1	147.6	122.4	96.1	71.3	56.6	149.9
1886	1936	1,000.0	216.4	143.1	147.4	124.5	97.0	70.6	56.2	144.8
1887	1937	1,000.0	213.2	148.8	147.1	126.8	98.6	69.5	55.9	140.1
1888	1938	1,000.0	210.4	149.4	151.1	129.3	100.0	67.5	57.0	135.3
1889	1939	1,000.0	207.7	149.8	157.0	132.8	100.5	66.8	54.7	130.7
1890	1940	1,000.0	204.1	151.4	163.4	135.4	101.1	65.9	53.3	125.4
1891	1941	1,000.0	199.7	157.6	167.7	137.3	100.6	64.3	51.8	121.0
1892	1942	1,000.0	193.9	165.7	173.9	138.4	99.6	62.9	49.7	115.9
1893	1943	1,000.0	190.8	173.1	176.2	139.7	99.0	62.0	48.6	110.6
1894	1944	1,000.0	190.0	178.9	181.4	140.7	96.3	60.0	46.5	106.2
1895	1945	1,000.0	189.1	184.6	186.8	140.5	93.7	58.0	45.2	102.1
1896	1946	1,000.0	188.8	192.6	189.8	140.2	91.3	56.4	43.8	97.1
1897	1947	1,000.0	189.4	198.8	193.9	138.6	89.7	54.9	42.0	92.7
1898	1948	1,000.0	193.9	200.0	197.2	136.9	88.4	52.9	41.3	89.4
1899	1949	1,000.0	197.2	203.6	198.2	134.9	86.0	52.1	40.9	87.1
1900	1950	1,000.0	203.5	208.5	196.9	132.4	83.8	51.3	39.5	84.1
1901	1951	1,000.0	202.9	217.4	199.5	131.4	81.6	50.4	37.7	79.1
1902	1952	1,000.0	200.0	225.9	203.6	129.8	81.2	49.4	35.9	74.2
1903	1953	1,000.0	197.3	230.6	208.2	129.7	80.6	48.7	34.3	70.6
1904	1954	1,000.0	200.9	232.1	210.0	128.3	79.7	47.6	33.6	67.8
1905	1955	1,000.0	208.3	232.0	210.0	127.1	78.9	46.7	32.1	64.9
1906	1956	1,000.0	213.5	231.5	211.6	127.5	77.4	45.8	30.7	62.0
1907	1957	1,000.0	215.4	228.5	215.2	129.9	76.8	44.7	30.2	59.3
1908	1958	1,000.0	217.8	225.8	218.9	130.6	76.7	44.2	29.1	56.9
1909	1959	1,000.0	216.1	221.7	222.8	133.0	78.0	43.7	28.5	56.2
1910	1960	1,000.0	215.0	218.1	224.9	136.3	78.7	44.2	27.5	55.3
1911	1961	1,000.0	207.9	216.0	228.6	140.4	79.8	44.7	27.9	54.7
1912	1962	1,000.0	201.2	213.3	233.5	143.6	82.0	44.5	28.3	53.6
1913	1963	1,000.0	190.9	210.3	238.3	149.0	84.6	45.9	28.7	52.3
1914	1964	1,000.0	180.0	204.8	243.3	155.4	87.6	47.3	29.2	52.4
1915	1965	1,000.0	170.7	198.4	246.7	160.9	91.6	49.2	29.9	52.6
1916	1966	1,000.0	166.7	191.5	248.0	164.5	94.7	51.5	29.9	53.2
1917	1967	1,000.0	161.2	182.4	249.9	169.5	99.0	53.9	30.6	53.5
1918	1968	1,000.0	156.5	175.5	251.0	173.9	102.3	55.3	31.3	54.2
1919	1969	1,000.0	136.9	173.5	254.5	180.6	106.8	58.2	33.0	56.5
1920	1970	1,000.0	123.6	172.0	255.3	184.7	111.1	60.2	35.0	58.1
1921	1971	1,000.0	114.1	167.0	254.1	189.4	116.0	63.1	36.6	59.7
1922	1972	1,000.0	115.2	158.4	250.9	193.3	119.4	64.6	37.8	60.4
1923	1973	1,000.0	109.7	152.3	248.6	197.3	123.5	67.5	39.3	61.8
1924	1974	1,000.0	102.9	145.0	247.0	201.1	127.6	70.9	40.9	64.6

TABLE 8B. DISTRIBUTIONS OF WHITE WOMEN BY PARITY AS OF THE BEGINNING OF EACH YEAR 1917-74 BY AGE FOR EACH COHORT FROM 1867 TO 1959

(BASED ON CUMULATIVE BIRTH RATES)

EXACT AGE AND COHORT	AS OF JANUARY 1	TOTAL	PARITY							
			0	1	2	3	4	5	6	7 AND HIGHER
15 YEARS										
1902	1917	1,000.0	998.0	2.0	*	*	*	*	*	*
1903	1918	1,000.0	998.0	2.0	*	*	*	*	*	*
1904	1919	1,000.0	997.9	2.1	*	*	*	*	*	*
1905	1920	1,000.0	998.4	1.6	*	*	*	*	*	*
1906	1921	1,000.0	998.0	2.0	*	*	*	*	*	*
1907	1922	1,000.0	997.8	2.2	*	*	*	*	*	*
1908	1923	1,000.0	998.0	2.0	*	*	*	*	*	*
1909	1924	1,000.0	998.0	2.0	*	*	*	*	*	*
1910	1925	1,000.0	997.9	2.1	*	*	*	*	*	*
1911	1926	1,000.0	997.9	2.1	*	*	*	*	*	*
1912	1927	1,000.0	997.9	2.1	*	*	*	*	*	*
1913	1928	1,000.0	997.6	2.4	*	*	*	*	*	*
1914	1929	1,000.0	997.9	2.1	*	*	*	*	*	*
1915	1930	1,000.0	997.8	2.2	*	*	*	*	*	*
1916	1931	1,000.0	997.7	2.3	*	*	*	*	*	*
1917	1932	1,000.0	998.0	2.0	*	*	*	*	*	*
1918	1933	1,000.0	998.2	1.8	*	*	*	*	*	*
1919	1934	1,000.0	998.2	1.8	*	*	*	*	*	*
1920	1935	1,000.0	998.1	1.9	*	*	*	*	*	*
1921	1936	1,000.0	997.9	2.1	*	*	*	*	*	*
1922	1937	1,000.0	998.1	1.9	*	*	*	*	*	*
1923	1938	1,000.0	998.0	2.0	*	*	*	*	*	*
1924	1939	1,000.0	998.0	2.0	*	*	*	*	*	*
1925	1940	1,000.0	998.1	1.9	*	*	*	*	*	*
1926	1941	1,000.0	998.1	1.9	*	*	*	*	*	*
1927	1942	1,000.0	997.9	2.1	*	*	*	*	*	*
1928	1943	1,000.0	997.9	2.1	*	*	*	*	*	*
1929	1944	1,000.0	997.9	2.1	*	*	*	*	*	*
1930	1945	1,000.0	998.1	1.9	*	*	*	*	*	*
1931	1946	1,000.0	998.1	1.9	*	*	*	*	*	*
1932	1947	1,000.0	998.1	1.9	*	*	*	*	*	*
1933	1948	1,000.0	997.2	2.8	*	*	*	*	*	*
1934	1949	1,000.0	996.8	3.2	*	*	*	*	*	*
1935	1950	1,000.0	997.0	3.0	*	*	*	*	*	*
1936	1951	1,000.0	996.9	3.1	*	*	*	*	*	*
1937	1952	1,000.0	996.8	3.2	*	*	*	*	*	*
1938	1953	1,000.0	996.9	3.1	*	*	*	*	*	*
1939	1954	1,000.0	996.8	3.2	*	*	*	*	*	*
1940	1955	1,000.0	996.5	3.5	*	*	*	*	*	*
1941	1956	1,000.0	996.5	3.5	*	*	*	*	*	*
1942	1957	1,000.0	996.4	3.6	*	*	*	*	*	*
1943	1958	1,000.0	996.4	3.6	*	*	*	*	*	*
1944	1959	1,000.0	996.5	3.5	*	*	*	*	*	*
1945	1960	1,000.0	996.4	3.6	*	*	*	*	*	*
1946	1961	1,000.0	996.4	3.6	*	*	*	*	*	*
1947	1962	1,000.0	996.8	3.2	*	*	*	*	*	*
1948	1963	1,000.0	997.0	3.0	*	*	*	*	*	*
1949	1964	1,000.0	997.1	2.9	*	*	*	*	*	*
1950	1965	1,000.0	997.2	2.8	*	*	*	*	*	*
1951	1966	1,000.0	997.3	2.7	*	*	*	*	*	*
1952	1967	1,000.0	997.2	2.8	*	*	*	*	*	*
1953	1968	1,000.0	997.3	2.7	*	*	*	*	*	*
1954	1969	1,000.0	997.1	2.9	*	*	*	*	*	*
1955	1970	1,000.0	996.8	3.2	*	*	*	*	*	*
1956	1971	1,000.0	996.4	3.6	*	*	*	*	*	*
1957	1972	1,000.0	996.3	3.7	*	*	*	*	*	*
1958	1973	1,000.0	995.9	4.1	*	*	*	*	*	*
1959	1974	1,000.0	995.7	4.3	*	*	*	*	*	*

TABLE 8B. DISTRIBUTIONS OF WHITE WOMEN BY PARITY AS OF THE BEGINNING OF EACH YEAR 1917-74 BY AGE FOR EACH COHORT FROM 1867 TO 1959--CON.

(BASED ON CUMULATIVE BIRTH RATES)

EXACT AGE AND COHORT	AS OF JANUARY 1	TOTAL	PARITY							
			0	1	2	3	4	5	6	7 AND HIGHER
16 YEARS										
1901---------------	1917	1,000.0	990.6	9.1	0.3	0.0	0.0	*	*	*
1902---------------	1918	1,000.0	990.6	9.0	0.4	0.0	0.0	*	*	*
1903---------------	1919	1,000.0	990.5	9.1	0.4	0.0	0.0	*	*	*
1904---------------	1920	1,000.0	991.8	7.9	0.3	0.0	0.0	*	*	*
1905---------------	1921	1,000.0	990.5	9.2	0.3	0.0	0.0	*	*	*
1906---------------	1922	1,000.0	989.5	10.2	0.3	0.0	0.0	*	*	*
1907---------------	1923	1,000.0	990.3	9.3	0.4	0.0	0.0	*	*	*
1908---------------	1924	1,000.0	990.6	9.0	0.4	0.0	0.0	*	*	*
1909---------------	1925	1,000.0	990.1	9.5	0.4	0.0	0.0	*	*	*
1910---------------	1926	1,000.0	990.0	9.6	0.4	0.0	0.0	*	*	*
1911---------------	1927	1,000.0	990.2	9.4	0.4	0.0	0.0	*	*	*
1912---------------	1928	1,000.0	989.4	10.2	0.4	0.0	0.0	*	*	*
1913---------------	1929	1,000.0	989.9	9.7	0.4	0.0	0.0	*	*	*
1914---------------	1930	1,000.0	990.0	9.6	0.4	0.0	0.0	*	*	*
1915---------------	1931	1,000.0	989.6	10.0	0.4	0.0	0.0	*	*	*
1916---------------	1932	1,000.0	990.2	9.4	0.4	0.0	0.0	*	*	*
1917---------------	1933	1,000.0	991.1	8.5	0.4	0.0	0.0	*	*	*
1918---------------	1934	1,000.0	991.8	7.9	0.3	0.0	0.0	*	*	*
1919---------------	1935	1,000.0	991.3	8.4	0.3	0.0	0.0	*	*	*
1920---------------	1936	1,000.0	990.9	8.8	0.3	0.0	0.0	*	*	*
1921---------------	1937	1,000.0	990.9	8.7	0.4	0.0	0.0	*	*	*
1922---------------	1938	1,000.0	990.9	8.7	0.4	0.0	0.0	*	*	*
1923---------------	1939	1,000.0	990.8	8.9	0.3	0.0	0.0	*	*	*
1924---------------	1940	1,000.0	991.1	8.5	0.4	0.0	0.0	*	*	*
1925---------------	1941	1,000.0	991.1	8.5	0.4	0.0	0.0	*	*	*
1926---------------	1942	1,000.0	990.5	9.1	0.4	0.0	0.0	*	*	*
1927---------------	1943	1,000.0	990.2	9.3	0.5	0.0	0.0	*	*	*
1928---------------	1944	1,000.0	990.2	9.2	0.6	0.0	0.0	*	*	*
1929---------------	1945	1,000.0	991.2	8.3	0.5	0.0	0.0	*	*	*
1930---------------	1946	1,000.0	991.7	7.9	0.4	0.0	0.0	*	*	*
1931---------------	1947	1,000.0	991.3	8.3	0.4	0.0	0.0	*	*	*
1932---------------	1948	1,000.0	988.0	11.5	0.5	0.0	0.0	*	*	*
1933---------------	1949	1,000.0	985.9	13.4	0.7	0.0	0.0	*	*	*
1934---------------	1950	1,000.0	985.6	13.4	0.9	0.1	0.0	*	*	*
1935---------------	1951	1,000.0	985.7	13.4	0.8	0.1	0.0	*	*	*
1936---------------	1952	1,000.0	985.1	14.0	0.9	0.0	0.0	*	*	*
1937---------------	1953	1,000.0	985.1	14.1	0.8	0.0	0.0	*	*	*
1938---------------	1954	1,000.0	984.9	14.3	0.8	0.0	0.0	*	*	*
1939---------------	1955	1,000.0	984.2	14.8	1.0	0.0	0.0	*	*	*
1940---------------	1956	1,000.0	983.9	15.1	1.0	0.0	0.0	*	*	*
1941---------------	1957	1,000.0	983.1	15.8	1.0	0.1	0.0	*	*	*
1942---------------	1958	1,000.0	982.8	16.1	1.0	0.1	0.0	*	*	*
1943---------------	1959	1,000.0	983.6	15.3	1.0	0.1	0.0	*	*	*
1944---------------	1960	1,000.0	984.0	14.9	1.0	0.1	0.0	*	*	*
1945---------------	1961	1,000.0	984.0	14.9	1.0	0.1	0.0	*	*	*
1946---------------	1962	1,000.0	984.3	14.5	1.1	0.1	0.0	*	*	*
1947---------------	1963	1,000.0	985.8	13.2	0.9	0.1	0.0	*	*	*
1948---------------	1964	1,000.0	986.5	12.6	0.8	0.1	0.0	*	*	*
1949---------------	1965	1,000.0	986.9	12.3	0.8	0.0	0.0	*	*	*
1950---------------	1966	1,000.0	987.4	11.9	0.7	0.0	0.0	*	*	*
1951---------------	1967	1,000.0	987.5	11.8	0.7	0.0	0.0	*	*	*
1952---------------	1968	1,000.0	987.7	11.7	0.6	0.0	0.0	*	*	*
1953---------------	1969	1,000.0	987.4	12.0	0.6	0.0	0.0	*	*	*
1954---------------	1970	1,000.0	986.6	12.8	0.6	0.0	0.0	*	*	*
1955---------------	1971	1,000.0	985.0	14.3	0.6	0.1	0.0	*	*	*
1956---------------	1972	1,000.0	984.7	14.6	0.7	0.0	0.0	*	*	*
1957---------------	1973	1,000.0	983.7	15.7	0.6	0.0	0.0	*	*	*
1958---------------	1974	1,000.0	983.0	16.3	0.7	0.0	0.0	*	*	*

TABLE 8B. DISTRIBUTIONS OF WHITE WOMEN BY PARITY AS OF THE BEGINNING OF EACH YEAR 1917-74 BY AGE FOR EACH COHORT FROM 1867 TO 1959--CON.

(BASED ON CUMULATIVE BIRTH RATES)

EXACT AGE AND COHORT	AS OF JANUARY 1	TOTAL	PARITY							
			0	1	2	3	4	5	6	7 AND HIGHER
17 YEARS										
1900---------------	1917	1,000.0	971.2	26.7	2.0	0.1	0.0	*	*	*
1901---------------	1918	1,000.0	971.2	26.7	2.0	0.1	0.0	*	*	*
1902---------------	1919	1,000.0	971.5	26.3	2.1	0.1	0.0	*	*	*
1903---------------	1920	1,000.0	974.2	23.7	2.0	0.1	0.0	*	*	*
1904---------------	1921	1,000.0	970.6	27.4	1.9	0.1	0.0	*	*	*
1905---------------	1922	1,000.0	967.8	30.1	2.0	0.1	0.0	*	*	*
1906---------------	1923	1,000.0	969.5	28.3	2.1	0.1	0.0	*	*	*
1907---------------	1924	1,000.0	970.8	26.8	2.3	0.1	0.0	*	*	*
1908---------------	1925	1,000.0	969.6	28.1	2.2	0.1	0.0	*	*	*
1909---------------	1926	1,000.0	969.2	28.4	2.3	0.1	0.0	*	*	*
1910---------------	1927	1,000.0	969.9	27.6	2.4	0.1	0.0	*	*	*
1911---------------	1928	1,000.0	969.1	28.4	2.3	0.2	0.0	*	*	*
1912---------------	1929	1,000.0	969.6	28.0	2.3	0.1	0.0	*	*	*
1913---------------	1930	1,000.0	970.1	27.5	2.3	0.1	0.0	*	*	*
1914---------------	1931	1,000.0	969.5	28.2	2.2	0.1	0.0	*	*	*
1915---------------	1932	1,000.0	970.7	27.1	2.1	0.1	0.0	*	*	*
1916---------------	1933	1,000.0	972.5	25.4	2.0	0.1	0.0	*	*	*
1917---------------	1934	1,000.0	974.8	23.3	1.8	0.1	0.0	*	*	*
1918---------------	1935	1,000.0	974.5	23.7	1.7	0.1	0.0	*	*	*
1919---------------	1936	1,000.0	973.5	24.7	1.7	0.1	0.0	*	*	*
1920---------------	1937	1,000.0	973.6	24.4	1.9	0.1	0.0	*	*	*
1921---------------	1938	1,000.0	972.4	25.4	2.1	0.1	0.0	*	*	*
1922---------------	1939	1,000.0	972.2	25.6	2.1	0.1	0.0	*	*	*
1923---------------	1940	1,000.0	973.4	24.5	2.0	0.1	0.0	*	*	*
1924---------------	1941	1,000.0	973.7	23.9	2.2	0.2	0.0	*	*	*
1925---------------	1942	1,000.0	972.3	25.3	2.2	0.2	0.0	*	*	*
1926---------------	1943	1,000.0	971.3	26.2	2.3	0.2	0.0	*	*	*
1927---------------	1944	1,000.0	970.9	26.3	2.6	0.2	0.0	*	*	*
1928---------------	1945	1,000.0	973.6	23.8	2.4	0.2	0.0	*	*	*
1929---------------	1946	1,000.0	975.5	22.3	2.0	0.2	0.0	*	*	*
1930---------------	1947	1,000.0	974.4	23.4	2.0	0.2	0.0	*	*	*
1931---------------	1948	1,000.0	965.0	32.3	2.5	0.2	0.0	*	*	*
1932---------------	1949	1,000.0	960.2	36.3	3.3	0.2	0.0	*	*	*
1933---------------	1950	1,000.0	958.2	37.3	4.2	0.3	0.0	*	*	*
1934---------------	1951	1,000.0	958.1	37.1	4.4	0.4	0.0	*	*	*
1935---------------	1952	1,000.0	956.4	38.8	4.4	0.4	0.0	*	*	*
1936---------------	1953	1,000.0	956.3	38.9	4.5	0.3	0.0	*	*	*
1937---------------	1954	1,000.0	955.3	39.9	4.5	0.3	0.0	*	*	*
1938---------------	1955	1,000.0	954.4	40.6	4.7	0.3	0.0	*	*	*
1939---------------	1956	1,000.0	953.7	40.9	5.1	0.3	0.0	*	*	*
1940---------------	1957	1,000.0	951.5	42.8	5.3	0.4	0.0	*	*	*
1941---------------	1958	1,000.0	949.7	44.2	5.6	0.5	0.0	*	*	*
1942---------------	1959	1,000.0	951.3	42.6	5.6	0.5	0.0	*	*	*
1943---------------	1960	1,000.0	953.5	40.6	5.4	0.5	0.0	*	*	*
1944---------------	1961	1,000.0	954.8	39.3	5.4	0.5	0.0	*	*	*
1945---------------	1962	1,000.0	955.1	39.0	5.4	0.5	0.0	*	*	*
1946---------------	1963	1,000.0	957.1	37.1	5.3	0.5	0.0	*	*	*
1947---------------	1964	1,000.0	959.8	35.1	4.6	0.5	0.0	*	*	*
1948---------------	1965	1,000.0	961.5	34.1	4.0	0.4	0.0	*	*	*
1949---------------	1966	1,000.0	963.1	33.0	3.6	0.3	0.0	*	*	*
1950---------------	1967	1,000.0	964.0	32.5	3.3	0.2	0.0	*	*	*
1951---------------	1968	1,000.0	964.6	32.0	3.2	0.2	0.0	*	*	*
1952---------------	1969	1,000.0	964.6	32.4	2.8	0.2	0.0	*	*	*
1953---------------	1970	1,000.0	963.6	33.3	2.9	0.2	0.0	*	*	*
1954---------------	1971	1,000.0	960.4	36.4	3.0	0.2	0.0	*	*	*
1955---------------	1972	1,000.0	959.2	37.5	3.0	0.3	0.0	*	*	*
1956---------------	1973	1,000.0	957.8	39.1	2.9	0.2	0.0	*	*	*
1957---------------	1974	1,000.0	956.8	40.2	2.8	0.2	0.0	*	*	*

TABLE 8B. DISTRIBUTIONS OF WHITE WOMEN BY PARITY AS OF THE BEGINNING OF EACH YEAR 1917-74 BY AGE FOR EACH COHORT FROM 1867 TO 1959--CON.

(BASED ON CUMULATIVE BIRTH RATES)

EXACT AGE AND COHORT	AS OF JANUARY 1	TOTAL	PARITY							
			0	1	2	3	4	5	6	7 AND HIGHER
18 YEARS										
1899	1917	1,000.0	932.2	59.4	7.8	0.6	0.0	*	*	*
1900	1918	1,000.0	931.9	59.7	7.7	0.7	0.0	*	*	*
1901	1919	1,000.0	933.2	58.6	7.5	0.7	0.0	*	*	*
1902	1920	1,000.0	939.1	52.8	7.5	0.6	0.0	*	*	*
1903	1921	1,000.0	931.3	60.7	7.4	0.6	0.0	*	*	*
1904	1922	1,000.0	924.3	67.2	7.8	0.7	0.0	*	*	*
1905	1923	1,000.0	927.0	63.9	8.5	0.5	0.1	*	*	*
1906	1924	1,000.0	929.6	61.0	8.7	0.6	0.1	*	*	*
1907	1925	1,000.0	928.1	62.8	8.4	0.6	0.1	*	*	*
1908	1926	1,000.0	927.9	63.0	8.4	0.7	0.0	*	*	*
1909	1927	1,000.0	928.7	61.9	8.7	0.6	0.1	*	*	*
1910	1928	1,000.0	929.2	61.4	8.6	0.7	0.1	*	*	*
1911	1929	1,000.0	930.2	60.7	8.3	0.7	0.1	*	*	*
1912	1930	1,000.0	931.6	59.5	8.2	0.6	0.1	*	*	*
1913	1931	1,000.0	930.8	60.3	8.2	0.6	0.1	*	*	*
1914	1932	1,000.0	933.4	58.3	7.7	0.6	0.0	*	*	*
1915	1933	1,000.0	936.2	55.9	7.3	0.6	0.0	*	*	*
1916	1934	1,000.0	940.7	52.0	6.8	0.5	0.0	*	*	*
1917	1935	1,000.0	941.0	52.1	6.4	0.5	0.0	*	*	*
1918	1936	1,000.0	940.2	53.2	6.1	0.5	0.0	*	*	*
1919	1937	1,000.0	940.2	52.8	6.5	0.5	0.0	*	*	*
1920	1938	1,000.0	938.5	54.0	6.9	0.6	0.0	*	*	*
1921	1939	1,000.0	935.8	56.3	7.2	0.7	0.0	*	*	*
1922	1940	1,000.0	938.3	53.8	7.2	0.7	0.0	*	*	*
1923	1941	1,000.0	940.1	51.5	7.6	0.7	0.1	*	*	*
1924	1942	1,000.0	938.0	53.5	7.6	0.8	0.1	*	*	*
1925	1943	1,000.0	934.4	56.9	7.8	0.8	0.1	*	*	*
1926	1944	1,000.0	933.6	57.2	8.3	0.8	0.1	*	*	*
1927	1945	1,000.0	938.2	53.1	7.8	0.8	0.1	*	*	*
1928	1946	1,000.0	942.9	49.4	6.9	0.8	0.0	*	*	*
1929	1947	1,000.0	939.5	52.7	7.0	0.8	0.0	*	*	*
1930	1948	1,000.0	921.7	69.4	8.0	0.9	0.0	*	*	*
1931	1949	1,000.0	911.5	77.1	10.4	0.9	0.1	*	*	*
1932	1950	1,000.0	908.5	77.5	12.7	1.2	0.1	*	*	*
1933	1951	1,000.0	907.4	77.3	13.8	1.4	0.1	*	*	*
1934	1952	1,000.0	902.9	80.8	14.6	1.6	0.1	*	*	*
1935	1953	1,000.0	902.3	81.2	14.8	1.6	0.1	*	*	*
1936	1954	1,000.0	900.4	82.6	15.2	1.7	0.1	*	*	*
1937	1955	1,000.0	898.4	84.4	15.4	1.7	0.1	*	*	*
1938	1956	1,000.0	898.2	83.9	16.0	1.8	0.1	*	*	*
1939	1957	1,000.0	893.9	86.8	17.3	1.9	0.1	*	*	*
1940	1958	1,000.0	889.8	90.1	17.9	2.0	0.2	*	*	*
1941	1959	1,000.0	890.8	88.3	18.5	2.2	0.2	*	*	*
1942	1960	1,000.0	894.6	84.9	18.0	2.3	0.2	*	*	*
1943	1961	1,000.0	899.4	80.7	17.5	2.2	0.2	*	*	*
1944	1962	1,000.0	901.4	79.2	17.0	2.2	0.2	*	*	*
1945	1963	1,000.0	904.0	77.0	16.6	2.2	0.2	*	*	*
1946	1964	1,000.0	907.7	74.4	15.7	2.0	0.2	*	*	*
1947	1965	1,000.0	912.6	71.7	13.7	1.8	0.2	*	*	*
1948	1966	1,000.0	916.1	70.5	11.9	1.4	0.1	*	*	*
1949	1967	1,000.0	918.9	69.2	10.6	1.2	0.1	*	*	*
1950	1968	1,000.0	921.2	67.7	10.0	1.0	0.1	*	*	*
1951	1969	1,000.0	921.8	67.8	9.4	0.9	0.1	*	*	*
1952	1970	1,000.0	921.2	68.8	9.1	0.8	0.1	*	*	*
1953	1971	1,000.0	917.1	72.8	9.2	0.8	0.1	*	*	*
1954	1972	1,000.0	916.0	74.0	9.2	0.8	0.0	*	*	*
1955	1973	1,000.0	914.9	75.5	8.7	0.9	0.0	*	*	*
1956	1974	1,000.0	914.6	76.1	8.5	0.8	0.0	*	*	*

TABLE 8B. DISTRIBUTIONS OF WHITE WOMEN BY PARITY AS OF THE BEGINNING OF EACH YEAR 1917-74 BY AGE FOR EACH COHORT FROM 1867 TO 1959--CON.

(BASED ON CUMULATIVE BIRTH RATES)

EXACT AGE AND COHORT	AS OF JANUARY 1	TOTAL	PARITY							
			0	1	2	3	4	5	6	7 AND HIGHER
19 YEARS										
1898	1917	1,000.0	872.9	103.5	20.8	2.8	0.0	*	*	*
1899	1918	1,000.0	872.0	104.3	20.9	2.6	0.2	*	*	*
1900	1919	1,000.0	873.3	103.2	20.6	2.7	0.2	*	*	*
1901	1920	1,000.0	883.9	93.8	19.6	2.5	0.2	*	*	*
1902	1921	1,000.0	873.6	104.1	19.7	2.4	0.2	*	*	*
1903	1922	1,000.0	859.5	116.7	21.0	2.6	0.2	*	*	*
1904	1923	1,000.0	860.7	113.6	22.9	2.5	0.3	*	*	*
1905	1924	1,000.0	864.9	108.2	23.9	2.6	0.4	*	*	*
1906	1925	1,000.0	863.1	111.0	22.8	2.7	0.4	*	*	*
1907	1926	1,000.0	864.2	110.5	22.2	2.7	0.4	*	*	*
1908	1927	1,000.0	865.9	108.6	22.5	2.7	0.3	*	*	*
1909	1928	1,000.0	867.7	106.6	22.6	2.7	0.4	*	*	*
1910	1929	1,000.0	870.6	104.9	21.5	2.6	0.4	*	*	*
1911	1930	1,000.0	874.2	102.0	20.9	2.5	0.4	*	*	*
1912	1931	1,000.0	873.6	102.9	20.7	2.4	0.4	*	*	*
1913	1932	1,000.0	877.1	100.0	20.3	2.3	0.3	*	*	*
1914	1933	1,000.0	882.0	96.3	19.3	2.2	0.2	*	*	*
1915	1934	1,000.0	888.4	91.6	17.7	2.1	0.2	*	*	*
1916	1935	1,000.0	889.7	91.2	17.0	1.9	0.2	*	*	*
1917	1936	1,000.0	889.2	92.5	16.3	1.8	0.2	*	*	*
1918	1937	1,000.0	889.9	91.6	16.5	1.8	0.2	*	*	*
1919	1938	1,000.0	887.8	92.9	17.2	1.9	0.2	*	*	*
1920	1939	1,000.0	884.2	95.6	17.9	2.2	0.1	*	*	*
1921	1940	1,000.0	884.2	94.9	18.4	2.3	0.2	*	*	*
1922	1941	1,000.0	888.4	89.5	19.0	2.8	0.3	*	*	*
1923	1942	1,000.0	886.8	90.9	19.2	2.7	0.4	*	*	*
1924	1943	1,000.0	877.6	99.7	19.6	2.7	0.4	*	*	*
1925	1944	1,000.0	874.7	101.8	20.3	2.8	0.4	*	*	*
1926	1945	1,000.0	882.1	95.7	19.1	2.7	0.4	*	*	*
1927	1946	1,000.0	889.2	90.9	17.2	2.4	0.3	*	*	*
1928	1947	1,000.0	883.2	96.2	17.9	2.5	0.2	*	*	*
1929	1948	1,000.0	855.0	122.2	20.0	2.6	0.2	*	*	*
1930	1949	1,000.0	840.7	131.3	24.8	2.9	0.3	*	*	*
1931	1950	1,000.0	833.8	132.4	29.6	3.7	0.5	*	*	*
1932	1951	1,000.0	833.9	129.1	32.1	4.4	0.5	*	*	*
1933	1952	1,000.0	824.6	135.8	34.1	4.9	0.6	*	*	*
1934	1953	1,000.0	821.5	137.1	35.4	5.3	0.7	*	*	*
1935	1954	1,000.0	818.4	138.9	36.5	5.6	0.6	*	*	*
1936	1955	1,000.0	814.6	141.7	37.1	5.9	0.7	*	*	*
1937	1956	1,000.0	813.5	141.6	38.2	6.0	0.7	*	*	*
1938	1957	1,000.0	808.6	144.1	40.1	6.5	0.7	*	*	*
1939	1958	1,000.0	801.0	149.2	42.3	6.7	0.8	*	*	*
1940	1959	1,000.0	800.1	148.4	43.6	6.9	1.0	*	*	*
1941	1960	1,000.0	803.2	144.8	43.4	7.6	1.0	*	*	*
1942	1961	1,000.0	810.5	138.8	42.1	7.6	1.0	*	*	*
1943	1962	1,000.0	817.1	134.4	40.3	7.2	1.0	*	*	*
1944	1963	1,000.0	822.4	130.7	39.1	6.9	0.9	*	*	*
1945	1964	1,000.0	826.8	128.6	37.1	6.6	0.9	*	*	*
1946	1965	1,000.0	833.7	125.4	34.1	5.9	0.9	*	*	*
1947	1966	1,000.0	842.5	122.1	29.8	4.9	0.7	*	*	*
1948	1967	1,000.0	846.6	122.7	26.3	4.0	0.4	*	*	*
1949	1968	1,000.0	853.1	118.5	24.6	3.4	0.4	*	*	*
1950	1969	1,000.0	855.7	118.2	22.8	2.9	0.4	*	*	*
1951	1970	1,000.0	856.2	118.6	22.1	2.7	0.4	*	*	*
1952	1971	1,000.0	853.0	122.2	21.9	2.6	0.3	*	*	*
1953	1972	1,000.0	853.8	121.9	21.6	2.4	0.3	*	*	*
1954	1973	1,000.0	856.2	121.0	20.4	2.2	0.2	*	*	*
1955	1974	1,000.0	857.9	120.2	19.5	2.3	0.1	*	*	*

TABLE 8B. DISTRIBUTIONS OF WHITE WOMEN BY PARITY AS OF THE BEGINNING OF EACH YEAR 1917-74 BY AGE FOR EACH COHORT FROM 1867 TO 1959--CON.

(BASED ON CUMULATIVE BIRTH RATES)

EXACT AGE AND COHORT	AS OF JANUARY 1	TOTAL	PARITY							
			0	1	2	3	4	5	6	7 AND HIGHER
20 YEARS										
1897---------------	1917	1,000.0	800.7	147.8	42.4	7.9	1.2	*	*	*
1898---------------	1918	1,000.0	794.8	152.1	43.9	8.2	1.0	*	*	*
1899---------------	1919	1,000.0	794.9	152.2	43.7	8.0	1.2	*	*	*
1900---------------	1920	1,000.0	811.2	137.6	42.2	7.9	1.1	*	*	*
1901---------------	1921	1,000.0	801.8	149.2	40.5	7.4	1.1	*	*	*
1902---------------	1922	1,000.0	785.3	164.3	41.7	7.6	1.1	*	*	*
1903---------------	1923	1,000.0	780.9	164.9	45.8	7.3	1.1	*	*	*
1904---------------	1924	1,000.0	784.3	158.9	47.9	7.6	1.3	*	*	*
1905---------------	1925	1,000.0	784.4	159.5	46.8	8.0	1.3	*	*	*
1906---------------	1926	1,000.0	786.2	159.8	44.8	7.9	1.3	*	*	*
1907---------------	1927	1,000.0	789.8	156.8	44.4	7.6	1.4	*	*	*
1908---------------	1928	1,000.0	792.5	154.1	44.4	7.7	1.3	*	*	*
1909---------------	1929	1,000.0	797.4	150.5	43.2	7.6	1.3	*	*	*
1910---------------	1930	1,000.0	803.9	146.4	41.3	7.1	1.3	*	*	*
1911---------------	1931	1,000.0	805.1	146.0	40.7	6.9	1.3	*	*	*
1912---------------	1932	1,000.0	809.0	143.6	39.7	6.5	1.2	*	*	*
1913---------------	1933	1,000.0	814.9	139.2	38.7	6.2	1.0	*	*	*
1914---------------	1934	1,000.0	823.9	133.4	36.0	5.9	0.8	*	*	*
1915---------------	1935	1,000.0	825.6	133.6	34.3	5.7	0.8	*	*	*
1916---------------	1936	1,000.0	825.5	135.4	33.0	5.3	0.8	*	*	*
1917---------------	1937	1,000.0	826.7	134.3	33.2	5.0	0.8	*	*	*
1918---------------	1938	1,000.0	826.1	134.3	33.6	5.2	0.8	*	*	*
1919---------------	1939	1,000.0	821.4	137.4	34.8	5.6	0.8	*	*	*
1920---------------	1940	1,000.0	820.8	137.2	35.5	5.8	0.7	*	*	*
1921---------------	1941	1,000.0	820.3	134.8	37.2	6.8	0.9	*	*	*
1922---------------	1942	1,000.0	819.8	134.5	37.7	7.0	1.0	*	*	*
1923---------------	1943	1,000.0	807.8	146.5	37.7	6.8	1.2	*	*	*
1924---------------	1944	1,000.0	801.5	150.5	39.5	7.2	1.3	*	*	*
1925---------------	1945	1,000.0	808.0	146.0	37.6	7.1	1.3	*	*	*
1926---------------	1946	1,000.0	818.4	140.2	34.1	6.2	1.1	*	*	*
1927---------------	1947	1,000.0	808.0	148.6	36.2	6.1	1.1	*	*	*
1928---------------	1948	1,000.0	772.7	179.9	39.9	6.6	0.9	*	*	*
1929---------------	1949	1,000.0	754.4	189.8	47.5	7.3	1.0	*	*	*
1930---------------	1950	1,000.0	746.0	188.8	55.0	8.8	1.4	*	*	*
1931---------------	1951	1,000.0	743.5	184.4	59.8	10.6	1.7	*	*	*
1932---------------	1952	1,000.0	733.4	189.5	63.2	12.0	1.9	*	*	*
1933---------------	1953	1,000.0	724.8	193.4	66.5	13.0	2.3	*	*	*
1934---------------	1954	1,000.0	718.4	195.7	69.6	13.9	2.4	*	*	*
1935---------------	1955	1,000.0	713.0	199.2	70.7	14.6	2.5	*	*	*
1936---------------	1956	1,000.0	710.1	199.2	72.8	15.2	2.7	*	*	*
1937---------------	1957	1,000.0	703.2	202.5	75.6	15.9	2.8	*	*	*
1938---------------	1958	1,000.0	695.7	206.4	77.9	17.1	2.9	*	*	*
1939---------------	1959	1,000.0	690.9	207.0	81.7	17.3	3.1	*	*	*
1940---------------	1960	1,000.0	691.1	203.9	82.9	18.6	3.5	*	*	*
1941---------------	1961	1,000.0	698.0	198.5	80.7	19.2	3.6	*	*	*
1942---------------	1962	1,000.0	707.1	193.2	77.6	18.5	3.6	*	*	*
1943---------------	1963	1,000.0	717.9	186.8	74.5	17.4	3.4	*	*	*
1944---------------	1964	1,000.0	725.4	184.0	71.2	16.3	3.1	*	*	*
1945---------------	1965	1,000.0	733.6	182.0	66.6	14.9	2.9	*	*	*
1946---------------	1966	1,000.0	745.9	179.1	59.9	12.6	2.5	*	*	*
1947---------------	1967	1,000.0	755.1	179.2	53.5	10.3	1.9	*	*	*
1948---------------	1968	1,000.0	763.5	176.9	49.5	8.7	1.4	*	*	*
1949---------------	1969	1,000.0	771.0	174.4	45.9	7.4	1.3	*	*	*
1950---------------	1970	1,000.0	774.3	173.8	43.8	6.9	1.2	*	*	*
1951---------------	1971	1,000.0	773.2	175.8	43.4	6.5	1.1	*	*	*
1952---------------	1972	1,000.0	777.8	173.3	41.9	6.2	0.8	*	*	*
1953---------------	1973	1,000.0	785.9	168.4	39.6	5.3	0.8	*	*	*
1954---------------	1974	1,000.0	792.9	164.0	37.6	4.9	0.6	*	*	*

TABLE 8B. DISTRIBUTIONS OF WHITE WOMEN BY PARITY AS OF THE BEGINNING OF EACH YEAR 1917-74 BY AGE FOR EACH COHORT FROM 1867 TO 1959--CON.

(BASED ON CUMULATIVE BIRTH RATES)

EXACT AGE AND COHORT	AS OF JANUARY 1	TOTAL	PARITY							
			0	1	2	3	4	5	6	7 AND HIGHER
21 YEARS										
1896	1917	1,000.0	721.9	185.6	70.4	18.2	3.4	0.4	0.1	0.0
1897	1918	1,000.0	716.0	189.8	71.9	18.6	3.2	0.4	0.0	0.1
1898	1919	1,000.0	709.7	194.8	73.2	18.7	3.2	0.3	0.0	0.1
1899	1920	1,000.0	728.6	178.2	71.5	18.0	3.3	0.3	0.1	0.0
1900	1921	1,000.0	723.2	186.6	69.0	17.6	3.1	0.4	0.1	0.0
1901	1922	1,000.0	709.9	202.1	67.5	16.9	3.1	0.4	0.1	0.0
1902	1923	1,000.0	703.4	204.4	72.3	16.5	3.0	0.3	0.0	0.1
1903	1924	1,000.0	700.9	201.7	77.0	16.9	3.0	0.4	0.0	0.1
1904	1925	1,000.0	700.7	201.4	76.5	17.7	3.2	0.4	0.0	0.1
1905	1926	1,000.0	704.9	199.8	73.9	17.6	3.3	0.4	0.0	0.1
1906	1927	1,000.0	709.5	197.8	72.0	16.9	3.3	0.4	0.1	0.0
1907	1928	1,000.0	713.9	194.4	71.3	16.6	3.3	0.4	0.0	0.1
1908	1929	1,000.0	720.0	190.3	69.6	16.6	3.1	0.3	0.1	0.0
1909	1930	1,000.0	728.2	184.8	67.7	15.9	3.0	0.3	0.1	0.0
1910	1931	1,000.0	732.7	183.4	65.4	15.1	3.0	0.3	0.0	0.1
1911	1932	1,000.0	737.9	180.3	64.0	14.6	2.8	0.3	0.1	0.0
1912	1933	1,000.0	744.5	176.2	62.5	13.8	2.7	0.2	0.1	0.0
1913	1934	1,000.0	754.1	170.6	59.6	13.0	2.4	0.2	0.1	0.0
1914	1935	1,000.0	757.9	169.9	57.1	12.6	2.2	0.2	0.1	0.0
1915	1936	1,000.0	757.4	173.4	54.7	12.0	2.2	0.2	0.1	0.0
1916	1937	1,000.0	758.0	173.7	54.5	11.4	2.1	0.2	0.1	0.0
1917	1938	1,000.0	758.1	173.2	55.1	11.3	2.0	0.2	0.1	0.0
1918	1939	1,000.0	755.8	174.0	56.1	11.8	2.0	0.2	0.1	0.0
1919	1940	1,000.0	753.5	175.0	57.1	12.1	2.0	0.2	0.1	0.0
1920	1941	1,000.0	751.5	174.2	58.8	13.1	2.1	0.2	0.1	0.0
1921	1942	1,000.0	743.2	178.9	61.2	14.1	2.3	0.2	0.1	0.0
1922	1943	1,000.0	730.7	191.3	61.3	13.9	2.5	0.2	0.1	0.0
1923	1944	1,000.0	724.5	194.6	63.3	14.4	2.8	0.3	0.1	0.0
1924	1945	1,000.0	726.9	193.3	61.7	14.7	3.0	0.3	0.1	0.0
1925	1946	1,000.0	736.3	190.3	57.2	13.1	2.7	0.3	0.1	0.0
1926	1947	1,000.0	723.1	199.7	61.4	12.8	2.6	0.3	0.1	0.0
1927	1948	1,000.0	683.4	233.2	67.1	13.4	2.5	0.3	0.1	0.0
1928	1949	1,000.0	664.2	241.2	76.8	15.0	2.4	0.3	0.1	0.0
1929	1950	1,000.0	653.3	238.9	87.1	17.3	2.9	0.4	0.0	0.1
1930	1951	1,000.0	650.9	231.2	93.4	20.4	3.7	0.3	0.1	0.0
1931	1952	1,000.0	637.3	234.9	99.2	23.6	4.5	0.4	0.1	0.0
1932	1953	1,000.0	627.2	237.5	104.1	25.6	5.0	0.5	0.1	0.0
1933	1954	1,000.0	616.4	239.9	110.1	27.3	5.6	0.6	0.1	0.0
1934	1955	1,000.0	606.3	244.0	113.6	29.3	6.0	0.7	0.1	0.0
1935	1956	1,000.0	601.3	244.8	116.3	30.4	6.4	0.7	0.1	0.0
1936	1957	1,000.0	592.7	247.7	120.0	31.9	6.8	0.8	0.1	0.0
1937	1958	1,000.0	584.1	250.5	123.8	33.7	7.0	0.8	0.1	0.0
1938	1959	1,000.0	579.9	250.2	126.7	34.9	7.3	0.8	0.2	0.0
1939	1960	1,000.0	575.6	248.1	130.8	36.7	7.7	0.9	0.2	0.0
1940	1961	1,000.0	578.6	244.0	129.8	38.1	8.4	0.9	0.1	0.1
1941	1962	1,000.0	587.4	239.4	125.6	37.9	8.5	1.0	0.2	0.0
1942	1963	1,000.0	601.0	232.8	120.8	36.1	8.1	1.0	0.2	0.0
1943	1964	1,000.0	614.4	228.1	115.6	33.4	7.5	0.9	0.1	0.0
1944	1965	1,000.0	624.8	227.6	109.4	30.6	6.7	0.8	0.1	0.0
1945	1966	1,000.0	640.5	225.5	101.0	26.5	5.7	0.7	0.1	0.0
1946	1967	1,000.0	652.0	228.4	92.2	22.0	4.8	0.5	0.1	0.0
1947	1968	1,000.0	665.8	226.0	85.4	18.6	3.7	0.4	0.1	0.0
1948	1969	1,000.0	674.3	226.7	79.7	16.0	3.0	0.2	0.1	0.0
1949	1970	1,000.0	683.3	223.6	75.6	14.4	2.8	0.2	0.1	0.0
1950	1971	1,000.0	686.0	223.8	73.7	13.7	2.5	0.2	0.1	0.0
1951	1972	1,000.0	694.4	219.0	71.3	12.9	2.1	0.3	0.0	0.0
1952	1973	1,000.0	709.0	211.2	66.6	11.3	1.7	0.2	0.0	0.0
1953	1974	1,000.0	722.5	202.8	63.0	10.0	1.5	0.2	0.0	0.0

TABLE 8B. DISTRIBUTIONS OF WHITE WOMEN BY PARITY AS OF THE BEGINNING OF EACH YEAR 1917-74 BY AGE FOR EACH COHORT FROM 1867 TO 1959--CON.

(BASED ON CUMULATIVE BIRTH RATES)

EXACT AGE AND COHORT	AS OF JANUARY 1	TOTAL	PARITY 0	1	2	3	4	5	6	7 AND HIGHER
22 YEARS										
1895	1917	1,000.0	643.9	212.8	100.1	33.6	7.9	1.3	0.3	0.1
1896	1918	1,000.0	637.6	217.4	101.7	34.2	7.5	1.2	0.3	0.1
1897	1919	1,000.0	631.0	222.9	102.8	34.3	7.5	1.1	0.2	0.2
1898	1920	1,000.0	645.3	209.6	102.7	33.6	7.4	1.1	0.1	0.2
1899	1921	1,000.0	642.4	216.6	99.6	32.5	7.4	1.1	0.3	0.1
1900	1922	1,000.0	635.3	227.7	96.2	31.8	7.4	1.2	0.3	0.1
1901	1923	1,000.0	632.8	230.5	98.8	29.6	6.8	1.2	0.2	0.1
1902	1924	1,000.0	627.9	229.4	104.3	30.1	6.8	1.1	0.2	0.2
1903	1925	1,000.0	622.4	231.1	106.2	31.9	6.8	1.2	0.2	0.2
1904	1926	1,000.0	625.2	230.1	103.9	32.0	7.2	1.3	0.1	0.2
1905	1927	1,000.0	632.2	226.6	101.4	30.7	7.4	1.3	0.2	0.2
1906	1928	1,000.0	637.5	224.9	99.0	29.7	7.3	1.2	0.3	0.1
1907	1929	1,000.0	645.3	220.2	96.7	29.4	6.8	1.2	0.2	0.2
1908	1930	1,000.0	653.6	215.4	94.5	28.6	6.5	1.1	0.3	0.0
1909	1931	1,000.0	660.0	212.4	92.4	27.4	6.4	1.1	0.2	0.1
1910	1932	1,000.0	668.8	208.6	89.0	26.1	6.2	1.0	0.1	0.2
1911	1933	1,000.0	676.3	204.2	87.4	25.1	5.8	0.9	0.3	0.0
1912	1934	1,000.0	686.4	199.1	84.1	23.8	5.5	0.8	0.3	0.0
1913	1935	1,000.0	690.7	198.5	81.7	22.9	5.2	0.7	0.2	0.1
1914	1936	1,000.0	691.8	202.0	78.4	21.9	4.9	0.7	0.3	0.0
1915	1937	1,000.0	691.4	204.4	77.6	20.8	4.8	0.7	0.3	0.0
1916	1938	1,000.0	690.5	205.3	78.2	20.4	4.6	0.7	0.3	0.0
1917	1939	1,000.0	688.6	205.6	79.6	20.8	4.4	0.7	0.3	0.0
1918	1940	1,000.0	689.4	204.5	79.8	21.0	4.4	0.7	0.2	0.0
1919	1941	1,000.0	684.3	206.4	81.7	21.9	4.7	0.7	0.3	0.0
1920	1942	1,000.0	673.5	213.5	84.3	23.0	4.7	0.7	0.3	0.0
1921	1943	1,000.0	651.3	231.2	87.5	23.7	5.2	0.8	0.3	0.0
1922	1944	1,000.0	647.7	230.9	90.1	24.5	5.6	0.9	0.3	0.0
1923	1945	1,000.0	649.2	230.6	88.0	24.9	6.0	1.0	0.3	0.0
1924	1946	1,000.0	654.8	231.6	83.5	23.2	5.7	0.9	0.3	0.0
1925	1947	1,000.0	636.2	243.6	90.7	22.8	5.5	0.9	0.2	0.1
1926	1948	1,000.0	597.4	273.9	98.6	23.7	5.2	0.9	0.3	0.0
1927	1949	1,000.0	577.3	281.1	109.4	25.6	5.4	0.9	0.3	0.0
1928	1950	1,000.0	566.8	275.7	121.3	29.1	5.7	1.1	0.2	0.1
1929	1951	1,000.0	562.3	266.5	129.5	33.5	6.7	1.2	0.2	0.1
1930	1952	1,000.0	550.6	265.1	136.2	38.1	8.4	1.3	0.2	0.1
1931	1953	1,000.0	536.1	266.3	143.9	42.0	9.7	1.6	0.4	0.0
1932	1954	1,000.0	525.5	265.4	151.2	45.1	10.6	1.8	0.3	0.1
1933	1955	1,000.0	511.1	268.2	158.0	48.4	11.8	2.1	0.4	0.0
1934	1956	1,000.0	500.7	269.8	162.7	51.5	12.5	2.3	0.5	0.0
1935	1957	1,000.0	491.1	272.3	166.5	53.8	13.4	2.4	0.4	0.1
1936	1958	1,000.0	481.9	273.0	171.1	56.8	14.0	2.7	0.4	0.1
1937	1959	1,000.0	477.0	271.8	174.8	58.5	14.7	2.7	0.4	0.1
1938	1960	1,000.0	474.4	267.7	178.3	60.8	15.4	2.7	0.6	0.1
1939	1961	1,000.0	471.8	265.1	179.7	63.5	16.2	3.0	0.6	0.1
1940	1962	1,000.0	476.3	262.0	177.0	63.8	17.1	3.1	0.5	0.2
1941	1963	1,000.0	489.0	257.0	170.7	62.7	16.6	3.3	0.6	0.1
1942	1964	1,000.0	505.4	252.0	164.8	58.8	15.3	3.1	0.5	0.1
1943	1965	1,000.0	520.6	251.6	157.3	53.6	13.8	2.6	0.5	0.0
1944	1966	1,000.0	537.5	252.9	148.2	47.1	11.7	2.2	0.4	0.0
1945	1967	1,000.0	552.7	256.4	138.7	40.3	9.8	1.7	0.4	0.0
1946	1968	1,000.0	567.3	258.5	129.9	34.3	8.3	1.4	0.3	0.0
1947	1969	1,000.0	581.1	259.5	121.9	29.6	6.6	1.0	0.3	0.0
1948	1970	1,000.0	589.6	260.6	116.4	26.7	5.6	0.8	0.3	0.0
1949	1971	1,000.0	598.6	258.1	112.4	24.7	5.2	0.8	0.2	0.0
1950	1972	1,000.0	610.6	252.8	107.8	23.4	4.5	0.7	0.2	0.0
1951	1973	1,000.0	629.6	243.7	101.7	20.5	3.8	0.6	0.1	0.0
1952	1974	1,000.0	649.4	233.4	95.3	18.3	3.0	0.5	0.1	0.0

TABLE 8B. DISTRIBUTIONS OF WHITE WOMEN BY PARITY AS OF THE BEGINNING OF EACH YEAR 1917-74 BY AGE FOR EACH COHORT FROM 1867 TO 1959--CON.

(BASED ON CUMULATIVE BIRTH RATES)

EXACT AGE AND COHORT	AS OF JANUARY 1	TOTAL	PARITY							
			0	1	2	3	4	5	6	7 AND HIGHER
23 YEARS										
1894	1917	1,000.0	572.0	229.8	126.5	52.1	15.5	3.2	0.7	0.2
1895	1918	1,000.0	566.8	233.4	128.1	52.9	14.8	3.1	0.6	0.3
1896	1919	1,000.0	560.0	239.4	129.1	53.1	14.6	2.9	0.6	0.3
1897	1920	1,000.0	572.5	228.5	128.8	52.1	14.5	2.7	0.5	0.4
1898	1921	1,000.0	565.9	237.3	127.7	51.1	14.4	2.8	0.4	0.4
1899	1922	1,000.0	561.3	247.0	123.8	49.5	14.5	2.9	0.7	0.3
1900	1923	1,000.0	564.3	245.8	125.2	47.2	13.7	2.9	0.6	0.3
1901	1924	1,000.0	563.7	245.5	128.2	45.8	13.1	2.9	0.5	0.3
1902	1925	1,000.0	555.2	248.9	130.6	48.3	13.2	2.8	0.6	0.4
1903	1926	1,000.0	552.2	250.2	130.7	49.5	13.6	2.9	0.6	0.3
1904	1927	1,000.0	557.0	248.2	128.7	48.0	14.1	3.1	0.5	0.4
1905	1928	1,000.0	565.2	245.4	125.3	46.0	14.1	3.1	0.5	0.4
1906	1929	1,000.0	573.5	243.3	121.5	44.7	13.2	2.8	0.8	0.2
1907	1930	1,000.0	583.5	237.7	119.0	43.7	12.5	2.7	0.6	0.3
1908	1931	1,000.0	590.2	235.2	116.8	42.3	12.2	2.5	0.7	0.1
1909	1932	1,000.0	600.4	230.2	114.0	40.5	11.7	2.4	0.6	0.2
1910	1933	1,000.0	612.0	225.1	110.0	38.6	11.3	2.3	0.4	0.3
1911	1934	1,000.0	622.5	219.9	107.2	37.1	10.5	2.1	0.6	0.1
1912	1935	1,000.0	628.1	218.8	104.6	35.7	10.2	1.9	0.6	0.1
1913	1936	1,000.0	629.4	222.8	101.6	34.0	9.7	1.9	0.4	0.2
1914	1937	1,000.0	629.7	226.3	99.8	32.6	9.2	1.8	0.5	0.1
1915	1938	1,000.0	627.0	229.5	100.4	31.8	8.9	1.7	0.6	0.1
1916	1939	1,000.0	624.0	231.2	101.9	31.8	8.7	1.8	0.5	0.1
1917	1940	1,000.0	624.7	230.0	102.6	32.0	8.4	1.7	0.5	0.1
1918	1941	1,000.0	624.9	228.5	103.0	32.4	8.8	1.8	0.5	0.1
1919	1942	1,000.0	610.1	238.5	106.2	33.6	9.1	1.8	0.6	0.1
1920	1943	1,000.0	583.0	257.8	112.2	35.2	9.2	2.0	0.5	0.1
1921	1944	1,000.0	570.8	261.7	117.5	37.1	10.1	2.1	0.6	0.1
1922	1945	1,000.0	575.2	258.5	115.4	37.3	10.6	2.3	0.6	0.1
1923	1946	1,000.0	580.0	260.8	110.5	35.5	10.3	2.2	0.6	0.1
1924	1947	1,000.0	555.9	275.2	120.6	35.3	10.2	2.1	0.6	0.1
1925	1948	1,000.0	516.1	303.0	131.7	36.7	9.8	2.0	0.5	0.2
1926	1949	1,000.0	498.2	307.4	142.7	39.2	9.7	2.1	0.6	0.1
1927	1950	1,000.0	486.7	301.6	155.1	43.0	10.6	2.2	0.7	0.1
1928	1951	1,000.0	483.0	289.3	164.3	48.7	11.4	2.6	0.5	0.2
1929	1952	1,000.0	471.0	284.5	172.3	54.9	13.6	2.9	0.6	0.2
1930	1953	1,000.0	458.6	281.2	179.9	60.1	16.0	3.4	0.6	0.2
1931	1954	1,000.0	445.6	276.4	189.7	65.3	18.0	4.0	0.8	0.2
1932	1955	1,000.0	431.5	275.6	197.4	70.4	19.6	4.4	0.9	0.2
1933	1956	1,000.0	416.5	276.7	204.4	74.9	21.4	4.9	1.1	0.1
1934	1957	1,000.0	403.4	277.4	209.7	80.0	22.9	5.2	1.2	0.2
1935	1958	1,000.0	393.8	276.9	214.5	83.5	24.3	5.5	1.2	0.3
1936	1959	1,000.0	388.8	274.0	217.6	86.7	25.4	6.0	1.2	0.3
1937	1960	1,000.0	386.2	269.5	221.0	89.1	26.5	6.1	1.3	0.3
1938	1961	1,000.0	384.8	265.0	222.0	92.2	27.8	6.4	1.4	0.4
1939	1962	1,000.0	383.9	262.9	221.4	94.2	29.0	6.7	1.5	0.4
1940	1963	1,000.0	392.2	259.7	216.4	93.5	29.3	7.0	1.4	0.5
1941	1964	1,000.0	407.2	256.2	210.0	90.3	27.6	6.9	1.5	0.3
1942	1965	1,000.0	423.7	256.6	203.3	83.8	24.9	6.1	1.3	0.3
1943	1966	1,000.0	444.0	259.0	195.1	74.1	21.6	4.9	1.2	0.1
1944	1967	1,000.0	458.8	267.1	186.4	64.7	18.0	4.0	0.9	0.1
1945	1968	1,000.0	477.2	269.2	177.8	56.4	15.2	3.3	0.8	0.1
1946	1969	1,000.0	491.1	274.7	169.0	49.0	12.9	2.6	0.6	0.1
1947	1970	1,000.0	503.9	277.0	161.5	44.0	10.9	2.0	0.6	0.1
1948	1971	1,000.0	511.3	279.6	156.3	41.0	9.5	1.7	0.6	0.0
1949	1972	1,000.0	528.6	273.3	149.7	37.7	8.6	1.7	0.4	0.0
1950	1973	1,000.0	550.5	265.2	141.7	33.7	7.3	1.2	0.4	0.0
1951	1974	1,000.0	574.0	254.7	134.0	30.0	5.9	1.2	0.2	0.0

TABLE 8B. DISTRIBUTIONS OF WHITE WOMEN BY PARITY AS OF THE BEGINNING OF EACH YEAR 1917-74 BY AGE FOR EACH COHORT FROM 1867 TO 1959--CON.

(BASED ON CUMULATIVE BIRTH RATES)

EXACT AGE AND COHORT	AS OF JANUARY 1	TOTAL	PARITY							
			0	1	2	3	4	5	6	7 AND HIGHER
24 YEARS										
1893	1917	1,000.0	507.4	237.4	148.4	71.2	26.4	7.1	1.8	0.3
1894	1918	1,000.0	501.8	241.1	150.4	72.5	25.4	6.7	1.6	0.5
1895	1919	1,000.0	496.4	246.0	151.4	72.6	25.2	6.5	1.3	0.6
1896	1920	1,000.0	507.1	237.4	151.2	71.4	24.8	6.1	1.4	0.6
1897	1921	1,000.0	501.1	246.6	149.7	70.0	24.5	6.0	1.4	0.7
1898	1922	1,000.0	491.8	258.3	148.2	68.6	24.7	6.3	1.4	0.7
1899	1923	1,000.0	496.3	256.5	149.8	65.3	23.8	6.1	1.6	0.6
1900	1924	1,000.0	501.2	252.1	151.2	64.1	22.9	6.3	1.6	0.6
1901	1925	1,000.0	497.7	256.4	150.7	64.8	22.3	6.1	1.4	0.6
1902	1926	1,000.0	491.6	260.4	150.9	66.6	22.5	5.8	1.5	0.7
1903	1927	1,000.0	490.3	261.1	151.5	65.9	23.0	6.1	1.5	0.6
1904	1928	1,000.0	496.1	260.1	148.6	63.4	23.5	6.2	1.4	0.7
1905	1929	1,000.0	506.6	257.7	144.2	60.9	22.5	6.1	1.3	0.7
1906	1930	1,000.0	517.5	254.4	140.4	59.0	21.0	5.7	1.5	0.5
1907	1931	1,000.0	525.8	251.1	137.9	57.7	20.2	5.4	1.3	0.6
1908	1932	1,000.0	535.9	247.2	135.4	55.4	19.4	5.0	1.4	0.3
1909	1933	1,000.0	548.6	241.1	132.1	53.1	18.7	4.7	1.3	0.4
1910	1934	1,000.0	563.6	234.9	127.1	50.8	17.7	4.4	1.0	0.5
1911	1935	1,000.0	569.9	233.2	124.9	49.3	17.0	4.2	1.2	0.3
1912	1936	1,000.0	572.8	236.6	121.8	47.1	16.2	4.0	1.2	0.3
1913	1937	1,000.0	573.1	240.8	120.6	44.8	15.5	3.9	0.9	0.4
1914	1938	1,000.0	570.6	245.7	120.1	43.7	14.9	3.7	1.0	0.3
1915	1939	1,000.0	565.3	249.6	122.0	43.7	14.4	3.6	1.1	0.3
1916	1940	1,000.0	564.5	250.0	123.1	43.4	14.1	3.7	0.9	0.3
1917	1941	1,000.0	564.9	248.3	123.7	43.8	14.2	3.7	1.1	0.3
1918	1942	1,000.0	557.3	253.6	125.0	44.3	14.6	3.9	1.0	0.3
1919	1943	1,000.0	524.9	273.2	134.6	47.0	15.0	3.9	1.1	0.3
1920	1944	1,000.0	507.0	279.0	142.7	50.0	15.7	4.2	1.1	0.3
1921	1945	1,000.0	503.4	280.6	142.4	51.1	16.6	4.4	1.2	0.3
1922	1946	1,000.0	511.3	280.1	137.6	48.9	16.3	4.3	1.2	0.3
1923	1947	1,000.0	487.7	293.5	147.9	48.9	16.3	4.2	1.2	0.3
1924	1948	1,000.0	446.4	318.7	162.5	51.0	15.9	4.1	1.1	0.3
1925	1949	1,000.0	426.8	323.0	174.6	54.4	15.7	4.0	1.1	0.4
1926	1950	1,000.0	416.5	315.8	187.0	58.4	16.5	4.2	1.3	0.3
1927	1951	1,000.0	411.8	303.2	196.6	64.3	18.0	4.5	1.3	0.3
1928	1952	1,000.0	403.0	293.4	205.1	71.6	20.1	5.2	1.2	0.4
1929	1953	1,000.0	390.5	287.3	212.6	78.6	23.2	6.0	1.4	0.4
1930	1954	1,000.0	380.6	278.2	221.0	85.1	26.3	6.9	1.4	0.5
1931	1955	1,000.0	365.3	272.6	230.2	92.3	29.4	7.8	1.9	0.5
1932	1956	1,000.0	350.7	270.9	236.8	98.8	31.6	8.5	2.2	0.5
1933	1957	1,000.0	334.7	269.5	243.6	105.5	34.5	9.3	2.4	0.5
1934	1958	1,000.0	322.0	267.1	249.0	111.7	37.1	9.9	2.5	0.7
1935	1959	1,000.0	316.4	263.1	252.5	115.3	38.7	10.6	2.6	0.8
1936	1960	1,000.0	314.4	257.5	253.8	119.0	40.6	11.2	2.7	0.8
1937	1961	1,000.0	312.7	252.9	255.0	121.7	42.2	11.8	2.8	0.9
1938	1962	1,000.0	312.7	249.6	253.5	124.1	44.1	12.1	3.0	0.9
1939	1963	1,000.0	315.5	247.9	250.5	124.8	44.6	12.5	3.3	0.9
1940	1964	1,000.0	325.4	245.9	246.0	122.6	43.8	12.2	3.1	1.0
1941	1965	1,000.0	340.0	246.8	240.4	117.1	40.3	11.7	2.9	0.8
1942	1966	1,000.0	359.2	251.2	234.9	106.6	35.3	9.7	2.4	0.7
1943	1967	1,000.0	376.4	260.2	229.2	94.2	29.9	7.7	2.0	0.4
1944	1968	1,000.0	393.1	266.6	222.9	83.7	25.4	6.4	1.6	0.3
1945	1969	1,000.0	411.2	271.6	214.6	74.0	21.7	5.2	1.4	0.3
1946	1970	1,000.0	423.2	278.5	207.0	66.5	19.0	4.4	1.1	0.3
1947	1971	1,000.0	434.3	282.4	200.3	61.7	16.4	3.6	1.1	0.2
1948	1972	1,000.0	447.4	284.1	193.2	56.9	14.3	3.1	0.9	0.1
1949	1973	1,000.0	473.2	276.3	184.1	50.5	12.5	2.7	0.6	0.1
1950	1974	1,000.0	498.7	267.7	175.2	45.3	10.4	2.1	0.5	0.1

TABLE 8B. DISTRIBUTIONS OF WHITE WOMEN BY PARITY AS OF THE BEGINNING OF EACH YEAR 1917-74 BY AGE FOR EACH COHORT FROM 1867 TO 1959--CON.

(BASED ON CUMULATIVE BIRTH RATES)

EXACT AGE AND COHORT	AS OF JANUARY 1	TOTAL	PARITY							
			0	1	2	3	4	5	6	7 AND HIGHER
25 YEARS										
1892	1917	1,000.0	454.6	236.8	164.8	88.5	38.4	12.4	3.3	1.2
1893	1918	1,000.0	447.7	241.6	166.1	89.5	38.2	12.5	3.4	1.0
1894	1919	1,000.0	441.6	246.7	167.9	90.1	37.5	12.0	3.1	1.1
1895	1920	1,000.0	450.4	239.8	168.4	88.8	37.0	11.6	2.8	1.2
1896	1921	1,000.0	445.8	247.5	167.3	87.4	36.5	11.3	3.0	1.2
1897	1922	1,000.0	437.3	259.6	165.2	85.7	36.3	11.4	3.2	1.3
1898	1923	1,000.0	434.5	262.0	169.2	83.1	35.6	11.2	3.1	1.3
1899	1924	1,000.0	440.9	257.2	171.1	80.7	34.3	11.3	3.2	1.3
1900	1925	1,000.0	444.1	256.2	169.2	81.4	33.4	11.2	3.2	1.3
1901	1926	1,000.0	442.6	261.1	166.9	81.6	32.9	10.7	3.0	1.2
1902	1927	1,000.0	438.2	265.2	167.5	81.3	33.0	10.5	3.0	1.3
1903	1928	1,000.0	437.1	267.2	167.3	79.7	33.7	10.8	3.0	1.2
1904	1929	1,000.0	444.3	266.9	164.1	76.8	33.1	10.7	2.9	1.2
1905	1930	1,000.0	457.2	263.7	159.7	73.7	31.4	10.4	2.7	1.2
1906	1931	1,000.0	466.7	262.4	155.9	71.6	29.8	9.8	2.8	1.0
1907	1932	1,000.0	477.2	258.4	153.7	69.6	28.4	9.1	2.5	1.1
1908	1933	1,000.0	489.9	253.5	150.6	66.9	27.3	8.5	2.6	0.7
1909	1934	1,000.0	505.5	246.6	146.5	64.4	26.0	7.9	2.3	0.8
1910	1935	1,000.0	517.4	243.0	142.1	61.7	25.2	7.7	2.0	0.9
1911	1936	1,000.0	521.1	245.3	139.8	59.6	23.9	7.4	2.2	0.7
1912	1937	1,000.0	522.3	249.9	138.0	57.2	22.9	6.9	2.2	0.6
1913	1938	1,000.0	519.9	255.4	138.4	55.0	22.1	6.6	1.8	0.8
1914	1939	1,000.0	514.8	260.8	139.3	54.8	21.2	6.5	2.0	0.6
1915	1940	1,000.0	510.5	264.0	141.4	54.7	20.6	6.2	2.0	0.6
1916	1941	1,000.0	508.8	264.1	142.8	54.7	20.6	6.5	1.8	0.7
1917	1942	1,000.0	501.9	268.1	144.7	55.4	20.8	6.5	2.0	0.6
1918	1943	1,000.0	479.3	281.4	151.8	57.3	21.0	6.6	1.9	0.7
1919	1944	1,000.0	455.4	287.2	164.0	61.6	22.1	6.9	2.1	0.7
1920	1945	1,000.0	447.0	289.2	166.8	64.1	22.8	7.3	2.1	0.7
1921	1946	1,000.0	446.3	293.0	164.3	63.2	23.0	7.4	2.1	0.7
1922	1947	1,000.0	427.8	302.3	173.8	62.8	23.3	7.1	2.2	0.7
1923	1948	1,000.0	390.7	322.5	188.6	65.5	23.0	6.9	2.1	0.7
1924	1949	1,000.0	368.1	327.2	202.6	69.7	22.8	6.8	2.1	0.7
1925	1950	1,000.0	355.4	320.9	215.8	74.5	23.6	6.9	2.1	0.8
1926	1951	1,000.0	351.1	307.3	225.9	80.3	25.2	7.2	2.3	0.7
1927	1952	1,000.0	342.9	296.0	234.2	88.1	27.7	8.0	2.4	0.7
1928	1953	1,000.0	334.8	284.8	240.8	96.3	30.9	9.2	2.4	0.8
1929	1954	1,000.0	324.6	273.9	248.3	104.2	34.9	10.5	2.7	0.9
1930	1955	1,000.0	313.9	264.1	254.9	112.3	38.9	11.9	2.9	1.1
1931	1956	1,000.0	298.9	257.6	261.7	120.8	43.1	13.0	3.7	1.2
1932	1957	1,000.0	284.2	253.2	267.5	129.0	46.4	14.3	4.1	1.3
1933	1958	1,000.0	268.9	249.1	273.6	136.4	50.7	15.5	4.4	1.4
1934	1959	1,000.0	260.0	244.0	276.6	142.9	53.6	16.6	4.7	1.6
1935	1960	1,000.0	257.0	238.5	277.2	147.1	56.1	17.4	4.9	1.8
1936	1961	1,000.0	256.6	232.5	276.5	150.5	58.5	18.4	5.2	1.8
1937	1962	1,000.0	256.0	229.6	275.0	152.4	60.2	19.5	5.4	1.9
1938	1963	1,000.0	259.0	227.2	271.8	153.1	61.8	19.5	5.7	1.9
1939	1964	1,000.0	262.8	226.9	269.4	152.5	61.3	19.4	5.8	1.9
1940	1965	1,000.0	272.2	228.1	266.3	148.8	58.7	18.6	5.4	1.9
1941	1966	1,000.0	288.6	232.5	263.0	140.1	52.8	16.7	4.8	1.5
1942	1967	1,000.0	303.8	243.3	261.3	127.6	45.4	13.5	3.8	1.3
1943	1968	1,000.0	321.4	251.4	258.8	114.6	38.8	11.1	3.0	0.9
1944	1969	1,000.0	336.4	259.9	254.6	103.3	33.5	9.1	2.6	0.6
1945	1970	1,000.0	354.1	265.3	246.7	93.8	29.4	7.8	2.3	0.6
1946	1971	1,000.0	363.6	273.8	240.5	86.7	26.2	6.8	1.8	0.6
1947	1972	1,000.0	378.2	278.6	233.0	79.9	22.6	5.6	1.7	0.4
1948	1973	1,000.0	397.2	280.2	225.6	71.7	19.2	4.6	1.3	0.2
1949	1974	1,000.0	425.8	272.3	216.6	63.7	16.6	3.9	0.9	0.2

TABLE 88. DISTRIBUTIONS OF WHITE WOMEN BY PARITY AS OF THE BEGINNING OF EACH YEAR 1917-74 BY AGE FOR EACH COHORT FROM 1867 TO 1959--CON.

(BASED ON CUMULATIVE BIRTH RATES)

EXACT AGE AND COHORT	AS OF JANUARY 1	TOTAL	PARITY							
			0	1	2	3	4	5	6	7 AND HIGHER
26 YEARS										
1891---------------	1917	1,000.0	412.5	229.1	175.6	102.6	51.5	20.0	6.2	2.5
1892---------------	1918	1,000.0	404.3	235.5	177.4	103.6	50.9	19.7	6.2	2.4
1893---------------	1919	1,000.0	396.6	241.9	178.7	104.0	50.9	19.7	6.1	2.1
1894---------------	1920	1,000.0	402.0	237.6	180.6	103.4	49.6	18.9	5.7	2.2
1895---------------	1921	1,000.0	398.3	243.6	180.6	102.1	49.0	18.7	5.4	2.3
1896---------------	1922	1,000.0	391.3	254.1	178.8	100.6	48.5	18.4	5.9	2.4
1897---------------	1923	1,000.0	388.1	259.0	181.5	97.8	47.4	17.9	5.9	2.4
1898---------------	1924	1,000.0	386.3	258.6	186.2	96.3	46.4	17.9	5.8	2.5
1899---------------	1925	1,000.0	392.0	256.3	185.6	95.3	44.8	17.7	5.8	2.5
1900---------------	1926	1,000.0	397.3	256.1	182.0	95.3	43.9	17.3	5.7	2.4
1901---------------	1927	1,000.0	397.2	261.5	179.8	93.9	43.3	16.6	5.4	2.3
1902---------------	1928	1,000.0	393.0	266.7	180.0	92.5	43.7	16.3	5.5	2.3
1903---------------	1929	1,000.0	392.8	269.4	179.9	90.7	43.3	16.5	5.2	2.2
1904---------------	1930	1,000.0	401.4	268.9	177.2	87.2	41.9	16.1	5.2	2.1
1905---------------	1931	1,000.0	413.0	267.3	172.8	84.4	40.0	15.5	4.8	2.2
1906---------------	1932	1,000.0	424.5	265.7	169.2	81.6	37.8	14.6	4.7	1.9
1907---------------	1933	1,000.0	436.9	261.0	166.6	79.4	36.3	13.5	4.4	1.9
1908---------------	1934	1,000.0	452.1	255.6	163.1	76.3	34.6	12.7	4.2	1.4
1909---------------	1935	1,000.0	465.0	250.6	159.5	73.8	33.5	12.2	3.9	1.5
1910---------------	1936	1,000.0	475.0	250.7	155.0	70.4	32.1	11.6	3.6	1.6
1911---------------	1937	1,000.0	476.8	254.4	153.8	68.2	30.7	10.9	3.8	1.4
1912---------------	1938	1,000.0	475.5	260.3	153.6	65.9	29.4	10.4	3.7	1.2
1913---------------	1939	1,000.0	470.5	266.2	155.4	64.7	28.5	10.0	3.3	1.4
1914---------------	1940	1,000.0	465.7	271.3	156.8	64.6	27.4	9.7	3.3	1.2
1915---------------	1941	1,000.0	459.5	274.4	160.0	65.1	26.9	9.6	3.2	1.3
1916---------------	1942	1,000.0	451.5	279.0	162.8	65.4	27.1	9.8	3.1	1.3
1917---------------	1943	1,000.0	431.8	289.8	169.7	67.2	27.2	9.7	3.4	1.2
1918---------------	1944	1,000.0	417.2	289.1	179.6	71.0	28.2	10.2	3.3	1.4
1919---------------	1945	1,000.0	403.2	289.8	187.1	75.1	29.3	10.5	3.6	1.4
1920---------------	1946	1,000.0	397.6	293.1	188.2	76.1	29.4	10.7	3.6	1.3
1921---------------	1947	1,000.0	373.1	305.5	198.1	77.1	30.4	10.8	3.6	1.4
1922---------------	1948	1,000.0	344.0	319.1	211.6	79.6	30.3	10.5	3.6	1.3
1923---------------	1949	1,000.0	323.8	322.1	224.7	84.1	30.2	10.2	3.5	1.4
1924---------------	1950	1,000.0	307.1	317.6	239.4	89.8	31.0	10.2	3.5	1.4
1925---------------	1951	1,000.0	299.9	305.2	250.6	96.1	32.7	10.5	3.5	1.5
1926---------------	1952	1,000.0	293.0	292.0	259.2	103.8	35.4	11.4	3.7	1.5
1927---------------	1953	1,000.0	285.9	279.4	264.7	112.8	39.0	12.7	4.1	1.4
1928---------------	1954	1,000.0	280.5	264.8	270.3	121.3	43.1	14.2	4.2	1.6
1929---------------	1955	1,000.0	270.6	253.0	275.1	130.5	48.1	16.0	4.9	1.8
1930---------------	1956	1,000.0	261.1	242.6	278.4	139.6	53.0	17.9	5.2	2.2
1931---------------	1957	1,000.0	246.2	234.5	283.4	149.1	58.4	19.7	6.2	2.5
1932---------------	1958	1,000.0	232.3	228.2	287.6	157.7	63.2	21.4	6.9	2.7
1933---------------	1959	1,000.0	220.4	222.2	291.2	164.9	67.8	23.3	7.4	2.8
1934---------------	1960	1,000.0	213.9	216.0	291.1	171.3	72.1	24.5	7.9	3.2
1935---------------	1961	1,000.0	212.6	210.5	289.2	175.2	75.0	25.8	8.2	3.5
1936---------------	1962	1,000.0	213.4	206.1	286.3	177.5	77.1	27.4	8.7	3.5
1937---------------	1963	1,000.0	214.8	204.8	283.4	177.7	78.6	28.1	9.0	3.6
1938---------------	1964	1,000.0	218.6	203.7	280.9	177.4	79.2	27.5	9.1	3.6
1939---------------	1965	1,000.0	221.7	205.8	280.2	175.8	77.1	27.1	8.9	3.4
1940---------------	1966	1,000.0	232.3	210.0	279.5	170.1	72.3	24.7	7.9	3.2
1941---------------	1967	1,000.0	245.7	218.9	280.5	160.1	63.9	21.6	6.8	2.5
1942---------------	1968	1,000.0	260.0	229.7	281.9	148.0	55.3	17.6	5.4	2.1
1943---------------	1969	1,000.0	274.5	240.1	282.3	134.6	48.1	14.6	4.3	1.5
1944---------------	1970	1,000.0	289.1	247.2	279.6	124.1	42.6	12.5	3.7	1.2
1945---------------	1971	1,000.0	305.5	253.5	272.6	114.9	38.1	11.0	3.3	1.1
1946---------------	1972	1,000.0	316.4	264.0	267.0	105.8	33.7	9.5	2.6	1.0
1947---------------	1973	1,000.0	334.6	269.7	260.9	95.9	28.4	7.5	2.4	0.6
1948---------------	1974	1,000.0	354.7	271.6	255.3	86.1	24.0	6.2	1.7	0.4

TABLE 8B. DISTRIBUTIONS OF WHITE WOMEN BY PARITY AS OF THE BEGINNING OF EACH YEAR 1917-74 BY AGE FOR EACH COHORT FROM 1867 TO 1959--CON.

(BASED ON CUMULATIVE BIRTH RATES)

EXACT AGE AND COHORT	AS OF JANUARY 1	TOTAL	PARITY 0	1	2	3	4	5	6	7 AND HIGHER
27 YEARS										
1890	1917	1,000.0	377.4	219.0	182.8	113.4	63.4	28.9	10.5	4.6
1891	1918	1,000.0	372.0	224.2	183.2	114.2	63.1	28.3	10.4	4.6
1892	1919	1,000.0	362.4	232.2	185.4	114.9	62.6	27.9	10.3	4.3
1893	1920	1,000.0	363.6	231.5	187.4	114.1	61.9	27.7	9.8	4.0
1894	1921	1,000.0	359.4	236.8	189.1	113.7	60.5	27.0	9.4	4.1
1895	1922	1,000.0	353.4	245.5	188.2	112.8	59.6	26.7	9.5	4.3
1896	1923	1,000.0	350.4	250.8	190.4	110.4	58.4	25.7	9.6	4.3
1897	1924	1,000.0	348.5	253.4	194.1	108.1	56.7	25.2	9.6	4.4
1898	1925	1,000.0	346.1	254.2	197.3	107.9	55.7	24.9	9.5	4.4
1899	1926	1,000.0	353.0	252.1	196.0	106.8	54.1	24.4	9.2	4.4
1900	1927	1,000.0	359.8	252.7	192.2	105.2	53.1	23.7	9.1	4.2
1901	1928	1,000.0	359.5	259.2	189.7	103.0	52.7	23.1	8.8	4.0
1902	1929	1,000.0	356.5	264.9	190.3	101.3	52.0	22.5	8.6	3.9
1903	1930	1,000.0	356.7	268.3	190.5	99.4	50.7	22.5	8.2	3.7
1904	1931	1,000.0	363.9	269.0	188.3	96.0	49.3	21.8	8.1	3.6
1905	1932	1,000.0	376.8	267.4	184.1	92.8	47.0	20.7	7.6	3.6
1906	1933	1,000.0	390.3	265.3	179.8	89.8	44.7	19.6	7.3	3.2
1907	1934	1,000.0	404.4	260.4	177.0	87.3	43.0	18.2	6.6	3.1
1908	1935	1,000.0	417.4	256.4	174.3	84.2	41.3	17.4	6.5	2.5
1909	1936	1,000.0	428.4	254.5	171.0	81.2	39.6	16.5	6.1	2.7
1910	1937	1,000.0	437.0	256.2	167.0	77.8	38.1	15.5	5.7	2.7
1911	1938	1,000.0	436.1	261.2	167.3	75.9	36.5	14.7	5.8	2.5
1912	1939	1,000.0	432.4	267.5	168.7	74.2	35.2	14.1	5.6	2.3
1913	1940	1,000.0	427.1	273.4	171.3	73.3	34.1	13.4	5.1	2.3
1914	1941	1,000.0	419.6	278.7	174.3	74.0	33.1	13.1	5.0	2.2
1915	1942	1,000.0	407.7	285.1	179.3	75.0	32.7	13.0	5.0	2.2
1916	1943	1,000.0	389.2	295.7	185.7	76.0	33.1	13.2	4.8	2.3
1917	1944	1,000.0	377.3	292.3	195.4	80.0	34.0	13.5	5.3	2.2
1918	1945	1,000.0	372.9	285.5	201.0	83.9	35.1	14.0	5.2	2.4
1919	1946	1,000.0	361.0	286.1	207.9	87.2	35.9	14.0	5.5	2.4
1920	1947	1,000.0	335.2	297.6	218.7	89.7	36.6	14.4	5.4	2.4
1921	1948	1,000.0	301.7	312.5	232.0	94.0	37.5	14.5	5.3	2.5
1922	1949	1,000.0	287.9	312.0	243.3	97.6	37.4	14.1	5.3	2.4
1923	1950	1,000.0	273.2	306.9	256.5	103.5	38.3	13.8	5.3	2.5
1924	1951	1,000.0	260.6	297.3	269.5	110.8	40.0	14.1	5.2	2.5
1925	1952	1,000.0	251.7	284.9	278.7	118.8	43.0	14.9	5.4	2.6
1926	1953	1,000.0	246.2	270.0	284.1	128.1	46.8	16.4	5.8	2.6
1927	1954	1,000.0	241.3	255.5	287.8	136.9	51.5	17.9	6.5	2.6
1928	1955	1,000.0	237.4	240.2	290.0	146.2	56.4	20.1	6.7	3.0
1929	1956	1,000.0	228.9	228.4	291.2	155.9	62.3	22.3	7.7	3.3
1930	1957	1,000.0	220.1	217.4	292.1	165.2	68.2	24.9	8.2	3.9
1931	1958	1,000.0	205.5	208.4	295.0	175.0	74.8	27.3	9.5	4.5
1932	1959	1,000.0	194.4	201.4	296.4	182.8	80.2	29.5	10.5	4.8
1933	1960	1,000.0	184.7	195.1	296.9	189.1	86.0	31.9	11.2	5.1
1934	1961	1,000.0	179.9	189.0	294.1	195.2	90.7	33.5	12.0	5.6
1935	1962	1,000.0	179.9	184.9	290.5	197.6	93.1	35.5	12.4	6.1
1936	1963	1,000.0	181.9	182.0	287.1	198.4	94.8	36.7	13.1	6.0
1937	1964	1,000.0	184.2	181.7	284.7	197.7	95.4	37.2	13.0	6.1
1938	1965	1,000.0	187.0	182.8	283.8	196.8	95.0	35.9	12.9	5.8
1939	1966	1,000.0	191.0	187.3	285.4	194.1	90.8	34.1	12.0	5.3
1940	1967	1,000.0	199.9	194.5	288.5	187.7	83.9	30.4	10.4	4.7
1941	1968	1,000.0	212.4	203.5	292.2	178.4	74.4	26.5	8.8	3.8
1942	1969	1,000.0	223.0	216.1	297.0	166.6	65.3	21.8	7.1	3.1
1943	1970	1,000.0	237.0	224.6	298.7	154.7	58.1	18.7	5.8	2.4
1944	1971	1,000.0	250.5	231.3	297.7	144.7	52.5	16.3	5.1	1.9
1945	1972	1,000.0	267.8	239.7	291.7	133.7	46.7	14.2	4.5	1.7
1946	1973	1,000.0	280.3	251.5	289.4	121.7	40.3	11.9	3.5	1.4
1947	1974	1,000.0	298.6	257.4	286.1	110.6	34.0	9.3	3.1	0.9

TABLE 8B. DISTRIBUTIONS OF WHITE WOMEN BY PARITY AS OF THE BEGINNING OF EACH YEAR 1917-74 BY AGE FOR EACH COHORT FROM 1867 TO 1959--CON.

(BASED ON CUMULATIVE BIRTH RATES)

EXACT AGE AND COHORT	AS OF JANUARY 1	TOTAL	PARITY							
			0	1	2	3	4	5	6	7 AND HIGHER
28 YEARS										
1889	1917	1,000.0	346.9	209.5	184.1	121.8	74.5	38.5	16.5	8.2
1890	1918	1,000.0	342.1	211.0	187.7	123.0	73.9	37.8	16.4	8.1
1891	1919	1,000.0	335.3	217.6	188.6	123.5	73.9	37.2	16.1	7.8
1892	1920	1,000.0	333.5	219.6	191.5	123.2	72.6	36.6	15.5	7.5
1893	1921	1,000.0	326.8	227.2	193.3	122.4	71.7	36.5	15.0	7.1
1894	1922	1,000.0	320.9	234.9	194.2	122.3	69.7	35.6	15.0	7.4
1895	1923	1,000.0	318.5	239.1	197.1	120.6	68.4	34.4	14.5	7.4
1896	1924	1,000.0	316.7	242.3	200.2	118.8	66.4	33.4	14.6	7.6
1897	1925	1,000.0	314.4	246.2	202.6	117.7	64.6	32.4	14.6	7.5
1898	1926	1,000.0	313.3	247.3	205.3	117.3	63.7	31.8	13.9	7.4
1899	1927	1,000.0	321.0	245.7	204.1	115.2	62.4	30.6	13.6	7.4
1900	1928	1,000.0	328.3	247.3	199.9	112.6	61.1	30.3	13.4	7.1
1901	1929	1,000.0	328.8	254.5	197.8	110.4	59.7	29.3	12.8	6.7
1902	1930	1,000.0	326.3	260.9	198.8	108.6	58.3	28.5	12.3	6.3
1903	1931	1,000.0	325.2	265.3	199.5	107.0	56.8	28.2	11.9	6.1
1904	1932	1,000.0	333.1	266.4	197.7	102.9	55.4	27.1	11.5	5.9
1905	1933	1,000.0	347.7	264.5	192.6	99.8	53.0	25.7	10.9	5.8
1906	1934	1,000.0	362.6	262.5	188.3	96.2	50.8	24.3	10.2	5.1
1907	1935	1,000.0	374.4	258.7	186.4	94.2	48.9	22.9	9.5	5.0
1908	1936	1,000.0	385.9	257.3	184.2	90.7	46.5	21.8	9.2	4.4
1909	1937	1,000.0	395.9	256.5	181.6	87.6	44.8	20.4	8.7	4.5
1910	1938	1,000.0	402.2	259.6	178.9	84.4	42.9	19.4	8.2	4.4
1911	1939	1,000.0	398.5	265.3	180.6	83.2	41.5	18.6	8.1	4.2
1912	1940	1,000.0	394.7	271.5	182.8	81.7	40.1	17.6	7.8	3.8
1913	1941	1,000.0	387.2	277.4	186.7	81.7	39.1	16.9	7.1	3.9
1914	1942	1,000.0	374.6	285.5	191.4	82.8	38.4	16.5	7.1	3.7
1915	1943	1,000.0	354.3	294.4	200.5	85.3	38.4	16.5	6.9	3.7
1916	1944	1,000.0	342.3	292.2	209.5	88.5	39.6	17.1	7.0	3.8
1917	1945	1,000.0	339.3	284.0	215.0	92.6	40.5	17.4	7.5	3.7
1918	1946	1,000.0	337.0	275.9	221.0	96.0	41.4	17.5	7.4	3.8
1919	1947	1,000.0	308.4	283.9	234.6	100.9	42.9	17.8	7.6	3.9
1920	1948	1,000.0	275.4	297.0	248.4	106.1	43.6	18.2	7.4	3.9
1921	1949	1,000.0	254.7	300.9	259.0	111.3	44.5	18.2	7.4	4.0
1922	1950	1,000.0	245.8	293.9	269.8	116.0	45.4	17.7	7.4	4.0
1923	1951	1,000.0	234.7	284.6	281.2	123.3	47.2	17.7	7.2	4.1
1924	1952	1,000.0	220.9	274.6	291.9	132.2	50.3	18.6	7.4	4.1
1925	1953	1,000.0	213.1	261.0	297.7	141.9	54.3	20.0	7.8	4.2
1926	1954	1,000.0	210.2	244.8	300.5	150.8	59.2	21.8	8.4	4.3
1927	1955	1,000.0	206.9	229.9	300.6	160.1	64.7	24.0	9.3	4.5
1928	1956	1,000.0	204.4	215.4	299.4	169.1	70.3	26.6	9.8	5.0
1929	1957	1,000.0	196.9	203.5	297.7	178.9	77.1	29.2	11.1	5.6
1930	1958	1,000.0	188.5	192.6	296.3	187.8	84.0	32.5	11.9	6.4
1931	1959	1,000.0	175.8	184.0	296.9	196.1	91.0	35.5	13.4	7.3
1932	1960	1,000.0	166.5	176.8	295.8	202.7	97.4	38.3	14.7	7.8
1933	1961	1,000.0	158.3	171.2	293.5	208.3	103.7	40.9	15.7	8.4
1934	1962	1,000.0	155.0	165.9	289.2	213.3	107.6	43.3	16.7	9.0
1935	1963	1,000.0	156.1	163.5	285.4	213.8	109.5	45.0	17.2	9.5
1936	1964	1,000.0	158.8	161.4	282.6	213.8	110.4	46.0	17.7	9.3
1937	1965	1,000.0	159.9	163.0	281.6	212.9	110.2	45.9	17.3	9.2
1938	1966	1,000.0	163.5	166.0	282.9	211.6	108.0	43.1	16.5	8.4
1939	1967	1,000.0	166.7	172.3	287.7	208.7	102.0	40.3	14.9	7.4
1940	1968	1,000.0	175.2	179.4	292.9	203.0	94.4	35.7	13.0	6.4
1941	1969	1,000.0	184.6	190.0	299.0	194.5	84.5	31.2	10.9	5.3
1942	1970	1,000.0	194.6	199.5	306.1	184.2	75.7	26.5	9.0	4.4
1943	1971	1,000.0	207.4	207.3	309.4	173.4	68.5	23.0	7.6	3.4
1944	1972	1,000.0	221.4	215.4	310.2	161.9	61.7	20.1	6.6	2.7
1945	1973	1,000.0	239.9	224.8	307.9	148.5	53.9	17.1	5.6	2.3
1946	1974	1,000.0	251.4	236.9	309.1	135.9	46.4	14.1	4.3	1.9

TABLE 8B. DISTRIBUTIONS OF WHITE WOMEN BY PARITY AS OF THE BEGINNING OF EACH YEAR 1917-74 BY AGE FOR EACH COHORT FROM 1867 TO 1959--CON.

(BASED ON CUMULATIVE BIRTH RATES)

EXACT AGE AND COHORT	AS OF JANUARY 1	TOTAL	PARITY							
			0	1	2	3	4	5	6	7 AND HIGHER
29 YEARS										
1888	1917	1,000.0	320.6	200.5	181.7	128.0	84.0	48.2	23.6	13.4
1889	1918	1,000.0	317.3	200.0	186.1	129.4	83.4	47.2	23.3	13.3
1890	1919	1,000.0	311.3	202.7	190.2	130.4	83.1	46.5	23.0	12.8
1891	1920	1,000.0	311.0	204.3	191.9	129.9	82.5	45.8	22.2	12.4
1892	1921	1,000.0	302.6	213.3	194.5	129.7	81.0	45.3	21.5	12.1
1893	1922	1,000.0	294.8	223.0	195.6	129.1	79.4	44.7	21.5	11.9
1894	1923	1,000.0	292.1	227.0	200.1	128.3	77.0	43.0	20.6	11.9
1895	1924	1,000.0	290.7	229.5	203.8	127.2	74.9	41.7	20.1	12.1
1896	1925	1,000.0	288.7	233.9	205.6	126.5	72.9	40.2	20.1	12.1
1897	1926	1,000.0	287.3	237.7	208.3	125.5	71.1	38.7	19.6	11.8
1898	1927	1,000.0	287.3	239.2	210.9	124.2	70.6	37.4	18.8	11.6
1899	1928	1,000.0	295.1	238.5	209.7	121.4	68.8	36.6	18.4	11.5
1900	1929	1,000.0	303.1	240.9	205.6	118.9	66.7	36.0	17.9	10.9
1901	1930	1,000.0	303.9	248.7	204.1	116.7	64.8	34.7	16.9	10.2
1902	1931	1,000.0	300.4	256.0	205.7	114.8	63.3	33.7	16.4	9.7
1903	1932	1,000.0	299.7	260.8	206.7	113.0	61.8	33.0	15.7	9.3
1904	1933	1,000.0	308.9	261.8	204.3	108.8	60.3	31.6	15.3	9.0
1905	1934	1,000.0	324.8	260.0	199.3	104.9	58.2	30.1	14.1	8.6
1906	1935	1,000.0	337.6	259.0	195.7	102.2	55.6	28.6	13.5	7.8
1907	1936	1,000.0	348.0	257.1	194.6	99.9	53.3	26.9	12.5	7.7
1908	1937	1,000.0	358.7	256.6	193.1	96.5	50.8	25.4	12.1	6.8
1909	1938	1,000.0	366.4	257.4	191.5	93.6	48.8	23.9	11.5	6.9
1910	1939	1,000.0	370.5	260.9	190.3	90.8	47.1	22.9	10.7	6.8
1911	1940	1,000.0	366.3	266.5	192.8	90.0	45.7	21.8	10.6	6.3
1912	1941	1,000.0	360.7	272.5	196.3	89.3	44.3	20.8	10.1	6.0
1913	1942	1,000.0	349.0	280.8	201.5	89.6	43.6	20.1	9.4	6.0
1914	1943	1,000.0	329.8	289.2	210.2	92.5	43.8	19.7	9.2	5.6
1915	1944	1,000.0	314.8	286.8	221.6	97.3	44.4	20.2	9.2	5.7
1916	1945	1,000.0	310.3	280.8	226.8	100.5	45.7	20.8	9.3	5.8
1917	1946	1,000.0	308.6	270.5	233.4	104.7	46.6	20.8	9.7	5.7
1918	1947	1,000.0	293.3	269.3	243.7	109.3	47.9	21.2	9.6	5.7
1919	1948	1,000.0	258.8	278.5	259.3	116.7	49.6	21.5	9.7	5.9
1920	1949	1,000.0	236.7	283.1	270.4	122.3	50.3	21.8	9.5	5.9
1921	1950	1,000.0	219.9	281.8	280.4	128.0	52.4	21.8	9.6	6.1
1922	1951	1,000.0	214.2	271.1	289.3	134.3	54.1	21.5	9.4	6.1
1923	1952	1,000.0	202.6	261.5	298.3	142.7	57.3	21.9	9.6	6.1
1924	1953	1,000.0	189.6	250.3	305.7	153.4	61.3	23.7	9.8	6.2
1925	1954	1,000.0	184.0	236.6	307.8	163.1	66.1	25.5	10.6	6.3
1926	1955	1,000.0	182.6	219.9	307.7	171.8	72.1	27.8	11.4	6.7
1927	1956	1,000.0	180.6	206.3	304.4	180.5	78.2	30.4	12.6	7.0
1928	1957	1,000.0	179.3	192.3	300.8	188.6	84.6	33.3	13.4	7.7
1929	1958	1,000.0	171.9	181.0	296.8	198.1	92.0	36.8	14.7	8.7
1930	1959	1,000.0	165.1	171.2	293.4	205.1	99.1	40.5	15.9	9.7
1931	1960	1,000.0	154.0	162.8	291.5	212.3	106.7	44.0	17.8	10.9
1932	1961	1,000.0	145.8	156.1	288.7	217.9	113.3	47.1	19.4	11.7
1933	1962	1,000.0	138.9	151.5	284.9	222.2	119.0	50.4	20.5	12.6
1934	1963	1,000.0	136.8	147.6	280.7	225.4	122.1	52.4	21.9	13.1
1935	1964	1,000.0	138.5	145.9	277.6	224.9	123.5	53.9	22.1	13.6
1936	1965	1,000.0	139.8	145.9	275.5	225.0	123.8	54.5	22.4	13.1
1937	1966	1,000.0	141.8	148.7	276.6	224.0	122.1	53.1	21.3	12.4
1938	1967	1,000.0	145.2	152.7	280.6	223.0	118.5	49.2	19.7	11.1
1939	1968	1,000.0	148.4	158.7	287.2	220.5	112.1	45.8	17.6	9.7
1940	1969	1,000.0	154.7	166.9	294.1	215.8	104.1	40.7	15.4	8.3
1941	1970	1,000.0	163.9	175.0	301.5	208.6	94.6	36.2	13.2	7.0
1942	1971	1,000.0	172.4	183.3	310.4	199.8	85.9	31.3	11.1	5.8
1943	1972	1,000.0	185.6	191.9	315.8	187.9	77.7	27.2	9.4	4.5
1944	1973	1,000.0	200.3	200.3	320.7	174.9	69.1	23.3	7.8	3.6
1945	1974	1,000.0	218.1	209.8	321.5	161.1	60.3	19.6	6.6	3.0

TABLE 8B. DISTRIBUTIONS OF WHITE WOMEN BY PARITY AS OF THE BEGINNING OF EACH YEAR 1917-74 BY AGE FOR EACH COHORT FROM 1867 TO 1959--CON.

(BASED ON CUMULATIVE BIRTH RATES)

EXACT AGE AND COHORT	AS OF JANUARY 1	TOTAL	PARITY							
			0	1	2	3	4	5	6	7 AND HIGHER
30 YEARS										
1887	1917	1,000.0	299.5	191.6	178.3	131.9	90.7	56.0	30.5	21.5
1888	1918	1,000.0	296.3	190.8	181.5	133.2	90.8	55.9	30.8	20.7
1889	1919	1,000.0	291.9	191.6	186.4	134.4	90.2	54.8	30.4	20.3
1890	1920	1,000.0	290.6	190.5	191.3	134.9	89.7	53.9	29.6	19.5
1891	1921	1,000.0	285.4	196.9	193.0	134.7	88.9	53.4	28.7	19.0
1892	1922	1,000.0	276.4	207.2	195.0	134.4	87.3	52.4	28.3	19.0
1893	1923	1,000.0	270.9	214.5	198.9	133.8	85.1	51.1	27.4	18.3
1894	1924	1,000.0	269.1	217.3	203.8	133.5	82.2	49.2	26.5	18.4
1895	1925	1,000.0	267.5	220.5	206.5	133.4	80.2	47.6	25.9	18.4
1896	1926	1,000.0	266.0	225.2	208.7	132.7	78.2	45.7	25.5	18.0
1897	1927	1,000.0	265.4	228.9	211.7	131.5	76.8	43.4	24.7	17.6
1898	1928	1,000.0	265.9	231.3	214.2	129.5	75.8	42.4	23.7	17.2
1899	1929	1,000.0	273.9	231.2	213.4	126.8	73.4	41.5	23.0	16.8
1900	1930	1,000.0	282.2	234.1	209.8	124.4	71.0	40.4	22.4	15.7
1901	1931	1,000.0	282.1	242.6	209.0	122.1	69.0	39.1	21.3	14.8
1902	1932	1,000.0	279.1	250.6	210.7	119.9	67.5	37.8	20.4	14.0
1903	1933	1,000.0	279.4	255.4	211.5	118.1	65.9	36.6	19.6	13.5
1904	1934	1,000.0	289.6	256.5	209.1	113.4	64.6	35.3	18.8	12.7
1905	1935	1,000.0	303.8	255.2	205.1	109.9	62.3	33.8	17.6	12.3
1906	1936	1,000.0	315.4	255.8	202.3	107.0	59.5	32.0	16.6	11.4
1907	1937	1,000.0	324.9	254.7	201.8	105.1	57.0	30.1	15.4	11.0
1908	1938	1,000.0	334.0	255.3	201.3	101.9	54.2	28.4	14.9	10.0
1909	1939	1,000.0	339.5	256.6	201.1	99.3	52.5	26.9	14.1	10.0
1910	1940	1,000.0	342.9	260.3	200.6	97.0	50.7	25.7	13.2	9.6
1911	1941	1,000.0	337.1	265.3	204.5	96.9	49.6	24.5	13.0	9.1
1912	1942	1,000.0	328.4	272.9	209.1	96.6	48.3	23.6	12.5	8.6
1913	1943	1,000.0	311.8	280.9	217.4	98.6	48.3	23.0	11.6	8.4
1914	1944	1,000.0	296.4	280.2	227.8	103.7	49.2	23.0	11.6	8.1
1915	1945	1,000.0	287.3	274.4	236.1	108.8	50.1	23.5	11.5	8.3
1916	1946	1,000.0	284.0	265.5	242.8	112.5	51.3	24.1	11.5	8.3
1917	1947	1,000.0	271.5	261.0	252.2	118.0	52.9	24.3	12.0	8.1
1918	1948	1,000.0	251.9	261.6	263.5	124.1	54.5	24.6	11.7	8.1
1919	1949	1,000.0	226.4	264.4	276.4	131.6	56.3	24.8	11.8	8.3
1920	1950	1,000.0	207.6	265.0	286.7	137.6	57.8	25.2	11.7	8.4
1921	1951	1,000.0	193.6	260.2	295.0	144.5	60.9	25.5	11.7	8.6
1922	1952	1,000.0	187.7	249.7	301.2	151.9	63.6	25.6	11.8	8.5
1923	1953	1,000.0	177.1	238.7	307.2	161.7	68.0	26.7	12.0	8.6
1924	1954	1,000.0	165.8	227.7	311.3	172.3	72.5	29.2	12.5	8.7
1925	1955	1,000.0	161.4	213.8	310.9	181.5	78.2	31.5	13.6	9.1
1926	1956	1,000.0	161.4	198.4	307.6	189.3	84.9	34.0	14.7	9.7
1927	1957	1,000.0	160.4	185.5	302.0	197.1	91.6	36.9	16.3	10.2
1928	1958	1,000.0	159.5	172.8	296.3	204.3	98.3	40.6	17.0	11.2
1929	1959	1,000.0	153.3	162.7	290.6	212.1	105.7	44.5	18.6	12.5
1930	1960	1,000.0	147.7	153.3	285.5	217.7	113.2	48.5	20.3	13.8
1931	1961	1,000.0	137.4	145.7	282.6	223.5	120.7	52.2	22.5	15.4
1932	1962	1,000.0	130.3	139.7	278.5	228.2	126.8	55.8	24.4	16.3
1933	1963	1,000.0	124.8	136.3	274.7	230.7	131.6	59.0	25.5	17.4
1934	1964	1,000.0	123.0	133.2	271.2	233.1	134.2	60.5	26.9	17.9
1935	1965	1,000.0	123.7	133.5	268.1	232.8	135.1	61.9	26.8	18.1
1936	1966	1,000.0	125.9	133.9	268.3	232.8	134.5	61.2	26.4	17.0
1937	1967	1,000.0	127.7	137.9	271.3	232.3	131.4	59.0	24.7	15.7
1938	1968	1,000.0	131.3	141.8	276.8	231.5	127.5	54.6	22.7	13.8
1939	1969	1,000.0	133.1	148.3	284.8	230.0	120.9	50.7	20.2	12.0
1940	1970	1,000.0	139.5	154.3	292.6	226.3	113.2	45.7	18.0	10.4
1941	1971	1,000.0	147.5	161.7	300.8	220.5	103.9	41.2	15.6	8.8
1942	1972	1,000.0	156.4	169.8	312.3	210.9	94.5	35.8	13.0	7.3
1943	1973	1,000.0	170.1	178.1	321.4	198.5	84.9	30.6	10.8	5.6
1944	1974	1,000.0	184.0	187.0	328.6	185.6	75.3	26.2	8.9	4.4

TABLE 8B. DISTRIBUTIONS OF WHITE WOMEN BY PARITY AS OF THE BEGINNING OF EACH YEAR 1917-74 BY AGE FOR EACH COHORT FROM 1867 TO 1959--CON.

(BASED ON CUMULATIVE BIRTH RATES)

EXACT AGE AND COHORT	AS OF JANUARY 1	TOTAL	PARITY 0	1	2	3	4	5	6	7 AND HIGHER
31 YEARS										
1886	1917	1,000.0	284.2	177.4	178.5	133.7	94.9	63.2	37.3	30.8
1887	1918	1,000.0	281.3	182.9	176.8	135.0	95.3	61.7	37.1	29.9
1888	1919	1,000.0	277.1	183.3	180.4	136.1	95.3	61.5	37.3	29.0
1889	1920	1,000.0	275.7	181.6	186.0	137.2	94.7	60.1	36.5	28.2
1890	1921	1,000.0	271.2	183.3	191.0	138.1	94.2	59.4	35.5	27.3
1891	1922	1,000.0	265.7	190.0	192.5	137.8	93.7	58.5	34.7	27.1
1892	1923	1,000.0	257.9	199.2	196.3	138.0	91.4	57.1	33.7	26.4
1893	1924	1,000.0	253.2	205.8	200.4	137.6	88.9	55.7	32.8	25.6
1894	1925	1,000.0	251.3	208.9	204.6	138.1	86.2	53.6	31.7	25.6
1895	1926	1,000.0	249.9	212.5	207.6	138.0	84.1	51.9	30.8	25.2
1896	1927	1,000.0	249.0	217.0	210.1	137.3	82.5	49.3	30.1	24.7
1897	1928	1,000.0	248.6	221.3	213.3	135.8	80.8	47.1	29.2	23.9
1898	1929	1,000.0	249.5	224.3	216.0	133.8	79.4	46.1	27.7	23.2
1899	1930	1,000.0	257.5	224.4	215.8	131.2	76.8	44.9	27.1	22.3
1900	1931	1,000.0	265.0	227.9	212.7	128.8	74.3	43.8	26.3	21.2
1901	1932	1,000.0	265.3	236.7	212.0	126.6	72.3	42.3	24.9	19.9
1902	1933	1,000.0	263.1	245.1	213.7	124.0	70.7	40.7	23.8	18.9
1903	1934	1,000.0	264.3	249.9	214.6	121.9	69.2	39.5	22.7	17.9
1904	1935	1,000.0	273.0	251.1	213.3	117.5	68.0	38.1	22.0	17.0
1905	1936	1,000.0	286.2	251.2	209.8	114.0	65.5	36.4	20.5	16.4
1906	1937	1,000.0	296.9	252.6	207.7	111.3	62.6	34.5	19.2	15.2
1907	1938	1,000.0	304.8	252.3	208.1	109.7	60.0	32.5	18.0	14.6
1908	1939	1,000.0	312.3	253.2	208.8	107.0	57.2	30.7	17.2	13.6
1909	1940	1,000.0	316.8	254.6	209.5	104.8	55.7	29.1	16.3	13.2
1910	1941	1,000.0	318.9	257.6	210.3	103.1	54.2	27.8	15.3	12.8
1911	1942	1,000.0	310.5	263.6	215.2	103.5	53.2	26.8	15.1	12.1
1912	1943	1,000.0	298.4	270.6	222.1	104.5	52.5	26.1	14.4	11.4
1913	1944	1,000.0	284.2	271.6	231.6	108.5	53.2	25.9	13.8	11.2
1914	1945	1,000.0	273.4	267.9	239.5	114.2	54.4	25.9	13.7	11.0
1915	1946	1,000.0	265.0	259.0	249.3	120.1	55.5	26.4	13.6	11.1
1916	1947	1,000.0	253.4	254.7	257.8	125.0	57.2	27.2	13.7	11.0
1917	1948	1,000.0	237.1	252.4	267.4	131.7	59.2	27.5	13.9	10.8
1918	1949	1,000.0	225.5	248.3	276.1	137.4	60.7	27.6	13.7	10.7
1919	1950	1,000.0	202.6	248.0	288.2	145.0	63.4	28.0	13.8	11.0
1920	1951	1,000.0	186.1	245.9	297.0	152.0	65.5	28.7	13.7	11.1
1921	1952	1,000.0	172.1	240.7	302.9	160.0	69.7	29.4	13.9	11.3
1922	1953	1,000.0	167.0	229.3	306.4	168.2	73.6	30.2	14.1	11.2
1923	1954	1,000.0	157.7	218.8	309.2	178.2	78.5	31.7	14.6	11.3
1924	1955	1,000.0	147.4	207.4	311.5	188.0	83.9	34.8	15.3	11.7
1925	1956	1,000.0	144.2	195.3	308.0	196.1	89.9	37.4	16.8	12.3
1926	1957	1,000.0	145.2	180.7	302.8	202.6	97.2	40.2	18.1	13.2
1927	1958	1,000.0	144.6	168.8	295.5	209.7	103.9	43.7	19.8	14.0
1928	1959	1,000.0	144.8	157.4	288.4	215.4	110.5	47.6	20.8	15.1
1929	1960	1,000.0	139.5	148.0	281.6	221.4	118.0	51.8	22.8	16.9
1930	1961	1,000.0	134.6	139.3	276.0	225.7	125.1	56.1	24.7	18.5
1931	1962	1,000.0	125.0	132.4	272.1	230.4	132.5	60.0	27.2	20.4
1932	1963	1,000.0	119.1	127.2	268.2	234.0	137.5	63.5	29.1	21.4
1933	1964	1,000.0	113.8	124.9	264.9	235.4	141.8	66.5	30.1	22.6
1934	1965	1,000.0	111.2	123.5	261.4	237.9	144.1	67.7	31.4	22.8
1935	1966	1,000.0	112.8	123.9	260.2	237.9	144.0	68.0	30.8	22.4
1936	1967	1,000.0	115.0	125.4	261.9	238.1	142.5	66.7	29.8	20.6
1937	1968	1,000.0	117.3	129.0	266.0	238.1	139.0	64.1	27.7	18.8
1938	1969	1,000.0	119.9	133.4	273.0	237.7	135.0	59.3	25.3	16.4
1939	1970	1,000.0	121.8	138.8	280.8	237.3	128.6	55.4	22.8	14.5
1940	1971	1,000.0	127.6	144.0	289.1	234.5	121.2	50.5	20.5	12.6
1941	1972	1,000.0	135.8	151.3	299.4	228.3	111.4	45.4	17.8	10.6
1942	1973	1,000.0	145.0	158.5	314.4	218.9	100.8	39.2	14.6	8.6
1943	1974	1,000.0	158.1	167.2	325.1	206.9	90.6	33.5	12.0	6.6

TABLE 8B. DISTRIBUTIONS OF WHITE WOMEN BY PARITY AS OF THE BEGINNING OF EACH YEAR 1917-74 BY AGE FOR EACH COHORT FROM 1867 TO 1959--CON.

(BASED ON CUMULATIVE BIRTH RATES)

EXACT AGE AND COHORT	AS OF JANUARY 1	TOTAL	PARITY							
			0	1	2	3	4	5	6	7 AND HIGHER
32 YEARS										
1885	1917	1,000.0	271.5	165.3	177.0	134.3	97.5	68.8	43.1	42.5
1886	1918	1,000.0	270.2	169.8	176.0	135.0	97.7	67.3	43.0	41.0
1887	1919	1,000.0	266.3	176.4	174.6	136.3	97.7	65.7	42.8	40.2
1888	1920	1,000.0	263.8	175.2	178.7	137.7	98.0	65.1	42.8	38.7
1889	1921	1,000.0	260.6	174.7	184.7	139.2	97.4	64.0	41.6	37.8
1890	1922	1,000.0	255.9	176.2	189.7	139.7	97.8	63.0	40.6	37.1
1891	1923	1,000.0	250.7	182.6	192.2	140.6	96.4	62.0	39.4	36.1
1892	1924	1,000.0	243.5	191.3	196.0	140.8	94.3	60.4	38.4	35.3
1893	1925	1,000.0	238.8	198.0	199.6	141.0	92.0	59.0	37.3	34.3
1894	1926	1,000.0	237.1	201.6	203.9	141.5	89.4	56.8	36.0	33.7
1895	1927	1,000.0	236.1	204.9	207.6	141.3	87.6	54.7	34.8	33.0
1896	1928	1,000.0	235.3	209.9	210.1	140.6	85.7	52.3	33.8	32.3
1897	1929	1,000.0	235.2	214.6	213.8	139.1	83.8	49.9	32.7	30.9
1898	1930	1,000.0	236.2	218.0	216.7	137.4	82.1	48.8	31.2	29.6
1899	1931	1,000.0	243.5	218.4	217.0	134.7	79.7	47.4	30.6	28.7
1900	1932	1,000.0	251.4	222.2	214.1	132.3	77.0	46.2	29.7	27.1
1901	1933	1,000.0	252.1	231.2	213.7	129.9	74.8	44.6	28.0	25.7
1902	1934	1,000.0	250.9	239.8	215.1	127.2	73.4	42.8	26.7	24.1
1903	1935	1,000.0	251.1	244.4	217.1	125.2	72.0	41.8	25.4	23.0
1904	1936	1,000.0	258.6	246.8	216.5	120.9	70.7	40.2	24.4	21.9
1905	1937	1,000.0	271.1	247.6	213.6	117.6	68.0	38.5	22.7	20.9
1906	1938	1,000.0	280.8	249.3	212.3	115.2	65.1	36.5	21.3	19.5
1907	1939	1,000.0	287.2	249.1	213.9	114.1	62.5	34.4	20.1	18.7
1908	1940	1,000.0	293.8	250.2	215.4	111.7	60.0	32.5	19.1	17.3
1909	1941	1,000.0	297.3	250.6	217.5	110.0	58.8	30.9	18.2	16.7
1910	1942	1,000.0	297.5	254.2	219.0	108.9	57.4	29.8	17.1	16.1
1911	1943	1,000.0	286.5	260.1	225.4	110.2	56.7	29.1	16.7	15.3
1912	1944	1,000.0	275.6	261.9	233.0	113.1	56.8	28.6	16.4	14.6
1913	1945	1,000.0	264.8	260.1	240.6	117.9	58.0	28.4	15.8	14.4
1914	1946	1,000.0	254.5	253.3	249.9	124.6	59.4	28.5	15.6	14.2
1915	1947	1,000.0	239.5	248.0	260.6	131.8	61.2	29.1	15.7	14.1
1916	1948	1,000.0	224.9	246.1	268.9	137.2	63.3	30.1	15.6	13.9
1917	1949	1,000.0	215.0	240.2	276.3	143.5	65.3	30.3	15.7	13.7
1918	1950	1,000.0	206.0	234.0	284.1	149.0	67.3	30.5	15.5	13.6
1919	1951	1,000.0	184.8	231.6	294.9	157.4	70.5	31.2	15.7	13.9
1920	1952	1,000.0	168.4	229.1	301.7	165.2	73.5	32.4	15.6	14.1
1921	1953	1,000.0	154.9	223.3	305.0	173.7	78.9	33.7	16.3	14.2
1922	1954	1,000.0	151.3	211.9	305.9	181.9	83.3	35.1	16.4	14.2
1923	1955	1,000.0	142.4	201.7	307.3	191.0	89.0	36.9	17.3	14.4
1924	1956	1,000.0	133.4	191.3	307.1	199.9	94.5	40.4	18.3	15.1
1925	1957	1,000.0	130.9	180.2	301.8	207.0	100.7	43.3	20.2	15.9
1926	1958	1,000.0	132.4	166.7	295.2	212.4	108.0	46.6	21.5	17.2
1927	1959	1,000.0	132.7	156.0	287.0	218.0	114.7	50.1	23.3	18.2
1928	1960	1,000.0	133.6	145.6	279.2	222.0	121.1	54.1	24.9	19.5
1929	1961	1,000.0	128.8	136.8	272.3	226.8	128.0	58.6	27.0	21.7
1930	1962	1,000.0	124.6	128.6	266.2	229.9	135.0	63.0	29.1	23.6
1931	1963	1,000.0	115.8	122.5	262.5	233.8	141.2	67.0	31.4	25.8
1932	1964	1,000.0	110.2	118.0	258.9	236.7	145.7	70.3	33.4	26.8
1933	1965	1,000.0	104.5	116.9	255.7	238.1	149.9	72.8	34.3	27.8
1934	1966	1,000.0	102.4	115.8	253.8	240.7	151.4	73.4	35.1	27.4
1935	1967	1,000.0	104.2	117.4	253.6	240.9	150.5	73.0	34.1	26.3
1936	1968	1,000.0	107.1	118.4	256.3	241.5	148.6	71.4	32.7	24.0
1937	1969	1,000.0	108.5	122.5	261.7	241.9	145.1	68.3	30.3	21.7
1938	1970	1,000.0	111.4	126.0	268.4	242.3	141.3	63.6	27.8	19.2
1939	1971	1,000.0	112.9	131.2	276.2	242.6	135.1	59.8	25.2	17.0
1940	1972	1,000.0	119.0	136.1	286.4	239.4	127.3	54.4	22.8	14.6
1941	1973	1,000.0	127.4	142.9	299.3	233.3	116.9	48.6	19.4	12.2
1942	1974	1,000.0	136.2	150.2	315.3	224.9	105.7	41.9	16.0	9.8

TABLE 8B. DISTRIBUTIONS OF WHITE WOMEN BY PARITY AS OF THE BEGINNING OF EACH YEAR 1917-74 BY AGE FOR EACH COHORT FROM 1867 TO 1959--CON.

(BASED ON CUMULATIVE BIRTH RATES)

EXACT AGE AND COHORT	AS OF JANUARY 1	TOTAL	PARITY							
			0	1	2	3	4	5	6	7 AND HIGHER
33 YEARS										
1884---------------	1917	1,000.0	260.3	157.1	172.5	134.0	99.5	73.2	48.0	55.4
1885---------------	1918	1,000.0	260.8	158.6	173.9	134.6	99.3	71.4	47.9	53.5
1886---------------	1919	1,000.0	258.7	164.0	173.2	135.2	99.2	69.9	47.7	52.1
1887---------------	1920	1,000.0	256.0	169.4	172.2	136.8	99.6	67.9	47.4	50.7
1888---------------	1921	1,000.0	252.1	169.1	176.6	138.5	99.8	67.8	47.0	49.1
1889---------------	1922	1,000.0	248.9	168.4	182.5	139.8	99.9	66.3	45.7	48.5
1890---------------	1923	1,000.0	244.3	169.6	188.5	141.3	99.7	65.2	44.5	46.9
1891---------------	1924	1,000.0	239.5	175.7	190.9	142.2	98.4	64.2	43.3	45.8
1892---------------	1925	1,000.0	232.3	184.5	194.2	143.1	96.4	62.6	42.1	44.8
1893---------------	1926	1,000.0	227.8	191.6	198.0	143.1	94.4	61.2	40.6	43.3
1894---------------	1927	1,000.0	226.6	195.1	202.5	143.7	92.0	58.9	39.0	42.2
1895---------------	1928	1,000.0	225.5	198.7	206.6	143.4	90.0	56.6	37.9	41.3
1896---------------	1929	1,000.0	225.0	203.8	209.5	143.0	87.9	54.4	36.6	39.8
1897---------------	1930	1,000.0	225.0	208.9	213.5	141.5	86.0	52.0	35.3	37.8
1898---------------	1931	1,000.0	225.5	212.7	216.5	139.9	84.4	50.6	34.1	36.3
1899---------------	1932	1,000.0	233.0	213.1	217.2	137.3	81.8	49.2	33.4	35.0
1900---------------	1933	1,000.0	241.4	216.9	214.5	134.6	79.0	48.0	32.2	33.4
1901---------------	1934	1,000.0	242.6	226.2	214.1	132.1	77.0	46.3	30.3	31.4
1902---------------	1935	1,000.0	240.7	234.8	216.2	129.6	75.6	44.6	28.9	29.6
1903---------------	1936	1,000.0	240.2	240.1	218.8	127.8	74.2	43.4	27.3	28.2
1904---------------	1937	1,000.0	247.0	242.9	218.8	123.8	72.7	41.8	26.3	26.7
1905---------------	1938	1,000.0	258.7	244.0	216.5	120.7	70.1	40.1	24.4	25.5
1906---------------	1939	1,000.0	267.3	245.6	216.3	118.7	67.2	38.0	23.0	23.9
1907---------------	1940	1,000.0	272.8	245.5	218.6	118.0	64.9	35.9	21.6	22.7
1908---------------	1941	1,000.0	278.8	245.7	221.2	116.0	62.6	34.0	20.7	21.0
1909---------------	1942	1,000.0	280.6	246.5	224.0	114.8	61.6	32.6	19.7	20.2
1910---------------	1943	1,000.0	277.7	250.5	226.9	114.7	60.4	31.8	18.4	19.6
1911---------------	1944	1,000.0	267.6	252.0	233.8	117.6	60.4	31.4	18.3	18.9
1912---------------	1945	1,000.0	259.5	251.5	239.7	121.2	61.0	30.9	18.0	18.2
1913---------------	1946	1,000.0	249.0	247.1	248.3	127.0	62.7	30.7	17.5	17.7
1914---------------	1947	1,000.0	233.6	242.9	258.4	134.7	64.6	31.0	17.4	17.4
1915---------------	1948	1,000.0	216.2	239.8	268.4	142.5	66.7	31.9	17.3	17.2
1916---------------	1949	1,000.0	206.9	235.5	274.7	147.2	68.8	32.8	17.3	16.8
1917---------------	1950	1,000.0	199.0	227.9	281.5	153.1	71.4	33.1	17.3	16.7
1918---------------	1951	1,000.0	191.7	220.2	288.2	159.1	73.6	33.4	17.3	16.5
1919---------------	1952	1,000.0	170.5	217.3	297.2	168.3	77.6	34.7	17.4	17.0
1920---------------	1953	1,000.0	154.3	214.7	302.0	176.1	81.6	36.4	17.7	17.2
1921---------------	1954	1,000.0	142.1	208.8	302.8	184.8	87.5	38.1	18.5	17.4
1922---------------	1955	1,000.0	139.0	197.5	302.6	192.0	92.8	39.7	19.0	17.4
1923---------------	1956	1,000.0	131.1	188.2	302.1	200.3	98.3	42.1	20.0	17.9
1924---------------	1957	1,000.0	122.6	178.6	300.6	208.0	104.1	46.0	21.2	18.9
1925---------------	1958	1,000.0	120.5	168.5	293.9	214.4	110.2	49.2	23.4	19.9
1926---------------	1959	1,000.0	122.8	156.1	287.0	218.2	117.2	52.5	24.8	21.4
1927---------------	1960	1,000.0	123.6	146.5	278.3	222.4	123.6	56.0	27.0	22.6
1928---------------	1961	1,000.0	125.1	136.5	270.6	225.3	129.5	60.1	28.6	24.3
1929---------------	1962	1,000.0	120.8	128.1	263.4	229.2	136.0	64.7	30.9	26.9
1930---------------	1963	1,000.0	117.2	120.5	257.8	231.8	141.9	68.9	33.0	28.9
1931---------------	1964	1,000.0	108.7	115.1	254.1	234.9	147.9	72.8	35.3	31.2
1932---------------	1965	1,000.0	102.7	111.5	251.0	237.6	152.2	75.7	37.2	32.1
1933---------------	1966	1,000.0	97.5	110.9	248.7	239.3	155.5	77.8	37.8	32.5
1934---------------	1967	1,000.0	95.6	110.6	247.8	242.1	156.6	77.8	38.0	31.5
1935---------------	1968	1,000.0	98.2	111.7	248.3	242.5	155.5	77.2	36.7	29.9
1936---------------	1969	1,000.0	100.3	113.6	251.9	243.5	153.4	75.2	35.0	27.1
1937---------------	1970	1,000.0	102.1	117.0	257.0	244.4	150.2	72.0	32.7	24.6
1938---------------	1971	1,000.0	104.8	120.3	264.0	245.2	146.3	67.5	30.1	21.8
1939---------------	1972	1,000.0	106.5	125.4	273.2	245.2	139.9	63.2	27.4	19.2
1940---------------	1973	1,000.0	112.8	130.0	285.2	242.3	131.6	57.3	24.4	16.4
1941---------------	1974	1,000.0	121.0	136.8	298.8	237.1	120.9	51.0	20.8	13.6

TABLE 8B. DISTRIBUTIONS OF WHITE WOMEN BY PARITY AS OF THE BEGINNING OF EACH YEAR 1917-74 BY AGE FOR EACH COHORT FROM 1867 TO 1959--CON.

(BASED ON CUMULATIVE BIRTH RATES)

EXACT AGE AND COHORT	AS OF JANUARY 1	TOTAL	PARITY							
			0	1	2	3	4	5	6	7 AND HIGHER
34 YEARS										
1883	1917	1,000.0	250.6	151.5	166.2	133.0	100.9	76.2	51.8	69.8
1884	1918	1,000.0	251.2	151.4	168.6	133.5	100.5	75.3	51.8	67.7
1885	1919	1,000.0	251.1	153.7	170.3	134.1	100.0	73.4	51.7	65.7
1886	1920	1,000.0	250.0	158.1	170.0	135.0	100.2	71.7	51.3	63.7
1887	1921	1,000.0	246.1	164.2	169.2	136.9	100.6	70.0	50.8	62.2
1888	1922	1,000.0	242.1	163.8	173.5	138.3	101.6	69.5	50.3	60.9
1889	1923	1,000.0	239.1	162.8	180.3	140.6	101.0	68.1	48.8	59.3
1890	1924	1,000.0	234.8	163.7	186.2	142.2	100.9	67.0	47.5	57.7
1891	1925	1,000.0	229.9	169.9	188.2	143.6	99.9	66.0	46.1	56.4
1892	1926	1,000.0	223.0	178.8	191.9	144.4	98.3	64.2	44.7	54.7
1893	1927	1,000.0	219.1	186.0	195.8	144.3	96.5	62.7	43.0	52.6
1894	1928	1,000.0	217.7	189.9	200.7	144.7	94.0	60.4	41.3	51.3
1895	1929	1,000.0	216.9	193.4	205.2	144.8	91.8	58.2	40.2	49.5
1896	1930	1,000.0	216.5	199.0	208.2	144.7	89.5	56.0	38.7	47.4
1897	1931	1,000.0	216.1	204.2	212.6	143.2	87.8	53.5	37.6	45.0
1898	1932	1,000.0	217.1	208.2	215.7	141.6	86.1	52.0	36.2	43.1
1899	1933	1,000.0	224.8	208.3	216.6	139.1	83.4	50.5	35.6	41.7
1900	1934	1,000.0	233.5	212.6	214.0	136.1	80.7	49.3	34.1	39.7
1901	1935	1,000.0	234.2	221.7	214.1	133.8	78.8	47.7	32.2	37.5
1902	1936	1,000.0	231.9	230.8	216.8	131.4	77.4	45.9	30.5	35.3
1903	1937	1,000.0	230.9	236.3	219.9	130.1	75.8	44.8	28.7	33.5
1904	1938	1,000.0	237.0	239.4	220.4	126.3	74.5	43.0	27.7	31.7
1905	1939	1,000.0	247.9	240.4	218.9	123.6	71.8	41.3	25.9	30.2
1906	1940	1,000.0	255.8	242.0	219.4	121.8	69.2	39.3	24.3	28.2
1907	1941	1,000.0	260.7	241.3	222.5	121.5	67.2	37.1	22.9	26.8
1908	1942	1,000.0	265.6	241.7	225.6	120.0	64.9	35.5	21.9	24.8
1909	1943	1,000.0	263.8	243.0	230.1	119.7	64.3	34.2	21.0	23.9
1910	1944	1,000.0	261.7	243.2	233.3	121.0	63.8	33.7	19.9	23.4
1911	1945	1,000.0	253.9	242.7	238.8	124.5	64.2	33.4	19.7	22.8
1912	1946	1,000.0	245.9	240.4	245.1	129.2	65.1	33.0	19.5	21.8
1913	1947	1,000.0	231.7	237.8	254.2	135.7	67.4	33.0	19.1	21.1
1914	1948	1,000.0	214.4	235.4	263.8	143.7	69.6	33.5	18.9	20.7
1915	1949	1,000.0	201.1	230.7	272.0	150.9	71.8	34.4	18.8	20.3
1916	1950	1,000.0	193.5	225.3	277.8	155.0	74.3	35.3	18.8	20.0
1917	1951	1,000.0	186.9	216.4	283.7	161.2	77.3	35.8	18.9	19.8
1918	1952	1,000.0	179.8	208.7	289.0	167.6	79.8	36.6	18.8	19.7
1919	1953	1,000.0	158.8	205.4	296.1	177.1	84.8	38.3	19.3	20.2
1920	1954	1,000.0	143.6	202.7	299.0	184.8	89.2	40.5	19.7	20.5
1921	1955	1,000.0	131.7	196.8	299.0	192.6	95.9	42.2	21.0	20.8
1922	1956	1,000.0	129.5	186.3	297.1	199.2	101.0	44.4	21.5	21.0
1923	1957	1,000.0	122.1	177.5	295.9	206.5	106.4	47.2	22.8	21.6
1924	1958	1,000.0	113.9	168.7	293.1	213.5	112.5	51.1	24.2	23.0
1925	1959	1,000.0	112.5	159.7	286.2	218.3	118.2	54.5	26.4	24.2
1926	1960	1,000.0	115.3	148.1	279.2	221.0	124.7	57.8	28.1	25.8
1927	1961	1,000.0	116.5	139.0	270.6	224.3	130.5	61.4	30.4	27.3
1928	1962	1,000.0	118.6	129.4	262.8	226.6	135.8	65.4	32.1	29.3
1929	1963	1,000.0	114.7	121.6	256.2	229.8	141.5	69.8	34.4	32.0
1930	1964	1,000.0	111.4	114.4	250.6	232.0	147.2	73.7	36.5	34.2
1931	1965	1,000.0	102.4	109.9	247.2	234.9	153.1	77.3	38.7	36.5
1932	1966	1,000.0	96.9	106.9	244.6	237.7	156.7	80.1	40.3	36.8
1933	1967	1,000.0	92.0	106.7	243.3	239.8	159.5	81.6	40.4	36.7
1934	1968	1,000.0	90.6	106.3	243.1	242.5	160.5	81.4	40.4	35.2
1935	1969	1,000.0	92.7	108.0	244.2	243.4	159.3	80.5	38.8	33.1
1936	1970	1,000.0	95.4	109.2	247.9	244.6	157.2	78.4	37.2	30.1
1937	1971	1,000.0	97.0	112.8	253.1	245.6	154.2	75.1	34.9	27.3
1938	1972	1,000.0	100.1	116.0	261.0	246.4	149.9	70.4	32.0	24.2
1939	1973	1,000.0	101.8	121.1	271.4	246.7	143.3	65.6	29.0	21.1
1940	1974	1,000.0	108.1	125.4	284.2	244.6	134.7	59.3	25.7	18.0

TABLE 8B. DISTRIBUTIONS OF WHITE WOMEN BY PARITY AS OF THE BEGINNING OF EACH YEAR 1917-74 BY AGE FOR EACH COHORT FROM 1867 TO 1959--CON.

(BASED ON CUMULATIVE BIRTH RATES)

EXACT AGE AND COHORT	AS OF JANUARY 1	TOTAL	PARITY							
			0	1	2	3	4	5	6	7 AND HIGHER
35 YEARS										
1882---------------	1917	1,000.0	243.8	145.2	160.6	131.2	101.2	77.1	55.8	85.1
1883---------------	1918	1,000.0	243.2	146.8	162.5	131.9	101.3	77.3	54.8	82.2
1884---------------	1919	1,000.0	243.4	147.3	165.1	132.3	100.8	76.5	54.7	79.9
1885---------------	1920	1,000.0	243.9	149.0	167.1	133.3	100.5	74.4	54.3	77.5
1886---------------	1921	1,000.0	242.0	153.9	166.9	134.4	100.7	72.9	53.9	75.3
1887---------------	1922	1,000.0	237.9	159.8	166.1	136.1	101.7	71.1	53.2	74.1
1888---------------	1923	1,000.0	234.1	159.3	171.0	138.3	102.2	70.6	52.7	71.8
1889---------------	1924	1,000.0	231.4	158.0	177.8	140.6	101.8	69.2	51.1	70.1
1890---------------	1925	1,000.0	227.0	159.0	183.3	142.7	101.8	68.2	49.7	68.3
1891---------------	1926	1,000.0	222.2	165.2	185.9	143.9	101.0	67.3	48.0	66.5
1892---------------	1927	1,000.0	215.8	174.3	189.4	144.8	99.8	65.2	46.5	64.2
1893---------------	1928	1,000.0	212.0	181.7	193.6	144.6	97.9	63.5	44.9	61.8
1894---------------	1929	1,000.0	210.8	185.6	198.8	145.4	95.3	61.5	43.0	59.6
1895---------------	1930	1,000.0	210.1	189.4	203.5	145.7	92.9	59.4	41.8	57.2
1896---------------	1931	1,000.0	209.3	195.1	206.8	145.7	90.8	57.2	40.3	54.8
1897---------------	1932	1,000.0	209.3	200.5	211.2	144.3	89.1	54.6	39.2	51.8
1898---------------	1933	1,000.0	210.8	204.3	214.4	142.8	87.2	53.0	37.9	49.6
1899---------------	1934	1,000.0	218.5	204.7	215.6	140.0	84.7	51.4	37.1	48.0
1900---------------	1935	1,000.0	226.8	208.8	213.3	137.3	82.1	50.2	35.6	45.9
1901---------------	1936	1,000.0	227.3	218.2	213.7	135.2	80.1	48.8	33.4	43.3
1902---------------	1937	1,000.0	224.7	227.4	217.0	133.0	78.8	46.8	31.7	40.6
1903---------------	1938	1,000.0	223.1	233.2	220.6	131.8	77.3	45.8	29.8	38.4
1904---------------	1939	1,000.0	228.5	236.2	221.7	128.4	76.0	44.0	28.7	36.5
1905---------------	1940	1,000.0	238.8	237.2	220.8	125.9	73.5	42.4	26.9	34.5
1906---------------	1941	1,000.0	246.2	238.4	221.9	124.5	71.0	40.4	25.3	32.3
1907---------------	1942	1,000.0	250.1	237.8	225.5	124.5	69.3	38.3	23.9	30.6
1908---------------	1943	1,000.0	252.4	238.5	229.7	123.9	67.2	36.8	23.0	28.5
1909---------------	1944	1,000.0	250.9	237.0	234.4	124.8	67.1	35.9	22.2	27.7
1910---------------	1945	1,000.0	250.2	235.6	236.7	126.7	67.1	35.3	21.2	27.2
1911---------------	1946	1,000.0	242.4	233.5	242.4	131.1	67.8	35.5	20.9	26.4
1912---------------	1947	1,000.0	231.6	232.5	249.1	136.5	69.1	35.1	20.8	25.3
1913---------------	1948	1,000.0	215.9	231.5	257.8	142.9	71.9	35.1	20.6	24.3
1914---------------	1949	1,000.0	201.8	227.8	266.1	150.5	74.0	35.8	20.2	23.8
1915---------------	1950	1,000.0	189.8	222.3	273.9	157.1	76.6	36.7	20.1	23.5
1916---------------	1951	1,000.0	183.3	216.1	278.8	161.3	79.4	37.8	20.3	23.0
1917---------------	1952	1,000.0	176.9	207.0	283.6	167.7	82.8	38.7	20.4	22.9
1918---------------	1953	1,000.0	170.1	199.3	287.2	174.5	85.9	39.7	20.5	22.8
1919---------------	1954	1,000.0	149.8	195.8	293.0	183.6	91.4	41.9	21.1	23.4
1920---------------	1955	1,000.0	135.1	192.9	295.0	190.8	96.2	44.2	22.0	23.8
1921---------------	1956	1,000.0	123.7	187.8	293.7	197.9	102.9	46.3	23.3	24.4
1922---------------	1957	1,000.0	122.1	177.5	291.3	203.8	107.7	49.0	23.9	24.7
1923---------------	1958	1,000.0	114.9	169.4	289.3	210.2	113.4	51.8	25.5	25.5
1924---------------	1959	1,000.0	107.3	161.5	286.1	216.2	119.0	55.8	27.0	27.1
1925---------------	1960	1,000.0	106.3	153.1	279.3	220.0	124.3	59.2	29.2	28.6
1926---------------	1961	1,000.0	109.5	141.9	272.5	221.7	130.5	62.5	31.0	30.4
1927---------------	1962	1,000.0	111.1	133.1	263.9	224.9	135.4	66.0	33.4	32.2
1928---------------	1963	1,000.0	113.6	124.3	256.5	226.6	140.1	69.6	35.2	34.1
1929---------------	1964	1,000.0	110.0	116.6	250.1	229.5	145.6	73.8	37.4	37.0
1930---------------	1965	1,000.0	106.1	110.4	244.9	231.3	151.2	77.6	39.4	39.1
1931---------------	1966	1,000.0	97.5	106.5	241.7	234.5	156.4	81.0	41.4	41.0
1932---------------	1967	1,000.0	92.4	103.5	240.1	237.5	159.7	83.3	42.6	40.9
1933---------------	1968	1,000.0	87.9	103.3	239.3	239.4	162.7	84.5	42.6	40.3
1934---------------	1969	1,000.0	86.2	103.6	239.4	242.5	163.4	84.2	42.3	38.4
1935---------------	1970	1,000.0	88.8	104.7	240.8	243.5	162.1	83.1	40.9	36.1
1936---------------	1971	1,000.0	91.4	106.1	244.6	244.9	160.1	80.9	39.2	32.8
1937---------------	1972	1,000.0	93.3	109.7	250.5	246.0	156.7	77.4	36.7	29.7
1938---------------	1973	1,000.0	96.5	113.0	259.1	247.2	152.2	72.4	33.5	26.1
1939---------------	1974	1,000.0	98.2	117.8	270.4	247.8	145.6	67.3	30.2	22.7

TABLE 8B. DISTRIBUTIONS OF WHITE WOMEN BY PARITY AS OF THE BEGINNING OF EACH YEAR 1917-74 BY AGE FOR EACH COHORT FROM 1867 TO 1959--CON.

(BASED ON CUMULATIVE BIRTH RATES)

EXACT AGE AND COHORT	AS OF JANUARY 1	TOTAL	PARITY							
			0	1	2	3	4	5	6	7 AND HIGHER
36 YEARS										
1881	1917	1,000.0	239.5	138.8	154.2	128.3	100.5	77.5	60.0	101.2
1882	1918	1,000.0	237.6	141.4	157.2	129.7	101.0	77.6	57.8	97.7
1883	1919	1,000.0	236.8	143.3	159.3	130.3	101.1	77.9	56.8	94.5
1884	1920	1,000.0	237.3	143.5	162.1	131.1	100.6	77.1	56.4	91.9
1885	1921	1,000.0	237.3	145.5	164.2	132.3	100.3	75.1	56.0	89.3
1886	1922	1,000.0	235.1	150.3	164.0	133.3	101.0	73.6	55.5	87.2
1887	1923	1,000.0	231.3	156.2	163.5	135.5	101.8	71.8	54.8	85.1
1888	1924	1,000.0	227.6	155.5	168.4	137.8	102.5	71.3	54.3	82.6
1889	1925	1,000.0	224.9	154.2	175.0	140.4	102.2	70.0	52.6	80.7
1890	1926	1,000.0	220.7	155.1	181.0	142.4	102.5	68.9	51.2	78.2
1891	1927	1,000.0	216.2	161.4	183.5	143.6	102.1	67.9	49.3	76.0
1892	1928	1,000.0	209.8	170.9	187.1	144.6	100.8	65.6	47.9	73.3
1893	1929	1,000.0	206.3	178.3	191.6	144.7	98.8	64.1	46.1	70.1
1894	1930	1,000.0	205.3	182.3	197.1	145.6	95.9	62.3	44.3	67.2
1895	1931	1,000.0	204.2	186.2	201.9	146.1	93.7	60.3	43.0	64.6
1896	1932	1,000.0	203.7	192.1	205.2	146.2	91.7	58.0	41.4	61.7
1897	1933	1,000.0	204.0	197.4	209.8	144.8	89.8	55.5	40.4	58.3
1898	1934	1,000.0	205.9	201.4	213.0	143.2	88.1	53.6	39.0	55.8
1899	1935	1,000.0	213.2	201.5	214.6	140.5	85.7	52.2	38.2	54.1
1900	1936	1,000.0	221.2	206.0	212.4	138.1	83.1	51.0	36.5	51.7
1901	1937	1,000.0	221.5	215.4	213.3	136.2	81.2	49.5	34.3	48.6
1902	1938	1,000.0	218.5	224.9	216.9	134.1	80.0	47.5	32.6	45.5
1903	1939	1,000.0	216.4	230.6	221.1	133.0	78.5	46.7	30.6	43.1
1904	1940	1,000.0	221.3	233.5	222.6	130.0	77.4	44.9	29.6	40.7
1905	1941	1,000.0	231.1	234.3	222.2	127.9	74.9	43.3	27.8	38.5
1906	1942	1,000.0	237.8	235.5	223.7	126.7	72.7	41.4	26.1	36.1
1907	1943	1,000.0	239.8	235.1	228.0	127.5	71.2	39.3	24.9	34.2
1908	1944	1,000.0	241.9	233.9	232.4	127.8	69.6	38.2	24.0	32.2
1909	1945	1,000.0	241.2	231.0	236.7	129.2	69.9	37.3	23.4	31.3
1910	1946	1,000.0	240.5	228.3	238.9	132.0	70.2	37.1	22.3	30.7
1911	1947	1,000.0	230.5	227.1	245.0	136.9	71.3	37.4	22.0	29.8
1912	1948	1,000.0	218.6	227.3	251.4	142.2	73.0	36.9	22.1	28.5
1913	1949	1,000.0	205.4	225.4	259.1	148.3	75.6	37.1	21.8	27.3
1914	1950	1,000.0	192.2	221.3	267.1	155.4	78.0	37.7	21.4	26.9
1915	1951	1,000.0	181.0	215.2	274.1	162.0	80.9	38.9	21.4	26.5
1916	1952	1,000.0	174.9	208.7	278.1	166.2	84.1	40.2	21.9	25.9
1917	1953	1,000.0	168.7	199.5	281.6	172.9	87.9	41.6	21.9	25.9
1918	1954	1,000.0	162.6	191.9	284.0	179.3	91.4	42.9	22.0	25.9
1919	1955	1,000.0	142.6	188.1	289.1	188.1	97.2	45.3	22.9	26.7
1920	1956	1,000.0	128.4	185.6	290.4	194.7	101.8	47.8	24.1	27.2
1921	1957	1,000.0	117.4	180.7	288.6	201.3	108.4	50.1	25.5	28.0
1922	1958	1,000.0	116.1	170.9	285.8	206.2	113.3	52.9	26.4	28.4
1923	1959	1,000.0	109.4	163.5	283.4	211.9	118.8	55.6	28.0	29.4
1924	1960	1,000.0	102.1	156.2	280.1	217.2	123.8	59.9	29.4	31.3
1925	1961	1,000.0	101.4	148.1	273.5	220.3	128.7	63.3	31.8	32.9
1926	1962	1,000.0	105.0	137.1	266.7	221.9	134.4	66.3	33.6	35.0
1927	1963	1,000.0	106.9	129.0	258.5	224.6	138.7	69.5	36.1	36.7
1928	1964	1,000.0	109.7	120.3	251.4	226.0	143.3	72.9	37.8	38.6
1929	1965	1,000.0	105.6	113.5	245.3	228.6	148.6	77.0	39.8	41.6
1930	1966	1,000.0	102.0	107.7	240.5	230.5	153.7	80.6	41.8	43.2
1931	1967	1,000.0	93.8	103.8	238.0	233.9	158.7	83.6	43.4	44.8
1932	1968	1,000.0	89.0	101.0	236.5	237.0	162.0	85.7	44.5	44.3
1933	1969	1,000.0	84.2	101.2	236.4	238.9	164.9	86.6	44.5	43.3
1934	1970	1,000.0	83.0	101.2	236.6	242.1	165.3	86.4	44.1	41.3
1935	1971	1,000.0	85.6	102.4	238.1	243.3	164.1	85.2	42.5	38.8
1936	1972	1,000.0	88.5	103.8	242.5	244.7	161.8	82.8	40.7	35.2
1937	1973	1,000.0	90.5	107.5	248.9	246.2	158.3	79.0	38.0	31.6
1938	1974	1,000.0	93.8	110.6	258.2	247.6	153.8	73.8	34.5	27.7

TABLE 8B. DISTRIBUTIONS OF WHITE WOMEN BY PARITY AS OF THE BEGINNING OF EACH YEAR 1917-74 BY AGE FOR EACH COHORT FROM 1867 TO 1959--CON.

(BASED ON CUMULATIVE BIRTH RATES)

EXACT AGE AND COHORT	AS OF JANUARY 1	TOTAL	PARITY							
			0	1	2	3	4	5	6	7 AND HIGHER
37 YEARS										
1880	1917	1,000.0	235.4	133.3	148.8	125.5	99.7	77.3	63.3	116.7
1881	1918	1,000.0	234.6	135.6	151.4	126.7	99.9	77.2	61.2	113.4
1882	1919	1,000.0	232.6	138.3	154.5	128.0	100.6	77.5	59.0	109.5
1883	1920	1,000.0	231.8	140.2	156.8	128.8	100.6	77.9	57.7	106.2
1884	1921	1,000.0	232.1	140.6	159.4	129.9	100.2	77.1	57.3	103.4
1885	1922	1,000.0	231.7	142.6	161.6	131.2	100.1	75.3	56.8	100.7
1886	1923	1,000.0	229.9	147.4	161.6	132.4	100.8	73.7	56.5	97.7
1887	1924	1,000.0	226.2	153.0	161.1	134.7	101.8	72.1	55.7	95.4
1888	1925	1,000.0	222.4	152.5	165.9	137.1	102.6	71.6	55.2	92.7
1889	1926	1,000.0	219.8	151.2	172.7	139.6	102.5	70.5	53.5	90.2
1890	1927	1,000.0	215.9	152.1	178.6	141.9	103.0	69.3	52.1	87.1
1891	1928	1,000.0	211.3	158.6	181.4	143.1	102.6	68.0	50.3	84.7
1892	1929	1,000.0	205.1	168.3	185.1	144.3	101.2	66.1	48.7	81.2
1893	1930	1,000.0	201.9	175.7	189.9	144.5	99.2	64.5	47.0	77.3
1894	1931	1,000.0	200.7	179.6	195.6	145.5	96.4	62.9	45.1	74.2
1895	1932	1,000.0	199.7	183.7	200.4	146.1	94.2	60.8	43.9	71.2
1896	1933	1,000.0	199.5	189.6	203.8	146.2	92.2	58.6	42.1	68.0
1897	1934	1,000.0	200.1	195.0	208.5	144.7	90.5	55.9	41.1	64.2
1898	1935	1,000.0	201.8	199.0	211.8	143.3	88.7	54.1	39.8	61.5
1899	1936	1,000.0	208.8	199.2	213.6	140.9	86.4	52.7	38.9	59.5
1900	1937	1,000.0	216.6	203.9	211.6	138.7	83.8	51.4	37.3	56.7
1901	1938	1,000.0	216.7	213.4	212.8	136.8	82.0	50.1	35.0	53.2
1902	1939	1,000.0	213.3	222.8	216.9	134.7	81.0	48.2	33.1	50.0
1903	1940	1,000.0	210.8	228.5	221.4	134.0	79.6	47.3	31.4	47.0
1904	1941	1,000.0	215.3	231.2	223.3	131.3	78.5	45.6	30.3	44.5
1905	1942	1,000.0	224.5	232.0	223.2	129.4	76.3	44.1	28.4	42.1
1906	1943	1,000.0	230.3	233.3	224.8	128.9	74.1	42.2	26.9	39.5
1907	1944	1,000.0	231.7	231.7	229.2	130.4	73.1	40.5	25.7	37.7
1908	1945	1,000.0	234.0	229.3	233.7	131.2	71.8	39.4	25.0	35.6
1909	1946	1,000.0	233.2	225.3	238.1	133.1	72.5	38.8	24.3	34.7
1910	1947	1,000.0	230.9	223.3	240.4	136.6	72.9	38.7	23.3	33.9
1911	1948	1,000.0	219.8	223.3	246.2	141.2	74.6	39.0	23.1	32.8
1912	1949	1,000.0	210.0	222.5	252.2	146.2	76.1	38.5	23.1	31.4
1913	1950	1,000.0	197.6	220.3	259.5	152.1	78.8	38.7	22.8	30.2
1914	1951	1,000.0	185.0	215.8	266.9	159.1	81.4	39.6	22.5	29.7
1915	1952	1,000.0	174.1	209.4	273.2	165.6	84.7	40.9	22.9	29.2
1916	1953	1,000.0	168.2	202.8	276.1	170.1	88.1	42.7	23.2	28.8
1917	1954	1,000.0	162.4	193.7	278.8	176.2	92.4	44.4	23.3	28.8
1918	1955	1,000.0	156.7	186.1	280.3	182.6	95.9	46.0	23.4	29.0
1919	1956	1,000.0	137.0	182.4	285.1	190.8	101.8	48.3	24.8	29.8
1920	1957	1,000.0	123.2	180.0	285.9	197.2	106.1	51.0	26.1	30.5
1921	1958	1,000.0	112.5	175.5	283.7	202.9	112.7	53.5	27.7	31.5
1922	1959	1,000.0	111.5	166.3	280.9	207.2	117.4	56.2	28.6	31.9
1923	1960	1,000.0	105.2	159.2	278.4	212.3	122.4	59.0	30.3	33.2
1924	1961	1,000.0	98.1	152.2	275.3	217.0	127.2	63.3	31.7	35.2
1925	1962	1,000.0	97.7	144.3	268.7	220.1	131.4	66.6	34.1	37.1
1926	1963	1,000.0	101.6	133.8	262.2	221.3	136.9	69.2	35.9	39.1
1927	1964	1,000.0	103.8	125.7	254.4	223.8	140.9	72.2	38.4	40.8
1928	1965	1,000.0	106.1	117.9	247.5	225.0	145.4	75.5	39.8	42.8
1929	1966	1,000.0	102.2	111.5	241.7	227.6	150.4	79.5	41.8	45.3
1930	1967	1,000.0	98.9	105.8	237.3	229.8	155.2	82.9	43.5	46.6
1931	1968	1,000.0	91.1	101.8	235.1	233.1	160.4	85.5	45.2	47.8
1932	1969	1,000.0	86.0	99.5	234.1	236.3	163.5	87.4	46.1	47.1
1933	1970	1,000.0	81.6	99.4	234.2	238.3	166.2	88.4	45.9	46.0
1934	1971	1,000.0	80.5	99.4	234.5	241.7	166.5	88.2	45.4	43.8
1935	1972	1,000.0	83.3	100.7	236.4	242.8	165.3	86.8	43.7	41.0
1936	1973	1,000.0	86.3	102.2	241.2	244.6	162.9	84.0	41.8	37.0
1937	1974	1,000.0	88.4	105.9	248.0	246.2	159.4	80.1	38.9	33.1

TABLE 8B. DISTRIBUTIONS OF WHITE WOMEN BY PARITY AS OF THE BEGINNING OF EACH YEAR 1917-74 BY AGE FOR EACH COHORT FROM 1867 TO 1959--CON.

(BASED ON CUMULATIVE BIRTH RATES)

EXACT AGE AND COHORT	AS OF JANUARY 1	TOTAL	PARITY							
			0	1	2	3	4	5	6	7 AND HIGHER
38 YEARS										
1879	1917	1,000.0	230.7	128.8	144.7	123.6	99.2	76.9	65.1	131.0
1880	1918	1,000.0	231.4	130.9	146.2	123.7	98.7	76.7	63.9	128.5
1881	1919	1,000.0	230.5	133.2	148.9	124.9	99.1	76.7	61.8	124.9
1882	1920	1,000.0	228.6	135.9	152.1	126.4	99.7	77.1	59.4	120.8
1883	1921	1,000.0	227.6	137.9	154.4	127.4	99.7	77.6	58.1	117.3
1884	1922	1,000.0	227.6	138.4	157.0	128.5	99.6	76.9	57.7	114.3
1885	1923	1,000.0	227.6	140.3	159.4	130.1	99.5	75.1	57.2	110.8
1886	1924	1,000.0	225.9	144.9	159.4	131.3	100.4	73.7	56.9	107.5
1887	1925	1,000.0	222.1	150.6	158.8	133.8	101.4	72.1	56.1	105.1
1888	1926	1,000.0	218.3	150.3	163.7	136.0	102.7	71.6	55.8	101.6
1889	1927	1,000.0	215.9	148.9	170.6	138.7	102.5	70.7	53.9	98.8
1890	1928	1,000.0	211.9	150.0	176.6	141.1	103.2	69.2	52.7	95.3
1891	1929	1,000.0	207.5	156.5	179.5	142.6	102.6	68.3	50.6	92.4
1892	1930	1,000.0	201.6	166.3	183.4	143.8	101.3	66.3	49.2	88.1
1893	1931	1,000.0	198.2	173.6	188.6	144.0	99.3	64.8	47.6	83.9
1894	1932	1,000.0	197.1	177.8	194.1	145.1	96.6	63.2	45.6	80.5
1895	1933	1,000.0	196.4	181.8	199.0	145.7	94.5	61.1	44.2	77.3
1896	1934	1,000.0	196.4	187.8	202.5	145.8	92.5	58.9	42.6	73.5
1897	1935	1,000.0	196.9	193.1	207.3	144.4	90.9	56.2	41.7	69.5
1898	1936	1,000.0	198.5	197.2	210.8	143.2	89.1	54.3	40.4	66.5
1899	1937	1,000.0	205.3	197.5	212.7	141.0	86.9	53.0	39.4	64.2
1900	1938	1,000.0	212.9	202.3	210.9	138.9	84.4	51.7	37.7	61.2
1901	1939	1,000.0	212.7	211.8	212.4	137.0	82.7	50.5	35.5	57.4
1902	1940	1,000.0	209.2	221.1	216.7	135.2	81.7	48.6	33.7	53.8
1903	1941	1,000.0	206.4	226.7	221.5	134.8	80.2	47.9	32.0	50.5
1904	1942	1,000.0	210.4	229.4	223.6	132.2	79.5	46.1	30.9	47.9
1905	1943	1,000.0	218.5	230.4	223.8	130.7	77.4	44.7	29.2	45.3
1906	1944	1,000.0	223.9	230.7	225.4	130.8	75.6	43.2	27.5	42.9
1907	1945	1,000.0	225.4	228.2	229.9	132.6	74.9	41.5	26.6	40.9
1908	1946	1,000.0	227.6	225.1	234.3	134.0	73.9	40.5	25.8	38.8
1909	1947	1,000.0	225.6	221.5	239.0	136.2	74.7	40.1	25.2	37.7
1910	1948	1,000.0	222.5	220.2	241.1	139.8	75.3	40.1	24.2	36.8
1911	1949	1,000.0	212.8	219.7	246.6	144.0	77.0	40.4	24.0	35.5
1912	1950	1,000.0	203.7	218.7	252.2	148.9	78.5	39.9	24.0	34.1
1913	1951	1,000.0	191.8	216.2	259.1	154.7	81.4	40.2	23.8	32.8
1914	1952	1,000.0	179.4	211.4	266.0	161.8	84.2	41.2	23.7	32.3
1915	1953	1,000.0	168.6	204.8	271.5	168.4	87.8	43.0	24.0	31.9
1916	1954	1,000.0	163.0	198.5	273.7	172.4	91.4	45.0	24.5	31.5
1917	1955	1,000.0	157.5	189.2	275.8	178.3	96.1	46.8	24.6	31.7
1918	1956	1,000.0	152.2	181.7	277.1	184.3	99.4	48.5	25.0	31.8
1919	1957	1,000.0	132.7	178.0	281.4	192.4	105.3	50.9	26.4	32.9
1920	1958	1,000.0	119.1	176.0	282.0	198.2	109.4	53.7	28.0	33.6
1921	1959	1,000.0	108.7	171.7	279.9	203.4	115.7	56.2	29.6	34.8
1922	1960	1,000.0	108.1	162.9	276.9	207.1	120.2	58.9	30.5	35.4
1923	1961	1,000.0	102.0	156.1	274.4	211.9	124.9	61.8	32.1	36.8
1924	1962	1,000.0	95.1	149.2	271.4	216.6	129.2	65.8	33.7	39.0
1925	1963	1,000.0	95.0	141.6	265.0	219.5	133.1	69.1	35.9	40.8
1926	1964	1,000.0	99.0	131.4	258.7	220.5	138.5	71.4	37.7	42.8
1927	1965	1,000.0	100.9	123.9	251.1	222.9	142.4	74.3	40.0	44.5
1928	1966	1,000.0	103.4	116.4	244.5	224.0	146.8	77.4	41.4	46.1
1929	1967	1,000.0	99.7	110.0	239.2	226.8	151.5	81.3	43.1	48.4
1930	1968	1,000.0	96.7	104.2	235.0	229.2	156.2	84.4	44.9	49.4
1931	1969	1,000.0	88.7	100.6	233.3	232.3	161.4	86.9	46.5	50.3
1932	1970	1,000.0	84.0	98.1	232.4	235.7	164.3	88.8	47.2	49.5
1933	1971	1,000.0	79.6	98.1	232.6	237.8	166.9	89.8	46.9	48.3
1934	1972	1,000.0	78.8	98.1	233.1	241.1	167.3	89.4	46.4	45.8
1935	1973	1,000.0	81.6	99.6	235.3	242.5	166.0	87.7	44.6	42.7
1936	1974	1,000.0	84.7	101.1	240.4	244.5	163.5	84.9	42.5	38.4

TABLE 8B. DISTRIBUTIONS OF WHITE WOMEN BY PARITY AS OF THE BEGINNING OF EACH YEAR 1917-74 BY AGE FOR EACH COHORT FROM 1867 TO 1959--CON.

(BASED ON CUMULATIVE BIRTH RATES)

EXACT AGE AND COHORT	AS OF JANUARY 1	TOTAL	PARITY							
			0	1	2	3	4	5	6	7 AND HIGHER
39 YEARS										
1878---------------	1917	1,000.0	225.6	125.3	141.7	122.0	98.9	76.7	65.8	144.0
1879---------------	1918	1,000.0	227.6	127.0	142.5	121.9	98.1	76.3	65.2	141.4
1880---------------	1919	1,000.0	228.2	129.1	144.1	122.0	97.7	76.2	64.0	138.7
1881---------------	1920	1,000.0	227.3	131.4	146.9	123.4	98.1	76.2	61.8	134.9
1882---------------	1921	1,000.0	225.3	134.2	150.0	125.1	98.7	76.7	59.4	130.6
1883---------------	1922	1,000.0	224.1	136.2	152.4	126.1	98.9	77.3	58.1	126.9
1884---------------	1923	1,000.0	224.4	136.7	155.1	127.4	98.9	76.6	57.7	123.2
1885---------------	1924	1,000.0	224.5	138.4	157.6	129.0	98.9	75.0	57.2	119.4
1886---------------	1925	1,000.0	222.7	143.1	157.5	130.3	99.9	73.6	56.9	116.0
1887---------------	1926	1,000.0	218.9	148.9	157.0	132.6	101.3	71.9	56.4	113.0
1888---------------	1927	1,000.0	215.3	148.6	162.0	135.0	102.4	71.7	56.0	109.0
1889---------------	1928	1,000.0	212.8	147.3	168.9	137.9	102.2	70.7	54.1	106.1
1890---------------	1929	1,000.0	208.9	148.4	175.0	140.5	103.0	69.4	52.7	102.1
1891---------------	1930	1,000.0	204.6	155.0	178.1	142.1	102.5	68.4	50.7	98.6
1892---------------	1931	1,000.0	198.7	164.7	182.2	143.1	101.3	66.3	49.6	94.1
1893---------------	1932	1,000.0	195.4	172.3	187.3	143.4	99.3	64.9	48.0	89.4
1894---------------	1933	1,000.0	194.5	176.5	192.8	144.7	96.6	63.2	45.8	85.9
1895---------------	1934	1,000.0	194.0	180.4	197.9	145.2	94.6	61.2	44.4	82.3
1896---------------	1935	1,000.0	193.9	186.4	201.5	145.3	92.7	58.9	43.0	78.3
1897---------------	1936	1,000.0	194.4	191.7	206.4	144.1	91.1	56.4	41.9	74.0
1898---------------	1937	1,000.0	195.9	196.0	209.9	143.0	89.4	54.5	40.7	70.6
1899---------------	1938	1,000.0	202.5	196.3	212.0	140.9	87.3	53.1	39.7	68.2
1900---------------	1939	1,000.0	209.9	201.1	210.3	139.0	84.7	51.9	38.0	65.1
1901---------------	1940	1,000.0	209.5	210.6	211.9	137.4	83.1	50.8	35.9	60.8
1902---------------	1941	1,000.0	205.9	219.7	216.5	135.8	82.0	49.0	34.1	57.0
1903---------------	1942	1,000.0	202.7	225.4	221.5	135.4	80.8	48.3	32.4	53.5
1904---------------	1943	1,000.0	205.8	228.3	223.8	133.0	80.3	46.5	31.5	50.8
1905---------------	1944	1,000.0	213.6	228.6	224.0	131.8	78.5	45.5	29.6	48.4
1906---------------	1945	1,000.0	219.1	228.2	225.6	132.2	76.9	44.0	28.2	45.8
1907---------------	1946	1,000.0	220.3	225.3	230.0	134.5	76.5	42.4	27.1	43.9
1908---------------	1947	1,000.0	221.7	222.4	234.7	136.1	75.6	41.5	26.5	41.5
1909---------------	1948	1,000.0	219.1	219.3	239.3	138.4	76.4	41.3	25.9	40.3
1910---------------	1949	1,000.0	217.0	217.6	241.3	141.6	77.2	41.2	24.8	39.3
1911---------------	1950	1,000.0	207.8	216.9	246.5	145.8	78.8	41.6	24.7	37.9
1912---------------	1951	1,000.0	199.1	215.6	251.9	150.6	80.5	41.1	24.7	36.5
1913---------------	1952	1,000.0	187.4	213.0	258.2	156.5	83.6	41.5	24.6	35.2
1914---------------	1953	1,000.0	175.0	208.0	264.6	163.7	86.5	42.8	24.7	34.7
1915---------------	1954	1,000.0	164.5	201.5	269.6	169.9	90.3	44.7	25.2	34.3
1916---------------	1955	1,000.0	159.0	195.2	271.5	173.6	94.1	46.9	25.7	34.0
1917---------------	1956	1,000.0	153.8	185.9	273.1	179.4	98.8	48.8	25.9	34.3
1918---------------	1957	1,000.0	148.9	178.4	274.2	185.3	101.8	50.6	26.3	34.5
1919---------------	1958	1,000.0	129.4	174.9	278.3	193.0	107.8	53.0	27.9	35.7
1920---------------	1959	1,000.0	116.1	173.1	279.0	198.4	111.6	55.8	29.4	36.6
1921---------------	1960	1,000.0	105.9	169.1	276.7	203.2	117.7	58.4	31.1	37.9
1922---------------	1961	1,000.0	105.5	160.6	273.7	206.7	121.9	61.1	31.9	38.6
1923---------------	1962	1,000.0	99.6	153.8	271.3	211.4	126.3	63.8	33.8	40.0
1924---------------	1963	1,000.0	92.9	147.2	268.5	215.8	130.5	67.8	35.1	42.2
1925---------------	1964	1,000.0	92.9	139.8	262.2	218.8	134.1	70.8	37.4	44.0
1926---------------	1965	1,000.0	96.7	130.0	256.1	219.5	139.7	73.0	39.0	46.0
1927---------------	1966	1,000.0	98.7	122.8	248.7	222.1	143.2	75.8	41.3	47.4
1928---------------	1967	1,000.0	101.4	115.4	242.4	223.2	147.6	78.8	42.4	48.8
1929---------------	1968	1,000.0	98.0	108.8	237.3	226.2	152.2	82.4	44.3	50.8
1930---------------	1969	1,000.0	94.8	103.4	233.4	228.6	156.9	85.5	45.8	51.6
1931---------------	1970	1,000.0	87.1	99.6	232.0	231.6	161.9	88.1	47.3	52.4
1932---------------	1971	1,000.0	82.4	97.2	231.2	235.1	164.7	89.9	48.0	51.5
1933---------------	1972	1,000.0	78.2	97.3	231.5	237.3	167.4	90.6	47.7	50.0
1934---------------	1973	1,000.0	77.5	97.3	232.2	240.8	167.8	90.0	47.1	47.3
1935---------------	1974	1,000.0	80.4	98.8	234.7	242.3	166.4	88.3	45.1	44.0

TABLE 8B. DISTRIBUTIONS OF WHITE WOMEN BY PARITY AS OF THE BEGINNING OF EACH YEAR 1917-74 BY AGE FOR EACH COHORT FROM 1867 TO 1959--CON.

(BASED ON CUMULATIVE BIRTH RATES)

EXACT AGE AND COHORT	AS OF JANUARY 1	TOTAL	PARITY							
			0	1	2	3	4	5	6	7 AND HIGHER
40 YEARS										
1877---------------	1917	1,000.0	221.8	122.2	138.4	120.1	98.1	77.7	65.6	156.1
1878---------------	1918	1,000.0	223.1	124.0	139.9	120.6	97.7	76.0	65.9	152.8
1879---------------	1919	1,000.0	225.1	125.7	140.6	120.6	96.9	75.7	65.3	150.1
1880---------------	1920	1,000.0	225.6	127.8	142.4	120.7	96.6	75.7	63.9	147.3
1881---------------	1921	1,000.0	224.6	130.2	145.2	122.2	97.0	75.7	61.7	143.4
1882---------------	1922	1,000.0	222.5	133.0	148.3	123.9	97.7	76.4	59.3	138.9
1883---------------	1923	1,000.0	221.5	135.0	150.8	125.1	98.1	76.9	58.0	134.6
1884---------------	1924	1,000.0	221.9	135.4	153.6	126.3	98.2	76.3	57.7	130.6
1885---------------	1925	1,000.0	221.9	137.2	156.0	128.1	98.2	74.7	57.2	126.7
1886---------------	1926	1,000.0	220.2	141.9	156.0	129.2	99.6	73.3	57.0	122.8
1887---------------	1927	1,000.0	216.5	147.6	155.6	131.7	100.9	71.8	56.3	119.6
1888---------------	1928	1,000.0	212.9	147.5	160.5	134.2	102.0	71.6	56.0	115.3
1889---------------	1929	1,000.0	210.4	146.2	167.7	137.1	101.8	70.7	54.1	112.0
1890---------------	1930	1,000.0	206.6	147.3	173.8	139.9	102.8	69.4	52.7	107.5
1891---------------	1931	1,000.0	202.3	153.9	177.0	141.4	102.3	68.3	50.9	103.9
1892---------------	1932	1,000.0	196.5	163.8	181.1	142.5	101.1	66.3	49.8	98.9
1893---------------	1933	1,000.0	193.4	171.3	186.4	142.7	99.2	64.7	48.2	94.1
1894---------------	1934	1,000.0	192.6	175.5	191.9	144.1	96.5	63.2	46.0	90.2
1895---------------	1935	1,000.0	192.1	179.3	197.1	144.6	94.6	61.2	44.6	86.5
1896---------------	1936	1,000.0	192.1	185.4	200.6	144.9	92.7	58.9	43.2	82.2
1897---------------	1937	1,000.0	192.5	190.8	205.5	143.9	91.2	56.5	42.1	77.5
1898---------------	1938	1,000.0	193.9	195.2	209.2	142.7	89.5	54.7	40.8	74.0
1899---------------	1939	1,000.0	200.3	195.4	211.4	140.9	87.3	53.3	39.9	71.5
1900---------------	1940	1,000.0	207.6	200.1	209.8	139.1	84.9	52.1	38.3	68.1
1901---------------	1941	1,000.0	207.1	209.6	211.6	137.7	83.1	51.1	36.2	63.6
1902---------------	1942	1,000.0	203.3	218.7	216.3	136.1	82.3	49.3	34.4	59.6
1903---------------	1943	1,000.0	199.4	224.6	221.4	135.8	81.4	48.6	32.8	56.0
1904---------------	1944	1,000.0	202.2	227.1	223.7	133.6	81.1	47.0	31.8	53.5
1905---------------	1945	1,000.0	210.0	226.9	224.0	132.6	79.4	46.1	30.0	51.0
1906---------------	1946	1,000.0	215.3	226.3	225.4	133.3	78.0	44.6	28.7	48.4
1907---------------	1947	1,000.0	215.8	223.5	230.2	135.7	77.7	43.2	27.6	46.3
1908---------------	1948	1,000.0	216.9	220.8	234.8	137.5	76.8	42.4	27.0	43.8
1909---------------	1949	1,000.0	214.9	217.5	239.3	139.6	77.7	42.2	26.4	42.4
1910---------------	1950	1,000.0	213.1	215.7	241.1	142.8	78.5	42.1	25.3	41.4
1911---------------	1951	1,000.0	204.2	214.8	246.2	146.9	80.1	42.6	25.2	40.0
1912---------------	1952	1,000.0	195.7	213.2	251.4	151.8	81.9	42.1	25.3	38.6
1913---------------	1953	1,000.0	184.0	210.7	257.1	157.6	85.3	42.6	25.5	37.2
1914---------------	1954	1,000.0	171.8	205.5	263.3	164.7	88.2	44.2	25.5	36.8
1915---------------	1955	1,000.0	161.4	199.1	267.9	170.6	92.2	46.1	26.2	36.5
1916---------------	1956	1,000.0	156.1	192.8	269.5	174.3	95.9	48.4	26.7	36.3
1917---------------	1957	1,000.0	151.2	183.4	271.0	179.9	100.5	50.4	26.9	36.7
1918---------------	1958	1,000.0	146.4	176.1	272.0	185.4	103.7	52.1	27.4	36.9
1919---------------	1959	1,000.0	127.1	172.7	276.0	193.1	109.3	54.5	29.0	38.3
1920---------------	1960	1,000.0	113.9	171.2	276.5	198.2	113.1	57.3	30.6	39.2
1921---------------	1961	1,000.0	103.9	167.4	274.1	202.7	119.1	60.0	32.2	40.6
1922---------------	1962	1,000.0	103.6	158.8	271.4	206.2	122.9	62.7	33.0	41.4
1923---------------	1963	1,000.0	97.9	152.3	269.0	210.8	127.2	65.2	34.9	42.7
1924---------------	1964	1,000.0	91.3	145.8	266.3	215.2	131.2	69.1	36.2	44.9
1925---------------	1965	1,000.0	91.0	138.8	260.2	218.0	134.9	72.0	38.5	46.6
1926---------------	1966	1,000.0	95.0	129.1	254.3	218.8	140.2	74.1	40.1	48.4
1927---------------	1967	1,000.0	97.1	122.1	247.0	221.5	143.8	76.7	42.1	49.7
1928---------------	1968	1,000.0	100.1	114.5	240.9	222.7	148.3	79.5	43.1	50.9
1929---------------	1969	1,000.0	96.5	108.2	236.2	225.7	152.5	83.2	45.1	52.6
1930---------------	1970	1,000.0	93.6	102.6	232.4	228.1	157.2	86.3	46.5	53.3
1931---------------	1971	1,000.0	85.9	99.0	231.0	231.1	162.1	88.9	47.9	54.1
1932---------------	1972	1,000.0	81.4	96.5	230.5	234.7	164.9	90.4	48.7	52.9
1933---------------	1973	1,000.0	77.2	96.8	230.9	237.0	167.6	91.1	48.1	51.3
1934---------------	1974	1,000.0	76.6	96.8	231.7	240.6	168.0	90.4	47.6	48.3

TABLE 8B. DISTRIBUTIONS OF WHITE WOMEN BY PARITY AS OF THE BEGINNING OF EACH YEAR 1917-74 BY AGE FOR EACH COHORT FROM 1867 TO 1959--CON.

(BASED ON CUMULATIVE BIRTH RATES)

EXACT AGE AND COHORT	AS OF JANUARY 1	TOTAL	PARITY							
			0	1	2	3	4	5	6	7 AND HIGHER
41 YEARS										
1876	1917	1,000.0	219.0	119.4	135.1	117.9	96.9	77.3	65.6	168.8
1877	1918	1,000.0	220.1	121.3	137.3	118.9	97.4	76.9	65.7	162.4
1878	1919	1,000.0	221.4	123.1	138.6	119.7	96.8	75.4	65.8	159.2
1879	1920	1,000.0	223.3	124.9	139.5	119.5	96.1	75.1	65.3	156.3
1880	1921	1,000.0	223.8	126.9	141.3	119.7	96.0	75.0	63.8	153.5
1881	1922	1,000.0	222.7	129.4	144.1	121.2	96.3	75.2	61.6	149.5
1882	1923	1,000.0	220.8	132.1	147.3	123.0	97.1	76.0	59.1	144.6
1883	1924	1,000.0	219.8	134.2	149.8	124.2	97.5	76.5	57.9	140.1
1884	1925	1,000.0	220.2	134.5	152.6	125.5	97.7	75.9	57.6	136.0
1885	1926	1,000.0	220.2	136.4	155.0	127.2	98.0	74.3	57.1	131.8
1886	1927	1,000.0	218.6	141.0	155.1	128.5	99.2	73.1	56.9	127.6
1887	1928	1,000.0	214.8	146.9	154.6	131.1	100.5	71.5	56.2	124.4
1888	1929	1,000.0	211.3	146.8	159.7	133.5	101.6	71.5	56.0	119.6
1889	1930	1,000.0	208.8	145.5	166.9	136.6	101.5	70.6	54.1	116.0
1890	1931	1,000.0	205.1	146.6	172.8	139.4	102.6	69.2	52.8	111.5
1891	1932	1,000.0	200.8	153.3	176.2	140.9	102.1	68.2	50.9	107.6
1892	1933	1,000.0	195.1	163.1	180.5	142.0	100.8	66.1	49.9	102.5
1893	1934	1,000.0	192.1	170.6	185.7	142.3	99.0	64.6	48.3	97.4
1894	1935	1,000.0	191.3	174.9	191.2	143.5	96.5	63.1	46.1	93.4
1895	1936	1,000.0	190.8	178.7	196.4	144.3	94.4	61.3	44.6	89.5
1896	1937	1,000.0	190.8	184.8	200.0	144.6	92.6	59.0	43.3	84.9
1897	1938	1,000.0	191.2	190.2	205.0	143.5	91.2	56.6	42.2	80.1
1898	1939	1,000.0	192.5	194.5	208.7	142.6	89.5	54.7	41.0	76.5
1899	1940	1,000.0	198.7	194.8	210.9	140.9	87.3	53.5	40.1	73.8
1900	1941	1,000.0	206.0	199.4	209.4	139.2	84.9	52.3	38.5	70.3
1901	1942	1,000.0	205.3	209.0	211.3	137.8	83.2	51.4	36.4	65.6
1902	1943	1,000.0	201.2	218.1	216.1	136.3	82.6	49.5	34.6	61.6
1903	1944	1,000.0	197.0	223.9	221.2	136.0	81.9	48.9	33.0	58.1
1904	1945	1,000.0	199.7	226.1	223.5	134.1	81.6	47.4	32.1	55.5
1905	1946	1,000.0	207.3	225.8	223.7	133.3	80.0	46.5	30.3	53.1
1906	1947	1,000.0	212.2	225.2	225.4	134.0	78.7	45.1	29.1	50.3
1907	1948	1,000.0	212.5	222.5	230.2	136.3	78.5	43.9	28.0	48.1
1908	1949	1,000.0	214.0	219.6	234.7	138.2	77.7	43.0	27.3	45.5
1909	1950	1,000.0	212.2	216.2	239.2	140.2	78.6	42.8	26.8	44.0
1910	1951	1,000.0	210.5	214.4	240.8	143.5	79.3	42.8	25.6	43.1
1911	1952	1,000.0	201.7	213.3	245.8	147.5	81.2	43.2	25.6	41.7
1912	1953	1,000.0	193.2	211.8	250.5	152.5	83.0	42.9	25.9	40.2
1913	1954	1,000.0	181.7	209.0	256.3	158.0	86.6	43.5	26.1	38.8
1914	1955	1,000.0	169.5	203.9	262.1	165.1	89.4	45.2	26.3	38.5
1915	1956	1,000.0	159.3	197.4	266.5	171.0	93.3	47.3	26.9	38.3
1916	1957	1,000.0	154.3	191.1	268.0	174.6	96.9	49.6	27.4	38.1
1917	1958	1,000.0	149.3	181.9	269.3	179.9	101.8	51.4	27.8	38.6
1918	1959	1,000.0	144.8	174.6	270.4	185.3	104.7	53.1	28.2	38.9
1919	1960	1,000.0	125.4	171.5	274.2	192.9	110.2	55.6	29.8	40.4
1920	1961	1,000.0	112.4	170.0	274.7	197.8	113.9	58.4	31.5	41.3
1921	1962	1,000.0	102.5	166.1	272.5	202.1	119.9	61.1	33.0	42.8
1922	1963	1,000.0	102.3	157.7	269.8	205.6	123.6	63.7	33.8	43.5
1923	1964	1,000.0	96.7	151.3	267.5	210.3	127.6	66.0	35.8	44.8
1924	1965	1,000.0	89.9	145.2	264.8	214.6	131.6	69.9	37.0	47.0
1925	1966	1,000.0	89.8	138.1	258.9	217.4	135.2	72.8	39.3	48.5
1926	1967	1,000.0	93.9	128.5	253.1	218.3	140.6	74.7	40.7	50.2
1927	1968	1,000.0	96.2	121.5	245.8	221.1	144.2	77.3	42.6	51.3
1928	1969	1,000.0	99.0	114.1	240.1	222.3	148.5	80.0	43.6	52.4
1929	1970	1,000.0	95.6	107.6	235.6	225.2	152.7	83.8	45.6	53.9
1930	1971	1,000.0	92.7	102.2	231.7	227.7	157.4	86.8	46.9	54.6
1931	1972	1,000.0	85.1	98.6	230.5	230.8	162.3	89.1	48.4	55.2
1932	1973	1,000.0	80.7	96.1	230.1	234.5	165.0	90.7	49.0	53.9
1933	1974	1,000.0	76.6	96.4	230.7	236.7	167.7	91.4	48.4	52.1

TABLE 8B. DISTRIBUTIONS OF WHITE WOMEN BY PARITY AS OF THE BEGINNING OF EACH YEAR 1917-74 BY AGE FOR EACH COHORT FROM 1867 TO 1959--CON.

(BASED ON CUMULATIVE BIRTH RATES)

EXACT AGE AND COHORT	AS OF JANUARY 1	TOTAL	PARITY							
			0	1	2	3	4	5	6	7 AND HIGHER
42 YEARS										
1875---------------	1917	1,000.0	216.2	116.9	132.3	116.1	96.1	77.0	65.8	179.6
1876---------------	1918	1,000.0	217.8	118.8	134.3	117.1	96.3	76.5	65.5	173.7
1877---------------	1919	1,000.0	218.9	120.7	136.4	118.2	96.7	76.3	65.5	167.3
1878---------------	1920	1,000.0	220.1	122.6	137.8	118.9	96.2	74.8	65.7	163.9
1879---------------	1921	1,000.0	222.0	124.4	138.6	118.7	95.7	74.4	65.1	161.1
1880---------------	1922	1,000.0	222.4	126.4	140.6	118.9	95.3	74.5	63.7	158.2
1881---------------	1923	1,000.0	221.5	128.8	143.4	120.4	95.9	74.7	61.3	154.0
1882---------------	1924	1,000.0	219.6	131.6	146.6	122.2	96.6	75.5	59.0	148.9
1883---------------	1925	1,000.0	218.6	133.6	149.1	123.5	97.1	76.1	57.7	144.3
1884---------------	1926	1,000.0	219.0	134.0	151.8	124.9	97.3	75.7	57.3	140.0
1885---------------	1927	1,000.0	219.0	135.9	154.4	126.6	97.6	74.0	56.9	135.6
1886---------------	1928	1,000.0	217.4	140.6	154.3	128.1	98.8	72.8	56.8	131.2
1887---------------	1929	1,000.0	213.6	146.5	154.0	130.6	100.1	71.4	56.0	127.8
1888---------------	1930	1,000.0	210.2	146.4	159.1	133.0	101.4	71.2	56.0	122.7
1889---------------	1931	1,000.0	207.7	145.1	166.2	136.2	101.2	70.4	54.2	119.0
1890---------------	1932	1,000.0	204.0	146.2	172.3	139.0	102.4	69.0	52.7	114.4
1891---------------	1933	1,000.0	199.8	152.8	175.8	140.4	101.9	68.0	50.9	110.4
1892---------------	1934	1,000.0	194.2	162.6	180.1	141.6	100.5	66.0	49.9	105.1
1893---------------	1935	1,000.0	191.2	170.3	185.1	141.9	98.8	64.5	48.3	99.9
1894---------------	1936	1,000.0	190.4	174.6	190.6	143.2	96.3	63.1	46.1	95.7
1895---------------	1937	1,000.0	189.9	178.4	195.9	144.0	94.3	61.2	44.7	91.6
1896---------------	1938	1,000.0	189.9	184.5	199.5	144.3	92.5	59.1	43.3	86.9
1897---------------	1939	1,000.0	190.3	189.7	204.7	143.3	91.1	56.6	42.2	82.1
1898---------------	1940	1,000.0	191.5	194.2	208.3	142.3	89.5	54.7	41.2	78.3
1899---------------	1941	1,000.0	197.6	194.5	210.6	140.7	87.3	53.6	40.2	75.5
1900---------------	1942	1,000.0	204.8	199.1	209.1	139.1	84.9	52.5	38.6	71.9
1901---------------	1943	1,000.0	204.1	208.6	211.0	137.8	83.3	51.6	36.5	67.1
1902---------------	1944	1,000.0	199.7	217.7	215.8	136.3	82.8	49.7	34.8	63.2
1903---------------	1945	1,000.0	195.3	223.4	220.9	136.3	82.0	49.2	33.2	59.7
1904---------------	1946	1,000.0	197.9	225.4	223.3	134.3	82.1	47.5	32.3	57.2
1905---------------	1947	1,000.0	205.3	225.1	223.6	133.7	80.3	46.9	30.5	54.6
1906---------------	1948	1,000.0	210.0	224.6	225.3	134.3	79.2	45.5	29.3	51.8
1907---------------	1949	1,000.0	210.6	221.7	230.0	136.7	79.0	44.3	28.2	49.5
1908---------------	1950	1,000.0	212.1	218.9	234.6	138.5	78.2	43.4	27.6	46.7
1909---------------	1951	1,000.0	210.4	215.5	238.9	140.5	79.1	43.3	27.0	45.3
1910---------------	1952	1,000.0	208.8	213.5	240.5	143.8	79.9	43.2	26.0	44.3
1911---------------	1953	1,000.0	200.0	212.4	245.2	147.9	81.8	43.8	25.9	43.0
1912---------------	1954	1,000.0	191.6	210.7	250.0	152.7	83.7	43.5	26.3	41.5
1913---------------	1955	1,000.0	180.1	208.0	255.4	158.3	87.3	44.1	26.7	40.1
1914---------------	1956	1,000.0	168.0	202.9	261.1	165.3	90.0	46.0	26.8	39.9
1915---------------	1957	1,000.0	158.0	196.2	265.4	171.2	94.0	48.1	27.3	39.8
1916---------------	1958	1,000.0	152.9	190.2	266.9	174.5	97.6	50.3	28.0	39.6
1917---------------	1959	1,000.0	148.1	180.9	268.3	179.7	102.3	52.2	28.4	40.1
1918---------------	1960	1,000.0	143.7	173.7	269.3	185.0	105.3	53.8	28.7	40.5
1919---------------	1961	1,000.0	124.3	170.7	273.1	192.5	110.7	56.3	30.4	42.0
1920---------------	1962	1,000.0	111.3	169.3	273.5	197.3	114.4	59.2	32.0	43.0
1921---------------	1963	1,000.0	101.6	165.3	271.4	201.6	120.4	61.8	33.5	44.4
1922---------------	1964	1,000.0	101.4	157.0	268.8	205.2	123.8	64.3	34.4	45.1
1923---------------	1965	1,000.0	95.7	150.9	266.4	210.0	127.7	66.6	36.3	46.4
1924---------------	1966	1,000.0	89.0	144.7	264.0	214.1	131.8	70.4	37.6	48.4
1925---------------	1967	1,000.0	89.0	137.7	258.1	217.1	135.3	73.2	39.8	49.8
1926---------------	1968	1,000.0	93.2	128.1	252.4	217.8	140.9	75.2	41.0	51.4
1927---------------	1969	1,000.0	95.4	121.3	245.2	220.8	144.3	77.6	43.0	52.4
1928---------------	1970	1,000.0	98.4	113.7	239.6	222.1	148.5	80.4	43.9	53.4
1929---------------	1971	1,000.0	95.0	107.3	235.1	225.0	152.8	84.1	45.8	54.9
1930---------------	1972	1,000.0	92.2	101.9	231.4	227.5	157.4	87.0	47.2	55.4
1931---------------	1973	1,000.0	84.6	98.4	230.2	230.6	162.4	89.2	48.6	56.0
1932---------------	1974	1,000.0	80.3	95.9	229.9	234.3	165.0	90.9	49.2	54.5

TABLE 8B. DISTRIBUTIONS OF WHITE WOMEN BY PARITY AS OF THE BEGINNING OF EACH YEAR 1917-74 BY AGE FOR EACH COHORT FROM 1867 TO 1959--CON.

(BASED ON CUMULATIVE BIRTH RATES)

EXACT AGE AND COHORT	AS OF JANUARY 1	TOTAL	PARITY							
			0	1	2	3	4	5	6	7 AND HIGHER
43 YEARS										
1874	1917	1,000.0	213.2	114.6	130.1	114.7	96.0	77.2	66.4	187.8
1875	1918	1,000.0	215.4	116.6	131.8	115.5	95.6	76.4	65.6	183.1
1876	1919	1,000.0	217.0	118.5	133.7	116.6	95.8	76.0	65.1	177.3
1877	1920	1,000.0	218.1	120.4	135.8	117.7	96.3	75.8	65.2	170.7
1878	1921	1,000.0	219.3	122.2	137.3	118.3	95.9	74.2	65.4	167.4
1879	1922	1,000.0	221.1	124.1	138.1	118.2	95.2	73.9	64.9	164.5
1880	1923	1,000.0	221.6	126.1	140.1	118.3	95.0	74.1	63.3	161.5
1881	1924	1,000.0	220.7	128.5	142.9	119.9	95.5	74.3	61.1	157.1
1882	1925	1,000.0	218.8	131.3	146.1	121.7	96.3	75.1	58.7	152.0
1883	1926	1,000.0	217.9	133.1	148.7	123.1	96.8	75.8	57.4	147.2
1884	1927	1,000.0	218.2	133.8	151.4	124.3	97.1	75.4	57.1	142.7
1885	1928	1,000.0	218.2	135.6	154.0	126.3	97.2	73.8	56.8	138.1
1886	1929	1,000.0	216.6	140.4	153.9	127.8	98.5	72.6	56.6	133.6
1887	1930	1,000.0	212.9	146.3	153.6	130.2	99.9	71.2	55.8	130.1
1888	1931	1,000.0	209.5	146.2	158.6	132.7	101.2	70.9	56.1	124.8
1889	1932	1,000.0	207.0	144.9	165.8	135.9	101.0	70.2	54.1	121.1
1890	1933	1,000.0	203.3	146.0	171.9	138.7	102.2	68.9	52.6	116.4
1891	1934	1,000.0	199.2	152.5	175.5	140.1	101.6	68.0	50.8	112.3
1892	1935	1,000.0	193.6	162.4	179.7	141.3	100.3	65.9	49.9	106.9
1893	1936	1,000.0	190.6	170.2	184.7	141.6	98.6	64.5	48.2	101.6
1894	1937	1,000.0	189.8	174.4	190.3	143.0	96.2	63.0	46.0	97.3
1895	1938	1,000.0	189.3	178.3	195.5	143.8	94.2	61.1	44.8	93.0
1896	1939	1,000.0	189.3	184.3	199.2	144.1	92.4	59.0	43.4	88.3
1897	1940	1,000.0	189.6	189.6	204.4	143.1	91.1	56.5	42.3	83.4
1898	1941	1,000.0	190.8	194.1	208.0	142.1	89.5	54.7	41.3	79.5
1899	1942	1,000.0	196.8	194.4	210.4	140.5	87.3	53.7	40.2	76.7
1900	1943	1,000.0	204.0	199.0	208.9	139.0	84.8	52.6	38.7	73.0
1901	1944	1,000.0	203.2	208.4	210.8	137.7	83.3	51.7	36.6	68.3
1902	1945	1,000.0	198.7	217.4	215.6	136.3	82.8	49.9	34.9	64.4
1903	1946	1,000.0	194.2	223.0	220.7	136.4	82.2	49.3	33.2	61.0
1904	1947	1,000.0	196.6	225.1	223.1	134.5	82.3	47.7	32.4	58.3
1905	1948	1,000.0	204.0	224.7	223.5	133.8	80.5	47.2	30.6	55.7
1906	1949	1,000.0	208.8	224.2	225.1	134.5	79.4	45.7	29.5	52.8
1907	1950	1,000.0	209.4	221.4	229.8	136.8	79.3	44.6	28.3	50.4
1908	1951	1,000.0	211.0	218.5	234.4	138.6	78.4	43.7	27.8	47.6
1909	1952	1,000.0	209.3	215.1	238.6	140.6	79.4	43.6	27.2	46.2
1910	1953	1,000.0	207.7	212.9	240.2	144.0	80.2	43.6	26.1	45.3
1911	1954	1,000.0	198.9	211.9	244.8	147.9	82.3	44.1	26.2	43.9
1912	1955	1,000.0	190.6	210.1	249.4	152.9	84.0	43.9	26.6	42.5
1913	1956	1,000.0	179.1	207.4	254.8	158.4	87.6	44.6	27.1	41.0
1914	1957	1,000.0	167.1	202.2	260.4	165.5	90.3	46.5	27.1	40.9
1915	1958	1,000.0	157.1	195.6	264.7	171.1	94.4	48.6	27.7	40.8
1916	1959	1,000.0	152.1	189.7	266.2	174.3	97.9	50.8	28.3	40.7
1917	1960	1,000.0	147.3	180.4	267.6	179.4	102.7	52.6	28.8	41.2
1918	1961	1,000.0	143.0	173.2	268.5	184.8	105.5	54.3	29.1	41.6
1919	1962	1,000.0	123.6	170.2	272.4	192.1	111.0	56.8	30.7	43.2
1920	1963	1,000.0	110.7	168.8	272.8	196.9	114.7	59.6	32.4	44.1
1921	1964	1,000.0	101.0	164.9	270.7	201.3	120.5	62.2	33.9	45.5
1922	1965	1,000.0	100.7	156.9	268.1	204.9	123.8	64.6	34.8	46.2
1923	1966	1,000.0	95.1	150.6	265.8	209.7	127.8	67.0	36.6	47.4
1924	1967	1,000.0	88.5	144.4	263.5	213.8	131.9	70.7	37.8	49.4
1925	1968	1,000.0	88.6	137.4	257.7	216.7	135.4	73.5	40.0	50.7
1926	1969	1,000.0	92.7	128.0	252.0	217.5	141.0	75.4	41.2	52.2
1927	1970	1,000.0	95.0	121.1	244.8	220.7	144.2	77.9	43.2	53.1
1928	1971	1,000.0	98.0	113.5	239.3	221.9	148.6	80.6	44.0	54.1
1929	1972	1,000.0	94.7	107.1	234.9	224.8	152.8	84.3	45.9	55.5
1930	1973	1,000.0	91.9	101.7	231.3	227.3	157.5	87.0	47.4	55.9
1931	1974	1,000.0	84.3	98.3	230.1	230.5	162.4	89.2	48.8	56.4

TABLE 8B. DISTRIBUTIONS OF WHITE WOMEN BY PARITY AS OF THE BEGINNING OF EACH YEAR 1917-74 BY AGE FOR EACH COHORT FROM 1867 TO 1959--CON.

(BASED ON CUMULATIVE BIRTH RATES)

EXACT AGE AND COHORT	AS OF JANUARY 1	TOTAL	PARITY							
			0	1	2	3	4	5	6	7 AND HIGHER
44 YEARS										
1873	1917	1,000.0	210.3	112.3	128.3	113.6	96.3	77.9	67.2	194.1
1874	1918	1,000.0	212.7	114.3	129.8	114.2	95.7	76.7	66.1	190.5
1875	1919	1,000.0	214.9	116.3	131.4	115.1	95.2	76.1	65.2	185.8
1876	1920	1,000.0	216.4	118.3	133.4	116.1	95.5	75.7	64.8	179.8
1877	1921	1,000.0	217.5	120.2	135.4	117.3	96.0	75.4	64.9	173.3
1878	1922	1,000.0	218.7	122.0	136.9	117.9	95.6	73.8	65.1	170.0
1879	1923	1,000.0	220.5	123.9	137.8	117.8	94.9	73.6	64.5	167.0
1880	1924	1,000.0	221.0	125.9	139.8	117.9	94.7	73.8	63.0	163.9
1881	1925	1,000.0	220.1	128.3	142.6	119.5	95.2	74.1	60.8	159.4
1882	1926	1,000.0	218.3	131.0	145.8	121.4	96.1	74.8	58.4	154.2
1883	1927	1,000.0	217.4	132.9	148.4	122.8	96.6	75.5	57.2	149.2
1884	1928	1,000.0	217.7	133.6	151.1	124.1	96.8	75.2	57.0	144.5
1885	1929	1,000.0	217.7	135.4	153.7	126.1	97.0	73.6	56.6	139.9
1886	1930	1,000.0	216.2	140.2	153.7	127.5	98.3	72.4	56.4	135.3
1887	1931	1,000.0	212.5	146.1	153.3	129.9	99.7	71.0	55.8	131.7
1888	1932	1,000.0	209.1	146.0	158.3	132.5	101.1	70.7	56.0	126.3
1889	1933	1,000.0	206.5	144.8	165.6	135.6	100.9	70.0	54.0	122.6
1890	1934	1,000.0	202.9	145.8	171.7	138.5	102.0	68.7	52.6	117.8
1891	1935	1,000.0	198.8	152.4	175.2	139.9	101.4	67.9	50.7	113.7
1892	1936	1,000.0	193.2	162.3	179.5	141.0	100.2	65.8	49.8	108.2
1893	1937	1,000.0	190.2	170.1	184.5	141.4	98.5	64.4	48.1	102.8
1894	1938	1,000.0	189.4	174.4	190.0	142.8	96.2	62.9	46.0	98.3
1895	1939	1,000.0	188.9	178.2	195.3	143.6	94.1	61.1	44.7	94.1
1896	1940	1,000.0	188.9	184.2	199.0	143.9	92.4	58.9	43.4	89.3
1897	1941	1,000.0	189.2	189.5	204.2	143.0	91.1	56.5	42.2	84.3
1898	1942	1,000.0	190.3	194.1	207.8	142.0	89.5	54.7	41.3	80.3
1899	1943	1,000.0	196.3	194.3	210.3	140.4	87.2	53.7	40.2	77.6
1900	1944	1,000.0	203.4	198.9	208.8	138.9	84.8	52.6	38.7	73.9
1901	1945	1,000.0	202.6	208.3	210.5	137.7	83.3	51.8	36.6	69.2
1902	1946	1,000.0	198.0	217.3	215.4	136.2	83.0	49.9	34.9	65.3
1903	1947	1,000.0	193.4	222.9	220.5	136.5	82.2	49.4	33.3	61.8
1904	1948	1,000.0	195.8	224.9	222.9	134.7	82.3	47.8	32.5	59.1
1905	1949	1,000.0	203.3	224.5	223.3	133.9	80.6	47.3	30.7	56.4
1906	1950	1,000.0	208.1	224.0	224.9	134.6	79.6	45.8	29.6	53.4
1907	1951	1,000.0	208.7	221.2	229.6	136.9	79.4	44.7	28.5	51.0
1908	1952	1,000.0	210.4	218.2	234.2	138.6	78.6	43.9	27.9	48.2
1909	1953	1,000.0	208.6	214.8	238.4	140.7	79.5	43.8	27.4	46.8
1910	1954	1,000.0	207.0	212.6	240.0	143.9	80.5	43.8	26.3	45.9
1911	1955	1,000.0	198.3	211.5	244.5	148.0	82.4	44.4	26.3	44.6
1912	1956	1,000.0	190.0	209.8	249.0	152.9	84.1	44.2	26.9	43.1
1913	1957	1,000.0	178.5	207.0	254.4	158.5	87.8	44.8	27.3	41.7
1914	1958	1,000.0	166.5	201.9	260.0	165.4	90.5	46.8	27.3	41.6
1915	1959	1,000.0	156.6	195.3	264.3	170.9	94.6	48.9	27.9	41.5
1916	1960	1,000.0	151.6	189.4	265.8	174.1	98.1	51.0	28.6	41.4
1917	1961	1,000.0	146.9	180.1	267.1	179.3	102.8	52.8	29.1	41.9
1918	1962	1,000.0	142.6	172.9	268.0	184.6	105.6	54.7	29.3	42.3
1919	1963	1,000.0	123.2	169.9	272.0	191.8	111.2	57.0	30.9	44.0
1920	1964	1,000.0	110.3	168.6	272.4	196.7	114.7	59.9	32.6	44.8
1921	1965	1,000.0	100.6	164.8	270.3	201.0	120.6	62.3	34.1	46.3
1922	1966	1,000.0	100.3	156.8	267.7	204.7	123.8	64.9	34.9	46.9
1923	1967	1,000.0	94.8	150.4	265.5	209.5	127.8	67.2	36.8	48.0
1924	1968	1,000.0	88.2	144.3	263.2	213.5	132.0	70.9	37.9	50.0
1925	1969	1,000.0	88.3	137.3	257.5	216.5	135.4	73.6	40.1	51.3
1926	1970	1,000.0	92.5	127.8	251.8	217.4	140.9	75.6	41.3	52.7
1927	1971	1,000.0	94.8	121.0	244.6	220.5	144.2	78.1	43.3	53.5
1928	1972	1,000.0	97.8	113.4	239.2	221.8	148.5	80.7	44.1	54.5
1929	1973	1,000.0	94.5	107.0	234.8	224.7	152.8	84.4	46.0	55.8
1930	1974	1,000.0	91.7	101.7	231.2	227.2	157.5	87.0	47.5	56.2

TABLE 8B. DISTRIBUTIONS OF WHITE WOMEN BY PARITY AS OF THE BEGINNING OF EACH YEAR 1917-74 BY AGE FOR EACH COHORT FROM 1867 TO 1959--CON.

(BASED ON CUMULATIVE BIRTH RATES)

EXACT AGE AND COHORT	AS OF JANUARY 1	TOTAL	PARITY: 0	1	2	3	4	5	6	7 AND HIGHER
45 YEARS										
1872	1917	1,000.0	207.7	110.3	126.5	112.7	96.4	78.4	67.8	200.2
1873	1918	1,000.0	210.0	112.1	128.1	113.4	96.0	77.6	67.0	195.8
1874	1919	1,000.0	212.4	114.1	129.6	114.0	95.3	76.5	66.0	192.1
1875	1920	1,000.0	214.6	116.2	131.1	114.9	94.9	75.9	65.1	187.3
1876	1921	1,000.0	216.1	118.1	133.2	115.8	95.3	75.4	64.7	181.4
1877	1922	1,000.0	217.2	120.1	135.1	117.1	95.7	75.2	64.8	174.8
1878	1923	1,000.0	218.4	121.9	136.6	117.7	95.4	73.6	64.9	171.5
1879	1924	1,000.0	220.2	123.8	137.6	117.5	94.7	73.4	64.3	168.5
1880	1925	1,000.0	220.7	125.8	139.5	117.7	94.5	73.6	62.9	165.3
1881	1926	1,000.0	219.8	128.2	142.4	119.3	95.0	73.9	60.6	160.8
1882	1927	1,000.0	218.0	130.9	145.6	121.2	96.0	74.6	58.3	155.4
1883	1928	1,000.0	217.1	132.8	148.2	122.7	96.4	75.4	57.1	150.3
1884	1929	1,000.0	217.4	133.5	151.0	123.9	96.6	75.1	56.9	145.6
1885	1930	1,000.0	217.4	135.4	153.5	125.9	96.9	73.5	56.5	140.9
1886	1931	1,000.0	215.9	140.2	153.5	127.3	98.2	72.3	56.3	136.3
1887	1932	1,000.0	212.3	145.9	153.2	129.8	99.5	70.9	55.8	132.6
1888	1933	1,000.0	208.9	145.9	158.2	132.3	101.0	70.6	55.9	127.2
1889	1934	1,000.0	206.3	144.7	165.5	135.4	100.8	69.8	54.1	123.4
1890	1935	1,000.0	202.7	145.7	171.6	138.3	101.9	68.6	52.5	118.7
1891	1936	1,000.0	198.5	152.5	175.0	139.7	101.4	67.8	50.6	114.5
1892	1937	1,000.0	193.0	162.3	179.3	140.9	100.1	65.7	49.7	109.0
1893	1938	1,000.0	190.0	170.1	184.3	141.3	98.5	64.2	48.1	103.5
1894	1939	1,000.0	189.2	174.3	189.9	142.7	96.1	62.9	45.9	99.0
1895	1940	1,000.0	188.7	178.2	195.1	143.5	94.1	61.0	44.7	94.7
1896	1941	1,000.0	188.7	184.2	198.8	143.8	92.4	58.9	43.4	89.8
1897	1942	1,000.0	188.9	189.5	204.1	143.0	91.1	56.4	42.2	84.8
1898	1943	1,000.0	190.0	194.1	207.7	141.9	89.4	54.7	41.3	80.9
1899	1944	1,000.0	196.0	194.2	210.3	140.3	87.1	53.7	40.2	78.2
1900	1945	1,000.0	203.1	198.8	208.7	138.8	84.8	52.6	38.7	74.5
1901	1946	1,000.0	202.2	208.3	210.3	137.7	83.3	51.9	36.6	69.7
1902	1947	1,000.0	197.6	217.2	215.3	136.2	83.0	50.0	34.9	65.8
1903	1948	1,000.0	193.0	222.8	220.4	136.5	82.2	49.4	33.5	62.2
1904	1949	1,000.0	195.4	224.8	222.8	134.7	82.4	47.9	32.5	59.5
1905	1950	1,000.0	202.9	224.4	223.2	133.9	80.7	47.4	30.7	56.8
1906	1951	1,000.0	207.7	223.9	224.9	134.5	79.7	45.9	29.6	53.8
1907	1952	1,000.0	208.3	221.1	229.5	136.9	79.5	44.8	28.5	51.4
1908	1953	1,000.0	210.0	218.1	234.1	138.6	78.6	44.1	27.9	48.6
1909	1954	1,000.0	208.2	214.7	238.2	140.7	79.6	43.9	27.5	47.2
1910	1955	1,000.0	206.6	212.5	239.8	144.0	80.5	43.9	26.4	46.3
1911	1956	1,000.0	197.9	211.4	244.3	148.0	82.4	44.6	26.4	45.0
1912	1957	1,000.0	189.7	209.6	248.7	153.0	84.2	44.3	27.0	43.5
1913	1958	1,000.0	178.2	206.8	254.2	158.4	88.0	44.8	27.5	42.1
1914	1959	1,000.0	166.2	201.8	259.7	165.3	90.6	47.0	27.4	42.0
1915	1960	1,000.0	156.3	195.2	264.0	170.8	94.7	49.0	28.1	41.9
1916	1961	1,000.0	151.4	189.2	265.5	174.0	98.2	51.1	28.8	41.8
1917	1962	1,000.0	146.7	179.9	266.9	179.1	102.9	52.9	29.2	42.4
1918	1963	1,000.0	142.4	172.7	267.8	184.5	105.7	54.8	29.4	42.7
1919	1964	1,000.0	123.0	169.7	271.8	191.7	111.2	57.2	31.0	44.4
1920	1965	1,000.0	110.1	168.5	272.2	196.5	114.8	59.9	32.8	45.2
1921	1966	1,000.0	100.4	164.7	270.1	200.9	120.6	62.4	34.2	46.7
1922	1967	1,000.0	100.1	156.8	267.5	204.5	123.8	65.0	35.0	47.3
1923	1968	1,000.0	94.6	150.4	265.3	209.3	127.9	67.3	36.8	48.4
1924	1969	1,000.0	88.0	144.3	263.0	213.4	132.1	70.9	37.9	50.4
1925	1970	1,000.0	88.2	137.2	257.4	216.4	135.3	73.7	40.2	51.6
1926	1971	1,000.0	92.4	127.7	251.7	217.3	140.9	75.7	41.4	52.9
1927	1972	1,000.0	94.7	121.0	244.5	220.4	144.2	78.1	43.4	53.7
1928	1973	1,000.0	97.7	113.4	239.1	221.8	148.5	80.7	44.1	54.7
1929	1974	1,000.0	94.4	107.0	234.7	224.7	152.8	84.4	46.0	56.0

TABLE 8B. DISTRIBUTIONS OF WHITE WOMEN BY PARITY AS OF THE BEGINNING OF EACH YEAR 1917-74 BY AGE FOR EACH COHORT FROM 1867 TO 1959--CON.

(BASED ON CUMULATIVE BIRTH RATES)

EXACT AGE AND COHORT	AS OF JANUARY 1	TOTAL	PARITY							
			0	1	2	3	4	5	6	7 AND HIGHER
46 YEARS										
1871---------------	1917	1,000.0	205.3	108.5	125.0	111.6	96.5	78.9	68.3	205.9
1872---------------	1918	1,000.0	207.5	110.2	126.4	112.5	96.3	78.2	67.7	201.2
1873---------------	1919	1,000.0	209.8	112.0	128.0	113.2	95.8	77.5	66.9	196.8
1874---------------	1920	1,000.0	212.2	114.1	129.4	113.9	95.1	76.3	66.0	193.0
1875---------------	1921	1,000.0	214.4	116.1	131.0	114.7	94.8	75.7	65.0	188.3
1876---------------	1922	1,000.0	215.9	118.1	133.0	115.7	95.1	75.2	64.7	182.3
1877---------------	1923	1,000.0	217.0	120.1	134.9	117.0	95.6	75.1	64.6	175.7
1878---------------	1924	1,000.0	218.2	121.9	136.4	117.6	95.3	73.4	64.8	172.4
1879---------------	1925	1,000.0	220.0	123.8	137.4	117.4	94.6	73.3	64.2	169.3
1880---------------	1926	1,000.0	220.5	125.8	139.4	117.5	94.4	73.5	62.8	166.1
1881---------------	1927	1,000.0	219.6	128.1	142.4	119.2	94.9	73.7	60.6	161.5
1882---------------	1928	1,000.0	217.8	130.9	145.5	121.1	95.9	74.5	58.2	156.1
1883---------------	1929	1,000.0	216.9	132.8	148.1	122.6	96.3	75.3	57.1	150.9
1884---------------	1930	1,000.0	217.2	133.5	150.9	123.8	96.5	75.1	56.8	146.2
1885---------------	1931	1,000.0	217.2	135.4	153.4	125.8	96.8	73.5	56.4	141.5
1886---------------	1932	1,C00.0	215.8	140.1	153.4	127.3	98.1	72.2	56.2	136.9
1887---------------	1933	1,000.0	212.2	145.8	153.1	129.7	99.5	70.8	55.8	133.1
1888---------------	1934	1,000.0	208.8	145.8	158.2	132.2	100.9	70.5	55.9	127.7
1889---------------	1935	1,000.0	206.2	144.7	165.4	135.3	100.7	69.8	54.0	123.9
1890---------------	1936	1,000.0	202.6	145.7	171.5	138.2	101.9	68.5	52.4	119.2
1891---------------	1937	1,000.0	198.4	152.5	174.9	139.6	101.3	67.8	50.6	114.9
1892---------------	1938	1,000.0	192.9	162.3	179.2	140.8	100.1	65.6	49.7	109.4
1893---------------	1939	1,000.0	189.9	170.1	184.2	141.2	98.5	64.1	48.1	103.9
1894---------------	1940	1,000.0	189.1	174.3	189.8	142.6	96.1	62.9	45.8	99.4
1895---------------	1941	1,000.0	188.6	178.2	195.0	143.4	94.1	61.0	44.7	95.0
1896---------------	1942	1,000.0	188.6	184.1	198.8	143.8	92.4	58.8	43.4	90.1
1897---------------	1943	1,000.0	188.8	189.4	204.1	143.0	91.0	56.4	42.2	85.1
1898---------------	1944	1,000.0	189.8	194.1	207.7	141.8	89.4	54.7	41.3	81.2
1899---------------	1945	1,000.0	195.8	194.2	210.2	140.3	87.1	53.7	40.2	78.5
1900---------------	1946	1,000.0	202.9	198.8	208.6	138.8	84.8	52.6	38.7	74.8
1901---------------	1947	1,000.0	202.0	208.3	210.2	137.7	83.3	51.9	36.6	70.0
1902---------------	1948	1,000.0	197.4	217.2	215.2	136.2	83.0	50.0	35.0	66.0
1903---------------	1949	1,000.0	192.8	222.8	220.3	136.5	82.2	49.5	33.5	62.4
1904---------------	1950	1,000.0	195.2	224.8	222.7	134.7	82.4	48.0	32.5	59.7
1905---------------	1951	1,000.0	202.7	224.4	223.1	133.9	80.7	47.5	30.7	57.0
1906---------------	1952	1,000.0	207.5	223.9	224.8	134.5	79.7	46.0	29.6	54.0
1907---------------	1953	1,000.0	208.1	221.1	229.4	136.9	79.5	44.9	28.5	51.6
1908---------------	1954	1,000.0	209.8	218.1	234.0	138.6	78.6	44.2	27.9	48.8
1909---------------	1955	1,000.0	208.0	214.7	238.1	140.7	79.6	44.0	27.5	47.4
1910---------------	1956	1,000.0	206.4	212.5	239.7	144.0	80.5	44.0	26.4	46.5
1911---------------	1957	1,000.0	197.7	211.3	244.2	148.1	82.4	44.6	26.5	45.2
1912---------------	1958	1,000.0	189.5	209.6	248.6	152.9	84.3	44.3	27.1	43.7
1913---------------	1959	1,000.0	178.0	206.8	254.1	158.3	88.1	44.8	27.6	42.3
1914---------------	1960	1,000.0	166.0	201.8	259.6	165.2	90.6	47.1	27.5	42.2
1915---------------	1961	1,000.0	156.2	195.1	263.9	170.7	94.8	49.0	28.2	42.1
1916---------------	1962	1,000.0	151.3	189.1	265.4	173.9	98.2	51.2	28.8	42.1
1917---------------	1963	1,000.0	146.6	179.8	266.8	179.0	103.0	52.9	29.3	42.6
1918---------------	1964	1,000.0	142.3	172.6	267.7	184.5	105.7	54.9	29.4	42.9
1919---------------	1965	1,000.0	122.9	169.7	271.6	191.7	111.2	57.2	31.1	44.6
1920---------------	1966	1,000.0	110.0	168.5	272.1	196.4	114.8	60.0	32.8	45.4
1921---------------	1967	1,C00.0	100.3	164.7	270.0	200.8	120.6	62.5	34.2	46.9
1922---------------	1968	1,000.0	100.0	156.8	267.4	204.4	123.8	65.1	35.0	47.5
1923---------------	1969	1,000.0	94.5	150.4	265.2	209.3	127.9	67.3	36.8	48.6
1924---------------	1970	1,000.0	87.9	144.3	263.0	213.3	132.1	70.9	38.0	50.5
1925---------------	1971	1,000.0	88.1	137.2	257.4	216.3	135.3	73.7	40.3	51.7
1926---------------	1972	1,000.0	92.3	127.7	251.7	217.3	140.9	75.6	41.5	53.0
1927---------------	1973	1,000.0	94.7	120.9	244.5	220.4	144.2	78.1	43.4	53.8
1928---------------	1974	1,000.0	97.7	113.3	239.1	221.8	148.5	80.7	44.1	54.8

TABLE 8B. DISTRIBUTIONS OF WHITE WOMEN BY PARITY AS OF THE BEGINNING OF EACH YEAR 1917-74 BY AGE FOR EACH COHORT FROM 1867 TO 1959--CON.

(BASED ON CUMULATIVE BIRTH RATES)

EXACT AGE AND COHORT	AS OF JANUARY 1	TOTAL	PARITY 0	1	2	3	4	5	6	7 AND HIGHER
47 YEARS										
1870	1917	1,000.0	203.0	106.9	123.4	110.8	96.6	79.4	68.8	211.1
1871	1918	1,000.0	205.2	108.4	125.0	111.5	96.4	78.8	68.2	206.5
1872	1919	1,000.0	207.4	110.1	126.4	112.4	96.1	78.1	67.7	201.8
1873	1920	1,000.0	209.7	112.0	127.9	113.1	95.6	77.5	66.9	197.3
1874	1921	1,000.0	212.1	114.0	129.4	113.8	94.9	76.2	66.0	193.6
1875	1922	1,000.0	214.3	116.1	130.9	114.6	94.7	75.6	65.0	188.8
1876	1923	1,000.0	215.8	118.1	132.9	115.6	95.1	75.1	64.6	182.8
1877	1924	1,000.0	216.9	120.1	134.8	116.9	95.6	74.9	64.6	176.2
1878	1925	1,000.0	218.1	121.9	136.3	117.5	95.3	73.3	64.7	172.9
1879	1926	1,000.0	219.9	123.8	137.3	117.3	94.6	73.2	64.1	169.8
1880	1927	1,000.0	220.4	125.8	139.3	117.4	94.4	73.4	62.8	166.5
1881	1928	1,000.0	219.5	128.1	142.3	119.2	94.8	73.6	60.6	161.9
1882	1929	1,000.0	217.7	130.9	145.4	121.1	95.8	74.5	58.1	156.5
1883	1930	1,000.0	216.8	132.8	148.0	122.6	96.2	75.3	57.1	151.2
1884	1931	1,000.0	217.1	133.5	150.9	123.7	96.4	75.1	56.8	146.5
1885	1932	1,000.0	217.1	135.4	153.3	125.8	96.8	73.4	56.4	141.8
1886	1933	1,000.0	215.7	140.1	153.4	127.2	98.0	72.2	56.2	137.2
1887	1934	1,000.0	212.1	145.8	153.1	129.6	99.5	70.7	55.8	133.4
1888	1935	1,000.0	208.8	145.7	158.2	132.1	100.9	70.5	55.8	128.0
1889	1936	1,000.0	206.1	144.7	165.4	135.2	100.7	69.8	53.9	124.2
1890	1937	1,000.0	202.6	145.6	171.5	138.2	101.8	68.5	52.4	119.4
1891	1938	1,000.0	198.4	152.5	174.8	139.5	101.4	67.7	50.6	115.1
1892	1939	1,000.0	192.9	162.3	179.1	140.7	100.1	65.6	49.7	109.6
1893	1940	1,000.0	189.8	170.2	184.1	141.2	98.4	64.1	48.1	104.1
1894	1941	1,000.0	189.0	174.4	189.7	142.6	96.0	62.9	45.8	99.6
1895	1942	1,000.0	188.5	178.2	195.0	143.4	94.1	60.9	44.7	95.2
1896	1943	1,000.0	188.5	184.1	198.8	143.8	92.4	58.8	43.3	90.3
1897	1944	1,000.0	188.7	189.4	204.1	143.0	91.0	56.4	42.1	85.3
1898	1945	1,000.0	189.7	194.1	207.7	141.7	89.5	54.7	41.2	81.4
1899	1946	1,000.0	195.7	194.2	210.2	140.3	87.0	53.7	40.2	78.7
1900	1947	1,000.0	202.8	198.8	208.6	138.7	84.8	52.6	38.7	75.0
1901	1948	1,C00.0	201.9	208.3	210.1	137.8	83.3	51.8	36.7	70.1
1902	1949	1,000.0	197.3	217.2	215.2	136.2	83.0	50.0	35.0	66.1
1903	1950	1,000.0	192.7	222.8	220.3	136.5	82.2	49.5	33.5	62.5
1904	1951	1,000.0	195.1	224.8	222.7	134.6	82.5	48.0	32.5	59.8
1905	1952	1,000.0	202.6	224.4	223.1	133.9	80.7	47.5	30.7	57.1
1906	1953	1,000.0	207.4	223.9	224.8	134.5	79.7	46.0	29.6	54.1
1907	1954	1,000.0	208.0	221.1	229.4	136.8	79.5	45.0	28.5	51.7
1908	1955	1,000.0	209.7	218.1	234.0	138.5	78.6	44.3	27.9	48.9
1909	1956	1,000.0	207.9	214.7	238.1	140.7	79.5	44.1	27.5	47.5
1910	1957	1,000.0	206.3	212.5	239.6	144.0	80.5	44.1	26.4	46.6
1911	1958	1,000.0	197.6	211.3	244.2	148.1	82.3	44.7	26.5	45.3
1912	1959	1,000.0	189.4	209.6	248.6	152.8	84.4	44.3	27.1	43.8
1913	1960	1,000.0	177.9	206.8	254.1	158.2	88.1	44.8	27.7	42.4
1914	1961	1,000.0	165.9	201.8	259.6	165.1	90.6	47.2	27.5	42.3
1915	1962	1,000.0	156.1	195.1	263.9	170.6	94.8	49.1	28.2	42.2
1916	1963	1,000.0	151.3	189.0	265.3	173.9	98.2	51.3	28.8	42.2
1917	1964	1,000.0	146.6	179.7	266.8	179.0	102.9	53.0	29.3	42.7
1918	1965	1,000.0	142.3	172.6	267.6	184.5	105.7	54.9	29.4	43.0
1919	1966	1,000.0	122.9	169.7	271.5	191.7	111.2	57.2	31.1	44.7
1920	1967	1,000.0	110.0	168.5	272.0	196.4	114.8	60.0	32.8	45.5
1921	1968	1,000.0	100.3	164.7	269.9	200.8	120.6	62.5	34.2	47.0
1922	1969	1,000.0	100.0	156.8	267.3	204.4	123.8	65.1	35.0	47.6
1923	1970	1,000.0	94.5	150.4	265.2	209.2	127.9	67.3	36.8	48.7
1924	1971	1,000.0	87.9	144.3	262.9	213.3	132.1	70.9	38.0	50.6
1925	1972	1,000.0	88.1	137.2	257.4	216.2	135.4	73.6	40.3	51.8
1926	1973	1,000.0	92.3	127.7	251.6	217.4	140.8	75.7	41.5	53.0
1927	1974	1,000.0	94.7	120.9	244.5	220.4	144.1	78.2	43.4	53.8

TABLE 8B. DISTRIBUTIONS OF WHITE WOMEN BY PARITY AS OF THE BEGINNING OF EACH YEAR 1917-74 BY AGE FOR EACH COHORT FROM 1867 TO 1959--CON.

(BASED ON CUMULATIVE BIRTH RATES)

EXACT AGE AND COHORT	AS OF JANUARY 1	TOTAL	PARITY							
			0	1	2	3	4	5	6	7 AND HIGHER
48 YEARS										
1869	1917	1,000.0	200.8	105.2	122.0	110.1	96.7	79.9	69.4	215.9
1870	1918	1,000.0	203.0	106.8	123.4	110.7	96.6	79.4	68.7	211.4
1871	1919	1,000.0	205.1	108.4	125.0	111.4	96.3	78.9	68.1	206.8
1872	1920	1,000.0	207.4	110.0	126.4	112.4	96.0	78.1	67.7	202.0
1873	1921	1,000.0	209.7	111.9	127.9	113.0	95.6	77.5	66.8	197.6
1874	1922	1,000.0	212.1	114.0	129.3	113.8	94.8	76.2	66.0	193.8
1875	1923	1,000.0	214.2	116.1	130.9	114.6	94.6	75.6	65.0	189.0
1876	1924	1,000.0	215.8	118.0	132.9	115.6	95.0	75.1	64.6	183.0
1877	1925	1,000.0	216.9	120.0	134.8	116.9	95.5	74.9	64.6	176.4
1878	1926	1,000.0	218.0	122.0	136.2	117.5	95.3	73.2	64.7	173.1
1879	1927	1,000.0	219.9	123.8	137.2	117.3	94.5	73.2	64.1	170.0
1880	1928	1,000.0	220.4	125.8	139.2	117.4	94.3	73.4	62.8	166.7
1881	1929	1,000.0	219.5	128.1	142.2	119.2	94.8	73.5	60.6	162.1
1882	1930	1,000.0	217.6	131.0	145.3	121.1	95.8	74.4	58.1	156.7
1883	1931	1,000.0	216.7	132.9	148.0	122.5	96.2	75.2	57.1	151.4
1884	1932	1,000.0	217.1	133.5	150.8	123.7	96.4	75.0	56.8	146.7
1885	1933	1,000.0	217.1	135.4	153.2	125.8	96.8	73.4	56.4	141.9
1886	1934	1,000.0	215.7	140.1	153.3	127.2	98.0	72.2	56.2	137.3
1887	1935	1,000.0	212.1	145.8	153.1	129.5	99.5	70.7	55.8	133.5
1888	1936	1,000.0	208.8	145.7	158.2	132.0	100.9	70.5	55.8	128.1
1889	1937	1,000.0	206.1	144.7	165.4	135.1	100.7	69.8	53.9	124.3
1890	1938	1,000.0	202.6	145.6	171.5	138.1	101.9	68.4	52.4	119.5
1891	1939	1,000.0	198.4	152.5	174.8	139.4	101.4	67.7	50.6	115.2
1892	1940	1,000.0	192.9	162.3	179.1	140.7	100.0	65.6	49.7	109.7
1893	1941	1,000.0	189.8	170.2	184.1	141.2	98.3	64.1	48.1	104.2
1894	1942	1,000.0	189.0	174.4	189.7	142.6	95.9	62.9	45.8	99.7
1895	1943	1,000.0	188.5	178.2	195.0	143.4	94.1	60.9	44.6	95.3
1896	1944	1,000.0	188.5	184.1	198.8	143.7	92.5	58.8	43.2	90.4
1897	1945	1,000.0	188.7	189.4	204.1	142.9	91.1	56.4	42.0	85.4
1898	1946	1,000.0	189.7	194.1	207.7	141.6	89.5	54.7	41.2	81.5
1899	1947	1,000.0	195.7	194.2	210.2	140.2	87.0	53.7	40.2	78.8
1900	1948	1,000.0	202.8	198.8	208.5	138.8	84.8	52.5	38.7	75.1
1901	1949	1,000.0	201.9	208.3	210.1	137.8	83.3	51.8	36.6	70.2
1902	1950	1,000.0	197.3	217.2	215.2	136.2	83.0	49.9	35.1	66.1
1903	1951	1,000.0	192.7	222.8	220.3	136.4	82.3	49.5	33.5	62.5
1904	1952	1,000.0	195.1	224.8	222.7	134.6	82.5	48.0	32.5	59.8
1905	1953	1,000.0	202.6	224.4	223.1	133.9	80.7	47.5	30.7	57.1
1906	1954	1,000.0	207.4	223.9	224.8	134.4	79.7	46.0	29.7	54.1
1907	1955	1,000.0	208.0	221.1	229.4	136.7	79.5	45.1	28.5	51.7
1908	1956	1,000.0	209.7	218.1	234.0	138.5	78.5	44.4	27.9	48.9
1909	1957	1,000.0	207.9	214.7	238.1	140.6	79.5	44.2	27.5	47.5
1910	1958	1,000.0	206.3	212.5	239.6	144.0	80.4	44.2	26.4	46.6
1911	1959	1,000.0	197.6	211.3	244.2	148.0	82.4	44.6	26.6	45.3
1912	1960	1,000.0	189.4	209.6	248.6	152.7	84.4	44.3	27.2	43.8
1913	1961	1,000.0	177.9	206.8	254.1	158.1	88.1	44.9	27.7	42.4
1914	1962	1,000.0	165.9	201.8	259.6	165.1	90.5	47.3	27.5	42.3
1915	1963	1,000.0	156.1	195.1	263.8	170.6	94.8	49.2	28.2	42.2
1916	1964	1,000.0	151.3	189.0	265.3	173.9	98.1	51.4	28.8	42.2
1917	1965	1,000.0	146.6	179.7	266.8	179.0	102.9	52.9	29.4	42.7
1918	1966	1,000.0	142.3	172.6	267.6	184.5	105.7	54.8	29.5	43.0
1919	1967	1,000.0	122.9	169.7	271.5	191.7	111.2	57.2	31.1	44.7
1920	1968	1,000.0	110.0	168.5	272.0	196.4	114.8	60.0	32.8	45.5
1921	1969	1,000.0	100.3	164.7	269.9	200.8	120.6	62.5	34.2	47.0
1922	1970	1,000.0	100.0	156.8	267.3	204.4	123.8	65.1	35.0	47.6
1923	1971	1,000.0	94.5	150.4	265.2	209.2	127.9	67.3	36.8	48.7
1924	1972	1,000.0	87.9	144.3	262.9	213.3	132.1	70.9	38.0	50.6
1925	1973	1,000.0	88.1	137.2	257.4	216.2	135.4	73.6	40.3	51.8
1926	1974	1,000.0	92.3	127.7	251.6	217.4	140.8	75.7	41.5	53.0

TABLE 8B. DISTRIBUTIONS OF WHITE WOMEN BY PARITY AS OF THE BEGINNING OF EACH YEAR 1917-74 BY AGE FOR EACH COHORT FROM 1867 TO 1959--CON.

(BASED ON CUMULATIVE BIRTH RATES)

EXACT AGE AND COHORT	AS OF JANUARY 1	TOTAL	PARITY							
			0	1	2	3	4	5	6	7 AND HIGHER
49 YEARS										
1868----------------	1917	1,000.0	198.7	103.5	120.6	109.4	96.7	80.5	70.1	220.5
1869----------------	1918	1,000.0	200.8	105.2	122.0	110.0	96.7	79.9	69.4	216.0
1870----------------	1919	1,000.0	203.0	106.8	123.4	110.6	96.6	79.4	68.7	211.5
1871----------------	1920	1,000.0	205.1	108.4	125.0	111.3	96.3	78.9	68.1	206.9
1872----------------	1921	1,000.0	207.4	110.0	126.4	112.3	96.0	78.1	67.6	202.2
1873----------------	1922	1,000.0	209.7	111.9	127.9	112.9	95.6	77.5	66.8	197.7
1874----------------	1923	1,000.0	212.1	114.0	129.3	113.7	94.8	76.2	66.0	193.9
1875----------------	1924	1,000.0	214.2	116.1	130.9	114.5	94.6	75.6	65.0	189.1
1876----------------	1925	1,000.0	215.8	118.0	132.9	115.5	95.0	75.1	64.6	183.1
1877----------------	1926	1,000.0	216.9	120.0	134.8	116.8	95.5	74.9	64.6	176.5
1878----------------	1927	1,000.0	218.0	122.0	136.2	117.5	95.2	73.2	64.7	173.2
1879----------------	1928	1,000.0	219.9	123.8	137.2	117.2	94.5	73.2	64.1	170.1
1880----------------	1929	1,000.0	220.4	125.8	139.2	117.4	94.2	73.4	62.8	166.8
1881----------------	1930	1,000.0	219.5	128.1	142.2	119.2	94.8	73.4	60.6	162.2
1882----------------	1931	1,000.0	217.6	131.0	145.3	121.1	95.8	74.3	58.1	156.8
1883----------------	1932	1,000.0	216.7	132.9	148.0	122.5	96.2	75.1	57.1	151.5
1884----------------	1933	1,000.0	217.1	133.5	150.8	123.7	96.4	74.9	56.8	146.8
1885----------------	1934	1,000.0	217.1	135.4	153.2	125.8	96.7	73.4	56.4	142.0
1886----------------	1935	1,000.0	215.7	140.1	153.3	127.2	97.9	72.3	56.1	137.4
1887----------------	1936	1,000.0	212.1	145.8	153.1	129.5	99.5	70.7	55.7	133.6
1888----------------	1937	1,000.0	208.8	145.7	158.2	132.0	100.9	70.5	55.7	128.2
1889----------------	1938	1,000.0	206.1	144.7	165.4	135.1	100.7	69.8	53.8	124.4
1890----------------	1939	1,000.0	202.6	145.6	171.5	138.1	101.8	68.5	52.4	119.5
1891----------------	1940	1,000.0	198.4	152.5	174.8	139.4	101.3	67.8	50.5	115.3
1892----------------	1941	1,000.0	192.9	162.3	179.1	140.7	100.0	65.6	49.7	109.7
1893----------------	1942	1,000.0	189.8	170.2	184.1	141.2	98.3	64.1	48.1	104.2
1894----------------	1943	1,000.0	189.0	174.4	189.7	142.6	95.9	62.9	45.8	99.7
1895----------------	1944	1,000.0	188.5	178.2	195.0	143.4	94.1	60.9	44.6	95.3
1896----------------	1945	1,000.0	188.5	184.1	198.8	143.7	92.5	58.8	43.2	90.4
1897----------------	1946	1,000.0	188.7	189.4	204.1	142.9	91.1	56.4	42.0	85.4
1898----------------	1947	1,000.0	189.7	194.1	207.7	141.6	89.5	54.7	41.2	81.5
1899----------------	1948	1,000.0	195.7	194.2	210.2	140.2	87.0	53.7	40.2	78.8
1900----------------	1949	1,000.0	202.8	198.8	208.5	138.8	84.8	52.5	38.7	75.1
1901----------------	1950	1,000.0	201.9	208.3	210.1	137.8	83.3	51.8	36.6	70.2
1902----------------	1951	1,000.0	197.3	217.2	215.2	136.2	83.0	49.9	35.1	66.1
1903----------------	1952	1,000.0	192.7	222.8	220.3	136.4	82.3	49.5	33.5	62.5
1904----------------	1953	1,000.0	195.1	224.8	222.7	134.6	82.5	48.0	32.5	59.8
1905----------------	1954	1,000.0	202.6	224.4	223.1	133.9	80.7	47.5	30.7	57.1
1906----------------	1955	1,000.0	207.4	223.9	224.8	134.4	79.7	46.0	29.7	54.1
1907----------------	1956	1,000.0	208.0	221.1	229.4	136.7	79.5	45.1	28.5	51.7
1908----------------	1957	1,000.0	209.7	218.1	234.0	138.5	78.5	44.4	27.9	48.9
1909----------------	1958	1,000.0	207.9	214.7	238.1	140.6	79.5	44.2	27.5	47.5
1910----------------	1959	1,000.0	206.3	212.5	239.6	144.0	80.4	44.2	26.4	46.6
1911----------------	1960	1,000.0	197.6	211.3	244.2	148.0	82.4	44.6	26.6	45.3
1912----------------	1961	1,000.0	189.4	209.6	248.6	152.7	84.4	44.3	27.2	43.8
1913----------------	1962	1,000.0	177.9	206.8	254.1	158.1	88.1	44.9	27.7	42.4
1914----------------	1963	1,000.0	165.9	201.8	259.6	165.1	90.5	47.3	27.5	42.3
1915----------------	1964	1,000.0	156.1	195.1	263.8	170.6	94.8	49.2	28.2	42.2
1916----------------	1965	1,000.0	151.3	189.0	265.3	173.9	98.1	51.4	28.8	42.2
1917----------------	1966	1,000.0	146.6	179.7	266.8	179.0	102.9	52.9	29.4	42.7
1918----------------	1967	1,000.0	142.3	172.6	267.6	184.5	105.7	54.8	29.5	43.0
1919----------------	1968	1,000.0	122.9	169.7	271.5	191.7	111.2	57.2	31.1	44.7
1920----------------	1969	1,000.0	110.0	168.5	272.0	196.4	114.8	60.0	32.8	45.5
1921----------------	1970	1,000.0	100.3	164.7	269.9	200.8	120.6	62.5	34.2	47.0
1922----------------	1971	1,000.0	100.0	156.8	267.3	204.4	123.8	65.1	35.0	47.6
1923----------------	1972	1,000.0	94.5	150.4	265.2	209.2	127.9	67.3	36.8	48.7
1924----------------	1973	1,000.0	87.9	144.3	262.9	213.3	132.1	70.9	38.0	50.6
1925----------------	1974	1,000.0	88.1	137.2	257.4	216.2	135.4	73.6	40.3	51.8

TABLE 8B. DISTRIBUTIONS OF WHITE WOMEN BY PARITY AS OF THE BEGINNING OF EACH YEAR 1917-74 BY AGE FOR EACH COHORT FROM 1867 TO 1959--CON.

(BASED ON CUMULATIVE BIRTH RATES)

EXACT AGE AND COHORT	AS OF JANUARY 1	TOTAL	PARITY							
			0	1	2	3	4	5	6	7 AND HIGHER
50 YEARS										
1867	1917	1,000.0	196.7	101.7	119.2	108.7	96.8	81.1	70.8	225.0
1868	1918	1,000.0	198.7	103.5	120.6	109.3	96.8	80.5	70.0	220.6
1869	1919	1,000.0	200.8	105.2	122.0	109.9	96.8	79.9	69.3	216.1
1870	1920	1,000.0	203.0	106.8	123.4	110.5	96.7	79.4	68.7	211.5
1871	1921	1,000.0	205.1	108.4	125.0	111.2	96.4	78.9	68.0	207.0
1872	1922	1,000.0	207.4	110.0	126.4	112.2	96.1	78.1	67.6	202.2
1873	1923	1,000.0	209.7	111.9	127.9	112.8	95.7	77.5	66.8	197.7
1874	1924	1,000.0	212.1	114.0	129.3	113.7	94.8	76.2	66.0	193.9
1875	1925	1,000.0	214.2	116.1	130.9	114.5	94.6	75.6	65.0	189.1
1876	1926	1,000.0	215.8	118.0	132.9	115.5	95.0	75.1	64.6	183.1
1877	1927	1,000.0	216.9	120.0	134.8	116.8	95.5	74.9	64.6	176.5
1878	1928	1,000.0	218.0	122.0	136.2	117.5	95.2	73.2	64.7	173.2
1879	1929	1,000.0	219.9	123.8	137.2	117.2	94.5	73.2	64.1	170.1
1880	1930	1,000.0	220.4	125.8	139.2	117.4	94.2	73.4	62.8	166.8
1881	1931	1,000.0	219.5	128.1	142.2	119.2	94.8	73.4	60.6	162.2
1882	1932	1,000.0	217.6	131.0	145.3	121.1	95.8	74.3	58.1	156.8
1883	1933	1,000.0	216.7	132.9	148.0	122.5	96.2	75.1	57.1	151.5
1884	1934	1,000.0	217.1	133.5	150.8	123.7	96.4	74.9	56.8	146.8
1885	1935	1,000.0	217.1	135.4	153.2	125.8	96.7	73.4	56.4	142.0
1886	1936	1,000.0	215.7	140.1	153.3	127.2	97.9	72.3	56.1	137.4
1887	1937	1,000.0	212.1	145.8	153.1	129.5	99.5	70.7	55.7	133.6
1888	1938	1,000.0	208.8	145.7	158.2	132.0	100.9	70.5	55.7	128.2
1889	1939	1,000.0	206.1	144.7	165.4	135.1	100.7	69.8	53.8	124.4
1890	1940	1,000.0	202.6	145.6	171.5	138.1	101.8	68.5	52.4	119.5
1891	1941	1,000.0	198.4	152.5	174.8	139.4	101.3	67.8	50.5	115.3
1892	1942	1,000.0	192.9	162.3	179.1	140.7	100.0	65.6	49.7	109.7
1893	1943	1,000.0	189.8	170.2	184.1	141.2	98.3	64.1	48.1	104.2
1894	1944	1,000.0	189.0	174.4	189.7	142.6	95.9	62.9	45.8	99.7
1895	1945	1,000.0	188.5	178.2	195.0	143.4	94.1	60.9	44.6	95.3
1896	1946	1,000.0	188.5	184.1	198.8	143.7	92.5	58.8	43.2	90.4
1897	1947	1,000.0	188.7	189.4	204.1	142.9	91.1	56.4	42.0	85.4
1898	1948	1,000.0	189.7	194.1	207.7	141.6	89.5	54.7	41.2	81.5
1899	1949	1,000.0	195.7	194.2	210.2	140.2	87.0	53.7	40.2	78.8
1900	1950	1,000.0	202.8	198.8	208.5	138.8	84.8	52.5	38.7	75.1
1901	1951	1,000.0	201.9	208.3	210.1	137.8	83.3	51.8	36.6	70.2
1902	1952	1,000.0	197.3	217.2	215.2	136.2	83.0	49.9	35.1	66.1
1903	1953	1,000.0	192.7	222.8	220.3	136.4	82.3	49.5	33.5	62.5
1904	1954	1,000.0	195.1	224.8	222.7	134.6	82.5	48.0	32.5	59.8
1905	1955	1,000.0	202.6	224.4	223.1	133.9	80.7	47.5	30.7	57.1
1906	1956	1,000.0	207.4	223.9	224.8	134.4	79.7	46.0	29.7	54.1
1907	1957	1,000.0	208.0	221.1	229.4	136.7	79.5	45.1	28.5	51.7
1908	1958	1,000.0	209.7	218.1	234.0	138.5	78.5	44.4	27.9	48.9
1909	1959	1,000.0	207.9	214.7	238.1	140.6	79.5	44.2	27.5	47.5
1910	1960	1,000.0	206.3	212.5	239.6	144.0	80.4	44.2	26.4	46.6
1911	1961	1,000.0	197.6	211.3	244.2	148.0	82.4	44.6	26.6	45.3
1912	1962	1,000.0	189.4	209.6	248.6	152.7	84.4	44.3	27.2	43.8
1913	1963	1,000.0	177.9	206.8	254.1	158.1	88.1	44.9	27.7	42.4
1914	1964	1,000.0	165.9	201.8	259.6	165.1	90.5	47.3	27.5	42.3
1915	1965	1,000.0	156.1	195.1	263.8	170.6	94.8	49.2	28.2	42.2
1916	1966	1,000.0	151.3	189.0	265.3	173.9	98.1	51.4	28.8	42.2
1917	1967	1,000.0	146.6	179.7	266.8	179.0	102.9	52.9	29.4	42.7
1918	1968	1,000.0	142.3	172.6	267.6	184.5	105.7	54.8	29.5	43.0
1919	1969	1,000.0	122.9	169.7	271.5	191.7	111.2	57.2	31.1	44.7
1920	1970	1,000.0	110.0	168.5	272.0	196.4	114.8	60.0	32.8	45.5
1921	1971	1,000.0	100.3	164.7	269.9	200.8	120.6	62.5	34.2	47.0
1922	1972	1,000.0	100.0	156.8	267.3	204.4	123.8	65.1	35.0	47.6
1923	1973	1,000.0	94.5	150.4	265.2	209.2	127.9	67.3	36.8	48.7
1924	1974	1,000.0	87.9	144.3	262.9	213.3	132.1	70.9	38.0	50.6

TABLE 8C. DISTRIBUTIONS OF ALL OTHER WOMEN BY PARITY AS OF THE BEGINNING OF EACH YEAR 1917-74 BY AGE FOR EACH COHORT FROM 1867 TO 1959

(BASED ON CUMULATIVE BIRTH RATES)

EXACT AGE AND COHORT	AS OF JANUARY 1	TOTAL	PARITY							
			0	1	2	3	4	5	6	7 AND HIGHER
15 YEARS										
1902----------------	1917	1,000.0	988.7	11.3	*	*	*	*	*	*
1903----------------	1918	1,000.0	987.2	12.8	*	*	*	*	*	*
1904----------------	1919	1,000.0	987.9	12.1	*	*	*	*	*	*
1905----------------	1920	1,C00.0	988.8	11.2	*	*	*	*	*	*
1906----------------	1921	1,000.0	987.0	13.0	*	*	*	*	*	*
1907----------------	1922	1,000.0	986.4	13.6	*	*	*	*	*	*
1908----------------	1923	1,000.0	987.7	12.3	*	*	*	*	*	*
1909----------------	1924	1,000.0	986.8	13.2	*	*	*	*	*	*
1910----------------	1925	1,C00.0	985.7	14.3	*	*	*	*	*	*
1911----------------	1926	1,000.0	984.4	15.6	*	*	*	*	*	*
1912----------------	1927	1,000.0	983.6	16.4	*	*	*	*	*	*
1913----------------	1928	1,C00.0	983.9	16.1	*	*	*	*	*	*
1914----------------	1929	1,000.0	985.3	14.7	*	*	*	*	*	*
1915----------------	1930	1,000.0	985.8	14.2	*	*	*	*	*	*
1916----------------	1931	1,000.0	985.5	14.5	*	*	*	*	*	*
1917----------------	1932	1,000.0	986.1	13.9	*	*	*	*	*	*
1918----------------	1933	1,000.0	985.8	14.2	*	*	*	*	*	*
1919----------------	1934	1,000.0	986.4	13.6	*	*	*	*	*	*
1920----------------	1935	1,000.0	986.1	13.9	*	*	*	*	*	*
1921----------------	1936	1,000.0	984.5	15.5	*	*	*	*	*	*
1922----------------	1937	1,000.0	985.2	14.8	*	*	*	*	*	*
1923----------------	1938	1,000.0	984.3	15.7	*	*	*	*	*	*
1924----------------	1939	1,C00.0	983.6	16.4	*	*	*	*	*	*
1925----------------	1940	1,000.0	983.2	16.8	*	*	*	*	*	*
1926----------------	1941	1,000.0	983.0	17.0	*	*	*	*	*	*
1927----------------	1942	1,000.0	982.1	17.9	*	*	*	*	*	*
1928----------------	1943	1,000.0	981.8	18.2	*	*	*	*	*	*
1929----------------	1944	1,000.0	981.5	18.5	*	*	*	*	*	*
1930----------------	1945	1,000.0	982.9	17.1	*	*	*	*	*	*
1931----------------	1946	1,000.0	982.5	17.5	*	*	*	*	*	*
1932----------------	1947	1,000.0	983.6	16.4	*	*	*	*	*	*
1933----------------	1948	1,000.0	979.6	20.4	*	*	*	*	*	*
1934----------------	1949	1,000.0	977.9	22.1	*	*	*	*	*	*
1935----------------	1950	1,000.0	977.4	22.6	*	*	*	*	*	*
1936----------------	1951	1,000.0	976.8	23.2	*	*	*	*	*	*
1937----------------	1952	1,000.0	975.7	24.3	*	*	*	*	*	*
1938----------------	1953	1,000.0	977.9	22.1	*	*	*	*	*	*
1939----------------	1954	1,000.0	978.0	22.0	*	*	*	*	*	*
1940----------------	1955	1,000.0	976.2	23.8	*	*	*	*	*	*
1941----------------	1956	1,000.0	977.3	22.7	*	*	*	*	*	*
1942----------------	1957	1,000.0	977.3	22.7	*	*	*	*	*	*
1943----------------	1958	1,000.0	977.0	23.0	*	*	*	*	*	*
1944----------------	1959	1,000.0	978.5	21.5	*	*	*	*	*	*
1945----------------	1960	1,000.0	977.7	22.3	*	*	*	*	*	*
1946----------------	1961	1,000.0	978.7	21.3	*	*	*	*	*	*
1947----------------	1962	1,000.0	978.8	21.2	*	*	*	*	*	*
1948----------------	1963	1,000.0	979.9	20.1	*	*	*	*	*	*
1949----------------	1964	1,000.0	980.1	19.9	*	*	*	*	*	*
1950----------------	1965	1,000.0	980.1	19.9	*	*	*	*	*	*
1951----------------	1966	1,000.0	979.6	20.4	*	*	*	*	*	*
1952----------------	1967	1,000.0	979.5	20.5	*	*	*	*	*	*
1953----------------	1968	1,000.0	978.7	21.3	*	*	*	*	*	*
1954----------------	1969	1,000.0	978.1	21.9	*	*	*	*	*	*
1955----------------	1970	1,000.0	977.6	22.4	*	*	*	*	*	*
1956----------------	1971	1,000.0	976.2	23.8	*	*	*	*	*	*
1957----------------	1972	1,000.0	976.4	23.6	*	*	*	*	*	*
1958----------------	1973	1,000.0	975.9	24.1	*	*	*	*	*	*
1959----------------	1974	1,000.0	975.5	24.5	*	*	*	*	*	*

TABLE 8C. DISTRIBUTIONS OF ALL OTHER WOMEN BY PARITY AS OF THE BEGINNING OF EACH YEAR 1917-74 BY AGE FOR EACH COHORT FROM 1867 TO 1959--CON.

(BASED ON CUMULATIVE BIRTH RATES)

EXACT AGE AND COHORT	AS OF JANUARY 1	TOTAL	PARITY							
			0	1	2	3	4	5	6	7 AND HIGHER
16 YEARS										
1901	1917	1,000.0	960.2	37.7	2.0	0.1	0.0	*	*	*
1902	1918	1,000.0	956.3	41.7	1.9	0.1	0.0	*	*	*
1903	1919	1,000.0	956.2	42.0	1.7	0.1	0.0	*	*	*
1904	1920	1,000.0	959.1	39.2	1.6	0.1	0.0	*	*	*
1905	1921	1,000.0	955.2	43.0	1.7	0.1	0.0	*	*	*
1906	1922	1,000.0	952.6	45.2	2.1	0.1	0.0	*	*	*
1907	1923	1,000.0	955.9	42.0	2.0	0.1	0.0	*	*	*
1908	1924	1,000.0	955.1	42.7	2.1	0.1	0.0	*	*	*
1909	1925	1,000.0	951.8	46.0	2.1	0.1	0.0	*	*	*
1910	1926	1,000.0	948.3	49.3	2.2	0.2	0.0	*	*	*
1911	1927	1,000.0	945.5	51.9	2.5	0.1	0.0	*	*	*
1912	1928	1,000.0	946.0	51.2	2.6	0.2	0.0	*	*	*
1913	1929	1,000.0	948.3	49.3	2.2	0.2	0.0	*	*	*
1914	1930	1,000.0	951.6	46.1	2.1	0.2	0.0	*	*	*
1915	1931	1,000.0	951.2	46.4	2.3	0.1	0.0	*	*	*
1916	1932	1,000.0	952.5	45.1	2.2	0.2	0.0	*	*	*
1917	1933	1,000.0	952.3	45.4	2.2	0.1	0.0	*	*	*
1918	1934	1,000.0	954.0	43.8	2.0	0.2	0.0	*	*	*
1919	1935	1,000.0	953.6	44.0	2.2	0.2	0.0	*	*	*
1920	1936	1,000.0	949.8	47.5	2.5	0.2	0.0	*	*	*
1921	1937	1,000.0	948.1	48.9	2.8	0.2	0.0	*	*	*
1922	1938	1,000.0	947.1	49.9	2.8	0.2	0.0	*	*	*
1923	1939	1,000.0	945.2	51.8	2.8	0.2	0.0	*	*	*
1924	1940	1,000.0	945.5	51.4	2.9	0.2	0.0	*	*	*
1925	1941	1,000.0	944.7	51.5	3.5	0.2	0.1	*	*	*
1926	1942	1,000.0	942.2	53.9	3.5	0.3	0.1	*	*	*
1927	1943	1,000.0	940.8	52.8	5.9	0.5	0.0	*	*	*
1928	1944	1,000.0	940.1	53.2	6.1	0.6	0.0	*	*	*
1929	1945	1,000.0	943.4	50.4	5.6	0.6	0.0	*	*	*
1930	1946	1,000.0	944.9	49.0	5.6	0.5	0.0	*	*	*
1931	1947	1,000.0	945.2	48.4	5.8	0.5	0.1	*	*	*
1932	1948	1,000.0	939.3	52.9	7.0	0.7	0.1	*	*	*
1933	1949	1,000.0	931.6	59.8	7.7	0.8	0.1	*	*	*
1934	1950	1,000.0	928.7	61.9	8.3	1.0	0.1	*	*	*
1935	1951	1,000.0	927.5	63.4	8.2	0.8	0.1	*	*	*
1936	1952	1,000.0	925.4	65.6	8.0	0.9	0.1	*	*	*
1937	1953	1,000.0	926.4	65.1	7.6	0.9	0.0	*	*	*
1938	1954	1,000.0	928.8	63.3	7.0	0.8	0.1	*	*	*
1939	1955	1,000.0	926.6	65.0	7.6	0.7	0.1	*	*	*
1940	1956	1,000.0	927.1	64.1	8.0	0.7	0.1	*	*	*
1941	1957	1,000.0	927.0	63.8	8.2	0.9	0.1	*	*	*
1942	1958	1,000.0	926.2	65.2	7.8	0.7	0.1	*	*	*
1943	1959	1,000.0	930.2	61.3	7.5	0.9	0.1	*	*	*
1944	1960	1,000.0	930.6	60.8	7.7	0.8	0.1	*	*	*
1945	1961	1,000.0	931.7	59.9	7.5	0.8	0.1	*	*	*
1946	1962	1,000.0	933.0	58.7	7.4	0.8	0.1	*	*	*
1947	1963	1,000.0	935.1	56.7	7.3	0.8	0.1	*	*	*
1948	1964	1,000.0	936.4	55.8	6.9	0.8	0.1	*	*	*
1949	1965	1,000.0	936.6	55.5	7.1	0.7	0.1	*	*	*
1950	1966	1,000.0	935.8	56.8	6.6	0.7	0.1	*	*	*
1951	1967	1,000.0	934.9	57.8	6.6	0.7	0.0	*	*	*
1952	1968	1,000.0	933.1	59.9	6.3	0.6	0.1	*	*	*
1953	1969	1,000.0	931.4	62.1	6.0	0.5	0.0	*	*	*
1954	1970	1,000.0	930.3	63.6	5.6	0.5	0.0	*	*	*
1955	1971	1,000.0	926.4	67.3	5.8	0.5	0.0	*	*	*
1956	1972	1,000.0	925.2	68.7	5.6	0.5	0.0	*	*	*
1957	1973	1,000.0	924.0	70.6	5.0	0.4	0.0	*	*	*
1958	1974	1,000.0	924.4	70.4	4.9	0.3	0.0	*	*	*

TABLE 8C. DISTRIBUTIONS OF ALL CTHER WOMEN BY PARITY AS OF THE BEGINNING OF EACH YEAR 1917-74 BY AGE FOR EACH COHORT FROM 1867 TO 1959--CON.

(BASED ON CUMULATIVE BIRTH RATES)

EXACT AGE AND COHORT	AS OF JANUARY 1	TOTAL	PARITY							
			0	1	2	3	4	5	6	7 AND HIGHER
17 YEARS										
1900	1917	1,000.0	911.3	79.8	8.1	0.7	0.1	*	*	*
1901	1918	1,000.0	904.4	87.1	7.8	0.6	0.1	*	*	*
1902	1919	1,000.0	902.1	89.8	7.4	0.7	0.0	*	*	*
1903	1920	1,000.0	905.8	86.7	6.8	0.6	0.1	*	*	*
1904	1921	1,000.0	899.9	92.5	6.9	0.7	0.0	*	*	*
1905	1922	1,000.0	895.3	95.7	8.2	0.7	0.1	*	*	*
1906	1923	1,000.0	900.2	90.7	8.3	0.7	0.1	*	*	*
1907	1924	1,000.0	900.3	90.6	8.2	0.8	0.1	*	*	*
1908	1925	1,000.0	895.5	95.1	8.5	0.8	0.1	*	*	*
1909	1926	1,000.0	888.5	101.3	9.2	0.9	0.1	*	*	*
1910	1927	1,000.0	885.3	104.3	9.3	1.0	0.1	*	*	*
1911	1928	1,000.0	883.9	104.4	10.7	0.9	0.1	*	*	*
1912	1929	1,000.0	887.8	101.4	9.7	1.0	0.1	*	*	*
1913	1930	1,000.0	892.7	97.0	9.2	1.0	0.1	*	*	*
1914	1931	1,000.0	894.4	95.7	8.9	0.9	0.1	*	*	*
1915	1932	1,000.0	895.7	94.2	9.2	0.8	0.1	*	*	*
1916	1933	1,000.0	895.9	94.1	9.0	0.9	0.1	*	*	*
1917	1934	1,000.0	899.7	90.9	8.6	0.7	0.1	*	*	*
1918	1935	1,000.0	899.0	91.2	8.8	0.9	0.1	*	*	*
1919	1936	1,000.0	894.8	94.3	9.9	0.9	0.1	*	*	*
1920	1937	1,000.0	891.2	97.2	10.5	1.0	0.1	*	*	*
1921	1938	1,000.0	884.8	102.4	11.6	1.0	0.2	*	*	*
1922	1939	1,000.0	883.0	104.2	11.6	1.1	0.1	*	*	*
1923	1940	1,000.0	884.0	102.9	11.8	1.2	0.1	*	*	*
1924	1941	1,000.0	885.8	99.8	12.8	1.4	0.2	*	*	*
1925	1942	1,000.0	881.6	102.4	14.2	1.5	0.3	*	*	*
1926	1943	1,000.0	877.0	103.3	17.0	2.4	0.3	*	*	*
1927	1944	1,000.0	875.2	101.7	20.2	2.7	0.2	*	*	*
1928	1945	1,000.0	880.9	96.9	19.3	2.7	0.2	*	*	*
1929	1946	1,000.0	884.4	94.0	18.8	2.6	0.2	*	*	*
1930	1947	1,000.0	887.0	91.3	18.8	2.6	0.3	*	*	*
1931	1948	1,000.0	874.2	100.8	21.6	3.0	0.4	*	*	*
1932	1949	1,000.0	864.6	106.9	24.6	3.5	0.4	*	*	*
1933	1950	1,000.0	857.1	111.0	27.6	3.8	0.5	*	*	*
1934	1951	1,000.0	853.1	114.2	27.9	4.3	0.5	*	*	*
1935	1952	1,000.0	849.7	117.9	27.7	4.2	0.5	*	*	*
1936	1953	1,000.0	849.5	119.1	26.6	4.3	0.5	*	*	*
1937	1954	1,000.0	849.8	119.5	26.2	4.0	0.5	*	*	*
1938	1955	1,000.0	850.7	118.7	26.1	4.0	0.5	*	*	*
1939	1956	1,000.0	850.2	118.4	26.9	3.9	0.6	*	*	*
1940	1957	1,000.0	849.8	117.8	27.7	4.1	0.6	*	*	*
1941	1958	1,000.0	848.8	118.4	27.9	4.2	0.7	*	*	*
1942	1959	1,000.0	853.4	114.5	27.3	4.2	0.6	*	*	*
1943	1960	1,000.0	856.9	112.1	26.1	4.3	0.6	*	*	*
1944	1961	1,000.0	860.3	108.6	26.3	4.2	0.6	*	*	*
1945	1962	1,000.0	861.7	108.2	25.2	4.3	0.6	*	*	*
1946	1963	1,000.0	865.2	104.9	25.2	4.1	0.6	*	*	*
1947	1964	1,000.0	867.2	103.6	24.4	4.2	0.6	*	*	*
1948	1965	1,000.0	868.4	102.9	24.2	3.9	0.6	*	*	*
1949	1966	1,000.0	867.5	105.1	23.2	3.7	0.5	*	*	*
1950	1967	1,000.0	866.2	107.3	22.7	3.4	0.4	*	*	*
1951	1968	1,000.0	863.5	110.5	22.4	3.3	0.3	*	*	*
1952	1969	1,000.0	860.6	115.3	21.1	2.6	0.4	*	*	*
1953	1970	1,000.0	858.0	119.6	19.7	2.4	0.3	*	*	*
1954	1971	1,000.0	852.7	124.8	19.9	2.4	0.2	*	*	*
1955	1972	1,000.0	849.2	128.6	19.7	2.3	0.2	*	*	*
1956	1973	1,000.0	846.1	133.2	18.5	2.0	0.2	*	*	*
1957	1974	1,000.0	847.4	133.5	17.2	1.8	0.1	*	*	*

TABLE 8C. DISTRIBUTIONS OF ALL OTHER WOMEN BY PARITY AS OF THE BEGINNING OF EACH YEAR 1917-74 BY AGE FOR EACH COHORT FROM 1867 TO 1959--CON.

(BASED ON CUMULATIVE BIRTH RATES)

EXACT AGE AND COHORT	AS OF JANUARY 1	TOTAL	PARITY							
			0	1	2	3	4	5	6	7 AND HIGHER
18 YEARS										
1899---------------	1917	1,000.0	837.0	136.1	23.2	3.2	0.5	*	*	*
1900---------------	1918	1,000.0	825.5	148.7	22.6	2.8	0.4	*	*	*
1901---------------	1919	1,000.0	822.0	153.8	21.1	2.8	0.3	*	*	*
1902---------------	1920	1,000.0	825.0	151.9	20.1	2.7	0.3	*	*	*
1903---------------	1921	1,000.0	815.0	162.0	19.9	2.8	0.3	*	*	*
1904---------------	1922	1,000.0	807.8	165.6	23.3	3.0	0.3	*	*	*
1905---------------	1923	1,000.0	814.9	157.8	23.9	3.0	0.4	*	*	*
1906---------------	1924	1,000.0	815.1	157.7	23.4	3.3	0.5	*	*	*
1907---------------	1925	1,000.0	809.5	162.5	24.0	3.4	0.6	*	*	*
1908---------------	1926	1,000.0	801.7	169.4	25.0	3.3	0.6	*	*	*
1909---------------	1927	1,000.0	796.8	172.3	26.7	3.5	0.7	*	*	*
1910---------------	1928	1,000.0	798.3	170.2	27.0	3.9	0.6	*	*	*
1911---------------	1929	1,000.0	800.1	168.8	26.7	3.8	0.6	*	*	*
1912---------------	1930	1,000.0	807.8	161.9	26.1	3.7	0.5	*	*	*
1913---------------	1931	1,000.0	809.9	160.9	25.3	3.3	0.6	*	*	*
1914---------------	1932	1,000.0	814.9	156.4	24.8	3.3	0.6	*	*	*
1915---------------	1933	1,000.0	815.3	156.0	24.9	3.3	0.5	*	*	*
1916---------------	1934	1,000.0	821.3	150.9	24.0	3.2	0.6	*	*	*
1917---------------	1935	1,000.0	820.2	151.9	24.0	3.4	0.5	*	*	*
1918---------------	1936	1,000.0	816.4	154.0	25.6	3.5	0.5	*	*	*
1919---------------	1937	1,000.0	813.4	154.9	27.4	3.7	0.6	*	*	*
1920---------------	1938	1,000.0	803.8	162.4	29.2	4.0	0.6	*	*	*
1921---------------	1939	1,000.0	795.0	169.4	30.6	4.2	0.8	*	*	*
1922---------------	1940	1,000.0	797.2	166.1	31.3	4.7	0.7	*	*	*
1923---------------	1941	1,000.0	802.4	158.9	32.1	5.6	1.0	*	*	*
1924---------------	1942	1,000.0	801.2	157.1	34.6	6.0	1.1	*	*	*
1925---------------	1943	1,000.0	793.8	159.7	38.0	7.2	1.3	*	*	*
1926---------------	1944	1,000.0	788.7	159.3	42.4	8.2	1.4	*	*	*
1927---------------	1945	1,000.0	795.5	151.5	43.3	8.3	1.4	*	*	*
1928---------------	1946	1,000.0	803.2	145.4	42.1	7.9	1.4	*	*	*
1929---------------	1947	1,000.0	804.8	144.1	41.7	8.1	1.3	*	*	*
1930---------------	1948	1,000.0	789.6	155.3	44.9	8.6	1.6	*	*	*
1931---------------	1949	1,000.0	773.7	162.4	52.3	9.9	1.7	*	*	*
1932---------------	1950	1,000.0	767.5	161.3	57.7	11.7	1.8	*	*	*
1933---------------	1951	1,000.0	760.4	163.7	61.4	12.3	2.2	*	*	*
1934---------------	1952	1,000.0	753.7	169.7	60.9	13.4	2.3	*	*	*
1935---------------	1953	1,000.0	752.2	172.2	59.9	13.3	2.4	*	*	*
1936---------------	1954	1,000.0	750.4	174.3	59.6	13.2	2.5	*	*	*
1937---------------	1955	1,000.0	747.9	177.9	58.6	13.2	2.4	*	*	*
1938---------------	1956	1,000.0	751.8	173.7	58.9	13.2	2.4	*	*	*
1939---------------	1957	1,000.0	748.7	174.6	60.5	13.6	2.6	*	*	*
1940---------------	1958	1,000.0	748.5	174.1	60.9	13.9	2.6	*	*	*
1941---------------	1959	1,000.0	753.4	168.5	61.3	14.0	2.8	*	*	*
1942---------------	1960	1,000.0	758.2	165.9	59.1	14.1	2.7	*	*	*
1943---------------	1961	1,000.0	765.1	161.6	57.1	13.5	2.7	*	*	*
1944---------------	1962	1,000.0	769.3	158.3	55.8	13.8	2.8	*	*	*
1945---------------	1963	1,000.0	773.6	155.6	54.4	13.8	2.6	*	*	*
1946---------------	1964	1,000.0	776.3	154.0	54.2	13.0	2.5	*	*	*
1947---------------	1965	1,000.0	776.6	154.6	53.3	13.0	2.5	*	*	*
1948---------------	1966	1,000.0	778.0	156.0	51.5	12.1	2.4	*	*	*
1949---------------	1967	1,000.0	775.4	161.1	50.6	10.9	2.0	*	*	*
1950---------------	1968	1,000.0	773.1	165.8	49.4	10.1	1.6	*	*	*
1951---------------	1969	1,000.0	768.2	173.8	47.4	9.2	1.4	*	*	*
1952---------------	1970	1,000.0	763.5	181.8	45.4	8.0	1.3	*	*	*
1953---------------	1971	1,000.0	757.0	189.2	45.0	7.7	1.1	*	*	*
1954---------------	1972	1,000.0	753.2	194.4	44.1	7.4	0.9	*	*	*
1955---------------	1973	1,000.0	748.5	201.8	42.3	6.6	0.8	*	*	*
1956---------------	1974	1,000.0	750.3	203.3	39.7	6.0	0.7	*	*	*

TABLE 8C. DISTRIBUTIONS OF ALL OTHER WOMEN BY PARITY AS OF THE BEGINNING OF EACH YEAR 1917-74 BY AGE FOR EACH COHORT FROM 1867 TO 1959--CON.

(BASED ON CUMULATIVE BIRTH RATES)

EXACT AGE AND COHORT	AS OF JANUARY 1	TOTAL	PARITY							
			0	1	2	3	4	5	6	7 AND HIGHER
19 YEARS										
1898----------------	1917	1,000.0	751.2	187.9	49.6	9.4	1.9	*	*	*
1899----------------	1918	1,000.0	735.9	205.5	48.7	8.5	1.4	*	*	*
1900----------------	1919	1,000.0	727.8	216.4	46.3	8.4	1.1	*	*	*
1901----------------	1920	1,000.0	731.5	216.4	43.1	7.7	1.3	*	*	*
1902----------------	1921	1,000.0	717.8	230.0	43.0	8.2	1.0	*	*	*
1903----------------	1922	1,000.0	706.1	235.0	49.0	8.6	1.3	*	*	*
1904----------------	1923	1,000.0	712.5	226.3	51.2	8.6	1.4	*	*	*
1905----------------	1924	1,000.0	714.2	224.3	50.1	9.6	1.8	*	*	*
1906----------------	1925	1,000.0	707.9	229.3	50.9	9.9	2.0	*	*	*
1907----------------	1926	1,000.0	701.1	236.0	51.2	9.4	2.3	*	*	*
1908----------------	1927	1,000.0	698.5	235.9	53.2	10.1	2.3	*	*	*
1909----------------	1928	1,000.0	699.7	233.8	53.9	10.4	2.2	*	*	*
1910----------------	1929	1,000.0	706.7	228.3	52.3	10.4	2.3	*	*	*
1911----------------	1930	1,000.0	710.9	224.4	52.6	10.1	2.0	*	*	*
1912----------------	1931	1,000.0	715.6	220.9	52.0	9.5	2.0	*	*	*
1913----------------	1932	1,000.0	720.5	217.6	50.7	9.1	2.1	*	*	*
1914----------------	1933	1,000.0	724.6	213.6	50.5	9.3	2.0	*	*	*
1915----------------	1934	1,000.0	731.2	208.4	49.4	9.1	1.9	*	*	*
1916----------------	1935	1,000.0	731.2	208.9	48.5	9.5	1.9	*	*	*
1917----------------	1936	1,000.0	729.2	208.5	50.6	9.8	1.9	*	*	*
1918----------------	1937	1,000.0	729.6	205.7	52.3	10.4	2.0	*	*	*
1919----------------	1938	1,000.0	719.8	210.8	56.3	11.0	2.1	*	*	*
1920----------------	1939	1,000.0	707.7	219.9	58.7	11.4	2.3	*	*	*
1921----------------	1940	1,000.0	701.1	221.8	61.7	12.8	2.6	*	*	*
1922----------------	1941	1,000.0	709.2	209.6	62.6	15.2	3.4	*	*	*
1923----------------	1942	1,000.0	712.1	201.9	65.6	16.6	3.8	*	*	*
1924----------------	1943	1,000.0	707.1	205.8	65.9	17.2	4.0	*	*	*
1925----------------	1944	1,000.0	699.3	206.2	71.6	18.5	4.4	*	*	*
1926----------------	1945	1,000.0	703.5	200.0	72.7	19.2	4.6	*	*	*
1927----------------	1946	1,000.0	712.4	191.7	73.1	18.3	4.5	*	*	*
1928----------------	1947	1,000.0	715.0	189.2	72.8	18.7	4.3	*	*	*
1929----------------	1948	1,000.0	694.4	204.1	77.1	19.9	4.5	*	*	*
1930----------------	1949	1,000.0	679.6	206.8	86.7	21.9	5.0	*	*	*
1931----------------	1950	1,000.0	669.4	202.7	96.2	26.0	5.7	*	*	*
1932----------------	1951	1,000.0	666.3	197.9	100.8	28.6	6.4	*	*	*
1933----------------	1952	1,000.0	655.8	203.9	103.4	29.8	7.1	*	*	*
1934----------------	1953	1,000.0	651.9	208.2	100.9	31.1	7.9	*	*	*
1935----------------	1954	1,000.0	646.9	213.0	101.1	30.9	8.1	*	*	*
1936----------------	1955	1,000.0	639.9	220.0	100.2	31.6	8.3	*	*	*
1937----------------	1956	1,000.0	639.5	219.4	101.4	31.5	8.2	*	*	*
1938----------------	1957	1,000.0	641.1	215.8	102.8	31.7	8.6	*	*	*
1939----------------	1958	1,000.0	638.9	216.0	103.7	32.6	8.8	*	*	*
1940----------------	1959	1,000.0	642.7	212.0	103.1	33.1	9.1	*	*	*
1941----------------	1960	1,000.0	648.6	206.9	101.9	33.3	9.3	*	*	*
1942----------------	1961	1,000.0	656.3	203.5	98.7	32.3	9.2	*	*	*
1943----------------	1962	1,000.0	664.9	200.5	94.1	31.4	9.1	*	*	*
1944----------------	1963	1,000.0	670.8	196.4	92.5	31.3	9.0	*	*	*
1945----------------	1964	1,000.0	674.2	195.6	91.2	30.6	8.4	*	*	*
1946----------------	1965	1,000.0	673.7	197.8	90.6	29.9	8.0	*	*	*
1947----------------	1966	1,000.0	674.9	200.4	88.5	28.3	7.9	*	*	*
1948----------------	1967	1,000.0	673.3	207.8	86.1	26.0	6.8	*	*	*
1949----------------	1968	1,000.0	670.1	216.0	84.4	23.6	5.9	*	*	*
1950----------------	1969	1,000.0	665.5	225.7	82.8	21.3	4.7	*	*	*
1951----------------	1970	1,000.0	658.3	237.0	80.6	19.9	4.2	*	*	*
1952----------------	1971	1,000.0	650.2	247.9	79.8	18.3	3.8	*	*	*
1953----------------	1972	1,000.0	647.0	254.1	78.3	17.3	3.3	*	*	*
1954----------------	1973	1,000.0	645.5	260.3	75.7	15.8	2.7	*	*	*
1955----------------	1974	1,000.0	646.4	264.6	72.2	14.5	2.3	*	*	*

TABLE 8C. DISTRIBUTIONS OF ALL OTHER WOMEN BY PARITY AS OF THE BEGINNING OF EACH YEAR 1917-74 BY AGE FOR EACH COHORT FROM 1867 TO 1959--CON.

(BASED ON CUMULATIVE BIRTH RATES)

EXACT AGE AND COHORT	AS OF JANUARY 1	TOTAL	PARITY 0	1	2	3	4	5	6	7 AND HIGHER
20 YEARS										
1897----------------	1917	1,000.0	636.0	253.4	81.8	22.8	6.0	*	*	*
1898----------------	1918	1,000.0	644.9	244.7	84.7	20.5	5.2	*	*	*
1899----------------	1919	1,000.0	631.9	262.9	80.3	20.3	4.6	*	*	*
1900----------------	1920	1,000.0	631.4	267.8	77.1	19.3	4.4	*	*	*
1901----------------	1921	1,000.0	617.9	283.6	75.4	18.9	4.2	*	*	*
1902----------------	1922	1,000.0	604.6	290.3	80.1	20.4	4.6	*	*	*
1903----------------	1923	1,000.0	607.4	281.3	86.3	20.1	4.9	*	*	*
1904----------------	1924	1,000.0	611.0	276.9	85.3	21.4	5.4	*	*	*
1905----------------	1925	1,000.0	605.7	280.7	84.6	23.0	6.0	*	*	*
1906----------------	1926	1,000.0	600.9	286.8	83.6	22.2	6.5	*	*	*
1907----------------	1927	1,000.0	599.7	285.1	86.4	22.0	6.8	*	*	*
1908----------------	1928	1,000.0	603.8	281.5	85.2	23.0	6.5	*	*	*
1909----------------	1929	1,000.0	610.8	276.3	83.5	22.7	6.7	*	*	*
1910----------------	1930	1,000.0	619.6	268.6	83.1	22.3	6.4	*	*	*
1911----------------	1931	1,000.0	620.5	267.4	84.0	22.0	6.1	*	*	*
1912----------------	1932	1,000.0	629.1	261.8	81.8	21.3	6.0	*	*	*
1913----------------	1933	1,000.0	632.7	258.2	81.8	21.3	6.0	*	*	*
1914----------------	1934	1,000.0	643.2	249.7	80.7	20.5	5.9	*	*	*
1915----------------	1935	1,000.0	643.5	250.0	79.7	21.0	5.8	*	*	*
1916----------------	1936	1,000.0	643.8	248.9	79.6	21.7	6.0	*	*	*
1917----------------	1937	1,000.0	646.3	243.2	82.3	22.2	6.0	*	*	*
1918----------------	1938	1,000.0	642.4	242.2	85.5	23.7	6.2	*	*	*
1919----------------	1939	1,000.0	630.3	248.8	89.6	24.7	6.6	*	*	*
1920----------------	1940	1,000.0	620.0	254.2	93.2	25.8	6.8	*	*	*
1921----------------	1941	1,000.0	616.1	250.0	96.0	29.4	8.5	*	*	*
1922----------------	1942	1,000.0	623.3	236.6	98.7	32.1	9.3	*	*	*
1923----------------	1943	1,000.0	625.3	233.0	97.7	33.6	10.4	*	*	*
1924----------------	1944	1,000.0	620.5	234.0	100.2	34.4	10.9	*	*	*
1925----------------	1945	1,000.0	620.0	231.1	102.0	35.3	11.6	*	*	*
1926----------------	1946	1,000.0	626.4	224.9	103.0	34.0	11.7	*	*	*
1927----------------	1947	1,000.0	626.3	221.8	105.9	34.7	11.3	*	*	*
1928----------------	1948	1,000.0	607.5	233.8	110.3	36.7	11.7	*	*	*
1929----------------	1949	1,000.0	589.6	235.2	122.3	40.2	12.7	*	*	*
1930----------------	1950	1,000.0	581.8	226.4	132.0	46.0	13.8	*	*	*
1931----------------	1951	1,000.0	576.7	216.9	138.3	52.1	16.0	*	*	*
1932----------------	1952	1,000.0	571.2	215.8	139.9	55.4	17.7	*	*	*
1933----------------	1953	1,000.0	563.2	220.6	141.0	55.6	19.6	*	*	*
1934----------------	1954	1,000.0	554.2	228.8	139.7	56.5	20.8	*	*	*
1935----------------	1955	1,000.0	542.4	239.3	139.3	57.7	21.3	*	*	*
1936----------------	1956	1,000.0	537.0	240.3	142.3	58.6	21.8	*	*	*
1937----------------	1957	1,000.0	532.7	240.3	145.6	59.3	22.1	*	*	*
1938----------------	1958	1,000.0	535.4	237.2	144.4	60.2	22.8	*	*	*
1939----------------	1959	1,000.0	537.8	234.4	143.5	60.7	23.6	*	*	*
1940----------------	1960	1,000.0	542.3	229.8	143.2	60.6	24.1	*	*	*
1941----------------	1961	1,000.0	549.8	225.6	140.4	60.1	24.1	*	*	*
1942----------------	1962	1,000.0	558.6	224.4	135.1	58.2	23.7	*	*	*
1943----------------	1963	1,000.0	568.1	223.5	129.4	56.2	22.8	*	*	*
1944----------------	1964	1,000.0	572.7	221.1	128.9	54.8	22.5	*	*	*
1945----------------	1965	1,000.0	573.2	224.6	127.4	54.0	20.8	*	*	*
1946----------------	1966	1,000.0	573.5	229.1	126.2	51.4	19.8	*	*	*
1947----------------	1967	1,000.0	570.7	239.4	124.3	47.8	17.8	*	*	*
1948----------------	1968	1,000.0	568.5	250.4	121.7	44.2	15.2	*	*	*
1949----------------	1969	1,000.0	563.0	264.4	119.7	40.1	12.8	*	*	*
1950----------------	1970	1,000.0	556.3	276.6	119.3	36.9	10.9	*	*	*
1951----------------	1971	1,000.0	547.2	288.5	118.9	35.5	9.9	*	*	*
1952----------------	1972	1,000.0	543.5	297.6	117.6	32.5	8.8	*	*	*
1953----------------	1973	1,000.0	545.3	303.4	113.8	30.2	7.3	*	*	*
1954----------------	1974	1,000.0	550.2	306.3	109.3	27.8	6.4	*	*	*

TABLE 8C. DISTRIBUTIONS OF ALL OTHER WOMEN BY PARITY AS OF THE BEGINNING OF EACH YEAR 1917-74 BY AGE FOR EACH COHORT FROM 1867 TO 1959--CON.

(BASED ON CUMULATIVE BIRTH RATES)

EXACT AGE AND COHORT	AS OF JANUARY 1	TOTAL	PARITY							
			0	1	2	3	4	5	6	7 AND HIGHER
21 YEARS										
1896	1917	1,000.0	553.7	274.9	113.5	42.9	12.7	1.7	0.4	0.2
1897	1918	1,000.0	546.4	285.3	116.1	39.6	11.1	1.0	0.3	0.2
1898	1919	1,000.0	555.0	280.1	114.5	38.6	10.4	1.0	0.3	0.1
1899	1920	1,000.0	549.4	292.2	110.5	36.9	9.5	1.1	0.2	0.2
1900	1921	1,000.0	533.6	309.7	109.6	36.4	9.2	1.1	0.3	0.1
1901	1922	1,000.0	523.4	318.9	109.5	37.1	9.5	1.2	0.3	0.1
1902	1923	1,000.0	522.2	312.6	116.1	37.6	9.9	1.1	0.4	0.1
1903	1924	1,000.0	525.0	305.9	118.0	38.9	10.4	1.3	0.3	0.2
1904	1925	1,000.0	522.4	306.9	116.1	41.5	11.3	1.2	0.4	0.2
1905	1926	1,000.0	518.8	311.4	115.3	39.9	12.3	1.5	0.5	0.3
1906	1927	1,000.0	518.0	312.3	115.4	39.1	12.8	1.5	0.6	0.3
1907	1928	1,000.0	523.6	307.5	114.6	39.4	12.5	1.6	0.5	0.3
1908	1929	1,000.0	534.0	301.3	110.6	39.5	12.2	1.6	0.5	0.3
1909	1930	1,000.0	541.2	296.0	109.9	38.5	12.3	1.4	0.4	0.3
1910	1931	1,000.0	547.8	289.7	109.8	39.0	11.5	1.5	0.5	0.2
1911	1932	1,000.0	550.6	287.8	109.9	38.1	11.6	1.3	0.5	0.2
1912	1933	1,000.0	558.2	280.7	109.7	38.0	11.3	1.5	0.5	0.1
1913	1934	1,000.0	567.0	274.7	108.5	36.7	11.1	1.4	0.5	0.1
1914	1935	1,000.0	572.3	270.3	107.5	36.6	11.3	1.5	0.3	0.2
1915	1936	1,000.0	573.5	268.8	106.8	37.3	11.4	1.6	0.4	0.2
1916	1937	1,000.0	578.0	262.9	107.2	37.9	11.7	1.7	0.4	0.2
1917	1938	1,000.0	577.2	258.3	110.5	40.0	11.7	1.6	0.5	0.2
1918	1939	1,000.0	573.1	257.2	113.5	41.7	12.4	1.4	0.5	0.2
1919	1940	1,000.0	561.9	261.7	118.5	43.0	12.7	1.5	0.5	0.2
1920	1941	1,000.0	552.6	264.4	120.8	45.4	14.1	1.8	0.7	0.2
1921	1942	1,000.0	546.4	259.9	125.4	49.7	15.8	1.9	0.7	0.2
1922	1943	1,000.0	554.2	249.4	123.9	51.8	17.3	2.6	0.6	0.2
1923	1944	1,000.0	557.1	242.7	124.5	53.4	18.7	2.7	0.7	0.2
1924	1945	1,000.0	557.2	242.8	123.2	53.6	19.4	2.9	0.7	0.2
1925	1946	1,000.0	557.5	242.0	124.7	52.5	19.7	2.6	0.7	0.3
1926	1947	1,000.0	552.8	239.1	130.9	53.7	19.8	2.7	0.7	0.3
1927	1948	1,000.0	532.7	248.5	138.5	56.5	19.8	2.9	0.8	0.3
1928	1949	1,000.0	519.2	244.3	149.1	61.7	21.5	3.1	0.8	0.3
1929	1950	1,000.0	507.2	236.2	159.6	68.6	23.6	3.7	0.8	0.3
1930	1951	1,000.0	505.4	223.0	163.3	77.3	25.9	3.9	0.8	0.4
1931	1952	1,000.0	499.4	215.5	166.3	83.3	29.6	4.7	0.8	0.4
1932	1953	1,000.0	494.9	217.0	164.8	84.1	32.7	5.1	1.0	0.4
1933	1954	1,000.0	481.7	224.8	168.1	83.7	35.6	4.7	1.1	0.3
1934	1955	1,000.0	466.8	235.5	167.8	86.3	36.3	5.4	1.4	0.5
1935	1956	1,000.0	453.7	242.0	171.8	87.6	37.1	5.9	1.4	0.5
1936	1957	1,000.0	445.2	241.7	176.7	89.7	38.6	6.2	1.5	0.4
1937	1958	1,000.0	440.7	242.7	176.7	92.1	39.1	6.5	1.8	0.4
1938	1959	1,000.0	448.0	237.8	174.1	91.2	40.1	6.7	1.7	0.4
1939	1960	1,000.0	450.9	234.2	173.9	90.9	41.4	6.6	1.6	0.5
1940	1961	1,000.0	455.7	231.8	171.7	91.1	41.0	6.5	1.6	0.6
1941	1962	1,000.0	463.3	229.8	168.7	88.0	41.3	6.7	1.7	0.5
1942	1963	1,000.0	471.8	231.7	162.5	85.8	39.5	6.4	1.9	0.4
1943	1964	1,000.0	480.8	232.7	158.1	82.4	37.7	6.3	1.5	0.5
1944	1965	1,000.0	483.0	234.1	158.3	80.2	36.8	5.6	1.6	0.4
1945	1966	1,000.0	483.6	240.9	157.0	77.9	33.8	5.1	1.4	0.3
1946	1967	1,000.0	480.7	252.6	156.1	74.0	30.8	4.5	1.1	0.2
1947	1968	1,000.0	477.3	265.7	156.0	68.4	27.8	3.7	0.8	0.3
1948	1969	1,000.0	472.6	282.9	154.3	63.0	23.5	3.0	0.5	0.2
1949	1970	1,000.0	466.0	298.1	153.8	58.6	20.3	2.5	0.5	0.2
1950	1971	1,000.0	457.9	310.0	154.9	56.1	18.4	2.1	0.4	0.2
1951	1972	1,000.0	453.8	318.8	155.4	53.3	16.4	1.8	0.4	0.1
1952	1973	1,000.0	457.3	326.0	152.0	48.7	14.2	1.5	0.2	0.1
1953	1974	1,000.0	464.6	329.1	147.2	45.4	12.3	1.1	0.2	0.1

TABLE 8C. DISTRIBUTIONS OF ALL OTHER WOMEN BY PARITY AS OF THE BEGINNING OF EACH YEAR 1917-74 BY AGE FOR EACH COHORT FROM 1867 TO 1959--CON.

(BASED ON CUMULATIVE BIRTH RATES)

EXACT AGE AND COHORT	AS OF JANUARY 1	TOTAL	PARITY							
			0	1	2	3	4	5	6	7 AND HIGHER
22 YEARS										
1895---------------	1917	1,000.0	486.2	276.4	136.4	68.2	24.6	5.7	1.7	0.8
1896---------------	1918	1,000.0	479.9	287.6	140.8	64.0	21.7	4.2	1.2	0.6
1897---------------	1919	1,000.0	471.2	303.2	137.7	62.4	20.5	3.3	1.2	0.5
1898---------------	1920	1,000.0	485.7	292.0	138.6	59.6	19.0	3.6	1.0	0.5
1899---------------	1921	1,000.0	467.4	314.0	137.0	58.3	18.2	3.6	1.0	0.5
1900---------------	1922	1,000.0	456.8	325.9	133.6	59.3	18.9	3.8	1.2	0.5
1901---------------	1923	1,000.0	457.1	323.5	137.5	58.1	18.3	3.9	1.1	0.5
1902---------------	1924	1,000.0	458.3	317.4	138.8	60.5	19.1	4.0	1.4	0.5
1903---------------	1925	1,000.0	455.5	316.1	138.2	63.7	20.2	4.2	1.4	0.7
1904---------------	1926	1,000.0	454.1	317.7	138.1	61.5	22.2	4.0	1.6	0.8
1905---------------	1927	1,000.0	453.4	319.4	138.5	58.7	22.6	4.7	1.9	0.8
1906---------------	1928	1,000.0	458.5	318.2	135.1	58.6	22.1	4.8	1.8	0.9
1907---------------	1929	1,000.0	468.4	313.8	131.3	57.9	21.0	5.0	1.7	0.9
1908---------------	1930	1,000.0	479.8	307.0	128.1	57.4	20.7	4.7	1.5	0.8
1909---------------	1931	1,000.0	485.0	302.9	127.7	57.0	20.7	4.6	1.4	0.7
1910---------------	1932	1,000.0	493.0	295.7	128.0	56.8	20.0	4.3	1.6	0.6
1911---------------	1933	1,000.0	494.7	292.2	129.3	57.0	20.5	4.3	1.5	0.5
1912---------------	1934	1,000.0	507.5	283.3	127.7	55.8	19.3	4.4	1.6	0.4
1913---------------	1935	1,000.0	512.2	279.8	126.9	54.8	20.1	4.3	1.4	0.5
1914---------------	1936	1,000.0	517.8	275.1	125.8	54.3	20.3	4.8	1.3	0.6
1915---------------	1937	1,000.0	521.5	270.6	125.9	54.8	20.2	5.0	1.4	0.6
1916---------------	1938	1,000.0	523.9	264.8	126.5	56.9	20.7	5.1	1.4	0.7
1917---------------	1939	1,000.0	523.9	259.8	128.5	59.7	21.2	4.7	1.5	0.7
1918---------------	1940	1,000.0	521.1	257.9	131.8	60.6	21.6	4.8	1.5	0.7
1919---------------	1941	1,000.0	509.4	263.1	134.6	62.0	23.0	5.4	1.7	0.8
1920---------------	1942	1,000.0	498.5	266.3	137.9	64.7	23.9	5.9	2.0	0.8
1921---------------	1943	1,000.0	492.0	262.0	141.1	68.6	26.8	6.7	2.1	0.7
1922---------------	1944	1,000.0	501.2	248.7	140.4	70.9	28.5	7.4	2.1	0.8
1923---------------	1945	1,000.0	507.1	242.8	137.7	71.5	30.1	7.8	2.2	0.8
1924---------------	1946	1,000.0	508.4	244.5	136.5	69.9	29.9	7.8	2.1	0.9
1925---------------	1947	1,000.0	497.6	244.9	145.1	71.3	30.4	7.6	2.2	0.9
1926---------------	1948	1,000.0	475.3	251.9	155.4	75.3	30.9	7.9	2.3	1.0
1927---------------	1949	1,000.0	460.7	245.8	167.3	81.7	32.6	8.5	2.3	1.1
1928---------------	1950	1,000.0	452.8	234.1	174.8	89.4	35.7	9.7	2.5	1.0
1929---------------	1951	1,000.0	445.6	223.0	178.4	99.3	39.3	10.8	2.5	1.1
1930---------------	1952	1,000.0	444.5	211.2	177.9	106.5	44.0	12.0	2.7	1.2
1931---------------	1953	1,000.0	438.6	206.8	178.3	109.1	49.2	13.5	3.2	1.3
1932---------------	1954	1,000.0	430.7	210.8	179.3	108.7	51.2	14.3	3.8	1.2
1933---------------	1955	1,000.0	412.4	219.3	184.1	110.3	53.7	14.6	4.2	1.4
1934---------------	1956	1,000.0	395.5	226.7	186.9	113.6	55.3	15.8	4.6	1.6
1935---------------	1957	1,000.0	379.2	231.1	192.7	116.3	57.7	16.8	4.6	1.6
1936---------------	1958	1,000.0	370.7	231.7	193.8	120.5	58.7	17.8	5.2	1.6
1937---------------	1959	1,000.0	369.9	230.4	193.3	121.0	59.7	18.8	5.4	1.5
1938---------------	1960	1,000.0	378.3	225.5	191.6	117.6	61.7	18.2	5.4	1.7
1939---------------	1961	1,000.0	381.0	224.7	189.0	118.8	61.4	17.8	5.4	1.9
1940---------------	1962	1,000.0	385.1	223.1	188.7	116.5	61.2	18.0	5.5	1.9
1941---------------	1963	1,000.0	392.9	224.0	184.3	113.9	59.4	18.2	5.5	1.8
1942---------------	1964	1,000.0	400.8	227.3	181.2	109.4	57.1	17.1	5.4	1.7
1943---------------	1965	1,000.0	408.5	231.2	178.1	105.8	54.1	16.0	4.7	1.6
1944---------------	1966	1,000.0	410.0	236.9	179.0	102.2	51.6	14.5	4.4	1.4
1945---------------	1967	1,000.0	409.0	248.3	179.4	99.2	46.9	12.3	4.0	0.9
1946---------------	1968	1,000.0	405.6	262.6	181.4	93.7	42.2	10.8	2.9	0.8
1947---------------	1969	1,000.0	399.6	281.8	181.2	87.3	38.3	8.9	2.0	0.9
1948---------------	1970	1,000.0	392.9	300.0	182.7	81.7	33.0	7.4	1.6	0.7
1949---------------	1971	1,000.0	386.5	312.7	183.9	78.7	29.9	6.2	1.5	0.6
1950---------------	1972	1,000.0	383.1	321.3	186.6	75.1	26.8	5.4	1.2	0.5
1951---------------	1973	1,000.0	385.4	329.7	184.9	70.4	23.9	4.4	1.0	0.3
1952---------------	1974	1,000.0	393.6	334.7	180.8	65.5	20.9	3.6	0.7	0.2

TABLE 8C. DISTRIBUTIONS OF ALL OTHER WOMEN BY PARITY AS OF THE BEGINNING OF EACH YEAR 1917-74 BY AGE FOR EACH COHORT FROM 1867 TO 1959--CON.

(BASED ON CUMULATIVE BIRTH RATES)

EXACT AGE AND COHORT	AS OF JANUARY 1	TOTAL	PARITY							
			0	1	2	3	4	5	6	7 AND HIGHER
23 YEARS										
1894	1917	1,000.0	436.3	264.1	146.7	92.5	41.0	12.6	4.6	2.2
1895	1918	1,000.0	430.2	276.3	152.9	88.7	36.9	9.9	3.3	1.8
1896	1919	1,000.0	422.9	292.0	151.6	86.3	34.7	8.1	3.0	1.4
1897	1920	1,000.0	419.1	303.0	151.2	82.8	32.2	7.6	2.6	1.5
1898	1921	1,000.0	423.3	298.8	154.5	80.6	31.1	7.8	2.6	1.3
1899	1922	1,000.0	409.4	316.5	149.7	80.4	31.7	8.0	3.0	1.3
1900	1923	1,000.0	406.6	319.3	150.4	79.6	31.3	8.3	3.1	1.4
1901	1924	1,000.0	409.0	317.9	149.3	80.2	30.7	8.5	2.9	1.5
1902	1925	1,000.0	405.7	315.6	147.5	84.7	32.4	8.9	3.6	1.6
1903	1926	1,000.0	403.1	316.0	150.0	81.9	35.1	8.6	3.5	1.8
1904	1927	1,000.0	403.8	316.5	150.3	78.2	36.3	9.3	3.6	2.0
1905	1928	1,000.0	409.4	315.8	147.2	76.6	35.4	9.9	3.8	1.9
1906	1929	1,000.0	418.0	315.8	142.0	74.9	33.6	9.8	3.8	2.1
1907	1930	1,000.0	428.7	311.4	139.4	73.4	31.9	10.0	3.4	1.8
1908	1931	1,000.0	438.6	305.9	136.5	72.4	32.0	9.8	3.1	1.7
1909	1932	1,000.0	444.2	301.0	137.2	71.9	31.9	9.1	3.2	1.5
1910	1933	1,000.0	451.4	292.7	137.9	73.0	31.5	8.9	3.3	1.3
1911	1934	1,000.0	456.7	288.3	137.1	72.8	31.8	8.9	3.2	1.2
1912	1935	1,000.0	466.6	281.2	135.5	72.0	31.2	9.1	3.2	1.2
1913	1936	1,000.0	471.1	278.3	135.0	69.7	32.2	9.2	3.2	1.3
1914	1937	1,000.0	478.6	270.6	135.5	69.2	31.8	9.9	3.0	1.4
1915	1938	1,000.0	481.0	265.8	135.1	71.0	32.3	10.1	3.2	1.5
1916	1939	1,000.0	484.2	259.7	134.1	74.1	33.0	10.0	3.3	1.6
1917	1940	1,000.0	484.3	254.2	136.8	76.4	33.3	10.0	3.4	1.6
1918	1941	1,000.0	482.4	252.7	137.3	76.3	35.2	10.6	3.6	1.9
1919	1942	1,000.0	468.7	258.2	141.1	78.3	36.0	11.6	4.2	1.9
1920	1943	1,000.0	454.6	264.1	145.2	79.9	37.4	12.6	4.4	1.8
1921	1944	1,000.0	449.5	257.4	148.9	83.9	40.4	13.4	4.6	1.9
1922	1945	1,000.0	461.5	245.0	145.3	84.9	42.3	14.3	4.8	1.9
1923	1946	1,000.0	468.9	240.7	142.8	84.1	42.2	14.5	4.8	2.0
1924	1947	1,000.0	459.8	241.7	149.6	84.9	42.8	14.4	4.7	2.1
1925	1948	1,000.0	434.3	249.9	162.1	89.0	43.3	14.4	4.9	2.1
1926	1949	1,000.0	416.8	243.6	174.3	96.9	46.1	14.9	5.0	2.4
1927	1950	1,000.0	406.7	231.8	182.5	104.9	49.7	16.5	5.4	2.5
1928	1951	1,000.0	403.0	218.3	183.1	114.9	54.0	18.7	5.6	2.4
1929	1952	1,000.0	396.9	207.5	183.2	122.0	60.9	20.9	6.1	2.5
1930	1953	1,000.0	396.2	198.9	180.0	125.8	66.2	23.1	7.0	2.8
1931	1954	1,000.0	388.2	195.1	183.4	126.1	69.3	26.8	7.9	3.2
1932	1955	1,000.0	376.6	199.7	185.2	127.9	71.3	26.7	9.2	3.4
1933	1956	1,000.0	356.1	206.3	191.9	130.1	74.5	27.6	9.7	3.8
1934	1957	1,000.0	336.7	210.7	196.2	134.8	77.7	29.7	9.9	4.3
1935	1958	1,000.0	320.1	214.7	199.7	139.7	79.6	30.9	11.1	4.2
1936	1959	1,000.0	313.9	213.9	200.2	142.2	81.5	32.4	11.7	4.2
1937	1960	1,000.0	314.2	213.6	198.7	140.9	82.7	33.6	11.9	4.4
1938	1961	1,000.0	323.1	211.2	195.3	138.5	83.1	32.3	11.8	4.7
1939	1962	1,000.0	325.9	209.8	195.0	137.0	83.5	31.9	12.0	4.9
1940	1963	1,000.0	330.6	209.8	193.4	136.7	81.2	31.5	12.1	4.7
1941	1964	1,000.0	338.0	212.3	192.0	131.9	78.3	31.4	11.5	4.6
1942	1965	1,000.0	344.0	218.2	191.3	127.5	75.2	28.6	11.0	4.2
1943	1966	1,000.0	351.5	225.4	190.2	122.9	70.4	26.7	9.2	3.7
1944	1967	1,000.0	351.8	234.8	193.2	119.8	65.9	22.9	8.6	3.0
1945	1968	1,000.0	350.7	248.0	197.0	115.8	58.9	20.2	7.0	2.4
1946	1969	1,000.0	345.3	266.3	199.9	110.2	53.8	17.3	5.3	1.9
1947	1970	1,000.0	337.2	286.3	201.9	104.7	49.5	14.5	4.2	1.7
1948	1971	1,000.0	328.9	303.2	205.8	100.7	44.6	12.0	3.4	1.4
1949	1972	1,000.0	326.1	312.8	208.6	97.9	40.0	10.5	3.0	1.1
1950	1973	1,000.0	328.3	322.5	209.9	91.3	35.8	9.1	2.3	0.8
1951	1974	1,000.0	334.4	328.4	208.7	86.9	31.9	7.3	1.8	0.6

TABLE 8C. DISTRIBUTIONS OF ALL OTHER WOMEN BY PARITY AS OF THE BEGINNING OF EACH YEAR 1917-74 BY AGE FOR EACH COHORT FROM 1867 TO 1959--CON.

(BASED ON CUMULATIVE BIRTH RATES)

EXACT AGE AND COHORT	AS OF JANUARY 1	TOTAL	PARITY							
			0	1	2	3	4	5	6	7 AND HIGHER
24 YEARS										
1893	1917	1,000.0	396.1	245.3	146.1	112.4	60.7	23.8	10.6	5.0
1894	1918	1,000.0	390.4	258.0	154.8	109.6	56.1	19.1	7.8	4.2
1895	1919	1,000.0	383.5	274.2	155.3	107.7	53.2	15.7	7.0	3.4
1896	1920	1,000.0	380.2	286.3	157.0	103.5	49.0	14.8	5.9	3.3
1897	1921	1,000.0	368.4	302.7	158.6	100.5	46.9	14.0	5.9	3.0
1898	1922	1,000.0	375.6	294.8	158.5	99.2	47.8	14.6	6.6	2.9
1899	1923	1,000.0	368.4	305.1	158.0	97.0	46.7	14.9	6.8	3.1
1900	1924	1,000.0	367.2	308.8	153.4	98.1	46.5	15.6	6.9	3.5
1901	1925	1,000.0	366.1	310.9	149.4	100.6	46.5	16.0	6.9	3.6
1902	1926	1,000.0	363.5	311.4	149.8	98.7	49.6	15.8	7.3	3.9
1903	1927	1,000.0	364.7	309.1	154.4	93.7	51.2	15.7	7.2	4.0
1904	1928	1,000.0	369.0	310.3	151.4	91.4	49.7	17.3	6.8	4.1
1905	1929	1,000.0	377.7	310.5	147.5	88.3	47.8	17.1	7.2	3.9
1906	1930	1,000.0	387.4	310.3	143.3	86.1	44.9	17.4	6.9	3.7
1907	1931	1,000.0	396.7	306.8	141.4	83.6	44.6	17.1	6.3	3.5
1908	1932	1,000.0	407.7	300.2	140.1	82.6	43.8	16.3	6.1	3.2
1909	1933	1,000.0	412.1	295.2	140.4	83.4	44.5	15.7	5.8	2.9
1910	1934	1,000.0	422.1	286.1	139.1	84.4	44.1	15.5	6.0	2.7
1911	1935	1,000.0	424.9	282.9	138.2	84.3	45.1	15.9	6.1	2.6
1912	1936	1,000.0	435.4	275.8	137.7	81.9	44.3	16.1	6.1	2.7
1913	1937	1,000.0	440.7	271.7	138.3	80.0	44.7	15.8	6.0	2.8
1914	1938	1,000.0	447.4	263.1	138.7	80.0	44.8	17.0	5.9	3.1
1915	1939	1,000.0	450.5	258.1	136.5	82.9	45.2	17.4	6.2	3.2
1916	1940	1,000.0	453.7	251.5	136.1	85.5	45.7	17.8	6.4	3.3
1917	1941	1,000.0	454.2	246.4	136.3	86.4	47.4	18.8	6.7	3.8
1918	1942	1,000.0	451.2	244.9	137.5	86.6	48.4	19.9	7.5	4.0
1919	1943	1,000.0	432.1	254.3	143.1	88.9	49.2	20.3	8.2	3.9
1920	1944	1,000.0	419.2	258.1	147.7	90.4	50.6	21.2	8.6	4.2
1921	1945	1,000.0	416.5	252.5	148.8	93.0	53.7	22.4	9.0	4.1
1922	1946	1,000.0	430.5	240.9	146.3	92.7	54.0	22.8	8.7	4.1
1923	1947	1,000.0	429.7	235.3	150.8	93.7	54.4	23.0	8.8	4.3
1924	1948	1,000.0	408.8	242.4	160.4	97.2	55.1	22.8	8.8	4.5
1925	1949	1,000.0	387.0	239.8	173.4	105.1	57.8	23.3	9.0	4.6
1926	1950	1,000.0	372.6	228.8	183.2	113.7	62.3	24.7	9.8	4.9
1927	1951	1,000.0	365.3	216.1	185.2	123.4	67.3	27.4	10.2	5.1
1928	1952	1,000.0	363.5	202.6	182.2	130.0	74.8	30.8	11.1	5.0
1929	1953	1,000.0	357.8	193.6	180.5	134.2	81.8	34.1	12.5	5.5
1930	1954	1,000.0	356.3	186.3	178.5	135.5	84.9	38.5	13.8	6.2
1931	1955	1,000.0	345.0	183.3	182.4	137.5	86.8	42.0	15.6	7.4
1932	1956	1,000.0	332.9	185.4	185.8	140.0	88.9	42.1	17.1	7.8
1933	1957	1,000.0	310.2	190.1	193.6	142.7	93.9	42.8	17.9	8.8
1934	1958	1,000.0	290.2	193.8	196.8	149.2	95.9	45.8	19.1	9.2
1935	1959	1,000.0	275.3	196.4	197.9	154.8	98.4	47.5	20.6	9.1
1936	1960	1,000.0	270.2	195.8	198.4	154.1	101.5	48.8	21.4	9.8
1937	1961	1,000.0	270.8	197.7	195.6	153.6	101.4	49.4	21.5	10.0
1938	1962	1,000.0	281.0	195.2	192.8	150.4	101.2	47.8	21.2	10.4
1939	1963	1,000.0	285.0	194.4	192.6	148.8	100.2	47.4	21.2	10.4
1940	1964	1,000.0	288.4	195.6	194.2	148.1	97.0	46.1	20.6	10.0
1941	1965	1,000.0	295.2	199.9	194.3	143.4	93.4	44.6	19.6	9.6
1942	1966	1,000.0	300.7	208.6	196.5	139.0	88.8	40.6	17.4	8.4
1943	1967	1,000.0	307.3	218.4	198.0	135.0	83.0	36.3	15.2	6.8
1944	1968	1,000.0	307.2	229.0	204.4	132.6	76.7	31.0	13.3	5.8
1945	1969	1,000.0	304.5	245.9	207.9	129.2	69.8	27.6	10.7	4.4
1946	1970	1,000.0	297.1	263.3	213.9	124.7	64.8	24.1	8.6	3.5
1947	1971	1,000.0	286.6	282.5	218.7	120.7	60.9	20.5	7.0	3.1
1948	1972	1,000.0	280.3	297.4	224.1	117.6	55.1	17.4	5.7	2.4
1949	1973	1,000.0	280.8	309.9	225.9	112.6	49.4	15.0	4.7	1.7
1950	1974	1,000.0	286.1	317.2	228.3	106.6	44.1	12.8	3.6	1.3

TABLE 8C. DISTRIBUTIONS OF ALL OTHER WOMEN BY PARITY AS OF THE BEGINNING OF EACH YEAR 1917-74 BY AGE FOR EACH COHORT FROM 1867 TO 1959--CON.

(BASED ON CUMULATIVE BIRTH RATES)

EXACT AGE AND COHORT	AS OF JANUARY 1	TOTAL	PARITY							
			0	1	2	3	4	5	6	7 AND HIGHER
25 YEARS										
1892	1917	1,000.0	365.4	230.7	164.6	112.5	71.8	31.0	15.0	9.0
1893	1918	1,000.0	360.2	238.5	147.4	123.8	74.4	31.7	15.5	8.5
1894	1919	1,000.0	353.5	254.9	151.5	122.9	70.8	26.2	13.1	7.1
1895	1920	1,000.0	349.9	267.1	155.1	119.4	66.1	24.1	11.5	6.8
1896	1921	1,000.0	340.1	283.0	158.1	115.6	62.9	23.0	11.1	6.2
1897	1922	1,000.0	331.3	296.6	156.6	112.9	62.1	22.6	11.5	6.4
1898	1923	1,000.0	343.5	282.7	160.5	110.3	61.6	23.0	12.1	6.3
1899	1924	1,000.0	338.0	294.3	155.7	109.4	60.0	23.8	12.1	6.7
1900	1925	1,000.0	334.7	300.7	147.2	111.6	60.8	24.8	12.9	7.3
1901	1926	1,000.0	333.4	305.2	146.0	108.5	62.5	24.6	12.2	7.6
1902	1927	1,000.0	334.0	303.9	149.2	103.9	64.0	24.4	12.8	7.8
1903	1928	1,000.0	338.5	302.5	150.8	101.0	62.4	25.7	11.7	7.4
1904	1929	1,000.0	345.7	303.9	147.4	97.7	60.5	25.9	11.4	7.5
1905	1930	1,000.0	354.9	304.6	144.7	93.7	57.5	25.9	11.9	6.8
1906	1931	1,000.0	363.4	305.0	141.3	91.3	55.2	25.7	11.4	6.7
1907	1932	1,000.0	374.3	300.1	140.5	88.7	54.7	24.8	10.7	6.2
1908	1933	1,000.0	384.3	294.2	139.0	88.0	54.5	24.4	9.9	5.7
1909	1934	1,000.0	390.6	288.4	137.9	88.9	55.6	23.6	9.8	5.2
1910	1935	1,000.0	398.3	280.8	136.3	90.3	55.2	24.0	9.9	5.2
1911	1936	1,000.0	401.7	277.3	136.3	88.7	56.3	24.2	10.3	5.2
1912	1937	1,000.0	412.9	269.3	137.1	86.7	54.7	23.8	10.3	5.2
1913	1938	1,000.0	417.8	264.6	136.8	85.8	55.4	23.9	10.2	5.5
1914	1939	1,000.0	424.3	256.3	136.1	86.4	55.5	25.3	10.3	5.8
1915	1940	1,000.0	427.0	251.4	134.3	89.0	55.5	26.2	10.7	5.9
1916	1941	1,000.0	430.5	245.0	132.5	90.2	57.1	27.1	11.1	6.5
1917	1942	1,000.0	429.6	239.8	133.3	91.7	58.1	28.7	11.9	6.9
1918	1943	1,000.0	422.8	240.8	136.5	92.0	58.5	29.3	12.8	7.3
1919	1944	1,000.0	404.1	248.6	142.7	94.0	59.6	29.8	13.6	7.6
1920	1945	1,000.0	392.8	253.1	145.5	94.8	60.9	30.8	14.4	7.7
1921	1946	1,000.0	390.9	248.2	147.8	96.5	63.0	31.5	14.3	7.8
1922	1947	1,000.0	398.6	235.0	150.9	98.1	63.8	31.8	14.1	7.7
1923	1948	1,000.0	389.3	234.6	156.6	101.4	64.1	31.6	14.4	8.0
1924	1949	1,000.0	371.1	232.8	166.7	108.1	66.5	32.0	14.3	8.5
1925	1950	1,000.0	351.3	226.8	178.0	115.8	71.0	33.2	15.3	8.6
1926	1951	1,000.0	338.6	214.8	182.7	125.6	76.8	36.1	16.2	9.2
1927	1952	1,000.0	332.4	202.0	181.7	132.9	84.0	40.2	17.7	9.1
1928	1953	1,000.0	331.6	190.1	177.6	136.2	91.3	44.4	19.0	9.8
1929	1954	1,000.0	325.2	181.5	176.1	138.3	97.3	49.5	21.1	11.0
1930	1955	1,000.0	322.5	174.5	174.4	140.2	98.7	53.9	23.3	12.5
1931	1956	1,000.0	310.9	170.1	179.1	142.7	99.6	57.5	25.7	14.4
1932	1957	1,000.0	297.7	171.0	182.5	146.0	103.0	56.2	27.8	15.8
1933	1958	1,000.0	274.3	174.3	190.3	150.1	107.0	58.4	28.8	16.8
1934	1959	1,000.0	255.9	176.7	192.1	156.5	109.4	61.5	30.5	17.4
1935	1960	1,000.0	240.9	179.5	192.3	161.0	112.8	63.5	31.9	18.1
1936	1961	1,000.0	236.4	180.2	192.5	159.9	115.2	64.1	32.7	19.0
1937	1962	1,000.0	238.1	182.3	189.6	158.7	114.7	64.3	32.9	19.4
1938	1963	1,000.0	249.6	180.5	187.2	155.1	113.3	62.2	32.9	19.2
1939	1964	1,000.0	252.2	181.0	188.8	154.6	111.6	61.5	31.2	19.1
1940	1965	1,000.0	255.5	183.6	191.6	153.8	108.1	58.9	30.5	18.0
1941	1966	1,000.0	261.9	189.6	194.8	149.7	103.9	56.0	27.5	16.6
1942	1967	1,000.0	266.2	200.8	199.5	146.4	98.5	50.3	24.5	13.8
1943	1968	1,000.0	272.8	210.5	204.4	143.7	92.0	44.5	20.9	11.2
1944	1969	1,000.0	270.7	224.7	211.1	142.1	86.1	38.4	17.8	9.1
1945	1970	1,000.0	267.3	239.3	217.1	140.2	79.4	34.9	14.7	7.1
1946	1971	1,000.0	256.4	256.3	225.5	137.8	75.0	30.9	12.3	5.8
1947	1972	1,000.0	247.0	274.7	230.7	135.1	70.9	26.7	10.1	4.8
1948	1973	1,000.0	241.7	293.0	237.1	130.5	63.6	22.6	8.0	3.5
1949	1974	1,000.0	244.9	303.0	240.6	125.7	57.5	19.3	6.4	2.6

TABLE 8C. DISTRIBUTIONS OF ALL OTHER WOMEN BY PARITY AS OF THE BEGINNING OF EACH YEAR 1917-74 BY AGE FOR EACH COHORT FROM 1867 TO 1959—CON.

(BASED ON CUMULATIVE BIRTH RATES)

EXACT AGE AND COHORT	AS OF JANUARY 1	TOTAL	PARITY							
			0	1	2	3	4	5	6	7 AND HIGHER
26 YEARS										
1891---------------	1917	1,000.0	343.3	219.8	152.9	116.8	84.6	42.9	23.6	16.1
1892---------------	1918	1,000.0	336.9	225.1	161.8	119.2	82.7	38.8	21.4	14.1
1893---------------	1919	1,000.0	330.5	236.4	141.0	132.2	86.1	38.7	22.2	12.9
1894---------------	1920	1,000.0	326.6	248.4	148.0	130.0	81.0	34.8	19.0	12.2
1895---------------	1921	1,000.0	317.6	263.2	152.4	126.5	78.1	32.5	18.3	11.4
1896---------------	1922	1,000.0	310.6	276.8	152.7	123.1	75.3	31.8	17.8	11.9
1897---------------	1923	1,000.0	306.0	286.2	155.0	119.1	73.2	30.7	18.3	11.5
1898---------------	1924	1,000.0	319.5	273.1	155.2	117.6	72.4	31.8	18.7	11.7
1899---------------	1925	1,000.0	313.2	287.2	146.6	117.1	71.3	32.7	19.4	12.5
1900---------------	1926	1,000.0	309.3	294.5	141.9	114.3	73.7	33.2	19.5	13.6
1901---------------	1927	1,000.0	310.4	297.6	143.6	108.5	73.9	32.8	19.8	13.4
1902---------------	1928	1,000.0	313.9	298.1	144.5	105.8	71.3	34.4	18.9	13.1
1903---------------	1929	1,000.0	320.9	297.1	145.4	103.0	70.1	33.9	17.3	12.3
1904---------------	1930	1,000.0	328.6	299.0	142.9	98.7	67.1	34.3	17.5	11.9
1905---------------	1931	1,000.0	337.0	300.0	140.7	95.4	64.5	33.7	17.5	11.2
1906---------------	1932	1,000.0	346.4	299.3	138.5	92.5	62.4	33.0	17.0	10.9
1907---------------	1933	1,000.0	356.9	295.0	137.0	90.1	62.3	33.1	15.5	10.1
1908---------------	1934	1,000.0	368.5	288.9	134.8	89.5	61.8	32.1	15.2	9.2
1909---------------	1935	1,000.0	372.9	284.2	133.9	89.8	63.2	31.9	15.2	8.9
1910---------------	1936	1,000.0	381.4	275.5	133.6	90.6	62.8	32.1	14.9	9.1
1911---------------	1937	1,000.0	385.0	271.6	134.3	89.0	63.5	32.0	15.4	9.2
1912---------------	1938	1,000.0	395.9	263.6	134.4	87.8	61.8	31.6	15.6	9.3
1913---------------	1939	1,000.0	400.3	259.2	133.5	87.6	62.1	32.3	15.6	9.4
1914---------------	1940	1,000.0	406.2	251.5	132.9	87.9	62.1	33.8	15.8	9.8
1915---------------	1941	1,000.0	408.9	246.6	130.7	89.7	62.5	35.0	16.3	10.3
1916---------------	1942	1,000.0	411.3	240.0	129.6	91.4	63.5	36.3	17.0	10.9
1917---------------	1943	1,000.0	408.0	236.0	131.6	93.1	64.5	37.1	17.9	11.8
1918---------------	1944	1,000.0	400.8	235.8	135.6	93.1	65.2	38.1	18.8	12.6
1919---------------	1945	1,000.0	382.9	244.0	140.4	95.2	66.2	38.4	20.1	12.8
1920---------------	1946	1,000.0	372.2	248.9	144.1	95.4	66.9	38.8	20.5	13.2
1921---------------	1947	1,000.0	364.9	242.8	150.4	98.7	69.4	39.9	20.7	13.2
1922---------------	1948	1,000.0	366.4	233.6	153.6	102.7	70.5	39.8	20.2	13.2
1923---------------	1949	1,000.0	359.6	226.5	159.8	108.4	71.3	40.3	20.4	13.7
1924---------------	1950	1,000.0	342.3	222.1	168.9	114.8	75.5	40.8	21.4	14.2
1925---------------	1951	1,000.0	323.6	214.6	177.1	122.8	81.3	43.5	22.5	14.6
1926---------------	1952	1,000.0	311.0	203.1	178.8	131.2	88.5	47.5	24.5	15.4
1927---------------	1953	1,000.0	305.4	191.0	177.0	135.5	95.8	52.8	26.3	16.2
1928---------------	1954	1,000.0	305.1	179.2	172.2	138.2	101.4	57.7	28.8	17.4
1929---------------	1955	1,000.0	297.4	171.1	171.7	138.7	106.4	63.6	31.4	19.7
1930---------------	1956	1,000.0	295.6	162.8	170.2	141.2	106.5	67.4	34.1	22.2
1931---------------	1957	1,000.0	283.1	158.1	174.2	144.0	107.9	69.7	37.5	25.5
1932---------------	1958	1,000.0	270.0	157.8	177.4	148.9	110.8	69.0	38.9	27.2
1933---------------	1959	1,000.0	248.0	159.8	184.4	152.6	115.0	71.7	40.3	28.2
1934---------------	1960	1,000.0	229.1	161.8	186.1	157.8	118.9	74.8	41.6	29.9
1935---------------	1961	1,000.0	214.2	166.1	185.8	162.0	122.0	75.4	43.6	30.9
1936---------------	1962	1,000.0	210.0	167.7	185.6	161.0	123.0	76.3	44.5	31.9
1937---------------	1963	1,000.0	212.8	169.4	184.2	158.5	122.0	76.2	44.8	32.1
1938---------------	1964	1,000.0	223.9	168.7	183.0	156.3	120.2	73.3	43.1	31.5
1939---------------	1965	1,000.0	227.2	169.4	184.7	156.8	118.4	71.9	40.9	30.7
1940---------------	1966	1,000.0	229.6	174.3	189.7	156.6	114.6	68.4	39.0	27.8
1941---------------	1967	1,000.0	235.2	181.7	194.8	153.8	111.0	64.5	34.6	24.4
1942---------------	1968	1,000.0	239.1	192.9	202.3	152.1	105.9	56.8	30.8	20.1
1943---------------	1969	1,000.0	243.1	206.5	208.2	149.7	100.0	50.7	25.9	15.9
1944---------------	1970	1,000.0	240.5	217.5	217.6	150.0	94.1	45.0	22.3	13.0
1945---------------	1971	1,000.0	234.4	231.4	225.1	149.8	88.0	41.9	18.7	10.7
1946---------------	1972	1,000.0	224.4	247.9	233.4	148.9	83.8	37.3	16.0	8.3
1947---------------	1973	1,000.0	214.8	268.9	240.5	145.7	78.7	31.9	12.8	6.7
1948---------------	1974	1,000.0	210.8	285.6	248.9	141.8	70.8	27.1	10.1	4.9

TABLE 8C. DISTRIBUTIONS OF ALL CTHER WOMEN BY PARITY AS OF THE BEGINNING OF EACH YEAR 1917-74 BY AGE FOR EACH COHORT FROM 1867 TO 1959--CON.

(BASED ON CUMULATIVE BIRTH RATES)

EXACT AGE AND COHORT	AS OF JANUARY 1	TOTAL	PARITY							
			0	1	2	3	4	5	6	7 AND HIGHER
27 YEARS										
1890	1917	1,000.0	325.6	210.3	141.9	116.7	92.8	53.7	32.7	26.3
1891	1918	1,000.0	321.6	215.9	148.2	120.4	91.5	49.1	30.2	23.1
1892	1919	1,000.0	313.9	224.3	154.6	124.4	89.9	44.4	28.2	20.3
1893	1920	1,000.0	309.6	231.1	136.4	136.3	92.3	46.0	28.3	20.0
1894	1921	1,000.0	301.3	244.7	143.6	133.8	89.6	41.9	26.2	18.9
1895	1922	1,000.0	294.9	257.6	146.0	130.8	86.2	40.0	24.6	19.9
1896	1923	1,000.0	291.2	268.3	149.7	126.2	82.6	38.3	24.4	19.3
1897	1924	1,000.0	288.1	278.6	149.5	123.0	79.6	37.8	24.4	19.0
1898	1925	1,000.0	301.3	267.4	145.3	121.5	79.5	39.1	25.9	20.0
1899	1926	1,000.0	293.9	281.5	140.7	116.9	80.7	39.3	26.4	20.6
1900	1927	1,000.0	291.4	288.2	137.5	112.1	81.8	40.0	27.3	21.7
1901	1928	1,000.0	294.3	292.4	138.3	108.2	78.3	41.2	26.4	20.9
1902	1929	1,000.0	300.3	293.5	139.3	104.9	75.8	41.5	24.9	19.8
1903	1930	1,000.0	307.9	292.8	141.2	101.5	73.6	41.2	23.4	18.4
1904	1931	1,000.0	314.8	295.1	139.3	98.0	70.8	40.8	23.0	18.2
1905	1932	1,000.0	323.9	295.5	137.0	94.6	68.7	39.6	23.5	17.2
1906	1933	1,000.0	333.0	295.3	134.6	91.1	67.1	40.0	22.4	16.5
1907	1934	1,000.0	344.9	290.6	132.8	89.5	66.1	39.7	21.2	15.2
1908	1935	1,000.0	355.5	285.5	130.7	88.1	66.0	38.7	21.1	14.4
1909	1936	1,000.0	360.0	280.4	130.6	88.4	67.3	38.6	20.5	14.2
1910	1937	1,000.0	368.8	271.2	131.1	88.8	66.4	38.8	20.6	14.3
1911	1938	1,000.0	372.1	267.2	131.1	88.2	66.8	38.9	20.8	14.9
1912	1939	1,000.0	382.3	259.4	131.1	87.6	65.3	38.1	21.5	14.7
1913	1940	1,000.0	386.1	256.0	130.1	87.1	65.5	38.8	21.5	14.9
1914	1941	1,000.0	391.7	248.1	130.0	87.1	65.7	40.0	21.8	15.6
1915	1942	1,000.0	393.4	243.1	128.3	89.6	65.6	41.5	22.3	16.2
1916	1943	1,000.0	395.0	237.0	127.5	90.9	66.8	42.5	23.0	17.3
1917	1944	1,000.0	390.8	232.1	130.4	92.2	68.3	43.9	23.8	18.5
1918	1945	1,000.0	383.7	231.9	133.5	93.0	68.9	44.4	25.1	19.5
1919	1946	1,000.0	366.1	240.3	138.9	94.6	68.9	45.0	26.2	20.0
1920	1947	1,000.0	350.9	244.5	145.1	96.3	70.5	45.4	27.0	20.3
1921	1948	1,000.0	338.5	240.6	151.9	101.8	73.5	46.3	27.1	20.3
1922	1949	1,000.0	341.8	227.3	155.6	107.1	74.5	46.8	26.3	20.6
1923	1950	1,000.0	336.1	217.9	160.9	112.6	77.0	47.2	27.1	21.2
1924	1951	1,000.0	319.6	211.9	167.5	118.9	82.5	49.1	28.4	22.1
1925	1952	1,000.0	300.3	205.2	172.7	126.5	89.8	51.9	30.9	22.7
1926	1953	1,000.0	287.6	193.4	174.8	132.7	96.2	57.6	33.1	24.6
1927	1954	1,000.0	282.6	180.8	172.9	136.0	101.8	63.9	35.5	26.5
1928	1955	1,000.0	282.4	169.4	168.3	136.8	106.9	68.9	38.8	28.5
1929	1956	1,000.0	275.6	160.4	167.0	138.2	111.1	74.1	41.8	31.8
1930	1957	1,000.0	273.5	152.0	165.5	140.7	110.8	76.9	44.9	35.7
1931	1958	1,000.0	261.8	146.0	168.6	144.7	112.1	79.0	48.0	39.8
1932	1959	1,000.0	249.2	145.7	172.3	148.2	115.4	78.2	49.2	41.8
1933	1960	1,000.0	227.1	147.5	178.2	152.2	119.8	81.7	50.0	43.5
1934	1961	1,000.0	208.2	150.3	179.7	157.0	124.0	83.5	51.7	45.6
1935	1962	1,000.0	193.3	154.6	180.1	160.0	126.6	83.9	54.7	46.8
1936	1963	1,000.0	189.6	156.5	180.0	159.5	126.6	84.9	55.1	47.8
1937	1964	1,000.0	192.5	159.0	179.2	157.3	125.3	85.0	54.1	47.6
1938	1965	1,000.0	204.3	158.3	178.5	156.9	123.6	80.7	51.8	45.9
1939	1966	1,000.0	206.4	160.9	181.6	157.5	123.1	78.7	48.8	43.0
1940	1967	1,000.0	208.3	166.8	188.9	158.8	119.0	75.0	45.3	37.9
1941	1968	1,000.0	213.3	174.6	195.6	157.3	116.3	70.2	40.1	32.6
1942	1969	1,000.0	215.2	187.9	205.2	155.7	112.0	62.1	35.5	26.4
1943	1970	1,000.0	218.5	199.6	212.7	155.1	106.4	56.2	30.6	20.9
1944	1971	1,000.0	213.6	209.7	223.1	156.9	101.4	51.1	26.6	17.6
1945	1972	1,000.0	208.4	222.8	230.4	158.3	95.1	48.3	22.4	14.3
1946	1973	1,000.0	198.2	241.1	241.0	156.7	90.7	42.2	19.2	10.9
1947	1974	1,000.0	188.6	261.9	249.4	154.6	85.5	36.1	15.2	8.7

TABLE 8C. DISTRIBUTIONS OF ALL OTHER WOMEN BY PARITY AS OF THE BEGINNING OF EACH YEAR 1917-74 BY AGE FOR EACH COHORT FROM 1867 TO 1959--CON.

(BASED ON CUMULATIVE BIRTH RATES)

EXACT AGE AND COHORT	AS OF JANUARY 1	TOTAL	PARITY							
			0	1	2	3	4	5	6	7 AND HIGHER
28 YEARS										
1889----------------	1917	1,000.0	309.4	201.0	134.2	112.6	98.1	62.3	42.6	39.8
1890----------------	1918	1,000.0	307.7	206.3	137.5	118.1	97.9	57.7	39.4	35.4
1891----------------	1919	1,000.0	302.6	214.5	141.6	123.4	96.9	52.5	37.3	31.2
1892----------------	1920	1,000.0	296.6	219.1	150.3	126.2	94.3	49.5	34.4	29.6
1893----------------	1921	1,000.0	288.5	227.2	132.1	137.8	98.8	50.9	35.9	28.8
1894----------------	1922	1,000.0	282.4	239.2	137.5	135.7	95.6	47.0	32.6	30.0
1895----------------	1923	1,000.0	278.7	249.7	143.0	131.8	91.5	44.3	31.5	29.5
1896----------------	1924	1,000.0	276.3	261.2	144.5	127.9	87.1	43.2	30.7	29.1
1897----------------	1925	1,000.0	273.1	273.3	140.8	124.6	84.5	42.3	31.7	29.7
1898----------------	1926	1,000.0	286.2	262.2	139.6	118.9	86.4	44.1	32.3	30.3
1899----------------	1927	1,000.0	279.9	275.6	135.5	113.9	86.6	43.6	34.3	30.6
1900----------------	1928	1,000.0	278.1	283.6	132.5	109.6	84.1	46.0	34.1	32.0
1901----------------	1929	1,000.0	282.9	288.5	133.5	105.8	80.5	46.4	32.4	30.0
1902----------------	1930	1,000.0	289.5	289.8	135.7	102.6	76.4	46.9	31.1	28.0
1903----------------	1931	1,000.0	296.7	289.6	137.7	99.6	75.0	46.2	28.6	26.6
1904----------------	1932	1,000.0	304.0	291.9	135.3	95.9	73.0	45.1	28.6	26.2
1905----------------	1933	1,000.0	313.2	292.1	133.2	92.4	70.9	44.1	29.1	25.0
1906----------------	1934	1,000.0	323.2	291.8	130.6	89.2	68.4	44.8	28.1	23.9
1907----------------	1935	1,000.0	334.5	287.6	128.9	87.0	67.9	44.4	27.4	22.3
1908----------------	1936	1,000.0	345.3	282.6	127.6	85.8	67.7	43.5	26.2	21.3
1909----------------	1937	1,000.0	349.8	276.9	128.3	85.8	68.7	43.6	25.8	21.1
1910----------------	1938	1,000.0	358.3	267.6	128.5	86.8	67.5	43.8	25.9	21.6
1911----------------	1939	1,000.0	361.1	263.6	128.0	86.6	68.5	43.2	26.7	22.3
1912----------------	1940	1,000.0	370.9	256.5	128.0	85.8	67.0	42.2	27.5	22.1
1913----------------	1941	1,000.0	374.4	253.0	127.4	85.1	67.4	42.5	27.5	22.7
1914----------------	1942	1,000.0	379.1	245.0	127.7	85.7	67.0	44.1	27.8	23.6
1915----------------	1943	1,000.0	379.6	240.5	126.4	88.9	66.8	45.8	28.0	24.0
1916----------------	1944	1,000.0	380.4	233.5	126.4	90.0	68.2	47.4	28.6	25.5
1917----------------	1945	1,000.0	376.2	228.5	128.6	91.9	69.7	48.3	29.9	26.9
1918----------------	1946	1,000.0	369.5	229.0	132.0	92.0	69.6	48.9	30.6	28.4
1919----------------	1947	1,000.0	348.1	236.6	138.8	95.2	70.6	49.8	32.0	28.9
1920----------------	1948	1,000.0	328.8	241.8	146.5	97.7	73.1	50.2	32.5	29.4
1921----------------	1949	1,000.0	317.3	235.2	152.7	104.5	76.3	51.4	32.9	29.7
1922----------------	1950	1,000.0	321.7	219.7	156.4	110.0	78.1	51.9	32.2	30.0
1923----------------	1951	1,000.0	316.8	209.4	159.8	115.1	81.7	52.9	33.5	30.8
1924----------------	1952	1,000.0	300.0	203.6	163.6	121.4	88.7	54.6	35.7	32.4
1925----------------	1953	1,000.0	280.3	196.4	169.2	127.4	94.8	59.6	38.3	34.0
1926----------------	1954	1,000.0	267.9	183.5	171.4	132.6	100.6	65.8	41.2	37.0
1927----------------	1955	1,000.0	263.0	172.0	168.7	134.0	105.5	72.3	44.4	40.1
1928----------------	1956	1,000.0	264.2	159.4	163.7	135.7	109.8	76.3	48.2	42.7
1929----------------	1957	1,000.0	257.4	150.2	162.5	136.5	113.6	81.3	50.8	47.7
1930----------------	1958	1,000.0	256.1	141.2	160.5	140.2	112.6	82.9	54.9	51.6
1931----------------	1959	1,000.0	245.0	136.0	163.2	143.1	114.5	84.4	56.8	57.0
1932----------------	1960	1,000.0	232.3	135.4	166.8	146.5	117.6	84.8	57.3	59.3
1933----------------	1961	1,000.0	210.3	137.5	173.0	150.3	122.1	87.5	58.3	61.0
1934----------------	1962	1,000.0	191.3	140.2	174.2	154.7	126.2	88.8	61.2	63.4
1935----------------	1963	1,000.0	176.9	144.4	175.0	157.6	128.8	89.7	62.9	64.7
1936----------------	1964	1,000.0	173.3	147.3	175.1	157.8	127.5	91.1	62.1	65.8
1937----------------	1965	1,000.0	176.9	149.3	174.8	156.6	127.2	89.6	61.4	64.2
1938----------------	1966	1,000.0	187.5	150.8	174.9	156.6	126.6	85.4	58.1	60.1
1939----------------	1967	1,000.0	189.4	153.4	180.5	159.0	125.6	83.6	53.8	54.7
1940----------------	1968	1,000.0	190.9	159.2	189.1	161.0	122.9	79.1	50.3	47.5
1941----------------	1969	1,000.0	193.9	169.0	198.0	159.0	121.3	73.9	44.7	40.2
1942----------------	1970	1,000.0	195.0	181.5	207.8	159.4	117.1	66.5	40.3	32.4
1943----------------	1971	1,000.0	196.8	192.0	215.9	160.2	112.2	61.7	34.6	26.6
1944----------------	1972	1,000.0	192.0	201.7	226.7	163.4	107.2	56.5	30.4	22.1
1945----------------	1973	1,000.0	187.1	215.5	236.1	164.3	101.1	52.5	25.8	17.6
1946----------------	1974	1,000.0	176.3	234.0	247.7	164.1	96.6	46.0	22.0	13.3

TABLE 8C. DISTRIBUTIONS OF ALL OTHER WOMEN BY PARITY AS OF THE BEGINNING OF EACH YEAR 1917-74 BY AGE FOR EACH COHORT FROM 1867 TO 1959--CON.

(BASED ON CUMULATIVE BIRTH RATES)

EXACT AGE AND COHORT	AS OF JANUARY 1	TOTAL	PARITY							
			0	1	2	3	4	5	6	7 AND HIGHER
29 YEARS										
1888---------------	1917	1,000.0	294.7	191.8	131.2	105.2	100.5	69.3	51.6	55.7
1889---------------	1918	1,000.0	294.9	197.3	130.7	112.5	101.6	64.6	48.5	49.9
1890---------------	1919	1,000.0	292.3	204.7	132.3	119.2	101.8	59.6	45.7	44.4
1891---------------	1920	1,000.0	288.6	209.8	138.2	123.5	99.8	55.9	42.6	41.6
1892---------------	1921	1,000.0	279.5	215.3	146.9	126.1	99.0	52.6	41.2	39.4
1893---------------	1922	1,000.0	273.1	222.1	127.3	137.8	103.0	54.1	41.3	41.3
1894---------------	1923	1,000.0	269.2	232.2	135.1	135.2	99.3	49.6	38.6	40.8
1895---------------	1924	1,000.0	266.5	243.4	138.8	132.0	94.4	47.5	36.9	40.5
1896---------------	1925	1,000.0	264.1	256.4	137.4	127.7	90.4	45.8	37.1	41.1
1897---------------	1926	1,000.0	261.3	268.8	135.5	121.4	89.1	45.7	37.0	41.2
1898---------------	1927	1,000.0	275.7	257.4	134.5	115.7	90.0	46.3	38.7	41.7
1899---------------	1928	1,000.0	269.1	272.1	131.1	110.7	87.4	47.5	39.6	42.5
1900---------------	1929	1,000.0	269.0	280.3	128.5	106.2	84.2	50.0	39.1	42.7
1901---------------	1930	1,000.0	273.9	285.3	130.1	103.4	79.4	50.6	37.7	39.6
1902---------------	1931	1,000.0	280.3	286.8	132.9	100.0	76.2	50.2	35.8	37.8
1903---------------	1932	1,000.0	287.9	287.2	134.5	96.6	75.6	48.8	33.5	35.9
1904---------------	1933	1,000.0	295.2	289.4	132.4	92.7	73.4	47.9	33.5	35.5
1905---------------	1934	1,000.0	305.4	288.9	130.0	90.0	70.7	47.3	33.7	34.0
1906---------------	1935	1,000.0	315.0	288.8	127.8	86.2	68.5	48.0	33.0	32.7
1907---------------	1936	1,000.0	326.3	285.2	126.2	84.5	67.7	47.7	31.9	30.5
1908---------------	1937	1,000.0	337.1	280.1	125.4	83.4	67.6	46.4	30.9	29.1
1909---------------	1938	1,000.0	341.6	273.8	126.1	83.8	68.2	46.6	30.2	29.7
1910---------------	1939	1,000.0	349.7	264.3	126.1	84.7	68.2	46.2	30.5	30.3
1911---------------	1940	1,000.0	352.1	260.9	125.6	84.3	69.1	45.5	31.2	31.3
1912---------------	1941	1,000.0	361.7	253.8	125.9	83.3	67.8	44.1	31.9	31.5
1913---------------	1942	1,000.0	364.5	250.2	125.6	83.1	67.7	44.7	31.9	32.3
1914---------------	1943	1,000.0	367.5	242.8	126.2	84.6	67.2	46.7	32.5	32.5
1915---------------	1944	1,000.0	367.4	237.5	125.6	87.6	67.1	48.9	32.6	33.3
1916---------------	1945	1,000.0	368.1	230.4	125.0	89.3	68.4	50.0	33.7	35.1
1917---------------	1946	1,000.0	364.1	225.7	127.7	90.8	69.5	51.2	34.4	36.6
1918---------------	1947	1,000.0	354.9	225.8	131.7	92.2	70.2	52.0	34.9	38.3
1919---------------	1948	1,000.0	329.9	233.7	140.1	95.6	72.4	52.9	36.4	39.0
1920---------------	1949	1,000.0	310.7	237.0	147.4	99.1	74.9	53.7	37.3	39.9
1921---------------	1950	1,000.0	299.9	228.3	153.3	106.9	78.4	55.0	37.6	40.6
1922---------------	1951	1,000.0	305.1	212.8	155.3	111.7	81.3	55.4	37.5	40.9
1923---------------	1952	1,000.0	300.4	202.3	156.8	116.4	85.9	56.7	39.1	42.4
1924---------------	1953	1,000.0	283.0	196.4	160.6	121.6	92.4	59.9	41.5	44.6
1925---------------	1954	1,000.0	263.5	188.0	166.3	126.5	98.3	65.3	44.6	47.5
1926---------------	1955	1,000.0	251.1	175.0	167.9	131.0	102.9	71.9	48.3	51.9
1927---------------	1956	1,000.0	247.6	162.7	164.5	132.7	107.5	77.6	52.0	55.4
1928---------------	1957	1,000.0	249.6	150.2	159.3	133.8	111.8	80.5	55.2	59.6
1929---------------	1958	1,000.0	243.1	140.8	157.2	135.8	114.2	85.2	58.7	65.0
1930---------------	1959	1,000.0	242.1	133.1	155.5	138.5	113.5	85.6	61.7	70.0
1931---------------	1960	1,000.0	231.3	127.3	158.2	140.9	115.4	87.8	63.3	75.8
1932---------------	1961	1,000.0	218.7	126.8	161.9	145.6	117.5	88.3	63.5	77.7
1933---------------	1962	1,000.0	196.9	128.5	167.9	147.7	123.4	90.5	65.2	79.9
1934---------------	1963	1,000.0	178.3	131.2	169.1	152.9	126.8	92.8	67.2	81.7
1935---------------	1964	1,000.0	163.7	136.2	169.8	156.3	128.7	94.2	67.9	83.2
1936---------------	1965	1,000.0	160.5	139.2	170.7	156.3	128.2	93.8	68.6	82.7
1937---------------	1966	1,000.0	163.2	142.1	171.6	155.7	129.1	92.7	66.1	79.5
1938---------------	1967	1,000.0	174.1	143.4	174.0	157.3	128.0	88.3	62.4	72.5
1939---------------	1968	1,000.0	176.0	146.0	180.1	160.3	128.3	86.6	57.5	65.2
1940---------------	1969	1,000.0	175.4	153.5	190.2	162.6	126.3	81.7	54.4	55.9
1941---------------	1970	1,000.0	177.6	162.6	199.5	161.7	124.9	77.8	49.1	46.8
1942---------------	1971	1,000.0	178.0	173.8	209.5	163.3	121.4	71.2	44.3	38.5
1943---------------	1972	1,000.0	179.2	184.5	217.9	165.2	116.8	66.5	37.9	32.0
1944---------------	1973	1,000.0	174.7	194.0	231.3	168.0	112.3	60.1	33.7	25.9
1945---------------	1974	1,000.0	169.1	208.5	241.3	170.1	106.3	55.8	28.4	20.5

TABLE 8C. DISTRIBUTIONS OF ALL OTHER WOMEN BY PARITY AS OF THE BEGINNING OF EACH YEAR 1917-74 BY AGE FOR EACH COHORT FROM 1867 TO 1959--CON.

(BASED ON CUMULATIVE BIRTH RATES)

EXACT AGE AND COHORT	AS OF JANUARY 1	TOTAL	PARITY							
			0	1	2	3	4	5	6	7 AND HIGHER
30 YEARS										
1887---------------	1917	1,000.0	281.5	185.3	127.7	104.6	100.3	75.7	54.8	70.1
1888---------------	1918	1,000.0	281.9	188.5	128.2	103.7	102.7	69.7	56.5	68.8
1889---------------	1919	1,000.0	281.1	195.7	126.4	112.1	104.1	64.7	54.0	61.9
1890---------------	1920	1,000.0	279.7	200.7	129.1	118.1	103.7	61.4	50.1	57.2
1891---------------	1921	1,000.0	273.6	206.6	134.9	122.2	103.4	57.4	48.3	53.6
1892---------------	1922	1,000.0	265.8	210.7	143.0	124.7	101.9	54.0	46.1	53.8
1893---------------	1923	1,000.0	261.0	216.1	125.0	136.2	105.6	55.3	46.4	54.4
1894---------------	1924	1,000.0	257.9	227.1	131.2	133.9	101.4	51.0	43.4	54.1
1895---------------	1925	1,000.0	255.3	239.2	132.4	130.8	96.9	48.3	42.5	54.6
1896---------------	1926	1,000.0	253.3	252.8	132.4	124.4	93.3	47.3	41.5	55.0
1897---------------	1927	1,000.0	252.1	264.2	131.7	117.7	90.8	47.0	41.5	55.0
1898---------------	1928	1,000.0	266.9	254.7	130.3	111.8	89.7	48.8	42.3	55.5
1899---------------	1929	1,000.0	260.8	269.8	127.2	107.2	86.5	49.6	43.6	55.3
1900---------------	1930	1,000.0	260.9	277.7	125.1	103.6	81.9	52.2	43.8	54.8
1901---------------	1931	1,000.0	265.6	282.4	127.3	100.8	78.1	52.1	42.4	51.3
1902---------------	1932	1,000.0	272.3	284.9	130.1	96.7	75.7	51.3	39.7	49.3
1903---------------	1933	1,000.0	280.2	285.1	132.0	93.4	74.6	50.1	37.5	47.1
1904---------------	1934	1,000.0	288.5	286.6	129.3	90.1	72.3	49.5	37.4	46.3
1905---------------	1935	1,000.0	298.4	286.2	127.6	87.0	69.6	49.1	37.2	44.9
1906---------------	1936	1,000.0	308.0	286.7	125.0	83.8	67.5	49.6	36.8	42.6
1907---------------	1937	1,000.0	319.2	283.1	124.1	82.0	66.9	49.1	35.8	39.8
1908---------------	1938	1,000.0	330.3	277.3	123.5	81.2	66.6	47.7	34.6	38.8
1909---------------	1939	1,000.0	334.2	271.6	123.6	81.6	68.0	47.7	33.4	39.9
1910---------------	1940	1,000.0	342.0	262.5	123.6	82.4	68.2	47.1	33.8	40.4
1911---------------	1941	1,000.0	344.2	259.0	123.5	81.9	68.9	46.4	34.3	41.8
1912---------------	1942	1,000.0	353.1	251.8	124.0	81.4	67.5	45.0	35.1	42.1
1913---------------	1943	1,000.0	354.8	248.1	124.3	82.2	67.0	46.1	35.1	42.4
1914---------------	1944	1,000.0	356.9	240.4	125.3	83.5	66.7	48.4	35.8	43.0
1915---------------	1945	1,000.0	356.5	235.0	124.4	86.9	66.5	50.3	36.2	44.2
1916---------------	1946	1,000.0	357.4	227.9	124.2	88.0	68.0	51.3	37.2	46.0
1917---------------	1947	1,000.0	351.3	222.9	127.4	90.8	69.6	53.2	37.4	47.4
1918---------------	1948	1,000.0	339.8	223.5	132.1	92.3	71.4	53.7	37.8	49.4
1919---------------	1949	1,000.0	314.5	229.4	140.8	96.0	74.1	54.9	39.8	50.5
1920---------------	1950	1,000.0	295.6	231.5	147.2	100.7	76.3	56.1	40.7	51.9
1921---------------	1951	1,000.0	285.3	222.7	151.8	108.2	80.4	57.1	41.8	52.7
1922---------------	1952	1,000.0	290.9	206.4	153.1	112.4	83.7	58.2	41.9	53.4
1923---------------	1953	1,000.0	286.1	195.9	154.4	116.3	88.4	60.3	43.2	55.4
1924---------------	1954	1,000.0	269.1	188.8	157.5	121.0	94.9	63.6	46.5	58.6
1925---------------	1955	1,000.0	249.0	180.7	162.9	124.9	100.4	69.7	49.8	62.6
1926---------------	1956	1,000.0	237.8	166.6	164.2	129.3	104.4	75.3	54.5	67.9
1927---------------	1957	1,000.0	234.9	154.6	159.8	130.9	108.3	80.7	57.4	73.4
1928---------------	1958	1,000.0	237.2	142.1	154.3	133.3	111.5	83.0	60.9	77.7
1929---------------	1959	1,000.0	231.4	133.6	152.4	133.7	114.6	86.7	63.5	84.1
1930---------------	1960	1,000.0	230.5	125.8	150.9	135.8	113.9	87.5	66.4	89.2
1931---------------	1961	1,000.0	220.0	119.5	154.2	139.5	114.5	89.7	67.5	95.1
1932---------------	1962	1,000.0	207.7	118.9	157.1	143.8	117.5	90.1	68.5	96.4
1933---------------	1963	1,000.0	186.5	121.0	163.0	145.9	123.6	92.7	69.3	98.0
1934---------------	1964	1,000.0	167.5	124.1	164.3	151.6	126.4	95.6	70.6	99.9
1935---------------	1965	1,000.0	153.1	129.0	165.6	154.7	128.8	96.1	72.4	100.3
1936---------------	1966	1,000.0	149.5	132.6	167.5	155.3	128.9	95.7	72.2	98.3
1937---------------	1967	1,000.0	152.2	135.6	169.8	155.7	130.1	94.7	69.6	92.3
1938---------------	1968	1,000.0	163.7	136.5	172.8	158.4	129.5	90.3	65.8	83.0
1939---------------	1969	1,000.0	163.6	140.7	180.0	161.6	130.8	88.4	61.0	73.9
1940---------------	1970	1,000.0	162.3	147.4	190.4	164.6	129.2	84.8	58.0	63.3
1941---------------	1971	1,000.0	164.1	155.3	199.8	165.1	128.0	81.3	52.8	53.6
1942---------------	1972	1,000.0	164.0	166.5	210.3	167.0	125.3	74.9	47.5	44.5
1943---------------	1973	1,000.0	165.1	177.0	221.6	168.8	120.7	69.7	40.7	36.4
1944---------------	1974	1,000.0	160.3	186.7	235.3	172.8	116.4	63.2	36.1	29.2

TABLE 8C. DISTRIBUTIONS OF ALL OTHER WOMEN BY PARITY AS OF THE BEGINNING OF EACH YEAR 1917-74 BY AGE FOR EACH COHORT FROM 1867 TO 1959--CON.

(BASED ON CUMULATIVE BIRTH RATES)

EXACT AGE AND COHORT	AS OF JANUARY 1	TOTAL	PARITY							
			0	1	2	3	4	5	6	7 AND HIGHER
31 YEARS										
1886---------------	1917	1,000.0	275.2	177.3	122.1	110.3	97.8	69.2	59.6	88.5
1887---------------	1918	1,000.0	272.1	182.7	125.2	103.2	101.0	75.0	57.9	82.9
1888---------------	1919	1,000.0	271.7	187.0	124.8	103.2	103.4	69.0	60.2	80.7
1889---------------	1920	1,000.0	271.8	192.7	123.5	111.1	104.7	65.6	56.7	73.9
1890---------------	1921	1,000.0	268.8	198.5	125.8	117.3	105.6	61.9	53.6	68.5
1891---------------	1922	1,000.0	263.6	203.0	131.8	121.0	104.6	57.7	51.7	66.6
1892---------------	1923	1,000.0	256.7	206.3	140.7	123.6	102.9	54.5	49.3	66.0
1893---------------	1924	1,000.0	252.4	212.5	121.6	135.0	106.4	55.7	49.6	66.8
1894---------------	1925	1,000.0	249.4	224.0	126.0	133.0	102.6	50.8	47.2	67.0
1895---------------	1926	1,000.0	247.2	236.6	128.0	128.6	97.9	48.5	45.7	67.5
1896---------------	1927	1,000.0	246.2	249.4	129.7	120.9	93.4	48.1	43.8	68.5
1897---------------	1928	1,000.0	245.7	262.2	128.0	115.1	89.8	48.2	43.3	67.7
1898---------------	1929	1,000.0	261.0	253.1	127.4	108.9	88.3	49.4	44.8	67.1
1899---------------	1930	1,000.0	255.0	267.8	124.5	105.0	84.1	51.0	46.3	66.3
1900---------------	1931	1,000.0	254.5	275.6	122.9	101.1	80.4	52.4	46.9	66.2
1901---------------	1932	1,000.0	259.4	280.9	125.2	98.1	76.9	51.8	45.0	62.7
1902---------------	1933	1,000.0	266.4	283.5	128.2	93.9	74.2	51.6	42.2	60.0
1903---------------	1934	1,000.0	275.2	283.2	129.6	91.3	73.5	50.3	39.8	57.1
1904---------------	1935	1,000.0	283.2	284.6	127.6	87.7	70.8	50.2	39.3	56.6
1905---------------	1936	1,000.0	293.3	284.4	125.4	85.1	68.2	49.6	39.6	54.4
1906---------------	1937	1,000.0	302.8	285.1	123.2	81.8	66.5	49.8	39.2	51.6
1907---------------	1938	1,000.0	314.2	281.0	122.6	80.1	65.6	49.3	38.0	49.2
1908---------------	1939	1,000.0	324.8	275.8	121.6	79.5	65.9	47.9	36.3	48.2
1909---------------	1940	1,000.0	328.3	270.3	121.9	79.6	67.8	47.6	35.4	49.1
1910---------------	1941	1,000.0	335.9	261.1	122.1	80.6	67.5	47.4	35.4	50.0
1911---------------	1942	1,000.0	337.5	257.5	122.1	80.4	68.4	46.6	36.0	51.5
1912---------------	1943	1,000.0	345.6	250.1	123.0	80.3	66.7	45.4	37.0	51.9
1913---------------	1944	1,000.0	346.5	246.2	123.5	81.1	66.3	46.6	37.2	52.6
1914---------------	1945	1,000.0	348.1	238.4	124.5	82.5	66.2	48.6	38.2	53.5
1915---------------	1946	1,000.0	347.8	232.7	124.0	85.7	66.0	50.8	38.5	54.5
1916---------------	1947	1,000.0	347.3	225.3	123.9	87.8	68.1	52.3	38.9	56.4
1917---------------	1948	1,000.0	339.1	221.0	127.5	91.1	70.2	54.2	38.9	58.0
1918---------------	1949	1,000.0	327.9	219.7	132.8	92.8	72.2	54.7	39.8	60.1
1919---------------	1950	1,000.0	302.1	225.5	140.1	97.4	74.8	56.2	42.0	61.9
1920---------------	1951	1,000.0	283.4	227.2	145.6	102.0	77.5	57.4	43.4	63.5
1921---------------	1952	1,000.0	273.3	217.1	150.3	108.6	81.9	59.2	44.5	65.1
1922---------------	1953	1,000.0	279.1	200.5	151.6	112.4	85.1	60.8	45.1	65.4
1923---------------	1954	1,000.0	274.9	189.4	152.1	115.9	89.9	62.7	46.9	68.2
1924---------------	1955	1,000.0	256.9	182.3	155.2	119.9	96.7	66.4	49.9	72.7
1925---------------	1956	1,000.0	237.9	173.7	160.0	123.4	101.4	72.2	54.0	77.4
1926---------------	1957	1,000.0	227.1	160.1	159.9	128.1	104.4	77.4	58.6	84.4
1927---------------	1958	1,000.0	224.9	147.0	155.6	130.2	107.8	82.8	60.8	90.9
1928---------------	1959	1,000.0	227.7	135.8	150.4	131.0	112.0	83.6	64.0	95.5
1929---------------	1960	1,000.0	221.8	127.5	148.2	131.3	114.4	88.2	66.4	102.2
1930---------------	1961	1,000.0	221.3	119.2	146.9	134.6	113.2	88.5	69.1	107.2
1931---------------	1962	1,000.0	211.1	113.0	149.5	137.7	115.0	90.4	70.5	112.8
1932---------------	1963	1,000.0	199.2	112.8	152.8	142.6	117.0	90.8	71.4	113.4
1933---------------	1964	1,000.0	178.0	114.9	158.7	144.4	123.2	94.5	72.0	114.3
1934---------------	1965	1,000.0	159.2	118.1	160.6	150.0	126.2	96.8	73.4	115.7
1935---------------	1966	1,000.0	144.5	123.2	162.6	153.7	128.9	97.3	75.0	114.8
1936---------------	1967	1,000.0	141.0	126.9	165.4	154.4	130.0	96.6	75.6	110.1
1937---------------	1968	1,000.0	144.0	129.8	167.8	156.3	130.9	96.2	72.2	102.8
1938---------------	1969	1,000.0	154.3	131.7	171.7	159.6	130.9	92.0	68.4	91.4
1939---------------	1970	1,000.0	153.4	135.1	179.5	163.1	132.8	91.2	63.5	81.4
1940---------------	1971	1,000.0	151.9	140.7	190.0	166.8	131.6	87.5	61.4	70.1
1941---------------	1972	1,000.0	153.4	148.0	200.0	167.9	130.8	84.6	55.4	59.9
1942---------------	1973	1,000.0	153.2	159.4	212.5	170.0	128.2	77.5	50.1	49.1
1943---------------	1974	1,000.0	153.8	170.1	224.6	172.6	124.0	72.2	42.6	40.1

TABLE 8C. DISTRIBUTIONS OF ALL OTHER WOMEN BY PARITY AS OF THE BEGINNING OF EACH YEAR 1917-74 BY AGE FOR EACH COHORT FROM 1867 TO 1959--CON.

(BASED ON CUMULATIVE BIRTH RATES)

EXACT AGE AND COHORT	AS OF JANUARY 1	TOTAL	PARITY							
			0	1	2	3	4	5	6	7 AND HIGHER
32 YEARS										
1885	1917	1,000.0	268.7	170.1	117.5	114.8	95.1	61.2	63.1	109.5
1886	1918	1,000.0	267.6	174.9	119.4	109.1	97.3	67.1	61.6	103.0
1887	1919	1,000.0	263.7	181.0	122.1	102.6	100.5	73.0	60.6	96.5
1888	1920	1,000.0	264.1	184.4	121.7	102.4	103.1	68.6	61.9	93.8
1889	1921	1,000.0	263.2	190.9	119.7	110.8	105.6	64.9	58.9	86.0
1890	1922	1,000.0	260.8	195.3	122.9	116.4	105.6	60.8	56.4	81.8
1891	1923	1,000.0	256.2	199.3	129.1	120.3	104.6	57.2	53.8	79.5
1892	1924	1,000.0	249.6	203.5	137.0	122.6	102.8	53.6	51.6	79.3
1893	1925	1,000.0	245.4	209.7	116.6	134.6	106.9	54.1	52.4	80.3
1894	1926	1,000.0	242.3	221.8	122.4	130.7	103.2	49.8	49.5	80.3
1895	1927	1,000.0	241.2	233.6	125.6	125.3	97.6	48.8	46.7	81.2
1896	1928	1,000.0	240.9	247.4	126.3	118.7	92.4	48.0	44.7	81.6
1897	1929	1,000.0	240.6	260.9	125.5	112.8	88.0	47.8	45.1	79.3
1898	1930	1,000.0	256.3	251.5	125.3	106.6	86.3	49.3	46.7	78.0
1899	1931	1,000.0	249.6	266.3	122.7	102.8	82.0	50.4	48.3	77.9
1900	1932	1,000.0	249.4	274.2	120.9	98.8	79.1	51.0	48.3	78.3
1901	1933	1,000.0	254.2	279.6	123.3	95.7	75.5	50.8	46.8	74.1
1902	1934	1,000.0	262.0	282.1	126.0	92.0	72.7	50.8	43.8	70.6
1903	1935	1,000.0	270.8	281.7	127.7	89.7	71.6	50.1	40.8	67.6
1904	1936	1,000.0	279.0	283.1	125.6	85.8	69.9	49.7	40.7	66.2
1905	1937	1,000.0	289.1	283.1	123.8	83.5	66.7	49.3	41.1	63.4
1906	1938	1,000.0	298.6	283.4	121.8	80.2	65.2	49.4	40.6	60.8
1907	1939	1,000.0	309.6	279.9	120.8	78.6	64.7	48.6	39.1	58.7
1908	1940	1,000.0	320.0	274.7	120.0	77.9	65.5	47.0	37.7	57.2
1909	1941	1,000.0	323.2	269.1	120.6	78.2	66.6	47.4	36.4	58.5
1910	1942	1,000.0	330.1	259.9	120.8	79.4	66.9	46.9	36.6	59.4
1911	1943	1,000.0	331.5	255.8	121.2	79.8	67.3	46.4	36.8	61.2
1912	1944	1,000.0	338.6	248.6	122.0	79.8	65.8	45.0	38.3	61.9
1913	1945	1,000.0	339.0	244.5	122.6	80.6	65.6	46.2	38.5	63.0
1914	1946	1,000.0	340.6	236.5	123.8	81.5	65.6	48.7	39.4	63.9
1915	1947	1,000.0	339.1	230.5	123.4	85.4	66.4	51.0	39.4	64.8
1916	1948	1,000.0	336.9	223.7	123.8	88.1	68.3	52.6	39.7	66.9
1917	1949	1,000.0	329.2	217.8	127.6	91.7	70.6	54.3	40.3	68.5
1918	1950	1,000.0	317.5	216.9	131.8	93.7	72.9	55.4	41.0	70.8
1919	1951	1,000.0	291.9	221.9	138.4	98.4	75.4	57.2	43.7	73.1
1920	1952	1,000.0	273.0	222.6	144.2	102.1	79.0	58.2	45.4	75.5
1921	1953	1,000.0	263.1	211.7	148.9	108.6	82.7	61.2	46.8	77.0
1922	1954	1,000.0	269.2	195.3	148.6	113.1	85.6	63.0	47.4	77.8
1923	1955	1,000.0	264.8	183.9	150.0	114.8	91.2	64.6	49.3	81.4
1924	1956	1,000.0	247.4	176.4	152.2	119.0	97.4	68.2	52.9	86.5
1925	1957	1,000.0	228.5	168.1	156.0	122.6	101.0	74.1	57.0	92.7
1926	1958	1,000.0	218.5	153.5	156.1	127.2	104.0	78.9	61.2	100.6
1927	1959	1,000.0	216.7	141.3	151.8	128.2	108.2	83.1	63.2	107.5
1928	1960	1,000.0	219.7	130.3	146.4	129.7	111.0	84.7	65.7	112.5
1929	1961	1,000.0	214.2	121.6	144.6	129.7	114.0	89.1	67.7	119.1
1930	1962	1,000.0	213.9	113.5	142.8	133.0	113.1	89.1	71.2	123.4
1931	1963	1,000.0	204.1	107.7	145.8	136.1	114.4	90.5	72.7	128.7
1932	1964	1,000.0	192.2	107.3	149.5	140.7	116.8	91.8	73.0	128.7
1933	1965	1,000.0	171.2	109.7	155.0	143.2	122.9	95.1	73.7	129.2
1934	1966	1,000.0	152.2	113.1	157.4	149.1	126.2	97.6	75.0	129.4
1935	1967	1,000.0	137.4	118.6	160.1	152.8	129.4	98.2	77.7	125.8
1936	1968	1,000.0	134.4	121.9	163.2	154.4	130.4	98.0	77.5	120.2
1937	1969	1,000.0	136.4	125.5	166.5	156.9	131.9	97.6	74.0	111.2
1938	1970	1,000.0	146.3	127.0	170.4	160.5	132.5	93.9	70.2	99.2
1939	1971	1,000.0	145.1	129.4	178.6	164.6	134.6	93.1	66.1	88.5
1940	1972	1,000.0	143.6	134.3	189.8	168.7	133.5	89.9	63.5	76.7
1941	1973	1,000.0	144.8	142.0	200.9	170.7	132.6	86.6	57.7	64.7
1942	1974	1,000.0	144.7	153.1	214.2	173.0	130.4	79.7	51.9	53.0

TABLE 8C. DISTRIBUTIONS OF ALL OTHER WOMEN BY PARITY AS OF THE BEGINNING OF EACH YEAR 1917-74 BY AGE FOR EACH COHORT FROM 1867 TO 1959--CON.

(BASED ON CUMULATIVE BIRTH RATES)

EXACT AGE AND COHORT	AS OF JANUARY 1	TOTAL	PARITY							
			0	1	2	3	4	5	6	7 AND HIGHER
33 YEARS										
1884	1917	1,000.0	259.8	164.0	114.8	113.8	93.3	59.1	65.2	130.0
1885	1918	1,000.0	263.2	167.8	115.8	113.7	93.7	59.0	64.2	122.6
1886	1919	1,000.0	261.6	173.1	117.4	108.5	95.9	65.1	63.2	115.2
1887	1920	1,000.0	258.4	178.5	120.2	101.8	99.3	72.3	61.5	108.0
1888	1921	1,000.0	258.2	182.5	119.3	101.9	102.9	67.7	63.1	104.4
1889	1922	1,000.0	257.7	188.0	118.0	109.9	104.6	63.7	60.6	97.5
1890	1923	1,000.0	255.7	192.2	121.2	115.7	104.7	60.0	57.5	93.0
1891	1924	1,000.0	251.3	196.8	126.7	119.4	103.6	56.1	55.1	91.0
1892	1925	1,000.0	244.8	201.0	133.6	122.1	102.2	52.0	53.2	91.1
1893	1926	1,000.0	240.4	207.8	113.8	132.9	106.4	52.9	53.6	92.2
1894	1927	1,000.0	238.0	219.4	119.9	128.5	102.7	49.1	50.0	92.4
1895	1928	1,000.0	237.1	232.1	122.9	123.7	96.5	47.7	46.8	93.2
1896	1929	1,000.0	237.4	246.1	124.2	117.1	90.8	47.2	45.8	91.4
1897	1930	1,000.0	237.4	259.4	123.9	111.1	86.6	47.1	45.9	88.6
1898	1931	1,000.0	252.5	250.7	123.6	105.1	84.2	48.4	47.6	87.9
1899	1932	1,000.0	245.9	265.4	120.9	101.1	80.7	49.0	48.5	88.5
1900	1933	1,000.0	245.7	273.1	119.0	97.0	77.5	49.6	49.1	89.0
1901	1934	1,000.0	250.7	278.4	121.6	94.2	73.9	49.6	47.2	84.4
1902	1935	1,000.0	258.6	281.0	124.3	90.7	71.0	50.0	44.3	80.1
1903	1936	1,000.0	267.8	280.3	126.5	87.9	70.8	49.3	41.5	75.9
1904	1937	1,000.0	276.0	281.9	124.2	84.8	68.6	48.8	41.3	74.4
1905	1938	1,000.0	286.0	281.9	122.6	82.4	65.1	48.6	41.8	71.6
1906	1939	1,000.0	295.2	282.3	120.5	79.1	64.0	48.6	40.8	69.5
1907	1940	1,000.0	306.0	278.8	119.6	77.4	63.9	47.7	39.6	67.0
1908	1941	1,000.0	316.2	273.5	119.1	76.9	64.1	46.6	37.8	65.8
1909	1942	1,000.0	318.9	267.8	119.7	77.4	65.6	46.8	36.6	67.2
1910	1943	1,000.0	325.3	258.4	120.1	78.7	66.0	46.4	37.1	68.0
1911	1944	1,000.0	325.9	254.4	120.5	79.1	66.6	45.8	37.7	70.0
1912	1945	1,000.0	332.6	247.0	121.5	79.0	65.3	44.3	39.2	71.1
1913	1946	1,000.0	332.9	243.0	121.7	80.1	64.9	46.2	38.7	72.5
1914	1947	1,000.0	333.8	234.4	123.2	80.9	66.3	48.3	39.8	73.3
1915	1948	1,000.0	330.5	229.0	123.5	85.6	66.2	51.2	39.7	74.3
1916	1949	1,000.0	329.2	220.9	123.5	88.8	68.2	52.5	40.4	76.5
1917	1950	1,000.0	320.7	215.5	126.8	92.4	71.0	54.5	41.1	78.0
1918	1951	1,000.0	309.3	213.9	130.5	94.3	73.4	56.2	41.7	80.7
1919	1952	1,000.0	283.2	218.5	137.1	98.5	76.4	57.5	44.6	84.2
1920	1953	1,000.0	264.8	218.0	142.5	102.0	79.8	59.6	47.0	86.3
1921	1954	1,000.0	254.5	207.5	146.3	109.2	83.0	63.0	48.3	88.2
1922	1955	1,000.0	260.9	190.8	146.4	112.5	85.9	64.3	49.2	90.0
1923	1956	1,000.0	257.0	179.1	147.3	114.1	91.8	65.9	51.3	93.5
1924	1957	1,000.0	239.7	171.3	149.0	118.5	97.4	69.3	55.1	99.7
1925	1958	1,000.0	221.4	162.6	152.6	121.6	100.6	75.3	59.0	106.9
1926	1959	1,000.0	211.6	148.6	152.7	125.9	104.0	79.2	63.1	114.9
1927	1960	1,000.0	210.1	136.5	148.4	127.2	106.8	84.1	64.2	122.7
1928	1961	1,000.0	213.6	125.1	143.4	128.4	110.4	85.6	66.4	127.1
1929	1962	1,000.0	208.1	117.0	140.8	127.8	114.4	89.2	68.6	134.1
1930	1963	1,000.0	208.3	108.7	139.8	131.2	112.4	89.4	72.8	137.4
1931	1964	1,000.0	198.5	102.9	142.9	134.5	114.3	91.1	73.5	142.3
1932	1965	1,000.0	186.7	103.5	145.9	139.7	116.4	91.7	74.2	141.9
1933	1966	1,000.0	165.7	105.5	152.3	142.0	122.9	96.0	74.5	141.1
1934	1967	1,000.0	146.6	109.4	154.6	148.7	126.2	98.3	76.9	139.3
1935	1968	1,000.0	132.1	114.6	157.9	151.7	130.3	99.4	78.7	135.3
1936	1969	1,000.0	128.4	118.1	161.9	154.6	131.2	98.9	78.9	128.0
1937	1970	1,000.0	130.0	121.7	165.0	157.5	132.7	99.3	75.3	118.5
1938	1971	1,000.0	140.0	122.3	169.0	161.3	133.7	95.8	72.0	105.9
1939	1972	1,000.0	138.7	124.4	177.5	166.2	135.9	94.6	67.9	94.8
1940	1973	1,000.0	137.0	129.4	189.8	170.7	134.6	91.6	65.5	81.4
1941	1974	1,000.0	138.4	136.5	201.9	172.8	134.2	88.2	59.3	68.7

TABLE 8C. DISTRIBUTIONS OF ALL OTHER WOMEN BY PARITY AS OF THE BEGINNING OF EACH YEAR 1917-74 BY AGE FOR EACH COHORT FROM 1867 TO 1959--CON.

(BASED ON CUMULATIVE BIRTH RATES)

EXACT AGE AND COHORT	AS OF JANUARY 1	TOTAL	PARITY 0	1	2	3	4	5	6	7 AND HIGHER
34 YEARS										
1883---------------	1917	1,000.0	249.7	158.9	112.9	108.6	92.3	58.7	66.6	152.3
1884---------------	1918	1,000.0	254.7	162.0	113.2	112.0	92.0	56.2	66.1	143.8
1885---------------	1919	1,000.0	257.6	166.2	114.1	112.3	92.4	56.2	65.8	135.4
1886---------------	1920	1,000.0	256.7	171.0	115.6	106.9	95.0	63.6	64.0	127.2
1887---------------	1921	1,000.0	253.0	176.9	118.0	100.6	99.2	70.8	62.6	118.9
1888---------------	1922	1,000.0	253.2	180.0	117.8	100.4	102.0	65.8	64.6	116.2
1889---------------	1923	1,000.0	253.1	185.3	116.6	108.5	103.8	62.2	61.6	108.9
1890---------------	1924	1,000.0	251.3	190.1	119.1	114.1	103.9	58.2	58.6	104.7
1891---------------	1925	1,000.0	247.0	194.6	123.8	118.1	103.2	53.7	56.7	102.9
1892---------------	1926	1,000.0	240.1	199.3	131.1	120.7	101.1	50.1	54.2	103.4
1893---------------	1927	1,000.0	236.9	205.2	111.1	130.9	106.5	51.0	53.8	104.6
1894---------------	1928	1,000.0	234.1	218.1	117.7	126.6	101.7	47.7	49.9	104.2
1895---------------	1929	1,000.0	233.8	231.0	120.9	122.0	94.8	46.9	47.4	103.2
1896---------------	1930	1,000.0	234.3	244.9	122.5	115.2	89.8	45.8	46.5	101.0
1897---------------	1931	1,000.0	234.0	258.6	122.5	109.7	84.3	46.0	46.5	98.4
1898---------------	1932	1,000.0	249.4	249.8	121.9	103.6	83.1	46.8	47.3	98.1
1899---------------	1933	1,000.0	242.6	264.5	119.1	99.5	79.0	47.2	49.0	99.1
1900---------------	1934	1,000.0	242.5	272.0	117.4	95.5	75.6	48.2	48.9	99.9
1901---------------	1935	1,000.0	247.3	277.4	119.9	92.9	72.1	48.3	47.4	94.7
1902---------------	1936	1,000.0	255.7	279.7	123.4	88.9	70.0	48.8	44.6	88.9
1903---------------	1937	1,000.0	265.1	279.3	125.3	86.7	69.3	48.4	41.9	84.0
1904---------------	1938	1,000.0	273.2	281.0	122.7	84.0	66.9	48.2	41.2	82.8
1905---------------	1939	1,000.0	283.0	280.9	121.4	81.4	63.5	48.0	41.4	80.4
1906---------------	1940	1,000.0	292.0	281.4	119.3	78.0	62.9	47.8	40.8	77.8
1907---------------	1941	1,000.0	302.7	277.7	118.7	76.5	62.2	47.4	39.2	75.6
1908---------------	1942	1,000.0	312.4	272.4	118.3	76.1	62.8	46.1	37.5	74.4
1909---------------	1943	1,000.0	314.6	266.5	119.0	76.5	64.9	46.2	36.5	75.8
1910---------------	1944	1,000.0	320.3	257.2	119.3	77.8	65.5	45.8	37.3	76.8
1911---------------	1945	1,000.0	320.5	253.1	119.8	78.2	66.3	45.0	38.0	79.1
1912---------------	1946	1,000.0	327.1	245.6	120.6	78.6	64.4	44.3	39.1	80.3
1913---------------	1947	1,000.0	326.8	241.2	121.2	79.4	65.1	45.9	38.9	81.5
1914---------------	1948	1,000.0	326.2	233.1	123.2	80.7	66.2	48.0	40.1	82.5
1915---------------	1949	1,000.0	323.5	226.7	123.0	86.0	66.1	51.2	40.0	83.5
1916---------------	1950	1,000.0	321.7	218.6	122.9	89.4	68.3	52.5	40.9	85.7
1917---------------	1951	1,000.0	313.7	213.0	125.5	92.5	71.2	55.2	41.5	87.4
1918---------------	1952	1,000.0	302.0	211.3	128.9	94.2	74.2	56.4	42.2	90.8
1919---------------	1953	1,000.0	275.9	214.8	135.1	98.7	76.9	58.1	45.8	94.7
1920---------------	1954	1,000.0	257.2	214.5	140.0	102.4	80.1	60.7	48.1	97.0
1921---------------	1955	1,000.0	247.3	203.7	144.0	108.4	82.6	64.5	49.9	99.6
1922---------------	1956	1,000.0	254.0	186.7	143.8	111.9	86.0	65.5	50.9	101.2
1923---------------	1957	1,000.0	250.4	174.4	144.8	113.3	91.9	66.7	52.8	105.7
1924---------------	1958	1,000.0	233.5	166.7	145.8	117.5	97.3	70.0	56.4	112.8
1925---------------	1959	1,000.0	215.3	158.3	149.3	120.9	100.2	75.8	60.3	119.9
1926---------------	1960	1,000.0	205.8	144.4	149.3	125.4	102.5	79.6	63.9	129.1
1927---------------	1961	1,000.0	204.7	132.1	145.6	125.8	106.2	84.8	64.6	136.2
1928---------------	1962	1,000.0	208.6	121.1	140.2	126.5	110.2	85.8	66.9	140.7
1929---------------	1963	1,000.0	203.3	112.9	137.9	125.9	113.8	89.5	69.9	146.8
1930---------------	1964	1,000.0	203.6	104.7	137.0	129.9	112.1	89.9	73.4	149.4
1931---------------	1965	1,000.0	193.9	99.7	139.4	133.3	113.8	90.8	74.5	154.6
1932---------------	1966	1,000.0	182.2	99.9	143.4	138.5	116.3	92.4	74.5	152.8
1933---------------	1967	1,000.0	161.0	102.6	149.4	141.9	122.6	96.8	75.4	150.3
1934---------------	1968	1,000.0	142.3	106.1	152.6	147.7	126.7	99.0	77.7	147.9
1935---------------	1969	1,000.0	127.1	111.4	156.4	151.8	130.7	100.0	79.9	142.7
1936---------------	1970	1,000.0	123.3	114.9	160.1	155.0	131.7	99.9	80.2	134.9
1937---------------	1971	1,000.0	124.9	118.1	163.4	157.9	133.3	100.9	76.5	125.0
1938---------------	1972	1,000.0	135.1	118.3	167.7	162.3	134.5	96.8	73.4	111.9
1939---------------	1973	1,000.0	133.4	120.7	177.1	167.6	136.4	96.0	69.3	99.5
1940---------------	1974	1,000.0	132.0	125.1	190.0	172.0	135.7	93.1	66.7	85.4

TABLE 8C. DISTRIBUTIONS OF ALL OTHER WOMEN BY PARITY AS OF THE BEGINNING OF EACH YEAR 1917-74 BY AGE FOR EACH COHORT FROM 1867 TO 1959--CON.

(BASED ON CUMULATIVE BIRTH RATES)

EXACT AGE AND COHORT	AS OF JANUARY 1	TOTAL	PARITY							
			0	1	2	3	4	5	6	7 AND HIGHER
35 YEARS										
1882---------------	1917	1,000.0	241.7	153.9	109.6	101.3	91.9	61.8	67.5	172.3
1883---------------	1918	1,000.0	244.9	157.0	111.5	106.2	90.3	56.0	66.9	167.2
1884---------------	1919	1,000.0	249.3	160.6	111.3	110.1	90.5	52.5	68.1	157.6
1885---------------	1920	1,000.0	252.9	164.3	112.5	109.9	90.9	54.2	66.5	148.8
1886---------------	1921	1,000.0	251.6	169.4	113.5	105.0	94.3	61.8	65.3	139.1
1887---------------	1922	1,000.0	248.3	175.1	116.4	98.4	97.8	68.9	64.3	130.8
1888---------------	1923	1,000.0	248.9	177.9	116.4	98.6	100.5	64.6	65.2	127.9
1889---------------	1924	1,000.0	249.2	183.4	114.8	106.6	102.7	60.3	62.4	120.6
1890---------------	1925	1,000.0	247.3	188.5	116.6	112.4	102.7	56.5	59.4	116.6
1891---------------	1926	1,000.0	242.6	193.6	121.3	117.1	101.4	51.6	57.2	115.2
1892---------------	1927	1,000.0	236.7	197.6	128.3	119.0	100.3	48.2	54.2	115.7
1893---------------	1928	1,000.0	233.1	204.6	109.1	129.0	105.2	49.9	53.1	116.0
1894---------------	1929	1,000.0	231.1	217.3	115.8	125.1	100.0	46.6	50.2	113.9
1895---------------	1930	1,000.0	230.9	230.1	119.1	120.3	93.7	45.4	47.7	112.8
1896---------------	1931	1,000.0	231.4	244.2	120.9	114.0	87.5	45.1	46.4	110.5
1897---------------	1932	1,000.0	231.2	257.9	121.2	108.1	83.0	44.6	46.1	107.9
1898---------------	1933	1,000.0	246.9	249.1	120.4	102.1	81.5	45.0	47.3	107.7
1899---------------	1934	1,000.0	239.8	263.7	117.9	98.1	77.2	45.9	48.3	109.1
1900---------------	1935	1,000.0	239.7	271.0	116.0	94.1	74.1	46.6	48.7	109.8
1901---------------	1936	1,000.0	244.6	276.2	119.0	91.5	70.8	47.2	47.2	103.5
1902---------------	1937	1,000.0	253.2	279.0	122.2	87.6	68.9	47.7	44.5	96.9
1903---------------	1938	1,000.0	262.7	278.5	124.1	85.9	67.8	47.8	41.1	92.1
1904---------------	1939	1,000.0	270.6	280.3	121.5	83.2	65.5	47.6	40.6	90.7
1905---------------	1940	1,000.0	280.3	280.2	120.3	80.5	62.5	47.3	40.9	88.0
1906---------------	1941	1,000.0	289.2	280.6	118.4	77.3	61.4	47.5	40.3	85.3
1907---------------	1942	1,000.0	299.6	276.8	117.8	76.0	60.8	47.1	38.6	83.3
1908---------------	1943	1,000.0	308.8	271.4	117.7	75.1	62.2	45.5	37.4	81.9
1909---------------	1944	1,000.0	310.5	265.5	118.3	75.6	64.4	45.5	36.7	83.5
1910---------------	1945	1,000.0	315.8	256.2	118.7	76.8	65.3	44.9	37.5	84.8
1911---------------	1946	1,000.0	315.8	252.1	119.0	77.6	65.4	44.9	37.7	87.5
1912---------------	1947	1,000.0	321.9	244.4	120.1	78.0	64.3	43.8	39.1	88.4
1913---------------	1948	1,000.0	320.3	240.4	121.0	78.9	65.1	45.7	39.0	89.6
1914---------------	1949	1,000.0	320.3	231.2	122.7	80.9	66.0	48.2	39.9	90.8
1915---------------	1950	1,000.0	317.2	224.7	122.3	86.6	66.0	51.2	40.2	91.8
1916---------------	1951	1,000.0	315.6	216.8	121.7	89.2	68.7	53.1	40.8	94.1
1917---------------	1952	1,000.0	307.3	211.0	124.1	92.7	71.5	55.4	41.9	96.1
1918---------------	1953	1,000.0	295.8	208.5	127.6	94.2	74.4	56.7	43.0	99.8
1919---------------	1954	1,000.0	269.7	211.6	133.5	98.5	77.4	58.4	46.8	104.1
1920---------------	1955	1,000.0	251.0	211.6	137.5	102.0	79.8	61.7	49.3	107.1
1921---------------	1956	1,000.0	241.3	200.1	142.0	107.6	82.7	65.2	51.5	109.6
1922---------------	1957	1,000.0	248.6	182.8	141.6	111.1	85.9	66.2	51.6	112.2
1923---------------	1958	1,000.0	245.2	170.5	142.1	112.6	91.7	67.2	53.7	117.0
1924---------------	1959	1,000.0	228.5	162.8	143.0	117.2	96.7	70.7	57.2	123.9
1925---------------	1960	1,000.0	210.2	155.2	146.4	120.0	99.2	76.0	61.0	132.0
1926---------------	1961	1,000.0	201.2	140.7	146.9	124.0	102.0	80.1	64.3	140.8
1927---------------	1962	1,000.0	200.4	128.9	142.5	124.1	106.4	84.5	65.0	148.2
1928---------------	1963	1,000.0	204.6	117.6	137.5	125.3	109.6	86.0	68.0	151.4
1929---------------	1964	1,000.0	199.5	109.5	135.5	124.9	113.1	89.9	70.4	157.2
1930---------------	1965	1,000.0	199.8	102.1	134.0	129.1	111.5	89.5	73.8	160.2
1931---------------	1966	1,000.0	190.2	96.8	137.1	132.3	113.5	91.4	74.8	163.9
1932---------------	1967	1,000.0	178.2	97.8	140.7	138.6	115.8	93.1	74.7	161.1
1933---------------	1968	1,000.0	157.6	99.6	147.9	141.0	122.8	97.3	76.1	157.7
1934---------------	1969	1,000.0	138.3	103.6	150.9	147.8	126.8	99.5	78.6	154.5
1935---------------	1970	1,000.0	123.1	108.8	154.7	151.8	130.9	100.9	80.8	149.0
1936---------------	1971	1,000.0	119.3	112.1	158.3	155.1	132.1	101.1	81.2	140.8
1937---------------	1972	1,000.0	121.2	115.0	161.8	158.2	134.2	101.3	77.7	130.6
1938---------------	1973	1,000.0	131.0	115.6	167.0	163.0	134.6	98.2	74.5	116.1
1939---------------	1974	1,000.0	129.4	117.5	176.6	168.6	137.2	97.1	70.2	103.4

TABLE 8C. DISTRIBUTIONS OF ALL OTHER WOMEN BY PARITY AS OF THE BEGINNING OF EACH YEAR 1917-74 BY AGE FOR EACH COHORT FROM 1867 TO 1959--CON.

(BASED ON CUMULATIVE BIRTH RATES)

EXACT AGE AND COHORT	AS OF JANUARY 1	TOTAL	PARITY							
			0	1	2	3	4	5	6	7 AND HIGHER
36 YEARS										
1881	1917	1,000.0	235.1	149.3	107.0	97.9	89.5	63.2	68.0	190.0
1882	1918	1,000.0	237.2	152.4	107.9	98.9	90.4	58.8	67.0	187.4
1883	1919	1,000.0	239.6	156.0	109.3	104.4	89.4	51.1	68.9	181.3
1884	1920	1,000.0	244.7	159.2	109.3	107.6	89.6	49.3	68.5	171.8
1885	1921	1,000.0	247.9	163.0	109.9	108.1	90.6	51.6	67.6	161.3
1886	1922	1,000.0	247.0	168.3	111.5	102.7	93.5	59.3	66.9	150.8
1887	1923	1,000.0	244.2	173.5	114.7	96.7	96.7	67.2	64.6	142.4
1888	1924	1,000.0	245.3	176.4	114.5	96.9	99.8	62.2	65.6	139.3
1889	1925	1,000.0	245.5	182.4	112.2	105.0	101.7	58.7	62.4	132.1
1890	1926	1,000.0	243.1	187.8	114.4	111.3	101.3	54.6	58.9	128.6
1891	1927	1,000.0	239.4	192.4	118.8	115.3	100.5	49.2	57.2	127.2
1892	1928	1,000.0	233.2	197.1	126.6	117.3	99.0	46.8	53.5	126.5
1893	1929	1,000.0	230.4	204.0	107.3	127.8	103.3	48.7	52.9	125.6
1894	1930	1,000.0	228.4	216.4	114.5	123.5	98.7	45.2	50.3	123.0
1895	1931	1,000.0	228.3	229.5	117.8	118.9	91.7	44.4	47.6	121.8
1896	1932	1,000.0	228.9	243.5	119.8	112.5	86.5	43.5	45.9	119.4
1897	1933	1,000.0	228.9	257.4	120.0	106.8	81.4	42.8	45.9	116.8
1898	1934	1,000.0	244.7	248.4	119.5	100.8	80.0	43.7	46.4	116.5
1899	1935	1,000.0	237.5	262.8	116.7	96.9	75.7	44.4	47.8	118.2
1900	1936	1,000.0	237.2	270.3	114.9	93.0	72.7	45.4	48.0	118.5
1901	1937	1,000.0	242.2	275.7	118.0	89.9	69.9	46.3	46.4	111.6
1902	1938	1,000.0	251.0	278.3	121.1	86.9	67.7	46.7	43.7	104.6
1903	1939	1,000.0	260.5	277.8	123.0	85.2	66.7	47.0	40.5	99.3
1904	1940	1,000.0	268.2	279.7	120.6	82.4	64.7	46.6	40.2	97.6
1905	1941	1,000.0	277.9	279.6	119.4	79.9	61.2	46.8	40.5	94.7
1906	1942	1,000.0	286.5	279.9	117.6	77.0	60.0	47.1	39.8	92.1
1907	1943	1,000.0	296.6	276.1	117.2	75.1	60.1	46.6	38.2	90.1
1908	1944	1,000.0	305.5	270.6	116.9	74.5	61.5	44.9	37.1	89.0
1909	1945	1,000.0	306.8	264.8	117.5	74.9	64.0	44.8	36.3	90.9
1910	1946	1,000.0	311.8	255.3	118.1	76.1	64.6	44.6	37.3	92.2
1911	1947	1,000.0	311.2	251.3	118.2	77.3	65.1	44.5	37.4	95.0
1912	1948	1,000.0	316.5	243.6	119.8	77.5	64.4	43.3	39.2	95.7
1913	1949	1,000.0	315.2	238.9	120.6	78.9	64.7	45.9	38.8	97.0
1914	1950	1,000.0	314.9	229.6	122.2	81.2	65.7	48.2	39.9	98.3
1915	1951	1,000.0	311.8	223.6	121.1	86.2	66.3	51.6	40.0	99.4
1916	1952	1,000.0	310.1	215.2	120.1	89.5	68.7	53.5	41.0	101.9
1917	1953	1,000.0	302.0	208.9	123.2	92.4	71.6	55.5	42.4	104.0
1918	1954	1,000.0	290.6	206.0	126.3	94.0	74.7	56.5	43.9	108.0
1919	1955	1,000.0	264.2	209.2	131.7	98.0	77.3	59.0	47.8	112.8
1920	1956	1,000.0	245.8	208.6	135.8	101.5	79.7	62.1	50.5	116.0
1921	1957	1,000.0	236.4	197.2	140.0	106.7	82.6	65.6	51.7	119.8
1922	1958	1,000.0	244.3	179.6	139.2	110.3	85.8	66.3	52.2	122.3
1923	1959	1,000.0	240.9	167.5	139.8	112.0	91.2	67.7	54.3	126.6
1924	1960	1,000.0	224.1	160.5	140.2	116.5	95.8	70.6	57.9	134.4
1925	1961	1,000.0	206.2	152.5	144.0	118.6	99.2	75.9	61.6	142.0
1926	1962	1,000.0	197.5	138.1	144.0	122.6	102.0	80.1	64.5	151.2
1927	1963	1,000.0	197.0	125.8	140.1	123.4	105.8	84.2	65.9	157.8
1928	1964	1,000.0	201.3	115.1	135.3	124.5	108.8	86.4	68.2	160.4
1929	1965	1,000.0	196.4	107.1	133.0	123.8	113.0	89.6	70.7	166.4
1930	1966	1,000.0	196.7	99.8	132.0	128.1	111.2	89.6	74.3	168.3
1931	1967	1,000.0	187.0	94.9	134.9	132.1	113.1	91.8	75.0	171.2
1932	1968	1,000.0	175.5	95.2	139.4	138.0	115.6	93.4	75.4	167.5
1933	1969	1,000.0	154.3	97.7	146.2	141.0	122.5	98.0	76.8	163.5
1934	1970	1,000.0	135.0	101.6	149.2	147.8	126.8	100.3	79.0	160.3
1935	1971	1,000.0	119.9	106.6	153.1	151.6	131.1	101.9	81.5	154.3
1936	1972	1,000.0	116.2	109.9	156.9	154.9	132.8	101.4	81.8	146.1
1937	1973	1,000.0	118.0	112.6	161.1	158.7	134.3	102.2	78.4	134.7
1938	1974	1,000.0	127.8	113.3	166.3	163.5	135.3	99.0	75.1	119.7

TABLE 8C. DISTRIBUTIONS OF ALL OTHER WOMEN BY PARITY AS OF THE BEGINNING OF EACH YEAR 1917-74 BY AGE FOR EACH COHORT FROM 1867 TO 1959--CON.

(BASED ON CUMULATIVE BIRTH RATES)

EXACT AGE AND COHORT	AS OF JANUARY 1	TOTAL	PARITY							
			0	1	2	3	4	5	6	7 AND HIGHER
37 YEARS										
1880---------------	1917	1,000.0	228.7	144.7	104.9	94.9	87.2	64.1	68.2	207.3
1881---------------	1918	1,000.0	231.4	147.7	105.0	96.4	87.9	60.6	66.3	204.7
1882---------------	1919	1,000.0	232.5	151.4	105.3	98.0	89.6	53.7	68.3	201.2
1883---------------	1920	1,000.0	235.5	154.6	107.1	102.5	88.5	47.6	68.5	195.7
1884---------------	1921	1,000.0	240.3	157.7	106.3	106.6	89.1	46.6	68.8	184.6
1885---------------	1922	1,000.0	243.8	162.1	107.4	106.6	89.7	49.2	68.5	172.7
1886---------------	1923	1,000.0	243.3	166.9	109.4	101.8	92.3	57.8	66.2	162.3
1887---------------	1924	1,000.0	241.1	172.0	112.6	95.9	96.0	64.9	64.1	153.4
1888---------------	1925	1,000.0	242.1	175.5	111.8	96.2	98.6	61.1	64.3	150.4
1889---------------	1926	1,000.0	241.8	182.2	110.1	103.6	100.6	57.2	61.0	143.5
1890---------------	1927	1,000.0	240.0	187.3	112.2	109.8	100.0	52.5	58.6	139.6
1891---------------	1928	1,000.0	236.0	192.4	117.1	113.9	99.5	47.6	55.9	137.6
1892---------------	1929	1,000.0	230.8	196.8	125.0	116.1	97.4	45.5	53.0	135.4
1893---------------	1930	1,000.0	228.1	203.1	106.2	126.8	101.7	47.6	52.5	134.0
1894---------------	1931	1,000.0	226.1	215.9	113.3	122.5	96.8	44.3	50.0	131.1
1895---------------	1932	1,000.0	226.1	229.0	116.8	117.6	90.4	43.0	47.3	129.8
1896---------------	1933	1,000.0	226.9	243.1	118.6	111.6	84.8	41.8	45.4	127.8
1897---------------	1934	1,000.0	227.0	256.8	119.2	105.8	80.0	41.8	45.1	124.3
1898---------------	1935	1,000.0	242.9	247.9	118.5	99.7	78.7	42.5	45.6	124.2
1899---------------	1936	1,000.0	235.5	262.2	115.7	96.1	74.5	43.2	46.8	126.0
1900---------------	1937	1,000.0	235.1	269.9	113.9	91.8	71.9	44.3	47.2	125.9
1901---------------	1938	1,000.0	240.1	275.2	117.0	89.1	68.9	45.4	45.4	118.9
1902---------------	1939	1,000.0	249.1	277.7	120.2	86.1	66.8	45.8	42.9	111.4
1903---------------	1940	1,000.0	258.5	277.2	122.4	84.3	66.2	45.9	39.8	105.7
1904---------------	1941	1,000.0	266.2	279.2	119.9	81.6	63.8	46.0	39.7	103.6
1905---------------	1942	1,000.0	275.7	279.0	118.8	79.4	60.0	46.3	39.9	100.9
1906---------------	1943	1,000.0	284.0	279.5	117.1	76.2	59.2	46.8	39.3	97.9
1907---------------	1944	1,000.0	293.9	275.5	116.6	74.6	59.4	46.2	37.7	96.1
1908---------------	1945	1,000.0	302.4	270.1	116.3	74.0	61.1	44.4	36.4	95.3
1909---------------	1946	1,000.0	303.5	264.3	116.7	74.3	63.5	44.4	36.1	97.2
1910---------------	1947	1,000.0	308.1	254.6	117.4	75.8	64.3	44.2	36.8	98.8
1911---------------	1948	1,000.0	306.8	250.6	117.7	77.0	65.0	44.2	37.1	101.6
1912---------------	1949	1,000.0	312.3	242.4	119.4	77.6	63.8	43.3	39.1	102.1
1913---------------	1950	1,000.0	310.9	237.6	120.1	79.0	64.4	45.7	38.8	103.5
1914---------------	1951	1,000.0	310.4	228.6	121.3	80.8	65.8	48.5	39.5	105.1
1915---------------	1952	1,000.0	307.1	222.6	119.5	86.5	66.3	51.6	40.1	106.3
1916---------------	1953	1,000.0	305.7	213.5	119.7	88.5	69.1	53.5	41.3	108.7
1917---------------	1954	1,000.0	297.5	207.2	121.9	92.3	71.5	55.7	42.6	111.3
1918---------------	1955	1,000.0	286.3	203.8	124.7	93.9	74.7	56.6	44.6	115.4
1919---------------	1956	1,000.0	259.7	206.9	130.4	97.3	77.4	59.2	48.3	120.8
1920---------------	1957	1,000.0	241.7	206.4	134.1	100.7	79.3	62.5	50.4	124.9
1921---------------	1958	1,000.0	232.6	194.8	137.8	105.9	82.4	65.7	52.2	128.6
1922---------------	1959	1,000.0	240.7	177.1	137.3	109.9	85.1	66.8	52.6	130.5
1923---------------	1960	1,000.0	237.3	165.9	137.3	111.4	90.6	67.5	54.8	135.2
1924---------------	1961	1,000.0	220.9	158.3	138.0	115.4	96.0	70.3	58.1	143.0
1925---------------	1962	1,000.0	203.2	150.1	141.8	117.2	99.1	76.2	61.7	150.7
1926---------------	1963	1,000.0	194.7	135.6	141.9	121.9	101.3	80.2	65.2	159.2
1927---------------	1964	1,000.0	194.1	123.7	138.6	122.5	104.7	84.7	65.9	165.8
1928---------------	1965	1,000.0	198.6	113.4	133.2	123.6	108.6	86.2	68.4	168.0
1929---------------	1966	1,000.0	193.8	105.2	131.3	123.0	112.4	89.7	71.3	173.3
1930---------------	1967	1,000.0	194.0	98.4	130.2	127.6	110.8	89.9	74.4	174.7
1931---------------	1968	1,000.0	184.7	92.9	133.8	131.4	113.0	91.9	75.4	176.9
1932---------------	1969	1,000.0	172.8	93.9	137.9	138.0	115.2	93.6	76.1	172.5
1933---------------	1970	1,000.0	151.7	95.9	145.2	140.7	122.4	98.9	76.8	168.4
1934---------------	1971	1,000.0	132.4	99.9	147.9	147.5	127.0	101.0	79.3	165.0
1935---------------	1972	1,000.0	117.4	105.0	151.8	151.4	131.4	102.1	81.9	159.0
1936---------------	1973	1,000.0	113.8	107.9	156.1	155.0	133.0	102.0	82.4	149.8
1937---------------	1974	1,000.0	115.5	111.0	160.2	159.1	134.6	102.7	79.0	137.9

TABLE 8C. DISTRIBUTIONS OF ALL OTHER WOMEN BY PARITY AS OF THE BEGINNING OF EACH YEAR 1917-74 BY AGE FOR EACH COHORT FROM 1867 TO 1959--CON.

(BASED ON CUMULATIVE BIRTH RATES)

EXACT AGE AND COHORT	AS OF JANUARY 1	TOTAL	PARITY							
			0	1	2	3	4	5	6	7 AND HIGHER
38 YEARS										
1879----------------	1917	1,000.0	222.0	140.3	103.2	92.6	85.1	63.6	68.0	225.2
1880----------------	1918	1,000.0	225.6	143.5	103.4	93.9	85.9	61.8	65.9	220.0
1881----------------	1919	1,000.0	227.4	146.9	103.0	96.0	87.3	56.1	66.5	216.8
1882----------------	1920	1,000.0	229.0	150.2	103.5	96.9	88.8	50.4	67.0	214.2
1883----------------	1921	1,000.0	231.6	153.4	104.6	102.0	88.0	45.0	68.0	207.4
1884----------------	1922	1,000.0	236.6	157.0	104.3	105.6	88.3	44.2	68.8	195.2
1885----------------	1923	1,000.0	240.5	160.9	105.7	106.1	88.7	47.6	67.1	183.4
1886----------------	1924	1,000.0	240.6	165.6	107.7	101.4	91.7	55.5	65.1	172.4
1887----------------	1925	1,000.0	238.3	171.3	110.4	95.5	95.0	63.7	62.3	163.5
1888----------------	1926	1,000.0	239.3	175.4	109.7	94.9	97.9	59.7	62.5	160.6
1889----------------	1927	1,000.0	239.3	181.8	108.3	102.2	100.0	55.1	59.9	153.4
1890----------------	1928	1,000.0	237.2	187.3	110.8	108.7	98.8	51.1	57.5	148.6
1891----------------	1929	1,000.0	234.0	192.3	115.8	112.4	98.5	46.3	55.2	145.5
1892----------------	1930	1,000.0	229.0	196.0	124.4	114.8	96.1	44.6	52.3	142.8
1893----------------	1931	1,000.0	226.1	202.8	105.3	125.7	100.1	46.3	52.6	141.1
1894----------------	1932	1,000.0	224.3	215.4	112.4	121.5	95.7	43.1	49.3	138.3
1895----------------	1933	1,000.0	224.3	228.8	115.7	116.8	89.3	40.8	47.1	137.2
1896----------------	1934	1,000.0	225.4	242.6	117.8	110.5	83.9	40.7	44.6	134.5
1897----------------	1935	1,000.0	225.3	256.7	118.3	104.8	78.9	40.8	44.1	131.1
1898----------------	1936	1,000.0	241.5	247.5	117.7	98.8	77.8	41.4	44.4	130.9
1899----------------	1937	1,000.0	233.8	261.9	114.8	95.2	73.7	42.2	45.8	132.6
1900----------------	1938	1,000.0	233.4	269.5	112.9	91.1	70.9	43.5	46.3	132.4
1901----------------	1939	1,000.0	238.4	274.6	116.5	88.0	68.2	44.4	44.5	125.4
1902----------------	1940	1,000.0	247.3	277.2	119.8	85.1	66.4	44.6	42.1	117.5
1903----------------	1941	1,000.0	256.7	276.8	122.0	83.4	65.3	45.2	39.3	111.3
1904----------------	1942	1,000.0	264.2	278.7	119.6	81.0	62.6	45.5	38.9	109.5
1905----------------	1943	1,000.0	273.6	278.6	118.3	78.8	59.1	46.0	39.3	106.3
1906----------------	1944	1,000.0	281.8	278.9	116.5	75.8	58.4	46.5	38.6	103.5
1907----------------	1945	1,000.0	291.4	275.0	115.9	74.2	58.9	45.8	36.9	101.9
1908----------------	1946	1,000.0	299.8	269.6	115.6	73.5	60.7	43.9	36.2	100.7
1909----------------	1947	1,000.0	300.5	263.5	116.1	74.1	63.2	44.2	35.5	102.9
1910----------------	1948	1,000.0	304.8	253.8	116.8	75.8	63.9	43.9	36.5	104.5
1911----------------	1949	1,000.0	303.3	249.6	117.4	76.9	64.5	44.1	36.9	107.3
1912----------------	1950	1,000.0	308.5	241.7	118.9	77.5	63.5	42.9	39.1	107.9
1913----------------	1951	1,000.0	307.2	236.8	119.2	78.8	64.3	45.6	38.5	109.6
1914----------------	1952	1,000.0	306.5	227.8	120.0	80.6	65.8	48.5	39.7	111.1
1915----------------	1953	1,000.0	303.5	221.2	118.6	86.2	66.4	51.5	40.3	112.3
1916----------------	1954	1,000.0	301.7	212.4	118.4	88.4	68.9	53.7	41.3	115.2
1917----------------	1955	1,000.0	294.0	205.3	120.8	91.9	71.2	56.0	42.8	118.0
1918----------------	1956	1,000.0	282.7	202.1	123.6	93.2	74.6	56.7	44.5	122.6
1919----------------	1957	1,000.0	256.1	205.3	128.9	96.8	77.0	59.1	48.2	128.6
1920----------------	1958	1,000.0	238.6	204.4	132.4	99.5	79.1	62.7	50.6	132.7
1921----------------	1959	1,000.0	229.4	192.9	136.4	105.2	81.6	66.2	52.2	136.1
1922----------------	1960	1,000.0	237.8	175.8	135.0	109.5	84.1	66.7	53.0	138.1
1923----------------	1961	1,000.0	234.7	164.2	135.4	110.2	90.8	67.1	55.0	142.6
1924----------------	1962	1,000.0	218.3	156.4	136.3	114.1	95.8	70.6	58.0	150.5
1925----------------	1963	1,000.0	200.8	148.2	139.9	116.3	98.8	76.2	62.0	157.8
1926----------------	1964	1,000.0	192.2	134.2	140.3	121.2	100.4	80.5	65.2	166.0
1927----------------	1965	1,000.0	191.8	122.4	136.8	121.4	104.6	84.7	65.8	172.5
1928----------------	1966	1,000.0	196.5	111.9	131.7	123.1	108.0	86.0	68.8	174.0
1929----------------	1967	1,000.0	191.7	104.0	129.8	122.3	112.1	89.8	71.5	178.8
1930----------------	1968	1,000.0	192.1	97.0	128.7	127.2	110.7	90.0	74.5	179.8
1931----------------	1969	1,000.0	182.5	91.8	132.8	131.3	112.4	91.9	76.0	181.3
1932----------------	1970	1,000.0	170.7	92.6	137.0	137.6	114.9	94.6	75.9	176.7
1933----------------	1971	1,000.0	149.6	94.7	144.0	140.3	122.7	99.3	77.0	172.4
1934----------------	1972	1,000.0	130.3	98.8	146.9	147.3	126.9	101.3	79.4	169.1
1935----------------	1973	1,000.0	115.6	103.2	151.3	151.2	131.8	102.3	82.3	162.3
1936----------------	1974	1,000.0	111.9	106.7	155.4	155.1	133.1	102.4	82.9	152.5

TABLE 8C. DISTRIBUTIONS OF ALL OTHER WOMEN BY PARITY AS OF THE BEGINNING OF EACH YEAR 1917-74 BY AGE FOR EACH COHORT FROM 1867 TO 1959--CON.

(BASED ON CUMULATIVE BIRTH RATES)

EXACT AGE AND COHORT	AS OF JANUARY 1	TOTAL	PARITY							
			0	1	2	3	4	5	6	7 AND HIGHER
39 YEARS										
1878---------------	1917	1,000.0	215.4	135.9	101.8	90.8	83.2	61.9	67.8	243.2
1879---------------	1918	1,000.0	219.6	139.1	102.3	91.5	84.0	61.6	66.2	235.7
1880---------------	1919	1,000.0	222.5	142.7	102.0	93.3	85.3	58.0	66.2	230.0
1881---------------	1920	1,000.0	224.6	145.8	101.8	94.8	86.5	53.3	65.5	227.7
1882---------------	1921	1,000.0	225.8	149.0	101.9	96.0	88.3	48.1	66.7	224.2
1883---------------	1922	1,000.0	228.6	152.5	103.3	100.8	87.2	42.8	68.2	216.6
1884---------------	1923	1,000.0	233.9	155.8	103.1	104.9	87.3	42.7	67.7	204.6
1885---------------	1924	1,000.0	238.3	159.6	104.6	105.4	88.1	45.5	66.2	192.3
1886---------------	1925	1,000.0	238.3	164.9	106.1	100.8	90.7	54.4	63.6	181.2
1887---------------	1926	1,000.0	236.1	171.1	108.5	94.7	94.1	62.2	61.2	172.1
1888---------------	1927	1,000.0	237.2	175.2	108.2	93.6	97.6	58.2	61.3	168.7
1889---------------	1928	1,000.0	237.0	181.9	107.1	101.3	98.8	54.1	59.1	160.7
1890---------------	1929	1,000.0	235.5	187.2	109.9	107.5	97.9	50.0	57.0	155.0
1891---------------	1930	1,000.0	232.5	191.8	115.1	111.5	97.4	45.5	54.4	151.8
1892---------------	1931	1,000.0	227.2	195.9	123.7	113.7	94.6	43.8	51.9	149.2
1893---------------	1932	1,000.0	224.6	202.4	104.8	124.5	99.1	45.2	52.2	147.2
1894---------------	1933	1,000.0	222.8	215.3	111.5	120.5	95.1	41.0	49.2	144.6
1895---------------	1934	1,000.0	223.0	228.5	115.1	115.8	88.4	40.0	46.3	142.9
1896---------------	1935	1,000.0	224.0	242.6	117.0	109.7	83.0	39.7	43.5	140.5
1897---------------	1936	1,000.0	224.2	256.5	117.5	104.0	78.1	40.1	43.0	136.6
1898---------------	1937	1,000.0	240.2	247.4	116.9	98.2	77.1	40.5	43.7	136.0
1899---------------	1938	1,000.0	232.5	261.5	114.1	94.7	72.6	41.7	45.0	137.9
1900---------------	1939	1,000.0	232.0	269.1	112.3	90.1	70.3	42.6	45.5	138.1
1901---------------	1940	1,000.0	237.0	274.2	116.0	87.1	67.9	43.4	43.7	130.7
1902---------------	1941	1,000.0	245.9	276.9	119.3	84.3	65.8	44.0	41.4	122.4
1903---------------	1942	1,000.0	255.2	276.4	121.6	82.8	64.4	44.8	38.5	116.3
1904---------------	1943	1,000.0	262.5	278.3	119.3	80.4	61.9	45.0	38.6	114.0
1905---------------	1944	1,000.0	271.8	278.1	117.8	78.4	58.4	45.5	39.1	110.9
1906---------------	1945	1,000.0	279.8	278.5	115.9	75.4	58.0	45.8	38.3	108.3
1907---------------	1946	1,000.0	289.3	274.7	115.3	73.7	58.4	45.3	36.7	106.6
1908---------------	1947	1,000.0	297.6	268.9	115.3	73.2	60.3	43.7	35.8	105.2
1909---------------	1948	1,000.0	297.9	263.0	115.5	74.1	62.7	44.0	35.2	107.6
1910---------------	1949	1,000.0	302.1	253.2	116.3	75.6	63.6	43.7	36.3	109.2
1911---------------	1950	1,000.0	300.4	248.9	116.9	76.8	64.3	43.7	36.7	112.3
1912---------------	1951	1,000.0	305.6	241.0	118.1	77.4	63.5	42.5	39.0	112.9
1913---------------	1952	1,000.0	304.2	235.9	118.5	78.5	64.3	45.5	38.5	114.6
1914---------------	1953	1,000.0	303.6	226.6	119.2	80.4	65.8	48.5	39.9	116.0
1915---------------	1954	1,000.0	300.2	220.5	117.5	86.0	66.1	51.9	40.1	117.7
1916---------------	1955	1,000.0	298.9	210.9	117.6	87.7	68.8	54.0	41.3	120.8
1917---------------	1956	1,000.0	291.1	204.2	119.7	91.2	71.2	55.7	42.8	124.1
1918---------------	1957	1,000.0	279.9	200.8	122.4	92.9	74.1	56.6	44.5	128.8
1919---------------	1958	1,000.0	253.5	203.8	127.7	95.8	76.9	59.1	48.4	134.8
1920---------------	1959	1,000.0	236.1	202.7	131.2	99.0	78.4	63.1	50.4	139.1
1921---------------	1960	1,000.0	227.1	191.7	134.6	104.8	80.9	65.8	52.6	142.5
1922---------------	1961	1,000.0	235.6	174.5	133.5	108.6	84.1	66.2	53.2	144.3
1923---------------	1962	1,000.0	232.6	162.7	134.0	109.3	90.4	67.2	55.2	148.6
1924---------------	1963	1,000.0	216.4	154.9	134.8	113.3	95.6	70.6	58.1	156.3
1925---------------	1964	1,000.0	198.7	147.0	138.6	115.6	98.4	76.1	62.2	163.4
1926---------------	1965	1,000.0	190.3	133.1	138.8	120.7	99.9	80.5	65.0	171.7
1927---------------	1966	1,000.0	189.9	121.4	135.5	120.9	104.1	84.7	65.7	177.8
1928---------------	1967	1,000.0	194.8	111.1	130.4	122.6	107.4	86.2	69.0	178.5
1929---------------	1968	1,000.0	190.0	103.0	128.5	122.1	112.1	89.6	71.4	183.3
1930---------------	1969	1,000.0	190.3	96.3	127.8	127.0	110.4	89.6	74.8	183.8
1931---------------	1970	1,000.0	180.9	90.8	132.1	130.8	112.3	92.4	75.8	184.9
1932---------------	1971	1,000.0	169.0	91.8	136.1	137.2	114.9	94.8	76.0	180.2
1933---------------	1972	1,000.0	148.1	93.7	143.2	140.2	122.4	99.6	77.0	175.8
1934---------------	1973	1,000.0	128.9	97.7	146.3	147.0	127.2	101.3	79.9	171.7
1935---------------	1974	1,000.0	114.2	102.3	150.7	151.2	131.8	102.7	82.4	164.7

TABLE 8C. DISTRIBUTIONS OF ALL CTHER WOMEN BY PARITY AS OF THE BEGINNING OF EACH YEAR 1917-74 BY AGE FOR EACH COHORT FROM 1867 TO 1959--CON.

(BASED ON CUMULATIVE BIRTH RATES)

EXACT AGE AND COHORT	AS OF JANUARY 1	TOTAL	PARITY							
			0	1	2	3	4	5	6	7 AND HIGHER
40 YEARS										
1877---------------	1917	1,000.0	209.3	131.7	100.7	89.0	81.1	59.8	67.5	260.9
1878---------------	1918	1,000.0	213.4	135.1	101.4	89.2	82.2	60.1	66.7	251.9
1879---------------	1919	1,000.0	216.7	138.9	101.4	90.6	83.1	58.4	66.4	244.5
1880---------------	1920	1,000.0	220.2	141.9	101.5	91.7	84.4	55.9	65.1	239.3
1881---------------	1921	1,C00.0	221.8	145.1	100.8	93.4	85.8	51.6	65.2	236.3
1882---------------	1922	1,000.0	223.2	148.3	101.0	94.5	87.6	46.2	66.3	232.9
1883---------------	1923	1,000.0	226.1	151.8	102.5	99.8	86.2	41.3	67.1	225.2
1884---------------	1924	1,000.0	231.7	155.1	102.2	103.9	86.7	41.0	66.6	212.8
1885---------------	1925	1,C00.0	236.2	159.3	103.4	104.1	87.3	44.6	64.8	200.3
1886---------------	1926	1,000.0	236.5	164.6	104.6	100.0	90.5	52.3	63.3	188.2
1887---------------	1927	1,C00.0	234.3	170.8	107.6	93.4	93.7	61.2	59.8	179.2
1888---------------	1928	1,000.0	235.3	175.3	107.4	92.8	96.5	57.2	60.5	175.0
1889---------------	1929	1,000.0	235.5	181.7	106.5	100.3	97.9	53.2	59.0	165.9
1890---------------	1930	1,000.0	234.2	186.9	109.3	106.5	97.2	49.1	56.5	160.3
1891---------------	1931	1,000.0	230.9	191.9	114.4	110.4	96.1	45.0	53.8	157.5
1892---------------	1932	1,000.0	225.9	195.6	123.4	112.5	93.8	42.8	51.5	154.5
1893---------------	1933	1,C00.0	223.4	202.2	104.2	123.5	98.7	43.3	52.1	152.6
1894---------------	1934	1,000.0	221.7	215.1	110.9	119.5	94.5	40.1	48.6	149.6
1895---------------	1935	1,000.0	221.9	228.4	114.5	115.0	87.6	39.1	45.4	148.1
1896---------------	1936	1,000.0	223.0	242.6	116.2	109.1	82.1	39.2	42.7	145.1
1897---------------	1937	1,000.0	223.2	256.4	116.8	103.5	77.4	39.5	42.2	141.0
1898---------------	1938	1,000.0	239.3	247.0	116.5	97.6	76.4	39.9	43.3	140.0
1899---------------	1939	1,000.0	231.4	261.2	113.6	94.0	72.0	41.0	44.4	142.4
1900---------------	1940	1,000.0	230.8	268.9	111.8	89.5	69.8	41.8	45.0	142.4
1901---------------	1941	1,C00.0	235.8	274.0	115.6	86.5	67.2	43.0	43.2	134.7
1902---------------	1942	1,000.0	244.7	276.6	119.0	83.7	65.1	43.6	40.9	126.4
1903---------------	1943	1,C00.0	254.0	276.0	121.2	82.4	63.8	44.3	38.3	120.0
1904---------------	1944	1,000.0	261.2	277.8	118.9	80.1	61.4	44.4	38.3	117.9
1905---------------	1945	1,000.0	270.4	277.6	117.3	78.2	57.9	44.9	38.8	114.9
1906---------------	1946	1,000.0	278.2	278.3	115.3	74.9	57.6	45.4	38.1	112.2
1907---------------	1947	1,000.0	287.5	274.2	115.2	73.2	58.2	45.0	36.3	110.4
1908---------------	1948	1,C00.0	295.7	268.5	114.9	73.1	59.9	43.4	35.7	108.8
1909---------------	1949	1,C00.0	296.0	262.5	115.0	73.8	62.5	43.9	34.9	111.4
1910---------------	1950	1,000.0	299.7	252.9	116.0	75.3	63.3	43.6	35.9	113.3
1911---------------	1951	1,000.0	298.0	248.5	116.3	76.8	64.2	43.2	36.6	116.4
1912---------------	1952	1,000.0	303.2	240.2	117.9	77.0	63.3	42.5	38.9	117.0
1913---------------	1953	1,000.0	301.9	235.2	117.6	78.5	64.1	45.7	38.5	118.5
1914---------------	1954	1,000.0	301.2	225.8	118.6	80.0	65.6	48.6	39.8	120.4
1915---------------	1955	1,000.0	297.9	219.6	117.0	85.0	66.3	51.8	40.3	122.1
1916---------------	1956	1,000.0	296.8	209.9	116.8	87.1	68.7	53.8	41.4	125.5
1917---------------	1957	1,000.0	288.9	203.3	118.7	91.0	70.6	55.7	42.6	129.2
1918---------------	1958	1,C00.0	277.9	199.7	121.7	92.2	73.8	56.7	44.2	133.8
1919---------------	1959	1,000.0	251.5	202.8	126.9	94.9	76.5	59.5	47.9	140.0
1920---------------	1960	1,000.0	234.4	201.6	130.0	98.3	78.0	62.8	50.6	144.3
1921---------------	1961	1,000.0	225.3	190.9	133.3	104.1	80.7	65.5	52.8	147.4
1922---------------	1962	1,000.0	233.9	173.5	132.3	108.0	83.9	65.7	53.5	149.2
1923---------------	1963	1,000.0	231.1	161.5	132.9	108.7	90.3	67.1	55.1	153.3
1924---------------	1964	1,C00.0	215.0	153.9	133.8	112.4	95.5	70.3	58.4	160.7
1925---------------	1965	1,000.0	197.2	146.2	137.3	115.0	98.2	76.1	62.1	167.9
1926---------------	1966	1,000.0	188.8	132.2	137.9	120.1	99.7	80.4	64.9	176.0
1927---------------	1967	1,000.0	188.6	120.6	134.6	120.4	103.6	84.6	66.1	181.5
1928---------------	1968	1,000.0	193.6	110.3	129.1	122.7	107.2	85.9	69.1	182.1
1929---------------	1969	1,000.0	188.6	102.5	127.9	121.6	112.1	89.2	71.4	186.7
1930---------------	1970	1,000.0	189.0	95.8	127.0	126.3	110.5	89.9	74.7	186.8
1931---------------	1971	1,000.0	179.7	90.1	131.5	130.2	112.4	92.4	76.0	187.7
1932---------------	1972	1,C00.0	167.8	91.2	135.4	137.0	114.8	94.9	76.0	182.9
1933---------------	1973	1,000.0	147.1	92.9	142.7	140.0	122.5	99.7	77.2	177.9
1934---------------	1974	1,000.0	127.9	97.0	145.9	146.9	127.1	101.6	80.0	173.6

TABLE 8C. DISTRIBUTIONS OF ALL OTHER WOMEN BY PARITY AS OF THE BEGINNING OF EACH YEAR 1917-74 BY AGE FOR EACH COHORT FROM 1867 TO 1959--CON.

(BASED ON CUMULATIVE BIRTH RATES)

EXACT AGE AND COHORT	AS OF JANUARY 1	TOTAL	PARITY							
			0	1	2	3	4	5	6	7 AND HIGHER
41 YEARS										
1876	1917	1,000.0	203.7	127.8	99.7	87.3	78.8	58.8	66.7	277.2
1877	1918	1,000.0	208.1	131.3	100.5	87.7	80.6	58.4	67.2	266.2
1878	1919	1,000.0	211.4	135.2	100.7	88.7	81.5	58.0	66.9	257.6
1879	1920	1,000.0	215.3	138.4	101.2	89.5	82.5	57.1	65.7	250.3
1880	1921	1,000.0	218.4	141.7	100.7	90.7	84.0	54.9	64.9	244.7
1881	1922	1,000.0	220.1	144.7	100.1	92.4	85.6	50.2	64.6	242.3
1882	1923	1,000.0	221.5	148.0	100.3	94.0	87.0	45.0	65.6	238.6
1883	1924	1,000.0	224.5	151.6	101.7	99.2	85.8	40.2	66.3	230.7
1884	1925	1,000.0	230.3	155.0	101.3	102.8	86.4	40.3	65.7	218.2
1885	1926	1,000.0	235.0	159.1	102.3	103.4	87.5	43.1	64.9	204.7
1886	1927	1,000.0	235.3	164.4	104.0	99.3	90.1	51.5	62.5	192.9
1887	1928	1,000.0	233.1	170.9	107.0	92.9	93.1	60.4	59.3	183.3
1888	1929	1,000.0	234.3	175.2	107.1	92.4	95.6	56.8	60.5	178.1
1889	1930	1,000.0	234.6	181.6	106.0	99.9	97.4	52.6	58.5	169.4
1890	1931	1,000.0	233.2	186.9	108.8	105.9	96.5	48.9	55.6	164.2
1891	1932	1,000.0	230.1	191.8	114.2	109.6	95.4	44.4	53.5	161.0
1892	1933	1,000.0	225.1	195.5	123.0	111.9	93.3	41.7	51.4	158.1
1893	1934	1,000.0	222.7	202.1	103.8	122.8	98.3	42.7	51.7	155.9
1894	1935	1,000.0	221.1	214.9	110.5	119.0	94.0	39.4	48.1	153.0
1895	1936	1,000.0	221.2	228.4	114.0	114.6	86.9	38.7	45.1	151.1
1896	1937	1,000.0	222.4	242.4	115.9	108.8	81.5	38.8	42.2	148.0
1897	1938	1,000.0	222.6	256.1	116.7	103.0	77.1	38.8	42.1	143.6
1898	1939	1,000.0	238.7	246.8	116.1	97.3	75.8	39.6	42.9	142.8
1899	1940	1,000.0	230.7	261.2	113.1	93.8	71.4	40.7	44.1	145.0
1900	1941	1,000.0	230.0	268.9	111.4	89.2	69.2	41.6	44.6	145.1
1901	1942	1,000.0	235.0	273.9	115.3	86.2	66.6	42.8	42.9	137.3
1902	1943	1,000.0	243.9	276.3	118.9	83.4	64.7	43.3	40.6	128.9
1903	1944	1,000.0	253.1	275.8	121.0	82.1	63.5	43.9	38.0	122.6
1904	1945	1,000.0	260.2	277.6	118.7	79.8	61.1	44.0	38.1	120.5
1905	1946	1,000.0	269.3	277.5	116.9	77.9	57.5	44.6	38.7	117.6
1906	1947	1,000.0	277.0	278.1	115.3	74.3	57.7	44.8	37.8	115.0
1907	1948	1,000.0	286.2	274.0	114.9	73.0	58.0	44.7	36.3	112.9
1908	1949	1,000.0	294.4	268.3	114.6	72.9	59.8	43.2	35.5	111.3
1909	1950	1,000.0	294.4	262.4	114.8	73.5	62.3	43.8	34.7	114.1
1910	1951	1,000.0	298.1	252.6	115.8	75.2	63.1	43.3	35.8	116.1
1911	1952	1,000.0	296.3	247.9	116.3	76.6	63.9	43.2	36.4	119.4
1912	1953	1,000.0	301.7	239.6	117.6	76.5	63.5	42.4	39.0	119.7
1913	1954	1,000.0	300.3	234.6	117.3	78.2	63.9	45.6	38.6	121.5
1914	1955	1,000.0	299.6	225.2	118.1	79.4	65.8	48.5	39.9	123.5
1915	1956	1,000.0	296.5	218.8	116.5	84.5	66.3	51.6	40.6	125.2
1916	1957	1,000.0	295.2	209.4	116.1	86.9	68.2	53.8	41.5	128.9
1917	1958	1,000.0	287.5	202.6	118.2	90.6	70.3	55.7	42.5	132.6
1918	1959	1,000.0	276.6	199.0	121.2	91.5	73.6	57.1	43.7	137.3
1919	1960	1,000.0	250.2	202.1	126.0	94.5	76.3	59.5	47.8	143.6
1920	1961	1,000.0	233.0	201.3	129.0	97.7	77.8	62.7	50.5	148.0
1921	1962	1,000.0	224.2	190.2	132.2	103.8	80.5	65.0	53.2	150.9
1922	1963	1,000.0	232.9	172.6	131.6	107.5	83.8	65.6	53.5	152.5
1923	1964	1,000.0	230.1	160.8	132.2	107.8	90.3	67.1	55.0	156.7
1924	1965	1,000.0	214.0	153.2	132.9	112.0	95.2	70.4	58.3	164.0
1925	1966	1,000.0	196.1	145.7	136.6	114.4	98.0	76.1	62.0	171.1
1926	1967	1,000.0	187.8	131.7	137.1	119.8	99.2	80.5	65.1	178.8
1927	1968	1,000.0	187.6	119.9	134.0	120.4	103.5	84.1	66.2	184.3
1928	1969	1,000.0	192.6	110.0	128.6	122.2	107.3	85.7	68.9	184.7
1929	1970	1,000.0	187.6	102.1	127.4	121.1	112.3	89.1	71.4	189.0
1930	1971	1,000.0	188.2	95.3	126.7	125.7	110.3	90.0	74.9	188.9
1931	1972	1,000.0	178.9	89.6	131.0	129.9	112.6	92.2	76.1	189.7
1932	1973	1,000.0	167.1	90.6	135.0	136.9	114.8	94.9	76.2	184.5
1933	1974	1,000.0	146.4	92.4	142.4	139.9	122.4	99.9	77.2	179.4

TABLE 8C. DISTRIBUTIONS OF ALL OTHER WOMEN BY PARITY AS OF THE BEGINNING OF EACH YEAR 1917-74 BY AGE FOR EACH COHORT FROM 1867 TO 1959--CON.

(BASED ON CUMULATIVE BIRTH RATES)

EXACT AGE AND COHORT	AS OF JANUARY 1	TOTAL	PARITY							
			0	1	2	3	4	5	6	7 AND HIGHER
42 YEARS										
1875	1917	1,000.0	198.2	124.2	98.4	85.7	77.3	58.1	66.1	292.0
1876	1918	1,000.0	203.0	127.5	99.5	86.4	78.4	57.8	66.7	280.7
1877	1919	1,000.0	206.7	131.4	99.9	87.6	79.8	57.0	67.3	270.3
1878	1920	1,000.0	210.7	134.5	100.8	88.0	80.9	57.4	66.2	261.5
1879	1921	1,000.0	214.1	138.3	100.6	88.9	82.0	56.8	65.4	253.9
1880	1922	1,000.0	217.4	141.1	100.2	90.2	83.8	54.0	64.1	249.2
1881	1923	1,000.0	219.0	144.4	99.6	92.3	85.1	49.2	64.1	246.3
1882	1924	1,000.0	220.3	147.9	99.6	93.9	86.6	44.4	64.7	242.6
1883	1925	1,000.0	223.6	151.5	101.0	98.3	85.7	39.8	65.5	234.6
1884	1926	1,000.0	229.4	154.9	100.8	101.9	86.6	39.2	65.9	221.3
1885	1927	1,000.0	234.1	159.0	102.0	102.9	87.0	42.5	64.4	208.1
1886	1928	1,000.0	234.4	164.5	103.6	98.9	89.8	50.9	61.9	196.0
1887	1929	1,000.0	232.4	170.8	106.9	92.4	92.6	60.2	59.0	185.7
1888	1930	1,000.0	233.7	175.1	106.8	92.1	95.3	56.4	60.1	180.5
1889	1931	1,000.0	234.0	181.6	105.6	99.5	96.9	52.4	57.8	172.2
1890	1932	1,000.0	232.6	187.0	108.6	105.3	96.1	48.3	55.4	166.7
1891	1933	1,000.0	229.5	191.8	113.9	109.4	94.7	43.9	53.3	163.5
1892	1934	1,000.0	224.6	195.5	122.6	111.5	93.0	41.3	51.0	160.5
1893	1935	1,000.0	222.2	202.0	103.6	122.4	98.0	42.2	51.4	158.2
1894	1936	1,000.0	220.6	214.8	110.3	118.6	93.6	39.1	47.8	155.2
1895	1937	1,000.0	220.7	228.4	113.8	114.3	86.5	38.4	44.6	153.3
1896	1938	1,000.0	222.0	242.3	115.7	108.4	81.5	38.3	41.8	150.0
1897	1939	1,000.0	222.2	256.0	116.5	102.8	76.8	38.5	41.8	145.4
1898	1940	1,000.0	238.3	246.7	115.9	97.1	75.4	39.3	42.9	144.4
1899	1941	1,000.0	230.1	261.2	113.0	93.5	71.0	40.5	43.9	146.8
1900	1942	1,000.0	229.5	268.8	111.2	88.9	68.9	41.4	44.4	146.9
1901	1943	1,000.0	234.5	273.7	115.2	86.0	66.4	42.7	42.5	139.0
1902	1944	1,000.0	243.4	276.1	118.8	83.0	64.7	43.0	40.2	130.8
1903	1945	1,000.0	252.5	275.7	120.8	81.8	63.4	43.7	37.7	124.4
1904	1946	1,000.0	259.4	277.6	118.5	79.5	60.9	43.7	38.0	122.4
1905	1947	1,000.0	268.5	277.4	116.9	77.5	57.4	44.3	38.4	119.6
1906	1948	1,000.0	276.2	277.9	115.1	74.1	57.6	44.7	37.5	116.9
1907	1949	1,000.0	285.3	273.9	114.7	72.7	58.1	44.6	36.1	114.6
1908	1950	1,000.0	293.3	268.3	114.5	72.7	59.6	43.2	35.3	113.1
1909	1951	1,000.0	293.4	262.1	114.8	73.4	62.0	43.7	34.6	116.0
1910	1952	1,000.0	296.9	252.3	115.7	75.0	63.0	43.3	35.6	118.2
1911	1953	1,000.0	295.3	247.5	116.0	76.4	64.0	43.0	36.4	121.4
1912	1954	1,000.0	300.7	239.1	117.4	76.3	63.3	42.3	39.0	121.9
1913	1955	1,000.0	299.3	234.1	116.9	77.8	64.2	45.4	38.6	123.7
1914	1956	1,000.0	298.6	224.6	117.9	79.1	65.7	48.5	40.0	125.6
1915	1957	1,000.0	295.4	218.5	116.0	84.4	65.8	51.7	40.5	127.7
1916	1958	1,000.0	294.2	209.0	115.7	86.6	67.9	53.9	41.4	131.3
1917	1959	1,000.0	286.6	202.1	118.0	89.9	70.3	55.8	42.2	135.1
1918	1960	1,000.0	275.7	198.6	120.6	91.3	73.3	57.3	43.4	139.8
1919	1961	1,000.0	249.3	201.8	125.4	94.0	76.0	59.7	47.6	146.2
1920	1962	1,000.0	232.2	200.9	128.2	97.4	77.9	62.2	50.6	150.6
1921	1963	1,000.0	223.5	189.6	131.7	103.3	80.3	65.2	53.1	153.3
1922	1964	1,000.0	232.2	172.1	131.2	106.9	83.5	65.7	53.4	155.0
1923	1965	1,000.0	229.3	160.5	131.6	107.3	90.1	67.3	54.8	159.1
1924	1966	1,000.0	213.3	152.8	132.5	111.4	95.0	70.3	58.5	166.2
1925	1967	1,000.0	195.4	145.3	136.1	114.0	97.9	76.0	62.1	173.2
1926	1968	1,000.0	187.2	131.2	136.6	119.8	99.1	80.1	65.2	180.8
1927	1969	1,000.0	187.0	119.6	133.7	119.9	103.6	83.9	66.1	186.2
1928	1970	1,000.0	191.9	109.6	128.4	121.8	107.3	85.7	69.0	186.3
1929	1971	1,000.0	187.1	101.7	127.1	120.6	112.3	89.2	71.5	190.5
1930	1972	1,000.0	187.6	95.0	126.5	125.4	110.4	89.8	74.9	190.4
1931	1973	1,000.0	178.5	89.0	130.9	129.8	112.6	92.1	76.1	191.0
1932	1974	1,000.0	166.6	90.3	134.8	136.8	114.7	94.9	76.4	185.5

TABLE 8C. DISTRIBUTIONS OF ALL OTHER WOMEN BY PARITY AS OF THE BEGINNING OF EACH YEAR 1917-74 BY AGE FOR EACH COHORT FROM 1867 TO 1959--CON.

(BASED ON CUMULATIVE BIRTH RATES)

EXACT AGE AND COHORT	AS OF JANUARY 1	TOTAL	PARITY							
			0	1	2	3	4	5	6	7 AND HIGHER
43 YEARS										
1874	1917	1,000.0	192.8	120.9	96.6	84.2	76.7	58.0	65.9	304.9
1875	1918	1,000.0	197.8	123.9	98.4	85.2	77.0	57.4	66.3	294.0
1876	1919	1,000.0	202.2	127.3	99.4	86.4	77.9	56.8	67.0	283.0
1877	1920	1,000.0	206.3	130.8	100.2	87.2	79.5	56.5	67.0	272.5
1878	1921	1,000.0	210.1	134.1	100.8	87.7	80.6	57.0	66.2	263.5
1879	1922	1,000.0	213.6	137.6	100.7	88.6	81.9	56.1	65.2	256.3
1880	1923	1,000.0	216.8	140.7	100.2	90.2	83.5	53.3	63.9	251.4
1881	1924	1,000.0	218.4	144.0	99.5	92.3	84.8	48.7	63.8	248.5
1882	1925	1,000.0	219.8	147.7	99.3	93.5	86.5	44.0	64.4	244.8
1883	1926	1,000.0	223.1	151.3	100.7	97.9	85.3	39.6	65.4	236.7
1884	1927	1,000.0	228.9	154.9	100.5	101.7	86.2	38.7	65.8	223.3
1885	1928	1,000.0	233.6	159.1	101.6	102.6	86.8	42.3	64.1	209.9
1886	1929	1,000.0	234.0	164.4	103.6	98.5	89.6	50.7	61.7	197.5
1887	1930	1,000.0	232.0	170.8	106.7	92.3	92.4	59.8	58.8	187.2
1888	1931	1,000.0	233.4	175.1	106.6	91.9	94.9	56.3	59.6	182.2
1889	1932	1,000.0	233.7	181.6	105.5	99.2	96.7	52.0	57.5	173.8
1890	1933	1,000.0	232.2	187.0	108.5	105.1	95.7	48.1	55.2	168.2
1891	1934	1,000.0	229.2	191.8	113.7	109.2	94.5	43.7	52.8	165.1
1892	1935	1,000.0	224.3	195.5	122.4	111.2	92.9	41.1	50.7	161.9
1893	1936	1,000.0	221.9	201.9	103.5	122.2	97.7	42.1	51.2	159.5
1894	1937	1,000.0	220.3	214.8	110.2	118.3	93.4	38.9	47.6	156.5
1895	1938	1,000.0	220.4	228.4	113.7	114.0	86.5	38.1	44.3	154.6
1896	1939	1,000.0	221.7	242.3	115.6	108.2	81.4	38.1	41.5	151.2
1897	1940	1,000.0	221.9	256.0	116.4	102.7	76.6	38.2	41.8	146.4
1898	1941	1,000.0	238.0	246.7	115.8	96.9	75.2	39.1	42.7	145.6
1899	1942	1,000.0	229.8	261.2	112.9	93.3	70.8	40.3	43.7	148.0
1900	1943	1,000.0	229.1	268.8	111.2	88.6	68.8	41.3	44.2	148.0
1901	1944	1,000.0	234.1	273.7	115.2	85.6	66.5	42.4	42.4	140.1
1902	1945	1,000.0	242.9	276.2	118.7	82.7	64.7	42.8	40.1	131.9
1903	1946	1,000.0	252.0	275.7	120.7	81.6	63.2	43.6	37.5	125.7
1904	1947	1,000.0	258.9	277.6	118.4	79.2	60.9	43.5	37.8	123.7
1905	1948	1,000.0	268.0	277.3	116.7	77.4	57.3	44.2	38.3	120.8
1906	1949	1,000.0	275.6	277.9	114.9	74.0	57.6	44.7	37.3	118.0
1907	1950	1,000.0	284.6	273.9	114.6	72.6	58.1	44.4	36.1	115.7
1908	1951	1,000.0	292.8	268.1	114.5	72.5	59.5	43.1	35.2	114.3
1909	1952	1,000.0	292.7	261.9	114.7	73.3	62.0	43.7	34.4	117.3
1910	1953	1,000.0	296.3	252.0	115.5	75.1	62.9	43.1	35.6	119.5
1911	1954	1,000.0	294.5	247.4	115.8	76.3	63.7	43.1	36.4	122.8
1912	1955	1,000.0	300.0	238.9	117.1	76.0	63.4	42.4	38.8	123.4
1913	1956	1,000.0	298.5	233.9	116.8	77.5	64.2	45.3	38.7	125.1
1914	1957	1,000.0	297.9	224.4	117.6	79.0	65.5	48.4	40.0	127.2
1915	1958	1,000.0	294.8	218.2	115.7	84.2	65.6	51.6	40.8	129.1
1916	1959	1,000.0	293.7	208.5	115.7	86.2	67.9	53.8	41.5	132.7
1917	1960	1,000.0	285.9	201.8	117.7	89.9	69.9	56.1	41.9	136.8
1918	1961	1,000.0	275.1	198.4	120.3	90.9	73.1	57.4	43.3	141.5
1919	1962	1,000.0	248.7	201.6	124.9	93.7	76.1	59.5	47.6	147.9
1920	1963	1,000.0	231.6	200.7	128.0	97.0	77.5	62.4	50.5	152.3
1921	1964	1,000.0	223.0	189.3	131.4	102.9	80.2	65.3	52.9	155.0
1922	1965	1,000.0	231.7	171.9	130.7	106.8	83.3	65.6	53.4	156.6
1923	1966	1,000.0	228.8	160.3	131.3	106.9	90.0	67.2	54.9	160.6
1924	1967	1,000.0	212.9	152.5	132.2	111.1	94.9	70.2	58.6	167.6
1925	1968	1,000.0	195.0	145.0	135.8	113.8	97.9	75.9	62.0	174.6
1926	1969	1,000.0	186.8	130.9	136.4	119.6	99.0	80.1	65.1	182.1
1927	1970	1,000.0	186.6	119.2	133.7	119.6	103.5	83.9	66.2	187.3
1928	1971	1,000.0	191.5	109.4	128.2	121.5	107.3	85.7	69.1	187.3
1929	1972	1,000.0	186.8	101.3	127.2	120.2	112.4	89.1	71.5	191.5
1930	1973	1,000.0	187.3	94.7	126.4	125.3	110.3	89.8	74.9	191.3
1931	1974	1,000.0	178.1	88.9	130.7	129.8	112.5	92.1	76.2	191.7

TABLE 8C. DISTRIBUTIONS OF ALL OTHER WOMEN BY PARITY AS OF THE BEGINNING OF EACH YEAR 1917-74 BY AGE FOR EACH COHORT FROM 1867 TO 1959--CON.

(BASED ON CUMULATIVE BIRTH RATES)

EXACT AGE AND COHORT	AS OF JANUARY 1	TOTAL	PARITY							
			0	1	2	3	4	5	6	7 AND HIGHER
44 YEARS										
1873---------------	1917	1,000.0	187.5	117.8	94.6	82.8	76.7	58.4	65.8	316.4
1874---------------	1918	1,000.0	192.4	120.8	96.6	83.7	76.5	57.5	66.1	306.4
1875---------------	1919	1,000.0	197.2	123.8	98.3	85.1	76.7	56.6	66.5	295.8
1876---------------	1920	1,000.0	201.9	126.9	99.5	86.2	77.6	56.4	66.9	284.6
1877---------------	1921	1,000.0	205.8	130.6	100.1	87.0	79.3	56.2	67.0	274.0
1878---------------	1922	1,000.0	209.7	133.7	100.8	87.4	80.6	56.5	66.0	265.3
1879---------------	1923	1,000.0	213.2	137.3	100.7	88.5	81.7	55.6	65.1	257.9
1880---------------	1924	1,000.0	216.3	140.6	100.0	90.1	83.3	53.0	63.7	253.0
1881---------------	1925	1,000.0	218.0	143.9	99.3	91.9	84.7	48.4	63.7	250.1
1882---------------	1926	1,000.0	219.4	147.5	99.2	93.4	86.0	43.8	64.1	246.6
1883---------------	1927	1,000.0	222.7	151.4	100.4	97.5	85.2	39.1	65.3	238.4
1884---------------	1928	1,000.0	228.5	154.9	100.3	101.3	86.2	38.5	65.5	224.8
1885---------------	1929	1,000.0	233.3	159.0	101.6	102.3	86.6	42.1	63.8	211.3
1886---------------	1930	1,000.0	233.7	164.5	103.4	98.3	89.5	50.4	61.6	198.6
1887---------------	1931	1,000.0	231.7	170.9	106.6	92.0	92.1	59.7	58.4	188.6
1888---------------	1932	1,000.0	233.1	175.1	106.6	91.7	94.7	56.1	59.3	183.4
1889---------------	1933	1,000.0	233.4	181.6	105.4	99.0	96.5	51.9	57.3	174.9
1890---------------	1934	1,000.0	232.0	186.9	108.4	105.0	95.5	48.0	54.8	169.4
1891---------------	1935	1,000.0	228.9	191.9	113.5	109.0	94.4	43.6	52.5	166.2
1892---------------	1936	1,000.0	224.1	195.4	122.3	111.1	92.7	41.0	50.4	163.0
1893---------------	1937	1,000.0	221.7	201.9	103.4	122.0	97.5	42.0	51.0	160.5
1894---------------	1938	1,000.0	220.1	214.8	110.0	118.2	93.3	38.8	47.3	157.5
1895---------------	1939	1,000.0	220.2	228.4	113.7	113.8	86.5	37.8	44.1	155.5
1896---------------	1940	1,000.0	221.5	242.3	115.6	108.0	81.4	37.8	41.5	151.9
1897---------------	1941	1,000.0	221.7	256.0	116.4	102.5	76.5	38.0	41.6	147.3
1898---------------	1942	1,000.0	237.8	246.7	115.8	96.7	75.1	38.9	42.6	146.4
1899---------------	1943	1,000.0	229.6	261.1	112.9	93.0	70.7	40.3	43.6	148.8
1900---------------	1944	1,000.0	228.9	268.7	111.2	88.2	68.9	41.1	44.1	148.9
1901---------------	1945	1,000.0	233.8	273.7	115.1	85.3	66.5	42.3	42.4	140.9
1902---------------	1946	1,000.0	242.6	276.1	118.7	82.6	64.5	42.8	39.9	132.8
1903---------------	1947	1,000.0	251.7	275.6	120.7	81.4	63.1	43.5	37.5	126.5
1904---------------	1948	1,000.0	258.6	277.5	118.3	79.1	60.9	43.3	37.7	124.6
1905---------------	1949	1,000.0	267.7	277.2	116.6	77.3	57.3	44.2	38.1	121.6
1906---------------	1950	1,000.0	275.2	277.8	114.9	73.8	57.7	44.6	37.1	118.9
1907---------------	1951	1,000.0	284.2	273.8	114.6	72.4	58.1	44.3	36.0	116.6
1908---------------	1952	1,000.0	292.4	268.1	114.3	72.3	59.6	43.2	35.0	115.1
1909---------------	1953	1,000.0	292.2	261.8	114.6	73.3	62.0	43.5	34.5	118.1
1910---------------	1954	1,000.0	295.8	252.0	115.3	75.0	62.7	43.2	35.5	120.5
1911---------------	1955	1,000.0	294.1	247.2	115.7	76.0	63.8	43.1	36.3	123.8
1912---------------	1956	1,000.0	299.5	238.7	117.0	75.9	63.4	42.3	38.8	124.4
1913---------------	1957	1,000.0	298.1	233.7	116.7	77.4	63.9	45.3	38.7	126.2
1914---------------	1958	1,000.0	297.4	224.3	117.3	79.0	65.3	48.4	40.1	128.2
1915---------------	1959	1,000.0	294.4	218.0	115.7	84.0	65.5	51.5	40.8	130.1
1916---------------	1960	1,000.0	293.2	208.4	115.6	86.0	67.7	53.9	41.4	133.8
1917---------------	1961	1,000.0	285.5	201.7	117.5	89.8	69.7	56.0	41.9	137.9
1918---------------	1962	1,000.0	274.7	198.3	120.0	90.7	73.1	57.4	43.2	142.6
1919---------------	1963	1,000.0	248.3	201.5	124.8	93.4	75.9	59.6	47.4	149.1
1920---------------	1964	1,000.0	231.3	200.5	127.8	96.8	77.3	62.5	50.5	153.3
1921---------------	1965	1,000.0	222.6	189.2	131.1	102.9	80.1	65.1	52.9	156.1
1922---------------	1966	1,000.0	231.4	171.7	130.6	106.5	83.2	65.5	53.5	157.6
1923---------------	1967	1,000.0	228.6	160.0	131.1	106.8	90.0	67.0	55.1	161.4
1924---------------	1968	1,000.0	212.6	152.5	131.8	111.1	94.8	70.1	58.6	168.5
1925---------------	1969	1,000.0	194.8	144.7	135.7	113.7	97.9	75.8	61.9	175.5
1926---------------	1970	1,000.0	186.5	130.7	136.3	119.5	98.8	80.2	65.1	182.9
1927---------------	1971	1,000.0	186.4	119.0	133.6	119.4	103.5	83.9	66.2	188.0
1928---------------	1972	1,000.0	191.3	109.2	128.2	121.4	107.2	85.6	69.2	187.9
1929---------------	1973	1,000.0	186.6	101.1	127.2	120.1	112.3	89.2	71.3	192.2
1930---------------	1974	1,000.0	187.1	94.6	126.4	125.2	110.2	89.7	75.1	191.7

TABLE 8C. DISTRIBUTIONS OF ALL OTHER WOMEN BY PARITY AS OF THE BEGINNING OF EACH YEAR 1917-74 BY AGE FOR EACH COHORT FROM 1867 TO 1959--CON.

(BASED ON CUMULATIVE BIRTH RATES)

EXACT AGE AND COHORT	AS OF JANUARY 1	TOTAL	PARITY							
			0	1	2	3	4	5	6	7 AND HIGHER
45 YEARS										
1872---------------	1917	1,000.0	182.5	115.0	92.7	81.5	76.5	58.7	65.8	327.3
1873---------------	1918	1,000.0	187.1	117.5	94.7	82.5	76.5	57.9	65.7	318.1
1874---------------	1919	1,000.0	191.7	121.0	96.1	83.1	76.9	55.4	67.0	308.8
1875---------------	1920	1,000.0	196.9	123.6	98.3	84.8	76.5	56.2	66.2	297.5
1876---------------	1921	1,000.0	201.4	126.6	99.5	86.0	77.5	55.9	66.8	286.3
1877---------------	1922	1,000.0	205.4	130.5	100.0	86.7	79.4	55.7	66.9	275.4
1878---------------	1923	1,000.0	209.3	133.7	100.6	87.3	80.5	56.1	65.7	266.8
1879---------------	1924	1,000.0	212.8	137.2	100.7	88.3	81.4	55.2	64.9	259.5
1880---------------	1925	1,000.0	215.9	140.6	99.8	89.8	83.1	52.7	63.6	254.5
1881---------------	1926	1,000.0	217.6	143.8	99.1	92.0	84.2	48.4	63.1	251.8
1882---------------	1927	1,000.0	218.9	147.6	99.0	93.0	86.2	43.3	64.1	247.9
1883---------------	1928	1,000.0	222.3	151.5	100.2	97.2	85.2	39.0	64.9	239.7
1884---------------	1929	1,000.0	228.1	155.0	100.3	100.9	86.2	38.1	65.4	226.0
1885---------------	1930	1,000.0	233.1	159.0	101.5	102.1	86.4	41.7	64.0	212.2
1886---------------	1931	1,000.0	233.5	164.5	103.3	98.1	89.2	50.2	61.5	199.7
1887---------------	1932	1,000.0	231.4	171.0	106.5	91.8	91.9	59.7	58.0	189.7
1888---------------	1933	1,000.0	232.9	175.1	106.5	91.5	94.6	55.7	59.3	184.4
1889---------------	1934	1,000.0	233.2	181.6	105.3	98.8	96.5	51.7	57.1	175.8
1890---------------	1935	1,000.0	231.8	186.9	108.3	104.8	95.4	47.9	54.7	170.2
1891---------------	1936	1,000.0	228.7	191.9	113.5	108.8	94.2	43.6	52.3	167.0
1892---------------	1937	1,000.0	223.9	195.4	122.2	111.0	92.6	41.0	50.2	163.7
1893---------------	1938	1,000.0	221.5	201.9	103.4	121.8	97.4	42.0	50.8	161.2
1894---------------	1939	1,000.0	219.9	214.9	109.9	118.1	93.3	38.6	47.1	158.2
1895---------------	1940	1,000.0	220.1	228.4	113.6	113.8	86.4	37.6	44.0	156.1
1896---------------	1941	1,000.0	221.3	242.4	115.5	107.9	81.4	37.6	41.3	152.6
1897---------------	1942	1,000.0	221.6	256.0	116.3	102.4	76.5	37.9	41.5	147.8
1898---------------	1943	1,000.0	237.7	246.6	115.7	96.6	75.0	38.8	42.6	147.0
1899---------------	1944	1,000.0	229.5	261.0	112.9	92.8	70.6	40.2	43.6	149.4
1900---------------	1945	1,000.0	228.7	268.7	111.1	88.1	68.8	41.0	44.1	149.5
1901---------------	1946	1,000.0	233.6	273.7	115.0	85.2	66.5	42.2	42.3	141.5
1902---------------	1947	1,000.0	242.4	276.0	118.8	82.4	64.4	42.8	39.9	133.3
1903---------------	1948	1,000.0	251.5	275.6	120.6	81.3	63.2	43.3	37.5	127.0
1904---------------	1949	1,000.0	258.5	277.4	118.2	79.1	60.8	43.3	37.6	125.1
1905---------------	1950	1,000.0	267.4	277.2	116.6	77.2	57.3	44.1	38.1	122.1
1906---------------	1951	1,000.0	275.0	277.8	114.8	73.6	57.8	44.5	37.1	119.4
1907---------------	1952	1,000.0	284.0	273.8	114.5	72.2	58.2	44.3	35.9	117.1
1908---------------	1953	1,000.0	292.1	268.1	114.3	72.3	59.6	43.0	35.0	115.6
1909---------------	1954	1,000.0	291.9	261.8	114.5	73.2	61.9	43.6	34.4	118.7
1910---------------	1955	1,000.0	295.6	251.9	115.3	74.8	62.7	43.2	35.5	121.0
1911---------------	1956	1,000.0	293.8	247.2	115.5	75.9	63.9	43.0	36.3	124.4
1912---------------	1957	1,000.0	299.3	238.6	117.0	75.7	63.4	42.1	38.9	125.0
1913---------------	1958	1,000.0	297.8	233.6	116.7	77.4	63.7	45.4	38.7	126.7
1914---------------	1959	1,000.0	297.2	224.2	117.2	79.0	65.2	48.3	40.2	128.7
1915---------------	1960	1,000.0	294.1	218.0	115.6	83.8	65.5	51.5	40.8	130.7
1916---------------	1961	1,000.0	293.0	208.3	115.4	86.0	67.7	53.7	41.4	134.5
1917---------------	1962	1,000.0	285.3	201.6	117.4	89.6	69.8	55.9	41.8	138.6
1918---------------	1963	1,000.0	274.5	198.3	119.9	90.6	73.0	57.3	43.1	143.3
1919---------------	1964	1,000.0	248.1	201.4	124.7	93.3	75.8	59.7	47.4	149.6
1920---------------	1965	1,000.0	231.1	200.4	127.7	96.8	77.1	62.3	50.7	153.9
1921---------------	1966	1,000.0	222.4	189.1	131.0	102.8	80.0	65.1	52.9	156.7
1922---------------	1967	1,000.0	231.3	171.6	130.4	106.4	83.2	65.4	53.6	158.1
1923---------------	1968	1,000.0	228.5	159.9	130.8	106.9	90.0	66.9	55.1	161.9
1924---------------	1969	1,000.0	212.5	152.3	131.8	111.0	94.7	70.1	58.5	169.1
1925---------------	1970	1,000.0	194.6	144.6	135.6	113.7	97.8	75.8	61.9	176.0
1926---------------	1971	1,000.0	186.4	130.6	136.2	119.4	98.8	80.1	65.2	183.3
1927---------------	1972	1,000.0	186.3	118.9	133.6	119.2	103.4	84.0	66.2	188.4
1928---------------	1973	1,000.0	191.2	109.1	128.1	121.4	107.1	85.7	69.1	188.3
1929---------------	1974	1,000.0	186.4	101.1	127.2	120.1	112.2	89.2	71.3	192.5

TABLE 8C. DISTRIBUTIONS OF ALL OTHER WOMEN BY PARITY AS OF THE BEGINNING OF EACH YEAR 1917-74 BY AGE FOR EACH COHORT FROM 1867 TO 1959--CON.

(BASED ON CUMULATIVE BIRTH RATES)

EXACT AGE AND COHORT	AS OF JANUARY 1	TOTAL	PARITY 0	1	2	3	4	5	6	7 AND HIGHER
46 YEARS										
1871	1917	1,000.0	177.9	112.1	91.1	80.3	76.3	59.0	65.7	337.6
1872	1918	1,000.0	182.0	114.9	92.6	81.5	76.2	58.5	65.3	329.0
1873	1919	1,000.0	186.4	117.9	93.7	82.2	77.0	55.8	66.2	320.8
1874	1920	1,000.0	191.4	120.9	95.9	83.1	76.6	55.2	66.4	310.5
1875	1921	1,000.0	196.5	123.3	98.1	84.8	76.4	55.9	65.8	299.2
1876	1922	1,000.0	201.0	126.8	99.1	85.8	77.6	55.8	66.5	287.4
1877	1923	1,000.0	205.0	130.7	99.6	86.7	79.3	55.6	66.4	276.7
1878	1924	1,000.0	209.0	133.6	100.5	87.2	80.2	55.9	65.3	268.3
1879	1925	1,000.0	212.4	137.3	100.3	88.3	81.2	55.0	64.7	260.8
1880	1926	1,000.0	215.6	140.5	99.6	89.8	82.9	52.6	63.2	255.8
1881	1927	1,000.0	217.1	144.1	98.7	91.7	84.5	47.9	62.9	253.1
1882	1928	1,000.0	218.5	147.7	98.9	92.7	86.2	43.1	64.0	248.9
1883	1929	1,000.0	221.9	151.6	100.3	96.8	85.2	38.7	64.7	240.8
1884	1930	1,000.0	227.9	154.9	100.3	100.8	86.0	37.7	65.6	226.8
1885	1931	1,000.0	232.9	159.0	101.3	102.0	86.3	41.5	63.9	213.1
1886	1932	1,000.0	233.2	164.7	103.2	97.9	88.9	50.3	61.2	200.6
1887	1933	1,000.0	231.2	171.0	106.5	91.7	91.7	59.3	58.1	190.5
1888	1934	1,000.0	232.7	175.1	106.5	91.3	94.6	55.5	59.1	185.2
1889	1935	1,000.0	233.0	181.6	105.3	98.6	96.5	51.5	57.1	176.4
1890	1936	1,000.0	231.6	187.0	108.2	104.7	95.3	47.8	54.6	170.8
1891	1937	1,000.0	228.5	192.0	113.4	108.7	94.1	43.6	52.1	167.6
1892	1938	1,000.0	223.7	195.4	122.2	110.9	92.6	40.9	50.0	164.3
1893	1939	1,000.0	221.3	202.0	103.4	121.7	97.4	41.9	50.6	161.7
1894	1940	1,000.0	219.8	214.9	109.9	118.0	93.2	38.6	47.0	158.6
1895	1941	1,000.0	219.9	228.6	113.5	113.7	86.3	37.6	43.8	156.6
1896	1942	1,000.0	221.2	242.4	115.5	107.8	81.4	37.6	41.2	152.9
1897	1943	1,000.0	221.5	255.9	116.3	102.3	76.5	37.7	41.6	148.2
1898	1944	1,000.0	237.6	246.5	115.7	96.5	75.0	38.7	42.6	147.4
1899	1945	1,000.0	229.4	261.0	112.8	92.8	70.4	40.2	43.6	149.8
1900	1946	1,000.0	228.6	268.7	111.0	88.0	68.8	40.9	44.1	149.9
1901	1947	1,000.0	233.5	273.6	115.0	85.1	66.5	42.1	42.4	141.8
1902	1948	1,000.0	242.3	276.0	118.8	82.3	64.4	42.7	39.9	133.6
1903	1949	1,000.0	251.4	275.6	120.5	81.3	63.2	43.2	37.5	127.3
1904	1950	1,000.0	258.4	277.3	118.2	79.1	60.8	43.2	37.6	125.4
1905	1951	1,000.0	267.2	277.3	116.5	77.1	57.4	44.0	38.1	122.4
1906	1952	1,000.0	274.9	277.8	114.7	73.5	57.9	44.4	37.1	119.7
1907	1953	1,000.0	283.8	273.9	114.4	72.2	58.2	44.3	35.7	117.5
1908	1954	1,000.0	292.0	268.0	114.3	72.3	59.6	43.0	34.9	115.9
1909	1955	1,000.0	291.7	261.8	114.6	73.0	62.0	43.5	34.4	119.0
1910	1956	1,000.0	295.5	251.9	115.1	74.8	62.7	43.2	35.4	121.4
1911	1957	1,000.0	293.7	247.1	115.5	75.9	63.8	43.0	36.3	124.7
1912	1958	1,000.0	299.2	238.5	117.0	75.6	63.3	42.2	38.9	125.3
1913	1959	1,000.0	297.6	233.6	116.7	77.4	63.6	45.4	38.7	127.0
1914	1960	1,000.0	297.0	224.3	117.1	78.8	65.3	48.2	40.2	129.1
1915	1961	1,000.0	294.0	218.0	115.4	83.8	65.5	51.5	40.7	131.1
1916	1962	1,000.0	292.9	208.3	115.3	85.9	67.7	53.7	41.4	134.8
1917	1963	1,000.0	285.2	201.6	117.3	89.5	69.8	55.9	41.8	138.9
1918	1964	1,000.0	274.4	198.2	119.9	90.6	72.9	57.3	43.0	143.7
1919	1965	1,000.0	248.0	201.4	124.6	93.3	75.7	59.6	47.5	149.9
1920	1966	1,000.0	231.0	200.4	127.6	96.7	77.1	62.2	50.8	154.2
1921	1967	1,000.0	222.3	189.1	130.9	102.7	80.0	65.1	53.0	156.9
1922	1968	1,000.0	231.3	171.5	130.2	106.5	83.1	65.4	53.7	158.3
1923	1969	1,000.0	228.5	159.8	130.7	106.8	90.0	67.0	55.0	162.2
1924	1970	1,000.0	212.4	152.3	131.7	111.0	94.7	70.1	58.4	169.4
1925	1971	1,000.0	194.5	144.6	135.5	113.7	97.8	75.7	61.9	176.3
1926	1972	1,000.0	186.3	130.6	136.1	119.4	98.7	80.2	65.2	183.5
1927	1973	1,000.0	186.2	118.9	133.6	119.1	103.4	84.0	66.1	188.7
1928	1974	1,000.0	191.1	109.1	128.1	121.4	107.0	85.8	69.1	188.4

TABLE 8C. DISTRIBUTIONS OF ALL OTHER WOMEN BY PARITY AS OF THE BEGINNING OF EACH YEAR 1917-74 BY AGE FOR EACH COHORT FROM 1867 TO 1959--CON.

(BASED ON CUMULATIVE BIRTH RATES)

EXACT AGE AND COHORT	AS OF JANUARY 1	TOTAL	PARITY							
			0	1	2	3	4	5	6	7 AND HIGHER
47 YEARS										
1870	1917	1,000.0	173.6	109.5	89.4	79.1	76.1	59.5	65.5	347.3
1871	1918	1,000.0	177.4	112.0	91.0	80.3	76.1	58.9	65.3	339.0
1872	1919	1,000.0	181.2	115.5	91.5	81.0	76.8	56.6	66.0	331.4
1873	1920	1,000.0	186.1	117.9	93.5	82.1	76.8	55.7	65.7	322.2
1874	1921	1,000.0	191.0	120.7	95.7	83.1	76.4	55.1	66.1	311.9
1875	1922	1,000.0	196.1	123.5	97.8	84.6	76.5	55.9	65.6	300.0
1876	1923	1,000.0	200.6	127.1	98.7	85.8	77.5	55.8	66.0	288.5
1877	1924	1,000.0	204.7	130.7	99.5	86.6	78.9	55.6	66.1	277.9
1878	1925	1,000.0	208.6	133.7	100.2	87.2	79.9	55.9	65.1	269.4
1879	1926	1,000.0	212.1	137.2	100.2	88.3	81.0	55.0	64.3	261.9
1880	1927	1,000.0	215.1	140.7	99.4	89.6	83.0	52.2	63.1	256.9
1881	1928	1,000.0	216.7	144.2	98.6	91.6	84.4	47.7	62.9	253.9
1882	1929	1,000.0	218.2	147.7	99.0	92.4	86.2	42.9	63.7	249.9
1883	1930	1,000.0	221.8	151.4	100.3	96.7	85.1	38.3	64.9	241.5
1884	1931	1,000.0	227.7	154.9	100.2	100.7	85.9	37.5	65.6	227.5
1885	1932	1,000.0	232.7	159.1	101.1	101.9	86.0	41.6	63.8	213.8
1886	1933	1,000.0	233.1	164.7	103.1	97.8	88.8	49.9	61.3	201.3
1887	1934	1,000.0	231.0	171.0	106.5	91.6	91.7	59.1	57.9	191.2
1888	1935	1,000.0	232.5	175.2	106.4	91.2	94.6	55.2	59.2	185.7
1889	1936	1,000.0	232.9	181.6	105.3	98.4	96.5	51.4	57.0	176.9
1890	1937	1,000.0	231.5	187.0	108.1	104.7	95.2	47.8	54.4	171.3
1891	1938	1,000.0	228.3	192.1	113.4	108.6	94.0	43.5	52.0	168.1
1892	1939	1,000.0	223.5	195.5	122.2	110.8	92.7	40.7	49.8	164.8
1893	1940	1,000.0	221.2	202.0	103.4	121.6	97.4	41.8	50.5	162.1
1894	1941	1,000.0	219.6	215.1	109.8	117.9	93.2	38.5	46.9	159.0
1895	1942	1,000.0	219.8	228.6	113.5	113.7	86.2	37.6	43.7	156.9
1896	1943	1,000.0	221.1	242.4	115.5	107.7	81.4	37.5	41.2	153.2
1897	1944	1,000.0	221.4	255.9	116.3	102.3	76.4	37.7	41.5	148.5
1898	1945	1,000.0	237.5	246.5	115.7	96.5	74.9	38.6	42.6	147.7
1899	1946	1,000.0	229.3	261.0	112.8	92.7	70.4	40.1	43.6	150.1
1900	1947	1,000.0	228.5	268.7	110.9	88.0	68.8	40.8	44.1	150.2
1901	1948	1,000.0	233.4	273.7	114.9	85.1	66.4	42.1	42.4	142.0
1902	1949	1,000.0	242.2	276.0	118.8	82.3	64.4	42.6	39.9	133.8
1903	1950	1,000.0	251.3	275.6	120.5	81.3	63.1	43.2	37.5	127.5
1904	1951	1,000.0	258.3	277.3	118.2	79.0	60.9	43.1	37.6	125.6
1905	1952	1,000.0	267.2	277.2	116.5	77.1	57.4	43.9	38.1	122.6
1906	1953	1,000.0	274.8	277.8	114.7	73.5	57.9	44.4	37.0	119.9
1907	1954	1,000.0	283.7	273.9	114.3	72.3	58.2	44.2	35.8	117.6
1908	1955	1,000.0	291.9	268.0	114.3	72.2	59.7	43.0	34.9	116.0
1909	1956	1,000.0	291.7	261.8	114.5	72.9	62.0	43.5	34.4	119.2
1910	1957	1,000.0	295.4	251.9	115.1	74.8	62.6	43.2	35.5	121.5
1911	1958	1,000.0	293.7	247.0	115.5	75.9	63.7	43.1	36.2	124.9
1912	1959	1,000.0	299.1	238.5	117.0	75.6	63.3	42.1	39.0	125.4
1913	1960	1,000.0	297.5	233.6	116.7	77.3	63.6	45.4	38.7	127.2
1914	1961	1,000.0	296.9	224.3	117.0	78.9	65.2	48.3	40.1	129.3
1915	1962	1,000.0	293.9	218.0	115.4	83.8	65.5	51.4	40.7	131.3
1916	1963	1,000.0	292.9	208.2	115.3	85.9	67.6	53.7	41.4	135.0
1917	1964	1,000.0	285.1	201.6	117.3	89.5	69.8	55.8	41.7	139.2
1918	1965	1,000.0	274.4	198.2	119.8	90.6	72.8	57.3	43.1	143.8
1919	1966	1,000.0	247.9	201.5	124.5	93.3	75.6	59.6	47.6	150.0
1920	1967	1,000.0	231.0	200.3	127.6	96.7	77.0	62.3	50.8	154.3
1921	1968	1,000.0	222.3	189.0	130.9	102.7	80.0	65.1	53.0	157.0
1922	1969	1,000.0	231.3	171.4	130.2	106.5	83.1	65.4	53.6	158.5
1923	1970	1,000.0	228.4	159.9	130.6	106.8	90.0	67.0	55.0	162.3
1924	1971	1,000.0	212.4	152.3	131.6	111.0	94.7	70.0	58.5	169.5
1925	1972	1,000.0	194.5	144.6	135.4	113.7	97.8	75.7	61.9	176.4
1926	1973	1,000.0	186.3	130.6	136.0	119.4	98.7	80.2	65.2	183.6
1927	1974	1,000.0	186.1	119.0	133.5	119.1	103.4	84.0	66.1	188.8

TABLE 8C. DISTRIBUTIONS OF ALL OTHER WOMEN BY PARITY AS OF THE BEGINNING OF EACH YEAR 1917-74 BY AGE FOR EACH COHORT FROM 1867 TO 1959--CON.

(BASED ON CUMULATIVE BIRTH RATES)

EXACT AGE AND COHORT	AS OF JANUARY 1	TOTAL	PARITY 0	1	2	3	4	5	6	7 AND HIGHER
48 YEARS										
1869	1917	1,000.0	169.6	106.9	87.9	78.0	75.8	59.9	65.4	356.5
1870	1918	1,000.0	173.2	109.6	89.3	79.1	76.0	59.4	65.2	348.2
1871	1919	1,C00.0	176.8	112.5	90.4	80.0	76.4	57.8	65.6	340.5
1872	1920	1,000.0	181.0	115.6	91.3	81.0	76.7	56.5	65.6	332.3
1873	1921	1,000.0	185.8	117.9	93.3	82.2	76.6	55.7	65.4	323.1
1874	1922	1,000.0	190.7	120.9	95.5	83.1	76.3	55.2	65.9	312.4
1875	1923	1,000.0	195.8	123.7	97.6	84.7	76.3	55.9	65.3	300.7
1876	1924	1,000.0	200.4	127.2	98.6	85.8	77.2	55.8	65.7	289.3
1877	1925	1,000.0	204.4	130.9	99.3	86.6	78.7	55.6	66.0	278.5
1878	1926	1,000.0	208.3	133.8	100.2	87.1	80.0	55.8	65.0	269.8
1879	1927	1,000.0	211.8	137.4	99.9	88.3	81.0	54.9	64.1	262.6
1880	1928	1,000.0	214.8	140.8	99.5	89.5	82.8	52.0	63.4	257.2
1881	1929	1,000.0	216.5	144.2	98.6	91.6	84.2	47.7	62.8	254.4
1882	1930	1,000.0	218.1	147.6	99.1	92.3	86.0	42.8	63.7	250.4
1883	1931	1,000.0	221.7	151.4	100.3	96.6	85.0	38.3	64.7	242.0
1884	1932	1,000.0	227.6	154.9	100.1	100.8	85.7	37.4	65.7	227.8
1885	1933	1,000.0	232.6	159.1	101.1	101.8	86.0	41.4	63.9	214.1
1886	1934	1,000.0	233.0	164.7	103.1	97.7	88.8	49.9	61.2	201.6
1887	1935	1,000.0	230.9	171.1	106.3	91.6	91.7	59.0	57.9	191.5
1888	1936	1,000.0	232.4	175.2	106.4	91.2	94.5	55.2	59.1	186.0
1889	1937	1,000.0	232.8	181.6	105.3	98.3	96.5	51.4	56.9	177.2
1890	1938	1,000.0	231.4	187.0	108.1	104.7	95.2	47.6	54.4	171.6
1891	1939	1,000.0	228.2	192.1	113.4	108.6	94.0	43.4	51.9	168.4
1892	1940	1,000.0	223.4	195.5	122.2	110.8	92.6	40.7	49.7	165.1
1893	1941	1,000.0	221.1	202.1	103.3	121.6	97.3	41.8	50.5	162.3
1894	1942	1,000.0	219.5	215.2	109.7	117.9	93.1	38.6	46.8	159.2
1895	1943	1,000.0	219.7	228.6	113.5	113.7	86.2	37.5	43.7	157.1
1896	1944	1,C00.0	221.1	242.3	115.6	107.7	81.3	37.5	41.1	153.4
1897	1945	1,000.0	221.4	255.9	116.2	102.4	76.3	37.7	41.4	148.7
1898	1946	1,000.0	237.5	246.5	115.6	96.5	74.8	38.6	42.6	147.9
1899	1947	1,000.0	229.2	261.1	112.7	92.7	70.4	40.0	43.6	150.3
1900	1948	1,000.0	228.4	268.8	110.8	88.0	68.8	40.8	44.1	150.3
1901	1949	1,000.0	233.3	273.7	114.9	85.1	66.4	42.1	42.4	142.1
1902	1950	1,000.0	242.2	275.9	118.8	82.3	64.4	42.6	39.9	133.9
1903	1951	1,000.0	251.3	275.6	120.5	81.2	63.1	43.2	37.5	127.6
1904	1952	1,000.0	258.3	277.2	118.2	79.1	60.8	43.1	37.6	125.7
1905	1953	1,000.0	267.2	277.2	116.5	77.1	57.3	44.0	38.0	122.7
1906	1954	1,C00.0	274.7	277.9	114.6	73.5	57.9	44.4	37.1	119.9
1907	1955	1,000.0	283.7	273.9	114.3	72.2	58.3	44.1	35.8	117.7
1908	1956	1,000.0	291.9	268.0	114.2	72.2	59.7	43.0	34.9	116.1
1909	1957	1,000.0	291.7	261.8	114.4	73.0	61.9	43.5	34.5	119.2
1910	1958	1,000.0	295.4	251.9	115.0	74.9	62.5	43.2	35.5	121.6
1911	1959	1,000.0	293.6	247.0	115.5	75.9	63.8	43.0	36.2	125.0
1912	1960	1,000.0	299.0	238.6	117.0	75.5	63.3	42.1	39.0	125.5
1913	1961	1,000.0	297.4	233.7	116.7	77.3	63.5	45.4	38.7	127.3
1914	1962	1,000.0	296.9	224.3	117.0	78.9	65.2	48.2	40.1	129.4
1915	1963	1,000.0	293.9	218.0	115.4	83.7	65.5	51.4	40.7	131.4
1916	1964	1,000.0	292.8	208.3	115.3	85.9	67.5	53.7	41.4	135.1
1917	1965	1,000.0	285.1	201.6	117.3	89.4	69.8	55.8	41.8	139.2
1918	1966	1,000.0	274.4	198.2	119.8	90.6	72.7	57.3	43.1	143.9
1919	1967	1,000.0	247.9	201.5	124.4	93.4	75.5	59.7	47.5	150.1
1920	1968	1,000.0	231.0	200.3	127.6	96.6	77.0	62.4	50.8	154.3
1921	1969	1,000.0	222.3	189.0	130.9	102.7	80.0	65.0	53.0	157.1
1922	1970	1,000.0	231.2	171.5	130.1	106.5	83.1	65.5	53.5	158.6
1923	1971	1,000.0	228.4	159.9	130.6	106.8	89.9	67.0	55.0	162.4
1924	1972	1,C00.0	212.4	152.3	131.5	111.1	94.7	70.0	58.5	169.5
1925	1973	1,000.0	194.5	144.6	135.4	113.7	97.7	75.8	61.9	176.4
1926	1974	1,000.0	186.3	130.6	136.0	119.4	98.7	80.2	65.2	183.6

TABLE 8C. DISTRIBUTIONS OF ALL OTHER WOMEN BY PARITY AS OF THE BEGINNING OF EACH YEAR 1917-74 BY AGE FOR EACH COHORT FROM 1867 TO 1959--CON.

(BASED ON CUMULATIVE BIRTH RATES)

EXACT AGE AND COHORT	AS OF JANUARY 1	TOTAL	PARITY 0	1	2	3	4	5	6	7 AND HIGHER
49 YEARS										
1868	1917	1,000.0	166.0	104.4	86.5	77.0	75.3	60.3	65.3	365.2
1869	1918	1,000.0	169.3	106.9	88.0	77.8	75.8	59.8	65.3	357.1
1870	1919	1,000.0	172.7	110.0	89.0	78.6	76.4	58.5	65.7	349.1
1871	1920	1,000.0	176.6	112.6	90.3	79.9	76.4	57.7	65.4	341.1
1872	1921	1,000.0	180.8	115.5	91.3	80.9	76.7	56.4	65.5	332.9
1873	1922	1,000.0	185.6	118.0	93.3	82.0	76.6	55.7	65.4	323.4
1874	1923	1,000.0	190.5	121.0	95.5	83.0	76.2	55.2	65.8	312.8
1875	1924	1,000.0	195.6	123.8	97.6	84.6	76.1	55.9	65.2	301.2
1876	1925	1,000.0	200.2	127.3	98.5	85.7	77.2	55.7	65.7	289.7
1877	1926	1,000.0	204.2	130.9	99.3	86.6	78.7	55.5	66.1	278.7
1878	1927	1,000.0	208.1	133.8	100.1	87.1	80.0	55.8	64.8	270.3
1879	1928	1,000.0	211.7	137.3	100.0	88.3	80.9	54.8	64.1	262.9
1880	1929	1,000.0	214.7	140.8	99.5	89.5	82.7	51.9	63.4	257.5
1881	1930	1,000.0	216.4	144.2	98.6	91.5	84.1	47.6	62.8	254.8
1882	1931	1,000.0	218.0	147.6	99.2	92.1	86.0	42.8	63.7	250.6
1883	1932	1,000.0	221.6	151.4	100.2	96.7	84.8	38.3	64.7	242.3
1884	1933	1,000.0	227.5	154.9	100.0	100.7	85.8	37.3	65.7	228.1
1885	1934	1,000.0	232.5	159.1	101.1	101.7	86.1	41.3	63.8	214.4
1886	1935	1,000.0	232.9	164.8	102.9	97.8	88.7	49.8	61.2	201.9
1887	1936	1,000.0	230.8	171.1	106.3	91.6	91.6	58.9	58.0	191.7
1888	1937	1,000.0	232.3	175.1	106.5	91.1	94.6	55.1	59.0	186.3
1889	1938	1,000.0	232.6	181.7	105.3	98.3	96.4	51.3	57.0	177.4
1890	1939	1,000.0	231.3	187.0	108.1	104.7	95.2	47.5	54.3	171.9
1891	1940	1,000.0	228.2	192.0	113.4	108.6	93.9	43.4	51.8	168.7
1892	1941	1,000.0	223.3	195.6	122.1	110.8	92.5	40.7	49.7	165.3
1893	1942	1,000.0	221.1	202.0	103.3	121.6	97.3	41.8	50.4	162.5
1894	1943	1,000.0	219.4	215.3	109.6	117.9	93.1	38.6	46.8	159.3
1895	1944	1,000.0	219.7	228.6	113.5	113.7	86.2	37.4	43.7	157.2
1896	1945	1,000.0	221.1	242.3	115.5	107.8	81.2	37.5	41.1	153.5
1897	1946	1,000.0	221.4	255.9	116.1	102.4	76.3	37.7	41.4	148.8
1898	1947	1,000.0	237.4	246.6	115.5	96.5	74.8	38.6	42.6	148.0
1899	1948	1,000.0	229.1	261.2	112.6	92.7	70.4	40.0	43.6	150.4
1900	1949	1,000.0	228.3	268.8	110.8	88.1	68.7	40.8	44.1	150.4
1901	1950	1,000.0	233.3	273.6	114.9	85.1	66.4	42.1	42.4	142.2
1902	1951	1,000.0	242.2	275.8	118.9	82.3	64.3	42.6	39.9	134.0
1903	1952	1,000.0	251.3	275.5	120.5	81.3	63.0	43.2	37.5	127.7
1904	1953	1,000.0	258.3	277.2	118.2	79.0	60.8	43.2	37.5	125.8
1905	1954	1,000.0	267.1	277.3	116.4	77.2	57.3	43.9	38.1	122.7
1906	1955	1,000.0	274.7	277.8	114.7	73.4	58.0	44.3	37.1	120.0
1907	1956	1,000.0	283.7	273.9	114.2	72.2	58.3	44.1	35.8	117.8
1908	1957	1,000.0	291.9	268.0	114.1	72.3	59.7	43.0	34.9	116.1
1909	1958	1,000.0	291.7	261.8	114.4	73.0	61.9	43.4	34.5	119.3
1910	1959	1,000.0	295.3	251.9	115.0	74.9	62.6	43.1	35.6	121.6
1911	1960	1,000.0	293.6	247.0	115.5	75.9	63.8	42.9	36.2	125.1
1912	1961	1,000.0	298.9	238.7	117.0	75.5	63.2	42.2	38.9	125.6
1913	1962	1,000.0	297.4	233.7	116.7	77.3	63.5	45.3	38.8	127.3
1914	1963	1,000.0	296.9	224.3	117.0	78.9	65.1	48.2	40.2	129.4
1915	1964	1,000.0	293.9	218.0	115.4	83.7	65.4	51.5	40.7	131.4
1916	1965	1,000.0	292.8	208.3	115.3	85.9	67.4	53.8	41.4	135.1
1917	1966	1,000.0	285.1	201.6	117.3	89.4	69.8	55.8	41.8	139.2
1918	1967	1,000.0	274.4	198.2	119.8	90.6	72.7	57.3	43.0	144.0
1919	1968	1,000.0	247.9	201.5	124.4	93.3	75.6	59.7	47.5	150.1
1920	1969	1,000.0	231.0	200.3	127.6	96.6	77.0	62.4	50.8	154.3
1921	1970	1,000.0	222.2	189.1	130.9	102.7	79.9	65.1	53.0	157.1
1922	1971	1,000.0	231.2	171.5	130.1	106.5	83.1	65.5	53.5	158.6
1923	1972	1,000.0	228.4	159.9	130.6	106.8	89.9	67.0	54.9	162.5
1924	1973	1,000.0	212.4	152.3	131.5	111.1	94.7	70.0	58.5	169.5
1925	1974	1,000.0	194.5	144.6	135.4	113.7	97.7	75.8	61.9	176.4

TABLE 8C. DISTRIBUTIONS OF ALL OTHER WOMEN BY PARITY AS OF THE BEGINNING OF EACH YEAR 1917-74 BY AGE FOR EACH COHORT FROM 1867 TO 1959--CON.

(BASED ON CUMULATIVE BIRTH RATES)

EXACT AGE AND COHORT	AS OF JANUARY 1	TOTAL	PARITY							
			0	1	2	3	4	5	6	7 AND HIGHER
50 YEARS										
1867---------------	1917	1,000.0	162.7	102.0	85.3	76.0	74.5	60.7	65.2	373.6
1868---------------	1918	1,000.0	165.9	104.3	86.6	76.9	75.3	60.1	65.2	365.7
1869---------------	1919	1,000.0	169.0	107.1	87.9	77.5	76.1	58.8	65.6	358.0
1870---------------	1920	1,000.0	172.6	110.0	89.0	78.6	76.3	58.4	65.5	349.6
1871---------------	1921	1,000.0	176.5	112.5	90.4	79.8	76.4	57.5	65.3	341.6
1872---------------	1922	1,000.0	180.7	115.5	91.3	80.8	76.8	56.3	65.4	333.2
1873---------------	1923	1,000.0	185.5	118.0	93.3	82.0	76.6	55.5	65.3	323.8
1874---------------	1924	1,000.0	190.4	121.0	95.5	83.0	76.1	55.1	65.7	313.2
1875---------------	1925	1,000.0	195.5	123.8	97.6	84.6	76.0	55.8	65.2	301.5
1876---------------	1926	1,000.0	200.1	127.3	98.5	85.7	77.1	55.7	65.8	289.8
1877---------------	1927	1,000.0	204.1	130.9	99.2	86.6	78.8	55.4	66.0	279.0
1878---------------	1928	1,000.0	208.0	133.8	100.2	87.1	79.9	55.8	64.8	270.4
1879---------------	1929	1,000.0	211.6	137.4	99.9	88.3	80.8	54.8	64.2	263.0
1880---------------	1930	1,000.0	214.6	140.8	99.5	89.5	82.6	51.8	63.4	257.8
1881---------------	1931	1,000.0	216.4	144.2	98.6	91.4	84.0	47.6	62.8	255.0
1882---------------	1932	1,000.0	217.9	147.6	99.2	92.2	85.9	42.7	63.7	250.8
1883---------------	1933	1,000.0	221.5	151.5	100.1	96.6	84.8	38.4	64.6	242.5
1884---------------	1934	1,000.0	227.4	155.0	99.9	100.6	85.9	37.3	65.7	228.2
1885---------------	1935	1,000.0	232.4	159.2	101.0	101.7	86.1	41.2	63.8	214.6
1886---------------	1936	1,000.0	232.8	164.8	102.9	97.8	88.6	49.7	61.4	202.0
1887---------------	1937	1,000.0	230.7	171.1	106.3	91.5	91.7	58.8	58.0	191.9
1888---------------	1938	1,000.0	232.1	175.2	106.6	91.1	94.4	55.1	59.1	186.4
1889---------------	1939	1,000.0	232.6	181.6	105.3	98.3	96.4	51.2	57.0	177.6
1890---------------	1940	1,000.0	231.3	186.9	108.1	104.7	95.2	47.4	54.3	172.1
1891---------------	1941	1,000.0	228.2	192.0	113.3	108.6	93.9	43.4	51.8	168.8
1892---------------	1942	1,000.0	223.3	195.6	122.0	110.8	92.5	40.7	49.7	165.4
1893---------------	1943	1,000.0	221.0	202.1	103.3	121.5	97.3	41.8	50.4	162.6
1894---------------	1944	1,000.0	219.4	215.3	109.6	117.9	93.1	38.6	46.7	159.4
1895---------------	1945	1,000.0	219.7	228.6	113.5	113.7	86.1	37.5	43.6	157.3
1896---------------	1946	1,000.0	221.1	242.3	115.5	107.7	81.3	37.4	41.1	153.6
1897---------------	1947	1,000.0	221.3	256.0	116.1	102.3	76.3	37.7	41.4	148.9
1898---------------	1948	1,000.0	237.3	246.7	115.4	96.6	74.8	38.5	42.6	148.1
1899---------------	1949	1,000.0	229.0	261.2	112.6	92.8	70.4	40.0	43.5	150.5
1900---------------	1950	1,000.0	228.3	268.8	110.7	88.1	68.8	40.7	44.1	150.5
1901---------------	1951	1,000.0	233.3	273.6	114.9	85.1	66.3	42.2	42.4	142.2
1902---------------	1952	1,000.0	242.2	275.8	118.8	82.4	64.3	42.6	39.9	134.0
1903---------------	1953	1,000.0	251.3	275.5	120.5	81.3	63.0	43.2	37.5	127.7
1904---------------	1954	1,000.0	258.2	277.3	118.2	79.0	60.8	43.1	37.6	125.8
1905---------------	1955	1,000.0	267.1	277.3	116.4	77.1	57.4	43.8	38.1	122.8
1906---------------	1956	1,000.0	274.7	277.8	114.7	73.4	57.9	44.4	37.1	120.0
1907---------------	1957	1,000.0	283.7	273.9	114.2	72.2	58.3	44.1	35.8	117.8
1908---------------	1958	1,000.0	291.9	268.0	114.1	72.3	59.7	42.9	35.0	116.1
1909---------------	1959	1,000.0	291.7	261.8	114.4	72.9	62.0	43.3	34.6	119.3
1910---------------	1960	1,000.0	295.3	251.9	115.0	74.9	62.6	43.1	35.5	121.7
1911---------------	1961	1,000.0	293.6	247.0	115.5	75.9	63.7	43.0	36.2	125.1
1912---------------	1962	1,000.0	298.9	238.7	117.0	75.5	63.2	42.1	39.0	125.6
1913---------------	1963	1,000.0	297.4	233.7	116.7	77.3	63.5	45.3	38.8	127.3
1914---------------	1964	1,000.0	296.9	224.3	117.0	78.9	65.1	48.2	40.2	129.4
1915---------------	1965	1,000.0	293.9	218.0	115.4	83.7	65.4	51.5	40.7	131.4
1916---------------	1966	1,000.0	292.8	208.3	115.3	85.9	67.4	53.8	41.4	135.1
1917---------------	1967	1,000.0	285.1	201.6	117.3	89.4	69.8	55.8	41.8	139.2
1918---------------	1968	1,000.0	274.4	198.2	119.8	90.6	72.7	57.3	43.0	144.0
1919---------------	1969	1,000.0	247.9	201.5	124.4	93.3	75.6	59.7	47.5	150.1
1920---------------	1970	1,000.0	231.0	200.3	127.6	96.6	77.0	62.4	50.8	154.3
1921---------------	1971	1,000.0	222.2	189.1	130.9	102.7	79.9	65.1	53.0	157.1
1922---------------	1972	1,000.0	231.2	171.5	130.1	106.5	83.1	65.5	53.5	158.6
1923---------------	1973	1,000.0	228.4	159.9	130.6	106.8	89.9	67.0	54.9	162.5
1924---------------	1974	1,000.0	212.4	152.3	131.5	111.1	94.7	70.0	58.5	169.5

TABLE 9A. BIRTH PROBABILITIES FOR ALL WOMEN FOR EACH YEAR 1917-73 BY AGE AND PARITY FOR GROUPS OF COHORTS FROM 1868-72 TO 1954-58

(PROBABILITIES ARE THE NUMBER OF BIRTHS PER 1,000 WOMEN IN SPECIFIED PARITY AND EXACT AGE GROUP. FIGURES IN THE "0 PARITY" COLUMN SHOW THE PROBABILITY OF FIRST BIRTHS TO "0 PARITY" WOMEN,THOSE IN THE "1 PARITY" COLUMN SHOW THE PROBABILITY OF SECOND BIRTHS TO "1 PARITY" WOMEN, ETC. BASED ON CENTRAL BIRTH RATES AND PARITY DISTRIBUTIONS FOR GROUPS OF COHORTS)

EXACT AGE AND COHORT	AS OF JANUARY 1	PARITY							
		0	1	2	3	4	5	6	7 AND HIGHER
15-19 YEARS									
1898-1902-------------	1917	48.4	257.4	*	*	*	*	*	*
1899-1903-------------	1918	47.4	242.3	*	*	*	*	*	*
1900-1904-------------	1919	40.4	229.5	*	*	*	*	*	*
1901-1905-------------	1920	51.7	247.8	*	*	*	*	*	*
1902-1906-------------	1921	55.4	245.0	*	*	*	*	*	*
1903-1907-------------	1922	49.2	236.7	*	*	*	*	*	*
1904-1908-------------	1923	48.7	253.4	*	*	*	*	*	*
1905-1909-------------	1924	51.7	251.0	*	*	*	*	*	*
1906-1910-------------	1925	50.6	237.9	*	*	*	*	*	*
1907-1911-------------	1926	49.0	239.0	*	*	*	*	*	*
1908-1912-------------	1927	48.4	239.4	*	*	*	*	*	*
1909-1913-------------	1928	46.0	228.1	*	*	*	*	*	*
1910-1914-------------	1929	44.2	225.1	*	*	*	*	*	*
1911-1915-------------	1930	45.6	229.0	*	*	*	*	*	*
1912-1916-------------	1931	42.7	217.5	*	*	*	*	*	*
1913-1917-------------	1932	41.1	218.5	*	*	*	*	*	*
1914-1918-------------	1933	38.1	209.2	*	*	*	*	*	*
1915-1919-------------	1934	40.6	219.4	*	*	*	*	*	*
1916-1920-------------	1935	41.5	216.1	*	*	*	*	*	*
1917-1921-------------	1936	40.4	220.7	*	*	*	*	*	*
1918-1922-------------	1937	42.2	231.3	*	*	*	*	*	*
1919-1923-------------	1938	43.7	231.8	*	*	*	*	*	*
1920-1924-------------	1939	41.6	229.1	*	*	*	*	*	*
1921-1925-------------	1940	41.0	254.9	*	*	*	*	*	*
1922-1926-------------	1941	43.6	268.2	*	*	*	*	*	*
1923-1927-------------	1942	47.7	267.3	*	*	*	*	*	*
1924-1928-------------	1943	47.2	267.9	*	*	*	*	*	*
1925-1929-------------	1944	41.5	238.0	*	*	*	*	*	*
1926-1930-------------	1945	39.6	228.9	*	*	*	*	*	*
1927-1931-------------	1946	46.4	271.7	*	*	*	*	*	*
1928-1932-------------	1947	64.2	301.8	*	*	*	*	*	*
1929-1933-------------	1948	63.5	297.8	*	*	*	*	*	*
1930-1934-------------	1949	61.5	312.3	336.3	*	*	*	*	*
1931-1935-------------	1950	59.9	316.3	315.8	*	*	*	*	*
1932-1936-------------	1951	65.0	330.0	323.9	*	*	*	*	*
1933-1937-------------	1952	64.2	322.7	331.1	*	*	*	*	*
1934-1938-------------	1953	66.2	331.2	337.8	*	*	*	*	*
1935-1939-------------	1954	68.0	331.3	346.7	*	*	*	*	*
1936-1940-------------	1955	67.5	337.4	348.7	*	*	*	*	*
1937-1941-------------	1956	71.0	355.2	356.7	*	*	*	*	*
1938-1942-------------	1957	72.7	355.8	359.8	*	*	*	*	*
1939-1943-------------	1958	69.9	352.8	349.1	*	*	*	*	*
1940-1944-------------	1959	68.4	360.7	366.3	*	*	*	*	*
1941-1945-------------	1960	65.8	359.4	360.9	*	*	*	*	*
1942-1946-------------	1961	64.7	355.7	359.8	*	*	*	*	*
1943-1947-------------	1962	61.8	352.4	354.4	*	*	*	*	*
1944-1948-------------	1963	60.3	342.3	335.5	*	*	*	*	*
1945-1949-------------	1964	58.3	323.5	326.5	*	*	*	*	*
1946-1950-------------	1965	55.9	291.5	299.3	*	*	*	*	*
1947-1951-------------	1966	55.8	268.8	274.2	*	*	*	*	*
1948-1952-------------	1967	54.1	257.1	271.9	*	*	*	*	*
1949-1953-------------	1968	54.3	237.9	241.1	*	*	*	*	*
1950-1954-------------	1969	54.8	231.6	245.3	*	*	*	*	*
1951-1955-------------	1970	57.6	227.7	245.1	*	*	*	*	*
1952-1956-------------	1971	54.7	206.2	225.5	*	*	*	*	*
1953-1957-------------	1972	53.0	185.3	198.0	*	*	*	*	*
1954-1958-------------	1973	51.0	173.7	*	*	*	*	*	*

TABLE 9A. BIRTH PROBABILITIES FOR ALL WOMEN FOR EACH YEAR 1917-73 BY AGE AND PARITY FOR GROUPS OF COHORTS FROM 1868-72 TO 1954-58--CON.

(PROBABILITIES ARE THE NUMBER OF BIRTHS PER 1,000 WOMEN IN SPECIFIED PARITY AND EXACT AGE GROUP. FIGURES IN THE "0 PARITY" COLUMN SHOW THE PROBABILITY OF FIRST BIRTHS TO "0 PARITY" WOMEN,THOSE IN THE "1 PARITY" COLUMN SHOW THE PROBABILITY OF SECOND BIRTHS TO "1 PARITY" WOMEN, ETC. BASED ON CENTRAL BIRTH RATES AND PARITY DISTRIBUTIONS FOR GROUPS OF COHORTS)

EXACT AGE AND COHORT	AS OF JANUARY 1	PARITY							
		0	1	2	3	4	5	6	7 AND HIGHER
20-24 YEARS									
1893-1897-------------	1917	116.3	255.9	277.3	278.3	283.6	*	*	*
1894-1898-------------	1918	118.4	242.8	271.9	280.8	288.0	*	*	*
1895-1899-------------	1919	93.0	226.7	257.4	274.1	292.7	*	*	*
1896-1900-------------	1920	120.4	233.9	258.7	282.8	310.9	*	*	*
1897-1901-------------	1921	124.5	221.9	267.0	302.3	341.9	*	*	*
1898-1902-------------	1922	111.3	220.3	247.5	284.2	310.9	*	*	*
1899-1903-------------	1923	108.7	223.2	252.2	298.6	342.1	*	*	*
1900-1904-------------	1924	113.9	219.9	260.7	301.4	348.2	*	*	*
1901-1905-------------	1925	110.3	207.8	250.7	292.9	327.4	*	*	*
1902-1906-------------	1926	106.6	203.3	240.2	293.2	330.5	*	*	*
1903-1907-------------	1927	103.7	197.5	235.7	293.8	316.7	*	*	*
1904-1908-------------	1928	98.2	188.7	227.4	277.0	302.5	*	*	*
1905-1909-------------	1929	93.3	185.5	220.6	267.0	309.7	*	*	*
1906-1910-------------	1930	94.6	187.3	222.0	272.7	308.4	*	*	*
1907-1911-------------	1931	88.8	182.5	214.6	262.8	288.5	*	*	*
1908-1912-------------	1932	84.3	181.3	212.7	263.3	290.0	*	*	*
1909-1913-------------	1933	78.2	174.7	206.6	255.7	*	*	*	*
1910-1914-------------	1934	83.3	182.4	214.2	269.4	*	*	*	*
1911-1915-------------	1935	86.2	177.0	209.2	267.4	*	*	*	*
1912-1916-------------	1936	86.4	178.5	206.5	269.1	*	*	*	*
1913-1917-------------	1937	89.4	183.5	212.2	275.5	*	*	*	*
1914-1918-------------	1938	92.1	189.0	217.2	273.8	*	*	*	*
1915-1919-------------	1939	89.6	184.8	209.1	264.9	*	*	*	*
1916-1920-------------	1940	91.2	191.0	218.2	287.8	*	*	*	*
1917-1921-------------	1941	102.7	197.7	218.1	279.6	*	*	*	*
1918-1922-------------	1942	124.3	209.6	218.6	275.9	*	*	*	*
1919-1923-------------	1943	116.3	212.7	228.3	286.7	*	*	*	*
1920-1924-------------	1944	105.4	189.8	215.8	280.3	*	*	*	*
1921-1925-------------	1945	100.3	168.7	189.6	246.9	298.1	*	*	*
1922-1926-------------	1946	138.1	231.4	217.9	268.9	294.1	*	*	*
1923-1927-------------	1947	174.4	245.4	219.4	262.3	294.1	*	*	*
1924-1928-------------	1948	156.0	240.2	224.2	266.5	310.0	*	*	*
1925-1929-------------	1949	148.2	250.7	227.9	279.1	333.3	*	*	*
1926-1930-------------	1950	139.9	256.0	230.5	276.3	324.3	*	*	*
1927-1931-------------	1951	152.2	274.7	239.8	282.7	328.0	*	*	*
1928-1932-------------	1952	155.4	283.2	240.9	280.9	326.4	*	*	*
1929-1933-------------	1953	157.8	297.6	243.8	279.1	327.2	*	*	*
1930-1934-------------	1954	166.1	309.7	251.7	283.4	325.8	*	*	*
1931-1935-------------	1955	170.6	316.9	255.8	281.3	322.9	*	*	*
1932-1936-------------	1956	179.4	328.6	265.5	286.6	323.5	*	*	*
1933-1937-------------	1957	184.2	335.2	271.0	288.4	325.7	*	*	*
1934-1938-------------	1958	180.3	332.7	268.8	284.0	321.6	*	*	*
1935-1939-------------	1959	178.3	336.9	271.9	287.4	316.5	*	*	*
1936-1940-------------	1960	175.6	336.7	273.4	287.5	315.8	*	*	*
1937-1941-------------	1961	172.1	332.4	270.5	285.5	311.0	*	*	*
1938-1942-------------	1962	163.5	322.7	265.2	275.2	305.3	*	*	*
1939-1943-------------	1963	157.1	314.5	252.8	257.9	286.8	*	*	*
1940-1944-------------	1964	152.4	300.3	236.8	240.7	271.3	*	*	*
1941-1945-------------	1965	141.1	271.8	206.1	211.9	236.8	*	*	*
1942-1946-------------	1966	140.9	253.0	183.3	188.6	212.9	*	*	*
1943-1947-------------	1967	133.7	242.6	173.7	184.1	205.7	*	*	*
1944-1948-------------	1968	132.0	229.6	163.6	176.6	192.1	*	*	*
1945-1949-------------	1969	130.6	226.2	166.3	186.6	198.5	*	*	*
1946-1950-------------	1970	131.4	224.5	168.8	188.0	208.7	*	*	*
1947-1951-------------	1971	118.9	207.5	156.4	174.0	194.2	*	*	*
1948-1952-------------	1972	102.6	184.3	131.1	146.6	*	*	*	*
1949-1953-------------	1973	92.9	178.0	122.5	138.7	*	*	*	*

TABLE 9A. BIRTH PROBABILITIES FOR ALL WOMEN FOR EACH YEAR 1917-73 BY AGE AND PARITY FOR GROUPS OF COHORTS FROM 1868-72 TO 1954-58--CON.

(PROBABILITIES ARE THE NUMBER OF BIRTHS PER 1,000 WOMEN IN SPECIFIED PARITY AND EXACT AGE GROUP. FIGURES IN THE "0 PARITY" COLUMN SHOW THE PROBABILITY OF FIRST BIRTHS TO "0 PARITY" WOMEN,THOSE IN THE "1 PARITY" COLUMN SHOW THE PROBABILITY OF SECOND BIRTHS TO "1 PARITY" WOMEN, ETC. BASED ON CENTRAL BIRTH RATES AND PARITY DISTRIBUTIONS FOR GROUPS OF COHORTS)

EXACT AGE AND COHORT	AS OF JANUARY 1	PARITY							
		0	1	2	3	4	5	6	7 AND HIGHER
25-29 YEARS									
1888-1892-------------	1917	90.8	184.7	209.3	241.3	267.4	305.6	299.3	*
1889-1893-------------	1918	95.4	180.5	202.5	236.4	261.9	304.2	284.7	*
1890-1894-------------	1919	77.4	170.0	188.3	224.9	256.5	301.3	292.9	*
1891-1895-------------	1920	98.8	170.8	188.0	227.5	260.5	308.5	303.0	*
1892-1896-------------	1921	103.6	162.6	188.5	230.0	272.2	334.5	343.8	*
1893-1897-------------	1922	95.4	158.9	173.4	212.4	251.2	306.6	320.3	*
1894-1898-------------	1923	93.0	158.1	170.9	212.1	260.7	324.9	336.0	*
1895-1899-------------	1924	94.2	153.2	172.6	213.1	261.9	330.9	338.7	*
1896-1900-------------	1925	90.9	146.9	165.6	207.8	254.4	314.6	328.0	*
1897-1901-------------	1926	87.1	139.9	157.1	204.9	247.8	321.8	325.2	*
1898-1902-------------	1927	85.5	133.4	151.7	203.8	250.9	316.2	319.7	*
1899-1903-------------	1928	82.9	125.5	143.2	191.8	238.3	296.4	300.0	*
1900-1904-------------	1929	80.5	120.0	136.4	182.5	232.5	284.0	287.0	*
1901-1905-------------	1930	82.6	119.7	135.2	183.2	231.4	279.4	288.3	*
1902-1906-------------	1931	78.9	114.5	129.1	178.6	222.9	269.7	289.7	*
1903-1907-------------	1932	73.4	110.5	127.2	177.5	220.4	273.9	291.3	*
1904-1908-------------	1933	67.2	106.2	122.1	173.4	212.3	257.9	*	*
1905-1909-------------	1934	69.7	111.4	126.6	179.0	222.5	272.7	*	*
1906-1910-------------	1935	71.0	109.5	120.5	171.0	216.4	270.0	*	*
1907-1911-------------	1936	72.1	110.4	118.0	168.1	212.8	270.8	*	*
1908-1912-------------	1937	75.6	113.7	118.1	168.8	215.7	278.7	*	*
1909-1913-------------	1938	80.2	119.4	121.7	172.1	216.8	275.3	*	*
1910-1914-------------	1939	81.2	118.8	118.6	167.3	210.0	271.7	*	*
1911-1915-------------	1940	86.0	124.2	122.0	170.0	216.2	279.8	*	*
1912-1916-------------	1941	97.5	129.9	123.8	171.4	219.2	280.5	*	*
1913-1917-------------	1942	118.7	146.0	129.5	172.2	215.5	274.4	*	*
1914-1918-------------	1943	110.2	160.9	142.6	185.8	233.5	284.8	*	*
1915-1919-------------	1944	94.6	149.3	137.0	178.4	227.3	282.4	*	*
1916-1920-------------	1945	91.8	147.9	128.2	164.3	213.5	264.4	*	*
1917-1921-------------	1946	134.7	180.8	137.5	170.7	215.4	268.6	*	*
1918-1922-------------	1947	162.6	193.3	142.4	166.3	206.5	259.9	*	*
1919-1923-------------	1948	141.9	181.5	138.4	160.6	204.9	264.0	*	*
1920-1924-------------	1949	136.4	186.4	140.7	164.0	207.7	268.2	*	*
1921-1925-------------	1950	130.5	191.9	144.3	167.8	207.9	273.7	*	*
1922-1926-------------	1951	138.3	203.0	151.3	175.7	216.0	282.6	*	*
1923-1927-------------	1952	140.1	212.4	158.3	179.9	224.1	283.5	*	*
1924-1928-------------	1953	136.7	219.1	160.0	179.9	223.7	283.0	*	*
1925-1929-------------	1954	135.7	228.4	165.6	183.3	225.9	283.3	*	*
1926-1930-------------	1955	133.5	234.7	169.1	182.1	218.6	275.2	327.1	*
1927-1931-------------	1956	134.5	244.0	174.9	184.3	216.9	275.6	322.0	*
1928-1932-------------	1957	137.6	254.0	180.2	185.5	216.3	272.1	315.4	*
1929-1933-------------	1958	135.8	253.2	178.6	183.0	211.5	263.6	307.7	*
1930-1934-------------	1959	135.0	254.6	181.3	186.1	210.6	262.7	313.7	372.5
1931-1935-------------	1960	135.1	253.9	182.1	184.5	206.3	261.3	306.7	360.4
1932-1936-------------	1961	133.5	249.1	180.7	182.6	206.5	259.5	296.5	355.9
1933-1937-------------	1962	129.0	239.4	174.3	175.6	197.7	247.6	281.8	349.6
1934-1938-------------	1963	125.7	234.3	168.4	167.3	186.9	232.2	272.7	333.3
1935-1939-------------	1964	128.7	229.7	162.3	158.7	174.8	215.0	251.3	309.5
1936-1940-------------	1965	122.8	215.0	145.6	137.9	149.8	187.6	217.4	268.3
1937-1941-------------	1966	123.5	204.9	130.3	118.7	129.7	160.0	190.8	228.1
1938-1942-------------	1967	120.5	199.8	122.7	110.2	119.1	150.3	180.6	215.7
1939-1943-------------	1968	127.0	197.1	116.7	105.0	111.1	141.1	161.8	*
1940-1944-------------	1969	123.0	199.2	119.2	109.5	118.5	144.4	162.4	*
1941-1945-------------	1970	122.5	200.1	120.4	112.3	121.4	148.6	160.0	*
1942-1946-------------	1971	115.3	185.4	108.9	104.7	116.5	140.9	*	*
1943-1947-------------	1972	105.4	170.4	90.5	87.9	97.4	118.6	*	*
1944-1948-------------	1973	101.0	164.1	82.1	79.1	87.1	107.8	*	*

TABLE 9A. BIRTH PROBABILITIES FOR ALL WOMEN FOR EACH YEAR 1917-73 BY AGE AND PARITY FOR GROUPS OF COHORTS FROM 1868-72 TO 1954-58--CON.

(PROBABILITIES ARE THE NUMBER OF BIRTHS PER 1,000 WOMEN IN SPECIFIED PARITY AND EXACT AGE GROUP. FIGURES IN THE "0 PARITY" COLUMN SHOW THE PROBABILITY OF FIRST BIRTHS TO "0 PARITY" WOMEN, THOSE IN THE "1 PARITY" COLUMN SHOW THE PROBABILITY OF SECOND BIRTHS TO "1 PARITY" WOMEN, ETC. BASED ON CENTRAL BIRTH RATES AND PARITY DISTRIBUTIONS FOR GROUPS OF COHORTS)

EXACT AGE AND COHORT	AS OF JANUARY 1	PARITY							
		0	1	2	3	4	5	6	7 AND HIGHER
30-34 YEARS									
1883-1887-------------	1917	41.6	103.4	120.7	152.8	187.8	234.6	244.5	263.8
1884-1888-------------	1918	44.4	101.3	117.9	148.6	185.6	232.7	250.0	266.7
1885-1889-------------	1919	39.6	98.2	114.0	142.1	176.7	225.5	239.8	274.1
1886-1890-------------	1920	45.9	100.1	114.3	139.9	175.3	222.9	235.7	282.0
1887-1891-------------	1921	47.0	99.6	113.9	142.9	174.2	232.9	249.4	310.1
1888-1892-------------	1922	46.0	97.7	105.8	128.7	161.9	220.6	232.2	293.6
1889-1893-------------	1923	45.4	94.9	103.3	126.9	162.2	223.7	239.6	308.1
1890-1894-------------	1924	46.6	91.9	103.1	124.8	161.9	225.3	244.9	309.9
1891-1895-------------	1925	46.6	86.7	97.3	119.9	156.6	217.5	239.6	311.3
1892-1896-------------	1926	44.8	82.1	92.2	115.7	150.1	212.0	235.9	300.0
1893-1897-------------	1927	45.1	77.5	87.4	111.9	149.8	214.3	238.2	301.0
1894-1898-------------	1928	43.5	73.1	81.1	105.1	143.0	204.3	224.1	279.8
1895-1899-------------	1929	42.8	69.8	77.3	99.9	138.6	196.8	211.8	272.7
1896-1900-------------	1930	44.7	69.4	76.0	100.1	140.2	199.6	215.8	277.0
1897-1901-------------	1931	42.5	65.9	72.9	96.6	135.5	192.0	208.7	270.1
1898-1902-------------	1932	40.4	62.3	69.4	94.6	135.0	195.2	212.2	274.6
1899-1903-------------	1933	37.5	57.9	65.9	91.9	129.8	185.3	202.7	259.3
1900-1904-------------	1934	40.0	60.0	66.6	94.1	132.0	185.8	209.1	275.1
1901-1905-------------	1935	41.2	58.6	63.6	90.5	124.3	177.3	203.6	275.5
1902-1906-------------	1936	42.5	57.8	61.8	86.8	120.5	169.1	198.5	272.4
1903-1907-------------	1937	44.1	59.4	61.5	86.1	120.2	170.5	200.8	275.5
1904-1908-------------	1938	46.6	63.5	62.3	85.6	119.8	170.7	202.5	276.7
1905-1909-------------	1939	47.7	65.8	62.7	85.4	116.2	164.8	195.6	272.7
1906-1910-------------	1940	49.1	71.1	64.5	86.8	114.9	166.7	201.9	285.7
1907-1911-------------	1941	53.6	75.3	66.2	88.5	117.8	167.7	201.0	283.8
1908-1912-------------	1942	63.5	85.5	71.0	91.9	120.1	170.3	206.2	282.4
1909-1913-------------	1943	62.0	96.2	82.0	103.5	131.7	183.9	219.3	295.2
1910-1914-------------	1944	55.1	95.1	84.4	104.3	133.4	187.7	224.0	304.3
1911-1915-------------	1945	55.6	103.1	87.0	103.2	133.3	181.2	226.5	296.1
1912-1916-------------	1946	74.9	115.6	90.7	104.1	130.7	180.1	217.9	287.8
1913-1917-------------	1947	88.0	119.7	91.1	101.4	125.4	167.7	211.1	285.7
1914-1918-------------	1948	73.7	111.8	85.9	95.7	119.9	164.1	206.7	280.8
1915-1919-------------	1949	70.6	112.1	84.7	96.6	119.4	164.6	205.6	290.6
1916-1920-------------	1950	67.4	114.1	86.7	97.8	121.3	161.7	204.4	282.9
1917-1921-------------	1951	71.9	117.8	90.8	102.3	125.0	164.7	212.0	285.0
1918-1922-------------	1952	74.6	120.8	95.9	108.5	129.9	169.5	208.6	284.4
1919-1923-------------	1953	73.8	120.0	97.9	109.8	131.9	170.3	207.3	279.1
1920-1924-------------	1954	75.7	122.6	99.6	112.5	133.9	177.1	215.0	292.2
1921-1925-------------	1955	73.1	120.1	99.3	111.9	134.6	176.9	213.3	287.6
1922-1926-------------	1956	71.5	121.1	100.0	112.2	135.3	177.0	214.3	292.4
1923-1927-------------	1957	71.5	122.1	101.2	112.0	134.9	177.7	215.8	296.0
1924-1928-------------	1958	67.4	119.7	98.4	109.6	128.8	169.0	210.1	285.2
1925-1929-------------	1959	64.7	119.5	97.5	107.9	127.7	168.8	207.3	289.7
1926-1930-------------	1960	61.1	121.7	96.5	106.3	125.2	164.6	202.7	283.0
1927-1931-------------	1961	58.9	121.7	96.4	104.9	122.5	160.7	198.1	277.6
1928-1932-------------	1962	56.4	119.6	91.8	98.2	116.2	151.4	185.8	263.9
1929-1933-------------	1963	55.9	118.7	89.3	95.1	110.5	143.7	177.8	248.7
1930-1934-------------	1964	63.3	118.0	87.2	90.9	102.8	134.9	164.0	233.1
1931-1935-------------	1965	62.2	112.7	80.7	81.2	91.3	117.4	143.6	201.9
1932-1936-------------	1966	62.4	105.1	73.2	71.3	78.5	101.1	119.0	176.5
1933-1937-------------	1967	57.9	101.2	68.9	65.6	71.5	89.5	110.0	155.2
1934-1938-------------	1968	63.5	101.2	65.2	60.1	63.9	79.1	95.5	140.5
1935-1939-------------	1969	61.0	101.3	65.9	60.0	64.4	80.7	95.2	136.1
1936-1940-------------	1970	61.2	102.2	65.5	59.1	64.0	79.0	92.8	134.9
1937-1941-------------	1971	57.6	97.8	58.8	54.0	59.8	74.2	87.9	125.9
1938-1942-------------	1972	54.5	95.3	50.1	45.8	50.1	65.1	75.5	105.9
1939-1943-------------	1973	53.2	92.4	45.6	40.9	45.1	56.6	69.1	100.0

TABLE 9A. BIRTH PROBABILITIES FOR ALL WOMEN FOR EACH YEAR 1917-73 BY AGE AND PARITY FOR GROUPS OF COHORTS FROM 1868-72 TO 1954-58--CON.

(PROBABILITIES ARE THE NUMBER OF BIRTHS PER 1,000 WOMEN IN SPECIFIED PARITY AND EXACT AGE GROUP. FIGURES IN THE "0 PARITY" COLUMN SHOW THE PROBABILITY OF FIRST BIRTHS TO "0 PARITY" WOMEN,THOSE IN THE "1 PARITY" COLUMN SHOW THE PROBABILITY OF SECOND BIRTHS TO "1 PARITY" WOMEN, ETC. BASED ON CENTRAL BIRTH RATES AND PARITY DISTRIBUTIONS FOR GROUPS OF COHORTS)

EXACT AGE AND COHORT	AS OF JANUARY 1	PARITY							
		0	1	2	3	4	5	6	7 AND HIGHER
35-39 YEARS									
1878-1882	1917	17.1	47.2	61.4	84.6	114.8	155.7	180.2	230.5
1879-1883	1918	18.0	47.1	60.6	84.2	112.7	155.7	180.6	230.6
1880-1884	1919	17.6	46.4	58.4	81.3	110.3	149.7	182.9	238.3
1881-1885	1920	18.4	45.8	58.8	80.5	109.2	147.8	182.1	243.9
1882-1886	1921	19.3	46.3	58.8	80.4	108.0	146.5	181.5	254.5
1883-1887	1922	18.2	43.3	55.1	74.2	100.6	138.6	170.5	243.1
1884-1888	1923	17.8	43.2	55.1	72.4	98.2	137.1	165.5	249.3
1885-1889	1924	18.4	41.9	54.4	71.3	95.5	137.0	165.5	255.4
1886-1890	1925	18.2	40.6	51.6	68.5	90.9	132.4	159.1	254.8
1887-1891	1926	17.2	38.6	49.2	65.2	86.5	127.8	154.7	249.0
1888-1892	1927	18.5	37.3	46.0	60.7	82.5	127.6	151.5	251.1
1889-1893	1928	17.9	34.4	42.5	56.3	77.8	119.8	143.1	233.7
1890-1894	1929	16.8	32.1	39.2	51.6	72.6	113.2	136.2	223.9
1891-1895	1930	18.0	31.5	37.7	51.3	73.9	114.7	138.9	224.1
1892-1896	1931	17.8	28.7	35.3	49.1	70.4	109.5	132.6	217.1
1893-1897	1932	16.4	26.7	33.6	46.4	67.9	109.2	135.1	217.1
1894-1898	1933	15.4	24.5	30.8	44.5	65.4	104.4	127.9	206.7
1895-1899	1934	15.7	24.9	30.9	45.0	67.0	107.9	129.2	213.4
1896-1900	1935	16.4	24.3	29.6	43.6	65.2	103.6	125.6	213.9
1897-1901	1936	16.6	23.7	29.0	42.1	62.2	98.6	119.9	206.9
1898-1902	1937	16.8	23.6	28.3	41.3	61.3	95.4	118.7	211.3
1899-1903	1938	18.1	24.3	28.1	42.0	61.7	95.3	118.5	211.5
1900-1904	1939	19.3	24.9	28.3	41.2	59.2	91.5	112.7	203.4
1901-1905	1940	20.0	26.1	28.5	40.3	57.8	87.6	112.5	206.2
1902-1906	1941	21.4	27.4	29.2	41.6	57.8	88.1	115.0	206.6
1903-1907	1942	25.7	31.0	31.8	43.6	59.2	88.8	113.7	205.3
1904-1908	1943	26.5	36.3	37.1	49.6	66.1	96.9	121.5	217.9
1905-1909	1944	25.2	39.0	39.9	52.8	68.4	99.8	123.6	222.7
1906-1910	1945	25.4	42.7	43.0	54.8	71.6	100.3	127.8	225.8
1907-1911	1946	30.5	46.8	45.0	55.3	71.6	99.0	124.0	219.9
1908-1912	1947	33.9	47.4	45.0	56.4	71.0	99.2	123.5	215.0
1909-1913	1948	29.3	44.7	41.8	53.1	67.0	93.9	121.0	212.3
1910-1914	1949	28.2	43.5	40.8	52.1	66.9	93.4	122.4	216.6
1911-1915	1950	27.1	43.6	41.0	52.2	68.0	94.8	118.9	212.8
1912-1916	1951	27.8	45.0	42.5	54.3	68.4	97.8	119.8	213.0
1913-1917	1952	28.1	46.2	44.4	56.2	70.8	95.2	122.0	213.2
1914-1918	1953	27.7	45.9	44.5	58.4	72.7	96.8	125.0	205.3
1915-1919	1954	28.1	46.9	45.8	59.3	75.1	99.3	126.5	206.3
1916-1920	1955	27.4	46.2	45.0	59.0	74.9	99.2	126.9	202.6
1917-1921	1956	27.5	45.5	44.7	58.0	74.3	98.8	128.7	206.5
1918-1922	1957	28.8	44.7	43.8	58.3	74.8	102.1	126.8	203.4
1919-1923	1958	28.7	42.2	42.0	55.6	72.1	98.9	123.7	194.8
1920-1924	1959	28.0	40.3	40.4	54.1	71.6	97.6	123.4	200.0
1921-1925	1960	27.6	39.7	38.6	52.4	68.7	94.1	120.1	193.8
1922-1926	1961	26.5	39.4	38.0	50.0	66.8	92.6	119.7	191.2
1923-1927	1962	24.4	37.6	35.2	46.4	62.0	84.8	110.8	182.9
1924-1928	1963	22.8	37.7	33.6	43.5	58.4	80.9	102.6	173.3
1925-1929	1964	25.3	37.9	33.2	41.6	54.4	74.4	100.0	164.6
1926-1930	1965	24.5	37.1	30.7	38.0	49.1	66.1	83.7	146.8
1927-1931	1966	23.1	35.7	28.3	33.5	42.8	57.4	75.2	125.0
1928-1932	1967	20.2	35.6	27.0	30.8	37.6	51.7	66.1	109.1
1929-1933	1968	24.1	36.0	25.1	27.7	34.0	45.6	55.8	96.7
1930-1934	1969	21.3	35.7	23.8	26.0	32.0	42.5	52.7	89.2
1931-1935	1970	22.4	34.9	22.9	24.4	29.7	38.5	50.5	84.4
1932-1936	1971	20.9	31.7	20.5	21.9	27.0	36.2	44.8	77.7
1933-1937	1972	20.0	30.3	18.1	18.7	22.6	30.9	37.5	66.1
1934-1938	1973	18.7	29.7	16.4	15.9	19.7	25.8	34.7	57.9

TABLE 9A. BIRTH PROBABILITIES FOR ALL WOMEN FOR EACH YEAR 1917-73 BY AGE AND PARITY FOR GROUPS OF COHORTS FROM 1868-72 TO 1954-58--CON.

(PROBABILITIES ARE THE NUMBER OF BIRTHS PER 1,000 WOMEN IN SPECIFIED PARITY AND EXACT AGE GROUP. FIGURES IN THE "0 PARITY" COLUMN SHOW THE PROBABILITY OF FIRST BIRTHS TO "0 PARITY" WOMEN, THOSE IN THE "1 PARITY" COLUMN SHOW THE PROBABILITY OF SECOND BIRTHS TO "1 PARITY" WOMEN, ETC. BASED ON CENTRAL BIRTH RATES AND PARITY DISTRIBUTIONS FOR GROUPS OF COHORTS)

EXACT AGE AND COHORT	AS OF JANUARY 1	PARITY							
		0	1	2	3	4	5	6	7 AND HIGHER
40-44 YEARS									
1873-1877	1917	3.7	11.0	14.7	22.0	30.6	47.6	56.0	96.9
1874-1878	1918	4.2	10.8	15.3	21.9	31.7	46.9	57.7	99.1
1875-1879	1919	4.1	11.5	14.4	21.8	30.7	45.9	54.8	97.9
1876-1880	1920	4.6	11.3	14.2	21.6	30.7	46.3	55.0	102.2
1877-1881	1921	4.5	11.1	14.1	21.5	31.7	46.6	55.6	105.9
1878-1882	1922	4.1	10.1	13.9	20.5	29.6	42.6	53.7	100.4
1879-1883	1923	4.1	9.9	13.7	19.5	28.5	42.5	53.7	101.0
1880-1884	1924	4.1	9.8	13.5	19.3	28.3	41.0	53.4	104.5
1881-1885	1925	4.1	9.6	12.5	19.1	26.1	38.3	53.0	103.9
1882-1886	1926	4.1	8.7	11.7	17.2	24.8	37.1	50.3	100.7
1883-1887	1927	3.7	8.5	11.5	16.1	23.6	36.1	47.3	101.4
1884-1888	1928	3.7	8.3	10.7	15.1	22.4	33.9	43.8	96.2
1885-1889	1929	3.7	7.5	9.9	14.1	21.2	31.5	42.5	91.4
1886-1890	1930	3.8	7.4	10.4	14.5	21.0	33.4	41.3	92.4
1887-1891	1931	3.8	6.6	8.8	12.7	18.8	32.6	40.1	90.0
1888-1892	1932	3.4	6.4	8.6	12.5	18.8	31.8	41.1	89.2
1889-1893	1933	3.5	6.3	7.7	11.6	17.8	29.4	38.5	86.7
1890-1894	1934	3.5	5.4	7.5	11.5	18.0	30.0	37.9	89.4
1891-1895	1935	3.1	5.2	7.3	10.7	17.3	27.6	37.1	86.4
1892-1896	1936	3.6	5.0	6.6	10.0	16.6	26.6	36.2	82.4
1893-1897	1937	3.7	4.8	5.9	10.0	15.9	25.6	33.0	82.0
1894-1898	1938	3.6	5.2	6.3	10.0	15.2	26.5	34.2	82.4
1895-1899	1939	3.6	4.6	6.2	10.1	15.6	25.5	32.8	77.9
1896-1900	1940	3.6	5.0	6.1	9.5	15.9	24.3	31.3	78.7
1897-1901	1941	4.0	4.9	6.6	9.6	15.1	24.9	32.3	78.4
1898-1902	1942	4.5	5.2	6.5	10.5	15.4	25.4	30.8	78.3
1899-1903	1943	4.9	6.0	7.4	11.4	17.0	27.9	34.8	83.4
1900-1904	1944	5.9	6.7	8.3	12.3	18.5	28.5	36.1	85.1
1901-1905	1945	5.9	7.0	9.2	13.2	18.8	29.0	37.8	88.1
1902-1906	1946	6.8	7.8	9.1	13.3	19.0	27.6	36.4	86.3
1903-1907	1947	7.1	8.2	9.5	14.0	19.2	28.2	37.7	85.3
1904-1908	1948	6.1	7.8	9.4	13.2	18.1	26.6	35.7	80.7
1905-1909	1949	6.0	7.9	8.8	13.1	18.2	27.1	33.7	83.9
1906-1910	1950	5.9	8.0	8.7	12.9	19.5	27.5	34.7	81.5
1907-1911	1951	5.5	8.1	9.4	14.2	19.4	27.6	35.5	83.8
1908-1912	1952	5.6	8.2	9.7	14.6	20.5	30.0	39.9	81.7
1909-1913	1953	5.7	8.3	10.0	15.0	21.3	32.1	40.1	81.4
1910-1914	1954	5.5	8.4	10.2	15.9	23.2	31.7	40.1	80.7
1911-1915	1955	5.7	8.6	10.0	15.3	23.7	33.1	39.7	79.7
1912-1916	1956	5.4	8.3	9.8	15.5	22.9	32.2	42.6	82.3
1913-1917	1957	5.7	8.0	9.7	15.6	22.1	33.0	42.0	80.5
1914-1918	1958	5.3	7.8	9.2	14.5	22.2	29.8	41.2	77.8
1915-1919	1959	5.0	7.5	9.1	14.7	21.4	30.4	40.1	76.8
1916-1920	1960	5.3	7.2	8.7	13.7	20.5	31.0	38.8	77.1
1917-1921	1961	5.0	7.4	8.2	13.9	20.6	29.7	40.1	75.3
1918-1922	1962	5.4	7.0	7.5	12.4	19.0	28.6	38.3	73.3
1919-1923	1963	4.9	6.7	7.1	11.6	17.4	25.8	36.6	69.4
1920-1924	1964	6.1	6.3	6.7	10.8	15.9	24.8	32.3	67.2
1921-1925	1965	6.4	6.6	6.4	9.6	14.6	22.3	30.9	60.1
1922-1926	1966	5.6	5.5	5.7	9.0	12.6	19.9	27.2	53.2
1923-1927	1967	4.7	5.8	5.4	8.3	11.4	16.4	23.8	48.2
1924-1928	1968	5.7	6.2	4.6	6.8	9.6	14.5	20.6	40.6
1925-1929	1969	3.8	5.8	4.7	6.2	9.3	12.7	17.6	36.5
1926-1930	1970	3.8	6.1	4.4	5.7	8.4	12.2	16.9	34.3
1927-1931	1971	3.8	5.6	3.6	4.7	6.8	9.5	14.3	29.5
1928-1932	1972	3.9	5.8	3.2	4.2	5.3	8.1	11.9	25.0
1929-1933	1973	4.1	5.0	3.2	3.7	5.2	7.9	9.7	23.6

TABLE 9A. BIRTH PROBABILITIES FOR ALL WOMEN FOR EACH YEAR 1917-73 BY AGE AND PARITY FOR GROUPS OF COHORTS FROM 1868-72 TO 1954-58--CON.

(PROBABILITIES ARE THE NUMBER OF BIRTHS PER 1,000 WOMEN IN SPECIFIED PARITY AND EXACT AGE GROUP. FIGURES IN THE "0 PARITY" COLUMN SHOW THE PROBABILITY OF FIRST BIRTHS TO "0 PARITY" WOMEN,THOSE IN THE "1 PARITY" COLUMN SHOW THE PROBABILITY OF SECOND BIRTHS TO "1 PARITY" WOMEN, ETC. BASED ON CENTRAL BIRTH RATES AND PARITY DISTRIBUTIONS FOR GROUPS OF COHORTS)

EXACT AGE AND COHORT	AS OF JANUARY 1	PARITY							
		0	1	2	3	4	5	6	7 AND HIGHER
45-49 YEARS									
1868-1872	1917	0.5	0.9	0.8	2.8	3.2	5.2	7.3	15.6
1869-1873	1918	0.5	0.9	1.6	2.8	4.2	6.5	7.4	18.7
1870-1874	1919	0.5	0.9	0.8	1.8	3.2	5.3	5.9	15.8
1871-1875	1920	0.5	1.8	1.6	2.7	4.3	5.3	7.5	17.2
1872-1876	1921	0.5	0.9	0.8	2.7	3.2	4.0	6.1	16.6
1873-1877	1922	0.5	0.9	0.8	1.8	3.2	4.0	6.1	15.6
1874-1878	1923	0.5	0.8	0.8	1.8	3.2	5.4	6.2	15.5
1875-1879	1924	0.5	0.8	0.8	1.8	3.2	4.1	6.2	15.9
1876-1880	1925	0.5	0.8	1.5	1.8	3.2	4.2	4.6	15.8
1877-1881	1926	0.5	0.8	0.7	1.7	2.1	4.2	6.3	15.1
1878-1882	1927	0.5	0.8	0.7	1.7	2.1	4.2	4.8	14.3
1879-1883	1928	0.5	0.8	0.7	1.7	2.1	4.2	4.9	14.0
1880-1884	1929	0.5	0.8	0.7	0.8	2.1	4.2	5.1	13.2
1881-1885	1930	0.5	0.7	0.7	0.8	2.1	2.8	5.2	13.1
1882-1886	1931	0.5	0.7	0.7	0.8	2.1	2.8	3.5	12.9
1883-1887	1932	0.0	0.7	0.7	0.8	2.1	2.8	5.3	12.7
1884-1888	1933	0.0	0.7	0.7	0.8	2.1	2.8	3.5	12.4
1885-1889	1934	0.0	0.0	0.7	0.8	2.0	2.9	3.6	12.2
1886-1890	1935	0.5	0.0	0.7	0.8	2.0	2.9	3.6	11.9
1887-1891	1936	0.0	0.0	0.6	0.8	1.0	3.0	3.7	11.5
1888-1892	1937	0.0	0.0	0.6	0.7	1.0	3.1	3.7	11.2
1889-1893	1938	0.0	0.0	0.6	0.7	1.0	3.1	3.9	10.8
1890-1894	1939	0.0	0.0	0.6	0.7	1.0	1.6	4.0	10.4
1891-1895	1940	0.0	0.0	0.6	0.7	1.0	1.6	2.1	9.9
1892-1896	1941	0.0	0.6	0.6	0.7	1.0	1.7	2.1	9.4
1893-1897	1942	0.0	0.5	0.5	0.7	1.1	1.7	2.2	9.9
1894-1898	1943	0.5	0.5	0.5	0.7	1.1	1.8	2.3	9.2
1895-1899	1944	0.5	0.5	0.5	0.7	1.1	1.8	2.3	9.6
1896-1900	1945	0.5	0.5	0.5	0.7	1.1	1.9	2.4	10.0
1897-1901	1946	0.5	0.5	0.5	0.7	1.2	1.9	2.5	9.3
1898-1902	1947	0.5	0.5	0.5	0.8	1.2	2.0	2.6	9.7
1899-1903	1948	0.5	0.5	0.5	0.8	1.2	2.0	2.7	8.9
1900-1904	1949	0.5	0.4	0.5	0.8	1.2	2.0	2.8	9.3
1901-1905	1950	0.5	0.4	0.5	0.8	1.2	2.1	2.9	8.4
1902-1906	1951	0.5	0.4	0.5	0.8	1.3	2.1	3.0	7.4
1903-1907	1952	0.5	0.4	0.5	0.8	1.3	2.1	3.1	7.7
1904-1908	1953	0.5	0.4	0.5	0.8	1.3	2.2	3.2	8.1
1905-1909	1954	0.5	0.4	0.5	0.8	1.3	2.2	3.3	8.4
1906-1910	1955	0.5	0.4	0.5	0.8	1.3	2.3	3.4	6.9
1907-1911	1956	0.5	0.5	0.5	0.7	1.3	2.3	3.5	8.9
1908-1912	1957	0.5	0.5	0.4	0.7	1.3	2.3	3.5	9.0
1909-1913	1958	0.0	0.5	0.4	0.7	1.2	2.2	3.6	9.2
1910-1914	1959	0.5	0.5	0.4	0.7	1.2	2.2	3.5	7.5
1911-1915	1960	0.0	0.5	0.4	0.7	1.2	2.2	3.5	7.5
1912-1916	1961	0.0	0.5	0.4	0.6	1.1	2.1	3.4	7.6
1913-1917	1962	0.0	0.5	0.4	0.6	1.1	2.0	3.4	7.6
1914-1918	1963	0.0	0.5	0.4	0.6	1.1	1.9	3.3	7.5
1915-1919	1964	0.0	0.0	0.4	0.6	1.0	1.9	3.2	5.6
1916-1920	1965	0.0	0.0	0.4	0.6	1.0	1.8	3.1	5.5
1917-1921	1966	0.0	0.0	0.4	0.6	0.9	1.7	3.0	5.3
1918-1922	1967	0.0	0.0	0.4	0.5	0.9	1.7	2.9	5.2
1919-1923	1968	0.0	0.0	0.4	0.5	0.9	1.6	2.7	5.1
1920-1924	1969	0.0	0.0	0.0	0.5	0.8	1.5	2.6	4.9
1921-1925	1970	0.0	0.0	0.0	0.5	0.8	1.5	2.5	3.2
1922-1926	1971	0.0	0.0	0.0	0.5	0.0	1.4	0.0	3.1
1923-1927	1972	0.0	0.0	0.0	0.0	0.0	0.0	0.0	3.0
1924-1928	1973	0.0	0.0	0.0	0.0	0.0	0.0	0.0	1.5

TABLE 9B. BIRTH PROBABILITIES FOR WHITE WOMEN FOR EACH YEAR 1917-73 BY AGE AND PARITY FOR GROUPS OF COHORTS FROM 1868-72 TO 1954-58

(PROBABILITIES ARE THE NUMBER OF BIRTHS PER 1,000 WOMEN IN SPECIFIED PARITY AND EXACT AGE GROUP. FIGURES IN THE "0 PARITY" COLUMN SHOW THE PROBABILITY OF FIRST BIRTHS TO "0 PARITY" WOMEN, THOSE IN THE "1 PARITY" COLUMN SHOW THE PROBABILITY OF SECOND BIRTHS TO "1 PARITY" WOMEN, ETC. BASED ON CENTRAL BIRTH RATES AND PARITY DISTRIBUTIONS FOR GROUPS OF COHORTS)

EXACT AGE AND COHORT	AS OF JANUARY 1	PARITY							
		0	1	2	3	4	5	6	7 AND HIGHER
15-19 YEARS									
1898-1902-------------	1917	42.9	266.8	*	*	*	*	*	*
1899-1903-------------	1918	42.1	259.9	*	*	*	*	*	*
1900-1904-------------	1919	34.8	248.7	*	*	*	*	*	*
1901-1905-------------	1920	45.8	273.0	*	*	*	*	*	*
1902-1906-------------	1921	49.9	258.0	*	*	*	*	*	*
1903-1907-------------	1922	44.4	251.7	*	*	*	*	*	*
1904-1908-------------	1923	43.3	269.6	*	*	*	*	*	*
1905-1909-------------	1924	46.0	263.3	*	*	*	*	*	*
1906-1910-------------	1925	44.5	250.6	*	*	*	*	*	*
1907-1911-------------	1926	43.1	252.3	*	*	*	*	*	*
1908-1912-------------	1927	43.0	255.4	*	*	*	*	*	*
1909-1913-------------	1928	41.1	241.6	*	*	*	*	*	*
1910-1914-------------	1929	39.6	238.4	*	*	*	*	*	*
1911-1915-------------	1930	40.9	241.3	*	*	*	*	*	*
1912-1916-------------	1931	38.0	225.5	*	*	*	*	*	*
1913-1917-------------	1932	36.2	223.9	*	*	*	*	*	*
1914-1918-------------	1933	33.6	212.8	*	*	*	*	*	*
1915-1919-------------	1934	35.9	223.8	*	*	*	*	*	*
1916-1920-------------	1935	36.6	214.1	*	*	*	*	*	*
1917-1921-------------	1936	35.6	220.4	*	*	*	*	*	*
1918-1922-------------	1937	36.9	228.4	*	*	*	*	*	*
1919-1923-------------	1938	38.2	232.2	*	*	*	*	*	*
1920-1924-------------	1939	36.2	225.5	*	*	*	*	*	*
1921-1925-------------	1940	35.8	256.1	*	*	*	*	*	*
1922-1926-------------	1941	38.4	262.9	*	*	*	*	*	*
1923-1927-------------	1942	42.6	256.9	*	*	*	*	*	*
1924-1928-------------	1943	42.0	255.2	*	*	*	*	*	*
1925-1929-------------	1944	36.5	223.9	*	*	*	*	*	*
1926-1930-------------	1945	34.6	204.9	*	*	*	*	*	*
1927-1931-------------	1946	41.9	255.1	*	*	*	*	*	*
1928-1932-------------	1947	59.3	282.2	*	*	*	*	*	*
1929-1933-------------	1948	58.0	271.0	*	*	*	*	*	*
1930-1934-------------	1949	56.0	286.8	*	*	*	*	*	*
1931-1935-------------	1950	54.3	292.2	*	*	*	*	*	*
1932-1936-------------	1951	59.7	309.6	284.3	*	*	*	*	*
1933-1937-------------	1952	59.2	306.4	287.0	*	*	*	*	*
1934-1938-------------	1953	61.0	318.8	297.3	*	*	*	*	*
1935-1939-------------	1954	62.5	321.4	307.0	*	*	*	*	*
1936-1940-------------	1955	62.1	326.3	307.7	*	*	*	*	*
1937-1941-------------	1956	65.8	345.6	325.0	*	*	*	*	*
1938-1942-------------	1957	67.9	346.4	320.3	*	*	*	*	*
1939-1943-------------	1958	65.6	344.3	315.8	*	*	*	*	*
1940-1944-------------	1959	64.0	352.3	335.8	*	*	*	*	*
1941-1945-------------	1960	61.5	351.2	330.9	*	*	*	*	*
1942-1946-------------	1961	60.3	349.5	325.8	*	*	*	*	*
1943-1947-------------	1962	57.5	343.8	320.3	*	*	*	*	*
1944-1948-------------	1963	55.7	331.4	308.9	*	*	*	*	*
1945-1949-------------	1964	53.3	305.7	284.5	*	*	*	*	*
1946-1950-------------	1965	50.5	270.3	254.7	*	*	*	*	*
1947-1951-------------	1966	49.8	245.8	*	*	*	*	*	*
1948-1952-------------	1967	47.5	236.4	*	*	*	*	*	*
1949-1953-------------	1968	47.3	219.4	*	*	*	*	*	*
1950-1954-------------	1969	47.5	216.3	*	*	*	*	*	*
1951-1955-------------	1970	49.8	215.6	*	*	*	*	*	*
1952-1956-------------	1971	46.8	194.8	*	*	*	*	*	*
1953-1957-------------	1972	44.9	173.0	*	*	*	*	*	*
1954-1958-------------	1973	43.2	164.4	*	*	*	*	*	*

TABLE 9B. BIRTH PROBABILITIES FOR WHITE WOMEN FOR EACH YEAR 1917-73 BY AGE AND PARITY FOR GROUPS OF COHORTS FROM 1868-72 TO 1954-58--CON.

(PROBABILITIES ARE THE NUMBER OF BIRTHS PER 1,000 WOMEN IN SPECIFIED PARITY AND EXACT AGE GROUP. FIGURES IN THE "0 PARITY" COLUMN SHOW THE PROBABILITY OF FIRST BIRTHS TO "0 PARITY" WOMEN, THOSE IN THE "1 PARITY" COLUMN SHOW THE PROBABILITY OF SECOND BIRTHS TO "1 PARITY" WOMEN, ETC. BASED ON CENTRAL BIRTH RATES AND PARITY DISTRIBUTIONS FOR GROUPS OF COHORTS)

EXACT AGE AND COHORT	AS OF JANUARY 1	PARITY							
		0	1	2	3	4	5	6	7 AND HIGHER
20-24 YEARS									
1893-1897-------------	1917	115.6	264.5	277.9	277.9	302.8	*	*	*
1894-1898-------------	1918	117.7	253.9	270.2	276.9	298.1	*	*	*
1895-1899-------------	1919	90.2	236.9	255.0	270.8	288.5	*	*	*
1896-1900-------------	1920	118.4	245.1	253.8	276.0	303.9	*	*	*
1897-1901-------------	1921	123.4	232.1	259.0	290.5	326.7	*	*	*
1898-1902-------------	1922	110.7	229.6	239.8	272.2	297.0	*	*	*
1899-1903-------------	1923	107.9	235.4	243.1	286.1	*	*	*	*
1900-1904-------------	1924	112.6	231.3	249.8	288.8	*	*	*	*
1901-1905-------------	1925	108.8	218.3	242.7	278.6	*	*	*	*
1902-1906-------------	1926	105.4	213.1	233.1	276.7	*	*	*	*
1903-1907-------------	1927	103.5	208.6	228.9	281.1	*	*	*	*
1904-1908-------------	1928	98.4	200.2	222.1	266.1	*	*	*	*
1905-1909-------------	1929	93.4	196.8	215.8	257.9	*	*	*	*
1906-1910-------------	1930	94.8	197.8	216.0	259.7	*	*	*	*
1907-1911-------------	1931	88.6	191.6	207.5	250.8	*	*	*	*
1908-1912-------------	1932	83.7	188.6	203.6	248.3	*	*	*	*
1909-1913-------------	1933	77.7	181.6	197.2	241.8	*	*	*	*
1910-1914-------------	1934	83.0	188.9	204.1	252.9	*	*	*	*
1911-1915-------------	1935	86.3	181.9	198.5	250.0	*	*	*	*
1912-1916-------------	1936	87.0	183.0	196.4	249.0	*	*	*	*
1913-1917-------------	1937	90.0	186.8	198.4	253.3	*	*	*	*
1914-1918-------------	1938	93.3	192.8	204.1	253.3	*	*	*	*
1915-1919-------------	1939	90.4	187.4	195.2	242.3	*	*	*	*
1916-1920-------------	1940	92.2	194.2	206.0	262.0	*	*	*	*
1917-1921-------------	1941	104.5	201.1	204.0	254.2	*	*	*	*
1918-1922-------------	1942	127.6	214.9	207.5	250.0	*	*	*	*
1919-1923-------------	1943	119.0	217.3	218.0	264.8	*	*	*	*
1920-1924-------------	1944	107.6	192.1	205.1	255.6	*	*	*	*
1921-1925-------------	1945	102.4	168.6	177.3	225.9	*	*	*	*
1922-1926-------------	1946	142.4	234.8	207.1	248.0	*	*	*	*
1923-1927-------------	1947	179.7	246.4	206.8	239.0	*	*	*	*
1924-1928-------------	1948	159.6	236.9	208.0	239.5	*	*	*	*
1925-1929-------------	1949	151.3	247.3	211.4	250.9	*	*	*	*
1926-1930-------------	1950	142.9	252.6	213.9	246.0	*	*	*	*
1927-1931-------------	1951	156.6	272.7	223.8	253.5	*	*	*	*
1928-1932-------------	1952	160.3	283.0	226.3	251.9	*	*	*	*
1929-1933-------------	1953	162.4	297.4	230.6	253.4	283.2	*	*	*
1930-1934-------------	1954	170.7	310.2	238.7	257.4	285.7	*	*	*
1931-1935-------------	1955	174.7	316.7	243.0	256.9	287.8	*	*	*
1932-1936-------------	1956	183.4	328.7	252.2	262.0	288.6	*	*	*
1933-1937-------------	1957	187.9	336.4	258.1	263.1	285.7	*	*	*
1934-1938-------------	1958	183.9	334.4	256.6	260.7	286.5	*	*	*
1935-1939-------------	1959	181.6	339.7	260.7	264.0	284.9	*	*	*
1936-1940-------------	1960	179.0	340.4	263.1	266.6	288.8	*	*	*
1937-1941-------------	1961	175.6	335.8	261.2	264.2	285.7	*	*	*
1938-1942-------------	1962	166.4	325.6	255.0	255.5	278.0	*	*	*
1939-1943-------------	1963	159.2	317.0	243.2	237.7	254.9	*	*	*
1940-1944-------------	1964	153.8	301.9	226.6	219.3	241.0	*	*	*
1941-1945-------------	1965	141.2	271.7	194.3	190.0	209.0	*	*	*
1942-1946-------------	1966	140.6	253.0	171.9	168.5	183.0	*	*	*
1943-1947-------------	1967	132.4	243.4	164.3	168.5	187.5	*	*	*
1944-1948-------------	1968	130.1	231.8	155.5	163.4	175.9	*	*	*
1945-1949-------------	1969	127.9	229.1	159.3	176.1	*	*	*	*
1946-1950-------------	1970	127.9	227.9	161.4	176.7	*	*	*	*
1947-1951-------------	1971	114.5	209.9	148.5	162.2	*	*	*	*
1948-1952-------------	1972	97.9	187.1	123.3	138.2	*	*	*	*
1949-1953-------------	1973	88.3	181.5	115.3	127.6	*	*	*	*

TABLE 9B. BIRTH PROBABILITIES FOR WHITE WOMEN FOR EACH YEAR 1917-73 BY AGE AND PARITY FOR GROUPS OF COHORTS FROM 1868-72 TO 1954-58--CON.

(PROBABILITIES ARE THE NUMBER OF BIRTHS PER 1,000 WOMEN IN SPECIFIED PARITY AND EXACT AGE GROUP. FIGURES IN THE "0 PARITY" COLUMN SHOW THE PROBABILITY OF FIRST BIRTHS TO "0 PARITY" WOMEN,THOSE IN THE "1 PARITY" COLUMN SHOW THE PROBABILITY OF SECOND BIRTHS TO "1 PARITY" WOMEN, ETC. BASED ON CENTRAL BIRTH RATES AND PARITY DISTRIBUTIONS FOR GROUPS OF COHORTS)

EXACT AGE AND COHORT	AS OF JANUARY 1	PARITY							
		0	1	2	3	4	5	6	7 AND HIGHER
25-29 YEARS									
1888-1892	1917	94.1	195.0	211.1	247.5	277.1	307.7	314.0	*
1889-1893	1918	98.8	190.6	203.8	242.9	273.0	302.4	302.5	*
1890-1894	1919	79.3	178.7	188.9	230.0	264.6	289.2	299.1	*
1891-1895	1920	101.0	179.2	187.6	230.6	268.5	295.4	312.5	*
1892-1896	1921	106.9	171.2	187.1	232.2	278.1	316.5	333.3	*
1893-1897	1922	98.7	168.0	171.9	214.4	255.5	293.0	309.1	*
1894-1898	1923	96.7	168.8	170.0	213.9	264.8	306.8	327.1	*
1895-1899	1924	97.9	164.8	169.5	211.9	261.6	305.0	320.8	*
1896-1900	1925	94.4	158.0	163.5	204.4	252.3	292.5	301.9	*
1897-1901	1926	90.9	150.7	155.5	200.4	244.8	292.7	310.7	*
1898-1902	1927	89.5	144.7	150.9	202.1	247.6	294.1	*	*
1899-1903	1928	87.1	137.6	143.2	189.6	236.5	280.9	*	*
1900-1904	1929	84.9	131.5	136.5	180.7	227.9	265.2	*	*
1901-1905	1930	87.2	130.5	135.4	180.2	226.7	267.9	*	*
1902-1906	1931	83.5	125.0	129.0	174.2	217.1	256.9	*	*
1903-1907	1932	77.4	120.6	126.7	172.8	215.2	258.4	*	*
1904-1908	1933	70.9	116.0	121.4	168.5	205.4	237.4	*	*
1905-1909	1934	73.7	121.8	125.3	173.5	214.1	252.7	*	*
1906-1910	1935	75.3	119.5	119.5	165.9	207.8	252.8	*	*
1907-1911	1936	76.4	119.8	117.2	163.1	202.0	254.4	*	*
1908-1912	1937	80.6	122.8	116.4	162.8	205.3	259.5	*	*
1909-1913	1938	85.7	128.3	120.0	166.7	206.1	260.0	*	*
1910-1914	1939	86.9	126.8	116.9	160.3	198.8	250.0	*	*
1911-1915	1940	92.4	132.6	120.7	161.9	202.4	262.8	*	*
1912-1916	1941	105.1	137.9	121.5	164.4	204.3	263.2	*	*
1913-1917	1942	128.6	154.8	127.8	165.8	203.1	250.0	*	*
1914-1918	1943	119.2	169.9	142.2	179.9	220.2	272.7	*	*
1915-1919	1944	101.7	156.8	135.1	171.9	216.6	264.7	*	*
1916-1920	1945	98.5	155.6	126.4	158.5	198.8	250.0	*	*
1917-1921	1946	145.4	190.7	136.0	163.9	201.1	248.2	*	*
1918-1922	1947	176.1	202.9	140.3	158.1	193.4	237.8	*	*
1919-1923	1948	153.5	188.3	135.5	150.4	187.5	237.8	*	*
1920-1924	1949	147.9	192.5	137.5	154.6	191.9	244.8	*	*
1921-1925	1950	141.6	197.9	140.6	156.4	188.5	241.1	*	*
1922-1926	1951	150.3	209.8	147.7	165.1	198.5	253.5	*	*
1923-1927	1952	151.8	219.3	155.2	169.9	203.7	253.3	*	*
1924-1928	1953	148.1	225.9	157.2	170.0	202.2	250.0	*	*
1925-1929	1954	146.3	235.6	163.3	173.1	205.9	255.6	*	*
1926-1930	1955	144.4	241.1	167.0	173.5	201.4	251.3	*	*
1927-1931	1956	145.7	250.4	172.1	175.0	198.7	248.9	*	*
1928-1932	1957	150.0	260.7	177.9	178.2	198.8	242.8	*	*
1929-1933	1958	148.1	260.5	177.0	176.0	195.9	239.7	*	*
1930-1934	1959	146.7	261.5	179.8	179.4	195.4	237.1	278.8	*
1931-1935	1960	145.5	261.7	181.1	179.4	192.6	237.2	283.2	*
1932-1936	1961	142.2	257.4	180.0	177.4	193.7	232.6	272.7	*
1933-1937	1962	136.8	247.9	173.2	170.3	184.9	224.4	257.8	*
1934-1938	1963	132.3	242.7	167.6	162.6	174.5	212.1	246.3	*
1935-1939	1964	136.0	238.7	161.6	153.6	163.8	192.9	222.2	*
1936-1940	1965	128.5	222.6	144.5	132.4	138.9	164.8	194.0	*
1937-1941	1966	129.8	211.8	129.0	113.8	120.0	142.9	168.0	*
1938-1942	1967	126.2	206.3	121.6	105.8	111.1	132.3	162.2	*
1939-1943	1968	132.0	204.4	116.4	101.2	105.3	127.7	*	*
1940-1944	1969	127.0	206.4	119.1	106.7	113.3	136.2	*	*
1941-1945	1970	125.6	206.8	119.7	109.1	116.7	137.3	*	*
1942-1946	1971	117.0	191.5	107.7	101.5	110.5	129.9	*	*
1943-1947	1972	105.1	176.1	89.6	84.4	92.8	111.1	*	*
1944-1948	1973	100.2	170.8	80.5	75.9	82.9	100.8	*	*

TABLE 98. BIRTH PROBABILITIES FOR WHITE WOMEN FOR EACH YEAR 1917-73 BY AGE AND PARITY FOR GROUPS OF COHORTS FROM 1868-72 TO 1954-58--CON.

(PROBABILITIES ARE THE NUMBER OF BIRTHS PER 1,000 WOMEN IN SPECIFIED PARITY AND EXACT AGE GROUP. FIGURES IN THE "0 PARITY" COLUMN SHOW THE PROBABILITY OF FIRST BIRTHS TO "0 PARITY" WOMEN,THOSE IN THE "1 PARITY" COLUMN SHOW THE PROBABILITY OF SECOND BIRTHS TO "1 PARITY" WOMEN, ETC. BASED ON CENTRAL BIRTH RATES AND PARITY DISTRIBUTIONS FOR GROUPS OF COHORTS)

EXACT AGE AND COHORT	AS OF JANUARY 1	PARITY							
		0	1	2	3	4	5	6	7 AND HIGHER
30-34 YEARS									
1883-1887	1917	43.6	110.3	123.2	156.7	194.4	235.6	249.4	272.3
1884-1888	1918	46.3	107.8	119.8	152.6	192.3	233.8	256.5	281.7
1885-1889	1919	41.3	105.3	115.8	145.7	182.4	227.3	245.8	284.3
1886-1890	1920	47.9	106.9	115.3	143.8	181.3	226.1	245.8	293.5
1887-1891	1921	49.4	107.0	114.8	146.9	180.9	232.1	258.0	317.1
1888-1892	1922	48.9	104.9	107.1	131.9	167.7	217.7	240.6	296.1
1889-1893	1923	47.9	101.8	104.0	130.4	169.0	220.8	244.8	312.8
1890-1894	1924	49.2	99.1	103.9	128.5	167.9	219.2	246.7	308.7
1891-1895	1925	49.2	93.7	98.2	122.9	161.7	211.1	240.4	303.6
1892-1896	1926	47.3	88.7	93.6	117.9	154.3	205.4	236.6	291.4
1893-1897	1927	47.7	84.8	88.5	114.6	153.8	208.2	236.2	297.1
1894-1898	1928	46.5	80.9	82.8	107.3	146.5	199.2	222.9	280.1
1895-1899	1929	45.8	77.8	78.5	101.8	141.7	192.0	211.8	271.9
1896-1900	1930	47.6	77.5	77.5	102.4	143.0	196.3	213.6	274.5
1897-1901	1931	45.5	73.2	74.0	98.0	138.0	189.8	206.7	267.1
1898-1902	1932	42.9	69.4	70.6	95.8	136.4	189.0	207.6	269.8
1899-1903	1933	40.4	64.4	66.8	92.1	129.9	179.1	200.7	255.6
1900-1904	1934	42.9	67.1	67.5	94.4	131.5	180.8	203.8	265.9
1901-1905	1935	44.9	65.0	64.7	90.1	124.8	172.3	202.4	276.2
1902-1906	1936	46.2	64.9	63.0	86.5	119.6	166.7	196.7	269.9
1903-1907	1937	48.5	66.9	62.2	85.9	117.6	165.8	200.9	274.4
1904-1908	1938	50.9	71.0	63.3	85.4	117.3	166.2	202.8	275.9
1905-1909	1939	52.3	73.5	63.3	84.4	114.1	160.3	195.0	264.2
1906-1910	1940	54.0	79.0	65.4	85.8	113.1	163.1	195.8	280.2
1907-1911	1941	59.3	83.3	66.9	86.8	114.7	161.8	194.4	271.7
1908-1912	1942	70.2	93.8	71.8	91.1	119.1	161.6	197.7	268.3
1909-1913	1943	68.2	105.3	83.4	102.2	131.2	176.5	207.3	286.6
1910-1914	1944	60.3	103.1	85.4	103.7	130.7	181.8	218.8	289.5
1911-1915	1945	61.2	112.2	87.9	101.4	128.7	176.1	208.9	288.6
1912-1916	1946	83.6	124.9	91.9	102.7	127.6	175.4	205.1	280.8
1913-1917	1947	98.4	129.0	91.5	100.0	121.9	162.6	192.3	272.7
1914-1918	1948	82.1	119.0	85.6	93.5	114.8	155.9	187.1	269.5
1915-1919	1949	78.1	119.4	84.0	94.3	114.6	153.3	194.8	285.7
1916-1920	1950	75.4	121.6	85.7	95.3	113.8	154.6	187.1	273.4
1917-1921	1951	80.1	125.2	90.2	98.8	118.0	154.8	194.8	271.4
1918-1922	1952	83.7	128.3	95.2	105.2	123.6	160.4	193.5	269.5
1919-1923	1953	83.1	126.9	97.6	106.8	125.3	160.6	195.0	265.7
1920-1924	1954	85.5	129.4	99.1	109.8	126.5	166.2	195.1	277.8
1921-1925	1955	83.1	126.4	98.9	109.5	128.4	167.6	203.5	272.1
1922-1926	1956	80.8	126.6	99.2	109.6	129.1	166.7	202.2	276.3
1923-1927	1957	80.8	128.0	100.8	110.2	129.0	166.3	203.0	275.0
1924-1928	1958	76.0	124.8	98.4	107.2	124.8	159.8	194.3	269.0
1925-1929	1959	72.1	124.4	97.3	106.3	123.6	160.6	193.0	273.2
1926-1930	1960	68.2	125.4	96.2	104.6	120.7	156.4	191.1	269.0
1927-1931	1961	66.1	126.3	95.8	103.5	119.2	154.2	187.3	266.4
1928-1932	1962	63.0	123.1	91.6	97.0	112.6	145.6	177.7	253.2
1929-1933	1963	63.4	121.8	89.0	94.0	107.3	138.7	172.6	239.0
1930-1934	1964	70.5	121.4	86.9	90.0	99.7	129.5	156.9	222.6
1931-1935	1965	68.9	115.0	80.3	80.0	87.8	112.5	136.9	189.1
1932-1936	1966	68.2	108.2	72.9	69.8	76.1	95.7	117.3	169.1
1933-1937	1967	62.7	104.5	68.5	64.5	68.9	85.2	104.8	148.9
1934-1938	1968	68.0	103.8	64.7	58.9	62.2	76.0	93.5	139.9
1935-1939	1969	63.1	103.8	65.4	58.5	62.4	77.8	93.6	135.7
1936-1940	1970	64.0	104.6	64.6	57.7	62.3	76.2	90.3	136.4
1937-1941	1971	59.3	99.3	57.5	52.6	57.5	71.4	87.0	125.7
1938-1942	1972	55.8	96.6	49.2	44.4	49.0	61.3	75.2	111.8
1939-1943	1973	54.0	93.8	44.6	39.5	43.3	55.9	71.4	101.6

TABLE 9B. BIRTH PROBABILITIES FOR WHITE WOMEN FOR EACH YEAR 1917-73 BY AGE AND PARITY FOR GROUPS OF COHORTS FROM 1868-72 TO 1954-58--CON.

(PROBABILITIES ARE THE NUMBER OF BIRTHS PER 1,000 WOMEN IN SPECIFIED PARITY AND EXACT AGE GROUP. FIGURES IN THE "0 PARITY" COLUMN SHOW THE PROBABILITY OF FIRST BIRTHS TO "0 PARITY" WOMEN, THOSE IN THE "1 PARITY" COLUMN SHOW THE PROBABILITY OF SECOND BIRTHS TO "1 PARITY" WOMEN, ETC. BASED ON CENTRAL BIRTH RATES AND PARITY DISTRIBUTIONS FOR GROUPS OF COHORTS)

EXACT AGE AND COHORT	AS OF JANUARY 1	PARITY							
		0	1	2	3	4	5	6	7 AND HIGHER
35-39 YEARS									
1878-1882-------------	1917	17.4	49.1	61.3	85.6	116.1	155.6	180.6	231.8
1879-1883-------------	1918	17.9	49.2	59.9	85.2	115.2	151.9	179.9	234.5
1880-1884-------------	1919	17.9	48.5	58.3	81.6	111.1	146.9	180.4	237.4
1881-1885-------------	1920	18.8	47.9	58.0	80.1	110.1	145.1	181.3	242.7
1882-1886-------------	1921	20.2	49.2	58.5	80.9	110.1	144.9	182.8	254.8
1883-1887-------------	1922	18.6	46.1	54.9	74.8	101.7	136.4	170.5	242.5
1884-1888-------------	1923	18.3	46.0	54.9	73.9	100.4	135.9	168.5	249.7
1885-1889-------------	1924	18.9	45.3	54.6	72.0	97.9	135.5	167.3	253.7
1886-1890-------------	1925	18.8	43.4	51.8	70.1	92.6	130.8	159.0	248.4
1887-1891-------------	1926	18.2	41.5	48.8	66.2	88.2	124.3	154.7	241.4
1888-1892-------------	1927	19.0	40.1	46.4	62.5	84.3	124.8	153.1	244.8
1889-1893-------------	1928	18.4	37.7	43.0	57.7	79.9	115.7	146.0	230.4
1890-1894-------------	1929	17.8	34.6	39.8	53.7	74.9	109.3	139.0	219.5
1891-1895-------------	1930	19.1	34.5	38.9	53.3	75.3	110.6	139.5	218.8
1892-1896-------------	1931	18.3	31.1	35.9	50.4	72.7	105.9	133.0	212.7
1893-1897-------------	1932	17.4	29.1	33.6	47.6	70.1	104.5	133.0	211.6
1894-1898-------------	1933	15.9	26.8	30.9	45.5	67.4	101.2	128.3	200.6
1895-1899-------------	1934	16.7	27.9	30.8	45.9	68.8	103.2	127.5	205.2
1896-1900-------------	1935	16.9	27.3	30.0	43.6	65.8	99.4	123.7	210.0
1897-1901-------------	1936	17.6	26.7	29.3	42.1	62.9	96.8	117.8	203.4
1898-1902-------------	1937	18.3	26.4	28.7	41.9	60.7	93.9	117.2	206.8
1899-1903-------------	1938	19.6	27.6	28.4	41.8	62.0	92.7	117.1	206.4
1900-1904-------------	1939	20.8	28.1	28.7	40.9	58.4	89.0	111.4	196.4
1901-1905-------------	1940	22.0	29.2	28.8	40.0	58.2	85.5	111.1	198.3
1902-1906-------------	1941	23.5	30.9	29.4	41.3	56.9	84.1	110.4	195.1
1903-1907-------------	1942	28.0	34.5	32.2	43.2	59.4	87.2	109.2	195.2
1904-1908-------------	1943	29.2	40.3	37.6	49.7	66.2	93.1	121.8	209.1
1905-1909-------------	1944	28.0	43.5	40.2	52.7	68.7	98.5	120.2	211.6
1906-1910-------------	1945	28.2	47.7	43.9	55.3	70.6	98.7	125.0	212.7
1907-1911-------------	1946	33.9	51.9	45.2	55.6	70.6	97.9	120.3	209.2
1908-1912-------------	1947	38.1	52.8	45.1	55.7	70.2	95.9	118.6	205.4
1909-1913-------------	1948	32.8	48.6	42.1	52.5	66.0	90.9	112.1	196.9
1910-1914-------------	1949	31.0	47.2	40.7	50.7	64.5	90.7	114.5	206.3
1911-1915-------------	1950	30.3	47.3	40.8	51.4	65.2	90.0	115.0	200.0
1912-1916-------------	1951	30.3	48.2	42.1	52.7	65.7	93.4	111.1	202.0
1913-1917-------------	1952	31.4	49.5	44.1	55.0	69.1	93.8	114.5	202.7
1914-1918-------------	1953	31.2	48.8	44.2	57.1	71.0	93.1	113.5	194.4
1915-1919-------------	1954	31.2	49.9	45.4	58.5	72.2	93.6	120.7	194.4
1916-1920-------------	1955	31.3	48.9	44.6	58.0	71.9	96.1	117.6	193.1
1917-1921-------------	1956	30.9	48.2	44.4	57.0	72.3	95.8	122.0	193.2
1918-1922-------------	1957	32.6	47.0	43.3	57.1	72.8	97.4	120.6	196.0
1919-1923-------------	1958	32.1	44.4	41.2	54.4	70.1	96.2	121.8	184.5
1920-1924-------------	1959	32.5	42.5	39.7	53.0	69.5	94.8	119.3	190.6
1921-1925-------------	1960	31.3	41.2	38.1	51.4	67.4	91.4	116.3	186.2
1922-1926-------------	1961	30.0	40.8	37.2	48.7	65.6	91.3	116.7	183.9
1923-1927-------------	1962	27.5	39.0	34.6	45.2	60.9	83.7	106.8	177.1
1924-1928-------------	1963	26.5	38.5	33.6	42.9	56.7	79.6	101.1	171.0
1925-1929-------------	1964	29.1	39.5	32.5	41.1	53.4	73.4	97.9	160.1
1926-1930-------------	1965	27.2	37.8	30.1	37.3	48.1	66.2	83.3	144.9
1927-1931-------------	1966	25.8	36.3	27.9	32.9	41.3	55.8	74.7	121.1
1928-1932-------------	1967	23.7	36.2	26.3	30.0	36.9	50.0	62.8	106.8
1929-1933-------------	1968	27.0	35.6	24.1	27.0	32.8	45.0	56.4	94.6
1930-1934-------------	1969	23.9	35.4	22.9	25.5	30.9	40.7	53.2	88.9
1931-1935-------------	1970	24.7	34.8	22.1	23.5	28.7	37.9	48.9	84.3
1932-1936-------------	1971	22.6	31.8	19.5	21.2	25.5	34.6	42.8	76.7
1933-1937-------------	1972	21.3	29.4	17.2	17.7	21.4	29.3	37.1	67.0
1934-1938-------------	1973	19.7	28.9	15.2	15.1	18.6	25.4	34.1	59.6

TABLE 9B. BIRTH PROBABILITIES FOR WHITE WOMEN FOR EACH YEAR 1917-73 BY AGE AND PARITY FOR GROUPS OF COHORTS FROM 1868-72 TO 1954-58--CON.

(PROBABILITIES ARE THE NUMBER OF BIRTHS PER 1,000 WOMEN IN SPECIFIED PARITY AND EXACT AGE GROUP. FIGURES IN THE "0 PARITY" COLUMN SHOW THE PROBABILITY OF FIRST BIRTHS TO "0 PARITY" WOMEN, THOSE IN THE "1 PARITY" COLUMN SHOW THE PROBABILITY OF SECOND BIRTHS TO "1 PARITY" WOMEN, ETC. BASED ON CENTRAL BIRTH RATES AND PARITY DISTRIBUTIONS FOR GROUPS OF COHORTS)

EXACT AGE AND COHORT	AS OF JANUARY 1	PARITY							
		0	1	2	3	4	5	6	7 AND HIGHER
40-44 YEARS									
1873-1877-------------	1917	4.2	12.0	14.3	22.3	32.1	47.8	57.5	99.3
1874-1878-------------	1918	4.1	11.8	14.9	22.2	33.2	47.1	57.8	99.7
1875-1879-------------	1919	4.6	10.8	14.7	22.0	32.2	46.1	56.6	100.7
1876-1880-------------	1920	4.5	11.4	14.5	21.9	31.2	46.4	56.9	104.5
1877-1881-------------	1921	4.5	11.2	14.3	21.8	32.3	46.7	57.6	108.3
1878-1882-------------	1922	4.1	10.2	13.4	20.8	29.2	42.8	55.6	102.4
1879-1883-------------	1923	4.1	10.1	12.5	19.8	29.1	42.7	55.5	103.1
1880-1884-------------	1924	4.1	9.9	13.0	19.7	29.0	41.2	55.2	106.7
1881-1885-------------	1925	4.1	9.8	12.7	18.6	26.8	38.6	53.1	105.1
1882-1886-------------	1926	4.1	9.6	11.2	17.6	25.6	36.1	50.5	101.3
1883-1887-------------	1927	4.1	8.7	11.8	16.6	24.4	36.5	49.2	103.0
1884-1888-------------	1928	4.2	8.5	10.3	15.5	23.2	34.3	45.9	97.9
1885-1889-------------	1929	3.7	7.7	10.1	14.5	21.0	31.9	43.0	92.4
1886-1890-------------	1930	3.8	7.6	9.9	15.0	21.8	33.8	41.8	93.2
1887-1891-------------	1931	3.9	7.5	9.1	13.2	19.7	31.4	40.8	90.5
1888-1892-------------	1932	3.9	7.3	8.2	13.0	19.7	30.5	41.7	88.8
1889-1893-------------	1933	3.5	6.4	8.0	12.2	18.8	29.6	39.1	85.2
1890-1894-------------	1934	3.6	5.6	7.7	12.0	18.0	28.7	40.4	88.0
1891-1895-------------	1935	3.6	5.4	7.0	11.2	17.3	27.9	37.6	85.9
1892-1896-------------	1936	3.7	5.2	6.8	10.5	16.6	27.1	36.6	81.8
1893-1897-------------	1937	3.7	5.0	6.7	10.5	15.9	26.3	33.4	80.4
1894-1898-------------	1938	3.7	5.4	6.5	10.5	16.2	27.2	34.6	80.9
1895-1899-------------	1939	4.2	5.3	6.4	10.5	16.5	26.3	33.2	77.6
1896-1900-------------	1940	4.1	5.2	6.3	9.9	15.7	25.4	31.7	77.6
1897-1901-------------	1941	4.5	5.6	6.2	10.0	16.1	24.2	30.2	75.1
1898-1902-------------	1942	5.0	5.9	6.6	10.1	16.4	24.9	31.4	76.3
1899-1903-------------	1943	5.5	6.7	7.5	11.6	17.9	27.3	35.6	80.5
1900-1904-------------	1944	6.0	7.4	8.3	12.5	19.3	28.0	37.1	85.2
1901-1905-------------	1945	6.5	8.2	9.1	13.3	18.3	28.6	39.0	86.7
1902-1906-------------	1946	7.4	8.9	9.5	13.4	19.7	27.4	37.6	82.5
1903-1907-------------	1947	7.8	9.4	9.8	14.1	20.0	28.0	36.1	84.7
1904-1908-------------	1948	6.7	8.9	9.2	13.3	18.9	26.5	33.9	79.3
1905-1909-------------	1949	6.7	8.6	8.7	13.2	17.7	24.7	31.7	81.1
1906-1910-------------	1950	6.2	8.7	9.0	13.0	19.0	27.5	36.4	78.4
1907-1911-------------	1951	6.2	8.8	9.2	14.2	18.9	27.6	37.3	79.3
1908-1912-------------	1952	6.3	8.9	9.9	14.5	21.2	27.8	37.9	77.6
1909-1913-------------	1953	6.0	9.4	9.7	15.5	20.7	30.0	38.2	77.6
1910-1914-------------	1954	6.3	9.1	10.4	15.0	22.6	32.0	38.3	79.7
1911-1915-------------	1955	6.1	9.2	10.2	15.1	23.0	31.3	37.7	76.7
1912-1916-------------	1956	5.9	8.9	10.0	14.6	22.2	30.4	40.9	78.1
1913-1917-------------	1957	6.2	8.7	9.5	15.3	22.4	33.4	40.4	78.7
1914-1918-------------	1958	5.8	8.5	9.0	14.3	21.5	30.1	39.9	75.9
1915-1919-------------	1959	6.2	8.2	8.6	14.4	20.6	30.8	42.3	75.2
1916-1920-------------	1960	5.9	7.9	8.5	13.4	20.8	31.4	41.0	74.1
1917-1921-------------	1961	6.3	8.1	8.1	13.6	19.9	28.4	42.8	74.7
1918-1922-------------	1962	6.0	7.8	7.7	12.2	18.3	27.2	38.0	72.9
1919-1923-------------	1963	6.5	7.4	7.0	10.9	17.6	26.0	36.3	70.9
1920-1924-------------	1964	7.0	6.3	6.7	10.2	16.2	24.9	34.7	66.7
1921-1925-------------	1965	7.3	6.6	6.4	9.5	14.9	22.4	30.5	60.2
1922-1926-------------	1966	6.4	6.3	5.7	8.5	12.9	18.6	26.5	54.3
1923-1927-------------	1967	5.4	5.9	5.1	7.9	11.0	16.6	22.8	46.6
1924-1928-------------	1968	6.4	5.4	4.8	6.4	9.3	14.6	22.0	41.3
1925-1929-------------	1969	4.2	5.7	4.5	5.9	9.0	12.8	18.8	38.3
1926-1930-------------	1970	4.2	6.1	4.2	5.4	8.1	11.1	15.9	33.8
1927-1931-------------	1971	4.3	5.5	3.4	4.4	6.5	9.6	13.2	29.5
1928-1932-------------	1972	4.4	4.8	3.0	3.9	5.1	8.1	12.8	25.6
1929-1933-------------	1973	3.5	5.0	2.6	3.0	4.3	6.8	10.5	23.8

TABLE 9B. BIRTH PROBABILITIES FOR WHITE WOMEN FOR EACH YEAR 1917-73 BY AGE AND PARITY FOR GROUPS OF COHORTS FROM 1868-72 TO 1954-58--CON.

(PROBABILITIES ARE THE NUMBER OF BIRTHS PER 1,000 WOMEN IN SPECIFIED PARITY AND EXACT AGE GROUP. FIGURES IN THE "0 PARITY" COLUMN SHOW THE PROBABILITY OF FIRST BIRTHS TO "0 PARITY" WOMEN, THOSE IN THE "1 PARITY" COLUMN SHOW THE PROBABILITY OF SECOND BIRTHS TO "1 PARITY" WOMEN, ETC. BASED ON CENTRAL BIRTH RATES AND PARITY DISTRIBUTIONS FOR GROUPS OF COHORTS)

EXACT AGE AND COHORT	AS OF JANUARY 1	PARITY							
		0	1	2	3	4	5	6	7 AND HIGHER
45-49 YEARS									
1868-1872-------------	1917	0.5	0.9	0.8	2.7	3.1	3.8	5.8	14.2
1869-1873-------------	1918	0.5	0.9	0.8	2.7	3.1	5.1	5.9	14.5
1870-1874-------------	1919	0.5	0.9	0.8	1.8	3.1	3.8	4.4	14.4
1871-1875-------------	1920	0.5	0.9	0.8	2.7	3.1	5.2	6.0	15.2
1872-1876-------------	1921	0.5	0.9	0.8	1.8	3.1	3.9	4.5	15.6
1873-1877-------------	1922	0.5	0.9	0.8	1.7	2.1	3.9	4.6	14.4
1874-1878-------------	1923	0.5	0.8	0.8	1.7	2.1	4.0	4.6	14.2
1875-1879-------------	1924	0.5	0.8	0.7	1.7	2.1	4.0	4.6	14.6
1876-1880-------------	1925	0.5	0.8	0.7	1.7	2.1	4.1	4.7	14.4
1877-1881-------------	1926	0.5	0.8	0.7	1.7	2.1	4.1	4.7	13.6
1878-1882-------------	1927	0.5	0.8	0.7	1.7	2.1	4.1	4.8	13.3
1879-1883-------------	1928	0.5	0.8	0.7	0.8	2.1	2.7	5.0	12.4
1880-1884-------------	1929	0.5	0.8	0.7	0.8	2.1	2.7	3.4	12.1
1881-1885-------------	1930	0.5	0.8	0.7	0.8	2.1	2.7	3.5	11.9
1882-1886-------------	1931	0.0	0.7	0.7	0.8	1.0	2.7	3.5	11.6
1883-1887-------------	1932	0.0	0.7	0.7	0.8	2.1	2.7	3.5	11.3
1884-1888-------------	1933	0.0	0.7	0.7	0.8	2.0	2.8	3.6	10.9
1885-1889-------------	1934	0.0	0.0	0.6	0.8	2.0	1.4	3.6	11.3
1886-1890-------------	1935	0.0	0.0	0.6	0.8	1.0	1.4	3.6	10.9
1887-1891-------------	1936	0.0	0.0	0.6	0.7	1.0	1.4	3.7	10.5
1888-1892-------------	1937	0.0	0.0	0.6	0.7	1.0	1.5	3.8	10.1
1889-1893-------------	1938	0.0	0.0	0.6	0.7	1.0	1.5	2.0	9.6
1890-1894-------------	1939	0.0	0.0	0.6	0.7	1.0	1.5	4.0	9.1
1891-1895-------------	1940	0.0	0.0	0.5	0.7	1.0	1.6	2.1	8.6
1892-1896-------------	1941	0.0	0.6	0.5	0.7	1.0	1.6	2.2	8.0
1893-1897-------------	1942	0.0	0.6	0.5	0.7	1.1	1.6	2.2	8.4
1894-1898-------------	1943	0.5	0.5	0.5	0.7	1.1	1.7	2.3	8.9
1895-1899-------------	1944	0.5	0.5	0.5	0.7	1.1	1.8	2.4	8.1
1896-1900-------------	1945	0.5	0.5	0.5	0.7	1.1	1.8	2.4	8.5
1897-1901-------------	1946	0.5	0.5	0.5	0.7	1.1	1.9	2.5	9.0
1898-1902-------------	1947	0.5	0.5	0.5	0.7	1.2	1.9	2.6	9.4
1899-1903-------------	1948	0.5	0.5	0.5	0.7	1.2	1.9	2.7	8.5
1900-1904-------------	1949	0.5	0.5	0.5	0.7	1.2	2.0	2.8	9.0
1901-1905-------------	1950	0.5	0.5	0.5	0.7	1.2	2.0	3.0	7.9
1902-1906-------------	1951	0.5	0.4	0.5	0.7	1.2	2.1	3.1	8.4
1903-1907-------------	1952	0.5	0.4	0.4	0.7	1.2	2.1	3.2	7.0
1904-1908-------------	1953	0.5	0.4	0.4	0.7	1.2	2.2	3.3	7.4
1905-1909-------------	1954	0.5	0.5	0.4	0.7	1.3	2.2	3.5	7.7
1906-1910-------------	1955	0.5	0.5	0.4	0.7	1.3	2.2	3.6	8.0
1907-1911-------------	1956	0.5	0.5	0.4	0.7	1.2	2.3	3.6	8.4
1908-1912-------------	1957	0.5	0.5	0.4	0.7	1.2	2.3	3.7	8.6
1909-1913-------------	1958	0.5	0.5	0.4	0.7	1.2	2.2	3.7	6.7
1910-1914-------------	1959	0.5	0.5	0.4	0.7	1.2	2.2	3.7	6.8
1911-1915-------------	1960	0.0	0.5	0.4	0.6	1.1	2.2	3.6	7.0
1912-1916-------------	1961	0.0	0.5	0.4	0.6	1.1	2.1	3.6	7.1
1913-1917-------------	1962	0.0	0.5	0.4	0.6	1.1	2.0	3.5	7.1
1914-1918-------------	1963	0.0	0.5	0.4	0.6	1.0	2.0	3.5	7.1
1915-1919-------------	1964	0.0	0.0	0.4	0.6	1.0	1.9	3.4	7.0
1916-1920-------------	1965	0.0	0.0	0.4	0.5	0.9	1.8	3.3	4.6
1917-1921-------------	1966	0.0	0.0	0.4	0.5	0.9	1.7	3.2	6.7
1918-1922-------------	1967	0.0	0.0	0.4	0.5	0.9	1.7	3.1	4.4
1919-1923-------------	1968	0.0	0.0	0.4	0.5	0.8	1.6	2.9	4.3
1920-1924-------------	1969	0.0	0.0	0.0	0.5	0.8	1.5	0.0	4.2
1921-1925-------------	1970	0.0	0.0	0.0	0.5	0.8	1.5	0.0	2.0
1922-1926-------------	1971	0.0	0.0	0.0	0.0	0.0	1.4	0.0	2.0
1923-1927-------------	1972	0.0	0.0	0.0	0.0	0.0	0.0	0.0	1.9
1924-1928-------------	1973	0.0	0.0	0.0	0.0	0.0	0.0	0.0	1.9

TABLE 9C. BIRTH PROBABILITIES FOR ALL OTHER WOMEN FOR EACH YEAR 1917-73 BY AGE AND PARITY FOR GROUPS OF COHORTS FROM 1868-72 TO 1954-58

(PROBABILITIES ARE THE NUMBER OF BIRTHS PER 1,000 WOMEN IN SPECIFIED PARITY AND EXACT AGE GROUP. FIGURES IN THE "0 PARITY" COLUMN SHOW THE PROBABILITY OF FIRST BIRTHS TO "0 PARITY" WOMEN, THOSE IN THE "1 PARITY" COLUMN SHOW THE PROBABILITY OF SECOND BIRTHS TO "1 PARITY" WOMEN, ETC. BASED ON CENTRAL BIRTH RATES AND PARITY DISTRIBUTIONS FOR GROUPS OF COHORTS)

EXACT AGE AND COHORT	AS OF JANUARY 1	PARITY							
		0	1	2	3	4	5	6	7 AND HIGHER
15-19 YEARS									
1898-1902-------------	1917	85.7	236.7	283.1	*	*	*	*	*
1899-1903-------------	1918	83.8	201.8	302.5	*	*	*	*	*
1900-1904-------------	1919	78.0	185.8	300.7	*	*	*	*	*
1901-1905-------------	1920	91.7	194.9	328.7	*	*	*	*	*
1902-1906-------------	1921	93.4	216.5	363.6	*	*	*	*	*
1903-1907-------------	1922	82.2	206.1	303.0	*	*	*	*	*
1904-1908-------------	1923	85.9	212.5	335.3	*	*	*	*	*
1905-1909-------------	1924	91.7	219.5	351.2	*	*	*	*	*
1906-1910-------------	1925	94.2	209.3	333.3	*	*	*	*	*
1907-1911-------------	1926	92.0	210.8	342.9	*	*	*	*	*
1908-1912-------------	1927	87.7	202.2	327.9	*	*	*	*	*
1909-1913-------------	1928	83.0	190.3	313.8	*	*	*	*	*
1910-1914-------------	1929	79.8	195.6	307.7	*	*	*	*	*
1911-1915-------------	1930	82.1	201.5	300.0	*	*	*	*	*
1912-1916-------------	1931	79.0	198.7	305.1	*	*	*	*	*
1913-1917-------------	1932	79.9	206.6	316.1	*	*	*	*	*
1914-1918-------------	1933	74.2	198.9	298.9	*	*	*	*	*
1915-1919-------------	1934	78.5	209.9	327.4	*	*	*	*	*
1916-1920-------------	1935	81.1	221.6	335.3	*	*	*	*	*
1917-1921-------------	1936	79.1	223.1	333.3	*	*	*	*	*
1918-1922-------------	1937	84.6	236.8	333.3	*	*	*	*	*
1919-1923-------------	1938	87.2	232.0	325.0	*	*	*	*	*
1920-1924-------------	1939	84.9	235.1	336.5	*	*	*	*	*
1921-1925-------------	1940	81.9	254.0	395.3	*	*	*	*	*
1922-1926-------------	1941	84.3	278.4	396.4	*	*	*	*	*
1923-1927-------------	1942	86.8	288.7	398.3	*	*	*	*	*
1924-1928-------------	1943	87.5	300.0	383.4	*	*	*	*	*
1925-1929-------------	1944	79.7	279.5	341.6	*	*	*	*	*
1926-1930-------------	1945	77.8	282.9	312.1	*	*	*	*	*
1927-1931-------------	1946	80.6	305.5	333.3	*	*	*	*	*
1928-1932-------------	1947	99.3	353.4	370.5	*	*	*	*	*
1929-1933-------------	1948	102.4	375.8	382.1	*	*	*	*	*
1930-1934-------------	1949	100.1	389.8	391.8	*	*	*	*	*
1931-1935-------------	1950	99.0	392.3	381.6	*	*	*	*	*
1932-1936-------------	1951	102.4	387.6	382.9	*	*	*	*	*
1933-1937-------------	1952	100.2	367.5	387.5	*	*	*	*	*
1934-1938-------------	1953	102.9	367.4	394.9	*	*	*	*	*
1935-1939-------------	1954	107.5	367.4	409.8	*	*	*	*	*
1936-1940-------------	1955	105.2	371.9	415.6	*	*	*	*	*
1937-1941-------------	1956	107.7	388.8	424.6	*	*	*	*	*
1938-1942-------------	1957	107.6	386.9	423.6	460.0	*	*	*	*
1939-1943-------------	1958	101.9	382.2	426.4	466.0	*	*	*	*
1940-1944-------------	1959	101.4	387.5	427.1	457.1	*	*	*	*
1941-1945-------------	1960	98.0	382.9	423.1	457.1	*	*	*	*
1942-1946-------------	1961	96.5	377.5	430.1	460.8	*	*	*	*
1943-1947-------------	1962	93.9	373.9	430.1	445.5	*	*	*	*
1944-1948-------------	1963	94.2	377.3	419.0	440.0	*	*	*	*
1945-1949-------------	1964	95.8	376.2	415.3	*	*	*	*	*
1946-1950-------------	1965	95.7	356.3	387.5	*	*	*	*	*
1947-1951-------------	1966	98.1	335.2	352.9	*	*	*	*	*
1948-1952-------------	1967	99.5	312.0	328.3	*	*	*	*	*
1949-1953-------------	1968	101.9	282.5	292.3	*	*	*	*	*
1950-1954-------------	1969	104.1	263.2	282.5	*	*	*	*	*
1951-1955-------------	1970	108.4	257.8	283.8	*	*	*	*	*
1952-1956-------------	1971	106.8	235.8	259.1	*	*	*	*	*
1953-1957-------------	1972	106.4	211.4	230.5	*	*	*	*	*
1954-1958-------------	1973	101.8	192.8	222.6	*	*	*	*	*

TABLE 9C. BIRTH PROBABILITIES FOR ALL OTHER WOMEN FOR EACH YEAR 1917-73 BY AGE AND PARITY FOR GROUPS OF COHORTS FROM 1868-72 TO 1954-58--CON.

(PROBABILITIES ARE THE NUMBER OF BIRTHS PER 1,000 WOMEN IN SPECIFIED PARITY AND EXACT AGE GROUP. FIGURES IN THE "0 PARITY" COLUMN SHOW THE PROBABILITY OF FIRST BIRTHS TO "0 PARITY" WOMEN,THOSE IN THE "1 PARITY" COLUMN SHOW THE PROBABILITY OF SECOND BIRTHS TO "1 PARITY" WOMEN, ETC. BASED ON CENTRAL BIRTH RATES AND PARITY DISTRIBUTIONS FOR GROUPS OF COHORTS)

EXACT AGE AND COHORT	AS OF JANUARY 1	PARITY							
		0	1	2	3	4	5	6	7 AND HIGHER
20-24 YEARS									
1893-1897-------------	1917	119.1	210.7	282.6	282.3	277.8	*	*	*
1894-1898-------------	1918	122.6	187.2	295.6	299.2	290.1	*	*	*
1895-1899-------------	1919	113.6	178.4	279.9	292.1	319.8	*	*	*
1896-1900-------------	1920	135.0	184.6	287.6	309.6	342.1	*	*	*
1897-1901-------------	1921	130.3	178.9	311.0	349.7	390.9	*	*	*
1898-1902-------------	1922	114.8	177.9	291.4	330.5	377.8	*	*	*
1899-1903-------------	1923	111.8	169.6	300.7	342.5	399.1	*	*	*
1900-1904-------------	1924	120.6	172.2	324.3	353.9	419.6	*	*	*
1901-1905-------------	1925	119.9	164.1	294.8	352.5	390.6	*	*	*
1902-1906-------------	1926	113.9	161.0	278.6	355.3	373.0	*	*	*
1903-1907-------------	1927	102.8	148.1	270.5	341.3	361.5	*	*	*
1904-1908-------------	1928	93.3	136.0	257.3	325.3	355.7	*	*	*
1905-1909-------------	1929	90.1	135.4	252.0	313.9	355.4	*	*	*
1906-1910-------------	1930	91.6	139.3	257.5	322.5	362.1	*	*	*
1907-1911-------------	1931	88.0	140.2	251.3	315.7	339.1	*	*	*
1908-1912-------------	1932	88.7	149.0	261.3	322.9	340.7	*	*	*
1909-1913-------------	1933	80.4	143.4	253.8	316.8	334.8	*	*	*
1910-1914-------------	1934	85.5	151.6	266.4	332.7	352.7	*	*	*
1911-1915-------------	1935	84.0	153.2	263.6	342.6	361.2	*	*	*
1912-1916-------------	1936	79.5	157.0	260.7	335.8	350.9	*	*	*
1913-1917-------------	1937	81.8	166.8	274.8	348.5	362.4	*	*	*
1914-1918-------------	1938	80.8	169.2	279.1	344.4	363.6	*	*	*
1915-1919-------------	1939	80.4	172.2	274.7	332.2	371.3	*	*	*
1916-1920-------------	1940	80.3	171.9	283.0	362.5	406.6	*	*	*
1917-1921-------------	1941	84.3	178.5	284.0	353.9	406.3	*	*	*
1918-1922-------------	1942	89.8	179.7	278.7	348.3	397.0	*	*	*
1919-1923-------------	1943	88.7	185.7	278.0	345.2	386.5	*	*	*
1920-1924-------------	1944	83.4	174.9	269.8	340.8	375.8	*	*	*
1921-1925-------------	1945	80.4	168.0	248.1	311.7	343.9	*	*	*
1922-1926-------------	1946	97.6	209.6	269.3	322.8	342.9	*	*	*
1923-1927-------------	1947	127.0	238.0	279.1	324.0	345.9	*	*	*
1924-1928-------------	1948	123.7	264.2	302.6	341.3	357.1	*	*	*
1925-1929-------------	1949	119.0	276.0	307.7	350.2	372.4	510.0	*	*
1926-1930-------------	1950	113.3	281.2	317.9	347.9	370.3	481.8	*	*
1927-1931-------------	1951	113.0	289.7	324.3	357.6	377.8	467.2	*	*
1928-1932-------------	1952	112.7	287.4	319.0	358.8	372.2	477.9	*	*
1929-1933-------------	1953	119.3	296.0	315.0	358.5	376.8	473.7	*	*
1930-1934-------------	1954	130.3	307.4	325.7	361.4	380.5	491.1	*	*
1931-1935-------------	1955	137.2	316.0	330.8	364.4	384.8	488.8	*	*
1932-1936-------------	1956	147.5	329.2	340.9	376.4	383.8	502.7	*	*
1933-1937-------------	1957	153.7	327.2	344.9	374.8	389.7	513.1	*	*
1934-1938-------------	1958	150.2	320.5	343.4	371.9	391.9	495.0	*	*
1935-1939-------------	1959	149.4	318.5	339.9	375.8	387.1	492.9	*	*
1936-1940-------------	1960	147.8	311.2	335.7	365.2	370.8	488.4	*	*
1937-1941-------------	1961	144.9	309.8	330.7	367.4	371.4	500.0	*	*
1938-1942-------------	1962	141.0	301.3	324.8	356.4	365.0	497.6	*	*
1939-1943-------------	1963	140.6	297.6	313.8	342.6	353.1	463.8	*	*
1940-1944-------------	1964	141.6	290.6	301.3	328.6	334.5	452.7	*	*
1941-1945-------------	1965	140.7	273.5	276.0	301.7	304.8	394.7	*	*
1942-1946-------------	1966	143.7	254.7	250.9	267.5	270.3	367.8	*	*
1943-1947-------------	1967	144.4	237.5	225.0	237.4	245.9	335.5	*	*
1944-1948-------------	1968	150.0	215.5	205.7	218.9	221.7	297.7	*	*
1945-1949-------------	1969	155.6	208.0	199.9	215.4	219.1	300.9	*	*
1946-1950-------------	1970	162.5	205.7	201.4	216.5	212.9	*	*	*
1947-1951-------------	1971	157.9	192.7	187.6	199.0	198.8	*	*	*
1948-1952-------------	1972	147.7	168.0	159.7	174.0	173.5	*	*	*
1949-1953-------------	1973	137.0	158.7	150.6	159.8	157.1	*	*	*

TABLE 9C. BIRTH PROBABILITIES FOR ALL OTHER WOMEN FOR EACH YEAR 1917-73 BY AGE AND PARITY FOR GROUPS OF COHORTS FROM 1868-72 TO 1954-58--CON.

(PROBABILITIES ARE THE NUMBER OF BIRTHS PER 1,000 WOMEN IN SPECIFIED PARITY AND EXACT AGE GROUP. FIGURES IN THE "0 PARITY" COLUMN SHOW THE PROBABILITY OF FIRST BIRTHS TO "0 PARITY" WOMEN, THOSE IN THE "1 PARITY" COLUMN SHOW THE PROBABILITY OF SECOND BIRTHS TO "1 PARITY" WOMEN, ETC. BASED ON CENTRAL BIRTH RATES AND PARITY DISTRIBUTIONS FOR GROUPS OF COHORTS)

EXACT AGE AND COHORT	AS OF JANUARY 1	PARITY							
		0	1	2	3	4	5	6	7 AND HIGHER
25-29 YEARS									
1888-1892	1917	58.3	110.1	191.2	207.0	214.4	297.0	273.0	290.7
1889-1893	1918	62.3	100.2	190.2	203.7	200.9	297.5	254.8	278.6
1890-1894	1919	57.4	103.6	189.3	200.2	222.2	327.3	303.8	353.4
1891-1895	1920	70.6	110.2	202.6	215.0	233.0	361.0	308.8	359.1
1892-1896	1921	65.5	103.0	210.1	221.1	252.3	408.0	391.0	464.1
1893-1897	1922	57.6	97.5	192.4	203.0	237.0	396.4	359.4	397.3
1894-1898	1923	54.1	87.9	188.3	206.4	248.5	409.7	376.0	427.9
1895-1899	1924	54.8	80.3	201.1	226.2	277.0	459.2	414.6	443.9
1896-1900	1925	55.5	77.6	188.3	234.9	270.4	432.4	393.7	488.7
1897-1901	1926	50.2	73.6	177.0	236.2	270.1	446.5	385.8	480.2
1898-1902	1927	46.3	64.0	163.5	221.1	272.4	411.8	368.4	443.5
1899-1903	1928	40.2	54.9	147.7	207.5	254.2	364.1	337.2	418.1
1900-1904	1929	38.2	52.3	138.3	199.8	260.1	349.4	324.0	391.1
1901-1905	1930	38.9	53.0	136.1	202.0	254.2	332.5	332.0	392.3
1902-1906	1931	36.1	51.1	132.9	206.4	251.8	330.8	334.8	383.1
1903-1907	1932	35.4	50.9	133.4	214.7	258.6	326.4	336.3	378.2
1904-1908	1933	30.9	48.8	133.0	211.5	258.8	321.9	327.3	360.2
1905-1909	1934	32.6	50.1	135.0	221.5	266.7	328.0	328.7	405.7
1906-1910	1935	31.0	50.1	131.6	214.0	257.0	310.2	319.2	401.2
1907-1911	1936	30.3	52.1	128.3	212.3	253.1	311.8	318.8	391.3
1908-1912	1937	29.9	54.8	133.3	215.7	260.1	322.5	344.7	417.7
1909-1913	1938	30.8	57.6	139.3	220.8	261.3	327.0	346.3	401.2
1910-1914	1939	31.6	58.3	138.2	222.0	260.9	329.7	344.5	406.1
1911-1915	1940	31.7	60.3	139.0	224.7	264.5	337.8	356.8	440.5
1912-1916	1941	33.6	65.8	144.6	223.9	271.5	338.6	354.8	433.5
1913-1917	1942	36.9	71.0	147.4	219.7	268.6	325.6	342.3	411.1
1914-1918	1943	38.8	78.9	153.5	228.0	279.3	325.1	350.9	419.4
1915-1919	1944	39.1	79.2	155.2	225.4	280.1	329.3	348.9	410.3
1916-1920	1945	39.1	76.2	143.4	215.3	272.5	320.8	341.5	387.3
1917-1921	1946	49.7	94.0	158.6	224.9	275.1	315.5	333.3	386.8
1918-1922	1947	62.7	106.0	164.6	225.8	267.1	310.5	334.6	382.5
1919-1923	1948	62.2	116.6	174.2	229.5	274.4	319.0	341.0	400.0
1920-1924	1949	61.7	124.2	178.4	231.5	275.1	327.4	347.3	400.0
1921-1925	1950	61.2	129.7	184.1	238.4	280.3	334.8	348.3	393.0
1922-1926	1951	63.0	135.4	191.7	248.3	283.4	348.1	351.4	391.5
1923-1927	1952	65.7	142.6	190.4	250.6	289.8	348.6	358.1	393.4
1924-1928	1953	66.9	151.5	192.6	251.7	293.3	350.4	365.9	399.2
1925-1929	1954	70.3	159.9	192.8	256.0	298.6	347.1	371.3	412.2
1926-1930	1955	67.4	168.8	196.2	250.6	292.0	337.4	361.9	406.6
1927-1931	1956	68.5	178.4	200.1	251.3	290.9	339.0	373.8	420.4
1928-1932	1957	68.3	187.5	204.4	243.9	286.1	334.7	356.5	409.2
1929-1933	1958	68.6	186.2	196.1	238.4	278.3	328.4	351.5	406.5
1930-1934	1959	72.6	191.0	196.5	238.8	279.3	323.7	350.1	391.6
1931-1935	1960	77.1	187.0	189.9	226.3	266.9	315.5	342.2	373.1
1932-1936	1961	81.3	183.4	187.6	225.8	265.6	322.1	336.0	384.6
1933-1937	1962	83.1	176.5	181.1	217.4	254.1	306.1	321.1	372.7
1934-1938	1963	85.9	170.1	175.3	206.0	244.5	289.8	313.7	362.5
1935-1939	1964	83.0	164.7	169.7	195.5	229.0	280.2	295.9	342.1
1936-1940	1965	85.9	159.5	158.2	180.7	204.8	248.1	264.8	298.1
1937-1941	1966	85.4	154.0	143.6	157.9	177.4	212.6	229.6	253.3
1938-1942	1967	83.9	150.0	133.3	143.1	155.5	190.9	204.1	223.6
1939-1943	1968	92.5	143.2	119.9	131.8	136.2	170.4	177.9	204.0
1940-1944	1969	95.1	146.0	120.5	130.7	136.4	166.4	162.5	193.2
1941-1945	1970	101.9	150.4	124.7	133.7	140.8	167.6	172.0	200.0
1942-1946	1971	102.9	142.0	119.7	125.7	133.5	153.7	161.2	191.9
1943-1947	1972	105.6	129.0	101.0	106.4	110.8	134.0	136.8	159.5
1944-1948	1973	109.7	121.2	93.2	94.8	96.3	116.9	120.6	147.3

TABLE 9C. BIRTH PROBABILITIES FOR ALL OTHER WOMEN FOR EACH YEAR 1917-73 BY AGE AND PARITY FOR GROUPS OF COHORTS FROM 1868-72 TO 1954-58--CON.

(PROBABILITIES ARE THE NUMBER OF BIRTHS PER 1,000 WOMEN IN SPECIFIED PARITY AND EXACT AGE GROUP. FIGURES IN THE "0 PARITY" COLUMN SHOW THE PROBABILITY OF FIRST BIRTHS TO "0 PARITY" WOMEN,THOSE IN THE "1 PARITY" COLUMN SHOW THE PROBABILITY OF SECOND BIRTHS TO "1 PARITY" WOMEN, ETC. BASED ON CENTRAL BIRTH RATES AND PARITY DISTRIBUTIONS FOR GROUPS OF COHORTS)

EXACT AGE AND COHORT	AS OF JANUARY 1	PARITY							
		0	1	2	3	4	5	6	7 AND HIGHER
30-34 YEARS									
1883-1887-------------	1917	24.3	50.8	89.9	111.4	137.8	225.7	225.1	244.4
1884-1888-------------	1918	26.5	49.7	92.3	111.6	132.6	232.4	210.4	223.6
1885-1889-------------	1919	24.0	48.7	90.9	115.1	130.9	210.4	203.9	245.1
1886-1890-------------	1920	27.1	48.5	96.7	117.5	121.7	199.1	193.5	251.1
1887-1891-------------	1921	25.1	49.2	93.9	116.7	129.6	224.8	214.7	288.5
1888-1892-------------	1922	23.4	47.6	88.4	107.4	123.4	223.5	212.9	282.5
1889-1893-------------	1923	22.6	42.0	87.0	102.6	122.7	240.5	225.3	293.5
1890-1894-------------	1924	22.6	39.8	94.4	103.2	125.5	263.6	240.3	316.9
1891-1895-------------	1925	23.8	36.0	86.2	98.7	127.1	274.1	248.0	348.5
1892-1896-------------	1926	20.0	33.5	80.4	98.9	128.5	273.6	261.8	335.0
1893-1897-------------	1927	19.3	26.5	72.8	88.2	123.2	258.2	258.5	316.3
1894-1898-------------	1928	17.1	22.2	61.6	81.4	120.2	245.3	231.3	289.8
1895-1899-------------	1929	15.8	21.4	59.2	81.9	121.5	236.5	223.0	277.4
1896-1900-------------	1930	17.7	21.5	58.7	84.0	129.5	238.3	226.6	287.0
1897-1901-------------	1931	16.7	19.9	56.5	86.6	124.7	230.9	232.8	289.6
1898-1902-------------	1932	16.1	19.2	56.5	90.3	134.0	234.0	231.9	289.1
1899-1903-------------	1933	14.7	18.4	55.5	89.7	132.5	220.9	231.6	280.1
1900-1904-------------	1934	14.8	18.5	55.3	91.8	137.2	217.3	232.7	298.5
1901-1905-------------	1935	13.2	17.7	51.8	91.5	131.0	200.0	215.3	274.7
1902-1906-------------	1936	12.5	16.6	48.7	86.9	127.0	190.3	209.4	275.9
1903-1907-------------	1937	12.1	17.0	49.9	88.4	131.7	189.4	218.0	285.9
1904-1908-------------	1938	12.6	17.4	52.2	93.1	133.5	191.4	226.5	287.1
1905-1909-------------	1939	12.9	18.3	52.7	97.4	130.4	190.9	222.5	291.7
1906-1910-------------	1940	13.2	19.7	53.8	96.2	135.5	192.0	232.0	312.2
1907-1911-------------	1941	14.5	22.0	57.9	101.5	135.1	197.9	239.8	317.3
1908-1912-------------	1942	15.7	25.6	62.0	105.2	137.5	203.0	241.8	314.1
1909-1913-------------	1943	17.9	28.9	67.4	113.2	146.3	216.9	249.3	323.9
1910-1914-------------	1944	19.0	32.1	71.3	118.3	149.5	226.8	252.7	328.4
1911-1915-------------	1945	19.2	33.3	72.6	117.9	156.1	217.5	252.6	328.0
1912-1916-------------	1946	21.7	39.6	80.6	124.5	153.5	209.1	243.5	315.5
1913-1917-------------	1947	26.8	45.5	84.8	123.7	155.0	203.6	246.8	310.7
1914-1918-------------	1948	25.4	50.0	90.5	124.6	156.2	202.3	246.8	306.6
1915-1919-------------	1949	27.7	52.5	95.8	127.3	159.5	201.9	244.4	306.8
1916-1920-------------	1950	27.9	53.2	98.7	133.1	166.4	204.0	245.7	308.5
1917-1921-------------	1951	30.3	57.3	101.2	140.3	170.6	215.5	257.1	306.3
1918-1922-------------	1952	30.6	61.3	103.7	143.5	177.0	219.3	247.1	306.2
1919-1923-------------	1953	31.8	63.4	106.5	143.1	179.2	220.0	248.4	307.4
1920-1924-------------	1954	33.2	67.3	105.4	146.9	184.5	228.4	257.4	316.7
1921-1925-------------	1955	32.4	70.6	105.5	145.6	179.6	226.1	250.0	318.6
1922-1926-------------	1956	32.4	74.2	106.8	143.8	179.8	229.1	258.1	318.9
1923-1927-------------	1957	31.3	79.1	107.2	141.8	175.9	224.2	258.0	318.0
1924-1928-------------	1958	31.3	79.0	102.0	134.2	162.0	211.5	245.0	309.8
1925-1929-------------	1959	31.7	82.2	101.1	129.8	163.3	204.4	243.6	309.4
1926-1930-------------	1960	30.3	88.0	100.3	125.5	153.1	188.7	227.8	295.2
1927-1931-------------	1961	29.3	89.9	101.4	126.9	147.7	186.3	222.1	290.8
1928-1932-------------	1962	28.6	91.7	96.5	116.7	142.0	178.9	204.1	276.5
1929-1933-------------	1963	29.5	95.0	93.3	112.3	134.3	163.4	189.6	261.0
1930-1934-------------	1964	30.9	90.3	89.7	104.1	126.5	159.8	184.8	250.6
1931-1935-------------	1965	34.1	91.1	84.1	97.1	115.1	140.3	164.2	220.6
1932-1936-------------	1966	37.8	85.3	79.2	86.7	101.8	124.2	134.8	189.3
1933-1937-------------	1967	37.9	82.6	73.8	81.0	91.6	109.4	122.7	165.9
1934-1938-------------	1968	44.7	82.9	70.6	72.2	79.5	96.3	103.5	146.0
1935-1939-------------	1969	47.2	85.3	72.3	72.7	79.3	91.2	99.3	133.5
1936-1940-------------	1970	47.5	89.0	73.4	73.1	79.7	91.7	95.1	128.6
1937-1941-------------	1971	46.8	90.1	71.1	68.6	73.4	87.2	94.2	126.4
1938-1942-------------	1972	48.3	86.8	61.4	57.7	62.9	73.7	74.8	103.1
1939-1943-------------	1973	47.7	84.4	55.9	53.1	55.2	64.1	68.8	93.7

TABLE 9C. BIRTH PROBABILITIES FOR ALL OTHER WOMEN FOR EACH YEAR 1917-73 BY AGE AND PARITY FOR GROUPS OF COHORTS FROM 1868-72 TO 1954-58--CON.

(PROBABILITIES ARE THE NUMBER OF BIRTHS PER 1,000 WOMEN IN SPECIFIED PARITY AND EXACT AGE GROUP. FIGURES IN THE "0 PARITY" COLUMN SHOW THE PROBABILITY OF FIRST BIRTHS TO "0 PARITY" WOMEN,THOSE IN THE "1 PARITY" COLUMN SHOW THE PROBABILITY OF SECOND BIRTHS TO "1 PARITY" WOMEN, ETC. BASED ON CENTRAL BIRTH RATES AND PARITY DISTRIBUTIONS FOR GROUPS OF COHORTS)

EXACT AGE AND COHORT	AS OF JANUARY 1	PARITY							
		0	1	2	3	4	5	6	7 AND HIGHER
35-39 YEARS									
1878-1882-------------	1917	13.6	30.4	54.1	75.4	97.3	173.3	181.1	229.8
1879-1883-------------	1918	17.3	32.4	62.3	77.0	94.6	211.1	177.4	226.6
1880-1884-------------	1919	14.9	30.4	58.4	77.8	98.4	215.5	183.4	254.3
1881-1885-------------	1920	16.4	32.3	67.4	81.1	99.0	219.6	165.2	264.6
1882-1886-------------	1921	15.0	28.4	57.8	74.4	94.3	213.4	153.0	265.7
1883-1887-------------	1922	13.7	27.6	55.3	67.1	87.6	181.8	154.3	254.6
1884-1888-------------	1923	11.6	24.0	51.0	64.0	76.3	166.1	149.5	256.6
1885-1889-------------	1924	11.5	20.4	50.5	64.2	78.5	150.8	153.0	268.6
1886-1890-------------	1925	12.0	18.1	46.7	61.8	72.6	149.7	157.1	295.0
1887-1891-------------	1926	10.4	17.0	42.6	60.4	70.6	154.4	159.5	288.9
1888-1892-------------	1927	11.7	15.0	36.5	50.0	65.2	148.3	150.9	287.4
1889-1893-------------	1928	8.9	11.9	31.6	42.1	59.8	144.3	136.2	258.2
1890-1894-------------	1929	8.2	13.0	30.5	39.0	58.4	143.2	136.2	248.7
1891-1895-------------	1930	9.1	11.1	28.5	36.9	62.6	153.2	142.0	255.1
1892-1896-------------	1931	8.3	10.6	26.7	36.2	57.3	147.3	142.9	244.1
1893-1897-------------	1932	7.9	8.7	26.1	34.2	56.1	161.7	151.5	252.9
1894-1898-------------	1933	7.0	8.8	23.9	34.9	56.7	141.8	142.6	240.5
1895-1899-------------	1934	7.3	8.1	24.6	36.7	61.1	143.9	151.8	252.6
1896-1900-------------	1935	6.8	7.8	24.7	36.6	61.5	133.2	146.0	236.4
1897-1901-------------	1936	7.2	7.6	24.8	39.3	61.5	126.7	137.3	227.5
1898-1902-------------	1937	6.6	7.9	25.6	38.9	63.6	122.2	136.3	238.8
1899-1903-------------	1938	7.0	8.1	24.6	42.5	64.7	120.0	137.7	238.1
1900-1904-------------	1939	7.2	8.0	23.6	41.6	60.7	114.3	135.5	234.5
1901-1905-------------	1940	7.0	7.9	22.5	41.7	67.2	107.5	130.8	239.1
1902-1906-------------	1941	7.1	8.6	24.2	41.8	70.9	106.8	139.3	245.4
1903-1907-------------	1942	7.6	9.3	25.2	46.7	71.4	104.1	132.7	244.0
1904-1908-------------	1943	8.1	10.5	28.8	50.6	76.0	108.7	139.9	257.1
1905-1909-------------	1944	8.5	11.3	31.6	54.1	76.2	113.5	150.8	257.8
1906-1910-------------	1945	9.0	11.9	33.4	58.6	79.8	117.3	148.2	269.2
1907-1911-------------	1946	10.2	14.4	36.8	61.3	78.4	116.3	152.2	254.1
1908-1912-------------	1947	11.4	16.4	39.2	63.4	80.4	122.4	151.8	253.8
1909-1913-------------	1948	11.3	17.6	41.5	65.2	84.1	122.2	149.7	247.5
1910-1914-------------	1949	12.2	19.3	42.7	66.7	83.7	126.7	151.8	246.8
1911-1915-------------	1950	12.2	19.5	45.8	71.1	86.4	123.1	151.7	244.2
1912-1916-------------	1951	12.6	21.4	49.9	74.0	92.7	124.5	151.5	248.6
1913-1917-------------	1952	12.1	22.9	49.0	73.7	92.0	119.8	146.8	238.7
1914-1918-------------	1953	12.9	24.1	52.6	74.7	96.5	122.2	155.0	232.0
1915-1919-------------	1954	12.7	26.0	53.4	78.4	100.3	126.8	153.8	236.3
1916-1920-------------	1955	13.3	26.4	53.0	77.1	99.5	127.2	154.9	230.8
1917-1921-------------	1956	13.3	25.9	52.2	74.3	99.9	127.1	160.0	236.9
1918-1922-------------	1957	12.7	26.2	51.0	75.7	99.0	125.8	154.5	227.0
1919-1923-------------	1958	12.8	26.7	49.3	69.7	95.0	115.3	144.0	216.4
1920-1924-------------	1959	12.8	24.9	48.0	66.3	91.2	121.1	144.2	218.0
1921-1925-------------	1960	12.3	26.5	46.1	65.8	82.1	111.1	132.4	209.7
1922-1926-------------	1961	11.8	28.5	45.9	65.0	81.6	105.7	128.2	204.9
1923-1927-------------	1962	11.4	29.9	44.3	59.6	74.9	97.8	114.9	189.6
1924-1928-------------	1963	11.8	30.1	40.3	53.3	69.5	86.8	106.6	177.0
1925-1929-------------	1964	11.7	30.2	40.7	52.5	63.8	81.3	101.1	172.2
1926-1930-------------	1965	11.3	32.9	38.5	47.7	59.5	74.3	88.8	151.4
1927-1931-------------	1966	11.4	31.8	37.4	43.1	53.7	64.6	77.6	130.0
1928-1932-------------	1967	10.6	34.6	36.0	40.4	47.4	58.8	70.0	111.6
1929-1933-------------	1968	12.8	34.9	33.2	35.6	43.5	54.1	60.3	96.5
1930-1934-------------	1969	13.1	36.2	32.4	35.8	42.6	45.5	56.2	88.8
1931-1935-------------	1970	14.4	35.8	32.0	35.3	39.5	45.2	52.8	84.0
1932-1936-------------	1971	15.2	33.6	29.8	31.4	35.9	43.1	50.6	76.9
1933-1937-------------	1972	15.8	34.4	27.6	27.9	30.9	35.6	40.2	64.7
1934-1938-------------	1973	16.5	30.7	25.6	24.5	27.2	30.6	35.2	55.1

TABLE 9C. BIRTH PROBABILITIES FOR ALL OTHER WOMEN FOR EACH YEAR 1917-73 BY AGE AND PARITY FOR GROUPS OF COHORTS FROM 1868-72 TO 1954-58--CON.

(PROBABILITIES ARE THE NUMBER OF BIRTHS PER 1,000 WOMEN IN SPECIFIED PARITY AND EXACT AGE GROUP. FIGURES IN THE "0 PARITY" COLUMN SHOW THE PROBABILITY OF FIRST BIRTHS TO "0 PARITY" WOMEN, THOSE IN THE "1 PARITY" COLUMN SHOW THE PROBABILITY OF SECOND BIRTHS TO "1 PARITY" WOMEN, ETC. BASED ON CENTRAL BIRTH RATES AND PARITY DISTRIBUTIONS FOR GROUPS OF COHORTS)

EXACT AGE AND COHORT	AS OF JANUARY 1	PARITY							
		0	1	2	3	4	5	6	7 AND HIGHER
40-44 YEARS									
1873-1877	1917	3.0	7.2	10.2	19.8	25.6	47.8	42.2	84.1
1874-1878	1918	5.4	8.6	15.1	19.7	26.6	61.7	49.5	96.9
1875-1879	1919	2.9	8.4	10.0	18.2	25.1	45.4	44.8	85.9
1876-1880	1920	4.3	8.9	14.9	21.5	27.2	47.6	42.3	91.0
1877-1881	1921	3.7	8.7	14.9	22.3	24.3	50.6	48.7	97.1
1878-1882	1922	3.7	7.8	13.9	16.5	22.6	49.4	46.0	91.9
1879-1883	1923	4.1	6.9	13.9	17.2	22.4	51.1	46.1	93.9
1880-1884	1924	3.2	5.4	12.9	19.8	24.6	54.9	44.6	93.9
1881-1885	1925	3.1	5.3	12.9	17.3	22.0	57.6	40.1	100.2
1882-1886	1926	3.1	4.5	10.8	15.1	19.5	52.8	40.2	101.1
1883-1887	1927	3.0	3.7	9.7	13.1	18.1	40.8	37.8	96.4
1884-1888	1928	2.6	3.6	6.7	11.3	16.6	34.1	30.5	88.0
1885-1889	1929	2.1	2.9	7.6	10.3	14.1	32.3	31.3	89.0
1886-1890	1930	2.1	2.8	6.6	11.2	15.9	31.7	37.2	92.1
1887-1891	1931	2.1	2.2	5.5	10.0	13.6	32.4	35.0	90.8
1888-1892	1932	2.2	2.7	6.3	9.7	13.6	37.0	34.3	99.5
1889-1893	1933	1.7	2.1	6.3	9.1	12.5	32.8	35.3	94.8
1890-1894	1934	1.8	2.0	5.4	8.8	12.6	34.8	34.7	99.3
1891-1895	1935	1.8	1.9	5.3	7.8	12.8	34.1	34.3	95.9
1892-1896	1936	1.8	1.8	5.3	6.9	12.1	32.5	33.8	91.1
1893-1897	1937	1.4	1.7	4.5	7.1	10.3	32.9	33.0	92.2
1894-1898	1938	1.3	1.7	4.4	6.5	10.9	30.9	34.2	91.9
1895-1899	1939	1.3	1.6	4.3	6.8	11.5	30.8	30.3	85.4
1896-1900	1940	1.7	1.6	4.4	8.1	13.3	30.4	34.8	90.4
1897-1901	1941	1.7	1.5	5.2	8.5	13.9	29.7	32.4	89.6
1898-1902	1942	1.7	1.9	5.2	8.9	14.4	26.6	30.3	89.4
1899-1903	1943	1.7	1.8	5.2	10.4	15.0	28.3	33.4	94.2
1900-1904	1944	2.0	2.2	6.0	11.9	16.9	30.3	34.5	94.6
1901-1905	1945	2.4	2.2	6.8	12.3	19.1	29.8	38.1	98.0
1902-1906	1946	2.3	2.5	5.9	12.6	18.1	29.5	39.0	97.5
1903-1907	1947	2.2	2.5	7.7	14.3	18.5	29.4	37.2	95.0
1904-1908	1948	2.2	2.5	7.8	14.6	18.7	24.9	35.0	89.9
1905-1909	1949	2.8	3.3	7.8	14.8	20.3	29.5	38.5	93.6
1906-1910	1950	2.4	3.4	8.7	15.0	19.9	31.8	41.9	90.4
1907-1911	1951	2.7	4.2	10.4	17.5	22.8	32.2	42.1	94.9
1908-1912	1952	2.7	4.3	10.4	18.7	20.8	34.8	41.6	91.1
1909-1913	1953	2.7	4.4	11.2	18.4	25.3	36.7	43.5	93.0
1910-1914	1954	2.7	4.6	12.0	22.0	25.0	36.0	44.9	91.4
1911-1915	1955	2.7	5.2	12.0	20.3	24.7	36.8	41.2	88.4
1912-1916	1956	2.7	4.9	12.0	18.6	27.4	39.3	45.1	91.9
1913-1917	1957	2.7	5.0	12.0	19.1	26.9	35.3	41.8	90.0
1914-1918	1958	2.4	5.2	10.2	18.5	24.8	31.9	43.1	87.0
1915-1919	1959	2.5	4.9	11.7	17.9	26.8	30.6	43.9	83.0
1916-1920	1960	2.6	4.4	11.5	18.5	26.0	32.8	44.4	80.9
1917-1921	1961	2.4	4.5	12.0	17.8	22.5	33.2	40.3	79.8
1918-1922	1962	2.5	4.7	10.2	16.2	23.0	29.1	38.2	75.6
1919-1923	1963	2.1	4.9	9.2	16.7	22.1	26.6	34.7	71.0
1920-1924	1964	2.7	5.1	9.9	14.2	19.9	27.2	33.3	69.8
1921-1925	1965	2.7	4.9	9.0	14.7	19.0	26.1	30.2	61.0
1922-1926	1966	2.4	5.2	9.0	12.5	17.2	23.6	25.5	55.9
1923-1927	1967	2.5	5.6	8.9	10.5	13.4	19.8	24.4	49.3
1924-1928	1968	2.6	5.3	7.5	10.2	11.9	16.4	23.4	41.0
1925-1929	1969	2.6	6.6	7.5	10.9	12.5	15.7	19.5	36.1
1926-1930	1970	2.1	6.3	6.9	9.9	12.2	14.0	15.9	33.2
1927-1931	1971	2.1	6.8	6.2	8.9	9.2	12.5	15.4	31.3
1928-1932	1972	1.6	7.2	6.2	7.1	9.0	11.1	13.6	24.4
1929-1933	1973	2.3	6.4	5.3	6.1	7.9	9.7	10.7	20.8

TABLE 9C. BIRTH PROBABILITIES FOR ALL OTHER WOMEN FOR EACH YEAR 1917-73 BY AGE AND PARITY FOR GROUPS OF COHORTS FROM 1868-72 TO 1954-58--CON.

(PROBABILITIES ARE THE NUMBER OF BIRTHS PER 1,000 WOMEN IN SPECIFIED PARITY AND EXACT AGE GROUP. FIGURES IN THE "0 PARITY" COLUMN SHOW THE PROBABILITY OF FIRST BIRTHS TO "0 PARITY" WOMEN, THOSE IN THE "1 PARITY" COLUMN SHOW THE PROBABILITY OF SECOND BIRTHS TO "1 PARITY" WOMEN, ETC. BASED ON CENTRAL BIRTH RATES AND PARITY DISTRIBUTIONS FOR GROUPS OF COHORTS)

EXACT AGE AND COHORT	AS OF JANUARY 1	PARITY							
		0	1	2	3	4	5	6	7 AND HIGHER
45-49 YEARS									
1868-1872	1917	2.3	3.6	4.5	6.3	7.9	11.8	15.3	25.4
1869-1873	1918	3.4	1.8	8.8	15.0	9.2	35.7	26.0	45.8
1870-1874	1919	1.1	1.7	3.3	4.9	6.5	10.6	15.1	25.4
1871-1875	1920	1.6	3.4	5.3	6.1	7.8	14.2	15.2	31.2
1872-1876	1921	1.6	0.8	3.1	6.0	5.2	7.2	9.1	24.8
1873-1877	1922	1.5	0.8	3.1	3.6	5.2	9.0	12.1	22.7
1874-1878	1923	1.0	1.6	3.0	3.5	7.7	10.8	13.7	25.3
1875-1879	1924	1.5	1.5	4.0	4.6	7.6	10.8	10.7	24.0
1876-1880	1925	1.0	2.2	3.0	3.4	5.0	9.1	9.2	22.5
1877-1881	1926	1.4	1.5	4.0	5.6	4.9	11.2	12.4	23.9
1878-1882	1927	1.4	1.4	2.0	3.3	4.8	9.8	7.8	22.1
1879-1883	1928	0.9	1.4	2.0	3.3	4.8	10.6	9.4	23.0
1880-1884	1929	0.5	1.4	2.0	3.2	4.7	13.7	7.8	22.4
1881-1885	1930	0.4	0.7	2.0	3.1	4.7	9.6	7.8	22.8
1882-1886	1931	0.9	0.6	2.0	2.0	4.6	9.5	7.8	20.7
1883-1887	1932	0.4	0.6	2.0	3.1	3.4	11.0	8.0	22.3
1884-1888	1933	0.4	0.6	1.0	3.1	2.2	6.1	6.5	20.1
1885-1889	1934	0.4	0.6	1.9	2.1	2.2	7.8	6.7	21.2
1886-1890	1935	0.4	0.6	0.9	2.1	3.2	5.7	5.2	21.1
1887-1891	1936	0.4	0.6	0.9	2.0	2.1	5.8	7.1	21.3
1888-1892	1937	0.9	0.5	0.9	1.0	2.1	6.3	5.5	20.8
1889-1893	1938	0.4	0.5	0.9	0.9	1.1	4.4	7.6	20.8
1890-1894	1939	0.4	0.5	0.9	0.9	2.1	4.7	5.9	18.8
1891-1895	1940	0.4	0.0	0.9	0.9	2.2	5.0	6.2	19.1
1892-1896	1941	0.5	0.5	0.9	0.9	2.2	2.6	4.3	16.3
1893-1897	1942	0.5	0.4	0.9	1.8	2.3	5.2	4.5	15.4
1894-1898	1943	0.0	0.4	0.9	0.9	1.2	5.2	4.6	16.3
1895-1899	1944	0.0	0.0	0.9	1.0	2.6	5.2	4.7	13.9
1896-1900	1945	0.0	0.0	0.9	2.1	2.7	5.1	4.7	16.0
1897-1901	1946	0.4	0.4	0.9	2.2	2.8	5.0	4.7	13.6
1898-1902	1947	0.4	0.0	0.9	1.1	1.4	4.9	4.7	13.8
1899-1903	1948	0.4	0.4	0.9	1.2	1.5	2.4	4.8	11.4
1900-1904	1949	0.0	0.4	0.9	1.2	1.5	4.7	5.0	11.1
1901-1905	1950	0.4	0.4	0.8	1.2	1.6	2.3	2.6	11.5
1902-1906	1951	0.0	0.4	0.8	1.3	1.6	2.3	2.6	11.1
1903-1907	1952	0.4	0.0	0.9	1.3	1.7	2.3	5.4	10.6
1904-1908	1953	0.4	0.4	0.9	1.3	1.7	2.3	2.7	10.8
1905-1909	1954	0.4	0.4	0.0	2.7	1.7	2.3	2.8	10.1
1906-1910	1955	0.0	0.0	0.9	1.4	3.3	2.3	5.6	9.3
1907-1911	1956	0.0	0.4	0.9	1.4	1.6	2.3	2.8	10.0
1908-1912	1957	0.0	0.4	0.9	1.3	1.6	2.3	2.8	11.5
1909-1913	1958	0.3	0.4	0.9	1.3	1.6	4.6	2.7	9.7
1910-1914	1959	0.3	0.0	0.9	1.3	1.6	4.5	5.3	9.6
1911-1915	1960	0.3	0.0	0.9	1.3	3.1	2.2	5.1	8.6
1912-1916	1961	0.0	0.0	0.9	1.2	1.5	4.1	2.5	8.5
1913-1917	1962	0.0	0.0	0.9	1.2	1.5	2.0	2.5	8.3
1914-1918	1963	0.3	0.5	0.9	1.2	1.5	1.9	4.8	7.4
1915-1919	1964	0.0	0.0	0.8	1.1	1.4	1.8	2.3	7.9
1916-1920	1965	0.0	0.0	0.8	1.1	1.4	1.7	2.2	6.9
1917-1921	1966	0.0	0.0	0.8	1.1	1.3	1.7	2.1	6.7
1918-1922	1967	0.0	0.0	0.8	1.0	1.3	1.6	2.0	5.2
1919-1923	1968	0.0	0.0	0.8	1.0	1.2	1.6	1.9	4.5
1920-1924	1969	0.4	0.0	0.8	1.0	1.2	1.5	1.8	3.7
1921-1925	1970	0.0	0.0	0.8	0.9	1.1	1.5	1.8	4.3
1922-1926	1971	0.0	0.0	0.8	0.9	1.1	1.4	1.7	3.5
1923-1927	1972	0.0	0.0	0.0	0.9	1.0	1.3	1.6	2.8
1924-1928	1973	0.0	0.0	0.0	0.0	1.0	0.0	0.0	2.2

TABLE 10A. BIRTH PROBABILITIES FOR ALL WOMEN FOR EACH YEAR 1917-73 BY AGE AND PARITY FOR EACH COHORT FROM 1868 TO 1958

(PROBABILITIES ARE THE NUMBER OF BIRTHS PER 1,000 WOMEN IN SPECIFIED PARITY AND EXACT AGE GROUP. FIGURES FOR "0 PARITY" SHOW THE PROBABILITY OF FIRST BIRTHS TO "0 PARITY" WOMEN, THOSE FOR "1 PARITY" SHOW THE PROBABILITY OF SECOND BIRTHS TO "1 PARITY" WOMEN, ETC. BASED ON CENTRAL BIRTH RATES AND PARITY DISTRIBUTIONS)

PARITY AND COHORT	DIAGONAL LINE FOR JANUARY 1	EXACT AGE											
		15	16	17	18	19	20	21	22	23	24	25	26
0 PARITY													
1891-------													95.1
1892-------												108.0	100.8
1893-------											115.5	111.5	81.6
1894-------										121.5	118.1	88.7	103.8
1895-------									119.8	123.3	92.6	114.2	109.5
1896-------								118.7	121.9	95.5	120.1	119.6	101.3
1897-------							109.7	120.9	94.7	125.0	125.4	109.7	98.5
1898-------						95.5	110.6	94.4	123.7	129.4	113.8	107.1	99.8
1899-------					71.5	94.6	88.5	121.6	126.4	114.5	109.3	107.9	96.3
1900-------				47.4	69.7	78.2	113.6	124.1	111.9	110.8	112.0	103.0	91.4
1901-------			24.7	45.9	59.8	100.0	119.0	110.7	109.2	116.3	109.2	99.9	91.1
1902-------	1917	10.9	24.3	40.1	77.2	107.7	107.9	109.1	116.0	114.0	106.3	99.3	88.2
1903-------	1918	10.9	21.4	51.4	84.1	97.0	106.3	114.4	113.4	110.9	105.5	96.9	87.0
1904-------	1919	9.3	26.8	54.8	74.8	95.0	110.9	110.4	109.6	107.6	100.6	92.1	88.4
1905-------	1920	11.5	28.2	48.2	73.9	99.9	105.9	105.5	105.3	101.5	94.2	92.5	82.9
1906-------	1921	12.1	24.8	48.0	78.8	96.1	101.9	102.9	99.5	95.6	94.9	86.5	76.8
1907-------	1922	10.6	24.8	51.1	76.5	92.6	99.3	97.2	94.9	96.9	89.2	80.8	70.5
1908-------	1923	10.8	26.5	50.7	74.0	90.2	94.1	93.2	96.1	90.2	83.3	73.8	72.7
1909-------	1924	11.5	26.9	49.2	72.0	86.0	89.5	94.8	89.9	85.2	76.4	77.0	74.5
1910-------	1925	11.8	26.0	48.6	68.9	81.6	91.4	88.6	85.0	77.8	79.8	78.3	75.7
1911-------	1926	11.8	26.7	46.6	65.9	84.2	86.4	85.2	79.3	83.2	82.9	80.9	80.3
1912-------	1927	12.2	25.1	45.1	68.0	78.8	82.9	79.2	84.6	86.0	84.8	85.0	85.1
1913-------	1928	11.3	24.7	46.5	63.5	76.2	77.5	85.2	88.0	87.3	89.1	90.0	86.5
1914-------	1929	11.1	25.4	43.1	61.2	70.6	83.1	88.0	88.6	91.5	93.7	90.4	92.4
1915-------	1930	11.4	23.8	41.7	56.7	75.7	85.3	87.6	91.9	95.3	92.8	94.4	104.9
1916-------	1931	10.6	22.7	38.3	60.1	76.8	83.7	89.6	94.4	92.4	94.2	106.0	127.7
1917-------	1932	10.2	20.9	40.6	61.0	74.5	85.3	91.9	91.4	92.8	106.3	131.1	117.5
1918-------	1933	9.4	22.1	41.4	59.0	76.5	87.3	88.1	91.9	104.3	132.8	121.8	99.3
1919-------	1934	9.9	23.0	40.6	61.9	79.7	85.0	92.0	106.0	134.2	126.0	108.3	98.2
1920-------	1935	10.7	22.6	43.0	64.3	76.7	86.7	103.4	130.3	125.5	112.9	104.5	146.4
1921-------	1936	10.6	24.2	44.7	61.7	77.0	95.8	121.6	120.3	113.8	108.4	154.1	177.9
1922-------	1937	11.0	24.6	41.8	59.3	81.7	109.0	112.0	109.0	106.8	154.5	183.1	151.1
1923-------	1938	11.2	23.1	40.7	62.7	92.5	103.8	102.7	103.6	151.8	187.7	160.0	144.4
1924-------	1939	10.7	23.0	43.4	70.1	90.4	94.0	98.0	145.6	188.1	166.2	154.8	140.1
1925-------	1940	10.9	24.8	45.9	69.9	80.1	89.9	133.2	182.7	166.5	158.9	146.9	149.4
1926-------	1941	11.7	25.4	46.0	61.0	76.0	116.6	170.7	161.7	157.9	149.7	155.5	149.2
1927-------	1942	11.9	25.5	40.3	57.8	94.5	153.8	153.2	152.9	148.3	158.7	156.1	145.4
1928-------	1943	12.0	22.4	38.2	68.4	127.9	141.0	144.8	144.0	158.7	160.2	152.1	143.0
1929-------	1944	10.7	21.6	43.2	95.3	121.3	134.8	137.6	157.0	163.1	159.6	156.0	143.2
1930-------	1945	10.5	22.9	60.7	93.7	116.0	127.9	150.6	160.8	162.3	165.3	157.1	145.4
1931-------	1946	10.8	32.8	62.7	90.9	111.6	141.9	154.9	162.9	172.2	171.3	164.4	152.2
1932-------	1947	14.8	34.8	61.1	87.9	123.2	143.7	158.8	172.9	178.9	179.3	170.5	150.3
1933-------	1948	16.4	34.8	60.4	96.7	123.3	149.0	167.9	179.6	188.3	186.5	168.8	150.4
1934-------	1949	16.6	34.9	64.9	95.4	128.2	156.2	171.8	189.2	194.5	183.6	167.8	149.2
1935-------	1950	16.7	36.7	63.7	98.4	132.3	157.4	181.3	193.8	190.3	180.6	165.0	146.4
1936-------	1951	17.3	36.0	65.6	101.3	131.9	165.9	185.1	189.2	186.0	177.3	161.8	141.2
1937-------	1952	16.9	37.0	66.8	100.3	139.0	169.8	181.2	186.2	184.4	174.3	153.9	136.2
1938-------	1953	17.2	37.9	65.9	105.3	142.5	166.2	179.3	184.2	180.8	164.6	149.2	137.0
1939-------	1954	18.0	37.7	69.7	108.9	139.8	166.4	177.7	181.6	172.2	160.7	149.0	132.3
1940-------	1955	17.7	39.4	71.6	105.6	138.6	162.5	174.5	172.7	165.3	157.7	140.9	133.4
1941-------	1956	18.6	40.4	68.2	103.0	133.3	158.1	165.7	164.0	160.7	146.6	143.1	130.1
1942-------	1957	18.6	37.8	65.8	98.6	129.7	150.6	158.0	159.4	149.2	149.8	139.4	137.1
1943-------	1958	17.3	36.6	62.7	95.9	124.0	145.3	152.4	146.2	149.5	142.6	141.9	132.4
1944-------	1959	17.2	35.4	62.0	92.3	121.2	140.7	141.1	146.0	141.7	141.5	137.7	131.4
1945-------	1960	17.0	35.1	59.3	90.4	116.8	130.0	138.7	137.1	137.6	136.9	135.6	121.8
1946-------	1961	16.6	33.1	57.7	87.1	109.8	129.3	132.4	135.7	138.2	140.5	129.1	114.2
1947-------	1962	15.3	32.1	55.6	82.8	109.0	122.7	130.7	135.0	139.0	130.0	116.5	108.6
1948-------	1963	14.8	31.1	53.9	82.6	104.3	122.2	129.8	135.5	126.9	114.4	108.5	
1949-------	1964	14.8	30.5	53.4	79.1	103.3	120.0	128.5	120.8	107.8	102.5		
1950-------	1965	14.7	30.5	52.4	79.4	103.0	120.8	115.2	102.7	97.1			
1951-------	1966	14.8	30.3	52.8	79.9	105.0	109.1	98.9	92.3				
1952-------	1967	14.9	30.8	53.8	83.1	96.7	95.8	89.5					
1953-------	1968	15.3	31.5	57.3	78.4	88.2	87.8						
1954-------	1969	16.0	34.4	55.6	74.9	82.4							
1955-------	1970	17.7	34.2	55.9	71.5								
1956-------	1971	17.7	35.6	54.4									
1957-------	1972	18.7	35.3										
1958-------	1973	18.9											

TABLE 10A. BIRTH PROBABILITIES FOR ALL WOMEN FOR EACH YEAR 1917-73 BY AGE AND PARITY FOR EACH COHORT FROM 1868 TO 1958--CON.

(PROBABILITIES ARE THE NUMBER OF BIRTHS PER 1,000 WOMEN IN SPECIFIED PARITY AND EXACT AGE GROUP. FIGURES FOR "0 PARITY" SHOW THE PROBABILITY OF FIRST BIRTHS TO "C PARITY" WOMEN, THOSE FOR "1 PARITY" SHOW THE PROBABILITY OF SECOND BIRTHS TO "1 PARITY" WOMEN, ETC. BASED ON CENTRAL BIRTH RATES AND PARITY DISTRIBUTIONS)

PARITY AND COHORT	DIAGONAL LINE FOR JANUARY 1	EXACT AGE											
		27	28	29	30	31	32	33	34	35	36	37	38
0 PARITY--CON.													
1879-------													13.1
1880-------												16.7	13.9
1881-------											20.1	17.6	13.5
1882-------										25.1	21.1	17.3	14.5
1883-------									28.8	26.0	20.7	18.2	15.0
1884-------								33.5	29.9	24.7	21.5	19.0	14.1
1885-------							37.4	35.7	27.5	26.2	22.7	17.7	13.2
1886-------						46.8	40.5	32.2	30.8	27.7	21.2	16.9	13.7
1887-------					57.7	50.9	36.6	36.8	31.7	26.5	21.1	17.6	13.9
1888-------				72.4	61.7	46.1	41.9	37.4	31.0	26.0	21.9	17.9	13.2
1889-------			81.5	76.6	53.3	52.6	42.4	37.0	30.5	26.7	22.2	16.8	13.8
1890-------	1917	90.0	86.2	64.4	64.0	53.5	42.4	36.5	31.5	26.8	20.7	18.0	13.6
1891-------	1918	95.2	70.0	79.9	66.3	53.5	42.1	37.7	32.2	25.6	22.1	17.5	13.0
1892-------	1919	77.5	89.8	83.2	63.7	53.1	43.3	38.0	30.5	26.8	21.4	16.5	13.8
1893-------	1920	98.4	94.2	77.8	62.4	54.2	43.8	36.1	31.1	25.9	20.3	17.3	13.6
1894-------	1921	103.5	86.2	75.6	63.3	53.9	42.1	37.3	30.0	24.7	20.9	16.9	12.7
1895-------	1922	95.3	83.5	76.8	62.6	52.2	42.3	35.7	29.6	26.2	21.1	16.0	11.7
1896-------	1923	92.8	84.8	75.3	60.8	52.1	40.8	35.4	31.1	25.4	19.7	15.0	11.7
1897-------	1924	94.2	82.5	72.5	59.7	50.5	40.3	37.1	29.7	23.9	18.1	15.0	12.2
1898-------	1925	90.5	78.4	70.0	57.1	49.3	41.8	34.3	26.9	21.5	18.2	15.1	12.4
1899-------	1926	86.7	76.8	68.0	56.3	51.0	39.7	33.2	26.3	22.9	19.7	16.2	12.6
1900-------	1927	83.7	72.9	65.1	57.4	47.8	37.4	30.5	26.7	23.5	19.5	16.2	13.2
1901-------	1928	81.4	71.4	67.5	55.8	46.5	35.2	32.4	27.9	24.3	20.3	17.1	14.1
1902-------	1929	80.1	74.5	66.3	53.6	42.9	37.6	33.7	28.8	25.2	21.8	18.1	14.7
1903-------	1930	83.3	73.6	63.2	49.8	46.4	39.4	35.3	30.5	27.5	23.7	19.1	16.2
1904-------	1931	79.6	68.1	58.0	52.9	48.1	40.9	36.6	33.0	28.9	24.5	20.5	20.0
1905-------	1932	72.8	61.5	60.2	53.5	48.1	41.7	38.1	33.6	29.0	26.0	24.5	20.6
1906-------	1933	66.9	64.4	61.0	54.1	49.4	43.8	39.1	34.1	30.9	28.6	25.1	19.7
1907-------	1934	69.6	65.8	61.7	56.8	52.6	45.5	40.0	36.7	37.4	30.2	24.4	20.3
1908-------	1935	70.8	65.6	63.8	59.4	53.8	46.4	42.6	44.9	37.3	29.4	24.9	23.4
1909-------	1936	71.2	69.2	68.0	61.4	56.2	50.9	54.3	44.4	35.1	29.9	29.6	25.8
1910-------	1937	74.7	73.1	68.8	64.2	61.4	60.0	52.5	40.1	35.5	36.0	32.7	22.6
1911-------	1938	80.5	74.8	73.4	71.8	70.0	59.8	46.5	41.4	44.4	41.5	28.4	21.1
1912-------	1939	81.1	79.3	82.2	82.9	69.3	52.8	47.5	52.3	50.2	35.4	27.1	20.5
1913-------	1940	86.6	90.4	97.1	80.0	62.2	54.3	62.0	60.8	43.6	34.1	26.7	21.0
1914-------	1941	99.2	109.6	92.2	70.8	62.6	72.9	73.3	52.6	42.4	33.6	27.2	21.8
1915-------	1942	120.7	101.9	80.0	70.3	86.3	86.8	62.2	50.4	41.3	34.4	28.2	21.9
1916-------	1943	111.0	85.8	77.5	97.0	100.2	71.3	58.1	47.3	41.0	34.3	27.3	21.3
1917-------	1944	93.4	83.5	109.6	114.1	84.0	67.0	54.3	48.0	41.5	33.4	27.2	21.0
1918-------	1945	89.4	118.8	128.1	94.9	78.2	62.4	55.8	48.2	39.2	32.3	25.8	19.8
1919-------	1946	134.9	147.3	114.2	95.4	79.2	69.7	61.3	50.7	43.0	34.6	27.9	21.9
1920-------	1947	164.9	129.2	112.4	93.9	85.9	74.5	61.9	53.1	43.9	36.1	29.3	21.9
1921-------	1948	144.0	125.4	108.9	100.1	89.4	73.7	64.6	53.2	44.5	36.7	29.3	22.1
1922-------	1949	134.4	117.2	111.4	98.7	83.4	72.2	59.5	50.1	42.5	34.4	26.9	20.3
1923-------	1950	129.1	123.7	113.1	97.0	85.8	69.6	59.7	51.1	41.5	33.7	26.6	20.5
1924-------	1951	139.4	128.1	112.1	99.3	83.4	70.7	61.4	49.8	41.8	33.4	26.5	20.0
1925-------	1952	141.1	124.9	111.7	95.5	82.4	70.1	58.8	48.9	40.4	32.5	24.5	18.6
1926-------	1953	135.5	121.2	106.4	91.0	79.4	65.2	54.8	45.2	36.6	28.5	22.2	20.9
1927-------	1954	132.4	116.5	102.2	89.1	74.5	61.6	50.7	41.6	33.6	26.3	24.4	19.6
1928-------	1955	128.1	112.5	100.6	83.5	70.4	57.0	47.2	37.9	30.5	28.2	23.0	17.5
1929-------	1956	129.2	115.6	98.0	81.6	68.9	56.0	44.9	36.6	34.7	28.3	22.0	15.3
1930-------	1957	131.3	112.1	94.9	79.5	66.5	52.9	43.4	41.4	33.8	27.1	19.8	17.4
1931-------	1958	131.6	112.0	96.3	80.2	65.2	53.3	50.5	41.0	33.7	25.4	23.2	15.8
1932-------	1959	131.1	112.6	95.4	77.6	66.4	60.4	50.2	40.8	31.9	29.9	20.6	16.8
1933-------	1960	131.8	112.5	92.7	79.6	73.5	60.8	50.7	39.5	37.0	27.8	22.0	15.7
1934-------	1961	129.6	109.5	94.2	87.7	73.1	60.6	47.9	45.1	34.4	27.8	20.6	15.2
1935-------	1962	125.7	107.2	101.0	83.3	72.0	55.4	52.8	40.2	33.3	25.6	19.4	14.0
1936-------	1963	121.2	113.5	95.0	81.6	65.2	60.7	47.3	40.5	30.6	23.9	17.8	
1937-------	1964	124.7	108.0	94.7	77.2	71.2	57.0	48.2	36.7	28.9	22.3		
1938-------	1965	119.6	105.8	90.1	82.0	67.6	56.9	43.0	35.4	26.8			
1939-------	1966	120.3	103.8	98.0	81.7	69.9	54.7	43.4	34.0				
1940-------	1967	118.0	112.4	94.8	82.2	65.1	50.8	40.6					
1941-------	1968	125.6	108.1	96.5	77.4	60.8	49.3						
1942-------	1969	122.9	110.4	90.6	72.3	60.2							
1943-------	1970	121.5	103.4	82.8	70.2								
1944-------	1971	114.6	94.8	81.9									
1945-------	1972	104.1	91.3										
1946-------	1973	103.7											

TABLE 10A. BIRTH PROBABILITIES FOR ALL WOMEN FOR EACH YEAR 1917-73 BY AGE AND PARITY FOR EACH COHORT FROM 1868 TO 1958--CON.

(PROBABILITIES ARE THE NUMBER OF BIRTHS PER 1,000 WOMEN IN SPECIFIED PARITY AND EXACT AGE GROUP. FIGURES FOR "0 PARITY" SHOW THE PROBABILITY OF FIRST BIRTHS TO "C PARITY" WOMEN, THOSE FOR "1 PARITY" SHOW THE PROBABILITY OF SECOND BIRTHS TO "1 PARITY" WOMEN, ETC. BASED ON CENTRAL BIRTH RATES AND PARITY DISTRIBUTIONS)

PARITY AND COHORT	DIAGONAL LINE FOR JANUARY 1	EXACT AGE										
		39	40	41	42	43	44	45	46	47	48	49
0 PARITY--CON.												
1868												0.0
1869											0.5	0.0
1870										0.5	0.5	0.0
1871									0.5	0.5	0.0	0.0
1872								1.0	1.0	0.5	0.0	0.0
1873							1.4	1.0	0.5	0.5	0.0	0.0
1874						2.4	1.9	1.0	0.5	0.5	0.5	0.0
1875					3.3	2.3	1.4	0.9	0.5	0.5	0.0	0.0
1876				5.1	3.7	2.8	1.4	0.9	0.5	0.5	0.0	0.0
1877			7.3	5.5	3.7	2.8	1.4	0.9	0.5	0.5	0.5	0.0
1878	1917	10.7	7.7	5.5	3.7	2.8	1.4	0.9	0.5	0.5	0.0	0.0
1879	1918	11.5	7.6	5.9	3.6	2.7	1.4	0.9	0.5	0.0	0.0	0.0
1880	1919	11.4	8.0	5.8	3.6	2.7	1.4	0.9	0.5	0.0	0.0	0.0
1881	1920	11.9	8.5	5.4	3.6	2.7	1.4	0.9	0.5	0.0	0.5	0.0
1882	1921	12.5	7.7	5.5	3.7	2.3	1.4	0.9	0.5	0.5	0.0	0.0
1883	1922	11.6	7.7	5.5	3.2	2.3	1.4	0.9	0.5	0.5	0.0	0.0
1884	1923	11.1	7.7	5.4	3.7	2.3	1.4	0.9	0.5	0.0	0.0	0.0
1885	1924	11.1	7.6	5.0	3.2	2.3	1.4	0.9	0.5	0.0	0.0	0.0
1886	1925	11.2	7.2	5.0	3.2	1.8	1.4	0.9	0.5	0.0	0.0	0.0
1887	1926	10.5	7.4	5.1	3.3	1.9	1.4	0.5	0.5	0.0	0.0	0.0
1888	1927	11.1	7.0	4.7	3.3	1.9	0.9	0.5	0.0	0.0	0.0	0.0
1889	1928	10.7	7.1	4.8	3.3	1.9	1.0	0.5	0.5	0.0	0.0	0.0
1890	1929	10.5	7.2	4.8	2.9	2.0	1.0	1.0	0.5	0.0	0.0	0.0
1891	1930	10.7	6.9	5.0	3.0	2.0	1.0	0.5	0.0	0.0	0.0	0.0
1892	1931	10.5	7.1	4.6	3.1	2.1	1.0	0.5	0.5	0.0	0.0	0.0
1893	1932	10.2	6.2	4.7	2.6	2.1	1.0	0.5	0.5	0.0	0.0	0.0
1894	1933	9.2	6.2	4.2	2.6	2.1	1.1	0.5	0.5	0.0	0.0	0.0
1895	1934	9.3	6.2	4.7	3.1	2.1	1.1	0.5	0.5	0.0	0.0	0.0
1896	1935	9.3	6.8	4.7	3.2	2.1	1.1	0.5	0.5	0.0	0.0	0.0
1897	1936	9.7	6.7	4.7	3.1	2.1	1.1	0.5	0.5	0.0	0.0	0.0
1898	1937	9.5	6.6	4.6	3.1	2.1	1.0	1.0	0.5	0.0	0.0	0.0
1899	1938	9.8	7.4	5.0	3.5	2.0	1.5	1.0	0.5	0.0	0.0	0.0
1900	1939	10.5	7.2	5.3	3.4	2.4	1.5	1.0	0.5	0.0	0.0	0.0
1901	1940	10.5	8.2	5.8	3.9	2.9	2.0	1.0	0.5	0.0	0.0	0.0
1902	1941	12.0	9.7	6.9	4.9	3.5	2.0	1.0	0.5	0.0	0.0	0.0
1903	1942	15.0	10.8	7.9	5.0	3.5	2.0	1.0	0.5	0.0	0.0	0.0
1904	1943	15.7	11.1	7.8	5.4	3.5	1.5	1.0	0.5	0.0	0.0	0.0
1905	1944	15.1	11.2	8.5	5.7	3.3	1.9	1.0	0.5	0.0	0.0	0.0
1906	1945	15.6	12.7	9.2	5.1	3.3	1.9	0.9	0.5	0.0	0.0	0.0
1907	1946	18.1	13.9	8.2	5.0	3.2	1.9	0.9	0.5	0.0	0.0	0.0
1908	1947	19.2	12.5	8.1	4.5	2.7	1.8	0.9	0.5	0.0	0.0	0.0
1909	1948	17.2	11.7	7.7	4.6	3.2	1.8	0.9	0.5	0.0	0.0	0.0
1910	1949	16.4	11.3	7.3	5.1	3.2	1.9	0.9	0.5	0.0	0.0	0.0
1911	1950	15.6	11.2	7.6	5.2	2.9	1.9	1.0	0.5	0.0	0.0	0.0
1912	1951	15.7	11.6	7.8	4.9	3.0	1.5	1.0	0.0	0.0	0.0	0.0
1913	1952	16.5	11.2	7.7	5.2	3.1	1.6	0.5	0.5	0.0	0.0	0.0
1914	1953	16.4	11.8	7.6	4.9	3.3	1.7	1.1	0.6	0.0	0.0	0.0
1915	1954	16.8	11.4	7.5	5.2	2.9	1.8	0.6	0.6	0.0	0.0	0.0
1916	1955	16.1	10.5	7.7	4.8	3.0	1.2	0.6	0.0	0.0	0.0	0.0
1917	1956	14.9	10.9	7.3	4.3	2.5	1.2	0.6	0.0	0.0	0.0	0.0
1918	1957	15.3	10.0	6.9	4.4	2.5	1.3	0.6	0.0	0.0	0.0	0.0
1919	1958	16.1	11.4	7.2	4.3	2.9	1.5	0.7	0.0	0.0	0.0	0.0
1920	1959	16.2	11.8	7.9	4.8	2.4	1.6	0.8	0.0	0.0	0.0	0.0
1921	1960	16.7	11.9	7.7	5.2	3.5	1.7	0.9	0.0	0.0	0.0	0.0
1922	1961	15.8	10.1	6.8	5.2	3.5	1.7	0.9	0.0	0.0	0.0	0.0
1923	1962	14.8	10.6	8.9	5.4	2.7	1.8	0.9	0.0	0.0	0.0	0.0
1924	1963	14.8	12.2	8.6	4.8	2.9	1.9	1.0	0.0	0.0	0.0	0.0
1925	1964	17.1	11.6	7.8	3.9	3.0	1.0	1.0	0.0	0.0	0.0	
1926	1965	15.8	10.4	6.7	4.8	1.9	1.0	1.0	0.0	0.0		
1927	1966	13.7	9.2	7.5	3.8	1.9	0.9	0.0	0.0			
1928	1967	11.6	9.9	5.4	3.7	1.8	0.9	0.0				
1929	1968	13.7	8.3	5.6	2.8	1.9	0.9					
1930	1969	11.2	8.5	4.8	2.9	1.9						
1931	1970	12.1	8.1	5.1	3.1							
1932	1971	10.7	7.6	5.4								
1933	1972	11.4	8.1									
1934	1973	10.7										

TABLE 10A. BIRTH PROBABILITIES FOR ALL WOMEN FOR EACH YEAR 1917-73 BY AGE AND PARITY FOR EACH COHORT FROM 1868 TO 1958--CON.

(PROBABILITIES ARE THE NUMBER OF BIRTHS PER 1,000 WOMEN IN SPECIFIED PARITY AND EXACT AGE GROUP. FIGURES FOR "0 PARITY" SHOW THE PROBABILITY OF FIRST BIRTHS TO "0 PARITY" WOMEN, THOSE FOR "1 PARITY" SHOW THE PROBABILITY OF SECOND BIRTHS TO "1 PARITY" WOMEN, ETC. BASED ON CENTRAL BIRTH RATES AND PARITY DISTRIBUTIONS)

PARITY AND COHORT	DIAGONAL LINE FOR JANUARY 1	EXACT AGE											
		15	16	17	18	19	20	21	22	23	24	25	26
1 PARITY													
1891-------													188.6
1892-------												210.3	182.9
1893-------											227.3	201.8	171.9
1894-------										248.1	217.3	189.1	174.7
1895-------									255.2	236.7	202.9	192.1	167.2
1896-------								270.8	242.9	218.9	205.5	183.2	163.7
1897-------							275.2	258.5	225.7	222.0	195.3	181.0	162.6
1898-------						281.1	268.5	246.1	237.6	215.9	199.7	186.7	161.7
1899-------					250.0	266.5	250.9	255.4	223.1	214.6	201.1	181.1	156.9
1900-------				223.8	236.5	251.9	265.1	238.5	220.9	217.8	197.5	170.9	148.2
1901-------			179.1	209.0	221.9	264.9	248.4	231.0	221.9	212.8	184.8	161.6	141.0
1902-------	1917	*	167.9	203.4	244.0	258.6	243.4	235.3	220.7	198.7	176.0	152.6	131.3
1903-------	1918	*	165.5	223.2	248.0	250.6	249.4	232.9	210.8	193.5	168.7	145.4	126.5
1904-------	1919	*	185.5	224.0	242.0	261.4	247.6	222.9	207.3	185.9	160.9	141.1	127.4
1905-------	1920	*	178.6	216.3	259.7	259.6	234.7	220.0	201.0	176.8	156.6	141.9	124.0
1906-------	1921	*	172.2	235.8	255.7	243.5	231.9	215.8	190.5	172.8	156.6	137.3	119.6
1907-------	1922	*	195.7	233.8	245.1	244.9	231.3	207.8	188.8	174.5	153.5	135.6	116.4
1908-------	1923	*	191.2	229.1	245.8	244.2	222.7	205.7	190.5	169.8	150.7	130.2	121.5
1909-------	1924	*	194.4	231.0	245.8	235.2	220.4	209.1	187.2	169.0	146.4	137.3	120.1
1910-------	1925	*	194.6	234.0	232.1	231.8	223.9	202.4	185.5	163.2	153.0	133.7	120.2
1911-------	1926	*	200.0	216.7	229.2	237.0	216.6	203.0	179.1	171.0	149.0	134.6	124.2
1912-------	1927	*	181.8	217.2	233.1	225.6	217.5	194.4	187.0	165.0	149.9	137.5	129.2
1913-------	1928	*	183.7	220.4	223.3	226.5	206.4	203.0	180.6	165.8	153.1	142.8	127.9
1914-------	1929	*	183.1	207.7	224.4	215.7	216.5	196.8	182.3	170.6	158.6	141.0	134.6
1915-------	1930	*	172.4	206.2	212.6	224.7	210.3	198.6	187.9	175.7	156.0	146.3	141.6
1916-------	1931	*	173.9	198.2	221.9	219.9	213.8	204.8	193.1	172.3	160.4	153.6	155.0
1917-------	1932	*	167.9	209.5	220.0	225.4	220.6	212.0	189.4	176.2	168.2	172.6	170.7
1918-------	1933	*	180.3	207.5	223.9	232.9	226.7	205.3	193.8	181.8	190.2	185.1	158.5
1919-------	1934	*	182.5	215.2	235.4	237.4	220.8	212.5	199.3	204.6	195.4	165.4	151.0
1920-------	1935	*	185.2	225.2	235.1	231.3	233.3	217.7	210.0	205.6	172.0	151.1	187.8
1921-------	1936	*	205.9	224.8	234.6	253.2	243.4	218.3	211.5	181.0	155.1	199.2	201.9
1922-------	1937	*	202.9	221.6	264.8	266.5	239.0	224.8	191.4	161.2	212.1	214.1	192.1
1923-------	1938	*	197.2	251.5	277.8	261.7	242.2	202.3	168.2	223.4	225.6	204.0	198.5
1924-------	1939	*	231.9	264.3	273.0	260.6	215.2	178.0	235.1	236.5	217.0	211.7	205.1
1925-------	1940	*	240.9	267.2	271.6	230.8	194.1	244.0	247.7	229.0	225.4	217.9	218.0
1926-------	1941	*	260.3	273.7	241.1	214.7	257.1	259.4	242.8	238.7	231.7	233.9	229.2
1927-------	1942	*	278.9	249.3	233.9	267.2	274.7	256.5	252.7	243.6	248.2	243.7	239.1
1928-------	1943	*	250.0	247.7	272.7	290.5	272.9	267.1	257.4	261.2	257.9	255.1	248.9
1929-------	1944	*	255.5	276.2	302.8	287.7	285.0	271.8	276.0	271.3	272.1	267.7	256.0
1930-------	1945	*	274.8	314.6	300.6	301.9	290.3	292.5	286.8	286.0	286.7	276.4	266.8
1931-------	1946	*	328.4	307.5	315.6	307.7	311.6	300.5	302.2	302.4	295.1	289.3	278.9
1932-------	1947	*	317.6	323.1	321.7	325.6	313.0	312.3	314.8	308.4	306.7	298.0	276.1
1933-------	1948	*	324.9	322.8	333.3	321.6	324.4	322.3	320.6	319.2	314.9	295.7	274.9
1934-------	1949	*	321.8	332.6	325.5	333.3	330.0	328.9	332.3	327.4	313.1	296.7	273.6
1935-------	1950	*	325.1	322.6	335.5	332.9	336.3	340.0	338.6	325.4	313.1	294.8	267.7
1936-------	1951	*	304.8	331.3	334.4	339.9	349.9	345.2	335.3	326.7	313.6	289.8	260.0
1937-------	1952	*	306.2	327.4	340.2	357.0	354.0	342.5	339.0	327.6	308.1	278.7	252.7
1938-------	1953	*	319.0	333.3	360.7	358.4	351.0	350.5	340.1	323.6	297.3	273.2	248.6
1939-------	1954	*	322.6	353.4	360.3	356.1	360.4	348.2	336.0	311.8	290.7	265.9	231.3
1940-------	1955	*	334.9	350.9	357.6	366.0	357.1	344.9	326.7	305.5	282.3	247.2	220.8
1941-------	1956	*	334.8	348.1	361.9	361.9	353.5	337.3	318.8	294.9	261.0	236.2	215.6
1942-------	1957	*	331.9	351.9	363.7	357.6	346.2	327.9	304.2	269.4	246.6	229.5	212.3
1943-------	1958	*	334.9	355.4	360.0	352.0	335.2	309.4	274.7	252.6	239.3	223.3	212.7
1944-------	1959	*	334.9	352.6	354.1	341.0	314.8	275.7	254.7	243.4	230.4	223.2	212.9
1945-------	1960	*	336.5	349.3	344.0	321.0	281.1	255.9	243.7	231.4	226.9	220.9	197.0
1946-------	1961	*	338.2	342.0	325.9	286.6	257.3	241.7	229.9	228.2	224.7	201.8	177.9
1947-------	1962	*	336.9	326.5	295.6	262.9	244.1	227.7	226.8	226.2	206.5	182.4	171.9
1948-------	1963	*	316.7	294.4	269.0	248.3	228.4	223.8	224.2	208.1	184.5	175.4	
1949-------	1964	*	294.4	277.0	258.9	232.5	224.5	223.7	209.4	186.2	178.8		
1950-------	1965	*	276.2	265.1	240.8	228.1	223.6	206.8	184.8	179.6			
1951-------	1966	*	273.2	244.2	234.6	227.1	206.3	182.9	178.8				
1952-------	1967	*	243.2	233.0	228.2	206.0	182.1	175.7					
1953-------	1968	*	230.4	230.3	207.8	183.7	174.7						
1954-------	1969	*	227.7	206.9	186.7	174.1							
1955-------	1970	*	203.6	186.3	174.1								
1956-------	1971	*	185.0	171.1									
1957-------	1972	*	171.5										
1958-------	1973	*											

TABLE 10A. BIRTH PROBABILITIES FOR ALL WOMEN FOR EACH YEAR 1917-73 BY AGE AND PARITY FOR EACH COHORT FROM 1868 TO 1958--CON.

(PROBABILITIES ARE THE NUMBER OF BIRTHS PER 1,000 WOMEN IN SPECIFIED PARITY AND EXACT AGE GROUP. FIGURES FOR "0 PARITY" SHOW THE PROBABILITY OF FIRST BIRTHS TO "0 PARITY" WOMEN, THOSE FOR "1 PARITY" SHOW THE PROBABILITY OF SECOND BIRTHS TO "1 PARITY" WOMEN, ETC. BASED ON CENTRAL BIRTH RATES AND PARITY DISTRIBUTIONS)

PARITY AND COHORT	DIAGONAL LINE FOR JANUARY 1	EXACT AGE											
		27	28	29	30	31	32	33	34	35	36	37	38
1 PARITY--CON.													
1879-------													36.8
1880-------												46.0	37.0
1881-------											55.6	45.9	36.3
1882-------										65.5	55.2	45.0	35.6
1883-------									75.3	64.7	53.8	44.3	36.4
1884-------								88.4	74.5	63.7	54.3	45.5	34.1
1885-------							98.6	86.3	72.7	64.2	55.5	42.8	33.6
1886-------						114.1	95.4	83.4	72.5	64.1	51.1	42.0	32.5
1887-------					131.7	110.8	91.5	83.2	71.8	60.0	49.9	39.9	30.0
1888-------				159.2	130.6	108.9	94.3	84.0	70.9	60.5	49.2	38.6	28.6
1889-------			175.0	157.9	127.4	112.6	95.2	84.4	70.3	59.9	47.9	37.2	29.3
1890-------	1917	186.3	173.0	152.0	130.3	113.4	95.4	83.2	69.9	58.8	46.3	37.0	27.7
1891-------	1918	181.9	163.1	152.5	126.4	110.4	91.4	80.6	67.0	54.4	44.1	33.7	25.4
1892-------	1919	170.1	161.5	144.5	121.1	104.8	87.9	75.9	60.9	50.5	39.3	30.4	24.8
1893-------	1920	170.1	151.7	138.9	116.2	101.5	82.0	69.5	57.0	46.3	36.5	30.3	22.1
1894-------	1921	162.2	148.1	135.6	112.5	95.8	77.9	66.6	53.8	43.3	36.5	27.7	20.3
1895-------	1922	158.9	145.8	130.5	107.2	92.5	74.6	63.4	50.9	43.6	33.9	25.8	19.1
1896-------	1923	156.4	138.9	123.8	102.1	86.7	69.9	58.9	50.0	39.5	31.1	23.3	18.9
1897-------	1924	150.4	133.0	118.5	96.3	81.7	65.9	57.8	46.2	37.4	28.2	23.1	17.8
1898-------	1925	146.2	128.0	112.6	91.8	79.5	66.2	54.8	44.1	34.8	29.0	23.0	17.2
1899-------	1926	140.9	123.4	107.9	90.3	80.1	64.3	54.4	42.6	36.6	29.5	23.1	17.9
1900-------	1927	133.8	115.3	103.5	89.6	75.6	61.3	50.2	43.9	36.3	28.8	23.0	18.4
1901-------	1928	124.3	109.6	101.8	84.0	71.1	55.8	50.9	42.2	34.9	28.6	23.0	18.6
1902-------	1929	117.5	107.6	94.6	77.3	64.1	56.9	48.9	40.8	34.1	28.8	23.4	18.8
1903-------	1930	117.7	102.7	89.6	72.6	67.4	55.5	48.3	41.2	35.8	29.5	24.2	19.6
1904-------	1931	113.3	98.2	85.6	77.3	66.7	55.9	49.4	43.5	37.5	32.0	26.0	22.4
1905-------	1932	109.5	94.4	89.9	76.1	66.7	57.7	52.8	45.4	39.8	34.0	29.3	26.1
1906-------	1933	105.1	98.7	88.7	76.3	68.7	61.6	54.9	48.8	42.1	36.8	34.6	28.2
1907-------	1934	110.8	97.9	89.8	79.4	73.9	64.5	59.4	52.2	48.8	43.9	37.8	31.1
1908-------	1935	108.7	98.6	92.0	83.7	76.1	69.5	62.6	60.8	56.6	48.0	41.2	34.1
1909-------	1936	109.8	101.9	97.9	87.1	83.0	74.8	74.3	70.0	59.6	52.9	45.4	35.1
1910-------	1937	113.2	107.8	99.2	93.3	87.7	84.1	84.4	71.6	65.3	57.7	46.5	33.8
1911-------	1938	119.3	108.1	104.8	97.8	95.4	94.6	83.5	77.3	71.1	58.1	43.6	32.6
1912-------	1939	117.7	113.0	108.7	109.4	107.3	93.2	90.0	84.5	71.7	54.5	41.8	32.5
1913-------	1940	122.9	117.5	123.3	121.6	105.7	101.7	99.2	85.5	66.6	52.8	41.8	32.9
1914-------	1941	129.1	135.1	137.2	117.8	115.9	114.4	102.0	79.9	65.6	53.0	43.2	34.6
1915-------	1942	145.6	150.2	130.9	128.3	131.0	117.6	94.5	79.3	66.3	54.9	44.9	34.2
1916-------	1943	161.1	140.3	139.4	146.0	135.9	108.7	93.9	80.4	68.3	56.6	44.0	34.9
1917-------	1944	150.8	147.1	162.2	154.4	128.0	110.4	96.9	84.0	71.2	56.7	46.0	35.0
1918-------	1945	151.3	172.1	172.0	143.7	128.5	112.8	99.7	86.1	70.4	57.4	45.2	34.2
1919-------	1946	181.4	183.3	158.6	143.8	129.4	116.1	101.5	84.6	71.2	56.6	44.7	33.6
1920-------	1947	192.7	168.7	158.9	144.6	132.3	116.7	99.4	84.7	68.1	54.6	42.6	31.8
1921-------	1948	180.6	172.3	162.3	149.8	136.3	115.9	101.3	82.2	67.3	53.3	41.2	30.0
1922-------	1949	186.4	177.7	169.1	156.9	137.2	119.0	99.5	82.6	67.3	51.7	38.8	29.2
1923-------	1950	191.9	186.4	176.7	157.0	140.6	117.1	99.8	82.3	64.2	49.3	38.0	29.2
1924-------	1951	203.1	195.0	178.3	162.7	139.2	117.5	99.3	78.6	62.7	49.3	38.1	27.4
1925-------	1952	212.3	198.0	184.4	160.3	139.3	117.2	95.5	77.2	62.7	49.2	36.6	26.7
1926-------	1953	219.9	207.3	187.0	163.9	142.5	116.3	96.0	78.6	62.8	47.4	36.6	27.4
1927-------	1954	227.7	210.3	191.9	168.7	141.0	114.9	96.5	78.3	60.4	48.2	36.7	26.7
1928-------	1955	233.7	216.8	197.8	167.5	140.8	116.7	96.1	76.1	61.4	48.3	35.7	25.0
1929-------	1956	242.6	226.2	196.8	169.3	143.2	118.0	96.3	77.2	63.1	47.1	35.3	26.6
1930-------	1957	253.0	225.1	200.0	172.0	144.5	117.2	96.9	79.8	60.6	46.1	35.4	26.2
1931-------	1958	253.3	227.4	201.8	171.6	140.9	116.8	97.6	75.1	59.4	46.1	35.0	26.3
1932-------	1959	253.6	226.6	197.9	164.5	138.2	115.0	92.4	71.8	56.5	43.9	34.4	25.7
1933-------	1960	249.5	220.6	186.4	158.4	134.1	107.6	85.0	68.5	55.2	42.5	33.2	22.4
1934-------	1961	245.9	213.1	184.4	156.2	129.7	101.5	82.6	66.0	54.2	42.6	30.2	22.4
1935-------	1962	235.9	206.7	179.6	147.3	118.5	95.9	80.0	65.2	53.0	38.8	29.6	21.0
1936-------	1963	230.6	204.5	170.6	139.4	114.4	95.6	80.3	64.4	48.6	37.2	27.2	
1937-------	1964	227.1	191.6	161.6	135.1	115.3	95.2	79.1	60.0	46.2	35.2		
1938-------	1965	212.7	183.5	157.1	134.7	115.6	95.9	74.6	57.6	45.0			
1939-------	1966	202.8	179.0	156.7	137.1	117.1	92.4	71.9	57.0				
1940-------	1967	198.1	177.7	161.6	140.2	112.8	89.8	70.8					
1941-------	1968	196.0	181.7	164.5	134.4	109.5	87.0						
1942-------	1969	200.7	185.8	156.1	130.6	106.0							
1943-------	1970	201.3	173.2	148.0	125.1								
1944-------	1971	187.8	162.5	143.1									
1945-------	1972	172.5	157.6										
1946-------	1973	166.3											

TABLE 10A. BIRTH PROBABILITIES FOR ALL WOMEN FOR EACH YEAR 1917-73 BY AGE AND PARITY FOR EACH COHORT FROM 1868 TO 1958--CON.

(PROBABILITIES ARE THE NUMBER OF BIRTHS PER 1,000 WOMEN IN SPECIFIED PARITY AND EXACT AGE GROUP. FIGURES FOR "0 PARITY" SHOW THE PROBABILITY OF FIRST BIRTHS TO "0 PARITY" WOMEN, THOSE FOR "1 PARITY" SHOW THE PROBABILITY OF SECOND BIRTHS TO "1 PARITY" WOMEN, ETC. BASED ON CENTRAL BIRTH RATES AND PARITY DISTRIBUTIONS)

PARITY AND COHORT	DIAGONAL LINE FOR JANUARY 1	EXACT AGE										
		39	40	41	42	43	44	45	46	47	48	49
1 PARITY--CON.												
1868----------------												0.0
1869----------------											0.9	0.0
1870----------------										0.9	0.0	0.0
1871----------------									1.8	0.9	0.0	0.9
1872----------------								2.7	1.8	0.9	0.9	0.0
1873----------------							4.4	2.7	1.8	0.9	0.0	0.0
1874----------------						6.1	4.3	2.6	1.7	0.0	0.0	0.0
1875----------------					9.3	6.8	4.3	2.6	0.9	0.9	0.0	0.0
1876----------------				14.1	9.2	6.7	4.2	1.7	0.8	0.8	0.0	0.0
1877----------------			20.3	14.7	9.0	6.6	3.3	1.6	1.6	0.8	0.0	0.0
1878----------------	1917	29.2	20.0	14.5	8.9	6.5	3.2	2.4	1.6	0.0	0.8	0.0
1879----------------	1918	29.6	20.4	14.2	9.5	6.4	4.0	2.4	0.8	0.8	0.0	0.0
1880----------------	1919	29.1	20.1	14.0	8.6	5.5	3.9	1.6	1.6	0.8	0.0	0.0
1881----------------	1920	28.5	20.4	13.7	8.4	5.4	3.1	1.5	0.8	0.8	0.0	0.0
1882----------------	1921	28.6	18.5	12.7	8.2	6.0	3.0	1.5	0.8	0.8	0.0	0.0
1883----------------	1922	26.7	18.2	12.5	8.1	5.2	3.0	1.5	0.7	0.7	0.0	0.0
1884----------------	1923	26.6	18.1	12.4	7.3	4.4	2.9	1.5	0.7	0.0	0.0	0.0
1885----------------	1924	26.2	17.2	12.2	7.2	5.1	2.2	1.4	0.7	0.0	0.0	0.0
1886----------------	1925	24.0	16.6	10.4	7.0	4.2	2.1	1.4	0.7	0.0	0.0	0.0
1887----------------	1926	23.1	15.3	10.0	6.0	4.0	2.0	1.3	0.7	0.0	0.0	0.0
1888----------------	1927	22.4	14.6	9.3	6.0	3.3	2.0	1.3	0.7	0.0	0.0	0.0
1889----------------	1928	21.7	13.9	9.3	6.0	4.0	2.0	0.7	0.7	0.0	0.0	0.0
1890----------------	1929	20.8	13.8	9.2	5.3	3.3	1.3	0.7	0.7	0.0	0.0	0.0
1891----------------	1930	20.0	12.6	8.2	5.1	3.2	1.3	0.6	0.0	0.0	0.0	0.0
1892----------------	1931	17.9	11.4	7.8	4.2	3.0	1.2	0.6	0.6	0.0	0.0	0.0
1893----------------	1932	16.6	10.9	6.9	4.0	2.9	1.2	0.6	0.0	0.0	0.0	0.0
1894----------------	1933	14.9	10.0	6.7	3.9	2.2	1.7	0.6	0.0	0.0	0.0	0.0
1895----------------	1934	15.0	9.7	6.5	3.8	2.7	1.1	0.5	0.5	0.0	0.0	0.0
1896----------------	1935	13.4	8.8	6.2	4.1	2.1	1.0	1.0	0.5	0.0	0.0	0.0
1897----------------	1936	12.9	9.0	6.5	3.5	2.5	1.5	1.0	0.5	0.0	0.0	0.0
1898----------------	1937	13.4	9.4	6.0	4.0	2.5	1.5	1.0	0.5	0.0	0.0	0.0
1899----------------	1938	14.1	9.8	6.9	3.9	2.5	1.5	1.0	0.5	0.0	0.0	0.0
1900----------------	1939	14.2	10.5	6.7	4.3	2.9	1.9	1.0	0.5	0.0	0.0	0.0
1901----------------	1940	14.6	10.1	6.9	4.6	3.2	1.8	0.9	0.5	0.5	0.0	0.0
1902----------------	1941	14.5	11.0	7.9	5.3	3.1	2.2	0.9	0.4	0.0	0.0	0.0
1903----------------	1942	16.3	12.5	8.6	5.6	3.9	2.2	0.9	0.4	0.0	0.0	0.0
1904----------------	1943	19.1	13.7	9.9	6.0	3.9	2.2	0.9	0.4	0.0	0.0	0.0
1905----------------	1944	20.3	14.9	10.3	6.9	3.9	2.2	0.9	0.4	0.0	0.0	0.0
1906----------------	1945	22.1	16.3	11.2	6.5	3.9	2.2	0.9	0.4	0.0	0.0	0.0
1907----------------	1946	25.0	17.3	10.9	6.5	3.9	1.8	0.9	0.4	0.0	0.0	0.0
1908----------------	1947	25.7	16.2	10.6	6.2	3.5	2.2	0.9	0.4	0.0	0.0	0.0
1909----------------	1948	24.4	16.5	10.8	6.3	4.1	2.3	0.9	0.5	0.0	0.0	0.0
1910----------------	1949	24.2	16.7	11.4	7.3	4.1	2.3	0.9	0.5	0.0	0.0	0.0
1911----------------	1950	24.4	17.3	11.5	6.9	4.2	2.3	0.9	0.5	0.0	0.0	0.0
1912----------------	1951	25.1	17.1	11.6	7.5	4.2	2.3	0.9	0.5	0.0	0.0	0.0
1913----------------	1952	25.0	17.8	11.8	7.1	4.3	1.9	1.0	0.5	0.0	0.0	0.0
1914----------------	1953	25.7	17.8	11.6	7.3	3.9	2.0	1.0	0.5	0.0	0.0	0.0
1915----------------	1954	25.9	17.8	12.0	7.0	4.0	2.0	1.0	0.5	0.0	0.0	0.0
1916----------------	1955	25.8	17.4	11.4	6.7	4.2	2.1	1.0	0.5	0.0	0.0	0.0
1917----------------	1956	26.0	17.7	11.4	7.1	3.8	2.2	1.1	0.5	0.0	0.0	0.0
1918----------------	1957	26.0	16.8	10.7	6.8	4.0	2.3	1.1	0.0	0.0	0.0	0.0
1919----------------	1958	24.6	15.9	10.3	6.3	3.5	2.3	0.6	0.0	0.0	0.0	0.0
1920----------------	1959	22.6	14.9	10.4	6.4	3.5	1.7	0.6	0.0	0.0	0.0	0.0
1921----------------	1960	21.0	15.3	9.5	6.0	3.0	1.8	0.6	0.0	0.0	0.0	0.0
1922----------------	1961	22.2	14.3	9.4	5.0	3.2	1.3	0.6	0.0	0.0	0.0	0.0
1923----------------	1962	20.0	13.6	8.5	5.2	3.3	1.3	0.7	0.0	0.0	0.0	0.0
1924----------------	1963	19.6	13.7	8.9	4.8	2.8	1.4	0.7	0.0	0.0	0.0	0.0
1925----------------	1964	20.0	13.6	8.7	5.1	2.9	1.5	0.7	0.0	0.0	0.0	
1926----------------	1965	20.0	12.4	8.5	5.4	3.1	1.6	0.8	0.0	0.0		
1927----------------	1966	18.8	13.1	8.3	5.0	2.5	0.8	0.8	0.0			
1928----------------	1967	18.2	13.1	8.8	5.3	2.6	1.8	0.9				
1929----------------	1968	19.4	13.0	8.4	4.7	2.8	0.9					
1930----------------	1969	19.6	12.8	7.9	5.0	2.0						
1931----------------	1970	19.4	12.4	7.2	4.1							
1932----------------	1971	17.6	11.5	7.3								
1933----------------	1972	15.4	10.3									
1934----------------	1973	15.4										

TABLE 10A. BIRTH PROBABILITIES FOR ALL WOMEN FOR EACH YEAR 1917-73 BY AGE AND PARITY FOR EACH COHORT FROM 1868 TO 1958--CON.

(PROBABILITIES ARE THE NUMBER OF BIRTHS PER 1,000 WOMEN IN SPECIFIED PARITY AND EXACT AGE GROUP. FIGURES FOR "0 PARITY" SHOW THE PROBABILITY OF FIRST BIRTHS TO "0 PARITY" WOMEN, THOSE FOR "1 PARITY" SHOW THE PROBABILITY OF SECOND BIRTHS TO "1 PARITY" WOMEN, ETC. BASED ON CENTRAL BIRTH RATES AND PARITY DISTRIBUTIONS)

PARITY AND COHORT	DIAGONAL LINE FOR JANUARY 1	EXACT AGE 15	16	17	18	19	20	21	22	23	24	25	26
2 PARITY													
1891-------													213.5
1892-------												233.9	206.6
1893-------											256.2	231.5	195.6
1894-------										277.6	249.7	216.4	195.9
1895-------									283.3	272.9	235.3	217.3	198.3
1896-------								297.5	278.9	257.4	235.4	221.7	183.8
1897-------							304.0	292.7	263.9	255.9	241.1	206.4	181.8
1898-------						298.8	293.8	275.6	263.2	262.5	225.2	207.9	183.5
1899-------					270.0	306.5	285.4	281.3	273.2	245.7	229.5	212.4	180.0
1900-------				*	*	298.8	292.1	292.6	256.7	255.6	239.9	206.2	171.4
1901-------			*	*	*	302.6	304.6	266.4	258.2	264.8	232.3	195.3	168.8
1902-------	1917	*	*	*	*	324.6	275.1	266.9	268.6	250.8	216.9	187.8	156.3
1903-------	1918	*	*	*	*	278.2	271.0	271.2	257.7	236.9	209.7	177.6	147.9
1904-------	1919	*	*	*	*	283.6	273.6	262.5	249.5	231.4	200.9	170.6	148.4
1905-------	1920	*	*	*	304.8	285.7	268.3	258.5	246.7	223.1	195.4	172.7	144.3
1906-------	1921	*	*	*	299.1	283.0	268.0	257.4	238.0	217.8	197.0	165.8	143.0
1907-------	1922	*	*	*	298.1	284.6	267.1	251.3	232.4	217.9	188.6	164.4	137.4
1908-------	1923	*	*	*	292.5	279.2	257.0	242.3	231.1	208.2	185.6	157.3	140.9
1909-------	1924	*	*	*	281.8	269.7	249.5	244.5	225.8	207.5	180.8	163.5	134.8
1910-------	1925	*	*	*	270.3	261.7	251.6	238.1	224.8	203.7	187.7	156.7	132.9
1911-------	1926	*	*	*	259.3	262.9	245.7	237.1	218.8	210.6	180.6	154.7	134.6
1912-------	1927	*	*	*	257.1	255.1	244.4	227.7	224.1	202.2	177.1	154.6	137.1
1913-------	1928	*	*	*	252.4	254.2	232.3	236.6	219.9	198.5	179.8	159.8	132.8
1914-------	1929	*	*	*	*	242.4	246.4	235.8	219.7	204.4	185.3	155.2	137.3
1915-------	1930	*	*	*	*	259.3	248.7	236.1	226.6	210.5	180.3	160.0	139.2
1916-------	1931	*	*	*	*	265.7	250.0	242.2	230.3	203.6	186.2	162.4	142.2
1917-------	1932	*	*	*	*	261.1	253.8	245.1	221.3	210.9	188.3	165.9	155.9
1918-------	1933	*	*	*	*	270.5	260.1	234.4	230.8	212.3	194.0	178.8	149.7
1919-------	1934	*	*	*	*	270.6	247.0	243.8	228.1	217.2	199.6	165.1	136.4
1920-------	1935	*	*	*	*	263.2	271.2	238.7	228.2	223.8	185.5	148.4	148.0
1921-------	1936	*	*	*	284.3	303.8	261.3	233.3	235.9	208.1	165.7	167.1	156.0
1922-------	1937	*	*	*	366.3	292.2	253.3	251.5	227.7	183.2	188.2	171.8	152.3
1923-------	1938	*	*	*	349.1	289.2	272.7	244.0	199.6	209.6	190.8	171.1	155.4
1924-------	1939	*	*	*	333.3	302.0	260.6	212.9	229.5	209.2	191.5	172.4	157.6
1925-------	1940	*	*	*	324.8	283.6	227.6	246.6	229.7	212.5	193.6	175.1	165.5
1926-------	1941	*	*	*	296.0	249.0	267.0	249.6	235.6	215.4	196.7	183.6	172.9
1927-------	1942	*	*	*	262.3	279.8	270.5	257.2	238.7	217.7	204.5	189.0	174.7
1928-------	1943	*	*	*	289.5	297.2	284.3	261.6	241.2	226.5	208.0	191.3	180.5
1929-------	1944	*	*	*	310.3	309.1	288.5	263.2	250.7	228.7	212.2	197.9	185.3
1930-------	1945	*	*	*	325.6	316.1	287.3	273.9	251.1	231.4	219.2	203.4	191.5
1931-------	1946	*	*	*	343.8	307.3	296.3	271.7	253.0	239.6	223.1	211.2	197.3
1932-------	1947	*	*	*	320.9	312.3	295.2	272.5	261.8	243.1	232.5	216.2	196.0
1933-------	1948	*	*	*	326.7	316.4	296.2	282.1	264.9	253.5	236.9	215.0	198.3
1934-------	1949	*	*	*	330.1	318.3	306.8	288.4	275.9	258.8	236.9	218.8	200.1
1935-------	1950	*	*	*	339.7	329.6	312.9	297.5	281.8	258.0	240.8	220.3	197.7
1936-------	1951	*	*	*	350.7	334.1	320.3	304.3	279.3	259.8	241.6	218.8	192.6
1937-------	1952	*	*	*	350.7	342.6	325.9	298.2	279.8	261.5	239.8	211.5	185.9
1938-------	1953	*	*	*	362.4	345.7	319.5	301.1	282.3	258.9	232.2	203.4	177.2
1939-------	1954	*	*	*	355.0	336.6	325.9	303.8	279.2	252.2	223.0	193.0	158.6
1940-------	1955	*	*	*	354.4	348.8	326.0	298.9	275.5	241.9	210.0	170.9	140.6
1941-------	1956	*	*	*	366.3	348.9	324.3	297.6	263.2	227.0	184.1	151.4	133.2
1942-------	1957	*	*	*	361.7	344.1	318.1	281.9	244.5	196.3	161.4	143.0	126.3
1943-------	1958	*	*	*	361.2	338.3	303.9	262.8	211.9	173.3	153.3	135.1	129.5
1944-------	1959	*	*	*	357.8	323.1	286.3	230.8	189.3	165.5	145.2	138.3	130.8
1945-------	1960	*	*	*	342.6	310.0	253.4	207.6	180.4	156.4	148.3	141.3	120.2
1946-------	1961	*	*	*	331.7	279.5	230.7	197.2	169.2	159.1	151.6	128.8	99.4
1947-------	1962	*	*	*	306.9	254.0	220.4	185.4	172.2	162.0	139.2	107.4	90.2
1948-------	1963	*	*	*	284.0	247.1	204.1	186.8	174.3	149.2	115.5	97.2	
1949-------	1964	*	*	*	275.0	226.3	207.5	190.3	163.8	125.6	106.4		
1950-------	1965	*	*	*	251.6	230.8	209.6	176.3	136.2	117.1			
1951-------	1966	*	*	*	258.5	227.7	192.2	147.8	128.6				
1952-------	1967	*	*	*	251.7	209.3	165.1	142.1					
1953-------	1968	*	*	*	225.4	182.4	157.7						
1954-------	1969	*	*	*	197.2	175.4							
1955-------	1970	*	*	*	188.4								
1956-------	1971	*	*	*									
1957-------	1972	*	*										
1958-------	1973	*											

TABLE 10A. BIRTH PROBABILITIES FOR ALL WOMEN FOR EACH YEAR 1917-73 BY AGE AND PARITY FOR EACH COHORT FROM 1868 TO 1958--CON.

(PROBABILITIES ARE THE NUMBER OF BIRTHS PER 1,000 WOMEN IN SPECIFIED PARITY AND EXACT AGE GROUP. FIGURES FOR "0 PARITY" SHOW THE PROBABILITY OF FIRST BIRTHS TO "C PARITY" WOMEN, THOSE FOR "1 PARITY" SHOW THE PROBABILITY OF SECOND BIRTHS TO "1 PARITY" WOMEN, ETC. BASED ON CENTRAL BIRTH RATES AND PARITY DISTRIBUTIONS)

PARITY AND COHORT	DIAGONAL LINE FOR JANUARY 1	EXACT AGE											
		27	28	29	30	31	32	33	34	35	36	37	38
2 PARITY--CON.													
1879-------													49.3
1880-------												60.5	48.9
1881-------											71.2	60.2	47.4
1882-------										82.7	69.9	57.8	47.7
1883-------									93.6	81.0	67.7	58.2	47.1
1884-------								105.8	90.4	77.8	67.7	57.9	43.6
1885-------							113.3	102.7	87.1	78.2	67.6	53.9	43.0
1886-------						133.2	111.6	100.8	89.2	79.7	64.6	54.0	43.7
1887-------					155.7	132.0	110.5	103.1	91.4	76.9	65.4	54.8	41.9
1888-------				185.7	151.4	127.2	109.9	102.4	85.5	75.1	63.9	51.0	39.6
1889-------			198.8	178.8	142.1	125.4	108.3	95.3	82.6	73.7	59.4	48.7	37.6
1890-------	1917	208.3	192.9	166.7	140.1	123.6	100.9	92.7	82.1	68.0	56.2	45.2	34.4
1891-------	1918	204.0	179.3	165.5	138.8	116.8	99.3	93.6	77.3	64.9	52.8	41.9	31.9
1892-------	1919	188.0	175.6	161.8	126.6	112.9	98.6	86.9	72.4	59.8	48.4	37.8	30.3
1893-------	1920	189.6	175.7	149.4	124.9	114.9	94.1	82.3	68.9	56.2	45.3	36.9	28.3
1894-------	1921	188.5	158.7	144.8	124.8	107.9	89.0	77.4	64.0	52.1	44.0	34.8	26.4
1895-------	1922	172.8	155.5	145.2	118.3	101.9	84.5	72.3	59.6	51.4	40.9	32.8	24.7
1896-------	1923	170.8	155.5	138.2	112.8	97.4	78.6	68.4	58.8	48.1	39.3	30.3	23.8
1897-------	1924	171.2	148.3	131.0	106.6	90.4	74.1	66.4	54.9	45.8	36.1	29.8	22.8
1898-------	1925	162.3	139.5	122.7	99.2	86.0	72.7	62.2	52.2	42.2	36.1	28.3	22.0
1899-------	1926	156.2	135.1	117.7	96.5	85.9	70.9	61.7	49.7	44.1	36.0	28.2	22.4
1900-------	1927	153.3	128.6	114.0	96.6	83.2	68.5	58.6	51.8	43.1	34.8	28.5	23.1
1901-------	1928	143.5	122.3	111.9	92.6	79.2	64.9	59.5	49.7	41.4	34.1	27.7	22.8
1902-------	1929	134.7	119.4	104.7	86.6	74.3	64.6	55.6	46.7	39.9	33.1	27.3	22.4
1903-------	1930	132.8	113.5	100.5	81.7	73.9	61.0	53.4	46.0	39.3	33.0	27.2	22.4
1904-------	1931	127.7	111.5	96.7	84.3	71.5	59.9	53.6	46.1	40.1	33.8	28.5	24.6
1905-------	1932	127.7	107.3	100.0	81.2	70.1	60.2	54.1	46.8	41.2	35.3	31.3	28.9
1906-------	1933	122.7	111.4	95.9	79.8	70.4	61.1	54.7	48.2	42.5	38.0	36.8	31.1
1907-------	1934	126.5	106.0	93.5	79.6	71.4	61.3	56.2	49.6	46.2	44.3	39.5	33.8
1908-------	1935	119.0	102.7	92.0	80.3	70.7	62.8	57.5	53.7	53.7	47.7	42.0	34.6
1909-------	1936	116.8	103.4	94.8	80.9	73.5	65.2	62.5	62.8	56.8	51.3	43.9	35.3
1910-------	1937	117.8	106.9	94.1	84.0	76.0	70.4	73.3	66.4	61.5	53.8	44.7	32.7
1911-------	1938	122.0	104.3	96.8	85.1	79.8	81.2	76.2	70.3	64.1	53.9	41.6	32.4
1912-------	1939	117.3	107.0	97.2	91.3	91.6	84.0	79.2	72.8	63.1	49.9	40.1	32.1
1913-------	1940	120.6	107.8	105.3	103.0	93.6	86.3	82.2	72.4	59.1	48.5	39.8	32.9
1914-------	1941	122.7	117.2	117.1	103.1	95.8	90.5	81.9	67.8	56.9	48.3	41.2	34.9
1915-------	1942	129.3	129.3	115.0	103.1	100.5	90.3	77.1	65.9	57.7	50.3	43.5	34.7
1916-------	1943	143.7	125.6	113.1	108.3	100.7	85.3	75.1	67.0	59.9	52.8	43.4	35.2
1917-------	1944	137.6	120.3	119.1	110.4	95.4	84.0	76.9	69.6	62.9	53.1	45.2	35.2
1918-------	1945	127.8	125.7	120.8	103.4	94.3	85.1	79.2	72.7	63.5	54.9	43.8	34.7
1919-------	1946	136.5	130.1	114.8	103.9	96.2	89.5	83.9	73.8	64.8	53.1	43.8	34.1
1920-------	1947	142.3	125.2	116.1	106.9	101.0	94.2	85.7	75.2	63.6	52.9	42.5	32.5
1921-------	1948	138.6	127.5	120.3	113.0	107.5	97.1	87.0	75.0	63.3	52.3	40.8	31.1
1922-------	1949	141.2	131.4	125.8	119.8	110.4	98.5	87.0	74.6	62.9	49.9	39.0	30.0
1923-------	1950	143.8	137.7	133.4	121.9	111.6	98.2	86.5	74.6	60.4	48.2	37.5	29.1
1924-------	1951	151.2	144.6	134.9	124.3	111.4	98.1	87.1	71.5	58.4	46.3	36.7	27.0
1925-------	1952	158.4	147.1	138.3	124.6	113.1	99.6	83.8	69.0	56.6	45.8	34.3	25.6
1926-------	1953	160.0	152.1	140.1	126.3	114.3	96.4	81.7	67.6	55.6	42.5	32.7	25.0
1927-------	1954	165.8	154.7	143.8	129.7	112.5	95.4	80.5	67.0	52.7	41.0	32.1	23.2
1928-------	1955	169.2	157.5	146.9	128.1	112.1	94.1	79.7	63.1	50.9	40.1	29.6	21.7
1929-------	1956	175.1	163.5	145.7	129.2	111.0	94.4	75.8	62.1	50.1	37.6	27.7	20.9
1930-------	1957	180.5	161.7	147.7	128.3	111.0	89.9	74.6	60.6	46.4	34.9	26.4	19.0
1931-------	1958	178.1	163.5	146.3	127.9	105.4	87.3	72.6	56.6	42.5	32.9	23.9	17.3
1932-------	1959	180.1	163.6	145.6	122.0	102.0	84.7	67.1	51.4	40.1	30.4	22.6	16.8
1933-------	1960	181.2	162.3	138.9	117.4	100.1	78.7	61.3	48.3	37.6	28.7	21.7	15.0
1934-------	1961	179.9	155.7	134.0	114.9	92.4	71.4	56.9	45.4	36.5	28.0	19.7	13.5
1935-------	1962	173.5	150.9	132.0	105.8	83.8	67.2	54.2	44.4	34.9	25.2	17.3	12.1
1936-------	1963	168.1	147.0	120.6	96.2	78.8	62.8	53.8	43.2	31.3	22.1	15.7	
1937-------	1964	162.4	133.3	109.4	90.8	74.4	63.9	52.3	38.6	27.2	19.8		
1938-------	1965	145.9	120.2	102.0	85.5	75.5	63.0	46.9	33.4	24.7			
1939-------	1966	130.8	113.1	97.9	87.6	75.6	56.6	40.7	30.5				
1940-------	1967	123.2	108.2	99.6	88.2	67.4	48.6	37.1					
1941-------	1968	117.5	110.7	100.8	79.0	57.7	44.4						
1942-------	1969	120.4	111.2	89.8	66.6	52.5							
1943-------	1970	121.4	100.3	75.6	60.6								
1944-------	1971	109.8	83.5	68.6									
1945-------	1972	92.0	76.4										
1946-------	1973	83.4											

TABLE 10A. BIRTH PROBABILITIES FOR ALL WOMEN FOR EACH YEAR 1917-73 BY AGE AND PARITY FOR EACH COHORT FROM 1868 TO 1958--CON.

(PROBABILITIES ARE THE NUMBER OF BIRTHS PER 1,000 WOMEN IN SPECIFIED PARITY AND EXACT AGE GROUP. FIGURES FOR "0 PARITY" SHOW THE PROBABILITY OF FIRST BIRTHS TO "C PARITY" WOMEN, THOSE FOR "1 PARITY" SHOW THE PROBABILITY OF SECOND BIRTHS TO "1 PARITY" WOMEN, ETC. BASED ON CENTRAL BIRTH RATES AND PARITY DISTRIBUTIONS)

PARITY AND COHORT	DIAGONAL LINE FOR JANUARY 1	EXACT AGE										
		39	40	41	42	43	44	45	46	47	48	49
2 PARITY--CON.												
1868----------------												0.0
1869----------------											0.0	0.0
1870----------------										0.8	0.8	0.0
1871----------------									1.6	1.6	0.0	0.0
1872----------------								3.3	3.3	0.8	0.8	0.0
1873----------------							5.6	4.0	1.6	1.6	0.0	0.0
1874----------------						8.7	5.6	3.2	2.4	0.8	0.0	0.0
1875----------------					12.4	8.6	5.5	3.9	1.6	0.8	0.0	0.0
1876----------------				18.3	13.0	8.5	5.4	3.1	1.5	0.8	0.0	0.0
1877----------------			26.1	20.3	12.1	8.3	5.3	3.0	1.5	0.8	0.0	0.0
1878----------------	1917	38.6	27.3	18.6	12.0	8.3	5.3	3.0	1.5	0.8	0.8	0.0
1879----------------	1918	39.9	25.7	19.2	11.9	8.2	5.2	3.0	2.2	0.8	0.0	0.0
1880----------------	1919	38.8	26.9	19.0	11.8	8.1	5.2	3.0	1.5	0.7	0.7	0.0
1881----------------	1920	38.8	26.4	17.3	11.6	8.0	4.4	2.2	1.5	0.7	0.0	0.0
1882----------------	1921	38.8	24.5	16.9	11.3	7.1	4.3	2.1	1.4	0.7	0.0	0.0
1883----------------	1922	35.4	24.1	16.6	10.5	7.0	3.5	2.1	1.4	0.0	0.7	0.0
1884----------------	1923	34.8	23.6	16.3	9.6	6.2	3.4	2.1	0.7	0.7	0.0	0.0
1885----------------	1924	34.3	22.6	14.7	9.4	6.1	3.4	2.0	1.4	0.7	0.0	0.0
1886----------------	1925	33.0	21.3	15.4	9.4	5.4	3.4	2.0	0.7	0.7	0.0	0.0
1887----------------	1926	32.5	21.4	14.1	8.8	5.4	3.4	2.0	0.7	0.0	0.0	0.0
1888----------------	1927	31.0	19.6	13.1	8.6	5.3	2.6	1.3	0.7	0.7	0.0	0.0
1889----------------	1928	28.0	18.8	13.2	8.2	5.1	2.5	1.3	0.6	0.0	0.0	0.0
1890----------------	1929	25.7	18.7	11.5	7.3	4.9	2.4	1.2	0.6	0.0	0.0	0.0
1891----------------	1930	25.1	15.9	10.6	6.5	4.8	2.4	1.2	0.6	0.0	0.0	0.0
1892----------------	1931	22.6	14.8	10.3	6.3	4.0	2.3	1.1	0.6	0.0	0.0	0.0
1893----------------	1932	21.2	14.0	9.6	6.2	3.4	1.7	1.1	0.6	0.0	0.0	0.0
1894----------------	1933	20.1	13.6	9.3	5.5	3.3	2.2	1.1	0.6	0.0	0.0	0.0
1895----------------	1934	19.0	13.3	8.5	4.8	3.2	2.1	1.1	0.5	0.0	0.0	0.0
1896----------------	1935	18.2	12.5	7.9	5.3	3.2	2.1	1.1	0.5	0.0	0.0	0.0
1897----------------	1936	17.8	11.8	8.2	5.1	3.1	2.1	1.0	0.5	0.0	0.0	0.0
1898----------------	1937	17.1	12.1	8.1	5.1	3.0	2.0	1.0	0.5	0.0	0.0	0.0
1899----------------	1938	17.5	12.5	8.0	5.5	3.5	2.0	1.0	0.5	0.0	0.0	0.0
1900----------------	1939	17.6	12.6	8.6	5.6	4.1	2.5	1.5	0.5	0.5	0.0	0.0
1901----------------	1940	17.4	13.0	8.5	6.0	4.5	2.5	1.5	0.5	0.0	0.0	0.0
1902----------------	1941	17.6	13.2	9.8	6.9	4.9	2.5	1.0	0.5	0.0	0.0	0.0
1903----------------	1942	18.6	14.8	11.0	7.7	4.8	2.4	1.4	0.5	0.0	0.0	0.0
1904----------------	1943	21.8	16.1	11.9	7.6	5.2	2.9	1.4	0.5	0.0	0.0	0.0
1905----------------	1944	23.7	18.0	12.3	8.1	5.2	2.9	1.0	0.5	0.0	0.0	0.0
1906----------------	1945	25.4	17.9	12.7	8.0	4.7	2.4	1.4	0.5	0.0	0.0	0.0
1907----------------	1946	26.4	19.0	12.5	7.4	4.6	2.8	1.4	0.5	0.0	0.0	0.0
1908----------------	1947	26.8	17.7	11.8	7.3	5.0	2.7	1.4	0.5	0.0	0.0	0.0
1909----------------	1948	25.0	17.4	11.6	7.6	4.9	2.7	1.3	0.4	0.0	0.0	0.0
1910----------------	1949	25.1	17.7	12.4	8.4	5.3	3.1	1.3	0.4	0.4	0.0	0.0
1911----------------	1950	24.7	18.2	13.0	8.3	5.7	3.1	1.3	0.9	0.4	0.0	0.0
1912----------------	1951	25.4	19.1	13.2	8.9	5.1	3.0	1.3	0.9	0.0	0.0	0.0
1913----------------	1952	26.4	19.1	13.7	8.8	5.4	2.9	1.3	0.4	0.0	0.0	0.0
1914----------------	1953	26.6	19.4	13.4	8.6	5.3	2.9	1.2	0.4	0.0	0.0	0.0
1915----------------	1954	27.0	19.6	13.6	8.5	4.8	2.8	1.2	0.4	0.4	0.0	0.0
1916----------------	1955	27.2	18.7	13.2	7.6	4.8	2.8	1.2	0.8	0.0	0.0	0.0
1917----------------	1956	27.0	18.9	12.3	7.6	4.8	2.4	1.2	0.4	0.0	0.0	0.0
1918----------------	1957	25.7	17.6	11.8	7.1	4.4	2.4	1.2	0.4	0.0	0.0	0.0
1919----------------	1958	24.9	17.4	11.3	7.4	3.9	2.4	1.2	0.4	0.0	0.0	0.0
1920----------------	1959	24.1	16.6	11.2	6.6	3.9	2.0	0.8	0.4	0.0	0.0	0.0
1921----------------	1960	23.0	16.3	10.1	6.3	3.5	2.0	0.8	0.4	0.0	0.0	0.0
1922----------------	1961	22.2	14.9	9.9	5.9	3.6	1.6	0.8	0.4	0.0	0.0	0.0
1923----------------	1962	20.8	13.9	9.6	5.6	3.2	1.6	0.8	0.0	0.0	0.0	0.0
1924----------------	1963	19.4	13.6	8.4	4.8	2.8	1.6	0.4	0.4	0.0	0.0	0.0
1925----------------	1964	19.0	12.2	7.8	4.5	2.5	1.2	0.4	0.4	0.0	0.0	
1926----------------	1965	17.8	11.7	7.5	4.2	2.5	1.3	0.4	0.4	0.0		
1927----------------	1966	16.2	11.2	6.5	4.3	2.2	0.9	0.4	0.0			
1928----------------	1967	15.8	9.7	6.2	3.5	1.8	0.9	0.4				
1929----------------	1968	13.9	9.4	5.9	3.2	1.8	0.9					
1930----------------	1969	13.2	8.7	5.5	2.8	1.4						
1931----------------	1970	12.8	7.8	4.6	2.8							
1932----------------	1971	11.0	6.9	4.1								
1933----------------	1972	9.6	6.0									
1934----------------	1973	8.6										

TABLE 10A. BIRTH PROBABILITIES FOR ALL WOMEN FOR EACH YEAR 1917-73 BY AGE AND PARITY FOR EACH COHORT FROM 1868 TO 1958--CON.

(PROBABILITIES ARE THE NUMBER OF BIRTHS PER 1,000 WOMEN IN SPECIFIED PARITY AND EXACT AGE GROUP. FIGURES FOR "0 PARITY" SHOW THE PROBABILITY OF FIRST BIRTHS TO "C PARITY" WOMEN, THOSE FOR "1 PARITY" SHOW THE PROBABILITY OF SECOND BIRTHS TO "1 PARITY" WOMEN, ETC. BASED ON CENTRAL BIRTH RATES AND PARITY DISTRIBUTIONS)

PARITY AND COHORT	DIAGONAL LINE FOR JANUARY 1	EXACT AGE											
		15	16	17	18	19	20	21	22	23	24	25	26
3 PARITY													
1891-------													249.0
1892-------												267.1	243.7
1893-------											270.9	259.9	230.3
1894-------										281.5	268.5	250.3	235.0
1895-------									274.4	284.5	262.3	257.8	241.4
1896-------								287.7	277.8	278.0	270.6	268.4	226.1
1897-------							*	292.5	272.5	284.4	285.9	253.4	227.6
1898-------						*	*	287.7	281.8	306.0	271.0	261.5	230.8
1899-------					*	*	*	302.4	303.6	287.3	283.5	263.9	229.1
1900-------				*	*	*	*	326.6	284.1	306.6	288.0	257.3	225.4
1901-------			*	*	*	*	*	292.3	297.3	310.1	280.6	251.5	226.3
1902-------	1917	*	*	*	*	*	*	312.5	305.0	294.3	272.6	249.1	210.8
1903-------	1918	*	*	*	*	*	*	311.6	299.2	293.7	273.0	236.4	200.2
1904-------	1919	*	*	*	*	*	*	311.0	306.4	296.2	260.8	231.2	203.6
1905-------	1920	*	*	*	*	*	330.0	320.4	307.2	281.4	255.4	233.0	200.2
1906-------	1921	*	*	*	*	*	*	315.0	284.9	270.5	256.8	224.5	200.5
1907-------	1922	*	*	*	*	*	*	291.5	272.5	272.0	244.7	223.8	192.1
1908-------	1923	*	*	*	*	*	*	283.5	283.5	263.6	247.0	217.3	200.3
1909-------	1924	*	*	*	*	*	*	289.5	270.7	263.4	237.3	228.6	193.2
1910-------	1925	*	*	*	*	*	*	281.8	273.3	258.1	252.3	220.2	191.3
1911-------	1926	*	*	*	*	*	*	284.1	267.1	271.0	245.4	218.9	192.4
1912-------	1927	*	*	*	*	*	*	278.1	280.6	269.3	245.6	222.4	196.8
1913-------	1928	*	*	*	*	*	*	291.9	282.5	267.5	252.0	225.8	190.5
1914-------	1929	*	*	*	*	*	*	303.2	284.0	276.4	254.2	218.8	191.7
1915-------	1930	*	*	*	*	*	*	300.0	293.2	276.7	245.9	226.2	191.2
1916-------	1931	*	*	*	*	*	*	310.3	291.5	269.0	262.4	224.1	193.6
1917-------	1932	*	*	*	*	*	*	299.3	275.6	292.2	257.7	220.4	207.1
1918-------	1933	*	*	*	*	*	*	279.2	302.3	288.4	252.0	235.4	198.9
1919-------	1934	*	*	*	*	*	*	303.8	295.9	280.2	259.6	222.6	181.5
1920-------	1935	*	*	*	*	*	*	284.0	293.9	289.6	250.5	202.7	191.6
1921-------	1936	*	*	*	*	*	*	289.6	299.0	279.3	226.8	217.6	185.7
1922-------	1937	*	*	*	*	*	300.0	309.8	296.7	246.5	243.5	210.1	179.6
1923-------	1938	*	*	*	*	*	316.8	307.3	261.4	265.7	233.5	205.7	184.6
1924-------	1939	*	*	*	*	*	320.8	271.8	282.8	257.8	234.2	211.8	188.2
1925-------	1940	*	*	*	*	*	289.7	294.4	276.8	261.0	243.4	214.3	196.6
1926-------	1941	*	*	*	*	*	*	292.8	283.8	272.5	244.3	221.6	199.8
1927-------	1942	*	*	*	*	*	*	306.9	299.7	269.7	251.0	225.2	200.5
1928-------	1943	*	*	*	*	*	336.6	325.2	294.0	279.2	250.6	221.8	202.9
1929-------	1944	*	*	*	*	*	359.6	315.1	302.2	276.9	250.3	225.1	200.9
1930-------	1945	*	*	*	*	*	335.8	320.1	295.7	272.2	250.8	223.3	202.3
1931-------	1946	*	*	*	*	*	333.3	316.5	296.1	276.2	248.7	227.4	205.0
1932-------	1947	*	*	*	*	*	340.8	310.4	298.0	273.3	253.6	228.9	203.4
1933-------	1948	*	*	*	*	*	342.1	321.9	300.0	279.7	255.4	226.0	206.7
1934-------	1949	*	*	*	*	*	350.3	320.8	304.5	279.7	250.6	229.1	205.1
1935-------	1950	*	*	*	*	*	349.5	328.1	303.5	275.4	252.7	228.1	203.0
1936-------	1951	*	*	*	*	*	360.2	329.1	302.3	278.9	254.2	226.5	196.6
1937-------	1952	*	*	*	*	*	362.4	329.3	304.9	281.0	253.8	220.5	188.4
1938-------	1953	*	*	*	*	*	359.6	334.9	307.5	279.0	244.9	207.6	176.6
1939-------	1954	*	*	*	*	388.3	364.8	328.8	302.4	267.7	229.3	193.6	153.0
1940-------	1955	*	*	*	*	392.5	355.1	327.5	291.1	250.0	212.2	167.0	131.2
1941-------	1956	*	*	*	*	383.9	358.9	315.4	274.0	232.3	185.4	144.9	122.3
1942-------	1957	*	*	*	*	388.9	346.0	300.5	256.9	203.6	161.6	136.9	118.6
1943-------	1958	*	*	*	*	375.0	333.3	283.9	228.9	181.6	155.8	134.2	125.9
1944-------	1959	*	*	*	*	352.9	313.1	252.7	205.5	176.1	151.5	141.7	130.0
1945-------	1960	*	*	*	*	*	287.1	234.2	202.1	174.2	161.1	147.1	121.3
1946-------	1961	*	*	*	*	*	265.5	225.7	194.8	182.5	164.6	136.0	100.5
1947-------	1962	*	*	*	*	*	261.7	217.7	200.5	183.4	153.0	112.8	91.1
1948-------	1963	*	*	*	*	*	242.4	222.7	201.2	170.1	126.5	103.3	
1949-------	1964	*	*	*	*	*	252.1	229.3	189.4	145.3	118.2		
1950-------	1965	*	*	*	*	*	247.8	201.0	161.8	133.0			
1951-------	1966	*	*	*	*	*	220.2	179.9	151.1				
1952-------	1967	*	*	*	*	*	190.0	166.7					
1953-------	1968	*	*	*	*	*	*						
1954-------	1969	*	*	*	*	*							
1955-------	1970	*	*	*	*								
1956-------	1971	*	*	*									
1957-------	1972	*	*										
1958-------	1973	*											

TABLE 10A. BIRTH PROBABILITIES FOR ALL WOMEN FOR EACH YEAR 1917-73 BY AGE AND PARITY FOR EACH COHORT FROM 1868 TO 1958--CON.

(PROBABILITIES ARE THE NUMBER OF BIRTHS PER 1,000 WOMEN IN SPECIFIED PARITY AND EXACT AGE GROUP. FIGURES FOR "0 PARITY" SHOW THE PROBABILITY OF FIRST BIRTHS TO "0 PARITY" WOMEN, THOSE FOR "1 PARITY" SHOW THE PROBABILITY OF SECOND BIRTHS TO "1 PARITY" WOMEN, ETC. BASED ON CENTRAL BIRTH RATES AND PARITY DISTRIBUTIONS)

PARITY AND COHORT	DIAGONAL LINE FOR JANUARY 1	EXACT AGE 27	28	29	30	31	32	33	34	35	36	37	38
3 PARITY--CON.													
1879-------													69.8
1880-------												85.0	70.5
1881-------											97.6	84.3	68.1
1882-------										112.6	96.6	81.0	66.6
1883-------									125.5	110.4	92.8	79.6	66.7
1884-------								139.5	121.8	106.7	91.5	79.7	61.3
1885-------							145.7	135.0	117.3	105.2	92.2	73.5	59.9
1886-------						165.7	141.7	129.5	115.6	106.3	85.1	72.5	59.1
1887-------					186.0	161.3	136.0	128.2	117.8	96.8	83.7	71.3	58.1
1888-------				220.3	181.6	154.4	133.7	130.1	106.1	95.2	81.5	69.3	54.1
1889-------			234.0	214.1	171.8	151.7	136.0	116.8	104.0	92.6	78.3	65.0	50.7
1890-------	1917	246.1	228.8	204.0	170.5	155.4	122.8	115.2	102.6	87.5	74.2	61.0	46.9
1891-------	1918	242.2	218.5	204.3	173.4	140.9	122.0	113.6	97.2	84.4	69.8	56.7	42.7
1892-------	1919	230.1	219.5	205.2	157.2	139.9	120.3	108.8	94.0	79.9	64.7	51.4	43.1
1893-------	1920	230.4	216.3	184.4	153.6	138.4	115.6	103.7	89.2	73.8	59.3	51.0	40.7
1894-------	1921	231.8	197.9	181.3	152.1	133.1	111.3	100.2	83.0	68.8	59.1	48.7	37.7
1895-------	1922	215.5	195.7	181.3	146.9	128.9	107.9	93.9	77.8	68.4	56.5	46.1	36.4
1896-------	1923	214.2	194.7	174.8	143.0	125.1	101.1	87.7	76.9	65.3	54.0	44.1	36.5
1897-------	1924	215.1	188.4	170.5	138.9	118.1	96.0	87.4	73.7	63.3	51.8	44.7	34.9
1898-------	1925	210.2	184.9	166.5	131.4	112.6	96.8	84.4	71.2	60.6	52.6	42.5	33.2
1899-------	1926	209.6	184.9	160.3	128.3	115.4	95.3	84.8	71.3	63.6	51.6	41.9	33.1
1900-------	1927	209.4	175.4	152.6	129.7	111.7	94.5	83.1	74.0	62.2	50.6	41.5	34.6
1901-------	1928	195.4	164.5	151.9	124.6	108.8	90.6	83.9	69.8	59.2	48.9	42.7	33.5
1902-------	1929	183.3	163.7	145.8	120.2	103.6	90.9	79.9	67.1	57.2	49.8	41.1	32.5
1903-------	1930	182.2	159.1	141.3	116.2	105.6	86.8	75.5	64.9	57.8	48.7	39.8	32.7
1904-------	1931	181.3	160.3	141.9	120.9	103.3	83.8	75.4	65.8	57.7	48.2	41.4	35.6
1905-------	1932	181.5	158.6	146.3	117.5	99.5	84.6	75.8	65.0	57.3	50.0	43.8	40.9
1906-------	1933	177.2	159.9	139.2	112.8	98.9	83.5	75.2	65.8	58.7	51.2	50.4	43.3
1907-------	1934	180.7	152.5	133.0	111.9	97.6	82.5	74.8	66.8	60.4	57.4	52.3	45.1
1908-------	1935	173.3	148.6	132.6	112.7	97.5	84.7	77.3	70.7	69.6	61.8	54.8	45.0
1909-------	1936	170.9	149.2	135.8	110.7	98.7	86.1	82.0	79.9	72.0	64.8	56.0	46.3
1910-------	1937	171.1	153.9	132.6	113.9	101.1	90.7	92.9	83.4	75.1	65.2	56.3	44.5
1911-------	1938	175.9	148.6	134.7	115.1	102.8	101.8	94.3	84.4	75.8	66.0	52.9	43.2
1912-------	1939	170.0	151.9	136.4	120.1	116.0	104.4	94.6	85.2	75.7	61.7	51.4	42.7
1913-------	1940	171.8	153.1	139.2	130.9	116.5	101.9	96.1	84.3	70.7	59.8	51.5	44.5
1914-------	1941	173.3	156.1	150.2	128.9	113.7	103.4	92.4	78.9	68.6	60.5	53.2	46.5
1915-------	1942	173.2	167.6	146.4	124.1	114.5	99.6	87.5	78.0	70.4	62.6	55.5	47.8
1916-------	1943	188.5	162.9	138.6	125.3	111.5	94.7	87.2	79.7	72.9	65.2	57.6	49.0
1917-------	1944	181.2	150.9	142.0	122.4	105.2	95.7	88.7	81.9	75.1	68.1	59.2	48.5
1918-------	1945	165.3	153.3	137.4	115.1	107.1	95.9	91.5	85.3	77.9	68.4	57.9	47.1
1919-------	1946	171.9	150.2	131.0	118.2	107.4	100.8	96.6	87.9	79.3	68.5	57.7	47.4
1920-------	1947	168.1	144.6	134.7	120.2	113.7	107.9	99.2	90.3	78.8	67.0	57.6	45.0
1921-------	1948	162.1	148.4	136.9	126.8	120.7	108.9	101.7	90.2	77.9	68.3	54.8	43.8
1922-------	1949	165.0	150.8	142.7	133.1	121.2	111.0	100.6	88.8	78.2	64.0	53.0	42.3
1923-------	1950	167.9	159.3	148.3	132.4	123.5	110.9	100.4	89.4	74.9	62.4	51.3	40.0
1924-------	1951	176.9	162.6	149.0	136.5	123.3	111.3	100.8	86.1	72.9	60.9	48.8	37.2
1925-------	1952	180.7	163.7	152.8	136.1	124.2	111.1	97.8	83.7	71.1	58.1	45.2	34.7
1926-------	1953	181.1	168.3	153.0	137.6	123.8	108.1	95.0	82.0	68.4	54.2	42.5	33.5
1927-------	1954	184.8	166.9	153.9	136.9	121.4	106.2	92.9	79.1	63.4	51.3	40.7	29.9
1928-------	1955	183.7	168.2	153.7	134.7	120.7	104.6	91.1	73.4	60.8	48.8	36.8	27.0
1929-------	1956	184.2	168.8	150.9	135.5	118.5	103.9	85.5	71.0	58.7	44.5	33.1	24.3
1930-------	1957	185.5	165.9	152.9	133.0	118.1	96.9	82.6	68.4	53.1	39.5	30.0	22.2
1931-------	1958	183.8	168.3	150.0	132.9	110.7	94.4	79.2	61.3	46.5	36.7	27.2	20.5
1932-------	1959	187.2	166.8	148.8	124.9	107.3	89.3	71.2	53.9	42.8	32.6	25.1	18.9
1933-------	1960	186.4	165.8	141.6	120.6	102.0	80.2	62.2	50.2	39.3	30.9	23.5	16.4
1934-------	1961	182.9	157.6	135.3	115.2	91.1	70.5	57.5	45.3	37.0	29.2	21.4	14.4
1935-------	1962	176.7	151.9	130.5	101.5	80.2	65.8	52.1	44.1	35.4	26.4	18.2	12.1
1936-------	1963	169.5	145.3	114.9	89.8	73.5	59.1	51.4	42.5	31.8	22.3	15.5	
1937-------	1964	160.6	127.1	100.5	82.4	67.8	59.4	49.8	38.1	26.9	19.6		
1938-------	1965	139.2	109.4	92.1	76.8	68.3	58.4	44.9	32.4	23.8			
1939-------	1966	120.0	102.0	86.2	77.5	68.2	53.5	38.8	28.8				
1940-------	1967	110.9	96.2	88.6	78.9	62.5	45.2	34.3					
1941-------	1968	106.4	100.1	90.4	73.2	53.1	40.9						
1942-------	1969	112.7	102.9	84.7	61.5	48.0							
1943-------	1970	115.7	96.1	71.9	56.0								
1944-------	1971	107.8	81.3	64.9									
1945-------	1972	91.2	73.7										
1946-------	1973	81.6											

TABLE 10A. BIRTH PROBABILITIES FOR ALL WOMEN FOR EACH YEAR 1917-73 BY AGE AND PARITY FOR EACH COHORT FROM 1868 TO 1958--CON.

(PROBABILITIES ARE THE NUMBER OF BIRTHS PER 1,000 WOMEN IN SPECIFIED PARITY AND EXACT AGE GROUP. FIGURES FOR "0 PARITY" SHOW THE PROBABILITY OF FIRST BIRTHS TO "C PARITY" WOMEN, THOSE FOR "1 PARITY" SHOW THE PROBABILITY OF SECOND BIRTHS TO "1 PARITY" WOMEN, ETC. BASED ON CENTRAL BIRTH RATES AND PARITY DISTRIBUTIONS)

PARITY AND COHORT	DIAGONAL LINE FOR JANUARY 1	EXACT AGE										
		39	40	41	42	43	44	45	46	47	48	49
3 PARITY--CON.												
1868												0.9
1869											0.9	0.9
1870										1.9	1.9	0.9
1871									2.8	1.8	0.9	0.9
1872								5.5	3.6	0.9	0.9	0.9
1873							9.0	5.4	2.7	1.8	0.9	0.9
1874						13.4	9.0	4.5	3.6	1.8	0.9	0.9
1875					19.5	12.4	8.0	5.4	2.7	0.9	0.9	0.9
1876				28.7	18.4	13.2	8.8	5.3	2.7	0.9	0.9	0.0
1877			40.2	27.7	18.2	13.1	7.9	4.4	2.6	0.9	0.9	0.0
1878	1917	57.2	40.1	28.4	18.2	13.0	7.9	4.4	2.6	0.9	0.9	0.0
1879	1918	57.2	39.1	29.2	18.2	12.2	7.8	4.4	2.6	0.9	0.9	0.0
1880	1919	56.3	39.9	28.3	17.2	12.1	7.8	4.3	2.6	1.7	0.9	0.0
1881	1920	56.5	39.5	26.3	17.1	12.0	6.9	4.3	2.6	0.9	0.0	0.0
1882	1921	55.7	36.4	25.9	16.8	10.9	6.8	4.2	2.5	0.8	0.0	0.0
1883	1922	51.1	35.2	25.6	16.6	10.8	5.8	3.3	1.7	0.8	0.0	0.0
1884	1923	49.8	34.8	25.3	15.6	9.9	5.8	3.3	1.7	0.8	0.8	0.0
1885	1924	49.2	34.4	22.6	14.6	8.9	5.7	3.3	1.6	0.8	0.8	0.0
1886	1925	47.8	30.8	21.4	13.5	8.8	5.6	3.2	1.6	0.8	0.0	0.0
1887	1926	44.7	29.5	20.3	12.5	8.6	4.7	2.4	1.6	0.8	0.0	0.0
1888	1927	41.7	27.4	18.4	12.3	7.7	4.6	2.3	1.5	0.8	0.8	0.0
1889	1928	39.2	25.3	18.6	11.2	7.5	4.5	2.3	1.5	0.8	0.0	0.0
1890	1929	35.5	25.5	16.8	11.0	7.3	4.4	2.2	1.5	0.7	0.7	0.0
1891	1930	35.7	23.7	16.6	10.1	7.3	3.6	2.2	1.5	0.7	0.0	0.0
1892	1931	33.4	22.1	15.1	10.1	6.5	3.6	2.2	1.4	0.0	0.0	0.0
1893	1932	31.0	21.2	14.9	9.3	5.7	3.6	2.1	0.7	0.0	0.0	0.0
1894	1933	29.5	21.1	14.1	8.5	5.7	3.5	2.1	0.7	0.0	0.0	0.0
1895	1934	29.5	19.7	13.4	9.2	5.7	3.6	1.4	0.7	0.0	0.0	0.0
1896	1935	27.5	19.1	13.5	8.5	5.7	2.9	1.4	0.7	0.0	0.0	0.0
1897	1936	27.1	19.3	12.9	8.6	5.8	2.9	1.4	0.7	0.7	0.0	0.0
1898	1937	26.0	18.1	13.8	8.7	5.8	3.6	2.2	1.5	0.7	0.0	0.0
1899	1938	26.5	19.1	13.3	8.9	5.9	3.7	2.2	1.5	0.7	0.0	0.0
1900	1939	26.4	18.8	13.6	9.0	6.8	4.5	2.3	1.5	0.0	0.0	0.0
1901	1940	25.1	19.0	13.7	9.9	7.6	4.6	2.3	0.8	0.0	0.0	0.0
1902	1941	26.2	20.0	15.4	10.8	7.7	4.6	2.3	0.8	0.0	0.0	0.0
1903	1942	27.9	22.4	16.2	11.6	7.7	4.6	2.3	0.8	0.8	0.0	0.0
1904	1943	32.3	23.5	18.0	11.7	7.8	3.9	2.3	1.6	0.0	0.0	0.0
1905	1944	34.2	26.1	18.1	12.6	7.9	4.7	2.4	0.8	0.8	0.0	0.0
1906	1945	36.6	26.1	18.9	11.8	7.8	3.9	2.4	0.8	0.8	0.0	0.0
1907	1946	35.9	27.1	18.5	11.5	7.7	4.6	2.3	1.5	0.8	0.0	0.0
1908	1947	36.6	25.4	17.7	11.5	7.7	4.6	2.3	1.5	0.8	0.0	0.0
1909	1948	35.0	24.9	17.3	12.8	8.3	5.3	2.3	1.5	0.8	0.0	0.0
1910	1949	34.3	25.2	18.4	12.5	8.8	4.4	2.2	1.5	0.0	0.0	0.0
1911	1950	34.0	26.6	19.3	12.8	8.6	5.0	2.1	0.7	0.7	0.0	0.0
1912	1951	35.2	28.0	19.5	13.9	9.0	4.9	2.8	1.4	0.7	0.0	0.0
1913	1952	37.3	28.3	20.8	13.4	8.7	4.7	2.0	1.3	0.7	0.0	0.0
1914	1953	37.6	29.0	19.9	13.5	8.4	4.5	2.6	1.3	0.0	0.0	0.0
1915	1954	39.3	28.6	19.9	13.6	8.1	5.0	2.5	0.6	0.6	0.0	0.0
1916	1955	38.3	27.3	20.6	12.7	8.5	4.3	2.4	1.2	0.0	0.0	0.0
1917	1956	38.2	28.7	19.4	12.9	7.7	4.7	2.4	0.6	0.0	0.0	0.0
1918	1957	37.7	26.9	18.9	12.0	7.5	4.0	1.7	0.6	0.0	0.0	0.0
1919	1958	35.7	25.8	18.2	12.1	7.2	3.9	1.7	0.6	0.0	0.0	0.0
1920	1959	35.4	25.2	17.7	11.3	6.5	3.8	1.6	0.5	0.0	0.0	0.0
1921	1960	33.9	24.6	16.8	10.0	6.3	3.2	1.6	0.5	0.0	0.0	0.0
1922	1961	32.2	22.6	14.9	9.3	5.2	3.1	1.6	0.5	0.0	0.0	0.0
1923	1962	29.5	20.6	14.1	8.6	5.1	3.0	1.0	0.5	0.0	0.0	0.0
1924	1963	27.5	19.7	12.8	7.9	5.0	2.5	1.0	0.5	0.0	0.0	0.0
1925	1964	26.6	18.0	11.2	7.3	3.9	2.0	1.0	0.5	0.0	0.0	
1926	1965	24.1	15.9	10.6	5.8	3.4	1.9	1.0	0.0	0.0		
1927	1966	21.4	14.3	9.1	5.3	3.4	1.4	0.5	0.0			
1928	1967	19.5	12.9	8.1	5.3	2.4	1.0	0.5				
1929	1968	17.3	12.2	7.5	4.2	2.4	0.9					
1930	1969	16.2	11.2	6.1	3.7	1.9						
1931	1970	15.1	9.2	5.5	3.2							
1932	1971	12.6	7.7	4.5								
1933	1972	10.7	6.7									
1934	1973	9.2										

TABLE 10A. BIRTH PROBABILITIES FOR ALL WOMEN FOR EACH YEAR 1917-73 BY AGE AND PARITY FOR EACH COHORT FROM 1868 TO 1958--CON.

(PROBABILITIES ARE THE NUMBER OF BIRTHS PER 1,000 WOMEN IN SPECIFIED PARITY AND EXACT AGE GROUP. FIGURES FOR "0 PARITY" SHOW THE PROBABILITY OF FIRST BIRTHS TO "C PARITY" WOMEN, THOSE FOR "1 PARITY" SHOW THE PROBABILITY OF SECOND BIRTHS TO "1 PARITY" WOMEN, ETC. BASED ON CENTRAL BIRTH RATES AND PARITY DISTRIBUTIONS)

PARITY AND COHORT	DIAGONAL LINE FOR JANUARY 1	EXACT AGE											
		15	16	17	18	19	20	21	22	23	24	25	26
4 PARITY													
1891-------													273.9
1892-------												291.8	268.7
1893-------											281.6	275.1	259.5
1894-------										291.0	281.4	276.8	269.0
1895-------									274.5	292.1	287.2	289.2	285.4
1896-------								*	*	302.3	304.7	311.6	266.4
1897-------							*	*	*	315.5	328.5	291.1	274.7
1898-------						*	*	*	*	343.4	303.2	305.1	277.1
1899-------					*	*	*	*	*	319.5	327.1	306.9	272.2
1900-------				*	*	*	*	*	*	355.8	328.2	297.6	270.3
1901-------			*	*	*	*	*	*	*	363.6	322.8	297.0	275.4
1902-------	1917	*	*	*	*	*	*	*	*	331.3	311.8	288.8	252.1
1903-------	1918	*	*	*	*	*	*	*	*	331.3	304.8	270.6	246.8
1904-------	1919	*	*	*	*	*	*	*	*	323.5	290.0	273.2	246.7
1905-------	1920	*	*	*	*	*	*	*	*	305.9	289.6	269.3	240.2
1906-------	1921	*	*	*	*	*	*	*	*	312.5	293.4	265.1	243.3
1907-------	1922	*	*	*	*	*	*	*	*	313.3	279.0	264.2	232.3
1908-------	1923	*	*	*	*	*	*	*	*	290.5	278.8	250.0	243.5
1909-------	1924	*	*	*	*	*	*	*	*	288.7	264.8	266.0	235.9
1910-------	1925	*	*	*	*	*	*	*	*	277.4	285.7	259.5	234.6
1911-------	1926	*	*	*	*	*	*	*	*	305.3	284.3	259.0	240.6
1912-------	1927	*	*	*	*	*	*	*	*	307.1	275.5	264.9	241.0
1913-------	1928	*	*	*	*	*	*	*	*	300.8	285.7	266.4	232.2
1914-------	1929	*	*	*	*	*	*	*	*	310.9	293.5	261.9	238.9
1915-------	1930	*	*	*	*	*	*	*	*	316.2	287.3	278.2	240.4
1916-------	1931	*	*	*	*	*	*	*	*	307.7	311.1	274.9	238.9
1917-------	1932	*	*	*	*	*	*	*	*	368.4	314.9	276.0	258.8
1918-------	1933	*	*	*	*	*	*	*	*	355.9	308.1	292.5	250.0
1919-------	1934	*	*	*	*	*	*	*	*	344.3	322.8	285.2	236.5
1920-------	1935	*	*	*	*	*	*	*	*	354.3	311.6	259.1	238.2
1921-------	1936	*	*	*	*	*	*	*	*	335.8	281.0	262.6	230.8
1922-------	1937	*	*	*	*	*	*	*	*	296.6	278.8	251.8	227.3
1923-------	1938	*	*	*	*	*	*	*	*	293.7	270.1	256.2	232.3
1924-------	1939	*	*	*	*	*	*	*	*	295.8	285.0	266.9	239.0
1925-------	1940	*	*	*	*	*	*	*	*	311.6	302.9	266.2	246.1
1926-------	1941	*	*	*	*	*	*	*	*	338.0	298.6	279.4	253.6
1927-------	1942	*	*	*	*	*	*	*	*	318.2	305.8	278.7	248.9
1928-------	1943	*	*	*	*	*	*	*	*	327.5	300.4	270.6	248.5
1929-------	1944	*	*	*	*	*	*	*	345.5	328.3	301.9	275.1	241.4
1930-------	1945	*	*	*	*	*	*	*	346.2	330.4	302.7	268.8	242.1
1931-------	1946	*	*	*	*	*	*	*	351.4	327.9	298.1	271.8	241.9
1932-------	1947	*	*	*	*	*	*	*	343.8	324.5	297.7	268.0	236.7
1933-------	1948	*	*	*	*	*	*	*	337.1	317.1	295.1	263.7	234.2
1934-------	1949	*	*	*	*	*	*	366.3	338.8	322.4	292.7	261.4	230.9
1935-------	1950	*	*	*	*	*	*	371.4	349.0	323.8	292.5	261.4	235.8
1936-------	1951	*	*	*	*	*	*	381.8	341.7	316.1	288.9	259.8	224.2
1937-------	1952	*	*	*	*	*	*	371.7	341.3	319.6	288.8	251.1	213.0
1938-------	1953	*	*	*	*	*	*	361.3	334.9	307.0	275.0	230.8	195.8
1939-------	1954	*	*	*	*	*	*	362.9	334.8	304.9	259.1	219.1	169.3
1940-------	1955	*	*	*	*	*	*	359.4	324.7	283.7	243.6	189.9	147.6
1941-------	1956	*	*	*	*	*	*	361.5	312.5	269.6	212.6	167.2	138.0
1942-------	1957	*	*	*	*	*	*	341.5	291.9	234.2	188.7	156.8	130.9
1943-------	1958	*	*	*	*	*	*	321.7	256.5	207.1	179.3	148.8	138.7
1944-------	1959	*	*	*	*	*	*	298.1	233.5	204.2	173.0	160.0	144.9
1945-------	1960	*	*	*	*	*	*	*	229.7	194.3	180.9	165.7	135.9
1946-------	1961	*	*	*	*	*	*	*	216.0	205.6	186.2	154.8	115.0
1947-------	1962	*	*	*	*	*	*	*	213.0	201.3	171.2	127.6	99.7
1948-------	1963	*	*	*	*	*	*	*	*	192.9	142.9	120.0	
1949-------	1964	*	*	*	*	*	*	*	*	164.1	137.9		
1950-------	1965	*	*	*	*	*	*	*	*	163.6			
1951-------	1966	*	*	*	*	*	*	*	*				
1952-------	1967	*	*	*	*	*	*	*					
1953-------	1968	*	*	*	*	*	*						
1954-------	1969	*	*	*	*	*							
1955-------	1970	*	*	*	*								
1956-------	1971	*	*	*									
1957-------	1972	*	*										
1958-------	1973	*											

TABLE 10A. BIRTH PROBABILITIES FOR ALL WOMEN FOR EACH YEAR 1917-73 BY AGE AND PARITY FOR EACH COHORT FROM 1868 TO 1958--CON.

(PROBABILITIES ARE THE NUMBER OF BIRTHS PER 1,000 WOMEN IN SPECIFIED PARITY AND EXACT AGE GROUP. FIGURES FOR "0 PARITY" SHOW THE PROBABILITY OF FIRST BIRTHS TO "C PARITY" WOMEN, THOSE FOR "1 PARITY" SHOW THE PROBABILITY OF SECOND BIRTHS TO "1 PARITY" WOMEN, ETC. BASED ON CENTRAL BIRTH RATES AND PARITY DISTRIBUTIONS)

PARITY AND COHORT	DIAGONAL LINE FOR JANUARY 1	EXACT AGE 27	28	29	30	31	32	33	34	35	36	37	38
4 PARITY--CON.													
1879-------													98.5
1880-------												116.2	96.8
1881-------											129.0	113.6	95.1
1882-------										147.6	126.1	110.6	93.3
1883-------									160.5	144.3	123.8	109.4	92.2
1884-------								177.2	159.0	140.0	123.2	108.9	85.3
1885-------							182.0	175.4	151.6	139.1	122.4	100.6	83.0
1886-------						203.4	181.0	165.8	150.5	139.0	113.9	99.2	81.6
1887-------					219.2	202.5	170.8	164.1	149.7	127.7	110.9	96.1	77.5
1888-------				254.4	215.5	190.6	168.7	162.2	138.1	124.8	107.8	91.2	73.5
1889-------			264.2	248.2	204.8	188.7	167.7	150.1	135.8	122.3	103.4	87.6	71.2
1890-------	1917	275.7	256.2	239.8	205.2	189.1	155.7	150.2	135.0	115.5	98.3	82.5	66.0
1891-------	1918	269.2	251.6	242.3	208.4	177.7	157.9	149.3	129.6	110.8	94.2	78.3	60.7
1892-------	1919	265.6	256.3	249.7	193.9	179.6	157.1	142.9	122.5	105.9	88.2	73.1	62.3
1893-------	1920	265.6	261.3	227.3	194.3	177.9	151.5	133.8	119.0	99.6	82.9	72.8	58.8
1894-------	1921	280.6	241.1	232.9	197.4	174.7	146.3	134.2	114.0	98.3	85.6	71.0	55.5
1895-------	1922	259.5	248.6	235.5	193.7	169.4	146.7	130.3	111.1	99.5	83.0	68.9	55.1
1896-------	1923	268.7	250.7	229.0	188.5	170.4	140.9	124.4	111.5	94.9	81.1	66.6	55.6
1897-------	1924	271.8	241.4	218.3	186.8	162.0	134.8	125.1	106.2	94.8	77.4	68.2	53.5
1898-------	1925	258.1	229.0	218.3	178.4	155.9	134.9	119.1	105.6	88.6	77.6	63.6	50.9
1899-------	1926	254.3	237.1	214.0	176.2	159.8	132.9	122.7	103.0	93.5	76.3	63.0	51.2
1900-------	1927	260.9	228.3	207.5	178.3	154.6	134.6	119.3	106.3	90.2	74.9	62.4	51.4
1901-------	1928	246.9	221.2	208.4	172.1	154.6	129.0	122.2	102.3	87.1	72.5	63.3	50.6
1902-------	1929	236.0	217.7	196.9	166.4	145.0	128.7	112.6	94.8	83.1	70.9	58.9	48.5
1903-------	1930	233.8	208.4	192.2	158.8	146.9	120.3	108.0	92.8	82.4	67.1	58.6	48.1
1904-------	1931	226.9	209.7	187.1	163.1	139.1	116.1	106.6	92.5	79.0	67.2	58.6	50.3
1905-------	1932	227.5	201.4	193.0	155.7	135.7	117.1	107.3	89.9	78.6	67.8	60.2	55.5
1906-------	1933	219.7	208.3	187.8	153.2	137.7	116.6	104.6	90.5	80.0	70.0	67.5	58.2
1907-------	1934	230.4	202.7	183.0	154.6	136.7	114.6	103.6	91.7	82.1	77.4	70.0	60.4
1908-------	1935	222.5	196.8	183.0	153.8	131.6	113.3	104.6	95.2	91.0	79.6	71.7	60.4
1909-------	1936	217.6	200.4	182.9	148.4	130.9	115.2	107.7	103.7	92.4	83.5	72.5	59.8
1910-------	1937	222.2	203.1	177.4	149.6	132.6	119.5	119.3	105.9	96.9	83.2	70.7	56.5
1911-------	1938	225.6	197.3	180.1	152.8	135.0	131.5	121.1	110.2	96.4	82.4	68.3	57.1
1912-------	1939	217.1	199.1	182.6	154.2	149.4	133.0	121.8	107.5	93.3	77.8	66.9	57.3
1913-------	1940	220.2	203.3	179.3	168.7	150.2	131.2	119.8	103.3	89.0	75.6	67.6	58.2
1914-------	1941	225.5	199.5	196.5	166.7	145.7	128.1	115.7	99.7	87.6	77.1	69.2	61.0
1915-------	1942	220.7	214.8	192.4	160.6	143.6	125.4	110.4	97.9	88.5	79.2	71.3	63.1
1916-------	1943	236.6	211.1	183.5	161.0	138.2	118.8	108.9	97.7	90.7	81.3	74.4	63.0
1917-------	1944	235.4	201.4	184.0	153.8	132.7	117.2	109.6	100.8	92.3	83.9	74.6	63.4
1918-------	1945	215.4	199.1	174.3	146.9	130.4	117.3	111.0	103.0	92.9	85.6	73.5	62.9
1919-------	1946	222.2	193.5	170.5	149.2	134.5	123.9	118.9	106.3	98.2	85.6	74.0	62.9
1920-------	1947	212.7	189.9	171.6	150.4	138.0	131.2	119.7	109.4	97.0	85.2	75.3	61.0
1921-------	1948	210.5	190.1	170.9	154.8	145.9	130.8	121.6	109.0	97.3	86.3	72.2	60.7
1922-------	1949	209.5	187.9	177.1	160.1	146.3	131.3	121.6	108.8	96.9	81.7	71.2	57.8
1923-------	1950	213.0	195.7	182.0	161.5	147.7	133.4	122.1	108.9	93.0	81.5	68.4	56.3
1924-------	1951	223.5	205.8	188.0	166.7	150.2	134.2	122.2	106.0	93.0	79.0	66.6	52.0
1925-------	1952	232.0	206.4	190.3	165.6	150.1	134.8	118.1	104.1	90.6	77.5	61.9	48.8
1926-------	1953	229.6	209.4	186.3	164.0	149.0	128.5	115.2	100.9	86.8	71.4	57.4	44.9
1927-------	1954	228.0	202.9	182.9	161.9	140.5	126.1	112.5	97.9	81.1	67.5	53.4	40.6
1928-------	1955	221.9	196.8	179.7	155.2	140.3	123.0	109.0	91.0	76.1	62.5	47.6	35.9
1929-------	1956	219.0	198.0	176.0	156.2	138.6	122.0	103.7	87.1	71.5	56.3	42.7	31.5
1930-------	1957	219.8	194.1	175.6	153.7	136.1	115.2	98.7	81.5	64.5	49.4	37.5	28.0
1931-------	1958	213.3	192.1	171.3	150.0	128.9	109.7	91.3	73.0	55.7	43.2	33.7	25.8
1932-------	1959	212.7	188.2	169.1	142.3	123.7	102.0	82.7	62.7	49.4	39.1	31.2	24.1
1933-------	1960	207.3	187.2	160.4	136.3	114.1	91.0	70.2	56.3	45.2	37.1	28.7	21.1
1934-------	1961	209.3	179.1	153.2	127.7	100.9	78.4	63.6	50.6	43.5	35.0	26.7	17.9
1935-------	1962	202.7	172.9	145.5	111.3	88.3	71.3	57.3	50.3	41.2	32.0	22.5	15.5
1936-------	1963	192.5	161.2	124.3	97.0	80.1	63.5	56.4	48.0	37.7	26.6	19.5	
1937-------	1964	178.9	137.7	108.0	89.0	72.4	64.1	55.4	43.6	31.9	23.2		
1938-------	1965	151.5	117.5	98.4	79.8	72.8	64.1	50.4	37.2	27.3			
1939-------	1966	131.3	108.2	90.8	83.3	74.2	59.1	43.7	32.9				
1940-------	1967	122.0	103.0	96.3	85.9	70.2	51.6	38.7					
1941-------	1968	116.1	109.5	99.3	82.1	59.6	46.3						
1942-------	1969	124.6	112.2	94.9	68.0	53.6							
1943-------	1970	127.3	108.0	78.7	61.5								
1944-------	1971	121.4	90.8	72.7									
1945-------	1972	103.2	81.3										
1946-------	1973	92.3											

TABLE 10A. BIRTH PROBABILITIES FOR ALL WOMEN FOR EACH YEAR 1917-73 BY AGE AND PARITY FOR EACH COHORT FROM 1868 TO 1958--CON.

(PROBABILITIES ARE THE NUMBER OF BIRTHS PER 1,000 WOMEN IN SPECIFIED PARITY AND EXACT AGE GROUP. FIGURES FOR "0 PARITY" SHOW THE PROBABILITY OF FIRST BIRTHS TO "0 PARITY" WOMEN, THOSE FOR "1 PARITY" SHOW THE PROBABILITY OF SECOND BIRTHS TO "1 PARITY" WOMEN, ETC. BASED ON CENTRAL BIRTH RATES AND PARITY DISTRIBUTIONS)

PARITY AND COHORT	DIAGONAL LINE FOR JANUARY 1	EXACT AGE										
		39	40	41	42	43	44	45	46	47	48	49
4 PARITY--CON.												
1868												1.1
1869											1.1	1.1
1870										2.1	1.1	1.1
1871									5.3	3.2	1.1	1.1
1872								7.4	5.3	2.1	1.1	0.0
1873							12.7	8.5	5.3	3.2	1.1	0.0
1874						19.1	12.8	7.5	5.4	2.1	1.1	0.0
1875					26.5	20.2	12.8	8.6	4.3	2.2	1.1	0.0
1876				40.0	27.5	19.1	12.8	7.5	4.3	2.1	1.1	1.1
1877			56.1	41.9	26.4	19.1	12.8	6.4	4.3	2.1	1.1	0.0
1878	1917	81.4	57.4	40.0	26.4	20.2	11.7	7.5	4.3	2.1	1.1	0.0
1879	1918	82.0	56.7	40.3	27.7	18.2	11.8	7.5	4.3	2.2	1.1	0.0
1880	1919	81.1	55.7	41.3	25.6	18.2	11.8	6.5	3.2	2.2	1.1	0.0
1881	1920	79.5	56.3	38.9	25.4	18.0	10.6	5.3	3.2	1.1	1.1	0.0
1882	1921	78.9	51.7	37.5	25.1	16.8	9.5	5.3	3.2	1.1	1.1	0.0
1883	1922	72.5	50.5	36.3	22.9	15.6	9.4	5.2	3.1	2.1	0.0	0.0
1884	1923	71.6	49.5	34.2	22.8	15.6	9.4	5.2	3.1	1.0	1.0	0.0
1885	1924	69.2	46.1	32.9	21.6	14.5	8.3	5.2	3.1	1.0	1.0	0.0
1886	1925	64.8	43.7	30.6	19.4	13.3	8.2	4.1	3.1	1.0	1.0	1.0
1887	1926	61.8	42.0	29.1	18.1	13.1	7.1	4.0	2.0	1.0	1.0	0.0
1888	1927	59.0	39.5	26.8	17.9	12.0	7.0	4.0	2.0	1.0	0.0	0.0
1889	1928	55.8	36.3	27.6	16.8	11.9	6.9	4.0	2.0	1.0	1.0	0.0
1890	1929	51.6	37.1	25.5	16.7	11.8	6.9	4.0	2.0	1.0	1.0	0.0
1891	1930	52.0	34.4	24.6	16.8	10.9	5.9	4.0	2.0	1.0	1.0	0.0
1892	1931	48.6	32.8	23.9	16.0	10.0	6.0	3.0	2.0	1.0	1.0	0.0
1893	1932	44.9	32.0	24.0	15.1	10.1	5.0	3.0	2.0	1.0	0.0	0.0
1894	1933	44.2	32.9	22.7	14.5	9.3	5.2	3.1	2.1	1.0	0.0	0.0
1895	1934	45.6	31.8	22.3	13.8	9.6	5.3	3.2	1.1	0.0	0.0	0.0
1896	1935	43.5	30.5	21.8	14.2	9.8	5.5	2.2	1.1	0.0	0.0	0.0
1897	1936	41.2	30.0	21.1	14.5	8.9	4.5	3.3	1.1	0.0	0.0	0.0
1898	1937	40.7	29.4	21.5	13.6	9.0	6.8	3.4	1.1	1.1	0.0	0.0
1899	1938	41.8	30.2	20.9	13.9	9.3	7.0	3.5	2.3	1.2	0.0	0.0
1900	1939	41.7	29.8	21.5	14.3	10.7	7.2	3.6	2.4	1.2	0.0	0.0
1901	1940	40.5	29.5	20.9	15.9	11.0	7.3	3.7	2.4	0.0	0.0	0.0
1902	1941	39.7	29.7	23.4	17.2	11.1	7.4	3.7	1.2	1.2	0.0	0.0
1903	1942	40.3	31.3	23.7	17.4	12.4	6.2	3.7	2.5	0.0	0.0	0.0
1904	1943	43.5	33.0	25.3	17.6	11.3	6.3	3.8	1.3	1.3	0.0	0.0
1905	1944	45.7	34.9	25.6	17.9	10.2	6.4	3.8	1.3	0.0	0.0	0.0
1906	1945	49.3	35.6	26.1	16.9	10.4	6.5	3.9	1.3	0.0	0.0	0.0
1907	1946	49.9	37.3	25.1	17.0	11.8	6.5	3.9	1.3	1.3	0.0	0.0
1908	1947	48.6	34.6	25.0	17.0	11.8	6.5	3.9	2.6	1.3	0.0	0.0
1909	1948	46.5	34.1	26.0	16.8	11.6	7.7	3.8	2.6	1.3	0.0	0.0
1910	1949	46.1	35.0	25.7	17.9	12.7	7.6	3.8	2.5	1.3	0.0	0.0
1911	1950	46.8	35.9	27.9	18.9	13.8	8.8	3.8	2.5	0.0	0.0	0.0
1912	1951	47.2	37.6	27.3	20.9	14.7	7.3	3.7	1.2	1.2	0.0	0.0
1913	1952	50.6	37.6	29.9	21.4	13.0	7.1	3.5	2.4	1.2	0.0	0.0
1914	1953	51.1	39.7	30.0	20.6	12.6	8.0	4.6	2.3	1.1	0.0	0.0
1915	1954	52.4	40.2	29.8	19.8	13.1	7.7	3.3	2.2	1.1	0.0	0.0
1916	1955	52.6	39.9	28.8	19.1	12.7	7.4	4.2	2.1	1.1	0.0	0.0
1917	1956	51.4	38.2	28.5	19.3	12.1	7.1	3.0	2.0	1.0	0.0	0.0
1918	1957	50.5	37.7	27.6	18.6	12.7	5.9	2.9	2.0	0.0	0.0	0.0
1919	1958	50.0	37.0	27.3	18.8	11.2	6.6	2.8	0.9	0.0	0.0	0.0
1920	1959	48.9	36.5	26.3	17.1	10.8	5.4	2.7	0.9	0.0	0.0	0.0
1921	1960	46.7	34.8	24.2	16.4	9.5	5.2	2.6	0.9	0.0	0.0	0.0
1922	1961	45.9	32.1	22.7	14.2	8.4	5.0	2.5	0.8	0.0	0.0	0.0
1923	1962	41.8	30.2	21.1	13.8	7.3	4.1	1.6	0.8	0.0	0.0	0.0
1924	1963	39.7	28.4	19.7	11.8	6.3	3.1	1.6	0.8	0.0	0.0	0.0
1925	1964	36.9	26.0	16.8	9.9	6.1	3.8	1.5	0.0	0.0	0.0	
1926	1965	33.4	22.2	14.8	8.8	5.9	3.0	0.7	0.7	0.0		
1927	1966	28.9	19.4	12.9	8.6	4.3	2.2	0.7	0.7			
1928	1967	24.5	16.8	11.8	7.0	4.2	1.4	0.7				
1929	1968	22.5	16.3	10.9	6.1	3.4	1.4					
1930	1969	21.2	15.2	8.6	4.6	2.6						
1931	1970	19.3	11.6	7.7	4.5							
1932	1971	16.4	10.1	6.3								
1933	1972	14.3	9.3									
1934	1973	12.3										

TABLE 10A. BIRTH PROBABILITIES FOR ALL WOMEN FOR EACH YEAR 1917-73 BY AGE AND PARITY FOR EACH COHORT FROM 1868 TO 1958--CON.

(PROBABILITIES ARE THE NUMBER OF BIRTHS PER 1,000 WOMEN IN SPECIFIED PARITY AND EXACT AGE GROUP. FIGURES FOR "0 PARITY" SHOW THE PROBABILITY OF FIRST BIRTHS TO "0 PARITY" WOMEN, THOSE FOR "1 PARITY" SHOW THE PROBABILITY OF SECOND BIRTHS TO "1 PARITY" WOMEN, ETC. BASED ON CENTRAL BIRTH RATES AND PARITY DISTRIBUTIONS)

PARITY AND COHORT	DIAGONAL LINE FOR JANUARY 1	EXACT AGE											
		15	16	17	18	19	20	21	22	23	24	25	26
5 PARITY													
1891-------													322.9
1892-------												352.1	314.8
1893-------											*	317.6	296.8
1894-------										*	*	333.3	320.4
1895-------									*	*	*	359.4	355.0
1896-------								*	*	*	*	401.6	325.0
1897-------							*	*	*	*	*	367.2	341.8
1898-------						*	*	*	*	*	*	392.0	348.7
1899-------					*	*	*	*	*	*	*	393.7	336.8
1900-------				*	*	*	*	*	*	*	*	375.0	340.3
1901-------			*	*	*	*	*	*	*	*	*	387.1	335.1
1902-------	1917	*	*	*	*	*	*	*	*	*	*	365.9	306.5
1903-------	1918	*	*	*	*	*	*	*	*	*	*	322.8	292.6
1904-------	1919	*	*	*	*	*	*	*	*	*	*	322.8	284.9
1905-------	1920	*	*	*	*	*	*	*	*	*	*	317.1	286.5
1906-------	1921	*	*	*	*	*	*	*	*	*	*	316.2	285.7
1907-------	1922	*	*	*	*	*	*	*	*	*	*	311.9	276.7
1908-------	1923	*	*	*	*	*	*	*	*	*	*	295.2	291.4
1909-------	1924	*	*	*	*	*	*	*	*	*	*	*	296.6
1910-------	1925	*	*	*	*	*	*	*	*	*	*	*	292.9
1911-------	1926	*	*	*	*	*	*	*	*	*	*	*	301.5
1912-------	1927	*	*	*	*	*	*	*	*	*	*	*	297.7
1913-------	1928	*	*	*	*	*	*	*	*	*	*	*	294.6
1914-------	1929	*	*	*	*	*	*	*	*	*	*	*	296.9
1915-------	1930	*	*	*	*	*	*	*	*	*	*	*	289.1
1916-------	1931	*	*	*	*	*	*	*	*	*	*	*	294.6
1917-------	1932	*	*	*	*	*	*	*	*	*	*	*	305.3
1918-------	1933	*	*	*	*	*	*	*	*	*	*	*	301.5
1919-------	1934	*	*	*	*	*	*	*	*	*	*	*	295.0
1920-------	1935	*	*	*	*	*	*	*	*	*	*	320.0	295.0
1921-------	1936	*	*	*	*	*	*	*	*	*	*	323.5	281.7
1922-------	1937	*	*	*	*	*	*	*	*	*	*	316.8	292.9
1923-------	1938	*	*	*	*	*	*	*	*	*	*	*	302.2
1924-------	1939	*	*	*	*	*	*	*	*	*	*	340.0	305.0
1925-------	1940	*	*	*	*	*	*	*	*	*	*	339.8	315.1
1926-------	1941	*	*	*	*	*	*	*	*	*	*	336.4	310.6
1927-------	1942	*	*	*	*	*	*	*	*	*	*	338.8	310.7
1928-------	1943	*	*	*	*	*	*	*	*	*	*	333.3	307.7
1929-------	1944	*	*	*	*	*	*	*	*	*	*	329.0	297.3
1930-------	1945	*	*	*	*	*	*	*	*	*	351.4	321.8	296.3
1931-------	1946	*	*	*	*	*	*	*	*	*	354.8	331.6	299.2
1932-------	1947	*	*	*	*	*	*	*	*	*	376.9	333.3	296.0
1933-------	1948	*	*	*	*	*	*	*	*	*	375.0	327.0	293.9
1934-------	1949	*	*	*	*	*	*	*	*	*	367.3	324.4	291.7
1935-------	1950	*	*	*	*	*	*	*	*	*	361.3	327.7	293.2
1936-------	1951	*	*	*	*	*	*	*	*	*	362.5	321.0	281.9
1937-------	1952	*	*	*	*	*	*	*	*	*	353.3	312.3	261.6
1938-------	1953	*	*	*	*	*	*	*	*	*	351.2	293.7	246.3
1939-------	1954	*	*	*	*	*	*	*	*	382.4	321.8	268.8	212.6
1940-------	1955	*	*	*	*	*	*	*	*	359.2	307.7	240.7	185.7
1941-------	1956	*	*	*	*	*	*	*	*	333.3	260.9	209.1	171.5
1942-------	1957	*	*	*	*	*	*	*	*	*	246.4	206.5	166.7
1943-------	1958	*	*	*	*	*	*	*	*	*	238.9	197.4	178.9
1944-------	1959	*	*	*	*	*	*	*	*	*	*	201.6	179.6
1945-------	1960	*	*	*	*	*	*	*	*	*	*	205.4	167.8
1946-------	1961	*	*	*	*	*	*	*	*	*	*	*	137.4
1947-------	1962	*	*	*	*	*	*	*	*	*	*	*	130.8
1948-------	1963	*	*	*	*	*	*	*	*	*	*	*	
1949-------	1964	*	*	*	*	*	*	*	*	*	*		
1950-------	1965	*	*	*	*	*	*	*	*	*			
1951-------	1966	*	*	*	*	*	*	*	*				
1952-------	1967	*	*	*	*	*	*	*					
1953-------	1968	*	*	*	*	*	*						
1954-------	1969	*	*	*	*	*							
1955-------	1970	*	*	*	*								
1956-------	1971	*	*	*									
1957-------	1972	*	*										
1958-------	1973	*											

TABLE 10A. BIRTH PROBABILITIES FOR ALL WOMEN FOR EACH YEAR 1917-73 BY AGE AND PARITY FOR EACH COHORT FROM 1868 TO 1958--CON.

(PROBABILITIES ARE THE NUMBER OF BIRTHS PER 1,000 WOMEN IN SPECIFIED PARITY AND EXACT AGE GROUP. FIGURES FOR "0 PARITY" SHOW THE PROBABILITY OF FIRST BIRTHS TO "0 PARITY" WOMEN, THOSE FOR "1 PARITY" SHOW THE PROBABILITY OF SECOND BIRTHS TO "1 PARITY" WOMEN, ETC. BASED ON CENTRAL BIRTH RATES AND PARITY DISTRIBUTIONS)

PARITY AND COHORT	DIAGONAL LINE FOR JANUARY 1	EXACT AGE 27	28	29	30	31	32	33	34	35	36	37	38
5 PARITY--CON.													
1879-------													137.2
1880-------												161.2	137.5
1881-------											173.6	159.0	131.6
1882-------										190.1	171.4	153.1	129.5
1883-------									202.6	189.0	165.6	150.5	126.6
1884-------								219.5	204.0	183.5	165.8	148.9	117.6
1885-------							227.1	222.8	198.6	184.4	165.8	141.3	116.1
1886-------						248.4	230.1	214.6	196.4	185.3	156.6	138.7	115.7
1887-------					258.1	252.0	221.2	210.8	201.1	176.5	154.8	139.3	113.3
1888-------				303.0	264.7	246.7	222.0	223.4	194.1	178.8	157.5	135.6	108.4
1889-------			306.2	296.9	255.0	243.3	229.9	209.5	194.6	177.5	152.7	131.8	108.3
1890-------	1917	324.8	296.2	290.5	254.6	255.1	217.0	213.7	195.4	171.7	148.2	129.9	101.8
1891-------	1918	316.8	292.7	294.0	269.7	240.1	221.7	215.0	188.8	167.7	148.5	122.7	95.1
1892-------	1919	311.9	258.9	312.2	250.5	244.2	222.2	205.9	182.4	164.6	137.2	114.8	98.9
1893-------	1920	308.7	315.0	283.8	251.9	242.4	210.3	195.0	178.6	154.1	129.4	114.6	93.8
1894-------	1921	347.4	294.3	298.2	259.6	240.2	207.1	199.0	169.8	148.8	129.1	111.7	93.4
1895-------	1922	321.4	310.7	305.7	258.4	235.9	213.8	191.3	165.8	149.3	128.6	110.9	88.7
1896-------	1923	337.0	317.9	298.3	257.1	237.8	200.8	181.0	165.8	143.4	125.9	105.8	91.5
1897-------	1924	347.0	302.7	297.2	255.1	230.0	190.8	185.7	158.8	145.0	121.3	107.9	85.6
1898-------	1925	320.8	304.2	294.3	243.6	219.4	198.4	178.6	163.1	141.8	125.7	106.3	83.5
1899-------	1926	334.6	306.3	283.1	235.8	225.4	192.1	186.2	159.0	145.4	118.7	100.4	82.7
1900-------	1927	328.1	286.6	271.3	239.2	218.8	194.9	176.7	160.9	136.5	117.1	98.6	82.5
1901-------	1928	308.3	271.6	270.5	229.1	216.6	183.2	177.7	150.6	131.7	110.0	97.0	78.3
1902-------	1929	285.1	271.8	257.0	225.3	201.9	181.8	164.8	141.9	125.0	106.7	93.2	76.3
1903-------	1930	281.1	259.0	257.1	211.5	202.9	170.2	155.8	136.6	121.2	102.3	88.8	73.4
1904-------	1931	274.6	267.8	240.4	217.7	196.0	166.3	156.5	137.0	118.8	101.8	89.7	78.1
1905-------	1932	281.4	250.0	251.6	212.9	189.5	168.3	155.7	130.3	116.0	100.5	90.1	82.4
1906-------	1933	268.2	263.2	247.6	206.5	193.4	168.9	150.9	131.8	116.8	102.6	96.2	85.3
1907-------	1934	285.0	259.8	243.2	214.3	198.3	164.8	153.6	133.9	122.8	110.3	102.7	86.3
1908-------	1935	275.0	254.1	247.3	215.0	189.6	166.7	152.5	139.3	132.6	116.0	103.0	85.8
1909-------	1936	278.9	264.1	251.9	208.2	191.7	167.7	157.9	152.1	138.6	118.7	102.0	86.6
1910-------	1937	284.2	264.6	241.2	212.0	188.7	166.1	169.6	156.3	134.2	115.5	101.3	81.3
1911-------	1938	286.5	258.1	249.0	211.7	186.4	181.5	174.2	149.0	130.4	114.3	95.2	80.3
1912-------	1939	284.9	270.5	253.2	209.1	206.3	188.3	168.2	149.9	131.5	110.2	96.2	81.1
1913-------	1940	289.2	273.6	241.4	223.9	206.3	178.0	166.2	145.3	122.0	108.5	94.8	81.9
1914-------	1941	290.9	260.0	255.4	228.1	201.4	180.1	159.6	135.6	125.3	107.1	100.2	82.7
1915-------	1942	277.1	268.7	253.2	216.4	197.3	166.7	151.6	137.0	122.1	111.1	96.9	86.2
1916-------	1943	289.2	267.0	239.7	208.8	182.1	161.6	151.0	134.0	124.1	107.9	97.9	84.8
1917-------	1944	284.9	250.0	230.8	196.4	178.0	158.7	148.0	133.2	119.8	108.0	97.8	85.1
1918-------	1945	272.7	250.0	225.8	196.4	178.6	161.7	150.0	136.6	122.3	110.1	99.4	84.8
1919-------	1946	276.8	240.7	225.3	200.0	181.0	162.3	153.8	138.7	126.4	113.7	99.6	85.7
1920-------	1947	268.2	247.7	232.3	202.1	187.5	170.0	156.0	144.9	129.6	115.2	103.3	84.1
1921-------	1948	273.2	253.4	233.5	208.9	191.5	167.6	162.6	146.3	129.1	116.6	99.5	84.9
1922-------	1949	279.3	253.5	243.1	213.6	189.3	177.1	162.0	145.0	131.6	112.1	99.5	82.1
1923-------	1950	279.3	267.0	243.3	212.9	195.5	174.9	160.8	146.0	127.5	111.3	94.2	81.1
1924-------	1951	297.3	264.1	243.8	214.3	195.4	174.6	162.9	139.7	124.4	107.3	93.2	72.1
1925-------	1952	297.4	268.0	249.2	218.2	199.0	178.3	154.9	138.4	120.7	104.8	84.1	68.6
1926-------	1953	290.3	269.1	244.8	218.3	195.1	167.0	153.0	133.0	116.7	97.8	80.2	63.0
1927-------	1954	291.1	263.3	245.2	212.3	185.2	167.6	149.3	130.4	110.9	92.2	74.2	58.0
1928-------	1955	283.5	259.9	235.3	203.1	188.1	162.3	145.3	123.5	103.2	85.7	66.2	48.3
1929-------	1956	279.3	253.5	225.6	204.0	180.5	159.7	136.8	114.5	97.1	74.8	56.7	44.7
1930-------	1957	275.3	245.5	225.8	199.3	175.5	150.2	129.5	109.1	84.4	64.6	51.1	38.6
1931-------	1958	269.0	245.2	222.9	195.8	168.8	142.9	123.8	95.1	74.2	59.2	46.5	34.4
1932-------	1959	269.4	243.2	219.0	185.7	159.7	134.2	106.8	82.1	65.2	53.2	40.9	32.5
1933-------	1960	266.3	240.9	207.2	174.1	148.6	116.6	91.3	73.2	59.4	48.9	38.0	28.7
1934-------	1961	266.2	228.7	195.5	162.3	129.7	100.4	80.6	64.4	56.8	45.3	35.6	25.3
1935-------	1962	252.4	213.3	183.2	142.6	111.1	88.9	71.1	64.9	52.6	42.2	30.3	21.1
1936-------	1963	237.8	202.7	158.0	123.5	99.3	78.9	71.6	60.4	50.2	36.3	26.6	
1937-------	1964	221.2	172.5	137.5	110.2	89.4	79.1	70.1	57.3	42.2	30.5		
1938-------	1965	192.9	149.3	124.5	100.7	90.9	79.6	65.8	50.0	36.9			
1939-------	1966	163.8	136.4	115.0	103.9	93.0	76.3	57.9	44.6				
1940-------	1967	156.2	129.8	121.0	105.9	88.3	65.9	51.7					
1941-------	1968	145.1	132.4	119.3	98.5	74.7	59.4						
1942-------	1969	155.0	138.4	115.1	85.6	68.0							
1943-------	1970	159.5	133.6	96.9	76.3								
1944-------	1971	149.0	112.9	89.0									
1945-------	1972	129.7	101.9										
1946-------	1973	119.5											

TABLE 10A. BIRTH PROBABILITIES FOR ALL WOMEN FOR EACH YEAR 1917-73 BY AGE AND PARITY FOR EACH COHORT FROM 1868 TO 1958--CON.

(PROBABILITIES ARE THE NUMBER OF BIRTHS PER 1,000 WOMEN IN SPECIFIED PARITY AND EXACT AGE GROUP. FIGURES FOR "0 PARITY" SHOW THE PROBABILITY OF FIRST BIRTHS TO "C PARITY" WOMEN, THOSE FOR "1 PARITY" SHOW THE PROBABILITY OF SECOND BIRTHS TO "1 PARITY" WOMEN, ETC. BASED ON CENTRAL BIRTH PATES AND PARITY DISTRIBUTIONS)

PARITY AND COHORT	DIAGONAL LINE FOR JANUARY 1	EXACT AGE										
		39	40	41	42	43	44	45	46	47	48	49
5 PARITY--CON.												
1868----------------												1.3
1869----------------											2.6	1.3
1870----------------										3.9	2.6	1.3
1871----------------									7.8	5.2	2.6	1.3
1872----------------								11.7	10.5	3.9	2.6	1.3
1873----------------							19.7	14.5	7.9	4.0	1.3	0.0
1874----------------						30.5	21.3	12.1	8.1	2.7	1.3	1.3
1875----------------					42.6	29.5	18.9	12.2	6.8	2.7	2.7	1.4
1876----------------				62.3	41.6	28.3	19.0	10.9	6.8	4.1	2.7	0.0
1877----------------			82.8	61.2	40.2	28.3	19.0	10.9	6.8	2.7	1.4	1.4
1878----------------	1917	117.5	83.8	60.0	41.3	30.5	18.1	11.2	7.0	2.8	1.4	0.0
1879----------------	1918	118.3	81.6	61.7	42.9	27.9	18.2	9.8	5.6	2.8	1.4	0.0
1880----------------	1919	114.9	81.9	62.0	38.9	27.9	18.2	11.3	7.1	2.8	1.4	1.4
1881----------------	1920	112.6	81.2	55.9	38.4	27.6	16.6	9.7	5.6	2.8	1.4	1.4
1882----------------	1921	110.5	73.8	55.4	36.7	26.0	16.5	9.6	5.5	2.8	1.4	0.0
1883----------------	1922	100.9	72.2	53.8	33.9	24.5	13.7	8.2	5.5	2.7	1.4	0.0
1884----------------	1923	99.5	70.3	50.3	34.2	23.3	13.8	8.3	4.1	2.8	1.4	0.0
1885----------------	1924	98.8	67.6	49.9	32.1	21.0	12.6	7.0	4.2	1.4	1.4	0.0
1886----------------	1925	95.4	64.1	47.6	29.5	19.7	12.7	7.1	4.2	1.4	1.4	1.4
1887----------------	1926	89.9	64.8	43.9	28.4	21.4	12.9	7.2	4.3	1.4	1.4	1.4
1888----------------	1927	91.0	61.0	42.2	29.2	20.5	13.2	7.4	4.4	1.5	1.5	1.5
1889----------------	1928	85.0	57.3	44.2	29.5	20.8	11.9	7.5	4.5	3.0	1.5	0.0
1890----------------	1929	79.3	59.9	42.0	28.6	19.6	12.1	6.1	4.5	1.5	1.5	0.0
1891----------------	1930	84.4	56.9	41.7	26.3	20.1	10.9	6.2	3.1	1.6	1.6	0.0
1892----------------	1931	78.5	56.6	39.5	26.9	17.4	11.1	6.4	3.2	1.6	0.0	0.0
1893----------------	1932	77.9	52.8	38.5	25.6	17.7	9.6	6.4	3.2	1.6	0.0	0.0
1894----------------	1933	74.1	54.5	38.1	24.9	16.6	10.0	5.0	3.3	1.7	0.0	0.0
1895----------------	1934	75.1	51.3	35.9	23.9	17.1	10.3	5.2	3.4	1.7	0.0	0.0
1896----------------	1935	72.3	49.5	33.6	24.7	15.9	8.8	5.3	3.5	0.0	0.0	0.0
1897----------------	1936	67.3	47.3	36.3	23.6	14.5	9.1	5.5	1.8	0.0	0.0	0.0
1898----------------	1937	66.3	49.1	35.9	22.7	15.1	11.3	5.7	1.9	1.9	0.0	0.0
1899----------------	1938	69.1	48.0	34.5	23.0	17.2	11.5	5.8	3.8	1.9	0.0	0.0
1900----------------	1939	66.7	47.0	35.2	23.4	17.6	9.8	5.8	3.9	1.9	0.0	0.0
1901----------------	1940	62.0	45.8	31.8	25.8	17.9	9.9	5.9	4.0	2.0	0.0	0.0
1902----------------	1941	61.6	45.0	36.7	26.4	18.3	10.1	6.1	2.0	2.0	0.0	0.0
1903----------------	1942	62.5	47.7	37.2	26.8	18.5	12.3	4.1	2.1	2.0	0.0	0.0
1904----------------	1943	66.8	49.3	40.4	25.5	19.0	8.5	4.2	2.1	0.0	0.0	0.0
1905----------------	1944	68.3	52.4	39.0	25.9	17.2	8.6	4.3	2.1	0.0	0.0	0.0
1906----------------	1945	70.5	51.6	35.6	24.2	15.4	8.8	4.4	2.2	2.2	0.0	0.0
1907----------------	1946	70.6	50.9	36.5	24.9	18.1	9.0	4.5	2.2	0.0	0.0	0.0
1908----------------	1947	69.5	47.2	34.9	25.3	16.1	9.1	4.6	2.3	0.0	0.0	0.0
1909----------------	1948	65.4	49.9	37.6	25.6	18.5	11.5	4.6	2.3	0.0	0.0	0.0
1910----------------	1949	65.1	49.6	37.3	25.4	18.3	11.4	4.6	2.3	0.0	0.0	0.0
1911----------------	1950	66.5	51.3	39.1	29.5	18.1	11.2	6.7	2.2	2.2	0.0	0.0
1912----------------	1951	69.4	54.0	41.6	29.7	20.4	11.3	6.7	2.2	2.2	0.0	0.0
1913----------------	1952	70.3	54.8	42.7	28.8	19.7	13.1	6.6	4.4	0.0	0.0	0.0
1914----------------	1953	70.8	57.8	43.7	30.2	21.4	10.7	6.4	2.1	2.1	0.0	0.0
1915----------------	1954	74.4	57.6	41.8	30.9	18.4	12.2	6.1	4.1	2.0	0.0	0.0
1916----------------	1955	73.4	55.1	42.0	27.7	19.6	11.7	5.8	3.9	0.0	0.0	0.0
1917----------------	1956	70.0	54.5	38.2	28.2	18.7	11.2	5.6	1.9	1.9	0.0	0.0
1918----------------	1957	70.0	53.0	39.0	27.5	18.2	10.9	3.6	3.6	0.0	0.0	0.0
1919----------------	1958	69.9	53.8	38.8	27.9	17.3	8.6	5.2	1.7	0.0	0.0	0.0
1920----------------	1959	70.7	51.8	39.0	25.2	15.0	10.0	5.0	1.7	0.0	0.0	0.0
1921----------------	1960	67.1	50.9	35.6	24.0	15.9	7.9	3.2	1.6	0.0	0.0	0.0
1922----------------	1961	66.7	47.8	34.6	23.4	14.0	7.8	3.1	1.5	0.0	0.0	0.0
1923----------------	1962	60.4	45.6	31.6	20.9	11.9	5.9	3.0	1.5	0.0	0.0	0.0
1924----------------	1963	57.1	41.8	28.5	18.4	9.9	5.6	2.8	1.4	0.0	0.0	0.0
1925----------------	1964	53.1	38.6	26.0	15.0	9.5	5.4	2.7	1.4	0.0	0.0	
1926----------------	1965	48.4	33.2	21.1	14.4	7.9	5.2	2.6	1.3	0.0		
1927----------------	1966	41.5	28.2	19.1	11.4	7.6	3.8	1.3	0.0			
1928----------------	1967	36.3	24.8	17.3	11.1	6.2	2.5	1.2				
1929----------------	1968	32.3	22.6	15.3	8.2	4.7	2.3					
1930----------------	1969	29.0	20.7	12.6	8.0	4.6						
1931----------------	1970	27.2	18.0	11.2	6.7							
1932----------------	1971	24.4	15.5	9.9								
1933----------------	1972	19.7	13.0									
1934----------------	1973	17.5										

TABLE 10A. BIRTH PROBABILITIES FOR ALL WOMEN FOR EACH YEAR 1917-73 BY AGE AND PARITY FOR EACH COHORT FROM 1868 TO 1958--CON.

(PROBABILITIES ARE THE NUMBER OF BIRTHS PER 1,000 WOMEN IN SPECIFIED PARITY AND EXACT AGE GROUP. FIGURES FOR "0 PARITY" SHOW THE PROBABILITY OF FIRST BIRTHS TO "0 PARITY" WOMEN, THOSE FOR "1 PARITY" SHOW THE PROBABILITY OF SECOND BIRTHS TO "1 PARITY" WOMEN, ETC. BASED ON CENTRAL BIRTH RATES AND PARITY DISTRIBUTIONS)

PARITY AND COHORT	DIAGONAL LINE FOR JANUARY 1	EXACT AGE											
		15	16	17	18	19	20	21	22	23	24	25	26
6 PARITY													
1891-------													*
1892-------												*	*
1893-------											*	*	*
1894-------										*	*	*	*
1895-------									*	*	*	*	*
1896-------								*	*	*	*	*	*
1897-------							*	*	*	*	*	*	*
1898-------						*	*	*	*	*	*	*	*
1899-------					*	*	*	*	*	*	*	*	*
1900-------				*	*	*	*	*	*	*	*	*	*
1901-------			*	*	*	*	*	*	*	*	*	*	*
1902-------	1917	*	*	*	*	*	*	*	*	*	*	*	*
1903-------	1918	*	*	*	*	*	*	*	*	*	*	*	*
1904-------	1919	*	*	*	*	*	*	*	*	*	*	*	*
1905-------	1920	*	*	*	*	*	*	*	*	*	*	*	*
1906-------	1921	*	*	*	*	*	*	*	*	*	*	*	*
1907-------	1922	*	*	*	*	*	*	*	*	*	*	*	*
1908-------	1923	*	*	*	*	*	*	*	*	*	*	*	*
1909-------	1924	*	*	*	*	*	*	*	*	*	*	*	*
1910-------	1925	*	*	*	*	*	*	*	*	*	*	*	*
1911-------	1926	*	*	*	*	*	*	*	*	*	*	*	*
1912-------	1927	*	*	*	*	*	*	*	*	*	*	*	*
1913-------	1928	*	*	*	*	*	*	*	*	*	*	*	*
1914-------	1929	*	*	*	*	*	*	*	*	*	*	*	*
1915-------	1930	*	*	*	*	*	*	*	*	*	*	*	*
1916-------	1931	*	*	*	*	*	*	*	*	*	*	*	*
1917-------	1932	*	*	*	*	*	*	*	*	*	*	*	*
1918-------	1933	*	*	*	*	*	*	*	*	*	*	*	*
1919-------	1934	*	*	*	*	*	*	*	*	*	*	*	*
1920-------	1935	*	*	*	*	*	*	*	*	*	*	*	*
1921-------	1936	*	*	*	*	*	*	*	*	*	*	*	*
1922-------	1937	*	*	*	*	*	*	*	*	*	*	*	*
1923-------	1938	*	*	*	*	*	*	*	*	*	*	*	*
1924-------	1939	*	*	*	*	*	*	*	*	*	*	*	*
1925-------	1940	*	*	*	*	*	*	*	*	*	*	*	*
1926-------	1941	*	*	*	*	*	*	*	*	*	*	*	*
1927-------	1942	*	*	*	*	*	*	*	*	*	*	*	*
1928-------	1943	*	*	*	*	*	*	*	*	*	*	*	*
1929-------	1944	*	*	*	*	*	*	*	*	*	*	*	*
1930-------	1945	*	*	*	*	*	*	*	*	*	*	*	*
1931-------	1946	*	*	*	*	*	*	*	*	*	*	*	352.9
1932-------	1947	*	*	*	*	*	*	*	*	*	*	*	333.3
1933-------	1948	*	*	*	*	*	*	*	*	*	*	*	344.5
1934-------	1949	*	*	*	*	*	*	*	*	*	*	*	344.0
1935-------	1950	*	*	*	*	*	*	*	*	*	*	*	333.3
1936-------	1951	*	*	*	*	*	*	*	*	*	*	*	316.2
1937-------	1952	*	*	*	*	*	*	*	*	*	*	*	302.2
1938-------	1953	*	*	*	*	*	*	*	*	*	*	*	286.8
1939-------	1954	*	*	*	*	*	*	*	*	*	*	*	251.9
1940-------	1955	*	*	*	*	*	*	*	*	*	*	*	221.3
1941-------	1956	*	*	*	*	*	*	*	*	*	*	*	211.5
1942-------	1957	*	*	*	*	*	*	*	*	*	*	*	*
1943-------	1958	*	*	*	*	*	*	*	*	*	*	*	*
1944-------	1959	*	*	*	*	*	*	*	*	*	*	*	*
1945-------	1960	*	*	*	*	*	*	*	*	*	*	*	*
1946-------	1961	*	*	*	*	*	*	*	*	*	*	*	*
1947-------	1962	*	*	*	*	*	*	*	*	*	*	*	*
1948-------	1963	*	*	*	*	*	*	*	*	*	*	*	
1949-------	1964	*	*	*	*	*	*	*	*	*	*		
1950-------	1965	*	*	*	*	*	*	*	*	*			
1951-------	1966	*	*	*	*	*	*	*	*				
1952-------	1967	*	*	*	*	*	*	*					
1953-------	1968	*	*	*	*	*	*						
1954-------	1969	*	*	*	*	*							
1955-------	1970	*	*	*	*								
1956-------	1971	*	*	*									
1957-------	1972	*	*										
1958-------	1973	*											

TABLE 10A. BIRTH PROBABILITIES FOR ALL WOMEN FOR EACH YEAR 1917-73 BY AGE AND PARITY FOR EACH COHORT FROM 1868 TO 1958--CON.

(PROBABILITIES ARE THE NUMBER OF BIRTHS PER 1,000 WOMEN IN SPECIFIED PARITY AND EXACT AGE GROUP. FIGURES FOR "0 PARITY" SHOW THE PROBABILITY OF FIRST BIRTHS TO "0 PARITY" WOMEN, THOSE FOR "1 PARITY" SHOW THE PROBABILITY OF SECOND BIRTHS TO "1 PARITY" WOMEN, ETC. BASED ON CENTRAL BIRTH RATES AND PARITY DISTRIBUTIONS)

PARITY AND COHORT	DIAGONAL LINE FOR JANUARY 1	EXACT AGE											
		27	28	29	30	31	32	33	34	35	36	37	38
6 PARITY--CON.													
1879-------													157.3
1880-------												185.1	156.3
1881-------											204.6	187.0	162.6
1882-------										228.6	207.6	194.9	165.5
1883-------									243.8	228.1	209.5	194.4	165.8
1884-------								255.1	236.2	220.6	203.9	188.6	153.2
1885-------							251.7	250.0	225.8	213.8	200.4	175.0	148.3
1886-------						270.9	250.0	237.8	221.0	216.8	187.9	171.3	147.8
1887-------					268.9	269.7	239.4	233.6	229.3	203.0	186.4	171.7	140.8
1888-------				290.9	252.2	248.2	227.6	237.9	208.7	198.5	181.2	159.6	130.9
1889-------			286.4	282.0	250.7	250.0	245.5	225.9	215.0	202.7	179.3	158.8	134.3
1890-------	1917	308.3	269.4	286.8	251.6	269.1	231.3	234.9	219.5	197.3	175.2	156.0	125.0
1891-------	1918	292.3	281.9	290.3	274.8	253.4	238.0	238.9	215.0	197.2	175.2	149.2	119.5
1892-------	1919	312.0	292.1	322.2	259.0	263.3	244.4	234.5	213.5	195.8	164.6	140.0	122.7
1893-------	1920	314.0	320.0	297.1	265.1	263.6	237.2	227.5	214.0	183.0	155.0	139.9	115.7
1894-------	1921	365.2	302.3	315.8	272.7	258.9	236.1	232.7	200.0	175.0	157.1	139.4	118.8
1895-------	1922	339.1	325.3	319.8	267.9	259.1	239.0	214.3	190.8	177.2	152.6	138.7	111.1
1896-------	1923	350.9	319.3	304.9	267.1	255.5	219.1	204.2	189.5	170.7	152.9	129.9	112.6
1897-------	1924	350.9	311.4	308.8	264.9	242.7	209.9	204.9	183.5	170.0	146.3	132.2	109.5
1898-------	1925	336.2	308.6	305.2	252.9	233.3	213.9	201.1	183.5	166.2	147.5	127.8	102.2
1899-------	1926	327.6	303.0	286.4	239.4	235.7	206.1	203.4	179.1	168.0	143.9	122.5	101.7
1900-------	1927	336.3	289.3	273.2	247.0	228.4	211.8	197.7	185.6	166.2	139.8	122.1	103.1
1901-------	1928	312.5	271.0	277.8	243.8	235.5	206.6	203.1	181.3	159.1	136.1	123.3	97.8
1902-------	1929	295.2	282.8	276.6	245.6	222.2	208.3	198.1	173.9	156.6	138.6	116.6	97.7
1903-------	1930	301.0	281.7	281.8	231.8	228.0	202.9	191.1	173.2	158.7	130.8	116.2	99.7
1904-------	1931	297.0	282.6	258.4	234.7	221.3	197.8	193.7	172.3	147.5	131.0	116.4	96.3
1905-------	1932	*	270.7	269.5	236.5	220.8	202.4	194.0	167.9	149.3	132.2	116.7	104.9
1906-------	1933	*	272.0	273.3	233.2	224.8	205.0	189.0	169.8	150.2	132.1	125.9	106.5
1907-------	1934	*	283.3	263.2	235.0	224.9	195.7	188.5	168.6	152.1	140.2	126.4	109.2
1908-------	1935	*	274.3	277.8	248.6	219.4	200.0	187.8	170.8	164.0	142.9	131.1	106.2
1909-------	1936	*	289.7	292.0	237.8	225.8	201.0	197.2	187.8	170.8	148.0	127.9	109.4
1910-------	1937	*	298.1	280.3	248.4	224.7	210.3	212.6	195.5	172.4	149.4	128.5	105.1
1911-------	1938	*	284.3	294.6	248.4	225.4	222.2	215.7	192.7	166.7	147.1	125.5	106.3
1912-------	1939	*	*	290.3	243.2	239.5	225.8	212.9	186.9	159.3	138.7	125.5	106.3
1913-------	1940	*	*	272.7	256.9	242.4	222.8	202.0	178.4	154.9	139.8	122.4	106.7
1914-------	1941	*	*	293.1	262.4	243.9	214.3	196.0	173.7	160.7	136.2	122.4	105.5
1915-------	1942	*	*	304.3	264.3	242.2	211.1	194.9	177.0	157.7	136.8	125.5	108.9
1916-------	1943	*	*	299.1	257.1	236.0	207.9	195.9	177.0	157.7	139.8	129.0	112.0
1917-------	1944	*	*	276.4	246.6	224.2	202.2	191.0	172.9	153.5	140.5	129.4	112.4
1918-------	1945	*	*	276.4	241.4	230.3	203.3	196.0	172.9	160.9	147.5	128.4	110.7
1919-------	1946	*	284.3	272.0	250.0	226.2	213.9	197.0	176.5	167.4	145.1	132.4	111.9
1920-------	1947	*	291.3	283.5	246.7	233.9	209.4	194.3	177.5	158.7	143.4	127.6	107.5
1921-------	1948	*	301.0	281.3	250.0	228.6	207.1	196.3	177.0	161.7	143.4	124.2	105.3
1922-------	1949	*	301.0	283.5	248.4	230.3	213.9	194.7	179.3	164.2	138.5	123.4	104.8
1923-------	1950	*	303.9	284.6	248.4	233.7	208.5	197.5	181.8	155.7	140.6	120.1	102.9
1924-------	1951	*	302.8	284.7	257.5	234.7	216.8	204.7	173.8	159.1	136.0	119.3	94.6
1925-------	1952	*	307.0	294.5	257.0	235.8	216.3	192.0	174.3	151.5	132.8	109.3	89.5
1926-------	1953	*	319.7	293.0	264.2	236.8	206.1	191.1	170.3	151.9	123.7	104.3	85.6
1927-------	1954	*	308.3	292.4	261.9	232.7	205.0	185.9	169.1	140.9	117.0	99.3	74.9
1928-------	1955	339.6	312.5	288.0	255.6	231.7	202.0	184.3	154.7	130.8	111.4	83.5	65.0
1929-------	1956	336.1	306.3	282.2	252.1	226.1	202.5	171.3	146.9	125.6	94.0	74.9	57.9
1930-------	1957	323.1	297.1	274.0	242.4	215.0	184.4	161.9	137.7	104.5	82.4	65.1	49.2
1931-------	1958	317.2	293.2	268.9	235.1	206.1	175.7	153.1	117.0	93.5	71.1	54.7	45.4
1932-------	1959	320.5	290.6	257.9	221.9	193.1	165.4	130.6	102.4	80.9	63.7	51.8	41.0
1933-------	1960	315.2	288.4	248.1	212.7	181.6	143.6	112.1	90.5	71.9	61.2	49.7	37.1
1934-------	1961	312.1	269.9	237.4	196.9	158.0	119.4	102.1	79.6	70.2	57.6	44.2	31.5
1935-------	1962	289.6	258.5	218.3	172.2	130.1	109.7	89.4	76.6	66.8	52.3	38.8	28.1
1936-------	1963	281.9	236.3	188.8	144.2	119.4	95.6	85.6	74.4	62.6	45.6	34.0	
1937-------	1964	262.0	205.1	163.6	132.3	109.1	96.4	83.1	71.4	52.1	41.5		
1938-------	1965	227.8	181.8	150.2	120.1	110.0	96.1	81.7	61.7	49.1			
1939-------	1966	201.2	169.2	139.1	120.6	109.2	90.6	69.7	54.9				
1940-------	1967	184.2	154.7	135.3	119.1	103.4	77.7	63.3					
1941-------	1968	178.3	150.3	134.1	117.1	88.1	73.5						
1942-------	1969	175.9	152.7	135.5	102.3	82.9							
1943-------	1970	*	151.8	113.6	94.6								
1944-------	1971	*	*	107.1									
1945-------	1972	*	*										
1946-------	1973	*											

TABLE 10A. BIRTH PROBABILITIES FOR ALL WOMEN FOR EACH YEAR 1917-73 BY AGE AND PARITY FOR EACH COHORT FROM 1868 TO 1958--CON.

(PROBABILITIES ARE THE NUMBER OF BIRTHS PER 1,000 WOMEN IN SPECIFIED PARITY AND EXACT AGE GROUP. FIGURES FOR "0 PARITY" SHOW THE PROBABILITY OF FIRST BIRTHS TO "0 PARITY" WOMEN, THOSE FOR "1 PARITY" SHOW THE PROBABILITY OF SECOND BIRTHS TO "1 PARITY" WOMEN, ETC. BASED ON CENTRAL BIRTH RATES AND PARITY DISTRIBUTIONS)

PARITY AND COHORT	DIAGONAL LINE FOR JANUARY 1	EXACT AGE										
		39	40	41	42	43	44	45	46	47	48	49
6 PARITY--CON.												
1868												1.4
1869											2.9	1.4
1870										4.4	2.9	1.5
1871									10.3	5.9	2.9	1.5
1872								16.3	10.4	4.5	3.0	1.5
1873							25.4	16.5	9.0	4.5	3.0	1.5
1874						39.3	25.8	15.2	10.7	4.6	3.1	1.5
1875					51.7	39.6	24.5	16.9	9.3	4.6	3.1	1.5
1876				71.5	51.8	36.7	24.6	13.9	9.3	4.6	3.1	0.0
1877			94.2	72.8	48.7	38.2	23.0	13.8	9.2	4.6	1.5	1.5
1878	1917	132.3	94.7	69.3	49.8	37.9	22.9	13.8	7.7	3.1	3.1	1.5
1879	1918	131.8	92.3	71.2	50.2	35.1	23.0	13.8	7.7	4.6	1.5	0.0
1880	1919	132.7	94.3	72.8	48.1	35.9	21.9	14.1	7.9	3.1	1.6	1.6
1881	1920	137.3	97.1	71.2	50.4	35.9	23.0	13.2	8.2	3.3	1.7	1.7
1882	1921	140.2	96.3	72.9	51.0	35.9	20.6	12.0	6.9	3.4	1.7	0.0
1883	1922	134.7	95.3	72.9	48.8	35.0	19.3	12.3	7.1	3.5	1.8	0.0
1884	1923	129.3	91.5	69.2	45.2	31.4	19.2	10.5	7.0	3.5	1.8	1.8
1885	1924	126.1	88.2	66.0	41.8	31.4	17.5	10.5	5.3	3.5	1.8	1.8
1886	1925	120.2	83.6	62.9	40.4	28.2	17.7	10.6	7.1	3.6	1.8	1.8
1887	1926	116.0	82.9	58.3	39.0	28.5	16.0	10.7	5.4	3.6	1.8	1.8
1888	1927	109.9	73.3	52.4	36.7	26.3	15.8	8.8	5.3	1.8	1.8	1.8
1889	1928	107.1	72.7	54.6	36.4	27.3	16.4	9.1	5.5	1.8	1.8	1.8
1890	1929	100.6	74.6	52.2	37.3	26.2	15.0	9.4	3.8	1.9	1.9	1.9
1891	1930	102.1	69.1	53.6	36.5	25.0	15.4	7.7	3.9	1.9	1.9	0.0
1892	1931	96.2	71.9	51.9	36.0	24.0	14.1	8.0	4.0	2.0	2.0	0.0
1893	1932	98.6	67.6	51.2	32.9	22.6	14.4	8.2	4.1	2.1	0.0	0.0
1894	1933	92.5	68.5	49.1	34.2	21.4	15.0	8.6	4.3	2.2	0.0	0.0
1895	1934	95.1	66.2	48.6	31.0	22.1	13.3	6.6	4.4	2.2	0.0	0.0
1896	1935	91.3	61.5	45.5	31.9	20.5	11.4	6.8	4.6	2.3	0.0	0.0
1897	1936	85.5	61.6	45.0	30.7	21.3	11.8	7.1	4.7	2.4	0.0	0.0
1898	1937	84.7	63.0	43.6	29.0	19.3	14.5	7.2	4.8	2.4	0.0	0.0
1899	1938	84.0	59.0	41.7	29.3	22.0	14.7	7.3	4.9	2.4	0.0	0.0
1900	1939	79.5	58.5	43.1	27.8	22.7	15.2	7.6	5.1	2.5	0.0	0.0
1901	1940	78.2	56.3	40.0	31.9	23.9	13.3	8.0	5.3	2.7	0.0	0.0
1902	1941	79.8	56.7	45.1	33.6	25.1	14.0	8.4	2.8	0.0	0.0	0.0
1903	1942	81.1	62.5	47.3	38.2	23.5	14.7	5.8	2.9	0.0	0.0	0.0
1904	1943	85.6	63.6	51.2	32.9	23.9	11.9	6.0	3.0	0.0	0.0	0.0
1905	1944	87.1	66.9	50.5	34.5	21.9	12.5	6.2	3.1	0.0	0.0	0.0
1906	1945	90.9	66.4	49.3	32.8	22.9	13.1	6.5	3.3	0.0	0.0	0.0
1907	1946	90.0	64.8	47.3	30.2	20.0	13.2	6.6	3.3	0.0	0.0	0.0
1908	1947	86.0	63.4	45.5	31.3	20.7	13.7	6.9	3.4	0.0	0.0	0.0
1909	1948	84.9	61.8	46.6	35.5	24.7	14.1	7.0	3.5	0.0	0.0	0.0
1910	1949	87.5	67.4	51.9	36.8	25.6	14.6	7.3	3.6	0.0	0.0	0.0
1911	1950	88.5	67.9	52.0	36.8	25.5	14.5	7.2	3.6	0.0	0.0	0.0
1912	1951	88.5	67.7	51.7	36.4	25.2	14.3	7.1	3.5	0.0	0.0	0.0
1913	1952	84.6	67.2	51.1	35.8	24.8	14.1	7.0	3.5	3.5	0.0	0.0
1914	1953	90.9	70.1	50.4	38.7	27.9	13.8	6.9	3.4	0.0	0.0	0.0
1915	1954	89.9	68.6	56.1	38.1	27.3	13.6	6.8	3.4	0.0	0.0	0.0
1916	1955	92.9	71.7	55.9	37.8	27.2	13.5	10.1	3.4	0.0	0.0	0.0
1917	1956	97.1	73.4	54.6	40.4	23.3	16.5	6.6	3.3	0.0	0.0	0.0
1918	1957	95.4	71.9	53.5	36.2	26.0	12.9	6.4	3.2	0.0	0.0	0.0
1919	1958	93.6	71.2	53.6	37.3	24.5	12.2	6.1	3.0	0.0	0.0	0.0
1920	1959	90.6	69.5	53.3	35.0	23.1	11.5	5.7	2.9	0.0	0.0	0.0
1921	1960	88.8	69.0	47.9	33.3	22.0	11.0	5.5	2.7	0.0	0.0	0.0
1922	1961	86.2	64.1	46.4	29.6	18.7	10.6	5.3	2.6	0.0	0.0	0.0
1923	1962	79.5	58.7	41.8	28.4	15.3	10.2	5.1	2.5	0.0	0.0	0.0
1924	1963	75.7	56.0	37.5	24.7	14.7	9.8	4.9	2.4	0.0	0.0	0.0
1925	1964	71.8	50.8	33.3	21.2	14.1	7.0	4.7	2.3	0.0	0.0	
1926	1965	64.3	44.3	29.9	20.5	11.4	6.8	2.3	0.0	0.0		
1927	1966	54.7	40.3	26.6	15.4	11.0	4.4	2.2	2.2			
1928	1967	50.5	34.7	21.5	14.9	8.5	4.2	2.1				
1929	1968	42.0	29.0	20.5	12.2	8.1	4.1					
1930	1969	36.2	27.8	17.7	9.8	5.9						
1931	1970	35.0	23.1	15.3	7.6							
1932	1971	30.8	20.9	11.3								
1933	1972	27.0	17.2									
1934	1973	23.3										

TABLE 10A. BIRTH PROBABILITIES FOR ALL WOMEN FOR EACH YEAR 1917-73 BY AGE AND PARITY FOR EACH COHORT FROM 1868 TO 1958--CON.

(PROBABILITIES ARE THE NUMBER OF BIRTHS PER 1,000 WOMEN IN SPECIFIED PARITY AND EXACT AGE GROUP. FIGURES FOR "0 PARITY" SHOW THE PROBABILITY OF FIRST BIRTHS TO "0 PARITY" WOMEN, THOSE FOR "1 PARITY" SHOW THE PROBABILITY OF SECOND BIRTHS TO "1 PARITY" WOMEN, ETC. BASED ON CENTRAL BIRTH RATES AND PARITY DISTRIBUTIONS)

PARITY AND COHORT	DIAGONAL LINE FOR JANUARY 1	EXACT AGE											
		15	16	17	18	19	20	21	22	23	24	25	26
7 AND HIGHER PARITY													
1891-------													*
1892-------												*	*
1893-------											*	*	*
1894-------										*	*	*	*
1895-------									*	*	*	*	*
1896-------								*	*	*	*	*	*
1897-------							*	*	*	*	*	*	*
1898-------						*	*	*	*	*	*	*	*
1899-------					*	*	*	*	*	*	*	*	*
1900-------				*	*	*	*	*	*	*	*	*	*
1901-------			*	*	*	*	*	*	*	*	*	*	*
1902-------	1917	*	*	*	*	*	*	*	*	*	*	*	*
1903-------	1918	*	*	*	*	*	*	*	*	*	*	*	*
1904-------	1919	*	*	*	*	*	*	*	*	*	*	*	*
1905-------	1920	*	*	*	*	*	*	*	*	*	*	*	*
1906-------	1921	*	*	*	*	*	*	*	*	*	*	*	*
1907-------	1922	*	*	*	*	*	*	*	*	*	*	*	*
1908-------	1923	*	*	*	*	*	*	*	*	*	*	*	*
1909-------	1924	*	*	*	*	*	*	*	*	*	*	*	*
1910-------	1925	*	*	*	*	*	*	*	*	*	*	*	*
1911-------	1926	*	*	*	*	*	*	*	*	*	*	*	*
1912-------	1927	*	*	*	*	*	*	*	*	*	*	*	*
1913-------	1928	*	*	*	*	*	*	*	*	*	*	*	*
1914-------	1929	*	*	*	*	*	*	*	*	*	*	*	*
1915-------	1930	*	*	*	*	*	*	*	*	*	*	*	*
1916-------	1931	*	*	*	*	*	*	*	*	*	*	*	*
1917-------	1932	*	*	*	*	*	*	*	*	*	*	*	*
1918-------	1933	*	*	*	*	*	*	*	*	*	*	*	*
1919-------	1934	*	*	*	*	*	*	*	*	*	*	*	*
1920-------	1935	*	*	*	*	*	*	*	*	*	*	*	*
1921-------	1936	*	*	*	*	*	*	*	*	*	*	*	*
1922-------	1937	*	*	*	*	*	*	*	*	*	*	*	*
1923-------	1938	*	*	*	*	*	*	*	*	*	*	*	*
1924-------	1939	*	*	*	*	*	*	*	*	*	*	*	*
1925-------	1940	*	*	*	*	*	*	*	*	*	*	*	*
1926-------	1941	*	*	*	*	*	*	*	*	*	*	*	*
1927-------	1942	*	*	*	*	*	*	*	*	*	*	*	*
1928-------	1943	*	*	*	*	*	*	*	*	*	*	*	*
1929-------	1944	*	*	*	*	*	*	*	*	*	*	*	*
1930-------	1945	*	*	*	*	*	*	*	*	*	*	*	*
1931-------	1946	*	*	*	*	*	*	*	*	*	*	*	*
1932-------	1947	*	*	*	*	*	*	*	*	*	*	*	*
1933-------	1948	*	*	*	*	*	*	*	*	*	*	*	*
1934-------	1949	*	*	*	*	*	*	*	*	*	*	*	*
1935-------	1950	*	*	*	*	*	*	*	*	*	*	*	*
1936-------	1951	*	*	*	*	*	*	*	*	*	*	*	*
1937-------	1952	*	*	*	*	*	*	*	*	*	*	*	*
1938-------	1953	*	*	*	*	*	*	*	*	*	*	*	*
1939-------	1954	*	*	*	*	*	*	*	*	*	*	*	*
1940-------	1955	*	*	*	*	*	*	*	*	*	*	*	*
1941-------	1956	*	*	*	*	*	*	*	*	*	*	*	*
1942-------	1957	*	*	*	*	*	*	*	*	*	*	*	*
1943-------	1958	*	*	*	*	*	*	*	*	*	*	*	*
1944-------	1959	*	*	*	*	*	*	*	*	*	*	*	*
1945-------	1960	*	*	*	*	*	*	*	*	*	*	*	*
1946-------	1961	*	*	*	*	*	*	*	*	*	*	*	*
1947-------	1962	*	*	*	*	*	*	*	*	*	*	*	*
1948-------	1963	*	*	*	*	*	*	*	*	*	*	*	
1949-------	1964	*	*	*	*	*	*	*	*	*	*		
1950-------	1965	*	*	*	*	*	*	*	*	*			
1951-------	1966	*	*	*	*	*	*	*	*				
1952-------	1967	*	*	*	*	*	*	*					
1953-------	1968	*	*	*	*	*	*						
1954-------	1969	*	*	*	*	*							
1955-------	1970	*	*	*	*								
1956-------	1971	*	*	*									
1957-------	1972	*	*										
1958-------	1973	*											

TABLE 10A. BIRTH PROBABILITIES FOR ALL WOMEN FOR EACH YEAR 1917-73 BY AGE AND PARITY FOR EACH COHORT FROM 1868 TO 1958--CON.

(PROBABILITIES ARE THE NUMBER OF BIRTHS PER 1,000 WOMEN IN SPECIFIED PARITY AND EXACT AGE GROUP. FIGURES FOR "0 PARITY" SHOW THE PROBABILITY OF FIRST BIRTHS TO "0 PARITY" WOMEN, THOSE FOR "1 PARITY" SHOW THE PROBABILITY OF SECOND BIRTHS TO "1 PARITY" WOMEN, ETC. BASED ON CENTRAL BIRTH RATES AND PARITY DISTRIBUTIONS)

PARITY AND COHORT	DIAGONAL LINE FOR JANUARY 1	EXACT AGE											
		27	28	29	30	31	32	33	34	35	36	37	38
7 AND HIGHER PARITY--CON.													
1879-------													218.5
1880-------												241.1	218.3
1881-------											246.6	241.3	225.9
1882-------										258.4	247.2	250.8	231.1
1883-------									259.8	260.9	256.5	256.0	239.8
1884-------								256.3	264.1	268.9	263.2	266.3	228.1
1885-------							253.0	263.5	271.1	276.7	275.0	254.4	235.2
1886-------						274.2	261.0	269.0	279.7	293.7	263.0	262.2	240.6
1887-------					278.8	284.9	267.2	276.7	300.7	281.1	271.3	268.2	241.3
1888-------				329.7	275.5	286.9	271.5	301.6	284.4	287.9	275.2	265.1	233.7
1889-------			319.3	323.9	286.9	298.5	302.5	288.4	297.4	295.5	277.5	263.0	239.3
1890-------	1917	*	303.6	341.5	302.5	332.3	289.8	305.8	303.7	295.8	268.5	265.6	223.1
1891-------	1918	*	317.3	363.1	336.2	314.3	303.2	309.1	306.8	286.5	274.2	246.1	213.6
1892-------	1919	*	336.6	398.7	313.0	323.6	302.7	309.4	291.9	286.7	248.1	232.3	213.1
1893-------	1920	*	*	372.5	325.9	326.7	306.3	297.1	292.8	263.6	239.8	233.3	207.1
1894-------	1921	*	350.0	388.2	325.9	324.5	293.1	295.0	269.2	254.2	239.8	227.3	207.1
1895-------	1922	*	370.0	383.1	324.4	313.3	290.9	275.4	260.8	256.7	232.1	227.5	197.6
1896-------	1923	*	380.0	392.2	321.3	315.3	275.9	268.1	266.4	246.3	232.4	214.8	203.5
1897-------	1924	*	376.2	379.1	322.7	299.0	267.8	269.4	253.4	250.0	220.9	223.3	200.8
1898-------	1925	*	382.4	375.0	304.1	289.8	272.0	264.2	256.0	235.4	228.6	220.6	193.0
1899-------	1926	*	366.3	364.2	297.2	295.6	267.4	274.3	247.9	250.5	232.1	216.9	198.1
1900-------	1927	*	339.8	349.0	302.4	288.4	273.3	259.4	262.3	253.7	227.4	222.7	199.1
1901-------	1928	*	*	347.8	300.5	297.6	258.7	276.3	264.6	244.1	234.0	221.9	190.0
1902-------	1929	*	*	348.5	293.5	270.8	271.8	270.9	253.0	250.5	233.4	216.0	195.4
1903-------	1930	*	*	333.3	271.2	289.5	266.7	266.9	256.9	251.1	222.0	217.7	194.8
1904-------	1931	*	*	317.1	295.9	292.2	271.1	273.0	257.2	240.7	226.4	218.1	196.4
1905-------	1932	*	*	350.4	302.5	290.5	272.0	275.6	250.0	248.2	224.7	215.0	206.4
1906-------	1933	*	*	367.0	300.7	298.0	275.3	270.3	264.5	246.8	223.3	229.1	212.7
1907-------	1934	*	*	346.2	305.6	304.8	273.5	290.3	264.6	244.6	237.7	235.4	214.1
1908-------	1935	*	*	*	313.9	294.4	291.5	289.5	265.4	262.9	243.0	238.3	207.3
1909-------	1936	*	*	*	292.0	306.8	284.4	281.9	274.8	263.8	248.7	227.0	201.8
1910-------	1937	*	*	*	310.6	298.2	284.4	297.6	280.4	268.4	240.1	224.1	199.1
1911-------	1938	*	*	*	303.0	294.1	291.9	298.8	284.7	261.1	237.3	222.0	204.1
1912-------	1939	*	*	*	310.1	315.2	302.4	295.5	269.0	254.5	229.5	225.6	200.0
1913-------	1940	*	*	*	333.3	325.0	300.0	286.3	270.5	250.8	237.3	222.2	201.4
1914-------	1941	*	*	*	330.6	310.6	288.6	283.3	261.6	256.3	233.0	224.0	202.9
1915-------	1942	*	*	*	309.5	306.7	282.2	279.2	266.2	247.6	234.3	222.5	191.3
1916-------	1943	*	*	*	310.1	297.0	275.9	283.3	259.0	247.6	228.6	208.9	192.8
1917-------	1944	*	*	*	299.2	300.6	290.0	278.5	261.8	243.6	224.8	212.6	190.8
1918-------	1945	*	*	*	300.0	309.1	285.7	279.2	258.1	240.5	223.8	208.2	189.6
1919-------	1946	*	*	*	325.8	307.7	285.0	283.4	261.3	245.4	224.0	213.4	191.3
1920-------	1947	*	*	360.0	316.2	306.4	286.4	276.7	261.9	241.8	224.0	210.1	181.8
1921-------	1948	*	*	352.9	318.8	306.8	282.4	284.0	260.0	244.9	222.8	199.1	182.8
1922-------	1949	*	*	352.9	311.6	295.5	290.3	280.8	259.9	243.6	215.7	202.3	177.2
1923-------	1950	*	*	346.2	305.0	316.7	291.5	284.6	267.5	237.6	221.1	199.6	175.2
1924-------	1951	*	*	342.6	326.5	315.8	292.4	287.7	255.2	238.3	213.8	193.8	164.8
1925-------	1952	*	*	359.6	324.8	315.3	292.5	274.5	259.1	235.4	212.1	184.7	160.0
1926-------	1953	*	*	360.7	333.3	315.1	285.7	278.3	250.7	230.6	199.6	175.0	154.0
1927-------	1954	*	*	366.4	331.5	309.3	290.1	271.4	250.0	221.0	189.2	166.7	135.5
1928-------	1955	*	*	368.1	329.9	311.0	283.4	267.4	236.8	205.7	180.8	149.7	115.4
1929-------	1956	*	381.8	364.8	328.7	306.9	281.5	256.2	222.7	192.7	159.7	126.4	101.4
1930-------	1957	*	380.2	358.4	321.9	299.7	270.0	243.6	208.6	174.0	136.8	111.1	87.7
1931-------	1958	*	365.0	336.8	311.3	280.9	250.0	223.2	183.0	147.4	119.1	95.8	81.6
1932-------	1959	*	340.1	335.0	295.2	269.2	234.6	196.2	158.4	129.8	106.9	90.8	76.7
1933-------	1960	371.4	356.7	319.6	280.7	252.8	203.8	168.8	139.8	115.5	100.5	86.1	69.0
1934-------	1961	375.0	343.4	308.4	266.2	215.7	178.3	149.0	124.3	110.5	95.5	79.5	60.7
1935-------	1962	362.1	325.4	291.3	229.5	192.0	156.2	133.8	119.0	107.2	90.1	68.5	54.4
1936-------	1963	353.4	307.7	253.3	200.7	168.7	143.6	130.5	115.6	101.5	75.8	61.3	
1937-------	1964	319.0	266.7	216.0	182.2	157.2	139.9	126.7	111.7	83.3	68.3		
1938-------	1965	283.2	220.8	195.9	163.8	150.4	136.7	120.5	91.4	72.9			
1939-------	1966	240.4	210.1	180.2	161.8	153.2	131.6	102.0	82.0				
1940-------	1967	*	193.3	183.7	165.7	142.9	113.0	95.2					
1941-------	1968	*	200.0	187.0	156.5	128.7	104.7						
1942-------	1969	*	*	176.5	130.1	120.6							
1943-------	1970	*	*	*	*								
1944-------	1971	*	*	*									
1945-------	1972	*	*										
1946-------	1973	*											

TABLE 10A. BIRTH PROBABILITIES FOR ALL WOMEN FOR EACH YEAR 1917-73 BY AGE AND PARITY FOR EACH COHORT FROM 1868 TO 1958--CON.

(PROBABILITIES ARE THE NUMBER OF BIRTHS PER 1,000 WOMEN IN SPECIFIED PARITY AND EXACT AGE GROUP. FIGURES FOR "0 PARITY" SHOW THE PROBABILITY OF FIRST BIRTHS TO "C PARITY" WOMEN, THOSE FOR "1 PARITY" SHOW THE PROBABILITY OF SECOND BIRTHS TO "1 PARITY" WOMEN, ETC. BASED ON CENTRAL BIRTH RATES AND PARITY DISTRIBUTIONS)

PARITY AND COHORT	DIAGONAL LINE FOR JANUARY 1	EXACT AGE 39	40	41	42	43	44	45	46	47	48	49
7 AND HIGHER PARITY--CON.												
1868												3.0
1869											6.5	4.4
1870										12.5	8.5	3.1
1871									22.4	15.5	6.8	3.6
1872								35.2	27.6	12.6	7.4	3.3
1873							52.8	39.4	22.9	13.8	7.1	3.3
1874						74.6	55.9	35.3	24.9	13.6	6.3	2.9
1875					91.6	75.1	52.3	37.7	24.5	12.0	6.5	3.0
1876				124.9	93.6	74.9	55.6	38.0	22.8	12.4	6.2	3.1
1877			153.1	128.6	93.7	78.3	57.6	36.1	23.1	12.3	6.4	2.7
1878	1917	202.8	155.3	127.1	96.8	81.6	54.9	36.3	23.0	11.5	5.5	2.7
1879	1918	204.9	155.8	132.1	100.4	77.3	54.8	37.0	22.9	11.1	5.6	2.8
1880	1919	207.5	160.6	135.7	95.1	78.2	55.8	36.0	22.2	10.2	5.7	2.8
1881	1920	213.6	166.0	129.1	96.3	80.8	55.5	35.1	20.4	10.5	5.2	2.3
1882	1921	221.4	157.5	130.4	99.9	80.1	53.6	33.8	20.5	10.8	5.4	2.4
1883	1922	209.8	159.8	134.6	99.8	77.7	53.4	33.1	19.3	9.9	5.0	2.5
1884	1923	214.2	164.8	133.9	97.4	77.2	50.2	31.1	19.4	9.7	5.1	2.6
1885	1924	220.1	165.1	131.1	98.3	73.4	47.4	31.6	18.8	9.4	5.3	2.7
1886	1925	217.5	158.3	131.2	92.4	68.9	48.5	30.7	18.8	9.0	5.5	2.8
1887	1926	213.4	162.6	125.4	88.0	71.2	47.1	30.3	17.9	9.3	5.0	2.9
1888	1927	211.7	152.7	118.4	89.4	68.3	46.5	29.1	17.1	8.9	5.2	2.2
1889	1928	203.0	147.2	120.3	87.1	68.4	45.8	29.3	17.7	8.4	4.6	2.3
1890	1929	194.4	148.1	117.5	87.4	67.1	46.9	28.9	16.8	8.8	4.8	2.4
1891	1930	195.2	144.8	115.5	85.2	69.4	45.2	27.5	16.6	8.3	5.0	1.7
1892	1931	187.3	141.6	111.2	88.0	67.1	42.8	26.9	15.6	7.8	4.3	1.7
1893	1932	187.7	138.0	115.4	84.5	63.8	41.2	26.4	15.4	7.2	3.6	1.8
1894	1933	178.6	141.7	113.1	80.2	61.7	42.0	24.6	14.2	7.5	2.8	1.9
1895	1934	183.1	138.3	107.0	79.2	61.1	38.7	24.6	13.8	6.9	2.9	1.0
1896	1935	182.4	132.6	106.9	80.0	57.8	38.5	23.8	13.4	6.2	3.1	2.1
1897	1936	173.4	133.1	108.6	74.9	58.4	37.1	25.0	13.0	6.5	3.2	1.1
1898	1937	173.7	136.9	103.1	77.7	57.2	42.0	27.0	13.5	7.8	3.4	2.2
1899	1938	178.2	128.0	103.5	75.2	58.8	40.7	24.3	13.8	6.9	3.4	2.3
1900	1939	168.0	130.0	103.5	75.4	61.0	41.0	25.1	13.1	7.1	3.6	1.2
1901	1940	170.0	130.0	99.5	80.4	63.6	42.3	24.2	14.0	6.3	3.8	1.3
1902	1941	172.8	131.7	110.6	85.7	66.3	40.9	24.4	13.5	6.7	2.7	1.3
1903	1942	172.9	140.6	113.5	88.6	63.8	41.5	22.8	12.8	5.7	2.8	1.4
1904	1943	180.9	143.3	116.5	85.9	64.9	38.7	22.2	11.8	5.9	2.9	1.5
1905	1944	185.7	144.8	113.5	84.9	59.8	38.9	21.7	10.8	6.2	3.1	1.5
1906	1945	187.3	142.6	113.6	80.5	61.1	35.9	21.1	11.3	4.8	3.2	1.6
1907	1946	183.6	141.3	107.7	82.3	58.6	37.5	22.0	10.1	5.1	1.7	1.7
1908	1947	178.9	135.7	110.5	78.6	61.2	37.4	21.2	12.3	5.3	1.8	1.8
1909	1948	175.3	139.8	106.7	81.8	60.2	36.0	21.5	10.7	5.3	3.6	1.8
1910	1949	181.4	136.8	108.7	79.4	57.5	36.6	20.0	10.9	5.4	3.6	1.8
1911	1950	175.2	136.5	106.1	78.4	60.0	35.2	22.1	11.0	5.5	1.8	1.8
1912	1951	175.1	133.3	106.4	80.1	57.5	37.8	20.6	11.2	5.6	1.9	1.9
1913	1952	175.7	135.2	105.4	78.3	61.0	36.9	21.2	9.6	5.7	1.9	1.9
1914	1953	170.1	133.3	103.3	80.3	58.9	36.8	19.2	11.5	5.7	1.9	1.9
1915	1954	167.8	131.2	105.4	78.0	54.8	34.7	19.1	9.5	3.8	1.9	0.0
1916	1955	164.4	130.1	102.2	75.2	52.3	34.4	18.9	9.4	3.8	1.9	0.0
1917	1956	166.7	131.6	99.6	72.8	53.8	34.2	18.8	9.4	3.7	1.9	0.0
1918	1957	165.9	125.3	100.0	73.6	53.1	31.8	16.7	9.2	3.7	1.8	0.0
1919	1958	157.1	128.3	97.9	72.5	52.7	32.3	16.0	8.9	3.5	1.8	0.0
1920	1959	161.2	124.8	97.0	70.4	49.5	29.6	15.6	8.6	3.4	1.7	0.0
1921	1960	154.3	122.9	94.0	68.4	48.1	27.1	15.2	6.7	3.4	1.7	0.0
1922	1961	151.3	116.9	89.0	65.6	40.7	25.1	13.3	5.0	3.3	0.0	0.0
1923	1962	148.0	111.5	86.5	57.2	38.0	22.9	11.4	4.9	1.6	0.0	0.0
1924	1963	140.0	109.2	75.7	51.4	34.8	18.8	10.9	4.7	1.5	0.0	0.0
1925	1964	133.3	96.1	67.7	46.2	28.9	16.6	9.0	4.5	1.5	0.0	
1926	1965	119.1	84.4	59.2	40.2	26.4	14.6	7.3	2.9	1.4		
1927	1966	103.6	72.6	51.5	36.2	22.9	12.8	7.1	2.8			
1928	1967	88.8	63.6	46.2	32.8	21.2	11.2	5.6				
1929	1968	78.2	58.7	43.5	29.1	17.9	10.9					
1930	1969	71.5	54.1	37.7	24.8	16.4						
1931	1970	66.0	47.6	31.6	23.1							
1932	1971	59.8	41.3	29.5								
1933	1972	50.7	36.5									
1934	1973	45.2										

TABLE 10B. BIRTH PROBABILITIES FOR WHITE WOMEN FOR EACH YEAR 1917-73 BY AGE AND PARITY FOR EACH COHORT FROM 1868 TO 1958

(PROBABILITIES ARE THE NUMBER OF BIRTHS PER 1,000 WOMEN IN SPECIFIED PARITY AND EXACT AGE GROUP. FIGURES FOR "0 PARITY" SHOW THE PROBABILITY OF FIRST BIRTHS TO "0 PARITY" WOMEN, THOSE FOR "1 PARITY" SHOW THE PROBABILITY OF SECOND BIRTHS TO "1 PARITY" WOMEN, ETC. BASED ON CENTRAL BIRTH RATES AND PARITY DISTRIBUTIONS)

PARITY AND COHORT	DIAGONAL LINE FOR JANUARY 1	EXACT AGE											
		15	16	17	18	19	20	21	22	23	24	25	26
0 PARITY													
1891-------													98.2
1892-------												110.6	103.6
1893-------											117.7	114.1	83.2
1894-------										122.7	120.0	89.7	106.0
1895-------									119.7	124.2	92.7	115.7	112.7
1896-------								116.8	121.7	94.5	120.9	122.3	104.5
1897-------							105.8	118.7	92.7	124.7	127.3	112.5	102.0
1898-------						89.5	107.1	90.7	123.0	130.9	116.5	110.9	104.1
1899-------					64.6	88.4	83.4	118.3	126.2	115.8	111.6	110.9	99.5
1900-------				40.5	62.9	71.1	108.5	121.5	111.8	111.8	113.9	105.4	94.4
1901-------			19.6	39.1	52.8	92.9	114.6	108.6	109.2	117.1	110.7	102.6	94.9
1902-------	1917	7.4	19.3	33.4	69.7	101.1	104.3	107.3	115.8	114.6	108.6	103.1	92.9
1903-------	1918	7.5	16.5	44.0	77.1	91.4	102.4	112.0	112.8	112.1	108.5	101.3	91.9
1904-------	1919	6.1	21.4	47.7	68.8	88.8	106.6	107.7	109.1	109.3	104.4	96.6	93.4
1905-------	1920	7.9	22.9	42.2	67.0	93.1	101.4	103.1	106.0	103.7	97.5	96.7	87.7
1906-------	1921	8.5	20.2	41.2	71.5	89.1	97.6	101.5	100.4	97.6	98.2	90.4	80.6
1907-------	1922	7.5	19.7	44.0	68.9	86.1	96.1	96.1	95.8	98.9	92.4	84.5	74.4
1908-------	1923	7.4	21.2	43.0	66.8	84.8	91.5	92.2	97.0	92.0	85.8	77.2	76.8
1909-------	1924	7.9	21.1	41.8	65.7	81.0	86.8	93.7	90.3	86.3	78.6	80.1	78.7
1910-------	1925	7.9	20.3	42.0	63.1	76.6	88.6	87.2	84.9	79.1	82.0	81.9	80.0
1911-------	1926	7.7	21.3	40.1	60.2	79.0	83.5	83.5	79.6	84.5	85.6	85.0	85.4
1912-------	1927	8.5	20.0	39.2	62.3	73.9	79.7	78.0	84.9	88.0	88.2	89.6	90.6
1913-------	1928	7.7	20.0	40.5	57.7	70.9	74.6	84.1	88.8	89.5	92.8	95.0	92.2
1914-------	1929	7.9	20.7	37.2	55.1	65.9	80.1	87.2	89.8	93.9	97.8	95.4	99.0
1915-------	1930	8.2	19.1	35.5	51.1	70.7	82.6	87.1	93.1	98.4	96.9	99.9	112.7
1916-------	1931	7.5	17.9	32.7	54.2	72.2	81.8	89.1	96.3	95.4	98.7	112.6	138.0
1917-------	1932	6.9	16.4	34.7	55.0	70.3	83.0	91.7	92.8	95.7	111.5	139.7	126.2
1918-------	1933	6.4	17.4	35.2	53.5	71.7	85.1	87.9	93.6	108.2	140.0	129.6	106.2
1919-------	1934	6.9	18.0	34.2	55.7	74.8	82.7	91.8	108.4	139.6	132.4	114.6	104.7
1920-------	1935	7.2	17.5	36.1	57.9	71.7	84.4	103.8	134.4	130.4	118.3	110.5	156.9
1921-------	1936	7.0	18.7	37.6	55.1	72.3	94.0	123.7	123.6	118.1	113.4	164.0	191.4
1922-------	1937	7.2	18.9	34.9	53.2	77.2	108.7	113.6	111.9	111.1	163.3	195.9	163.1
1923-------	1938	7.2	17.6	34.2	56.7	89.1	103.1	103.9	106.6	159.1	198.9	171.2	156.3
1924-------	1939	6.9	17.6	36.7	64.4	86.7	93.1	99.2	151.0	197.0	175.4	165.7	151.4
1925-------	1940	7.0	19.0	39.0	63.9	76.3	88.7	136.0	188.8	173.0	167.3	156.2	160.7
1926-------	1941	7.6	19.4	38.8	55.2	72.2	116.4	173.8	166.1	164.0	157.0	165.5	159.7
1927-------	1942	7.7	19.5	33.7	52.2	91.3	154.2	155.3	156.9	153.9	167.3	166.2	156.0
1928-------	1943	7.7	16.8	31.5	63.3	125.1	140.4	146.6	147.8	165.6	169.2	162.2	153.7
1929-------	1944	6.7	15.8	36.9	89.9	117.7	134.0	139.3	162.4	170.9	168.8	166.4	154.1
1930-------	1945	6.4	17.4	54.1	87.9	112.6	127.5	154.1	167.1	170.1	175.2	168.2	157.0
1931-------	1946	6.8	26.5	55.4	85.2	108.3	142.8	158.8	168.8	180.2	181.8	176.3	165.3
1932-------	1947	10.1	28.1	53.8	82.1	120.5	144.8	162.1	178.9	187.3	189.6	182.6	163.2
1933-------	1948	11.3	28.1	53.0	91.2	121.0	149.6	170.8	185.1	196.4	196.6	180.4	162.0
1934-------	1949	11.2	27.9	57.6	90.2	125.5	156.0	174.2	194.3	201.8	192.5	177.3	159.0
1935-------	1950	11.3	29.7	56.6	93.0	128.8	156.7	183.3	198.1	196.5	187.7	172.8	153.8
1936-------	1951	11.8	29.2	58.5	95.3	128.3	165.3	186.9	193.2	191.4	183.8	168.4	147.6
1937-------	1952	11.7	30.3	59.6	94.5	135.6	169.4	183.4	190.4	190.3	181.3	160.9	142.5
1938-------	1953	12.0	31.0	58.9	99.8	139.6	166.5	181.9	188.9	187.4	171.7	156.0	144.6
1939-------	1954	12.6	31.0	62.7	103.9	137.5	166.9	180.3	186.3	178.2	167.0	156.4	138.5
1940-------	1955	12.6	32.9	64.8	100.8	136.2	162.8	176.8	176.6	170.3	163.5	146.6	139.5
1941-------	1956	13.4	34.0	62.0	98.3	131.0	158.5	167.5	167.3	165.0	151.2	148.6	135.5
1942-------	1957	13.6	32.1	59.6	94.0	127.6	150.0	159.1	161.7	152.2	154.2	144.2	142.3
1943-------	1958	12.8	30.6	56.7	91.5	121.4	144.2	152.7	147.1	152.3	146.1	145.9	136.6
1944-------	1959	12.5	29.7	55.9	87.6	117.9	138.7	139.7	146.4	143.2	144.2	140.6	133.5
1945-------	1960	12.4	29.4	53.5	85.4	112.7	126.9	137.1	136.6	138.3	138.9	137.2	123.4
1946-------	1961	12.1	27.6	51.6	81.5	105.3	125.9	129.9	134.3	138.3	140.8	129.8	114.1
1947-------	1962	11.0	26.4	49.2	76.8	103.7	118.3	127.2	132.9	138.1	129.2	115.3	107.6
1948-------	1963	10.5	25.3	47.2	75.9	98.2	116.8	125.6	132.8	125.0	112.2	107.0	
1949-------	1964	10.2	24.1	45.9	71.6	96.2	113.7	124.0	116.9	104.8	100.2		
1950-------	1965	9.8	23.7	44.4	71.1	95.1	114.0	109.9	98.4	94.1			
1951-------	1966	9.8	23.2	44.4	71.2	96.9	101.9	93.3	88.3				
1952-------	1967	9.5	23.4	45.0	74.0	88.2	88.5	84.1					
1953-------	1968	9.9	24.1	48.3	69.0	79.5	80.7						
1954-------	1969	10.5	26.6	46.2	65.3	73.9							
1955-------	1970	11.8	26.2	46.2	62.3								
1956-------	1971	11.7	27.3	45.1									
1957-------	1972	12.6	27.3										
1958-------	1973	13.0											

TABLE 10B. BIRTH PROBABILITIES FOR WHITE WOMEN FOR EACH YEAR 1917-73 BY AGE AND PARITY FOR EACH COHORT FROM 1868 TO 1958--CON.

(PROBABILITIES ARE THE NUMBER OF BIRTHS PER 1,000 WOMEN IN SPECIFIED PARITY AND EXACT AGE GROUP. FIGURES FOR "0 PARITY" SHOW THE PROBABILITY OF FIRST BIRTHS TO "0 PARITY" WOMEN, THOSE FOR "1 PARITY" SHOW THE PROBABILITY OF SECOND BIRTHS TO "1 PARITY" WOMEN, ETC. BASED ON CENTRAL BIRTH RATES AND PARITY DISTRIBUTIONS)

PARITY AND COHORT	DIAGONAL LINE FOR JANUARY 1	EXACT AGE											
		27	28	29	30	31	32	33	34	35	36	37	38
0 PARITY--CON.													
1879-------													13.4
1880-------												17.0	13.8
1881-------											20.5	17.5	13.9
1882-------										25.4	21.0	17.2	14.4
1883-------									29.5	26.3	21.1	18.1	15.4
1884-------								35.0	31.1	25.1	21.9	19.4	14.1
1885-------							39.4	37.2	28.7	27.1	23.6	17.7	13.6
1886-------						49.3	42.6	33.6	32.0	28.5	22.1	17.4	14.2
1887-------					60.8	53.3	38.7	38.7	33.3	27.7	22.0	18.1	14.4
1888-------				75.8	64.8	48.0	44.4	39.7	33.0	27.8	22.8	18.4	13.7
1889-------			85.3	80.1	55.5	54.8	44.9	39.4	32.2	28.1	22.7	17.7	14.4
1890-------	1917	93.5	90.0	66.5	66.8	56.4	45.3	38.9	33.2	27.8	21.7	18.5	14.2
1891-------	1918	98.7	72.5	82.3	69.0	56.5	44.7	40.1	33.5	27.0	22.7	18.0	14.0
1892-------	1919	79.7	92.7	86.6	66.9	55.8	46.0	40.0	32.3	27.8	22.4	17.1	14.4
1893-------	1920	101.2	97.9	81.1	65.3	56.9	46.1	38.2	32.4	26.9	21.3	18.3	14.1
1894-------	1921	107.1	89.7	78.7	66.1	56.5	44.3	39.3	31.7	26.1	22.4	17.9	13.2
1895-------	1922	98.8	87.3	79.8	65.8	55.2	44.9	38.1	31.4	28.1	22.0	16.5	12.2
1896-------	1923	96.2	88.4	78.6	63.9	55.0	43.8	37.8	33.3	26.8	20.6	15.5	12.7
1897-------	1924	97.8	86.2	76.2	63.3	53.9	43.4	39.6	31.5	25.3	19.1	16.0	12.7
1898-------	1925	94.8	83.0	74.5	61.7	53.3	45.3	37.3	29.0	23.2	19.9	16.4	13.1
1899-------	1926	90.7	80.7	71.8	59.9	54.4	43.1	35.2	28.0	24.3	20.6	16.8	13.6
1900-------	1927	87.5	76.8	69.0	60.9	51.3	39.8	32.7	28.7	24.7	20.8	17.1	14.1
1901-------	1928	85.4	75.7	71.7	59.6	49.8	37.7	34.6	29.5	25.5	21.7	18.5	15.0
1902-------	1929	84.7	79.4	70.9	57.3	46.4	40.7	36.6	31.0	27.6	23.8	19.2	15.8
1903-------	1930	88.3	78.4	67.7	54.0	49.9	43.4	38.7	33.8	30.0	25.9	20.9	17.9
1904-------	1931	84.6	72.7	62.5	57.3	52.7	44.9	40.5	35.9	31.5	27.1	22.8	21.9
1905-------	1932	77.2	65.9	64.7	57.9	52.8	45.7	41.7	36.7	32.2	28.6	26.7	22.4
1906-------	1933	71.0	68.9	65.8	58.7	54.2	48.1	43.0	37.5	34.1	31.5	27.8	21.4
1907-------	1934	74.2	70.5	66.4	61.9	57.7	50.1	44.4	40.7	41.2	33.8	27.2	22.6
1908-------	1935	75.5	70.5	68.9	65.0	59.2	51.1	47.3	49.7	41.6	32.7	27.4	25.9
1909-------	1936	75.9	74.5	73.4	66.9	61.6	56.2	59.9	48.9	38.7	33.2	32.6	28.8
1910-------	1937	79.6	78.8	74.5	70.0	67.1	66.6	57.6	43.9	38.8	39.9	36.4	24.7
1911-------	1938	86.2	80.8	79.7	78.9	77.3	66.0	51.2	45.3	49.1	46.4	31.8	23.5
1912-------	1939	87.2	86.1	89.5	91.4	76.4	58.4	52.4	58.2	56.1	39.3	30.0	22.6
1913-------	1940	93.4	98.7	106.6	88.5	68.3	59.7	69.5	68.2	48.6	38.0	29.4	22.9
1914-------	1941	107.2	119.6	101.3	77.6	69.1	82.1	82.2	58.8	47.6	37.5	30.3	24.5
1915-------	1942	131.0	111.5	87.4	77.6	96.2	97.3	69.8	56.2	46.4	38.1	31.6	24.3
1916-------	1943	120.5	93.5	84.8	107.7	112.5	80.0	64.8	52.7	45.8	38.3	30.9	24.5
1917-------	1944	100.7	90.5	120.2	126.7	93.2	74.4	60.8	53.5	46.4	37.3	30.2	23.5
1918-------	1945	96.3	129.7	141.2	104.8	86.5	69.4	62.1	53.9	44.1	36.3	28.7	21.7
1919-------	1946	145.7	160.8	125.2	105.1	87.9	77.4	68.6	56.7	48.1	39.3	31.4	24.9
1920-------	1947	178.4	140.5	122.9	103.6	95.1	83.7	69.3	59.2	49.6	40.5	33.3	25.2
1921-------	1948	155.8	136.6	119.6	111.1	99.9	82.6	73.2	60.7	50.9	41.7	33.8	25.8
1922-------	1949	146.2	128.6	123.7	110.3	94.0	81.3	68.3	57.1	49.1	39.6	30.5	24.1
1923-------	1950	140.9	136.8	125.9	109.5	97.0	79.4	68.6	59.0	47.9	38.4	30.4	23.5
1924-------	1951	152.3	141.7	125.5	111.0	95.0	81.0	71.0	57.9	48.5	39.2	30.6	23.1
1925-------	1952	153.4	136.6	122.8	106.6	92.2	79.4	66.4	55.1	46.1	36.5	27.6	22.1
1926-------	1953	146.2	131.3	116.1	100.4	88.2	72.5	61.1	50.3	41.1	32.4	25.6	23.2
1927-------	1954	142.6	127.1	111.8	98.5	82.3	68.6	57.4	46.4	37.8	29.0	27.9	21.8
1928-------	1955	139.0	122.8	110.4	92.2	77.3	63.6	52.0	42.2	34.3	32.8	25.4	19.3
1929-------	1956	139.8	127.0	108.2	90.0	76.7	62.1	50.5	41.0	40.0	32.2	24.5	17.1
1930-------	1957	143.6	124.1	105.4	88.7	74.3	59.4	49.5	47.6	38.6	30.4	22.2	19.6
1931-------	1958	144.5	124.0	107.8	90.2	73.6	61.3	58.0	47.9	37.9	28.8	26.3	18.0
1932-------	1959	143.5	124.3	106.3	86.0	74.7	68.1	56.5	46.4	36.8	33.7	23.3	19.0
1933-------	1960	142.9	122.6	101.5	88.1	81.7	67.0	56.4	44.6	42.1	30.9	24.5	17.6
1934-------	1961	138.4	117.4	100.9	95.9	79.1	66.4	52.3	48.6	37.1	30.1	21.1	16.5
1935-------	1962	132.3	112.7	106.9	88.1	76.2	57.6	56.0	42.1	36.0	26.9	20.4	14.7
1936-------	1963	127.0	119.6	99.4	86.6	68.7	63.5	48.9	41.9	31.7	24.9	18.5	
1937-------	1964	131.9	113.2	99.4	81.4	75.0	59.0	50.0	38.1	30.0	23.2		
1938-------	1965	125.7	111.9	95.7	86.8	70.9	59.2	44.8	36.0	28.0			
1939-------	1966	127.2	109.8	103.1	84.9	73.1	56.7	44.1	35.4				
1940-------	1967	123.6	117.0	98.3	85.3	67.4	52.1	41.7					
1941-------	1968	130.9	112.1	100.1	79.3	61.9	50.2						
1942-------	1969	127.4	114.1	92.8	72.9	60.7							
1943-------	1970	124.9	105.1	83.5	70.5								
1944-------	1971	116.2	95.3	81.4									
1945-------	1972	104.2	90.9										
1946-------	1973	103.1											

TABLE 108. BIRTH PROBABILITIES FOR WHITE WOMEN FOR EACH YEAR 1917-73 BY AGE AND PARITY FOR EACH COHORT FROM 1868 TO 1958--CON.

(PROBABILITIES ARE THE NUMBER OF BIRTHS PER 1,000 WOMEN IN SPECIFIED PARITY AND EXACT AGE GROUP. FIGURES FOR "0 PARITY" SHOW THE PROBABILITY OF FIRST BIRTHS TO "C PARITY" WOMEN, THOSE FOR "1 PARITY" SHOW THE PROBABILITY OF SECOND BIRTHS TO "1 PARITY" WOMEN, ETC. BASED ON CENTRAL BIRTH RATES AND PARITY DISTRIBUTIONS)

PARITY AND COHORT	DIAGONAL LINE FOR JANUARY 1	EXACT AGE										
		39	40	41	42	43	44	45	46	47	48	49
0 PARITY--CON.												
1868----------------												0.0
1869----------------											0.0	0.0
1870----------------										0.0	0.0	0.0
1871----------------									0.5	0.5	0.0	0.0
1872----------------								1.0	0.5	0.0	0.0	0.0
1873----------------							1.4	1.0	0.5	0.0	0.0	0.0
1874----------------						2.3	1.4	0.9	0.5	0.0	0.0	0.0
1875----------------					3.7	2.3	1.4	0.9	0.5	0.5	0.0	0.0
1876----------------				5.5	3.7	2.8	1.4	0.9	0.5	0.0	0.0	0.0
1877----------------			7.7	5.5	3.7	2.8	1.4	0.9	0.5	0.0	0.0	0.0
1878----------------	1917	11.1	7.6	5.9	3.6	2.7	1.4	0.9	0.5	0.5	0.0	0.0
1879----------------	1918	11.0	8.0	5.8	4.1	2.7	1.4	0.9	0.5	0.0	0.0	0.0
1880----------------	1919	11.4	8.0	6.3	3.6	2.7	1.4	0.9	0.5	0.0	0.0	0.0
1881----------------	1920	11.9	8.5	5.4	3.6	2.7	1.4	0.9	0.5	0.0	0.0	0.0
1882----------------	1921	12.4	7.6	5.4	3.6	2.3	1.4	0.9	0.5	0.5	0.0	0.0
1883----------------	1922	11.6	7.7	5.5	3.2	2.3	1.4	0.9	0.5	0.5	0.0	0.0
1884----------------	1923	11.1	7.7	5.4	3.7	2.3	1.4	0.9	0.5	0.0	0.0	0.0
1885----------------	1924	11.6	7.7	5.4	3.7	2.3	1.4	0.9	0.5	0.0	0.0	0.0
1886----------------	1925	11.2	7.3	5.5	3.7	1.8	1.4	0.5	0.5	0.0	0.0	0.0
1887----------------	1926	11.0	7.9	5.6	3.3	1.9	0.9	0.5	0.5	0.0	0.0	0.0
1888----------------	1927	11.1	7.5	5.2	3.3	1.9	1.0	0.5	0.0	0.0	0.0	0.0
1889----------------	1928	11.3	7.6	5.3	3.4	2.4	1.0	0.5	0.5	0.0	0.0	0.0
1890----------------	1929	11.0	7.3	5.4	3.4	2.0	1.0	0.5	0.0	0.0	0.0	0.0
1891----------------	1930	11.2	7.4	5.0	3.0	2.0	1.5	0.5	0.0	0.0	0.0	0.0
1892----------------	1931	11.1	7.1	4.6	3.1	2.1	1.0	0.5	0.0	0.0	0.0	0.0
1893----------------	1932	10.2	6.7	4.7	3.1	2.1	1.1	0.5	0.5	0.0	0.0	0.0
1894----------------	1933	9.8	6.7	4.7	3.2	2.1	1.1	0.5	0.5	0.0	0.0	0.0
1895----------------	1934	9.8	6.8	4.7	3.2	2.1	1.1	0.5	0.5	0.0	0.0	0.0
1896----------------	1935	9.3	6.8	4.7	3.2	2.1	1.1	0.5	0.5	0.0	0.0	0.0
1897----------------	1936	9.8	6.8	4.7	3.7	2.1	1.6	0.5	0.5	0.0	0.0	0.0
1898----------------	1937	10.2	7.2	5.2	3.7	2.6	1.6	1.1	0.5	0.0	0.0	0.0
1899----------------	1938	10.9	8.0	5.5	4.0	2.5	1.5	1.0	0.5	0.0	0.0	0.0
1900----------------	1939	11.0	7.7	5.8	3.9	2.9	1.5	1.0	0.5	0.0	0.0	0.0
1901----------------	1940	11.5	8.7	5.8	4.4	3.0	2.0	1.0	0.5	0.0	0.0	0.0
1902----------------	1941	12.6	10.3	7.5	5.0	3.5	2.0	1.0	0.5	0.0	0.0	0.0
1903----------------	1942	16.3	12.0	8.6	5.6	4.1	2.1	1.0	0.5	0.0	0.0	0.0
1904----------------	1943	17.5	12.4	9.0	6.6	4.1	2.0	1.0	0.5	0.0	0.0	0.0
1905----------------	1944	16.9	12.9	9.6	6.3	3.4	2.0	1.0	0.5	0.0	0.0	0.0
1906----------------	1945	17.3	14.4	10.4	5.7	3.4	1.9	1.0	0.5	0.0	0.0	0.0
1907----------------	1946	20.4	15.3	8.9	5.7	3.3	1.9	1.0	0.5	0.0	0.0	0.0
1908----------------	1947	21.7	13.4	8.9	5.2	2.8	1.9	1.0	0.5	0.0	0.0	0.0
1909----------------	1948	19.2	12.6	8.5	5.2	3.3	1.9	1.0	0.5	0.0	0.0	0.0
1910----------------	1949	18.0	12.2	8.1	5.3	3.4	1.9	1.0	0.5	0.0	0.0	0.0
1911----------------	1950	17.3	12.2	8.4	5.5	3.0	2.0	1.0	0.5	0.0	0.0	0.0
1912----------------	1951	17.1	12.8	8.3	5.2	3.1	1.6	1.1	0.5	0.0	0.0	0.0
1913----------------	1952	18.1	12.5	8.8	5.6	3.4	1.7	1.1	0.6	0.0	0.0	0.0
1914----------------	1953	18.3	13.4	8.8	5.4	3.6	1.8	1.2	0.6	0.0	0.0	0.0
1915----------------	1954	18.8	13.0	8.2	5.7	3.2	1.9	0.6	0.6	0.0	0.0	0.0
1916----------------	1955	18.2	11.5	9.1	5.2	3.3	1.3	0.7	0.0	0.0	0.0	0.0
1917----------------	1956	16.9	12.6	8.0	5.4	2.7	1.4	0.7	0.0	0.0	0.0	0.0
1918----------------	1957	16.8	10.9	7.6	4.9	2.8	1.4	0.7	0.0	0.0	0.0	0.0
1919----------------	1958	17.8	13.4	8.8	5.6	3.2	1.6	0.8	0.0	0.0	0.0	0.0
1920----------------	1959	18.9	13.2	9.8	5.4	3.6	1.8	0.9	0.0	0.0	0.0	0.0
1921----------------	1960	18.9	13.5	8.8	5.9	4.0	2.0	1.0	0.0	0.0	0.0	0.0
1922----------------	1961	18.0	12.5	8.8	6.9	4.0	2.0	1.0	0.0	0.0	0.0	0.0
1923----------------	1962	17.1	12.3	10.3	6.3	3.2	2.1	1.1	0.0	0.0	0.0	0.0
1924----------------	1963	17.2	15.3	10.0	5.6	3.4	2.3	1.1	0.0	0.0	0.0	0.0
1925----------------	1964	20.5	13.2	8.9	4.5	3.4	1.1	1.1	0.0	0.0	0.0	
1926----------------	1965	17.6	11.6	7.5	5.4	2.2	1.1	1.1	0.0	0.0		
1927----------------	1966	16.2	9.3	8.3	4.2	2.1	1.1	0.0	0.0			
1928----------------	1967	12.8	11.0	6.1	4.1	2.0	1.0	0.0				
1929----------------	1968	15.3	9.3	6.3	3.2	2.1	1.1					
1930----------------	1969	12.7	9.6	5.4	3.3	2.2						
1931----------------	1970	13.8	9.3	5.9	3.5							
1932----------------	1971	12.1	8.6	5.0								
1933----------------	1972	12.8	7.8									
1934----------------	1973	11.6										

TABLE 10B. BIRTH PROBABILITIES FOR WHITE WOMEN FOR EACH YEAR 1917-73 BY AGE AND PARITY FOR EACH COHORT FROM 1868 TO 1958--CON.

(PROBABILITIES ARE THE NUMBER OF BIRTHS PER 1,000 WOMEN IN SPECIFIED PARITY AND EXACT AGE GROUP. FIGURES FOR "0 PARITY" SHOW THE PROBABILITY OF FIRST BIRTHS TO "0 PARITY" WOMEN, THOSE FOR "1 PARITY" SHOW THE PROBABILITY OF SECOND BIRTHS TO "1 PARITY" WOMEN, ETC. BASED ON CENTRAL BIRTH RATES AND PARITY DISTRIBUTIONS)

PARITY AND COHORT	DIAGONAL LINE FOR JANUARY 1	EXACT AGE											
		15	16	17	18	19	20	21	22	23	24	25	26
1 PARITY													
1891-------													198.2
1892-------												217.9	191.9
1893-------											233.8	210.3	179.4
1894-------										256.3	226.5	197.4	182.7
1895-------									265.5	247.6	212.2	201.4	176.5
1896-------								282.9	255.7	229.3	215.7	193.5	173.9
1897-------							288.9	273.4	237.3	233.3	206.0	191.8	174.5
1898-------						285.0	278.8	254.6	246.7	223.8	207.5	196.9	172.5
1899-------					257.6	280.0	264.8	268.2	234.1	224.7	213.3	193.6	168.6
1900-------				236.0	252.9	268.4	283.4	250.8	232.3	231.1	210.2	183.1	159.7
1901-------			*	228.5	240.6	284.6	261.4	241.0	234.7	224.4	196.6	172.3	153.0
1902-------	1917	*	*	224.3	268.9	269.9	254.4	247.1	231.9	209.3	186.6	164.8	143.6
1903-------	1918	*	*	248.9	260.3	260.5	262.0	243.4	221.1	203.8	180.4	157.6	138.1
1904-------	1919	*	*	237.2	256.0	273.8	258.7	232.4	217.7	197.4	173.0	153.2	139.1
1905-------	1920	*	*	232.6	278.6	269.9	245.8	229.7	212.7	188.7	168.4	154.0	135.1
1906-------	1921	*	186.3	254.4	270.5	253.2	242.2	227.0	202.8	184.5	168.2	148.2	130.2
1907-------	1922	*	*	250.0	258.0	254.3	244.3	220.2	201.2	186.4	164.5	145.9	126.8
1908-------	1923	*	*	242.0	260.3	256.9	235.6	217.0	202.4	179.8	160.6	140.8	132.6
1909-------	1924	*	*	246.5	263.3	247.7	231.9	219.7	196.8	177.7	156.0	148.0	130.5
1910-------	1925	*	*	250.0	245.9	240.2	233.6	211.0	193.2	171.5	162.2	142.8	129.6
1911-------	1926	*	*	232.4	242.2	246.1	225.3	209.1	186.6	178.7	157.4	143.5	133.3
1912-------	1927	*	196.1	232.1	245.4	232.3	222.1	199.8	193.9	171.4	157.2	145.7	137.9
1913-------	1928	*	*	236.4	232.2	230.0	211.2	208.1	186.4	171.9	160.3	151.1	136.0
1914-------	1929	*	*	212.8	229.8	218.1	221.1	200.1	187.1	175.4	165.6	148.0	142.6
1915-------	1930	*	180.0	210.3	216.5	227.1	212.6	201.8	192.3	181.3	161.9	153.8	149.8
1916-------	1931	*	*	204.7	226.9	219.3	215.7	206.7	197.8	176.0	166.4	160.5	163.4
1917-------	1932	*	*	214.6	218.8	223.8	221.1	214.2	192.1	180.4	174.0	180.5	179.4
1918-------	1933	*	*	202.5	223.7	230.3	227.8	206.3	198.0	186.0	197.9	193.3	165.7
1919-------	1934	*	*	210.5	233.0	235.7	220.5	216.0	204.0	211.7	203.1	172.7	158.4
1920-------	1935	*	*	225.4	235.2	228.0	235.4	222.2	216.4	212.6	178.5	157.3	197.5
1921-------	1936	*	*	224.4	230.9	252.9	244.8	221.4	216.3	185.3	159.3	207.2	210.8
1922-------	1937	*	*	222.7	263.9	263.7	240.1	226.9	194.5	163.6	218.9	221.6	198.1
1923-------	1938	*	*	257.1	269.9	257.4	240.3	202.0	169.1	228.5	231.7	208.7	204.3
1924-------	1939	*	*	255.2	265.4	253.8	211.3	174.9	238.8	239.8	219.0	215.8	210.3
1925-------	1940	*	*	249.0	260.1	221.0	187.7	245.9	249.2	228.7	227.6	221.9	224.4
1926-------	1941	*	*	255.7	227.3	200.6	255.3	257.9	239.9	238.5	234.0	238.9	235.6
1927-------	1942	*	*	224.3	210.9	258.5	269.2	249.6	249.4	243.0	251.0	248.6	245.2
1928-------	1943	*	*	214.3	261.1	278.6	262.4	260.8	254.6	262.4	261.8	260.9	255.7
1929-------	1944	*	*	251.1	284.6	270.0	274.0	265.4	275.0	273.1	276.0	273.5	262.1
1930-------	1945	*	*	286.3	275.2	283.3	279.1	287.2	286.3	288.1	290.4	281.3	272.9
1931-------	1946	*	*	269.3	290.5	289.3	302.1	297.1	301.9	304.3	298.6	294.3	284.9
1932-------	1947	*	260.9	289.3	296.8	310.6	307.1	310.7	315.7	310.2	310.8	303.7	283.5
1933-------	1948	*	283.6	289.5	314.4	310.8	320.1	321.0	321.0	321.6	319.9	302.7	282.6
1934-------	1949	*	283.6	310.0	310.6	324.6	326.0	327.0	332.5	330.6	318.6	303.7	282.4
1935-------	1950	*	291.0	301.5	322.7	324.7	331.8	337.8	340.4	329.4	319.3	303.6	277.0
1936-------	1951	*	278.6	313.6	323.2	331.7	345.9	345.2	337.4	331.8	321.6	299.4	269.8
1937-------	1952	*	283.7	310.8	328.2	348.9	351.1	342.5	342.5	334.3	316.3	287.5	262.2
1938-------	1953	*	293.7	317.7	350.4	351.1	348.8	351.7	344.8	330.2	304.9	281.3	257.7
1939-------	1954	*	297.3	339.9	351.4	350.5	358.5	349.9	339.9	317.2	297.3	274.1	239.1
1940-------	1955	*	311.3	336.4	348.5	360.5	355.1	345.5	329.8	310.4	288.7	254.3	228.1
1941-------	1956	*	316.5	334.8	352.2	355.7	351.1	337.5	321.4	299.0	266.2	243.0	222.5
1942-------	1957	*	310.6	338.0	355.7	353.0	344.2	328.2	306.0	272.4	252.0	235.9	220.3
1943-------	1958	*	313.7	344.8	354.4	348.2	333.0	308.2	275.0	256.4	245.2	231.5	220.7
1944-------	1959	*	322.1	343.5	347.2	334.4	309.8	272.4	255.0	247.8	237.8	230.9	220.5
1945-------	1960	*	322.1	335.9	332.5	309.5	272.5	252.3	244.5	236.3	233.4	227.7	203.2
1946-------	1961	*	317.2	326.1	309.1	271.9	249.0	239.1	232.1	233.3	230.9	208.2	184.1
1947-------	1962	*	310.6	302.0	274.8	248.2	237.2	226.5	230.1	231.8	212.1	188.4	179.1
1948-------	1963	*	277.8	263.9	245.4	235.5	222.7	224.1	227.6	212.4	190.4	182.4	
1949-------	1964	*	252.0	242.4	238.4	221.1	220.8	224.5	212.3	191.7	186.0		
1950-------	1965	*	235.3	233.8	221.6	218.3	220.4	207.3	188.7	185.9			
1951-------	1966	*	228.8	218.8	218.3	217.5	202.5	183.1	183.0				
1952-------	1967	*	205.1	216.0	215.1	197.2	178.3	177.1					
1953-------	1968	*	208.3	210.2	195.1	175.6	172.2						
1954-------	1969	*	203.1	186.8	173.0	167.8							
1955-------	1970	*	181.8	168.0	162.9								
1956-------	1971	*	164.4	158.6									
1957-------	1972	*	152.9										
1958-------	1973	*											

TABLE 10B. BIRTH PROBABILITIES FOR WHITE WOMEN FOR EACH YEAR 1917-73 BY AGE AND PARITY FOR EACH COHORT FROM 1868 TO 1958--CON.

(PROBABILITIES ARE THE NUMBER OF BIRTHS PER 1,000 WOMEN IN SPECIFIED PARITY AND EXACT AGE GROUP FIGURES FOR "0 PARITY" SHOW THE PROBABILITY OF FIRST BIRTHS TO "C PARITY" WOMEN, THOSE FOR "1 PARITY" SHOW THE PROBABILITY OF SECOND BIRTHS TO "1 PARITY" WOMEN, ETC. BASED ON CENTRAL BIRTH RATES AND PARITY DISTRIBUTIONS)

PARITY AND COHORT	DIAGONAL LINE FOR JANUARY 1	EXACT AGE											
		27	28	29	30	31	32	33	34	35	36	37	38
1 PARITY--CON.													
1879-------													38.0
1880-------												48.0	38.2
1881-------											58.4	47.9	37.5
1882-------										68.9	57.3	46.3	36.8
1883-------									79.9	67.4	56.5	46.4	37.7
1884-------								94.2	78.6	67.2	56.4	47.7	35.4
1885-------							105.3	92.1	77.4	67.8	58.4	44.9	35.6
1886-------						121.8	101.9	89.0	77.2	68.2	53.9	44.1	34.5
1887-------					140.4	117.6	98.1	89.1	76.7	63.8	53.1	42.5	32.5
1888-------				169.6	139.9	116.7	101.6	90.5	76.3	64.7	52.7	41.3	31.3
1889-------			186.6	169.0	136.7	121.1	103.0	91.4	76.8	65.2	52.5	41.0	31.6
1890-------	1917	197.7	185.3	162.3	139.6	122.2	103.3	90.8	76.4	64.2	50.3	40.1	30.7
1891-------	1918	193.1	172.8	161.5	135.1	117.9	99.1	87.6	73.0	59.3	47.7	37.2	28.1
1892-------	1919	178.7	169.4	151.4	127.9	111.9	94.1	81.3	65.4	53.9	42.7	32.7	27.1
1893-------	1920	177.5	159.3	145.3	123.1	107.9	87.9	74.6	61.3	50.1	39.3	33.0	23.6
1894-------	1921	170.6	156.2	144.1	120.6	102.9	84.3	72.3	59.0	47.4	40.0	30.1	21.9
1895-------	1922	168.2	156.4	140.3	116.1	100.7	82.0	70.0	55.8	48.0	37.6	28.3	20.9
1896-------	1923	168.3	150.2	134.2	111.9	95.9	78.1	65.3	55.8	44.1	34.9	25.8	20.8
1897-------	1924	163.0	144.6	129.2	106.6	90.8	74.1	65.1	51.4	41.9	31.9	26.2	20.2
1898-------	1925	156.2	137.9	122.5	101.2	87.4	73.4	60.6	49.0	38.2	32.3	25.6	19.3
1899-------	1926	152.3	134.7	119.5	100.3	89.1	72.3	61.0	47.5	41.5	33.3	26.1	20.3
1900-------	1927	146.0	127.8	115.0	100.0	84.7	68.9	56.2	49.4	40.2	32.5	26.0	20.8
1901-------	1928	136.6	120.6	112.2	93.6	79.0	62.7	57.0	46.9	39.4	31.6	26.2	20.8
1902-------	1929	129.1	118.1	104.3	85.8	71.4	63.4	54.5	45.9	38.3	32.5	26.0	21.3
1903-------	1930	128.6	113.1	98.5	80.7	74.8	62.2	54.6	46.1	39.9	33.4	27.1	22.1
1904-------	1931	124.2	108.1	94.0	85.8	74.5	62.8	55.6	48.9	41.9	35.5	29.0	24.8
1905-------	1932	119.7	103.6	99.2	84.6	74.4	64.6	59.0	51.2	44.7	38.0	32.8	29.1
1906-------	1933	115.0	108.6	98.1	84.8	76.8	69.0	61.5	54.5	47.4	41.2	38.6	31.6
1907-------	1934	121.7	108.2	99.2	88.3	82.4	72.3	66.4	58.4	54.7	48.9	42.3	35.1
1908-------	1935	119.3	108.4	101.3	93.2	84.9	77.9	70.0	67.9	63.3	53.4	46.2	38.2
1909-------	1936	119.8	111.5	107.6	96.3	92.3	83.0	82.4	77.8	66.2	59.3	50.6	39.3
1910-------	1937	122.6	117.1	108.1	102.6	96.3	92.4	93.0	78.5	72.2	64.0	51.5	36.8
1911-------	1938	128.3	116.8	114.1	106.7	104.3	103.8	91.3	85.3	78.4	63.8	47.5	35.5
1912-------	1939	126.0	121.5	117.1	118.4	116.4	101.2	98.2	92.3	78.3	59.0	45.4	35.2
1913-------	1940	131.3	125.5	132.1	131.4	113.8	110.7	107.6	92.9	71.7	57.2	44.9	35.2
1914-------	1941	137.1	144.0	146.6	126.0	125.0	123.6	109.9	85.8	70.7	57.4	46.3	36.9
1915-------	1942	154.7	160.0	139.1	137.4	140.9	127.0	100.9	85.4	71.5	59.0	48.2	36.1
1916-------	1943	170.4	148.5	148.1	155.9	145.7	116.2	100.2	86.1	73.1	60.4	46.8	36.8
1917-------	1944	158.4	155.6	172.3	164.8	135.9	117.8	103.6	89.6	75.8	60.7	48.5	37.0
1918-------	1945	159.4	182.3	182.3	151.8	136.1	120.1	106.3	91.5	74.8	61.0	47.8	36.3
1919-------	1946	191.5	193.7	167.0	152.0	137.9	123.5	108.6	90.6	76.1	60.1	47.7	36.0
1920-------	1947	203.0	177.1	166.7	153.2	140.3	124.4	105.7	90.3	72.6	58.2	45.0	33.5
1921-------	1948	187.5	179.1	170.0	157.6	143.7	122.3	107.3	86.4	71.4	55.9	43.3	31.5
1922-------	1949	192.9	185.1	176.7	164.6	144.4	126.0	104.8	87.0	71.0	53.8	40.9	30.1
1923-------	1950	198.1	194.0	184.7	164.6	148.1	123.0	104.7	86.2	67.3	52.0	39.6	30.1
1924-------	1951	209.9	202.5	185.4	170.0	145.1	122.8	104.1	81.8	65.0	51.2	39.4	28.2
1925-------	1952	219.4	205.0	191.9	167.0	145.4	122.6	99.7	80.2	64.7	50.6	37.4	27.5
1926-------	1953	226.7	214.5	194.2	170.9	148.3	121.2	99.3	81.0	65.5	48.9	37.4	28.2
1927-------	1954	234.8	217.1	198.7	175.2	146.3	119.2	99.7	81.3	62.4	49.6	37.4	26.6
1928-------	1955	240.6	223.8	204.4	174.2	146.1	120.9	99.6	78.1	63.6	49.9	35.6	25.8
1929-------	1956	249.1	233.4	203.9	175.2	148.0	122.1	98.4	79.8	64.3	47.6	35.9	26.4
1930-------	1957	259.4	232.6	206.2	176.8	148.6	120.5	98.8	81.3	61.6	46.4	35.9	25.9
1931-------	1958	259.6	233.7	207.0	176.4	144.3	118.4	99.9	75.5	60.1	45.3	35.4	25.8
1932-------	1959	260.7	234.2	204.4	169.6	142.3	118.6	93.3	73.9	57.0	44.6	34.2	25.5
1933-------	1960	257.8	228.4	193.4	164.3	138.5	111.2	87.5	70.3	56.1	43.5	33.2	22.4
1934-------	1961	254.0	220.0	191.1	161.4	133.6	103.6	84.1	66.8	54.1	42.5	30.2	21.4
1935-------	1962	244.5	215.3	186.4	153.6	121.9	99.7	82.4	66.7	52.5	39.1	27.8	20.1
1936-------	1963	240.1	213.8	177.5	144.9	118.8	98.0	81.9	65.0	49.0	36.6	26.4	
1937-------	1964	236.7	198.8	167.5	140.0	118.6	97.1	79.5	60.3	45.6	34.4		
1938-------	1965	220.5	190.4	162.4	139.6	119.2	97.6	74.8	56.9	45.1			
1939-------	1966	209.8	185.1	161.9	140.3	118.9	93.0	71.8	57.0				
1940-------	1967	204.6	183.9	166.6	143.9	114.6	90.4	71.5					
1941-------	1968	202.9	187.9	169.7	136.7	111.0	87.5						
1942-------	1969	208.2	192.5	160.9	133.7	107.9							
1943-------	1970	208.8	179.5	152.7	128.6								
1944-------	1971	194.6	168.1	147.8									
1945-------	1972	178.6	163.7										
1946-------	1973	173.0											

TABLE 10B. BIRTH PROBABILITIES FOR WHITE WOMEN FOR EACH YEAR 1917-73 BY AGE AND PARITY FOR EACH COHORT FROM 1868 TO 1958--CON.

(PROBABILITIES ARE THE NUMBER OF BIRTHS PER 1,000 WOMEN IN SPECIFIED PARITY AND EXACT AGE GROUP. FIGURES FOR "0 PARITY" SHOW THE PROBABILITY OF FIRST BIRTHS TO "0 PARITY" WOMEN, THOSE FOR "1 PARITY" SHOW THE PROBABILITY OF SECOND BIRTHS TO "1 PARITY" WOMEN, ETC. BASED ON CENTRAL BIRTH RATES AND PARITY DISTRIBUTIONS)

PARITY AND COHORT	DIAGONAL LINE FOR JANUARY 1	EXACT AGE 39	40	41	42	43	44	45	46	47	48	49
1 PARITY--CON.												
1868												0.0
1869											0.0	0.0
1870										0.9	0.0	0.0
1871									1.8	0.9	0.0	0.0
1872								2.7	1.8	0.9	0.0	0.0
1873							4.5	2.7	0.9	0.9	0.0	0.0
1874						7.0	4.4	1.8	1.8	0.0	0.0	0.0
1875					9.4	6.9	3.4	2.6	0.9	0.9	0.0	0.0
1876				15.1	9.3	6.8	4.2	1.7	0.8	0.8	0.0	0.0
1877			21.3	14.8	9.1	6.6	3.3	1.7	0.8	0.8	0.0	0.0
1878	1917	30.3	21.0	14.6	9.8	6.5	3.3	1.6	0.8	0.0	0.0	0.0
1879	1918	29.9	20.7	14.4	9.6	6.4	3.2	1.6	0.8	0.0	0.0	0.0
1880	1919	30.2	21.1	15.0	8.7	6.3	3.2	1.6	0.8	0.0	0.0	0.0
1881	1920	29.7	20.7	13.9	8.5	6.2	3.1	2.3	0.8	0.0	0.0	0.0
1882	1921	29.8	19.5	12.9	8.4	6.1	3.1	1.5	0.8	0.0	0.0	0.0
1883	1922	27.9	18.5	13.4	9.0	5.3	3.0	1.5	0.8	0.0	0.0	0.0
1884	1923	27.8	19.2	12.6	7.5	5.2	3.0	1.5	0.7	0.0	0.0	0.0
1885	1924	27.5	18.2	12.5	8.1	5.2	2.2	1.5	0.7	0.0	0.0	0.0
1886	1925	25.9	17.6	11.3	7.1	4.3	2.1	1.4	0.7	0.0	0.0	0.0
1887	1926	24.8	16.3	10.9	6.1	4.1	2.7	1.4	0.7	0.0	0.0	0.0
1888	1927	23.6	15.6	10.2	6.1	4.1	2.1	1.4	0.7	0.0	0.0	0.0
1889	1928	23.8	15.7	10.3	6.2	4.1	2.1	0.7	0.7	0.0	0.0	0.0
1890	1929	22.9	14.9	10.2	6.2	4.1	2.1	0.7	0.7	0.0	0.0	0.0
1891	1930	21.9	13.6	9.8	5.9	3.3	1.3	0.7	0.0	0.0	0.0	0.0
1892	1931	18.8	12.8	8.6	4.9	3.1	1.2	0.6	0.0	0.0	0.0	0.0
1893	1932	17.4	11.7	7.0	4.1	2.9	1.2	0.6	0.0	0.0	0.0	0.0
1894	1933	16.4	10.8	6.9	4.6	2.3	1.7	0.6	0.0	0.0	0.0	0.0
1895	1934	16.6	10.6	6.7	3.9	2.8	1.1	0.6	0.6	0.0	0.0	0.0
1896	1935	15.0	10.2	6.5	4.3	2.7	1.1	1.1	0.5	0.0	0.0	0.0
1897	1936	14.6	10.0	7.4	4.2	2.6	1.6	1.1	0.5	0.0	0.0	0.0
1898	1937	14.3	10.8	6.7	4.1	2.6	1.5	1.0	0.5	0.0	0.0	0.0
1899	1938	15.8	11.3	7.2	4.6	3.1	2.1	1.0	0.5	0.0	0.0	0.0
1900	1939	16.4	11.5	7.5	4.5	3.5	2.0	1.0	0.5	0.0	0.0	0.0
1901	1940	16.1	11.5	7.7	5.3	3.4	1.9	1.0	0.5	0.0	0.0	0.0
1902	1941	16.4	12.3	8.7	6.0	3.7	2.3	0.9	0.5	0.0	0.0	0.0
1903	1942	18.2	13.8	9.8	6.7	4.0	2.2	0.9	0.4	0.0	0.0	0.0
1904	1943	21.0	15.4	11.1	7.1	4.4	2.2	0.9	0.4	0.0	0.0	0.0
1905	1944	23.2	16.7	12.0	7.6	4.0	2.2	0.9	0.4	0.0	0.0	0.0
1906	1945	25.0	18.6	12.4	7.1	4.0	2.2	0.9	0.4	0.0	0.0	0.0
1907	1946	28.0	19.2	12.1	6.8	4.1	2.3	0.9	0.5	0.0	0.0	0.0
1908	1947	28.8	18.6	11.8	6.9	4.1	2.3	0.9	0.5	0.0	0.0	0.0
1909	1948	27.4	18.4	11.6	7.0	4.6	2.3	0.9	0.5	0.0	0.0	0.0
1910	1949	26.7	18.1	12.1	8.0	4.7	2.4	0.9	0.5	0.0	0.0	0.0
1911	1950	26.3	18.6	12.2	7.5	4.7	2.4	1.4	0.5	0.0	0.0	0.0
1912	1951	26.9	18.3	12.7	7.6	4.3	2.4	1.0	0.5	0.0	0.0	0.0
1913	1952	26.8	19.0	12.4	7.7	4.8	2.4	1.0	0.5	0.0	0.0	0.0
1914	1953	27.4	19.0	12.3	7.9	4.5	2.0	1.0	0.5	0.0	0.0	0.0
1915	1954	27.3	19.1	12.7	7.6	4.1	2.0	1.0	0.5	0.0	0.0	0.0
1916	1955	27.2	18.2	12.0	6.8	4.2	2.1	1.1	0.5	0.0	0.0	0.0
1917	1956	27.4	18.5	12.1	7.2	3.9	2.2	1.1	0.6	0.0	0.0	0.0
1918	1957	26.9	17.6	11.5	6.9	4.0	2.3	1.2	0.0	0.0	0.0	0.0
1919	1958	25.7	16.8	11.1	7.0	4.1	2.4	0.6	0.0	0.0	0.0	0.0
1920	1959	23.7	15.8	10.6	6.5	3.6	1.8	0.6	0.0	0.0	0.0	0.0
1921	1960	21.9	16.1	10.2	6.0	3.0	1.8	0.6	0.0	0.0	0.0	0.0
1922	1961	23.0	15.1	10.1	5.1	3.2	1.3	0.6	0.0	0.0	0.0	0.0
1923	1962	20.8	14.4	9.3	6.0	3.3	1.3	0.7	0.0	0.0	0.0	0.0
1924	1963	20.4	13.7	9.6	5.5	2.8	1.4	0.7	0.0	0.0	0.0	0.0
1925	1964	20.7	13.7	8.7	5.1	2.9	1.5	0.7	0.0	0.0	0.0	
1926	1965	20.0	13.2	8.6	4.7	3.1	1.6	0.8	0.0	0.0		
1927	1966	18.7	12.3	8.2	4.9	2.5	0.8	0.8	0.0			
1928	1967	19.1	13.1	8.8	5.3	2.6	0.9	0.9				
1929	1968	19.3	13.9	8.4	4.7	2.8	0.9					
1930	1969	19.3	12.7	7.8	4.9	2.0						
1931	1970	18.1	12.1	7.1	4.1							
1932	1971	17.5	11.4	6.2								
1933	1972	15.4	10.3									
1934	1973	14.4										

TABLE 10B. BIRTH PROBABILITIES FOR WHITE WOMEN FOR EACH YEAR 1917-73 BY AGE AND PARITY FOR EACH COHORT FROM 1868 TO 1958--CON.

(PROBABILITIES ARE THE NUMBER OF BIRTHS PER 1,000 WOMEN IN SPECIFIED PARITY AND EXACT AGE GROUP. FIGURES FOR "0 PARITY" SHOW THE PROBABILITY OF FIRST BIRTHS TO "0 PARITY" WOMEN, THOSE FOR "1 PARITY" SHOW THE PROBABILITY OF SECOND BIRTHS TO "1 PARITY" WOMEN, ETC. BASED ON CENTRAL BIRTH RATES AND PARITY DISTRIBUTIONS)

PARITY AND COHORT	DIAGONAL LINE FOR JANUARY 1	EXACT AGE 15	16	17	18	19	20	21	22	23	24	25	26
2 PARITY													
1891-------													215.3
1892-------												236.7	209.7
1893-------											254.7	230.0	194.2
1894-------										276.7	246.7	214.4	193.2
1895-------									284.7	269.3	232.5	214.4	196.0
1896-------								301.1	277.3	254.1	232.1	217.6	182.3
1897-------							311.3	292.1	261.7	251.6	235.8	202.8	179.6
1898-------						307.7	298.4	274.6	260.0	255.3	220.0	204.5	179.9
1899-------					*	306.2	286.0	275.5	266.1	238.3	223.0	206.3	176.7
1900-------				*	*	296.1	289.1	284.1	248.4	246.0	231.5	201.5	168.7
1901-------			*	*	*	295.9	296.3	257.8	250.0	254.3	226.9	192.3	167.4
1902-------	1917	*	*	*	*	309.6	268.6	255.9	257.9	243.5	212.1	186.3	155.6
1903-------	1918	*	*	*	*	266.7	262.0	258.4	250.5	231.1	206.6	176.3	147.9
1904-------	1919	*	*	*	*	266.4	261.0	253.6	243.5	226.1	198.5	169.4	148.4
1905-------	1920	*	*	*	*	263.6	258.5	249.0	239.6	218.7	193.5	172.2	143.5
1906-------	1921	*	*	*	*	267.5	256.7	248.6	233.3	214.0	194.4	164.2	141.8
1907-------	1922	*	*	*	*	265.8	256.8	244.0	227.5	213.4	184.9	161.4	136.3
1908-------	1923	*	*	*	*	266.7	250.0	235.6	225.4	202.9	180.9	154.1	139.2
1909-------	1924	*	*	*	*	256.6	240.7	234.9	218.6	200.0	175.6	160.4	132.9
1910-------	1925	*	*	*	*	251.2	244.6	230.9	216.9	195.5	181.7	153.4	132.3
1911-------	1926	*	*	*	*	253.6	235.9	223.4	209.4	201.5	174.5	151.6	132.6
1912-------	1927	*	*	*	*	236.7	229.2	217.6	215.2	194.1	172.4	150.7	135.4
1913-------	1928	*	*	*	*	226.6	219.6	224.8	209.3	190.0	172.5	156.1	130.6
1914-------	1929	*	*	*	*	222.8	233.3	222.4	209.2	194.4	179.0	151.5	135.2
1915-------	1930	*	*	*	*	237.3	233.2	221.2	212.6	199.2	172.1	155.6	136.3
1916-------	1931	*	*	*	*	235.3	233.3	223.9	216.1	191.4	177.9	156.9	139.4
1917-------	1932	*	*	*	*	233.1	234.9	228.7	207.3	198.8	179.5	161.7	155.0
1918-------	1933	*	*	*	*	242.4	241.1	217.5	216.8	199.0	187.2	175.2	147.6
1919-------	1934	*	*	*	*	250.0	229.9	231.2	215.4	208.1	193.9	161.6	134.2
1920-------	1935	*	*	*	*	234.6	253.5	224.5	217.1	216.6	180.1	144.5	145.6
1921-------	1936	*	*	*	*	282.6	241.9	217.3	228.6	200.9	160.1	163.7	154.0
1922-------	1937	*	*	*	*	257.9	230.8	238.2	217.5	174.2	182.4	168.0	148.9
1923-------	1938	*	*	*	*	255.2	254.6	230.6	187.5	200.9	184.6	165.4	151.3
1924-------	1939	*	*	*	*	275.5	243.0	194.5	218.0	199.8	182.8	166.8	153.3
1925-------	1940	*	*	*	*	256.2	207.4	232.5	217.2	200.5	185.0	168.7	161.2
1926-------	1941	*	*	*	*	219.9	249.3	232.9	219.1	203.2	187.2	177.5	169.4
1927-------	1942	*	*	*	*	261.6	251.4	237.0	223.0	205.0	195.8	184.0	171.5
1928-------	1943	*	*	*	*	268.2	258.1	239.6	224.2	213.6	200.4	186.0	177.6
1929-------	1944	*	*	*	*	275.0	261.1	241.1	235.5	217.1	205.1	193.7	182.5
1930-------	1945	*	*	*	*	282.3	260.0	252.7	236.4	221.8	212.2	199.3	188.6
1931-------	1946	*	*	*	307.7	273.6	272.6	253.0	240.4	229.8	216.8	206.7	194.8
1932-------	1947	*	*	*	283.5	280.4	273.7	256.5	248.7	233.5	225.9	212.3	194.4
1933-------	1948	*	*	*	289.9	287.4	275.2	264.3	251.3	243.6	230.7	211.3	196.1
1934-------	1949	*	*	*	294.5	291.0	284.5	270.2	262.4	249.9	230.9	215.5	199.2
1935-------	1950	*	*	*	304.1	298.6	290.0	279.4	268.5	248.0	234.9	217.9	197.1
1936-------	1951	*	*	*	315.8	304.6	298.1	286.7	266.5	251.4	236.8	216.3	191.4
1937-------	1952	*	*	*	318.2	314.1	302.9	281.1	268.3	253.8	235.3	209.5	184.9
1938-------	1953	*	*	*	331.3	319.2	297.8	287.3	272.6	252.3	228.0	201.6	176.6
1939-------	1954	*	*	*	317.9	305.0	307.2	289.8	269.3	245.3	218.8	190.8	157.0
1940-------	1955	*	*	*	318.4	325.7	307.6	285.8	265.5	235.7	206.1	168.2	139.2
1941-------	1956	*	*	*	335.1	327.2	307.3	284.2	253.7	220.0	179.3	148.3	131.9
1942-------	1957	*	*	*	338.9	320.7	300.3	268.2	234.2	188.4	157.1	140.8	125.9
1943-------	1958	*	*	*	331.4	312.7	283.2	247.4	199.6	165.6	149.2	134.1	129.6
1944-------	1959	*	*	*	317.6	296.7	264.0	212.1	177.5	159.3	142.2	137.5	130.2
1945-------	1960	*	*	*	307.2	277.6	228.2	190.1	170.2	150.7	145.9	139.8	118.9
1946-------	1961	*	*	*	293.0	243.4	205.3	183.3	160.9	154.4	148.8	126.8	98.1
1947-------	1962	*	*	*	262.8	221.5	198.1	172.1	164.9	157.3	135.8	105.6	88.5
1948-------	1963	*	*	*	243.7	216.7	185.9	176.9	166.7	144.0	112.3	94.9	
1949-------	1964	*	*	*	235.8	199.2	191.7	177.2	155.7	120.2	102.7		
1950-------	1965	*	*	*	220.0	210.5	191.8	166.9	128.0	111.5			
1951-------	1966	*	*	*	*	203.6	177.4	136.0	120.9				
1952-------	1967	*	*	*	*	187.2	148.0	130.6					
1953-------	1968	*	*	*	*	157.4	141.4						
1954-------	1969	*	*	*	*	152.0							
1955-------	1970	*	*	*	*								
1956-------	1971	*	*	*									
1957-------	1972	*	*										
1958-------	1973	*											

TABLE 10B. BIRTH PROBABILITIES FOR WHITE WOMEN FOR EACH YEAR 1917-73 BY AGE AND PARITY FOR EACH COHORT FROM 1868 TO 1958--CON.

(PROBABILITIES ARE THE NUMBER OF BIRTHS PER 1,000 WOMEN IN SPECIFIED PARITY AND EXACT AGE GROUP. FIGURES FOR "0 PARITY" SHOW THE PROBABILITY OF FIRST BIRTHS TO "0 PARITY" WOMEN, THOSE FOR "1 PARITY" SHOW THE PROBABILITY OF SECOND BIRTHS TO "1 PARITY" WOMEN, ETC. BASED ON CENTRAL BIRTH RATES AND PARITY DISTRIBUTIONS)

PARITY AND COHORT	DIAGONAL LINE FOR JANUARY 1	EXACT AGE 27	28	29	30	31	32	33	34	35	36	37	38
2 PARITY--CON.													
1879-------													49.1
1880-------												60.5	48.6
1881-------											70.7	59.4	47.0
1882-------										83.4	68.7	57.0	46.7
1883-------									95.1	80.6	66.5	56.8	46.6
1884-------								108.4	91.3	78.1	66.6	57.1	43.3
1885-------							115.8	104.7	88.7	77.8	67.6	53.2	42.7
1886-------						135.0	114.2	102.8	90.0	80.3	64.0	53.8	43.3
1887-------					159.3	134.0	112.8	105.1	92.8	77.1	65.4	54.6	42.2
1888-------				188.2	153.2	128.0	111.4	104.2	86.5	75.4	63.5	51.2	39.1
1889-------			201.5	180.0	142.7	125.3	109.4	96.4	83.2	73.7	59.4	48.1	37.5
1890-------	1917	210.1	195.0	167.2	140.6	124.1	102.3	93.9	82.7	68.2	56.4	45.4	35.1
1891-------	1918	206.9	181.9	166.2	140.4	117.9	100.9	94.8	78.1	65.6	53.4	43.0	32.3
1892-------	1919	190.9	178.6	163.5	129.2	115.1	101.0	89.1	74.0	61.8	49.7	38.9	31.1
1893-------	1920	187.8	175.4	148.8	125.2	114.8	95.2	83.3	69.5	57.3	45.4	37.4	28.6
1894-------	1921	186.7	158.6	144.9	124.6	108.5	90.2	78.5	65.3	52.8	44.6	35.3	26.8
1895-------	1922	172.2	155.8	144.7	118.6	103.1	85.7	74.1	60.9	52.6	42.1	32.9	24.6
1896-------	1923	170.2	154.8	137.6	114.0	99.0	80.9	69.7	60.0	49.3	39.5	30.4	24.2
1897-------	1924	169.0	147.6	131.1	107.7	91.9	75.8	67.9	56.0	46.4	36.2	30.2	23.2
1898-------	1925	160.7	138.8	123.3	100.8	87.5	74.8	63.3	53.3	42.9	36.2	28.8	22.3
1899-------	1926	154.6	134.7	118.3	97.5	87.1	71.9	62.6	50.3	44.1	35.9	28.6	22.1
1900-------	1927	151.9	129.6	114.3	97.7	84.2	69.6	59.2	52.3	43.6	35.3	28.4	22.8
1901-------	1928	143.9	123.4	112.7	94.3	80.2	66.0	60.3	50.4	42.1	34.2	28.2	23.1
1902-------	1929	135.0	120.2	105.5	87.8	75.3	65.6	56.4	48.0	40.6	33.7	27.7	22.6
1903-------	1930	133.9	114.3	101.1	82.7	75.5	62.2	54.8	46.4	39.9	33.5	27.6	22.6
1904-------	1931	127.5	112.3	96.9	85.1	72.7	61.0	54.4	47.2	40.6	34.1	28.7	24.6
1905-------	1932	127.6	107.5	100.4	82.4	71.0	61.3	55.4	47.5	41.7	35.6	31.4	29.0
1906-------	1933	122.4	112.1	96.1	80.6	71.3	62.2	55.5	48.8	42.8	38.4	37.4	31.5
1907-------	1934	126.0	106.2	94.0	80.3	72.1	62.2	56.7	49.9	46.6	45.2	39.7	34.4
1908-------	1935	118.8	103.1	92.2	81.0	71.4	63.6	57.9	54.5	54.0	48.2	42.8	35.0
1909-------	1936	116.4	103.0	94.5	81.1	74.0	65.7	63.4	63.5	57.2	52.0	44.1	35.1
1910-------	1937	116.8	106.2	94.1	84.7	76.6	71.2	74.5	67.3	62.5	54.8	44.9	32.8
1911-------	1938	120.7	104.1	97.0	86.1	80.4	82.5	77.0	71.6	64.8	54.3	41.4	32.0
1912-------	1939	116.2	106.7	97.3	92.3	92.8	85.0	80.5	74.3	63.8	50.1	40.0	31.7
1913-------	1940	119.7	107.1	105.2	104.4	94.6	87.7	83.4	72.8	59.3	48.2	39.7	32.8
1914-------	1941	121.1	116.5	118.0	103.6	96.5	91.2	82.4	67.9	56.7	48.3	40.8	34.6
1915-------	1942	127.7	129.7	114.6	103.8	101.1	90.9	76.8	65.4	57.3	49.6	43.2	34.3
1916-------	1943	143.2	124.6	112.9	108.7	100.9	84.8	74.6	66.2	59.2	52.5	43.1	34.7
1917-------	1944	136.6	120.0	119.1	110.2	95.0	83.6	76.0	68.7	62.4	52.9	44.5	35.2
1918-------	1945	126.9	124.9	120.2	102.8	93.4	84.5	78.4	72.3	63.0	54.2	43.2	34.3
1919-------	1946	135.2	129.2	113.4	102.7	95.4	89.2	83.1	73.3	64.2	52.9	43.5	33.8
1920-------	1947	140.4	123.2	114.3	105.7	100.3	93.5	85.1	74.6	63.1	52.7	42.0	31.6
1921-------	1948	136.2	125.5	118.8	112.2	107.3	96.7	86.5	74.6	63.0	52.0	40.2	30.7
1922-------	1949	138.5	129.4	124.4	119.2	109.7	98.1	86.6	74.0	62.1	49.3	38.4	29.3
1923-------	1950	140.7	135.5	132.1	121.4	110.9	97.6	85.7	74.0	59.8	47.6	37.0	28.4
1924-------	1951	148.4	143.2	133.5	123.7	110.8	97.7	86.8	71.0	57.7	45.7	36.0	26.2
1925-------	1952	156.1	145.8	137.4	124.2	112.3	99.4	83.4	68.8	56.2	45.0	33.9	25.3
1926-------	1953	157.7	150.7	139.1	125.8	113.6	96.2	81.2	67.0	55.4	42.0	32.4	24.4
1927-------	1954	164.0	153.4	142.6	129.1	112.4	95.1	80.1	66.5	51.9	40.6	31.4	22.7
1928-------	1955	166.9	156.3	145.6	128.2	111.7	93.8	79.1	62.4	50.7	39.4	29.1	20.9
1929-------	1956	173.1	162.6	145.2	129.0	110.8	94.0	75.2	61.7	49.2	36.7	26.9	20.1
1930-------	1957	178.7	161.0	147.2	128.2	110.5	89.8	74.1	59.9	45.7	34.1	25.7	18.3
1931-------	1958	176.9	163.0	146.1	128.1	105.5	87.2	72.4	55.8	41.8	31.9	23.0	16.7
1932-------	1959	179.1	164.0	145.8	122.1	102.2	84.6	66.9	50.7	39.6	29.2	21.8	15.9
1933-------	1960	180.9	162.5	138.6	117.2	100.0	78.2	60.7	47.3	36.4	27.9	20.9	14.2
1934-------	1961	179.9	155.6	134.3	115.4	92.2	70.9	56.5	44.4	35.1	27.0	18.8	12.9
1935-------	1962	173.1	150.7	132.2	105.9	83.4	67.0	53.6	43.4	34.1	23.9	16.5	11.0
1936-------	1963	167.9	147.2	120.1	96.2	78.3	62.4	52.8	42.0	29.8	21.0	14.5	
1937-------	1964	161.9	132.8	109.2	90.7	73.7	63.4	51.4	37.1	26.3	18.5		
1938-------	1965	145.2	119.8	101.9	85.3	75.1	62.2	45.5	32.6	23.2			
1939-------	1966	129.6	112.6	97.8	87.1	75.1	55.0	39.5	29.1				
1940-------	1967	122.7	108.6	99.6	87.8	66.4	47.1	36.1					
1941-------	1968	118.1	111.0	100.8	78.1	56.4	43.4						
1942-------	1969	120.9	111.4	88.9	66.0	51.5							
1943-------	1970	121.2	99.5	75.0	59.7								
1944-------	1971	109.2	82.8	67.7									
1945-------	1972	91.2	75.3										
1946-------	1973	82.2											

TABLE 10B. BIRTH PROBABILITIES FOR WHITE WOMEN FOR EACH YEAR 1917-73 BY AGE AND PARITY FOR EACH COHORT FROM 1868 TO 1958--CON.

(PROBABILITIES ARE THE NUMBER OF BIRTHS PER 1,000 WOMEN IN SPECIFIED PARITY AND EXACT AGE GROUP. FIGURES FOR "0 PARITY" SHOW THE PROBABILITY OF FIRST BIRTHS TO "0 PARITY" WOMEN, THOSE FOR "1 PARITY" SHOW THE PROBABILITY OF SECOND BIRTHS TO "1 PARITY" WOMEN, ETC. BASED ON CENTRAL BIRTH RATES AND PARITY DISTRIBUTIONS)

PARITY AND COHORT	DIAGONAL LINE FOR JANUARY 1	EXACT AGE										
		39	40	41	42	43	44	45	46	47	48	49
2 PARITY--CON.												
1868----------------												0.0
1869----------------											0.0	0.0
1870----------------										0.8	0.0	0.0
1871----------------									1.6	0.8	0.0	0.0
1872----------------								3.2	1.6	0.8	0.0	0.0
1873----------------							5.5	3.1	1.6	0.8	0.0	0.0
1874----------------						8.5	5.4	3.1	1.5	0.8	0.0	0.0
1875----------------					12.1	9.1	5.3	3.1	1.5	0.8	0.0	0.0
1876----------------				19.2	12.7	8.2	5.2	3.0	1.5	0.8	0.0	0.0
1877----------------			26.7	19.7	12.5	8.8	5.2	3.0	1.5	0.7	0.0	0.0
1878----------------	1917	39.5	27.9	18.8	12.3	8.7	5.1	2.9	1.5	0.7	0.0	0.0
1879----------------	1918	40.0	26.3	19.4	12.3	8.0	4.4	2.9	1.5	0.7	0.0	0.0
1880----------------	1919	38.9	26.7	18.4	11.4	7.9	5.0	2.2	1.4	0.7	0.0	0.0
1881----------------	1920	38.1	26.2	17.3	11.2	7.7	4.2	2.1	1.4	0.7	0.0	0.0
1882----------------	1921	38.0	24.3	16.3	10.9	7.5	4.1	2.1	1.4	0.7	0.0	0.0
1883----------------	1922	35.4	23.2	16.7	10.7	6.7	4.0	2.0	1.4	0.0	0.0	0.0
1884----------------	1923	34.2	23.4	16.4	9.2	6.6	3.3	2.0	0.7	0.7	0.0	0.0
1885----------------	1924	34.3	22.4	14.8	9.7	6.5	3.3	2.0	1.3	0.7	0.0	0.0
1886----------------	1925	33.0	21.8	15.5	9.1	5.2	3.3	2.0	0.7	0.7	0.0	0.0
1887----------------	1926	32.5	21.9	14.2	8.4	5.9	3.3	2.0	0.7	0.0	0.0	0.0
1888----------------	1927	30.9	19.3	13.1	8.8	5.7	2.5	1.3	0.6	0.0	0.0	0.0
1889----------------	1928	27.8	18.5	13.2	7.8	4.8	2.4	1.2	0.6	0.0	0.0	0.0
1890----------------	1929	26.3	18.4	11.6	7.5	4.7	2.3	1.2	0.6	0.0	0.0	0.0
1891----------------	1930	25.3	16.4	10.8	6.8	4.6	2.3	1.1	0.6	0.0	0.0	0.0
1892----------------	1931	23.1	14.9	10.0	6.7	3.9	2.2	1.1	0.6	0.0	0.0	0.0
1893----------------	1932	20.8	14.5	9.7	5.9	3.8	2.2	1.1	0.5	0.0	0.0	0.0
1894----------------	1933	19.7	13.5	9.4	5.8	3.7	2.1	1.1	0.5	0.0	0.0	0.0
1895----------------	1934	19.2	13.2	8.7	5.6	3.6	2.0	1.0	0.5	0.0	0.0	0.0
1896----------------	1935	18.4	12.5	8.5	5.5	3.5	2.0	1.0	0.5	0.0	0.0	0.0
1897----------------	1936	17.9	11.7	8.3	5.4	3.4	2.0	1.0	0.5	0.0	0.0	0.0
1898----------------	1937	16.7	12.4	8.1	5.3	3.4	1.9	1.0	0.5	0.0	0.0	0.0
1899----------------	1938	17.5	12.8	8.1	5.2	3.3	1.9	1.4	0.5	0.0	0.0	0.0
1900----------------	1939	18.1	12.9	8.6	5.3	3.8	2.4	1.4	0.5	0.5	0.0	0.0
1901----------------	1940	17.5	12.8	9.0	6.2	4.7	2.9	1.4	1.0	0.0	0.0	0.0
1902----------------	1941	17.6	13.4	10.2	7.0	4.6	2.8	1.4	0.5	0.0	0.0	0.0
1903----------------	1942	19.0	14.9	11.3	7.7	5.0	2.7	1.4	0.5	0.0	0.0	0.0
1904----------------	1943	21.9	16.5	12.1	8.1	5.4	2.7	1.3	0.4	0.0	0.0	0.0
1905----------------	1944	23.7	18.3	12.5	8.1	4.9	2.7	1.3	0.4	0.0	0.0	0.0
1906----------------	1945	26.2	18.6	12.9	8.0	4.9	2.2	1.3	0.4	0.0	0.0	0.0
1907----------------	1946	26.5	18.7	12.6	7.4	4.8	2.6	1.3	0.4	0.0	0.0	0.0
1908----------------	1947	26.8	17.9	11.5	7.2	4.7	2.6	1.3	0.4	0.0	0.0	0.0
1909----------------	1948	25.1	17.1	11.7	7.5	5.0	2.9	1.3	0.4	0.0	0.0	0.0
1910----------------	1949	24.9	17.4	12.0	8.3	5.0	2.9	1.3	0.8	0.0	0.0	0.0
1911----------------	1950	24.3	17.9	13.0	8.2	5.3	2.9	1.6	0.4	0.0	0.0	0.0
1912----------------	1951	25.0	19.1	12.8	8.8	5.2	3.2	1.2	0.4	0.0	0.0	0.0
1913----------------	1952	26.3	18.7	13.7	8.6	5.5	2.8	1.2	0.4	0.0	0.0	0.0
1914----------------	1953	26.5	19.4	13.4	8.8	5.0	2.7	1.2	0.4	0.0	0.0	0.0
1915----------------	1954	26.7	19.4	13.5	8.3	4.5	2.6	1.1	0.4	0.4	0.0	0.0
1916----------------	1955	26.9	18.6	12.7	7.5	4.5	2.6	1.1	0.8	0.0	0.0	0.0
1917----------------	1956	26.4	18.8	11.9	7.5	4.5	2.2	1.1	0.4	0.0	0.0	0.0
1918----------------	1957	25.5	17.3	11.5	7.4	4.5	2.2	1.1	0.4	0.0	0.0	0.0
1919----------------	1958	24.4	17.0	10.9	7.0	4.0	2.2	1.1	0.4	0.0	0.0	0.0
1920----------------	1959	23.7	16.3	10.9	6.6	3.7	1.8	0.7	0.4	0.0	0.0	0.0
1921----------------	1960	22.8	15.7	10.3	6.3	3.3	1.8	0.7	0.4	0.0	0.0	0.0
1922----------------	1961	21.9	14.7	9.6	5.6	3.4	1.5	0.7	0.4	0.0	0.0	0.0
1923----------------	1962	20.3	13.8	9.3	5.6	3.0	1.5	0.8	0.0	0.0	0.0	0.0
1924----------------	1963	19.4	13.1	8.3	4.9	2.7	1.5	0.4	0.4	0.0	0.0	0.0
1925----------------	1964	18.7	12.3	7.7	4.3	2.3	1.2	0.4	0.0	0.0	0.0	
1926----------------	1965	17.2	11.4	7.1	4.0	2.4	1.2	0.4	0.4	0.0		
1927----------------	1966	16.1	10.9	6.5	4.1	2.0	0.8	0.4	0.0			
1928----------------	1967	15.3	9.5	6.2	3.8	1.7	0.8	0.4				
1929----------------	1968	13.5	8.9	5.9	3.0	1.7	0.9					
1930----------------	1969	12.9	8.6	4.7	2.6	1.3						
1931----------------	1970	12.1	7.4	4.3	2.2							
1932----------------	1971	10.4	6.5	3.5								
1933----------------	1972	9.1	5.2									
1934----------------	1973	8.2										

TABLE 10B. BIRTH PROBABILITIES FOR WHITE WOMEN FOR EACH YEAR 1917-73 BY AGE AND PARITY FOR EACH COHORT FROM 1868 TO 1958--CON.

(PROBABILITIES ARE THE NUMBER OF BIRTHS PER 1,000 WOMEN IN SPECIFIED PARITY AND EXACT AGE GROUP. FIGURES FOR "0 PARITY" SHOW THE PROBABILITY OF FIRST BIRTHS TO "0 PARITY" WOMEN, THOSE FOR "1 PARITY" SHOW THE PROBABILITY OF SECOND BIRTHS TO "1 PARITY" WOMEN, ETC. BASED ON CENTRAL BIRTH RATES AND PARITY DISTRIBUTIONS)

PARITY AND COHORT	DIAGONAL LINE FOR JANUARY 1	EXACT AGE											
		15	16	17	18	19	20	21	22	23	24	25	26
3 PARITY													
1891-------													255.4
1892-------												270.1	250.0
1893-------											273.9	264.8	236.5
1894-------										280.2	269.0	251.9	237.9
1895-------									273.8	279.8	261.7	256.8	241.9
1896-------								285.7	271.9	273.1	267.5	265.4	226.6
1897-------							*	284.9	265.3	278.3	280.0	249.7	228.0
1898-------						*	*	278.1	273.8	295.5	263.8	257.5	227.4
1899-------					*	*	*	288.9	292.3	276.8	275.7	256.5	223.5
1900-------				*	*	*	*	306.8	267.3	294.5	276.1	248.2	218.3
1901-------			*	*	*	*	*	278.1	287.2	296.9	268.5	242.6	223.6
1902-------	1917	*	*	*	*	*	*	297.0	289.0	279.5	259.8	246.0	207.6
1903-------	1918	*	*	*	*	*	*	289.9	282.1	278.8	265.6	232.1	197.4
1904-------	1919	*	*	*	*	*	*	288.1	290.6	285.4	253.9	226.6	200.7
1905-------	1920	*	*	*	*	*	*	301.1	293.2	271.7	247.9	228.0	194.3
1906-------	1921	*	*	*	*	*	*	301.8	272.7	261.7	249.2	217.9	193.6
1907-------	1922	*	*	*	*	*	*	277.1	261.9	260.9	235.7	215.5	186.4
1908-------	1923	*	*	*	*	*	*	265.1	265.7	250.6	234.7	206.3	194.0
1909-------	1924	*	*	*	*	*	*	276.7	259.1	251.9	224.1	218.9	187.0
1910-------	1925	*	*	*	*	*	*	271.5	260.5	240.9	240.2	212.3	186.1
1911-------	1926	*	*	*	*	*	*	260.3	251.0	253.4	233.3	211.4	186.2
1912-------	1927	*	*	*	*	*	*	260.9	260.5	249.3	231.4	211.5	189.7
1913-------	1928	*	*	*	*	*	*	269.2	262.0	250.0	236.6	216.4	180.8
1914-------	1929	*	*	*	*	*	*	269.8	260.3	254.6	238.0	206.2	182.7
1915-------	1930	*	*	*	*	*	*	275.0	264.4	254.7	228.8	212.1	182.8
1916-------	1931	*	*	*	*	*	*	280.7	269.6	248.4	244.2	213.9	185.0
1917-------	1932	*	*	*	*	*	*	274.3	254.8	268.8	242.0	209.4	200.9
1918-------	1933	*	*	*	*	*	*	254.2	281.0	265.4	234.8	225.1	191.5
1919-------	1934	*	*	*	*	*	*	281.0	269.4	258.9	244.7	211.0	173.1
1920-------	1935	*	*	*	*	*	*	251.9	265.2	269.9	232.0	188.8	181.3
1921-------	1936	*	*	*	*	*	*	262.4	278.5	258.8	209.4	205.7	176.4
1922-------	1937	*	*	*	*	*	*	287.8	277.6	227.9	229.0	197.5	169.6
1923-------	1938	*	*	*	*	*	*	284.7	236.9	247.9	218.8	192.4	173.6
1924-------	1939	*	*	*	*	*	*	238.1	262.9	238.0	215.7	196.6	174.8
1925-------	1940	*	*	*	*	*	*	274.8	254.4	237.1	224.3	198.7	184.2
1926-------	1941	*	*	*	*	*	*	265.6	257.4	250.0	224.3	206.7	188.8
1927-------	1942	*	*	*	*	*	*	276.1	273.4	244.2	228.6	208.9	188.8
1928-------	1943	*	*	*	*	*	*	286.7	261.2	250.5	229.1	205.6	190.4
1929-------	1944	*	*	*	*	*	*	277.5	271.6	249.5	229.0	209.2	190.0
1930-------	1945	*	*	*	*	*	*	289.2	267.7	247.9	231.5	209.3	192.7
1931-------	1946	*	*	*	*	*	311.3	283.9	269.0	254.2	231.9	213.6	196.5
1932-------	1947	*	*	*	*	*	308.3	281.3	272.7	251.4	235.8	217.8	195.3
1933-------	1948	*	*	*	*	*	307.7	293.0	272.7	256.3	239.8	214.8	199.5
1934-------	1949	*	*	*	*	*	316.5	290.1	275.7	258.8	235.5	218.3	199.1
1935-------	1950	*	*	*	*	*	321.9	299.3	278.8	256.3	238.5	219.6	197.5
1936-------	1951	*	*	*	*	*	328.9	297.8	276.4	258.4	240.3	217.9	191.0
1937-------	1952	*	*	*	*	*	320.8	296.7	278.6	263.7	240.8	211.9	182.3
1938-------	1953	*	*	*	*	*	315.8	300.9	282.9	261.4	232.1	199.2	170.2
1939-------	1954	*	*	*	*	*	329.5	302.5	278.7	251.6	217.1	184.3	146.2
1940-------	1955	*	*	*	*	*	322.6	299.2	271.2	234.2	199.8	157.9	125.2
1941-------	1956	*	*	*	*	*	317.7	287.6	250.4	214.8	171.6	135.6	116.8
1942-------	1957	*	*	*	*	*	308.1	268.7	231.3	185.0	149.2	128.5	114.2
1943-------	1958	*	*	*	*	*	293.1	251.5	203.4	164.6	146.5	128.3	122.6
1944-------	1959	*	*	*	*	*	276.1	219.0	184.7	165.4	144.6	137.5	127.3
1945-------	1960	*	*	*	*	*	241.6	203.8	186.1	163.1	155.4	142.9	118.4
1946-------	1961	*	*	*	*	*	230.2	209.1	180.8	175.5	159.4	131.5	97.4
1947-------	1962	*	*	*	*	*	223.3	198.9	192.6	175.0	145.9	107.6	87.6
1948-------	1963	*	*	*	*	*	*	212.5	191.0	161.0	121.3	97.6	
1949-------	1964	*	*	*	*	*	*	215.3	182.2	137.9	112.9		
1950-------	1965	*	*	*	*	*	*	189.8	149.6	124.6			
1951-------	1966	*	*	*	*	*	*	162.8	136.6				
1952-------	1967	*	*	*	*	*	*	150.4					
1953-------	1968	*	*	*	*	*	*						
1954-------	1969	*	*	*	*	*							
1955-------	1970	*	*	*	*								
1956-------	1971	*	*	*									
1957-------	1972	*	*										
1958-------	1973	*											

TABLE 10B. BIRTH PROBABILITIES FOR WHITE WOMEN FOR EACH YEAR 1917-73 BY AGE AND PARITY FOR EACH COHORT FROM 1868 TO 1958--CON.

(PROBABILITIES ARE THE NUMBER OF BIRTHS PER 1,000 WOMEN IN SPECIFIED PARITY AND EXACT AGE GROUP. FIGURES FOR "0 PARITY" SHOW THE PROBABILITY OF FIRST BIRTHS TO "0 PARITY" WOMEN, THOSE FOR "1 PARITY" SHOW THE PROBABILITY OF SECOND BIRTHS TO "1 PARITY" WOMEN, ETC. BASED ON CENTRAL BIRTH RATES AND PARITY DISTRIBUTIONS)

PARITY AND COHORT	DIAGONAL LINE FOR JANUARY 1	EXACT AGE											
		27	28	29	30	31	32	33	34	35	36	37	38
3 PARITY--CON.													
1879-------													71.2
1880-------												86.1	71.1
1881-------											97.4	85.2	68.1
1882-------										113.6	96.4	81.3	66.5
1883-------									127.1	111.4	92.9	80.0	66.7
1884-------								143.3	124.3	106.6	91.5	80.8	61.5
1885-------							150.4	138.9	118.6	105.0	92.2	73.9	60.7
1886-------						170.5	147.4	133.1	117.8	107.9	85.5	74.0	60.2
1887-------					191.8	165.9	140.9	131.6	120.5	98.5	84.9	72.0	59.0
1888-------				226.6	186.9	158.0	138.7	134.3	108.5	96.9	82.7	70.0	54.4
1889-------			242.2	220.2	177.1	155.2	140.8	120.2	106.7	94.6	79.8	65.9	51.9
1890-------	1917	254.0	237.4	209.4	175.7	160.0	127.4	118.9	104.8	89.7	75.1	62.7	48.2
1891-------	1918	250.4	225.9	208.6	178.2	144.4	126.6	117.4	100.3	86.9	71.7	58.0	44.2
1892-------	1919	235.9	224.8	208.9	160.7	143.5	124.3	111.8	95.6	82.2	66.4	53.4	44.5
1893-------	1920	235.8	222.2	189.0	157.7	142.4	119.9	106.9	92.2	76.1	61.5	52.6	41.7
1894-------	1921	234.8	202.8	185.5	155.8	136.1	114.5	103.7	85.7	70.8	61.1	50.2	38.6
1895-------	1922	218.1	199.8	183.2	149.2	131.2	111.1	96.9	80.1	70.7	58.2	47.9	37.1
1896-------	1923	217.4	196.1	174.7	144.7	127.5	103.8	90.2	79.5	66.6	55.4	45.1	37.0
1897-------	1924	214.6	187.8	169.7	140.7	120.0	99.2	90.5	75.4	64.4	53.2	45.6	35.3
1898-------	1925	206.7	184.1	166.7	133.6	114.3	99.7	85.8	72.7	61.6	53.1	43.3	34.2
1899-------	1926	205.1	184.9	159.8	129.3	116.6	96.5	85.9	71.9	64.3	52.0	42.6	34.0
1900-------	1927	207.2	174.1	151.4	129.4	111.8	95.2	83.2	73.5	61.9	50.0	41.8	33.8
1901-------	1928	193.2	163.9	150.8	124.5	108.2	91.6	84.8	70.3	59.2	49.2	42.4	32.8
1902-------	1929	181.6	163.0	144.6	120.1	104.0	92.0	80.2	67.0	57.9	50.0	40.8	31.8
1903-------	1930	180.1	157.0	139.8	116.0	105.8	87.1	75.9	65.3	57.7	48.1	39.6	32.6
1904-------	1931	178.1	158.4	139.7	120.8	103.0	85.2	75.9	65.7	57.6	48.5	41.9	35.6
1905-------	1932	177.8	156.3	143.0	116.5	99.1	85.0	75.4	65.5	57.2	50.0	44.0	41.3
1906-------	1933	173.7	157.0	137.0	112.1	97.9	84.2	75.0	65.7	58.6	50.5	50.4	43.6
1907-------	1934	176.4	149.7	131.1	110.4	96.6	82.4	75.4	66.7	60.2	58.0	52.9	45.2
1908-------	1935	168.6	145.5	128.5	109.9	95.3	84.2	75.9	70.0	68.6	61.0	54.9	45.5
1909-------	1936	166.3	145.0	132.5	108.8	98.3	86.4	81.0	79.4	72.1	65.0	55.6	45.5
1910-------	1937	165.8	149.3	128.9	112.4	99.9	90.0	92.4	82.6	75.0	64.4	55.6	43.6
1911-------	1938	170.0	144.2	131.1	113.5	102.4	101.6	94.4	84.3	75.5	65.7	52.4	42.4
1912-------	1939	163.1	145.7	132.1	118.0	114.8	103.4	93.2	84.4	74.7	60.5	50.6	42.3
1913-------	1940	165.1	148.1	136.2	129.8	115.2	101.8	94.5	83.3	69.3	58.7	50.6	43.3
1914-------	1941	166.2	152.2	147.0	126.3	111.2	101.9	91.3	77.2	67.8	59.2	51.5	45.1
1915-------	1942	168.0	164.1	142.9	121.3	112.4	98.6	85.6	76.9	68.7	61.7	54.3	46.3
1916-------	1943	185.5	159.3	135.3	123.6	110.4	93.3	86.3	78.1	71.9	64.4	56.4	48.1
1917-------	1944	176.3	147.9	138.5	119.5	103.3	94.1	86.9	80.6	74.5	67.1	58.5	48.2
1918-------	1945	159.7	149.0	132.7	111.2	103.3	93.3	88.6	83.5	76.2	67.5	57.0	46.1
1919-------	1946	165.1	143.7	124.3	114.0	104.1	97.8	94.5	85.8	77.9	67.0	56.6	46.3
1920-------	1947	159.4	135.7	127.6	115.6	109.2	104.7	96.5	88.2	77.0	65.7	55.8	43.9
1921-------	1948	152.1	142.0	131.3	121.8	117.5	105.9	99.6	88.3	76.3	66.6	53.7	43.3
1922-------	1949	156.8	143.1	137.0	129.0	118.3	109.4	99.0	87.3	77.0	63.5	52.6	41.0
1923-------	1950	157.5	151.7	143.0	128.6	120.7	108.4	98.4	88.1	74.2	61.8	50.4	39.2
1924-------	1951	167.9	155.8	142.8	132.3	120.2	109.6	99.0	84.8	71.7	59.9	47.5	36.5
1925-------	1952	171.7	156.4	146.5	132.2	120.9	109.2	96.1	82.5	70.0	56.7	44.1	33.7
1926-------	1953	172.5	161.1	147.3	134.2	121.4	106.4	94.0	81.4	67.2	53.2	42.0	33.1
1927-------	1954	175.3	160.5	148.5	133.9	118.7	105.0	91.7	77.6	62.2	50.3	39.8	29.2
1928-------	1955	174.4	161.4	149.0	131.7	118.8	103.2	89.2	72.4	60.0	48.2	36.4	26.3
1929-------	1956	175.8	163.2	146.9	133.0	116.5	102.3	83.8	70.1	57.5	43.7	32.1	23.8
1930-------	1957	179.2	161.9	149.2	131.4	116.5	95.7	81.5	67.7	51.9	38.6	29.2	21.4
1931-------	1958	177.7	164.2	147.9	131.1	109.8	93.2	78.3	60.5	45.6	35.9	26.6	19.8
1932-------	1959	181.6	164.3	145.9	123.6	105.6	88.7	70.3	53.0	42.1	32.1	24.1	18.2
1933-------	1960	182.4	162.3	139.5	119.2	101.1	79.0	61.0	49.6	38.4	30.1	22.7	16.0
1934-------	1961	178.3	154.2	133.1	113.7	89.5	69.0	56.2	44.5	36.3	28.1	20.7	13.7
1935-------	1962	172.6	149.2	128.1	100.1	78.6	63.9	51.1	43.1	34.5	25.5	17.3	11.5
1936-------	1963	165.3	142.2	112.4	88.1	71.8	58.0	50.1	41.3	30.6	21.3	14.7	
1937-------	1964	156.3	123.5	97.8	80.9	66.4	58.3	49.1	36.6	26.0	18.7		
1938-------	1965	134.1	106.3	90.1	75.2	66.9	57.0	44.0	31.3	22.7			
1939-------	1966	115.4	98.7	84.4	76.1	66.6	51.9	37.9	27.6				
1940-------	1967	107.1	93.6	87.1	77.3	61.0	44.3	33.0					
1941-------	1968	103.1	98.2	88.7	71.2	52.1	39.4						
1942-------	1969	109.8	100.4	82.6	59.7	46.6							
1943-------	1970	113.1	94.0	69.7	54.4								
1944-------	1971	105.7	78.4	62.9									
1945-------	1972	88.3	71.4										
1946-------	1973	78.9											

TABLE 10B. BIRTH PROBABILITIES FOR WHITE WOMEN FOR EACH YEAR 1917-73 BY AGE AND PARITY FOR EACH COHORT FROM 1868 TO 1958--CON.

(PROBABILITIES ARE THE NUMBER OF BIRTHS PER 1,000 WOMEN IN SPECIFIED PARITY AND EXACT AGE GROUP. FIGURES FOR "0 PARITY" SHOW THE PROBABILITY OF FIRST BIRTHS TO "0 PARITY" WOMEN, THOSE FOR "1 PARITY" SHOW THE PROBABILITY OF SECOND BIRTHS TO "1 PARITY" WOMEN, ETC. BASED ON CENTRAL BIRTH RATES AND PARITY DISTRIBUTIONS)

PARITY AND COHORT	DIAGONAL LINE FOR JANUARY 1	EXACT AGE										
		39	40	41	42	43	44	45	46	47	48	49
3 PARITY--CON.												
1868----------------												0.9
1869----------------											0.9	0.9
1870----------------										1.8	0.9	0.9
1871----------------									2.7	1.8	0.9	0.9
1872----------------								5.3	2.7	0.9	0.9	0.9
1873----------------							7.9	5.3	2.7	1.8	0.9	0.9
1874----------------						13.9	7.9	4.4	2.6	0.9	0.9	0.0
1875----------------					18.9	13.9	7.8	5.2	2.6	0.9	0.9	0.0
1876----------------				28.8	18.8	13.7	8.6	4.3	2.6	0.9	0.9	0.0
1877----------------			40.8	28.6	18.6	13.6	7.7	4.3	2.6	0.9	0.9	0.0
1878----------------	1917	57.4	39.8	28.4	19.3	13.5	7.6	4.2	2.6	0.9	0.0	0.0
1879----------------	1918	57.4	39.8	29.3	18.5	12.7	7.6	4.3	2.6	0.9	0.9	0.0
1880----------------	1919	56.6	39.8	28.4	18.5	12.7	7.6	4.2	2.6	0.9	0.0	0.0
1881----------------	1920	55.1	39.3	27.2	17.4	12.5	6.7	3.4	1.7	0.8	0.0	0.0
1882----------------	1921	55.2	36.3	26.0	17.2	11.5	6.6	3.3	1.7	0.8	0.0	0.0
1883----------------	1922	50.8	35.2	25.8	16.2	10.6	5.7	3.3	1.6	0.8	0.0	0.0
1884----------------	1923	50.2	34.8	24.7	16.0	9.7	5.6	3.2	1.6	0.8	0.0	0.0
1885----------------	1924	48.8	34.3	22.8	14.2	9.5	5.6	3.2	1.6	0.8	0.0	0.0
1886----------------	1925	48.3	31.7	21.8	13.3	8.6	5.5	2.4	1.6	0.8	0.0	0.0
1887----------------	1926	45.2	30.4	20.6	13.0	9.2	4.6	3.1	1.5	0.8	0.0	0.0
1888----------------	1927	43.0	28.3	19.5	12.8	8.3	4.5	2.3	1.5	0.8	0.0	0.0
1889----------------	1928	39.9	26.3	19.0	11.7	8.1	4.4	2.2	1.5	0.7	0.0	0.0
1890----------------	1929	37.0	26.4	17.2	11.5	7.2	4.3	2.2	0.7	0.7	0.0	0.0
1891----------------	1930	36.6	24.0	17.0	10.7	7.1	4.3	2.1	1.4	0.7	0.0	0.0
1892----------------	1931	33.5	22.5	15.5	10.6	7.1	3.5	2.1	1.4	0.0	0.0	0.0
1893----------------	1932	32.1	21.7	15.5	9.9	6.4	3.5	2.1	0.7	0.0	0.0	0.0
1894----------------	1933	30.4	22.2	14.6	9.1	6.3	3.5	2.1	0.7	0.0	0.0	0.0
1895----------------	1934	30.3	20.1	13.9	9.0	6.3	3.5	2.1	0.7	0.0	0.0	0.0
1896----------------	1935	28.2	19.3	13.8	9.0	6.2	3.5	1.4	0.7	0.7	0.0	0.0
1897----------------	1936	27.1	19.5	13.2	9.1	5.6	2.8	1.4	0.7	0.7	0.0	0.0
1898----------------	1937	26.6	18.9	14.0	9.1	5.6	3.5	2.1	1.4	0.7	0.0	0.0
1899----------------	1938	26.3	19.2	13.5	9.2	5.7	3.6	2.1	0.7	0.7	0.0	0.0
1900----------------	1939	26.6	18.7	13.6	8.6	6.5	4.3	2.2	1.4	0.0	0.0	0.0
1901----------------	1940	24.7	18.9	13.8	10.2	7.3	4.4	2.2	0.7	0.0	0.0	0.0
1902----------------	1941	25.8	19.8	16.1	11.0	8.1	4.4	2.2	0.7	0.0	0.0	0.0
1903----------------	1942	28.1	22.8	16.2	11.7	7.3	4.4	2.2	0.7	0.7	0.0	0.0
1904----------------	1943	32.3	24.0	18.6	11.9	7.4	4.5	2.2	1.5	0.0	0.0	0.0
1905----------------	1944	34.1	25.6	18.0	12.7	7.5	4.5	2.2	0.7	0.0	0.0	0.0
1906----------------	1945	36.3	26.3	19.4	11.9	7.4	4.5	2.2	0.7	0.7	0.0	0.0
1907----------------	1946	36.4	27.3	18.3	11.7	7.3	4.4	2.2	1.5	0.7	0.0	0.0
1908----------------	1947	36.0	25.5	17.4	11.6	7.9	4.3	2.2	1.4	0.0	0.0	0.0
1909----------------	1948	34.7	25.1	17.8	12.1	7.8	5.0	2.1	0.7	0.7	0.0	0.0
1910----------------	1949	33.9	24.5	18.1	12.5	9.0	4.2	2.1	1.4	0.0	0.0	0.0
1911----------------	1950	33.6	25.9	19.0	13.5	8.1	4.7	2.0	0.7	0.7	0.0	0.0
1912----------------	1951	33.9	27.0	19.7	13.1	8.5	4.6	2.6	1.3	0.7	0.0	0.0
1913----------------	1952	36.4	27.9	20.3	13.3	8.2	5.0	2.5	1.3	0.6	0.0	0.0
1914----------------	1953	36.7	28.5	20.0	12.7	8.5	4.8	2.4	1.2	0.0	0.0	0.0
1915----------------	1954	38.3	28.1	19.9	13.4	8.2	4.7	2.3	1.2	0.6	0.0	0.0
1916----------------	1955	38.0	27.0	20.0	12.6	8.0	4.6	2.3	1.2	0.0	0.0	0.0
1917----------------	1956	37.3	28.3	18.9	12.8	7.2	4.5	2.2	0.6	0.0	0.0	0.0
1918----------------	1957	37.2	25.9	18.3	11.9	7.6	3.8	1.6	0.5	0.0	0.0	0.0
1919----------------	1958	34.7	25.4	17.6	11.9	7.3	3.6	1.6	0.5	0.0	0.0	0.0
1920----------------	1959	34.3	24.7	17.7	11.2	6.1	3.6	1.5	0.5	0.0	0.0	0.0
1921----------------	1960	33.5	24.2	16.3	9.9	6.0	3.0	1.5	0.5	0.0	0.0	0.0
1922----------------	1961	31.4	22.3	14.6	8.8	5.4	2.9	1.5	0.5	0.0	0.0	0.0
1923----------------	1962	28.9	19.9	13.3	8.6	4.8	2.9	1.0	0.5	0.0	0.0	0.0
1924----------------	1963	26.9	19.1	12.6	7.5	4.7	2.3	0.9	0.5	0.0	0.0	0.0
1925----------------	1964	26.1	17.4	10.6	6.9	3.7	1.8	0.9	0.5	0.0	0.0	
1926----------------	1965	23.2	15.5	10.5	6.0	3.2	1.8	0.5	0.0	0.0		
1927----------------	1966	20.7	14.0	8.6	5.0	3.2	1.4	0.5	0.0			
1928----------------	1967	18.8	12.1	7.6	5.0	2.3	0.9	0.5				
1929----------------	1968	16.4	11.5	7.1	4.0	2.2	0.9					
1930----------------	1969	15.3	10.5	5.7	3.5	1.8						
1931----------------	1970	14.2	8.7	5.2	2.6							
1932----------------	1971	11.9	7.2	4.3								
1933----------------	1972	10.1	6.3									
1934----------------	1973	8.7										

TABLE 10B. BIRTH PROBABILITIES FOR WHITE WOMEN FOR EACH YEAR 1917-73 BY AGE AND PARITY FOR EACH COHORT FROM 1868 TO 1958--CON.

(PROBABILITIES ARE THE NUMBER OF BIRTHS PER 1,000 WOMEN IN SPECIFIED PARITY AND EXACT AGE GROUP. FIGURES FOR "0 PARITY" SHOW THE PROBABILITY OF FIRST BIRTHS TO "0 PARITY" WOMEN, THOSE FOR "1 PARITY" SHOW THE PROBABILITY OF SECOND BIRTHS TO "1 PARITY" WOMEN, ETC. BASED ON CENTRAL BIRTH RATES AND PARITY DISTRIBUTIONS)

PARITY AND COHORT	DIAGONAL LINE FOR JANUARY 1	EXACT AGE											
		15	16	17	18	19	20	21	22	23	24	25	26
4 PARITY													
1891-------													283.5
1892-------												296.9	279.0
1893-------											291.7	288.0	267.2
1894-------										303.2	291.3	282.7	276.2
1895-------									*	297.3	285.7	291.9	287.8
1896-------								*	*	294.5	298.4	306.8	266.0
1897-------							*	*	*	310.3	318.4	283.7	274.3
1898-------						*	*	*	*	333.3	291.5	297.8	271.6
1899-------					*	*	*	*	*	303.4	315.1	297.4	267.9
1900-------				*	*	*	*	*	*	343.1	314.4	290.4	264.2
1901-------			*	*	*	*	*	*	*	335.9	304.9	285.7	267.9
1902-------	1917	*	*	*	*	*	*	*	*	318.2	302.2	281.8	249.4
1903-------	1918	*	*	*	*	*	*	*	*	323.5	295.7	264.1	242.5
1904-------	1919	*	*	*	*	*	*	*	*	305.0	276.6	259.8	241.1
1905-------	1920	*	*	*	*	*	*	*	*	290.8	275.6	261.1	235.0
1906-------	1921	*	*	*	*	*	*	*	*	295.5	281.0	255.0	235.4
1907-------	1922	*	*	*	*	*	*	*	*	296.0	267.3	250.0	223.1
1908-------	1923	*	*	*	*	*	*	*	*	278.7	262.9	238.1	234.1
1909-------	1924	*	*	*	*	*	*	*	*	273.5	246.0	253.8	229.9
1910-------	1925	*	*	*	*	*	*	*	*	256.6	265.5	246.0	221.2
1911-------	1926	*	*	*	*	*	*	*	*	276.2	270.6	242.7	224.8
1912-------	1927	*	*	*	*	*	*	*	*	284.3	259.3	244.5	227.9
1913-------	1928	*	*	*	*	*	*	*	*	*	258.1	248.9	214.0
1914-------	1929	*	*	*	*	*	*	*	*	*	275.2	240.6	222.6
1915-------	1930	*	*	*	*	*	*	*	*	*	263.9	257.3	226.8
1916-------	1931	*	*	*	*	*	*	*	*	*	290.8	252.4	225.1
1917-------	1932	*	*	*	*	*	*	*	*	*	281.7	250.0	246.3
1918-------	1933	*	*	*	*	*	*	*	*	*	274.0	271.4	237.6
1919-------	1934	*	*	*	*	*	*	*	*	*	293.3	262.4	218.4
1920-------	1935	*	*	*	*	*	*	*	*	*	286.6	241.2	224.5
1921-------	1936	*	*	*	*	*	*	*	*	306.9	259.0	243.5	213.8
1922-------	1937	*	*	*	*	*	*	*	*	264.2	257.7	231.8	211.2
1923-------	1938	*	*	*	*	*	*	*	*	271.8	245.4	234.8	215.2
1924-------	1939	*	*	*	*	*	*	*	*	264.7	257.9	241.2	216.1
1925-------	1940	*	*	*	*	*	*	*	*	*	273.9	241.5	226.3
1926-------	1941	*	*	*	*	*	*	*	*	*	266.7	254.0	231.6
1927-------	1942	*	*	*	*	*	*	*	*	292.5	277.8	256.3	225.6
1928-------	1943	*	*	*	*	*	*	*	*	307.0	278.6	246.0	227.4
1929-------	1944	*	*	*	*	*	*	*	*	301.5	271.6	246.4	220.4
1930-------	1945	*	*	*	*	*	*	*	*	287.5	270.0	241.6	220.8
1931-------	1946	*	*	*	*	*	*	*	*	288.9	261.9	243.6	220.9
1932-------	1947	*	*	*	*	*	*	*	311.3	290.8	269.0	243.5	218.4
1933-------	1948	*	*	*	*	*	*	*	305.1	285.0	263.8	240.6	216.8
1934-------	1949	*	*	*	*	*	*	*	304.0	283.8	264.2	236.9	215.0
1935-------	1950	*	*	*	*	*	*	*	306.0	288.1	261.0	238.9	220.0
1936-------	1951	*	*	*	*	*	*	*	307.1	283.5	263.5	242.7	210.1
1937-------	1952	*	*	*	*	*	*	*	306.1	294.3	267.8	230.9	198.5
1938-------	1953	*	*	*	*	*	*	*	311.7	280.6	251.7	212.0	181.8
1939-------	1954	*	*	*	*	*	*	*	302.5	279.3	233.2	200.7	155.6
1940-------	1955	*	*	*	*	*	*	*	298.2	252.6	219.2	168.7	134.2
1941-------	1956	*	*	*	*	*	*	*	283.1	242.8	188.6	149.6	128.3
1942-------	1957	*	*	*	*	*	*	*	261.4	204.8	164.3	143.2	124.8
1943-------	1958	*	*	*	*	*	*	*	224.6	180.6	163.9	139.2	135.1
1944-------	1959	*	*	*	*	*	*	*	205.1	183.3	157.5	152.2	138.5
1945-------	1960	*	*	*	*	*	*	*	*	177.6	175.1	159.9	131.2
1946-------	1961	*	*	*	*	*	*	*	*	193.8	178.9	148.9	109.8
1947-------	1962	*	*	*	*	*	*	*	*	201.8	170.7	123.9	98.6
1948-------	1963	*	*	*	*	*	*	*	*	*	139.9	114.6	
1949-------	1964	*	*	*	*	*	*	*	*	*	128.0		
1950-------	1965	*	*	*	*	*	*	*	*	*			
1951-------	1966	*	*	*	*	*	*	*	*				
1952-------	1967	*	*	*	*	*	*	*					
1953-------	1968	*	*	*	*	*	*						
1954-------	1969	*	*	*	*	*							
1955-------	1970	*	*	*	*								
1956-------	1971	*	*	*									
1957-------	1972	*	*										
1958-------	1973	*											

TABLE 10B. BIRTH PROBABILITIES FOR WHITE WOMEN FOR EACH YEAR 1917-73 BY AGE, AND PARITY FOR EACH COHORT FROM 1868 TO 1958--CON.

(PROBABILITIES ARE THE NUMBER OF BIRTHS PER 1,000 WOMEN IN SPECIFIED PARITY AND EXACT AGE GROUP. FIGURES FOR "0 PARITY" SHOW THE PROBABILITY OF FIRST BIRTHS TO "C PARITY" WOMEN, THOSE FOR "1 PARITY" SHOW THE PROBABILITY OF SECOND BIRTHS TO "1 PARITY" WOMEN, ETC. BASED ON CENTRAL BIRTH RATES AND PARITY DISTRIBUTIONS)

PARITY AND COHORT	DIAGONAL LINE FOR JANUARY 1	EXACT AGE											
		27	28	29	30	31	32	33	34	35	36	37	38
4 PARITY--CON.													
1879-------													99.8
1880-------												118.4	99.3
1881-------											130.3	116.1	95.9
1882-------										149.2	127.7	112.3	94.3
1883-------									163.5	147.1	124.6	111.3	93.3
1884-------								182.9	162.2	141.9	123.3	110.8	86.3
1885-------							188.7	181.3	154.0	141.3	123.6	102.9	85.4
1886-------						210.7	188.3	171.4	153.7	141.0	114.9	101.2	83.7
1887-------					228.2	209.9	177.1	170.7	153.1	130.8	113.0	99.2	78.9
1888-------				264.3	224.7	197.3	176.5	168.3	141.7	128.2	110.2	92.6	75.0
1889-------			276.5	260.2	214.0	196.4	175.6	157.2	140.6	126.7	106.7	89.8	73.2
1890-------	1917	288.6	270.6	249.1	214.0	196.4	162.6	156.5	138.8	118.9	99.5	84.5	67.8
1891-------	1918	282.1	261.2	250.9	216.0	183.6	163.9	154.5	133.1	112.9	96.0	80.9	62.4
1892-------	1919	273.2	265.8	256.8	200.5	184.9	163.3	146.3	125.1	109.2	91.3	75.1	63.2
1893-------	1920	276.3	272.0	235.5	203.3	185.6	157.6	139.8	123.3	103.2	86.0	75.6	60.4
1894-------	1921	289.3	251.1	241.6	204.4	181.0	152.1	140.2	118.1	101.8	87.6	73.7	58.0
1895-------	1922	265.1	257.3	240.3	199.5	173.6	151.8	134.4	114.4	102.3	85.4	71.1	56.1
1896-------	1923	274.0	253.0	230.5	190.5	173.3	144.7	128.6	114.0	96.9	82.9	68.3	56.2
1897-------	1924	269.8	241.5	219.4	188.8	164.6	138.4	127.9	108.2	96.5	78.0	68.5	53.9
1898-------	1925	256.7	230.8	219.5	180.7	158.7	138.9	122.0	106.9	90.6	79.5	65.4	51.6
1899-------	1926	251.4	238.8	215.1	177.1	161.5	136.8	124.7	104.3	94.5	77.0	63.7	50.6
1900-------	1927	259.9	229.1	205.4	180.3	157.5	137.7	120.3	106.6	91.4	74.6	62.1	52.1
1901-------	1928	244.8	217.8	206.8	172.5	154.9	129.7	122.1	102.8	86.1	72.7	62.2	49.6
1902-------	1929	232.7	217.8	195.9	165.9	144.3	129.4	113.8	95.6	82.5	71.3	59.3	49.0
1903-------	1930	232.7	207.7	189.3	157.8	146.0	120.8	109.2	92.3	82.8	67.5	59.0	47.4
1904-------	1931	223.1	205.8	180.8	159.4	138.2	117.4	104.5	91.3	78.9	67.2	57.3	49.1
1905-------	1932	223.4	196.2	187.3	154.1	134.4	116.2	105.6	89.1	78.9	66.8	60.3	55.6
1906-------	1933	212.5	202.8	181.7	149.6	134.2	116.7	102.7	89.6	78.9	68.8	67.5	58.2
1907-------	1934	220.9	198.4	176.4	150.9	135.0	112.0	101.7	89.3	80.8	77.2	69.8	58.7
1908-------	1935	217.9	191.4	177.2	151.3	129.4	113.3	103.8	94.0	90.8	80.5	71.0	59.5
1909-------	1936	209.6	194.2	178.3	144.8	129.3	113.9	107.1	104.2	92.4	83.0	71.7	60.2
1910-------	1937	212.6	195.8	172.0	146.0	131.0	118.5	119.2	105.0	95.4	82.6	71.3	55.8
1911-------	1938	216.4	188.0	172.9	149.2	133.5	132.3	120.9	107.5	94.4	79.9	67.0	55.8
1912-------	1939	204.5	192.0	176.1	149.1	146.7	132.0	118.0	106.0	91.2	75.3	65.7	54.8
1913-------	1940	208.2	194.4	172.0	163.6	144.7	125.9	116.4	100.9	86.2	72.8	64.7	55.3
1914-------	1941	211.5	187.5	187.2	160.6	141.5	126.3	113.0	96.3	83.8	74.4	66.3	59.4
1915-------	1942	211.0	208.3	184.7	155.7	140.5	122.5	106.4	94.7	84.9	76.6	69.7	60.4
1916-------	1943	229.6	202.0	175.1	155.9	134.6	115.3	104.7	94.2	86.9	79.7	71.5	61.3
1917-------	1944	223.5	187.7	176.0	147.4	126.7	113.3	103.6	97.0	89.4	80.8	71.4	61.4
1918-------	1945	202.3	188.4	164.9	139.4	125.2	112.9	107.3	99.0	90.8	83.2	71.9	61.4
1919-------	1946	206.1	181.8	157.3	140.3	126.2	117.7	112.1	101.4	93.0	82.3	71.7	60.8
1920-------	1947	199.5	176.6	161.0	141.9	131.3	125.2	115.2	104.3	94.6	83.5	72.6	59.4
1921-------	1948	194.7	177.5	158.4	144.5	137.7	124.2	114.3	104.3	93.3	83.9	70.1	58.8
1922-------	1949	195.2	174.0	164.5	150.9	138.6	124.8	116.4	105.9	93.8	79.4	69.0	56.6
1923-------	1950	193.2	182.2	169.3	151.5	140.1	128.1	118.0	105.3	89.9	80.0	67.0	55.2
1924-------	1951	207.5	190.9	174.6	157.2	143.0	130.2	117.2	103.1	89.9	77.5	65.3	51.1
1925-------	1952	211.6	191.5	178.5	157.3	143.5	130.1	114.3	100.7	88.5	76.1	60.9	48.1
1926-------	1953	207.3	192.6	173.4	154.3	142.0	124.1	110.9	97.8	84.3	69.2	56.2	44.0
1927-------	1954	209.7	188.6	171.4	153.9	135.7	122.1	109.2	95.8	79.0	65.6	52.5	40.0
1928-------	1955	205.7	184.9	170.2	149.5	135.7	119.7	106.6	89.1	74.2	61.4	46.8	34.7
1929-------	1956	202.2	185.5	167.4	150.4	133.9	118.8	100.7	84.8	70.1	55.2	41.2	31.0
1930-------	1957	202.3	182.1	166.5	147.5	131.1	111.9	95.8	79.5	62.8	48.1	36.7	26.9
1931-------	1958	199.2	181.3	163.1	145.0	125.3	106.9	89.2	71.2	53.7	42.2	32.4	25.4
1932-------	1959	199.5	178.6	161.5	138.0	120.0	99.5	80.2	61.3	48.2	37.7	30.0	23.7
1933-------	1960	195.3	178.4	154.6	131.5	110.7	88.1	68.2	54.5	43.0	35.8	28.3	19.8
1934-------	1961	197.4	171.0	146.6	123.7	97.2	75.3	61.9	49.2	42.2	33.9	25.2	16.7
1935-------	1962	190.1	163.5	139.3	106.6	84.7	69.1	55.3	48.3	39.5	30.5	21.2	14.5
1936-------	1963	181.4	154.0	117.9	92.9	77.2	61.9	54.8	45.8	36.2	25.3	18.4	
1937-------	1964	168.8	130.7	103.2	85.2	69.8	62.0	53.3	42.2	30.6	22.1		
1938-------	1965	141.1	111.1	93.7	77.6	71.1	62.3	49.2	36.0	26.3			
1939-------	1966	123.3	102.9	87.4	81.1	72.3	57.7	42.2	31.4				
1940-------	1967	114.4	98.5	93.2	83.9	67.7	49.5	37.2					
1941-------	1968	111.6	106.5	97.3	78.9	57.5	44.5						
1942-------	1969	121.0	105.6	92.0	66.7	52.6							
1943-------	1970	122.2	103.6	75.9	60.1								
1944-------	1971	116.2	85.9	69.5									
1945-------	1972	98.5	77.9										
1946-------	1973	86.8											

TABLE 10B. BIRTH PROBABILITIES FOR WHITE WOMEN FOR EACH YEAR 1917-73 BY AGE AND PARITY FOR EACH COHORT FROM 1868 TO 1958--CON.

(PROBABILITIES ARE THE NUMBER OF BIRTHS PER 1,000 WOMEN IN SPECIFIED PARITY AND EXACT AGE GROUP. FIGURES FOR "0 PARITY" SHOW THE PROBABILITY OF FIRST BIRTHS TO "0 PARITY" WOMEN, THOSE FOR "1 PARITY" SHOW THE PROBABILITY OF SECOND BIRTHS TO "1 PARITY" WOMEN, ETC. BASED ON CENTRAL BIRTH RATES AND PARITY DISTRIBUTIONS)

PARITY AND COHORT	DIAGONAL LINE FOR JANUARY 1	EXACT AGE										
		39	40	41	42	43	44	45	46	47	48	49
4 PARITY--CON.												
1868												0.0
1869											1.0	0.0
1870										2.1	1.0	0.0
1871									4.1	3.1	1.0	0.0
1872								7.3	5.2	2.1	1.0	0.0
1873							12.5	8.3	5.2	2.1	1.0	0.0
1874						19.8	13.6	7.3	5.3	2.1	1.1	0.0
1875					28.1	20.9	12.6	7.4	4.2	2.1	1.1	0.0
1876				41.3	28.0	19.8	12.6	7.3	3.2	2.1	1.1	0.0
1877			57.1	42.1	26.9	19.7	12.5	6.3	3.1	2.1	1.0	0.0
1878	1917	82.9	58.3	41.3	27.0	19.8	11.5	6.3	3.1	1.0	1.0	0.0
1879	1918	83.6	57.8	40.6	28.2	18.9	11.6	6.3	3.2	2.1	1.1	0.0
1880	1919	81.9	55.9	42.7	26.2	18.9	11.6	6.3	3.2	2.1	1.1	0.0
1881	1920	80.5	56.7	38.4	26.1	18.8	10.5	5.3	3.2	1.1	0.0	0.0
1882	1921	80.0	52.2	38.1	24.8	16.6	9.4	5.2	3.1	1.0	0.0	0.0
1883	1922	72.8	51.0	36.9	23.7	15.5	9.3	5.2	3.1	1.0	0.0	0.0
1884	1923	71.8	49.9	35.8	22.6	15.4	9.3	5.2	3.1	1.0	0.0	0.0
1885	1924	70.8	46.8	33.7	22.5	14.4	8.2	5.2	2.1	1.0	1.0	0.0
1886	1925	66.1	45.2	32.3	20.2	13.2	8.1	4.1	3.1	1.0	1.0	0.0
1887	1926	63.2	43.6	30.8	19.0	14.0	8.0	4.0	2.0	1.0	0.0	0.0
1888	1927	60.5	41.2	27.6	18.7	11.9	6.9	4.0	2.0	1.0	0.0	0.0
1889	1928	57.7	38.3	28.6	17.8	11.9	6.9	4.0	2.0	1.0	0.0	0.0
1890	1929	52.4	37.9	25.3	17.6	11.7	6.9	2.9	2.0	0.0	1.0	0.0
1891	1930	52.7	35.2	25.5	17.7	11.8	5.9	3.9	1.0	1.0	1.0	0.0
1892	1931	49.4	34.6	24.8	16.9	11.0	6.0	3.0	2.0	1.0	0.0	0.0
1893	1932	47.3	33.3	24.2	16.2	10.1	5.1	3.0	2.0	1.0	0.0	0.0
1894	1933	46.6	33.2	23.8	14.5	9.4	6.2	3.1	2.1	1.0	0.0	0.0
1895	1934	46.5	32.8	22.2	14.8	10.6	5.3	3.2	1.1	0.0	0.0	0.0
1896	1935	44.2	31.3	22.7	15.1	9.7	5.4	2.2	1.1	0.0	0.0	0.0
1897	1936	41.7	30.7	21.9	14.3	8.8	4.4	3.3	1.1	0.0	0.0	0.0
1898	1937	41.4	30.2	22.3	14.5	8.9	6.7	3.4	1.1	1.1	0.0	0.0
1899	1938	42.4	30.9	21.8	14.9	10.3	6.9	3.4	2.3	1.1	0.0	0.0
1900	1939	41.3	30.6	22.4	15.3	10.6	7.1	3.5	2.4	0.0	0.0	0.0
1901	1940	40.9	30.1	21.6	16.8	12.0	7.2	3.6	1.2	0.0	0.0	0.0
1902	1941	39.0	29.2	24.2	18.1	10.9	7.2	3.6	1.2	0.0	0.0	0.0
1903	1942	39.6	31.9	25.6	17.1	12.2	7.3	3.6	1.2	0.0	0.0	0.0
1904	1943	43.6	33.3	24.5	17.1	12.2	6.1	3.6	1.2	0.0	0.0	0.0
1905	1944	45.9	35.3	26.3	18.7	11.2	6.2	3.7	1.2	0.0	0.0	0.0
1906	1945	48.1	35.9	26.7	17.7	10.1	6.3	3.8	1.3	1.3	0.0	0.0
1907	1946	48.4	37.3	25.5	16.5	11.3	6.3	3.8	2.5	1.3	0.0	0.0
1908	1947	48.9	33.9	24.5	17.9	11.5	7.6	3.8	2.5	1.3	0.0	0.0
1909	1948	45.8	33.5	25.4	17.7	12.6	7.5	3.8	2.5	1.3	0.0	0.0
1910	1949	45.3	34.4	25.2	18.8	12.5	7.5	3.7	2.5	1.2	0.0	0.0
1911	1950	45.7	33.7	27.1	18.3	13.4	8.5	3.6	2.4	0.0	0.0	0.0
1912	1951	46.0	36.6	27.7	20.3	14.3	7.1	3.6	1.2	1.2	0.0	0.0
1913	1952	47.8	36.3	28.9	20.6	12.6	6.8	3.4	2.3	1.1	0.0	0.0
1914	1953	49.7	39.7	30.2	20.0	13.3	7.7	4.4	2.2	1.1	0.0	0.0
1915	1954	50.9	40.1	28.9	20.2	12.7	7.4	3.2	2.1	1.1	0.0	0.0
1916	1955	51.0	38.6	28.9	19.5	12.3	7.1	4.1	2.0	1.0	0.0	0.0
1917	1956	50.6	37.8	28.5	18.6	11.7	6.8	2.9	1.9	0.0	0.0	0.0
1918	1957	49.1	36.6	26.7	19.0	12.3	5.7	2.8	0.9	0.0	0.0	0.0
1919	1958	48.2	36.6	26.3	18.1	10.8	6.3	2.7	0.9	0.0	0.0	0.0
1920	1959	47.5	36.3	26.3	16.6	10.5	5.2	2.6	0.9	0.0	0.0	0.0
1921	1960	45.9	34.4	23.4	15.8	9.1	5.0	2.5	0.8	0.0	0.0	0.0
1922	1961	45.1	31.7	22.7	14.5	8.9	4.8	2.4	0.8	0.0	0.0	0.0
1923	1962	41.2	29.9	21.2	13.3	7.8	3.9	1.6	0.8	0.0	0.0	0.0
1924	1963	39.1	28.2	19.0	11.4	6.8	3.0	1.5	0.8	0.0	0.0	0.0
1925	1964	36.5	25.9	16.3	10.3	5.9	3.7	1.5	0.0	0.0	0.0	
1926	1965	32.9	21.4	14.2	8.5	5.7	2.8	0.7	0.7	0.0		
1927	1966	27.9	18.8	12.5	8.3	4.9	2.1	0.7	0.7			
1928	1967	23.7	16.9	11.4	6.7	4.0	1.3	0.7				
1929	1968	22.3	15.7	9.8	5.9	3.3	1.3					
1930	1969	20.4	14.0	8.3	4.4	2.5						
1931	1970	19.1	11.1	6.8	3.7							
1932	1971	15.8	9.7	6.1								
1933	1972	13.1	8.4									
1934	1973	11.3										

TABLE 10B. BIRTH PROBABILITIES FOR WHITE WOMEN FOR EACH YEAR 1917-73 BY AGE AND PARITY FOR EACH COHORT FROM 1868 TO 1958–CON.

(PROBABILITIES ARE THE NUMBER OF BIRTHS PER 1,000 WOMEN IN SPECIFIED PARITY AND EXACT AGE GROUP. FIGURES FOR "0 PARITY" SHOW THE PROBABILITY OF FIRST BIRTHS TO "0 PARITY" WOMEN, THOSE FOR "1 PARITY" SHOW THE PROBABILITY OF SECOND BIRTHS TO "1 PARITY" WOMEN, ETC. BASED ON CENTRAL BIRTH RATES AND PARITY DISTRIBUTIONS)

PARITY AND COHORT	DIAGONAL LINE FOR JANUARY 1	EXACT AGE											
		15	16	17	18	19	20	21	22	23	24	25	26
5 PARITY													
1891-------													315.0
1892-------												330.6	304.6
1893-------											*	304.0	284.3
1894-------										*	*	308.3	296.3
1895-------									*	*	*	319.0	326.2
1896-------								*	*	*	*	362.8	304.3
1897-------							*	*	*	*	*	333.3	318.4
1898-------						*	*	*	*	*	*	348.2	312.8
1899-------					*	*	*	*	*	*	*	336.3	299.4
1900-------				*	*	*	*	*	*	*	*	321.4	300.6
1901-------			*	*	*	*	*	*	*	*	*	327.1	307.2
1902-------	1917	*	*	*	*	*	*	*	*	*	*	333.3	288.3
1903-------	1918	*	*	*	*	*	*	*	*	*	*	296.3	272.7
1904-------	1919	*	*	*	*	*	*	*	*	*	*	299.1	273.3
1905-------	1920	*	*	*	*	*	*	*	*	*	*	298.1	271.0
1906-------	1921	*	*	*	*	*	*	*	*	*	*	*	267.1
1907-------	1922	*	*	*	*	*	*	*	*	*	*	*	251.9
1908-------	1923	*	*	*	*	*	*	*	*	*	*	*	267.7
1909-------	1924	*	*	*	*	*	*	*	*	*	*	*	278.7
1910-------	1925	*	*	*	*	*	*	*	*	*	*	*	275.9
1911-------	1926	*	*	*	*	*	*	*	*	*	*	*	284.4
1912-------	1927	*	*	*	*	*	*	*	*	*	*	*	288.5
1913-------	1928	*	*	*	*	*	*	*	*	*	*	*	270.0
1914-------	1929	*	*	*	*	*	*	*	*	*	*	*	*
1915-------	1930	*	*	*	*	*	*	*	*	*	*	*	*
1916-------	1931	*	*	*	*	*	*	*	*	*	*	*	*
1917-------	1932	*	*	*	*	*	*	*	*	*	*	*	*
1918-------	1933	*	*	*	*	*	*	*	*	*	*	*	284.3
1919-------	1934	*	*	*	*	*	*	*	*	*	*	*	276.2
1920-------	1935	*	*	*	*	*	*	*	*	*	*	*	271.0
1921-------	1936	*	*	*	*	*	*	*	*	*	*	*	259.3
1922-------	1937	*	*	*	*	*	*	*	*	*	*	*	266.7
1923-------	1938	*	*	*	*	*	*	*	*	*	*	*	284.3
1924-------	1939	*	*	*	*	*	*	*	*	*	*	*	274.5
1925-------	1940	*	*	*	*	*	*	*	*	*	*	*	285.7
1926-------	1941	*	*	*	*	*	*	*	*	*	*	*	280.7
1927-------	1942	*	*	*	*	*	*	*	*	*	*	*	283.5
1928-------	1943	*	*	*	*	*	*	*	*	*	*	*	274.6
1929-------	1944	*	*	*	*	*	*	*	*	*	*	295.2	268.8
1930-------	1945	*	*	*	*	*	*	*	*	*	*	285.7	262.6
1931-------	1946	*	*	*	*	*	*	*	*	*	*	292.3	269.0
1932-------	1947	*	*	*	*	*	*	*	*	*	*	293.7	266.4
1933-------	1948	*	*	*	*	*	*	*	*	*	*	283.9	261.8
1934-------	1949	*	*	*	*	*	*	*	*	*	*	289.2	265.3
1935-------	1950	*	*	*	*	*	*	*	*	*	311.3	287.4	263.6
1936-------	1951	*	*	*	*	*	*	*	*	*	312.5	282.6	251.8
1937-------	1952	*	*	*	*	*	*	*	*	*	305.1	271.8	231.3
1938-------	1953	*	*	*	*	*	*	*	*	*	305.8	261.5	218.2
1939-------	1954	*	*	*	*	*	*	*	*	*	280.0	237.1	184.5
1940-------	1955	*	*	*	*	*	*	*	*	*	262.3	204.3	161.9
1941-------	1956	*	*	*	*	*	*	*	*	*	222.2	179.6	152.8
1942-------	1957	*	*	*	*	*	*	*	*	*	*	177.8	153.4
1943-------	1958	*	*	*	*	*	*	*	*	*	*	171.2	164.4
1944-------	1959	*	*	*	*	*	*	*	*	*	*	*	168.0
1945-------	1960	*	*	*	*	*	*	*	*	*	*	*	163.6
1946-------	1961	*	*	*	*	*	*	*	*	*	*	*	*
1947-------	1962	*	*	*	*	*	*	*	*	*	*	*	*
1948-------	1963	*	*	*	*	*	*	*	*	*	*	*	
1949-------	1964	*	*	*	*	*	*	*	*	*	*		
1950-------	1965	*	*	*	*	*	*	*	*	*			
1951-------	1966	*	*	*	*	*	*	*	*				
1952-------	1967	*	*	*	*	*	*	*					
1953-------	1968	*	*	*	*	*	*						
1954-------	1969	*	*	*	*	*							
1955-------	1970	*	*	*	*								
1956-------	1971	*	*	*									
1957-------	1972	*	*										
1958-------	1973	*											

TABLE 10B. BIRTH PROBABILITIES FOR WHITE WOMEN FOR EACH YEAR 1917–73 BY AGE AND PARITY FOR EACH COHORT FROM 1868 TO 1958--CON.

(PROBABILITIES ARE THE NUMBER OF BIRTHS PER 1,000 WOMEN IN SPECIFIED PARITY AND EXACT AGE GROUP. FIGURES FOR "0 PARITY" SHOW THE PROBABILITY OF FIRST BIRTHS TO "0 PARITY" WOMEN, THOSE FOR "1 PARITY" SHOW THE PROBABILITY OF SECOND BIRTHS TO "1 PARITY" WOMEN, ETC. BASED ON CENTRAL BIRTH RATES AND PARITY DISTRIBUTIONS)

PARITY AND COHORT	DIAGONAL LINE FOR JANUARY 1	EXACT AGE											
		27	28	29	30	31	32	33	34	35	36	37	38
5 PARITY--CON.													
1879-------													136.5
1880-------												160.4	134.3
1881-------											172.9	156.7	130.4
1882-------										189.4	167.5	151.0	127.1
1883-------									202.1	185.0	161.7	147.6	123.7
1884-------								219.9	200.5	179.1	160.8	146.6	115.7
1885-------							229.7	224.1	196.2	181.5	162.5	139.4	114.5
1886-------						251.6	234.8	217.5	198.0	185.2	156.3	138.4	115.3
1887-------					267.9	259.3	229.8	219.4	204.3	177.2	156.0	140.1	113.7
1888-------				300.8	264.8	247.2	224.3	222.7	191.4	175.6	154.3	132.7	106.1
1889-------			309.1	298.7	255.5	244.6	231.3	209.7	192.4	174.9	148.6	127.7	106.1
1890-------	1917	325.3	298.9	286.0	254.2	250.8	217.5	211.7	191.0	167.2	142.2	127.0	98.3
1891-------	1918	314.5	287.6	286.0	264.0	234.2	219.4	208.7	181.8	160.5	142.9	117.6	92.2
1892-------	1919	301.1	289.6	302.4	244.3	238.2	218.5	199.7	176.0	161.0	132.6	112.0	96.5
1893-------	1920	299.6	309.6	275.2	248.5	237.0	208.5	191.2	177.0	149.6	126.4	111.6	91.0
1894-------	1921	329.6	283.7	288.4	252.0	231.3	202.5	193.5	165.6	144.7	125.2	108.1	88.6
1895-------	1922	303.4	299.4	290.2	245.8	227.4	208.4	185.5	159.8	144.8	124.4	105.3	85.1
1896-------	1923	323.0	299.4	281.1	247.3	229.2	196.9	178.3	160.7	139.9	120.7	102.4	88.3
1897-------	1924	321.4	287.0	281.7	248.8	222.9	190.4	182.7	157.0	141.0	118.9	105.5	83.6
1898-------	1925	297.2	286.2	280.7	235.8	214.8	196.7	175.9	157.7	137.7	121.3	103.5	81.0
1899-------	1926	303.3	290.8	270.5	231.3	220.5	192.0	180.9	154.5	140.1	116.9	98.7	81.1
1900-------	1927	303.8	273.9	258.3	232.7	212.3	190.5	170.8	156.2	133.5	113.7	95.3	81.2
1901-------	1928	290.0	259.4	259.4	222.5	210.4	179.4	172.8	146.8	127.0	107.1	93.8	75.2
1902-------	1929	271.1	263.2	246.3	219.6	199.0	179.9	163.7	141.6	123.9	105.3	91.3	74.1
1903-------	1930	271.1	248.2	245.5	204.9	197.5	169.9	154.4	133.9	120.1	100.6	86.7	71.0
1904-------	1931	261.5	254.6	227.8	212.5	191.6	166.7	153.1	134.9	115.9	100.2	87.7	75.9
1905-------	1932	265.7	233.5	239.2	207.1	184.1	163.6	154.6	128.3	115.6	97.0	90.7	78.3
1906-------	1933	244.9	246.9	234.3	200.0	185.5	167.1	147.4	129.8	113.9	101.4	94.8	83.3
1907-------	1934	263.7	248.9	230.5	206.0	190.8	159.9	150.4	129.4	120.1	109.4	101.2	84.3
1908-------	1935	264.4	243.1	236.2	207.7	182.4	163.1	147.1	135.2	127.7	115.2	101.5	84.0
1909-------	1936	266.7	254.9	238.5	200.7	185.6	161.8	153.4	146.2	133.7	115.3	100.5	82.3
1910-------	1937	271.0	252.6	231.4	206.2	183.5	161.1	166.7	151.3	130.3	113.2	98.2	77.3
1911-------	1938	272.1	247.3	238.5	208.2	179.1	178.7	168.8	143.7	126.8	109.6	92.3	76.7
1912-------	1939	262.4	255.7	240.4	199.2	199.2	181.8	165.0	145.5	128.2	105.7	93.5	77.7
1913-------	1940	268.7	260.4	228.9	217.4	200.8	176.1	162.9	142.4	119.7	105.1	93.0	79.6
1914-------	1941	274.8	242.4	248.7	217.4	196.9	175.4	154.8	131.3	120.1	103.4	96.0	82.5
1915-------	1942	261.5	260.6	242.6	208.5	193.2	161.5	144.2	130.8	117.2	108.0	92.9	83.7
1916-------	1943	280.3	251.5	226.0	203.3	176.5	152.8	143.3	127.5	119.0	104.5	93.7	82.2
1917-------	1944	274.1	241.4	226.0	189.3	170.9	151.8	142.0	128.5	116.3	103.4	94.6	83.3
1918-------	1945	257.1	234.3	212.3	187.0	170.3	154.1	140.7	131.1	115.9	104.9	95.7	82.5
1919-------	1946	257.1	230.3	209.3	189.5	171.4	153.8	147.0	130.5	121.7	110.4	97.3	84.5
1920-------	1947	243.1	225.3	215.6	186.5	170.7	160.5	145.6	138.3	124.4	110.9	98.0	81.9
1921-------	1948	248.3	236.3	211.0	192.2	180.3	160.2	154.9	139.8	125.3	113.8	97.2	81.9
1922-------	1949	262.4	231.6	223.3	195.3	175.5	165.2	153.7	137.4	126.5	107.8	96.1	78.1
1923-------	1950	253.6	248.6	223.7	198.5	183.0	168.0	154.4	139.8	123.6	109.7	91.5	79.3
1924-------	1951	269.5	241.9	219.4	198.6	183.9	165.8	154.3	135.0	118.3	103.5	91.6	69.9
1925-------	1952	268.5	245.0	227.5	203.2	187.2	166.3	148.4	132.1	116.6	102.7	82.6	68.0
1926-------	1953	262.2	247.7	226.6	202.9	184.1	160.9	146.7	129.8	115.2	96.5	79.5	63.0
1927-------	1954	262.6	241.7	227.0	197.8	176.2	161.7	144.6	128.7	109.1	92.1	73.4	56.5
1928-------	1955	253.7	236.8	213.2	189.7	178.6	157.1	141.4	120.8	102.0	85.0	64.9	47.8
1929-------	1956	255.6	229.5	209.2	193.3	173.7	155.3	132.9	114.6	94.9	74.0	55.3	44.3
1930-------	1957	249.0	224.6	209.9	187.6	169.3	146.0	127.7	105.8	83.8	63.3	50.7	36.7
1931-------	1958	245.4	225.4	209.1	185.8	160.0	138.8	119.5	93.1	71.6	57.4	44.4	33.4
1932-------	1959	244.1	224.5	203.8	175.6	152.8	129.4	103.0	79.9	63.6	51.3	40.0	31.5
1933-------	1960	244.5	220.0	194.4	166.1	141.4	112.6	87.4	71.1	58.0	47.3	37.3	27.8
1934-------	1961	241.8	214.8	187.0	155.4	122.6	95.4	78.4	62.7	55.8	44.0	34.0	24.6
1935-------	1962	231.0	200.0	170.7	134.1	105.9	84.9	68.7	63.4	51.7	39.9	30.0	20.5
1936-------	1963	215.3	184.8	145.0	114.4	94.5	75.6	69.1	59.9	48.2	35.0	25.0	
1937-------	1964	198.9	156.9	126.2	103.4	85.8	77.6	68.1	55.9	41.3	30.4		
1938-------	1965	172.7	136.9	115.9	95.2	89.4	77.0	63.7	48.3	35.9			
1939-------	1966	146.6	124.1	107.0	100.6	88.4	73.6	55.4	42.7				
1940-------	1967	141.4	120.4	115.5	102.8	85.1	62.5	50.6					
1941-------	1968	135.8	128.2	116.0	97.1	70.5	57.6						
1942-------	1969	146.8	132.1	108.6	81.0	66.3							
1943-------	1970	149.7	126.1	91.9	71.9								
1944-------	1971	141.1	104.5	81.5									
1945-------	1972	119.7	99.4										
1946-------	1973	109.2											

TABLE 10B. BIRTH PROBABILITIES FOR WHITE WOMEN FOR EACH YEAR 1917-73 BY AGE AND PARITY FOR EACH COHORT FROM 1868 TO 1958--CON.

(PROBABILITIES ARE THE NUMBER OF BIRTHS PER 1,000 WOMEN IN SPECIFIED PARITY AND EXACT AGE GROUP. FIGURES FOR "0 PARITY" SHOW THE PROBABILITY OF FIRST BIRTHS TO "C PARITY" WOMEN, THOSE FOR "1 PARITY" SHOW THE PROBABILITY OF SECOND BIRTHS TO "1 PARITY" WOMEN, ETC. BASED ON CENTRAL BIRTH RATES AND PARITY DISTRIBUTIONS)

PARITY AND COHORT	DIAGONAL LINE FOR JANUARY 1	EXACT AGE										
		39	40	41	42	43	44	45	46	47	48	49
5 PARITY--CON.												
1868												0.0
1869											1.3	0.0
1870										2.5	1.3	0.0
1871									6.3	2.5	1.3	0.0
1872								11.5	7.7	2.6	1.3	0.0
1873							19.3	11.6	6.5	2.6	1.3	0.0
1874						31.1	19.6	11.8	7.9	2.6	1.3	0.0
1875					42.9	30.1	18.4	11.9	6.6	2.6	1.3	0.0
1876				62.1	41.8	28.9	19.8	11.9	5.3	2.7	1.3	0.0
1877			82.4	61.1	40.6	30.3	18.6	9.3	6.7	2.7	1.3	0.0
1878	1917	116.0	82.9	61.0	42.8	31.0	17.6	10.9	5.4	2.7	1.4	0.0
1879	1918	115.3	81.9	61.3	43.0	28.4	17.7	9.5	5.5	2.7	1.4	0.0
1880	1919	111.5	80.6	61.3	38.9	28.3	17.6	9.5	5.4	2.7	1.4	0.0
1881	1920	110.2	79.3	55.9	38.8	26.9	16.2	9.5	5.4	2.7	1.4	0.0
1882	1921	106.9	72.0	55.3	37.1	25.3	14.7	8.0	4.0	2.7	1.3	0.0
1883	1922	98.3	70.2	52.3	34.2	23.7	13.2	8.0	4.0	2.7	1.3	0.0
1884	1923	96.6	69.5	48.7	33.0	22.5	13.3	6.7	4.0	2.7	1.3	0.0
1885	1924	97.3	66.9	48.5	32.4	21.7	12.2	6.8	4.1	1.4	1.4	0.0
1886	1925	93.8	64.1	47.9	30.2	20.7	12.4	6.9	4.2	1.4	0.0	0.0
1887	1926	90.4	65.5	44.8	29.4	22.5	12.7	7.1	4.2	1.4	0.0	0.0
1888	1927	87.9	60.1	43.4	30.9	19.7	11.3	7.1	2.8	1.4	0.0	0.0
1889	1928	83.5	56.6	43.9	28.4	19.9	12.9	5.7	2.9	1.4	0.0	0.0
1890	1929	77.8	59.1	40.5	27.5	20.3	11.6	5.8	2.9	1.5	0.0	0.0
1891	1930	80.4	54.2	41.1	26.5	19.1	10.3	5.9	2.9	1.5	0.0	0.0
1892	1931	75.4	55.8	39.3	27.3	18.2	10.6	6.1	3.0	1.5	0.0	0.0
1893	1932	75.5	52.6	38.7	24.8	17.1	10.9	6.2	3.1	1.6	0.0	0.0
1894	1933	71.2	52.2	36.5	23.8	15.9	9.5	4.8	3.2	1.6	0.0	0.0
1895	1934	71.9	49.0	35.9	24.5	16.4	9.8	4.9	3.3	0.0	0.0	0.0
1896	1935	69.6	47.5	33.9	25.4	16.9	8.5	5.1	1.7	0.0	0.0	0.0
1897	1936	65.6	47.8	35.3	24.7	14.2	8.8	5.3	1.8	0.0	0.0	0.0
1898	1937	64.2	49.4	36.6	23.8	14.6	11.0	5.5	1.8	1.8	0.0	0.0
1899	1938	65.9	46.9	33.6	22.4	16.8	11.2	5.6	3.7	1.9	0.0	0.0
1900	1939	63.6	46.1	32.5	22.9	17.1	11.4	5.7	3.8	1.9	0.0	0.0
1901	1940	61.0	43.1	31.1	25.2	17.4	9.7	5.8	3.9	0.0	0.0	0.0
1902	1941	59.2	44.6	36.4	26.2	18.0	10.0	6.0	2.0	2.0	0.0	0.0
1903	1942	60.0	47.3	36.8	26.4	18.3	12.1	4.0	2.0	0.0	0.0	0.0
1904	1943	64.5	48.9	40.1	25.3	18.9	8.4	4.2	2.1	0.0	0.0	0.0
1905	1944	65.9	52.1	36.6	25.6	16.9	8.5	4.2	2.1	0.0	0.0	0.0
1906	1945	70.5	51.6	37.7	26.4	15.3	8.7	4.4	2.2	2.2	0.0	0.0
1907	1946	68.4	50.9	36.4	22.6	17.9	8.9	4.5	2.2	0.0	0.0	0.0
1908	1947	67.5	47.2	34.9	25.3	16.0	9.1	4.5	2.3	0.0	0.0	0.0
1909	1948	63.0	47.4	35.0	25.4	18.3	11.4	4.6	2.3	0.0	0.0	0.0
1910	1949	63.1	47.5	37.4	25.5	18.3	11.4	4.6	2.3	0.0	0.0	0.0
1911	1950	62.5	49.3	37.0	27.4	18.1	11.3	6.7	2.2	2.2	0.0	0.0
1912	1951	65.7	52.3	39.6	29.9	20.5	11.3	6.8	2.3	2.3	0.0	0.0
1913	1952	69.9	51.6	43.7	29.5	20.2	13.4	6.7	4.5	0.0	0.0	0.0
1914	1953	67.8	56.6	42.0	28.3	19.4	10.7	6.4	2.1	0.0	0.0	0.0
1915	1954	71.6	54.2	40.2	29.1	18.5	12.3	6.1	2.0	0.0	0.0	0.0
1916	1955	70.4	51.7	42.3	27.8	19.7	11.8	5.9	2.0	0.0	0.0	0.0
1917	1956	69.7	55.6	40.9	28.7	19.0	11.4	5.7	1.9	1.9	0.0	0.0
1918	1957	69.2	53.7	39.5	27.9	16.6	9.1	3.6	1.8	1.8	0.0	0.0
1919	1958	69.8	53.2	39.6	26.6	17.6	8.8	5.2	1.7	0.0	0.0	0.0
1920	1959	68.1	52.4	37.7	25.3	15.1	10.0	3.3	1.7	0.0	0.0	0.0
1921	1960	65.1	50.0	34.4	24.3	16.1	8.0	3.2	1.6	0.0	0.0	0.0
1922	1961	63.8	46.3	34.5	23.3	12.4	7.7	3.1	1.5	0.0	0.0	0.0
1923	1962	59.6	46.0	31.8	19.5	11.9	6.0	3.0	1.5	0.0	0.0	0.0
1924	1963	56.0	42.0	28.6	17.0	9.9	5.6	2.8	1.4	0.0	0.0	0.0
1925	1964	52.3	37.5	24.7	15.0	9.5	5.4	2.7	1.4	0.0	0.0	
1926	1965	47.9	32.4	20.1	13.3	8.0	4.0	2.6	0.0	0.0		
1927	1966	40.9	27.4	19.4	11.6	6.4	3.8	1.3	0.0			
1928	1967	35.5	25.2	16.3	10.0	6.2	2.5	1.2				
1929	1968	31.6	21.6	14.3	8.3	4.7	2.4					
1930	1969	28.1	19.7	12.7	8.0	4.6						
1931	1970	26.1	18.0	11.2	6.7							
1932	1971	23.4	14.4	8.8								
1933	1972	18.8	12.1									
1934	1973	16.7										

TABLE 10B. BIRTH PROBABILITIES FOR WHITE WOMEN FOR EACH YEAR 1917-73 BY AGE AND PARITY FOR EACH COHORT FROM 1868 TO 1958--CON.

(PROBABILITIES ARE THE NUMBER OF BIRTHS PER 1,000 WOMEN IN SPECIFIED PARITY AND EXACT AGE GROUP. FIGURES FOR "0 PARITY" SHOW THE PROBABILITY OF FIRST BIRTHS TO "0 PARITY" WOMEN, THOSE FOR "1 PARITY" SHOW THE PROBABILITY OF SECOND BIRTHS TO "1 PARITY" WOMEN, ETC. BASED ON CENTRAL BIRTH RATES AND PARITY DISTRIBUTIONS)

PARITY AND COHORT	DIAGONAL LINE FOR JANUARY 1	EXACT AGE											
		15	16	17	18	19	20	21	22	23	24	25	26
6 PARITY													
1891-------													*
1892-------												*	*
1893-------											*	*	*
1894-------										*	*	*	*
1895-------									*	*	*	*	*
1896-------								*	*	*	*	*	*
1897-------							*	*	*	*	*	*	*
1898-------						*	*	*	*	*	*	*	*
1899-------					*	*	*	*	*	*	*	*	*
1900-------				*	*	*	*	*	*	*	*	*	*
1901-------			*	*	*	*	*	*	*	*	*	*	*
1902-------	1917	*	*	*	*	*	*	*	*	*	*	*	*
1903-------	1918	*	*	*	*	*	*	*	*	*	*	*	*
1904-------	1919	*	*	*	*	*	*	*	*	*	*	*	*
1905-------	1920	*	*	*	*	*	*	*	*	*	*	*	*
1906-------	1921	*	*	*	*	*	*	*	*	*	*	*	*
1907-------	1922	*	*	*	*	*	*	*	*	*	*	*	*
1908-------	1923	*	*	*	*	*	*	*	*	*	*	*	*
1909-------	1924	*	*	*	*	*	*	*	*	*	*	*	*
1910-------	1925	*	*	*	*	*	*	*	*	*	*	*	*
1911-------	1926	*	*	*	*	*	*	*	*	*	*	*	*
1912-------	1927	*	*	*	*	*	*	*	*	*	*	*	*
1913-------	1928	*	*	*	*	*	*	*	*	*	*	*	*
1914-------	1929	*	*	*	*	*	*	*	*	*	*	*	*
1915-------	1930	*	*	*	*	*	*	*	*	*	*	*	*
1916-------	1931	*	*	*	*	*	*	*	*	*	*	*	*
1917-------	1932	*	*	*	*	*	*	*	*	*	*	*	*
1918-------	1933	*	*	*	*	*	*	*	*	*	*	*	*
1919-------	1934	*	*	*	*	*	*	*	*	*	*	*	*
1920-------	1935	*	*	*	*	*	*	*	*	*	*	*	*
1921-------	1936	*	*	*	*	*	*	*	*	*	*	*	*
1922-------	1937	*	*	*	*	*	*	*	*	*	*	*	*
1923-------	1938	*	*	*	*	*	*	*	*	*	*	*	*
1924-------	1939	*	*	*	*	*	*	*	*	*	*	*	*
1925-------	1940	*	*	*	*	*	*	*	*	*	*	*	*
1926-------	1941	*	*	*	*	*	*	*	*	*	*	*	*
1927-------	1942	*	*	*	*	*	*	*	*	*	*	*	*
1928-------	1943	*	*	*	*	*	*	*	*	*	*	*	*
1929-------	1944	*	*	*	*	*	*	*	*	*	*	*	*
1930-------	1945	*	*	*	*	*	*	*	*	*	*	*	*
1931-------	1946	*	*	*	*	*	*	*	*	*	*	*	*
1932-------	1947	*	*	*	*	*	*	*	*	*	*	*	*
1933-------	1948	*	*	*	*	*	*	*	*	*	*	*	*
1934-------	1949	*	*	*	*	*	*	*	*	*	*	*	*
1935-------	1950	*	*	*	*	*	*	*	*	*	*	*	*
1936-------	1951	*	*	*	*	*	*	*	*	*	*	*	*
1937-------	1952	*	*	*	*	*	*	*	*	*	*	*	*
1938-------	1953	*	*	*	*	*	*	*	*	*	*	*	*
1939-------	1954	*	*	*	*	*	*	*	*	*	*	*	*
1940-------	1955	*	*	*	*	*	*	*	*	*	*	*	*
1941-------	1956	*	*	*	*	*	*	*	*	*	*	*	*
1942-------	1957	*	*	*	*	*	*	*	*	*	*	*	*
1943-------	1958	*	*	*	*	*	*	*	*	*	*	*	*
1944-------	1959	*	*	*	*	*	*	*	*	*	*	*	*
1945-------	1960	*	*	*	*	*	*	*	*	*	*	*	*
1946-------	1961	*	*	*	*	*	*	*	*	*	*	*	*
1947-------	1962	*	*	*	*	*	*	*	*	*	*	*	*
1948-------	1963	*	*	*	*	*	*	*	*	*	*	*	
1949-------	1964	*	*	*	*	*	*	*	*	*	*		
1950-------	1965	*	*	*	*	*	*	*	*	*			
1951-------	1966	*	*	*	*	*	*	*	*				
1952-------	1967	*	*	*	*	*	*	*					
1953-------	1968	*	*	*	*	*	*						
1954-------	1969	*	*	*	*	*							
1955-------	1970	*	*	*	*								
1956-------	1971	*	*	*									
1957-------	1972	*	*										
1958-------	1973	*											

TABLE 10B. BIRTH PROBABILITIES FOR WHITE WOMEN FOR EACH YEAR 1917-73 BY AGE AND PARITY FOR EACH COHORT FROM 1868 TO 1958--CON.

(PROBABILITIES ARE THE NUMBER OF BIRTHS PER 1,000 WOMEN IN SPECIFIED PARITY AND EXACT AGE GROUP. FIGURES FOR "0 PARITY" SHOW THE PROBABILITY OF FIRST BIRTHS TO "0 PARITY" WOMEN, THOSE FOR "1 PARITY" SHOW THE PROBABILITY OF SECOND BIRTHS TO "1 PARITY" WOMEN, ETC. BASED ON CENTRAL BIRTH RATES AND PARITY DISTRIBUTIONS)

PARITY AND COHORT	DIAGONAL LINE FOR JANUARY 1	EXACT AGE 27	28	29	30	31	32	33	34	35	36	37	38
6 PARITY--CON.													
1879-------													159.8
1880-------												186.4	159.6
1881-------											203.3	187.9	161.8
1882-------										225.8	204.2	191.5	165.0
1883-------									239.4	224.5	206.0	192.4	165.2
1884-------								256.3	235.5	219.4	203.9	190.2	154.2
1885-------							255.2	254.7	228.2	217.3	203.6	177.8	150.3
1886-------						273.5	258.1	243.2	226.1	220.8	189.2	173.5	149.4
1887-------					275.4	277.6	245.3	242.6	234.3	206.8	188.0	174.1	140.8
1888-------				309.3	269.5	260.1	243.0	251.1	216.7	204.9	186.0	161.2	132.6
1889-------			309.1	300.4	259.9	263.0	257.2	236.3	221.3	207.4	180.6	160.7	135.4
1890-------	1917	333.3	286.6	291.3	263.5	276.1	241.4	242.7	223.2	199.2	173.8	157.4	129.0
1891-------	1918	307.7	285.7	297.3	282.2	259.4	246.2	244.8	219.1	197.9	176.5	153.1	122.5
1892-------	1919	310.7	296.8	320.9	261.5	264.1	247.4	235.2	212.5	195.7	164.9	141.7	122.0
1893-------	1920	*	320.0	297.7	266.4	265.2	241.3	229.1	214.0	184.9	156.2	140.4	115.5
1894-------	1921	*	300.0	315.5	271.7	255.5	236.1	233.3	201.0	176.7	158.0	139.7	118.4
1895-------	1922	*	324.1	313.4	262.5	253.2	238.5	216.4	191.5	177.0	153.5	139.0	113.1
1896-------	1923	*	308.2	293.5	262.7	252.5	221.9	207.7	191.2	171.2	152.2	130.6	112.7
1897-------	1924	*	294.5	295.9	255.1	239.7	211.0	204.0	180.9	165.8	146.0	129.0	107.9
1898-------	1925	*	302.2	297.9	253.2	231.0	214.7	199.4	179.6	163.6	146.2	125.6	101.5
1899-------	1926	*	301.5	288.0	239.1	236.2	205.9	200.6	177.0	164.4	141.4	120.8	101.5
1900-------	1927	*	283.6	268.2	245.5	224.3	212.1	195.7	181.8	162.9	137.0	120.6	103.4
1901-------	1928	*	273.4	272.2	239.4	232.9	203.6	201.3	180.1	158.7	134.1	120.0	95.8
1902-------	1929	*	276.4	262.2	240.2	218.5	206.0	197.2	173.8	154.6	138.0	114.8	95.0
1903-------	1930	*	268.9	267.5	224.5	224.7	204.7	194.1	170.7	157.7	127.5	111.5	93.8
1904-------	1931	*	269.6	241.8	228.7	222.7	196.7	190.1	173.3	146.3	128.4	112.2	93.9
1905-------	1932	*	256.9	262.4	233.0	219.5	202.6	192.6	166.0	148.7	129.5	112.7	106.2
1906-------	1933	*	264.7	266.7	228.9	224.0	206.6	187.0	168.7	150.2	130.3	126.4	105.5
1907-------	1934	*	*	264.0	233.8	227.8	199.0	189.8	165.9	150.6	140.6	124.5	112.8
1908-------	1935	*	*	264.5	241.6	215.1	193.7	183.6	168.9	160.9	141.7	128.0	104.7
1909-------	1936	*	*	269.6	227.0	214.7	192.3	187.8	181.0	162.2	145.3	123.5	103.2
1910-------	1937	*	*	261.7	242.4	215.7	204.7	206.5	191.0	165.1	143.5	124.5	103.3
1911-------	1938	*	*	264.2	230.8	211.9	215.6	213.1	182.7	162.7	136.4	116.9	100.0
1912-------	1939	*	*	257.4	224.0	222.2	219.5	200.0	179.5	153.8	131.2	116.9	100.0
1913-------	1940	*	*	*	241.4	231.9	208.9	194.3	167.5	145.6	133.0	114.0	100.8
1914-------	1941	*	*	*	250.0	233.6	205.1	189.7	164.0	153.5	130.8	115.6	101.3
1915-------	1942	*	*	*	243.5	220.6	197.5	179.2	170.2	149.3	126.2	117.9	100.0
1916-------	1943	*	*	*	234.8	211.7	185.9	185.0	159.6	142.9	132.4	116.4	102.0
1917-------	1944	*	*	*	225.0	208.6	191.1	179.2	164.0	147.1	132.4	124.5	105.7
1918-------	1945	*	*	*	222.2	211.7	187.1	185.0	164.9	151.2	140.9	119.7	108.0
1919-------	1946	*	*	*	228.8	210.1	197.5	183.9	165.8	156.4	135.4	125.0	106.1
1920-------	1947	*	*	*	230.8	219.0	198.7	186.4	167.5	154.5	136.9	118.8	107.1
1921-------	1948	*	*	*	230.8	208.6	196.3	183.8	171.4	154.5	137.3	119.1	104.7
1922-------	1949	*	*	*	228.8	212.8	195.1	189.5	172.1	154.8	132.6	122.4	104.9
1923-------	1950	*	*	*	225.0	212.3	202.3	185.0	171.1	152.9	135.7	118.8	99.7
1924-------	1951	*	*	*	240.0	222.2	207.7	193.4	169.4	155.6	132.7	119.9	95.0
1925-------	1952	*	*	264.2	235.3	214.3	198.0	183.8	166.7	147.3	132.1	108.5	89.1
1926-------	1953	*	*	263.2	238.1	221.0	195.3	177.4	163.7	148.4	122.0	103.1	84.9
1927-------	1954	*	*	254.0	233.1	212.1	188.8	174.1	161.2	134.7	113.6	96.4	72.5
1928-------	1955	*	*	261.2	229.4	211.5	192.8	174.8	149.5	127.8	111.1	82.9	65.2
1929-------	1956	*	279.3	258.5	236.6	210.5	192.6	165.0	145.3	123.0	93.0	74.2	55.7
1930-------	1957	*	277.3	257.9	231.5	206.5	182.1	160.6	134.2	104.1	81.3	64.4	49.0
1931-------	1958	*	268.7	252.8	222.2	198.5	172.0	150.1	116.3	91.8	69.1	55.3	45.2
1932-------	1959	285.7	265.3	237.1	209.0	185.6	158.7	126.3	101.7	79.8	62.9	52.1	42.4
1933-------	1960	294.6	267.5	234.1	203.9	172.8	137.0	111.1	89.1	70.4	60.7	50.1	36.2
1934-------	1961	283.3	245.5	219.2	182.2	146.5	116.8	97.4	79.2	68.6	56.7	44.1	32.3
1935-------	1962	274.2	238.4	203.6	160.4	126.6	105.6	87.2	77.3	66.0	51.8	38.9	29.1
1936-------	1963	251.9	214.7	174.1	136.4	114.1	94.8	85.7	72.6	61.2	44.2	33.5	
1937-------	1964	238.5	185.0	154.9	125.5	104.7	95.7	82.6	68.8	51.8	39.5		
1938-------	1965	201.6	163.6	137.1	114.5	110.7	93.5	79.7	59.4	47.8			
1939-------	1966	175.0	154.4	130.7	123.8	109.6	87.3	69.3	55.2				
1940-------	1967	163.5	146.2	136.4	122.2	97.6	78.9	65.6					
1941-------	1968	*	156.0	136.4	115.4	89.9	72.2						
1942-------	1969	*	*	135.1	100.0	82.2							
1943-------	1970	*	*	*	92.6								
1944-------	1971	*	*	*									
1945-------	1972	*	*										
1946-------	1973	*											

TABLE 10B. BIRTH PROBABILITIES FOR WHITE WOMEN FOR EACH YEAR 1917-73 BY AGE AND PARITY FOR EACH COHORT FROM 1868 TO 1958--CON.

(PROBABILITIES ARE THE NUMBER OF BIRTHS PER 1,000 WOMEN IN SPECIFIED PARITY AND EXACT AGE GROUP. FIGURES FOR "0 PARITY" SHOW THE PROBABILITY OF FIRST BIRTHS TO "C PARITY" WOMEN, THOSE FOR "1 PARITY" SHOW THE PROBABILITY OF SECOND BIRTHS TO "1 PARITY" WOMEN, ETC. BASED ON CENTRAL BIRTH RATES AND PARITY DISTRIBUTIONS)

PARITY AND COHORT	DIAGONAL LINE FOR JANUARY 1	EXACT AGE										
		39	40	41	42	43	44	45	46	47	48	49
6 PARITY--CON.												
1868												1.4
1869											1.4	1.4
1870										4.4	1.5	0.0
1871									8.8	4.4	1.5	1.5
1872								14.7	8.9	3.0	3.0	0.0
1873							25.3	14.9	7.5	4.5	1.5	0.0
1874						40.7	24.2	13.6	9.1	3.0	1.5	0.0
1875					53.2	41.2	23.0	15.4	7.7	3.1	1.5	0.0
1876				74.7	55.0	38.4	24.7	13.9	7.7	3.1	1.5	0.0
1877			96.0	74.6	51.9	39.9	23.1	13.9	7.7	3.1	1.5	0.0
1878	1917	133.7	97.1	71.4	53.3	39.8	23.0	13.9	7.7	3.1	1.5	0.0
1879	1918	133.4	94.9	73.5	52.2	38.5	23.3	12.4	7.8	3.1	1.6	0.0
1880	1919	134.4	97.0	73.7	51.8	37.9	22.2	12.7	6.4	3.2	1.6	0.0
1881	1920	137.5	98.9	73.1	50.6	37.6	23.0	11.6	6.6	3.3	1.7	0.0
1882	1921	139.7	96.1	72.8	52.5	37.5	20.5	12.0	6.9	3.4	1.7	0.0
1883	1922	132.5	94.8	72.5	50.3	34.8	19.2	10.5	5.3	3.5	1.8	0.0
1884	1923	128.2	93.6	69.4	47.1	31.5	19.3	10.5	5.3	3.5	1.8	0.0
1885	1924	127.6	89.2	66.5	43.9	31.7	17.7	10.6	5.3	1.8	1.8	0.0
1886	1925	119.5	84.2	63.3	42.3	30.0	17.7	10.7	5.3	1.8	1.8	0.0
1887	1926	117.0	85.3	60.5	41.1	28.7	16.1	9.0	5.4	1.8	1.8	0.0
1888	1927	112.5	76.8	55.4	37.5	26.7	16.1	8.9	5.4	1.8	1.8	0.0
1889	1928	109.1	73.9	55.5	38.7	27.7	14.8	9.2	5.6	1.9	1.9	0.0
1890	1929	102.5	75.9	54.9	38.0	26.6	17.1	9.5	3.8	1.9	0.0	0.0
1891	1930	104.5	72.7	55.0	37.3	27.6	15.8	7.9	4.0	2.0	2.0	0.0
1892	1931	96.8	72.3	52.1	36.1	26.1	16.1	8.0	4.0	2.0	0.0	0.0
1893	1932	97.9	68.5	51.8	35.2	24.9	14.6	8.3	4.2	2.1	0.0	0.0
1894	1933	93.9	69.6	49.9	34.7	21.7	15.2	8.7	4.4	2.2	0.0	0.0
1895	1934	94.6	67.3	47.1	31.3	24.6	13.4	6.7	4.5	2.2	0.0	0.0
1896	1935	90.7	62.5	46.2	32.3	23.0	11.5	6.9	4.6	2.3	0.0	0.0
1897	1936	83.5	61.8	47.4	30.8	21.3	11.8	7.1	4.7	2.4	0.0	0.0
1898	1937	83.5	61.3	43.9	29.1	19.4	14.5	7.3	4.8	2.4	0.0	0.0
1899	1938	83.1	57.6	42.4	29.9	22.4	14.9	7.5	5.0	2.5	0.0	0.0
1900	1939	78.9	57.4	41.6	28.5	23.3	15.5	7.8	5.2	2.6	0.0	0.0
1901	1940	78.0	55.2	41.2	32.9	24.6	13.7	8.2	2.7	2.7	0.0	0.0
1902	1941	76.2	58.1	46.2	34.5	25.8	14.3	5.7	2.9	0.0	0.0	0.0
1903	1942	77.2	64.0	48.5	39.2	24.1	12.0	6.0	3.0	0.0	0.0	0.0
1904	1943	85.7	62.9	53.0	34.1	24.7	12.3	6.2	3.1	0.0	0.0	0.0
1905	1944	87.8	70.0	49.5	36.1	22.9	13.0	6.5	3.3	0.0	0.0	0.0
1906	1945	92.2	66.2	51.5	34.1	20.3	13.5	6.8	3.4	0.0	0.0	0.0
1907	1946	88.6	65.2	50.0	31.9	21.2	14.0	7.0	3.5	0.0	0.0	0.0
1908	1947	86.8	63.0	44.0	32.6	21.6	14.3	7.2	3.6	0.0	0.0	0.0
1909	1948	81.1	60.6	48.5	33.3	22.1	14.6	7.3	3.6	0.0	0.0	0.0
1910	1949	84.7	67.2	46.9	38.5	23.0	15.2	7.6	3.8	0.0	0.0	0.0
1911	1950	85.0	67.5	50.8	34.7	26.7	15.2	7.6	3.8	0.0	0.0	0.0
1912	1951	85.0	63.2	50.2	38.0	22.6	14.9	7.4	3.7	0.0	0.0	0.0
1913	1952	81.3	62.7	49.8	33.7	25.8	14.7	7.3	3.6	0.0	0.0	0.0
1914	1953	85.0	66.7	53.2	37.3	25.8	14.7	7.3	3.6	0.0	0.0	0.0
1915	1954	87.3	68.7	55.8	36.6	25.3	14.3	7.1	3.5	0.0	0.0	0.0
1916	1955	89.5	67.4	54.7	39.3	24.7	14.0	10.4	3.5	0.0	0.0	0.0
1917	1956	92.7	70.6	54.0	38.7	24.3	17.2	6.8	3.4	0.0	0.0	0.0
1918	1957	91.3	73.0	56.7	38.3	24.1	13.7	6.8	3.4	0.0	0.0	0.0
1919	1958	93.2	72.4	53.7	39.5	26.1	12.9	6.5	3.2	0.0	0.0	0.0
1920	1959	88.4	68.6	54.0	34.4	21.6	12.3	6.1	3.0	0.0	0.0	0.0
1921	1960	86.8	68.3	48.5	32.8	23.6	11.7	5.8	2.9	0.0	0.0	0.0
1922	1961	87.8	63.6	47.3	32.0	20.1	11.5	5.7	2.9	0.0	0.0	0.0
1923	1962	79.9	60.2	44.7	27.5	16.4	10.9	5.4	2.7	0.0	0.0	0.0
1924	1963	76.9	58.0	37.8	26.6	15.9	10.6	2.6	2.6	0.0	0.0	0.0
1925	1964	69.5	49.4	33.1	22.6	15.0	7.5	2.5	2.5	0.0	0.0	
1926	1965	61.5	44.9	29.5	19.5	12.1	4.8	2.4	0.0	0.0		
1927	1966	55.7	38.0	25.8	16.3	9.3	4.6	2.3	0.0			
1928	1967	49.5	34.8	22.9	15.9	9.1	4.5	2.3				
1929	1968	40.6	28.8	21.9	13.1	6.5	4.3					
1930	1969	37.1	28.0	17.1	10.6	6.3						
1931	1970	35.9	23.0	16.5	8.2							
1932	1971	29.2	20.5	12.2								
1933	1972	27.3	16.6									
1934	1973	21.2										

TABLE 10B. BIRTH PROBABILITIES FOR WHITE WOMEN FOR EACH YEAR 1917-73 BY AGE AND PARITY FOR EACH COHORT FROM 1868 TO 1958--CON.

(PROBABILITIES ARE THE NUMBER OF BIRTHS PER 1,000 WOMEN IN SPECIFIED PARITY AND EXACT AGE GROUP. FIGURES FOR "0 PARITY" SHOW THE PROBABILITY OF FIRST BIRTHS TO "0 PARITY" WOMEN, THOSE FOR "1 PARITY" SHOW THE PROBABILITY OF SECOND BIRTHS TO "1 PARITY" WOMEN, ETC. BASED ON CENTRAL BIRTH RATES AND PARITY DISTRIBUTIONS)

PARITY AND COHORT	DIAGONAL LINE FOR JANUARY 1	EXACT AGE											
		15	16	17	18	19	20	21	22	23	24	25	26
7 AND HIGHER PARITY													
1891-------													*
1892-------												*	*
1893-------											*	*	*
1894-------										*	*	*	*
1895-------									*	*	*	*	*
1896-------								*	*	*	*	*	*
1897-------							*	*	*	*	*	*	*
1898-------						*	*	*	*	*	*	*	*
1899-------					*	*	*	*	*	*	*	*	*
1900-------				*	*	*	*	*	*	*	*	*	*
1901-------			*	*	*	*	*	*	*	*	*	*	*
1902-------	1917	*	*	*	*	*	*	*	*	*	*	*	*
1903-------	1918	*	*	*	*	*	*	*	*	*	*	*	*
1904-------	1919	*	*	*	*	*	*	*	*	*	*	*	*
1905-------	1920	*	*	*	*	*	*	*	*	*	*	*	*
1906-------	1921	*	*	*	*	*	*	*	*	*	*	*	*
1907-------	1922	*	*	*	*	*	*	*	*	*	*	*	*
1908-------	1923	*	*	*	*	*	*	*	*	*	*	*	*
1909-------	1924	*	*	*	*	*	*	*	*	*	*	*	*
1910-------	1925	*	*	*	*	*	*	*	*	*	*	*	*
1911-------	1926	*	*	*	*	*	*	*	*	*	*	*	*
1912-------	1927	*	*	*	*	*	*	*	*	*	*	*	*
1913-------	1928	*	*	*	*	*	*	*	*	*	*	*	*
1914-------	1929	*	*	*	*	*	*	*	*	*	*	*	*
1915-------	1930	*	*	*	*	*	*	*	*	*	*	*	*
1916-------	1931	*	*	*	*	*	*	*	*	*	*	*	*
1917-------	1932	*	*	*	*	*	*	*	*	*	*	*	*
1918-------	1933	*	*	*	*	*	*	*	*	*	*	*	*
1919-------	1934	*	*	*	*	*	*	*	*	*	*	*	*
1920-------	1935	*	*	*	*	*	*	*	*	*	*	*	*
1921-------	1936	*	*	*	*	*	*	*	*	*	*	*	*
1922-------	1937	*	*	*	*	*	*	*	*	*	*	*	*
1923-------	1938	*	*	*	*	*	*	*	*	*	*	*	*
1924-------	1939	*	*	*	*	*	*	*	*	*	*	*	*
1925-------	1940	*	*	*	*	*	*	*	*	*	*	*	*
1926-------	1941	*	*	*	*	*	*	*	*	*	*	*	*
1927-------	1942	*	*	*	*	*	*	*	*	*	*	*	*
1928-------	1943	*	*	*	*	*	*	*	*	*	*	*	*
1929-------	1944	*	*	*	*	*	*	*	*	*	*	*	*
1930-------	1945	*	*	*	*	*	*	*	*	*	*	*	*
1931-------	1946	*	*	*	*	*	*	*	*	*	*	*	*
1932-------	1947	*	*	*	*	*	*	*	*	*	*	*	*
1933-------	1948	*	*	*	*	*	*	*	*	*	*	*	*
1934-------	1949	*	*	*	*	*	*	*	*	*	*	*	*
1935-------	1950	*	*	*	*	*	*	*	*	*	*	*	*
1936-------	1951	*	*	*	*	*	*	*	*	*	*	*	*
1937-------	1952	*	*	*	*	*	*	*	*	*	*	*	*
1938-------	1953	*	*	*	*	*	*	*	*	*	*	*	*
1939-------	1954	*	*	*	*	*	*	*	*	*	*	*	*
1940-------	1955	*	*	*	*	*	*	*	*	*	*	*	*
1941-------	1956	*	*	*	*	*	*	*	*	*	*	*	*
1942-------	1957	*	*	*	*	*	*	*	*	*	*	*	*
1943-------	1958	*	*	*	*	*	*	*	*	*	*	*	*
1944-------	1959	*	*	*	*	*	*	*	*	*	*	*	*
1945-------	1960	*	*	*	*	*	*	*	*	*	*	*	*
1946-------	1961	*	*	*	*	*	*	*	*	*	*	*	*
1947-------	1962	*	*	*	*	*	*	*	*	*	*	*	*
1948-------	1963	*	*	*	*	*	*	*	*	*	*	*	
1949-------	1964	*	*	*	*	*	*	*	*	*	*		
1950-------	1965	*	*	*	*	*	*	*	*	*			
1951-------	1966	*	*	*	*	*	*	*	*				
1952-------	1967	*	*	*	*	*	*	*					
1953-------	1968	*	*	*	*	*	*						
1954-------	1969	*	*	*	*	*							
1955-------	1970	*	*	*	*								
1956-------	1971	*	*	*									
1957-------	1972	*	*										
1958-------	1973	*											

TABLE 10B. BIRTH PROBABILITIES FOR WHITE WOMEN FOR EACH YEAR 1917-73 BY AGE AND PARITY FOR EACH COHORT FROM 1868 TO 1958--CON.

(PROBABILITIES ARE THE NUMBER OF BIRTHS PER 1,000 WOMEN IN SPECIFIED PARITY AND EXACT AGE GROUP. FIGURES FOR "0 PARITY" SHOW THE PROBABILITY OF FIRST BIRTHS TO "C PARITY" WOMEN, THOSE FOR "1 PARITY" SHOW THE PROBABILITY OF SECOND BIRTHS TO "1 PARITY" WOMEN, ETC. BASED ON CENTRAL BIRTH RATES AND PARITY DISTRIBUTIONS)

PARITY AND COHORT	DIAGONAL LINE FOR JANUARY 1	EXACT AGE											
		27	28	29	30	31	32	33	34	35	36	37	38
7 AND HIGHER PARITY--CON.													
1879-------													222.1
1880-------												243.4	222.6
1881-------											247.0	245.1	226.6
1882-------										259.7	249.7	250.2	231.0
1883-------									262.2	265.2	254.0	255.2	242.1
1884-------								267.1	270.3	267.8	260.1	266.9	229.2
1885-------							268.2	280.4	272.5	274.8	272.1	254.2	235.6
1886-------						285.7	282.9	282.1	281.0	292.2	260.3	263.1	240.9
1887-------					293.0	301.0	283.6	289.9	302.3	278.0	269.1	267.3	236.0
1888-------				358.2	304.3	303.4	294.6	317.7	285.7	289.7	273.6	261.1	230.3
1889-------			*	345.9	295.6	312.1	317.5	294.8	298.5	291.0	267.7	256.1	233.8
1890-------	1917	*	*	343.8	312.8	337.0	296.5	313.4	299.8	284.0	258.3	259.5	220.4
1891-------	1918	*	*	362.9	336.8	313.7	313.0	310.0	294.3	275.2	265.8	242.0	210.0
1892-------	1919	*	*	388.4	310.5	329.5	308.8	305.8	281.5	278.8	244.2	230.3	208.9
1893-------	1920	*	*	361.3	327.9	328.1	306.1	295.6	287.1	260.5	235.4	229.0	203.8
1894-------	1921	*	*	378.2	320.7	312.5	293.8	293.8	269.0	250.0	235.1	223.7	201.2
1895-------	1922	*	*	371.9	309.8	305.6	293.9	278.5	258.6	253.5	229.1	223.3	192.8
1896-------	1923	*	*	363.6	300.0	307.7	278.6	268.8	261.6	242.7	226.9	208.8	197.3
1897-------	1924	*	*	347.5	312.5	297.1	271.8	272.5	251.1	245.2	217.8	215.0	197.1
1898-------	1925	*	*	353.4	296.5	284.5	273.6	264.5	250.6	231.9	222.2	217.9	191.0
1899-------	1926	*	*	339.1	285.7	287.0	264.8	271.4	239.8	239.6	229.2	213.4	193.1
1900-------	1927	*	*	330.3	293.0	283.0	276.8	254.5	251.9	252.7	224.4	216.9	194.4
1901-------	1928	*	*	323.5	290.5	291.5	256.8	270.7	264.0	244.8	230.5	218.0	184.7
1902-------	1929	*	*	*	285.7	269.8	269.7	273.6	255.0	246.3	228.6	208.0	187.7
1903-------	1930	*	*	*	266.7	284.9	273.9	269.5	253.7	247.4	215.8	208.5	184.2
1904-------	1931	*	*	*	283.5	294.1	274.0	273.4	258.7	235.6	218.7	206.7	185.8
1905-------	1932	*	*	*	300.8	286.6	277.5	274.5	245.0	240.6	215.6	204.3	196.5
1906-------	1933	*	*	*	289.5	302.6	282.1	267.8	258.9	238.4	216.1	217.7	202.8
1907-------	1934	*	*	*	300.0	294.5	267.4	277.5	253.7	232.0	228.1	222.8	200.5
1908-------	1935	*	*	*	310.0	286.8	289.0	281.0	254.0	252.6	236.0	224.7	198.5
1909-------	1936	*	*	*	280.0	295.5	275.4	267.3	263.6	252.7	233.2	216.1	191.0
1910-------	1937	*	*	*	*	281.3	267.1	280.6	265.0	250.0	228.0	209.4	184.8
1911-------	1938	*	*	*	*	281.0	287.6	285.7	267.5	246.2	224.8	207.3	194.4
1912-------	1939	*	*	*	*	307.0	301.4	291.2	261.5	245.1	217.5	216.6	190.6
1913-------	1940	*	*	*	*	312.5	298.6	276.8	260.7	234.6	227.1	208.6	189.0
1914-------	1941	*	*	*	*	300.0	281.7	275.9	251.2	247.9	223.0	208.8	192.0
1915-------	1942	*	*	*	*	297.3	276.6	267.4	261.1	238.3	222.6	212.3	181.8
1916-------	1943	*	*	*	*	281.8	266.2	279.8	255.0	239.1	223.9	201.4	181.0
1917-------	1944	*	*	*	*	287.0	284.7	269.5	252.5	235.8	216.2	201.4	183.0
1918-------	1945	*	*	*	*	308.4	279.4	272.7	248.7	232.5	212.4	196.6	179.2
1919-------	1946	*	*	*	*	290.9	273.4	270.6	247.5	230.8	209.7	198.0	182.4
1920-------	1947	*	*	*	*	288.3	276.6	267.4	248.8	226.9	209.6	200.0	172.6
1921-------	1948	*	*	*	*	292.0	274.6	270.1	250.0	229.5	210.7	190.5	175.3
1922-------	1949	*	*	*	*	285.7	281.7	264.4	247.6	234.8	204.2	194.4	169.5
1923-------	1950	*	*	*	*	300.9	277.8	268.2	250.0	227.5	210.9	192.8	168.5
1924-------	1951	*	*	*	*	290.6	278.1	269.8	243.5	225.1	207.7	187.5	161.5
1925-------	1952	*	*	*	*	300.8	283.0	261.3	247.9	227.3	206.7	180.6	156.9
1926-------	1953	*	*	*	*	295.5	267.4	261.7	240.3	223.7	194.3	173.9	149.5
1927-------	1954	*	*	*	313.7	300.0	280.2	261.1	245.4	214.3	188.0	164.2	132.6
1928-------	1955	*	*	*	321.4	298.0	276.9	259.3	232.1	205.3	178.8	149.5	115.0
1929-------	1956	*	*	*	312.0	289.9	271.9	249.1	218.8	186.5	158.7	123.6	99.2
1930-------	1957	*	*	*	304.3	281.1	258.5	235.3	201.8	168.8	131.9	109.4	87.0
1931-------	1958	*	*	321.1	298.7	269.6	240.3	214.7	175.3	141.5	118.3	96.2	81.5
1932-------	1959	*	*	316.2	282.2	257.0	227.6	186.9	154.9	127.1	106.1	91.3	74.7
1933-------	1960	*	*	301.6	264.4	234.5	190.6	163.1	136.2	114.1	99.3	84.8	68.3
1934-------	1961	*	*	290.1	245.8	201.8	171.5	142.9	122.2	112.0	94.4	79.9	61.1
1935-------	1962	*	*	264.7	209.9	178.6	152.1	130.4	120.8	108.0	90.2	68.3	53.9
1936-------	1963	*	*	229.0	188.2	160.2	141.7	132.8	119.6	103.7	79.5	64.9	
1937-------	1964	*	*	193.5	172.0	154.3	142.9	130.1	113.6	87.5	69.6		
1938-------	1965	*	*	189.2	166.7	152.4	135.4	123.9	95.0	80.5			
1939-------	1966	*	*	*	166.7	151.7	129.4	104.2	90.0				
1940-------	1967	*	*	*	173.1	142.9	116.4	97.6					
1941-------	1968	*	*	*	*	132.1	114.8						
1942-------	1969	*	*	*	*	*							
1943-------	1970	*	*	*	*								
1944-------	1971	*	*	*									
1945-------	1972	*	*										
1946-------	1973	*											

TABLE 10B. BIRTH PROBABILITIES FOR WHITE WOMEN FOR EACH YEAR 1917-73 BY AGE AND PARITY FOR EACH COHORT FROM 1868 TO 1958--CON.

(PROBABILITIES ARE THE NUMBER OF BIRTHS PER 1,000 WOMEN IN SPECIFIED PARITY AND EXACT AGE GROUP. FIGURES FOR "0 PARITY" SHOW THE PROBABILITY OF FIRST BIRTHS TO "C PARITY" WOMEN, THOSE FOR "1 PARITY" SHOW THE PROBABILITY OF SECOND BIRTHS TO "1 PARITY" WOMEN, ETC. BASED ON CENTRAL BIPTH RATES AND PARITY DISTRIBUTIONS)

PARITY AND COHORT	DIAGONAL LINE FOR JANUARY 1	EXACT AGE										
		39	40	41	42	43	44	45	46	47	48	49
7 AND HIGHER PARITY--CON.												
1868----------------												2.3
1869----------------											5.6	2.3
1870----------------										10.9	5.7	2.4
1871----------------									20.4	11.1	5.3	2.4
1872----------------								34.0	20.9	10.9	5.9	2.5
1873----------------							53.1	34.2	20.3	11.7	6.1	2.5
1874----------------						76.7	52.5	33.8	21.8	11.9	5.7	2.6
1875----------------					95.2	76.5	52.7	35.2	22.3	11.1	5.3	2.6
1876----------------				128.0	95.6	77.3	55.1	36.9	20.8	10.4	5.5	2.2
1877----------------			157.0	129.9	97.4	81.4	58.3	35.5	19.9	10.8	5.1	1.7
1878----------------	1917	205.6	158.4	131.3	101.3	84.2	55.3	34.4	20.9	10.4	4.6	2.3
1879----------------	1918	206.5	159.2	135.0	104.3	80.2	55.1	35.6	20.7	9.4	4.7	1.8
1880----------------	1919	208.4	162.9	138.8	98.6	80.5	56.7	35.1	19.9	9.6	4.2	1.8
1881----------------	1920	212.8	168.8	131.8	99.4	83.4	55.8	33.6	19.2	9.3	4.3	1.8
1882----------------	1921	222.1	160.5	133.5	103.4	82.2	53.2	32.8	18.6	8.9	3.8	1.9
1883----------------	1922	210.4	162.7	138.5	103.3	79.5	53.6	31.9	17.9	8.6	4.6	2.0
1884----------------	1923	215.1	167.7	135.3	99.3	79.9	50.5	30.2	17.1	8.9	4.1	2.0
1885----------------	1924	220.3	164.2	131.3	101.8	76.0	47.9	29.8	17.0	8.5	4.2	2.1
1886----------------	1925	213.8	158.0	132.4	96.0	71.1	48.0	29.3	16.1	8.0	4.4	1.5
1887----------------	1926	208.0	161.4	127.8	90.0	72.3	47.1	27.9	15.8	8.2	3.7	1.5
1888----------------	1927	209.2	154.4	120.4	92.1	69.7	45.9	27.5	15.7	7.8	3.9	1.6
1889----------------	1928	200.8	147.3	120.7	89.1	69.4	44.9	28.4	15.3	7.2	4.0	1.6
1890----------------	1929	191.0	147.0	117.5	88.3	67.0	45.8	27.0	14.3	7.5	4.2	1.7
1891----------------	1930	189.7	143.4	114.3	85.1	68.6	44.9	26.2	13.9	7.0	3.5	0.9
1892----------------	1931	183.8	138.5	110.2	88.5	67.4	42.5	24.8	14.6	6.4	2.7	0.9
1893----------------	1932	181.2	135.0	115.0	85.1	63.0	39.9	25.1	13.5	5.8	2.9	1.0
1894----------------	1933	172.3	139.7	111.3	80.5	60.6	40.7	23.2	12.1	6.0	2.0	1.0
1895----------------	1934	176.2	136.4	106.1	79.7	61.3	38.3	23.2	12.6	5.3	2.1	1.0
1896----------------	1935	176.2	130.2	104.8	79.4	57.8	37.0	21.2	12.2	5.5	2.2	1.1
1897----------------	1936	170.3	131.6	107.4	76.7	57.6	35.6	23.6	11.8	5.9	2.3	1.2
1898----------------	1937	168.6	133.8	102.0	77.9	55.3	39.9	24.7	12.3	6.1	2.5	1.2
1899----------------	1938	171.6	125.9	101.6	75.5	57.4	38.7	23.0	12.7	6.4	2.5	1.3
1900----------------	1939	162.8	126.3	101.0	75.1	60.3	40.6	24.2	12.0	6.7	2.7	1.3
1901----------------	1940	162.8	125.8	99.1	80.5	63.0	41.9	23.0	12.9	5.7	2.8	1.4
1902----------------	1941	161.4	127.5	107.1	87.0	65.2	39.8	24.3	12.1	6.1	3.0	1.5
1903----------------	1942	164.5	135.7	113.6	88.8	62.3	42.1	22.5	12.8	4.8	1.6	1.6
1904----------------	1943	173.2	138.3	113.5	83.9	65.2	38.9	21.8	11.7	5.0	1.7	1.7
1905----------------	1944	175.6	139.2	109.2	84.2	59.2	37.2	21.1	10.5	5.3	1.8	1.8
1906----------------	1945	176.9	138.4	111.3	79.2	58.7	35.6	22.3	11.1	5.5	1.8	1.8
1907----------------	1946	173.1	136.1	104.0	80.8	57.5	39.2	21.4	9.7	5.8	1.9	0.0
1908----------------	1947	171.1	130.1	107.7	79.2	58.8	37.3	20.6	10.2	4.1	2.0	2.0
1909----------------	1948	166.3	134.4	104.5	79.5	60.6	34.2	21.2	10.5	6.3	2.1	0.0
1910----------------	1949	170.5	130.4	104.4	76.7	55.2	37.0	19.4	10.8	4.3	2.1	2.1
1911----------------	1950	166.2	130.0	100.7	76.7	59.2	35.9	22.2	11.1	4.4	2.2	2.2
1912----------------	1951	164.4	126.9	102.0	79.5	56.5	37.1	20.7	11.4	4.6	2.3	2.3
1913----------------	1952	167.6	129.0	105.7	77.3	58.5	36.0	21.4	9.5	4.7	2.4	0.0
1914----------------	1953	158.5	127.7	101.3	77.7	56.2	36.1	19.0	9.5	4.7	2.4	0.0
1915----------------	1954	157.4	126.0	101.8	77.9	53.9	33.7	19.1	9.5	4.7	2.4	0.0
1916----------------	1955	158.8	126.7	99.7	75.8	54.1	33.8	19.1	9.5	4.7	2.4	0.0
1917----------------	1956	157.4	125.3	95.9	74.8	53.4	33.4	18.9	9.4	4.7	0.0	0.0
1918----------------	1957	159.4	119.2	97.7	74.1	52.9	33.1	16.4	7.0	2.3	2.3	0.0
1919----------------	1958	148.5	125.3	96.5	71.4	50.9	31.8	15.8	9.0	4.5	0.0	0.0
1920----------------	1959	155.7	119.9	94.4	69.8	49.9	29.0	15.5	6.6	2.2	0.0	0.0
1921----------------	1960	147.8	118.2	93.5	67.6	46.2	25.9	15.0	6.4	2.1	0.0	0.0
1922----------------	1961	145.1	115.9	89.7	64.3	41.1	25.6	12.7	6.3	2.1	0.0	0.0
1923----------------	1962	142.5	112.4	84.8	58.2	38.0	22.9	10.3	4.1	2.1	0.0	0.0
1924----------------	1963	137.4	106.9	76.6	51.7	34.4	20.0	9.9	4.0	2.0	0.0	0.0
1925----------------	1964	129.5	94.4	68.0	46.2	29.6	17.5	7.8	3.9	1.9	0.0	
1926----------------	1965	117.4	84.7	57.8	40.9	26.8	15.2	7.6	3.8	1.9		
1927----------------	1966	101.3	72.4	52.6	36.3	22.6	13.1	7.4	3.7			
1928----------------	1967	86.1	64.8	47.7	33.7	20.3	11.0	5.5				
1929----------------	1968	76.8	58.9	44.5	29.1	18.0	10.8					
1930----------------	1969	69.8	54.4	36.6	25.3	16.1						
1931----------------	1970	64.9	46.2	32.6	23.2							
1932----------------	1971	58.3	41.6	29.7								
1933----------------	1972	50.0	37.0									
1934----------------	1973	46.5										

TABLE 10C. BIRTH PROBABILITIES FOR ALL OTHER WOMEN FOR EACH YEAR 1917-73 BY AGE AND PARITY FOR EACH COHORT FROM 1868 TO 1958

(PROBABILITIES ARE THE NUMBER OF BIRTHS PER 1,000 WOMEN IN SPECIFIED PARITY AND EXACT AGE GROUP. FIGURES FOR "0 PARITY" SHOW THE PROBABILITY OF FIRST BIRTHS TO "C PARITY" WOMEN, THOSE FOR "1 PARITY" SHOW THE PROBABILITY OF SECOND BIRTHS TO "1 PARITY" WOMEN, ETC. BASED ON CENTRAL BIRTH RATES AND PARITY DISTRIBUTIONS)

PARITY AND COHORT	DIAGONAL LINE FOR JANUARY 1	EXACT AGE 15	16	17	18	19	20	21	22	23	24	25	26
0 PARITY													
1891-------													63.2
1892-------												78.0	68.3
1893-------											90.6	82.5	63.2
1894-------										105.2	94.5	76.1	77.5
1895-------									115.2	108.6	87.6	92.3	71.5
1896-------								133.3	118.8	101.0	105.5	86.7	62.5
1897-------							140.9	137.6	110.6	121.0	100.7	76.4	58.5
1898-------						141.5	139.4	124.9	128.5	112.7	85.5	69.9	57.0
1899-------					120.8	141.3	130.6	149.3	124.1	100.1	82.5	73.4	61.6
1900-------				94.2	118.4	132.5	154.9	143.9	109.9	96.9	88.5	75.9	57.9
1901-------			58.1	91.1	110.1	155.3	152.9	126.7	105.2	104.9	89.3	69.0	51.9
1902-------	1917	32.8	56.7	85.5	129.9	157.7	136.3	122.4	114.8	104.0	81.2	60.2	43.3
1903-------	1918	31.4	52.7	100.2	133.6	139.8	135.7	132.4	115.0	95.3	71.8	52.0	40.5
1904-------	1919	29.2	61.7	102.3	118.0	142.5	145.0	130.7	110.8	86.2	63.1	49.5	42.0
1905-------	1920	34.0	62.7	89.8	123.6	151.9	143.5	126.1	97.0	77.4	60.4	50.4	38.9
1906-------	1921	34.9	55.0	94.5	131.5	151.2	138.0	114.9	88.3	73.2	62.0	46.8	38.7
1907-------	1922	30.9	58.2	100.9	133.9	144.6	126.9	105.4	84.8	74.6	56.5	46.5	33.6
1908-------	1923	33.0	62.4	104.7	128.7	135.6	115.6	101.5	85.9	70.5	57.4	41.1	35.3
1909-------	1924	35.5	66.5	103.2	121.9	127.1	113.9	103.8	84.1	72.3	52.2	45.3	34.6
1910-------	1925	37.9	66.4	98.3	114.7	123.2	115.9	100.0	84.4	64.9	56.4	42.4	33.0
1911-------	1926	39.5	65.2	94.8	111.5	127.2	112.7	101.5	76.8	69.6	54.6	41.6	33.5
1912-------	1927	38.2	61.5	90.1	114.1	120.9	112.7	90.8	80.6	66.9	51.7	41.2	34.4
1913-------	1928	36.2	58.6	92.8	110.4	121.9	103.8	96.6	80.2	64.5	52.0	41.9	35.5
1914-------	1929	34.2	60.1	88.9	110.8	112.3	110.2	95.2	75.7	65.2	51.6	42.7	35.7
1915-------	1930	35.1	58.3	89.8	103.2	119.9	108.8	90.7	77.7	63.4	52.2	42.4	37.9
1916-------	1931	33.5	59.4	83.3	109.7	119.5	102.2	93.6	75.8	63.0	51.1	44.6	39.6
1917-------	1932	34.3	55.2	88.4	110.9	113.7	106.9	92.3	75.6	62.2	54.2	50.3	42.2
1918-------	1933	32.3	57.7	91.9	106.3	119.5	107.9	90.7	74.3	64.7	62.9	52.0	42.7
1919-------	1934	33.3	61.7	91.0	115.1	124.3	108.5	93.4	79.9	78.1	64.8	52.5	43.9
1920-------	1935	36.8	61.7	98.1	119.6	123.9	108.7	97.9	88.1	77.9	63.0	52.4	57.2
1921-------	1936	37.0	66.8	101.5	118.1	121.2	113.1	99.6	86.4	73.4	61.5	66.5	72.3
1922-------	1937	38.7	67.7	97.2	110.4	121.1	110.9	95.6	79.2	67.2	74.1	80.8	67.1
1923-------	1938	39.7	64.7	92.3	112.5	121.9	109.1	89.8	75.3	83.6	94.0	76.3	65.4
1924-------	1939	38.7	63.1	95.5	117.4	122.5	102.0	87.6	95.6	110.9	92.2	77.6	66.3
1925-------	1940	39.2	66.8	99.6	119.0	113.4	100.8	107.4	127.2	108.9	92.2	78.8	72.0
1926-------	1941	41.5	69.2	100.7	108.0	109.6	117.5	140.2	123.1	106.0	91.3	81.5	75.2
1927-------	1942	42.1	69.7	91.1	104.5	120.9	149.4	135.2	117.2	101.8	90.1	81.2	74.7
1928-------	1943	42.5	63.0	88.2	109.8	150.3	145.3	127.9	110.0	98.0	87.8	79.9	74.4
1929-------	1944	38.8	62.5	90.0	137.2	150.9	139.8	121.5	109.3	98.5	91.1	85.5	73.3
1930-------	1945	38.7	61.3	109.8	139.3	143.9	131.3	120.5	108.7	100.7	94.9	83.4	74.8
1931-------	1946	38.0	75.1	115.0	134.8	138.5	134.0	121.7	114.9	111.3	98.8	89.4	75.2
1932-------	1947	45.0	79.5	112.3	131.9	142.7	133.6	129.7	125.6	116.0	105.7	93.0	77.0
1933-------	1948	49.0	80.0	112.8	137.6	141.2	144.7	143.9	136.5	128.9	115.7	95.9	84.3
1934-------	1949	50.3	81.4	116.5	135.1	149.9	157.7	152.7	148.7	138.1	118.2	104.7	91.2
1935-------	1950	51.1	83.9	114.7	140.0	161.5	163.5	164.2	155.9	140.0	125.0	110.8	97.6
1936-------	1951	52.6	82.0	116.7	147.3	160.8	170.9	167.3	153.2	139.2	125.1	111.7	97.1
1937-------	1952	50.5	82.7	119.9	144.9	167.0	172.7	160.7	150.6	138.1	120.8	106.3	95.4
1938-------	1953	50.2	84.1	116.3	147.2	164.9	163.2	155.6	145.9	130.3	111.7	103.0	87.5
1939-------	1954	52.6	82.5	119.4	146.7	158.2	161.6	155.0	144.6	125.5	115.1	99.1	91.5
1940-------	1955	50.3	83.4	119.2	141.3	156.2	159.7	154.9	141.5	127.6	114.1	101.4	92.8
1941-------	1956	51.5	84.4	112.4	139.1	152.3	157.3	152.0	139.7	126.6	112.8	101.9	93.1
1942-------	1957	52.3	78.6	111.6	134.4	148.9	155.4	150.5	141.7	125.9	114.7	101.8	100.0
1943-------	1958	47.9	78.8	107.1	131.0	145.6	153.7	150.4	139.5	125.7	112.3	108.9	101.2
1944-------	1959	49.0	75.5	105.8	128.0	146.2	156.6	151.1	142.0	126.8	118.8	111.6	111.9
1945-------	1960	47.0	75.1	102.2	128.5	149.8	156.3	154.3	142.5	131.7	122.2	123.1	110.9
1946-------	1961	46.7	72.7	102.8	132.2	148.7	161.8	156.2	148.7	139.6	137.0	124.8	116.8
1947-------	1962	44.6	72.6	104.5	131.0	154.4	163.7	162.8	156.2	150.1	138.2	130.4	122.0
1948-------	1963	44.4	72.6	104.1	134.6	155.7	168.7	168.6	162.9	147.8	137.7	127.8	
1949-------	1964	44.4	73.8	106.2	135.8	159.8	172.3	170.6	156.3	138.9	127.8		
1950-------	1965	45.2	74.4	107.5	139.2	164.1	176.9	163.4	143.0	128.5			
1951-------	1966	45.6	76.4	110.4	143.1	168.8	170.7	150.7	132.3				
1952-------	1967	47.4	77.7	112.8	148.4	164.1	158.6	139.3					
1953-------	1968	48.3	78.8	117.7	145.3	157.2	148.0						
1954-------	1969	48.9	83.4	116.7	143.0	147.6							
1955-------	1970	52.4	83.3	118.6	136.4								
1956-------	1971	52.2	85.5	113.2									
1957-------	1972	53.7	82.9										
1958-------	1973	52.8											

TABLE 10C. BIRTH PROBABILITIES FOR ALL OTHER WOMEN FOR EACH YEAR 1917-73 BY AGE AND PARITY FOR EACH COHORT FROM 1868 TO 1958--CON.

(PROBABILITIES ARE THE NUMBER OF BIRTHS PER 1,000 WOMEN IN SPECIFIED PARITY AND EXACT AGE GROUP. FIGURES FOR "0 PARITY" SHOW THE PROBABILITY OF FIRST BIRTHS TO "C PARITY" WOMEN, THOSE FOR "1 PARITY" SHOW THE PROBABILITY OF SECOND BIRTHS TO "1 PARITY" WOMEN, ETC. BASED ON CENTRAL BIRTH RATES AND PARITY DISTRIBUTIONS)

PARITY AND COHORT	DIAGONAL LINE FOR JANUARY 1	EXACT AGE											
		27	28	29	30	31	32	33	34	35	36	37	38
0 PARITY--CON.													
1879-------													10.8
1880-------												13.6	13.7
1881-------											15.7	17.3	12.3
1882-------										18.6	19.8	15.1	14.0
1883-------									19.2	21.6	17.1	16.6	13.0
1884-------								19.6	21.2	18.5	18.0	15.4	11.4
1885-------							20.5	21.3	18.2	19.8	16.5	13.5	9.1
1886-------						27.6	22.4	18.7	19.9	18.3	15.0	11.1	9.6
1887-------					33.4	30.9	20.1	20.9	18.6	16.5	12.7	11.6	9.2
1888-------				43.4	36.2	28.0	22.3	19.4	17.0	14.5	13.0	11.6	8.8
1889-------			46.9	46.8	33.1	31.6	20.9	17.9	15.4	14.8	15.1	10.3	9.6
1890-------	1917	55.0	50.0	43.1	39.0	29.8	19.6	17.2	15.9	17.0	12.8	11.7	7.2
1891-------	1918	59.1	46.3	52.0	36.5	28.1	19.1	17.1	17.8	13.2	14.2	8.5	6.4
1892-------	1919	55.1	57.7	49.0	34.2	27.7	19.2	19.2	14.2	14.8	10.3	7.8	7.9
1893-------	1920	68.2	53.4	44.3	33.0	27.7	20.4	14.6	16.0	11.6	10.0	8.8	6.6
1894-------	1921	62.7	46.7	42.0	33.0	28.5	17.7	16.4	12.8	11.7	10.1	8.0	6.7
1895-------	1922	54.9	43.8	42.0	31.7	24.3	17.0	13.9	12.4	11.3	9.6	8.0	5.8
1896-------	1923	51.2	44.2	40.9	28.0	21.5	14.5	13.1	12.4	10.8	8.7	6.6	6.2
1897-------	1924	52.1	43.2	35.2	25.4	20.8	13.3	14.3	12.0	9.9	8.3	7.5	4.9
1898-------	1925	50.1	36.7	31.9	22.1	18.0	14.8	12.3	10.0	8.9	7.4	5.8	5.4
1899-------	1926	47.6	38.6	30.8	22.2	21.2	14.8	13.4	11.5	9.6	8.4	7.2	5.6
1900-------	1927	45.6	32.7	30.1	24.5	20.0	14.8	13.0	11.5	10.4	8.9	7.2	6.0
1901-------	1928	38.7	31.8	30.3	23.3	20.0	13.8	13.6	10.9	9.8	8.7	7.1	5.9
1902-------	1929	36.0	31.8	28.5	21.7	16.5	13.0	11.2	9.8	8.7	7.6	7.2	5.7
1903-------	1930	36.4	29.7	26.7	17.8	16.0	11.1	10.1	9.1	8.4	7.7	7.0	5.8
1904-------	1931	34.3	28.9	22.7	18.4	14.8	10.8	10.1	9.5	8.9	7.5	7.5	6.4
1905-------	1932	33.0	24.9	22.9	17.1	14.3	10.7	10.5	9.5	8.6	7.9	7.6	6.6
1906-------	1933	29.4	25.4	22.2	16.9	13.9	11.4	10.8	9.6	9.3	8.7	7.7	7.1
1907-------	1934	30.2	24.5	21.8	15.7	14.6	11.6	10.8	10.2	10.0	9.1	8.5	7.2
1908-------	1935	28.7	23.7	20.2	16.7	14.8	11.9	12.0	11.5	10.7	10.1	8.6	7.3
1909-------	1936	28.3	23.4	21.7	17.7	15.5	13.3	13.5	13.0	11.9	10.8	9.9	8.7
1910-------	1937	28.5	24.0	22.0	17.8	17.3	14.5	15.4	14.0	12.7	11.9	10.7	8.9
1911-------	1938	29.6	24.9	22.4	19.5	17.8	16.9	16.6	14.7	14.6	14.1	11.4	9.6
1912-------	1939	29.8	24.8	23.8	21.2	20.3	17.7	16.5	15.9	16.8	13.3	12.2	9.4
1913-------	1940	30.3	26.4	26.6	23.4	21.6	18.0	18.3	19.9	15.9	13.6	11.9	9.8
1914-------	1941	32.2	30.6	28.8	24.7	21.5	20.0	22.8	18.1	16.9	14.3	12.6	9.5
1915-------	1942	35.1	32.1	29.7	24.4	25.0	25.4	21.2	19.5	17.0	15.1	11.7	10.9
1916-------	1943	37.0	32.3	29.1	28.3	29.9	22.9	22.8	19.0	17.4	14.2	13.1	9.3
1917-------	1944	37.4	32.2	35.2	34.7	29.2	25.8	21.8	20.4	17.2	14.9	11.8	9.9
1918-------	1945	37.0	39.5	42.5	35.0	31.7	25.8	23.6	20.5	17.6	14.8	12.6	9.9
1919-------	1946	49.2	52.3	46.7	39.4	33.8	29.8	25.8	22.5	20.4	17.0	13.9	10.2
1920-------	1947	63.0	55.0	48.6	41.3	36.7	30.0	28.7	24.1	20.7	16.7	12.8	10.5
1921-------	1948	62.6	54.8	48.7	42.1	37.3	32.7	28.3	24.3	20.3	16.1	13.8	10.0
1922-------	1949	58.8	51.6	46.5	40.6	35.5	30.8	26.4	21.3	17.3	14.7	12.0	9.3
1923-------	1950	57.4	51.8	47.6	39.1	36.7	29.5	25.7	20.8	17.5	14.9	11.0	8.9
1924-------	1951	61.3	56.7	49.1	45.3	37.0	31.1	25.9	21.4	19.3	14.3	11.8	8.7
1925-------	1952	66.6	59.9	55.0	44.6	39.5	31.1	27.6	23.7	19.0	14.5	11.8	10.5
1926-------	1953	68.5	62.7	53.0	45.0	37.9	31.6	27.4	22.4	18.4	14.2	12.8	9.9
1927-------	1954	69.4	58.6	51.3	42.6	36.5	30.5	25.7	21.0	17.0	14.7	11.8	9.9
1928-------	1955	64.4	55.3	49.7	40.1	35.1	27.8	23.4	19.2	16.1	13.4	10.6	8.7
1929-------	1956	66.0	55.6	48.1	41.5	34.3	28.5	23.1	18.7	15.5	13.2	10.8	8.9
1930-------	1957	63.6	54.7	47.9	39.9	33.4	26.2	22.6	18.7	15.5	13.7	9.8	9.4
1931-------	1958	64.2	55.9	48.9	40.5	33.2	27.4	23.2	19.1	16.8	12.3	11.9	8.8
1932-------	1959	67.8	58.5	50.3	40.9	35.1	28.6	24.1	22.0	15.2	15.4	12.2	10.0
1933-------	1960	74.0	63.7	52.8	45.6	38.2	32.1	28.4	21.1	20.9	16.9	13.8	10.0
1934-------	1961	81.2	68.0	60.6	49.6	44.0	36.8	29.3	28.1	23.9	19.3	15.9	10.7
1935-------	1962	84.8	74.6	64.8	56.2	49.1	38.6	37.9	31.5	26.0	20.9	15.3	12.1
1936-------	1963	86.0	73.9	68.5	56.9	46.8	44.6	39.7	32.4	26.0	20.7	16.7	
1937-------	1964	81.0	77.4	67.4	53.9	52.8	46.9	39.2	29.6	26.4	21.2		
1938-------	1965	82.2	71.5	59.7	57.4	51.8	43.1	35.0	30.3	24.4			
1939-------	1966	82.4	70.7	70.5	62.3	54.1	44.1	38.2	30.0				
1940-------	1967	83.5	81.2	74.7	64.1	54.6	46.0	36.5					
1941-------	1968	91.0	84.1	76.0	65.2	56.1	44.2						
1942-------	1969	93.9	87.2	78.7	65.9	55.5							
1943-------	1970	99.3	89.4	78.7	68.4								
1944-------	1971	101.1	90.1	82.4									
1945-------	1972	102.2	96.2										
1946-------	1973	110.5											

TABLE 10C. BIRTH PROBABILITIES FOR ALL OTHER WOMEN FOR EACH YEAR 1917-73 BY AGE AND PARITY FOR EACH COHORT FROM 1868 TO 1958--CON.

(PROBABILITIES ARE THE NUMBER OF BIRTHS PER 1,000 WOMEN IN SPECIFIED PARITY AND EXACT AGE GROUP. FIGURES FOR "0 PARITY" SHOW THE PROBABILITY OF FIRST BIRTHS TO "C PARITY" WOMEN, THOSE FOR "1 PARITY" SHOW THE PROBABILITY OF SECOND BIRTHS TO "1 PARITY" WOMEN, ETC. BASED ON CENTRAL BIRTH RATES AND PARITY DISTRIBUTIONS)

PARITY AND COHORT	DIAGONAL LINE FOR JANUARY 1	EXACT AGE										
		39	40	41	42	43	44	45	46	47	48	49
0 PARITY--CON.												
1868----------------												0.6
1869----------------											1.8	1.8
1870----------------										2.3	2.9	0.6
1871----------------									2.8	3.4	1.1	0.6
1872----------------								2.7	4.4	1.1	1.1	0.6
1873----------------							2.1	3.7	1.6	1.6	1.1	0.5
1874----------------						2.1	3.6	1.6	2.1	1.6	1.0	0.5
1875----------------					2.0	3.0	1.5	2.0	2.0	1.5	1.0	0.5
1876----------------				3.4	3.9	1.5	2.5	2.0	2.0	1.0	1.0	0.5
1877----------------			5.7	6.7	1.9	2.4	1.9	1.9	1.5	1.5	1.0	0.5
1878----------------	1917	9.3	9.4	3.3	2.8	1.9	1.9	1.4	1.9	1.4	1.0	0.5
1879----------------	1918	13.2	6.5	5.6	2.3	1.9	1.9	1.9	1.4	1.4	0.5	0.5
1880----------------	1919	10.3	8.2	4.6	2.8	2.3	1.8	1.4	2.3	1.4	0.5	0.5
1881----------------	1920	12.5	7.7	5.0	2.7	1.8	1.8	2.3	1.8	0.9	0.5	0.0
1882----------------	1921	11.5	7.6	5.4	2.3	1.8	2.3	1.8	1.4	0.5	0.5	0.5
1883----------------	1922	10.9	7.1	4.0	2.2	1.8	1.8	1.8	0.5	0.5	0.5	0.5
1884----------------	1923	9.4	6.0	3.9	2.2	1.7	1.8	0.9	0.9	0.4	0.4	0.4
1885----------------	1924	8.8	5.1	3.8	2.1	1.3	0.9	0.9	0.9	0.4	0.4	0.4
1886----------------	1925	7.6	5.1	3.8	1.7	1.3	0.9	1.3	0.4	0.4	0.4	0.4
1887----------------	1926	7.6	5.1	3.0	1.7	1.3	1.3	0.9	0.9	0.4	0.4	0.4
1888----------------	1927	8.0	4.2	2.6	1.3	1.3	0.9	0.9	0.9	0.4	0.4	0.9
1889----------------	1928	6.3	3.8	2.6	1.3	1.3	0.9	0.9	0.4	0.4	0.9	0.0
1890----------------	1929	5.5	4.3	2.6	1.7	0.9	0.9	0.9	0.4	0.4	0.4	0.0
1891----------------	1930	6.9	3.5	2.6	1.3	1.3	0.9	0.9	0.9	0.4	0.0	0.0
1892----------------	1931	5.7	3.5	2.2	1.3	0.9	0.9	0.9	0.9	0.4	0.4	0.0
1893----------------	1932	5.3	3.1	2.2	1.4	0.9	0.9	0.9	0.5	0.5	0.0	0.5
1894----------------	1933	4.9	2.7	2.3	1.4	0.9	0.9	0.5	0.9	0.5	0.5	0.0
1895----------------	1934	4.9	3.2	2.3	1.4	0.9	0.5	0.9	0.5	0.5	0.0	0.0
1896----------------	1935	4.5	2.7	1.8	1.4	0.9	0.9	0.5	0.5	0.0	0.0	0.0
1897----------------	1936	4.5	2.7	1.8	1.4	0.9	0.5	0.5	0.5	0.0	0.0	0.5
1898----------------	1937	3.7	2.5	1.7	1.3	0.8	0.4	0.4	0.4	0.0	0.4	0.4
1899----------------	1938	4.7	3.0	2.6	1.3	0.9	0.4	0.4	0.4	0.4	0.4	0.4
1900----------------	1939	5.2	3.5	2.2	1.7	0.9	0.9	0.4	0.4	0.4	0.4	0.0
1901----------------	1940	5.1	3.4	2.1	1.7	1.3	0.9	0.4	0.4	0.4	0.0	0.0
1902----------------	1941	4.9	3.3	2.1	2.1	1.2	0.8	0.4	0.4	0.0	0.0	0.0
1903----------------	1942	4.7	3.5	2.4	2.0	1.2	0.8	0.4	0.4	0.0	0.0	0.0
1904----------------	1943	5.0	3.8	3.1	1.9	1.2	0.4	0.4	0.4	0.0	0.0	0.4
1905----------------	1944	5.2	4.1	3.0	1.9	1.1	1.1	0.7	0.0	0.0	0.4	0.0
1906----------------	1945	5.7	4.3	2.9	2.2	1.5	0.7	0.4	0.4	0.4	0.0	0.0
1907----------------	1946	6.2	4.5	3.1	2.5	1.4	0.7	0.7	0.4	0.0	0.0	0.0
1908----------------	1947	6.4	4.4	3.7	1.7	1.4	1.0	0.3	0.3	0.0	0.0	0.0
1909----------------	1948	6.4	5.4	3.4	2.4	1.7	1.0	0.7	0.0	0.0	0.0	0.0
1910----------------	1949	7.9	5.3	4.0	2.0	1.7	0.7	0.3	0.3	0.0	0.3	0.0
1911----------------	1950	8.0	5.7	3.4	2.7	1.4	1.0	0.3	0.0	0.3	0.0	0.0
1912----------------	1951	7.9	4.9	3.3	2.3	1.7	0.7	0.3	0.3	0.3	0.3	0.0
1913----------------	1952	7.6	5.3	3.3	2.7	1.3	1.0	0.7	0.3	0.3	0.0	0.0
1914----------------	1953	7.9	5.3	3.3	2.3	1.7	0.7	0.7	0.3	0.0	0.0	0.0
1915----------------	1954	7.7	4.7	3.7	2.0	1.4	1.0	0.3	0.3	0.0	0.0	0.0
1916----------------	1955	7.0	5.4	3.4	1.7	1.7	0.7	0.3	0.0	0.3	0.0	0.0
1917----------------	1956	7.6	4.8	3.1	2.4	1.4	0.7	0.4	0.4	0.0	0.0	0.0
1918----------------	1957	7.1	4.7	3.3	2.2	1.5	0.7	0.4	0.0	0.0	0.0	0.0
1919----------------	1958	7.9	5.2	3.6	2.4	1.6	0.8	0.4	0.4	0.0	0.0	0.0
1920----------------	1959	7.2	6.0	3.4	2.6	1.3	0.9	0.4	0.0	0.0	0.0	0.0
1921----------------	1960	7.9	4.9	3.1	2.2	1.8	0.9	0.4	0.0	0.0	0.4	0.0
1922----------------	1961	7.2	4.3	3.0	2.2	1.3	0.4	0.0	0.0	0.4	0.0	0.0
1923----------------	1962	6.4	4.3	3.5	2.2	0.9	0.4	0.0	0.4	0.0	0.0	0.0
1924----------------	1963	6.5	4.7	3.3	1.9	1.4	0.5	0.5	0.0	0.0	0.0	0.0
1925----------------	1964	7.5	5.6	3.6	2.0	1.0	1.0	0.5	0.0	0.0	0.0	
1926----------------	1965	7.9	5.3	3.2	2.1	1.6	0.5	0.5	0.0	0.0		
1927----------------	1966	6.8	5.3	3.2	2.1	1.1	0.5	0.5	0.5			
1928----------------	1967	6.2	5.2	3.6	2.1	1.0	0.5	0.5				
1929----------------	1968	7.4	5.3	2.7	1.6	1.1	1.1					
1930----------------	1969	6.8	4.2	3.2	1.6	1.1						
1931----------------	1970	6.6	4.5	2.2	2.2							
1932----------------	1971	7.1	4.2	3.0								
1933----------------	1972	6.8	4.8									
1934----------------	1973	7.8										

TABLE 10C. BIRTH PROBABILITIES FOR ALL OTHER WOMEN FOR EACH YEAR 1917-73 BY AGE AND PARITY FOR EACH COHORT FROM 1868 TO 1958--CON.

(PROBABILITIES ARE THE NUMBER OF BIRTHS PER 1,000 WOMEN IN SPECIFIED PARITY AND EXACT AGE GROUP. FIGURES FOR "0 PARITY" SHOW THE PROBABILITY OF FIRST BIRTHS TO "C PARITY" WOMEN, THOSE FOR "1 PARITY" SHOW THE PROBABILITY OF SECOND BIRTHS TO "1 PARITY" WOMEN, ETC. BASED ON CENTRAL BIRTH RATES AND PARITY DISTRIBUTIONS)

PARITY AND COHORT	DIAGONAL LINE FOR JANUARY 1	EXACT AGE											
		15	16	17	18	19	20	21	22	23	24	25	26
1 PARITY													
1891-------													116.5
1892-------												147.8	105.7
1893-------											174.1	133.3	110.8
1894-------										196.9	155.0	131.0	116.7
1895-------									203.0	176.6	148.4	135.5	107.5
1896-------								222.3	182.9	165.8	151.6	126.1	100.8
1897-------							227.7	200.8	172.5	168.3	142.7	120.4	89.1
1898-------						263.4	222.7	204.9	190.4	173.0	149.9	118.9	87.5
1899-------					232.9	226.8	202.4	206.0	176.8	165.6	135.0	108.4	87.0
1900-------				211.8	201.7	207.9	208.7	195.7	174.3	156.3	131.5	105.1	82.2
1901-------			169.8	180.3	181.4	214.4	208.7	193.5	166.0	157.0	123.5	100.3	71.6
1902-------	1917	177.0	146.3	167.0	191.6	230.0	207.0	189.1	171.4	147.0	118.8	85.2	61.1
1903-------	1918	140.6	135.7	178.8	221.6	223.0	205.5	193.9	166.1	143.4	106.1	76.0	58.2
1904-------	1919	140.5	150.5	205.4	208.9	224.9	211.6	187.4	162.1	129.5	95.7	72.4	59.2
1905-------	1920	160.7	167.4	191.2	216.7	232.3	200.2	184.3	149.0	117.2	92.4	73.9	58.7
1906-------	1921	169.2	152.7	199.6	225.7	215.9	200.1	171.6	134.8	114.3	94.4	74.4	58.1
1907-------	1922	154.4	166.7	208.6	214.8	221.6	188.4	159.0	134.2	117.5	94.9	75.0	55.6
1908-------	1923	178.9	168.6	205.0	216.6	208.1	177.6	161.0	137.8	119.6	97.9	71.7	56.8
1909-------	1924	166.7	173.9	204.3	206.6	198.5	180.6	166.6	141.0	125.9	95.9	75.9	58.8
1910-------	1925	167.8	162.3	202.3	196.8	205.0	188.8	168.5	150.8	122.7	101.7	79.1	61.3
1911-------	1926	166.7	175.3	185.8	199.1	211.2	185.1	178.9	143.4	129.0	101.8	80.8	63.7
1912-------	1927	170.7	156.3	192.3	205.1	206.4	198.6	171.4	151.8	130.2	105.1	84.3	67.5
1913-------	1928	149.1	160.2	194.8	203.2	216.9	190.5	180.9	152.3	133.0	110.4	86.5	67.1
1914-------	1929	156.5	164.9	196.4	211.6	212.1	201.4	183.9	158.9	143.0	113.6	89.3	71.2
1915-------	1930	169.0	165.9	197.5	203.2	221.2	204.8	186.8	167.4	143.7	117.0	91.1	77.0
1916-------	1931	165.5	168.5	189.2	212.7	226.9	208.1	198.6	169.2	149.0	118.1	98.8	80.4
1917-------	1932	165.5	156.4	203.5	226.5	231.2	222.0	200.5	174.0	149.1	126.6	105.9	89.4
1918-------	1933	154.9	173.5	217.1	227.9	246.5	224.2	199.5	170.2	154.3	132.7	112.1	89.1
1919-------	1934	176.5	193.2	220.6	243.4	244.3	223.1	195.3	173.3	156.9	132.5	103.8	84.0
1920-------	1935	194.2	187.4	228.4	237.7	242.8	225.0	197.4	173.1	156.8	121.7	98.0	103.3
1921-------	1936	193.5	200.4	222.7	245.0	256.1	239.2	201.2	179.8	147.2	118.4	126.5	117.8
1922-------	1937	202.7	196.4	229.4	267.9	281.0	238.0	215.3	174.5	143.3	156.9	143.0	132.3
1923-------	1938	191.1	195.0	248.8	297.7	275.9	251.1	205.6	166.0	185.3	174.7	161.1	141.7
1924-------	1939	189.0	219.8	273.5	289.0	283.8	232.9	194.0	210.2	208.1	195.1	169.7	148.1
1925-------	1940	226.2	236.9	297.9	300.6	263.8	223.3	235.5	238.1	229.7	203.1	175.9	152.4
1926-------	1941	229.4	293.1	312.7	279.3	261.0	264.1	270.6	265.2	242.2	209.8	183.0	163.0
1927-------	1942	357.5	316.3	294.0	283.2	292.1	301.6	300.6	276.6	246.3	217.5	188.1	172.8
1928-------	1943	368.1	291.4	301.3	305.4	332.5	332.8	313.5	280.2	252.9	219.2	196.7	181.4
1929-------	1944	335.1	305.6	313.8	349.8	361.1	346.1	316.7	287.9	255.4	230.9	210.5	189.9
1930-------	1945	356.7	318.4	365.8	376.7	378.1	352.5	326.0	286.9	264.0	244.8	221.2	202.1
1931-------	1946	365.7	384.3	385.9	394.1	387.3	362.8	322.5	300.3	281.9	258.0	234.0	211.3
1932-------	1947	475.6	391.3	399.4	400.5	390.1	348.0	324.4	309.3	290.4	267.5	239.2	208.5
1933-------	1948	421.6	389.6	396.4	393.4	372.2	350.4	332.7	316.0	301.0	272.0	234.1	207.8
1934-------	1949	425.3	376.4	384.4	373.0	370.3	352.7	340.1	330.0	300.9	265.2	236.0	200.2
1935-------	1950	402.7	367.5	366.4	374.6	367.1	359.4	352.9	326.7	293.9	261.2	223.4	195.1
1936-------	1951	387.9	341.5	368.6	371.8	375.5	376.2	349.6	322.0	288.9	252.3	215.9	188.4
1937-------	1952	349.8	341.0	364.0	376.1	391.5	372.9	342.4	314.7	277.6	243.3	209.5	181.2
1938-------	1953	357.5	358.6	369.8	394.9	390.6	365.9	344.8	308.2	275.1	236.2	207.8	177.8
1939-------	1954	381.8	353.8	382.6	391.8	382.9	371.6	339.0	311.5	268.4	237.7	202.2	173.0
1940-------	1955	369.7	368.2	382.0	390.0	389.6	368.1	342.1	303.9	268.8	229.6	191.7	165.2
1941-------	1956	405.3	369.9	382.6	394.1	387.1	364.8	331.6	297.3	260.0	218.1	182.5	159.6
1942-------	1957	378.9	360.4	382.5	387.6	377.4	354.3	325.4	289.9	242.4	202.8	174.3	149.8
1943-------	1958	369.6	367.0	377.3	379.3	368.1	349.4	317.1	271.6	227.2	194.1	160.1	152.5
1944-------	1959	400.0	370.1	380.3	381.6	373.7	346.9	299.9	254.5	214.7	178.2	166.4	159.5
1945-------	1960	376.7	362.3	376.2	381.7	368.1	326.4	279.0	236.0	194.8	178.1	170.5	149.5
1946-------	1961	389.7	368.0	379.4	381.8	348.3	302.5	257.7	215.5	192.3	181.2	157.6	133.1
1947-------	1962	386.8	370.4	382.2	361.6	325.3	280.3	231.8	205.5	190.0	167.8	138.3	123.5
1948-------	1963	388.1	374.6	362.5	339.1	299.3	253.2	221.3	202.7	179.4	144.6	130.7	
1949-------	1964	397.0	351.4	343.5	312.8	271.8	239.4	217.7	192.8	154.1	138.1		
1950-------	1965	371.9	336.3	322.5	287.7	258.3	235.0	204.8	166.8	147.3			
1951-------	1966	357.8	323.5	289.6	268.7	251.5	218.7	180.4	158.6				
1952-------	1967	341.5	285.5	265.4	259.6	229.9	194.2	168.7					
1953-------	1968	305.2	256.0	262.5	238.4	206.2	181.3						
1954-------	1969	278.5	257.9	239.6	215.0	189.4							
1955-------	1970	281.3	236.3	213.8	194.7								
1956-------	1971	256.3	212.5	192.9									
1957-------	1972	228.8	194.1										
1958-------	1973	215.8											

TABLE 10C. BIRTH PROBABILITIES FOR ALL OTHER WOMEN FOR EACH YEAR 1917-73 BY AGE AND PARITY FOR EACH COHORT FROM 1868 TO 1958--CON.

(PROBABILITIES ARE THE NUMBER OF BIRTHS PER 1,000 WOMEN IN SPECIFIED PARITY AND EXACT AGE GROUP. FIGURES FOR "0 PARITY" SHOW THE PROBABILITY OF FIRST BIRTHS TO "C PARITY" WOMEN, THOSE FOR "1 PARITY" SHOW THE PROBABILITY OF SECOND BIRTHS TO "1 PARITY" WOMEN, ETC. BASED ON CENTRAL BIRTH RATES AND PARITY DISTRIBUTIONS)

PARITY AND COHORT	DIAGONAL LINE FOR JANUARY 1	EXACT AGE											
		27	28	29	30	31	32	33	34	35	36	37	38
1 PARITY--CON.													
1879-------													25.7
1880-------												29.7	27.2
1881-------											35.5	32.5	26.5
1882-------										39.0	37.4	31.0	29.3
1883-------									42.2	40.1	35.3	33.0	25.4
1884-------								43.3	42.0	37.4	37.1	27.9	24.8
1885-------							45.9	42.9	39.7	38.3	30.7	27.8	21.8
1886-------						56.4	44.6	40.4	39.2	33.6	30.3	24.0	18.1
1887-------					64.8	55.3	43.1	39.2	36.7	32.6	26.5	20.3	14.0
1888-------				83.9	62.1	54.5	42.3	41.1	35.6	28.7	23.2	16.5	13.1
1889-------			90.5	78.1	62.9	54.0	44.0	38.8	31.3	25.6	21.4	15.9	12.1
1890-------	1917	104.1	82.4	81.1	65.3	56.4	42.0	33.8	29.5	26.0	19.2	14.9	9.6
1891-------	1918	94.5	87.2	86.7	65.8	54.7	37.1	33.0	27.7	22.7	17.7	10.9	10.4
1892-------	1919	100.3	95.4	85.0	64.1	48.0	35.9	31.8	25.6	20.2	13.7	13.2	9.7
1893-------	1920	108.2	90.2	81.5	56.5	46.1	32.9	29.4	21.4	16.1	15.7	11.3	9.4
1894-------	1921	99.7	84.4	70.6	51.1	41.5	30.2	23.7	17.4	16.6	12.9	10.7	7.4
1895-------	1922	93.6	74.1	63.3	44.7	38.0	24.0	19.0	16.5	13.9	11.8	8.7	7.0
1896-------	1923	82.0	65.1	56.2	41.5	29.3	19.4	17.5	14.7	13.1	9.9	8.2	5.8
1897-------	1924	72.9	59.6	51.3	31.8	24.4	18.0	16.2	13.5	10.9	9.7	7.0	5.1
1898-------	1925	75.9	58.4	44.7	29.4	24.9	18.3	16.0	12.8	11.6	9.3	7.3	5.7
1899-------	1926	70.7	51.9	39.0	28.9	25.8	17.3	15.8	13.6	12.1	9.9	7.6	6.5
1900-------	1927	62.1	43.7	38.2	30.6	23.6	17.5	15.7	14.0	11.8	9.2	7.8	6.7
1901-------	1928	52.3	42.3	39.3	27.3	23.1	16.8	15.8	14.1	10.5	9.4	8.4	6.6
1902-------	1929	49.4	42.1	34.5	25.6	20.5	16.0	14.9	11.4	10.4	9.0	8.3	6.1
1903-------	1930	49.2	38.7	34.1	24.2	20.8	15.6	13.2	11.5	10.4	9.4	7.9	6.9
1904-------	1931	47.4	38.7	32.8	25.5	20.0	14.8	13.1	11.7	10.7	8.9	9.0	7.5
1905-------	1932	47.7	37.7	33.6	24.1	19.3	15.2	14.2	12.1	10.7	10.0	9.0	8.3
1906-------	1933	45.0	38.4	31.5	23.7	20.7	15.9	14.5	12.8	12.1	10.4	10.0	8.6
1907-------	1934	46.1	36.9	32.3	25.1	20.3	16.8	15.8	14.4	13.4	12.0	10.9	8.7
1908-------	1935	45.9	37.9	34.3	25.2	21.4	18.2	17.9	16.9	15.1	13.3	11.5	10.8
1909-------	1936	48.9	40.8	35.1	26.5	23.3	20.8	20.9	19.1	16.6	14.4	14.4	11.8
1910-------	1937	52.0	44.5	35.9	28.6	26.8	24.2	24.0	21.4	19.1	17.2	16.1	13.0
1911-------	1938	54.6	44.4	37.6	31.7	29.9	27.4	26.3	22.5	21.4	20.3	18.0	14.4
1912-------	1939	55.1	46.4	41.8	36.5	34.0	30.6	27.9	26.1	25.4	22.2	18.6	14.9
1913-------	1940	57.4	50.2	47.2	41.1	37.4	31.1	32.5	30.3	27.5	23.4	18.9	16.5
1914-------	1941	63.3	56.3	53.5	44.9	39.4	37.6	38.0	33.5	30.3	24.0	20.6	18.0
1915-------	1942	67.5	63.2	56.4	46.8	46.8	43.8	40.6	36.6	28.9	25.5	22.5	18.1
1916-------	1943	76.4	66.0	57.3	55.7	53.3	46.9	44.4	36.1	32.7	28.3	23.9	20.2
1917-------	1944	78.4	65.2	69.1	63.3	59.3	49.6	44.1	39.4	35.1	29.7	26.1	19.5
1918-------	1945	73.7	77.7	77.1	70.2	60.1	51.6	46.3	42.6	36.9	31.6	26.0	20.3
1919-------	1946	90.3	89.2	84.3	71.1	61.2	54.5	50.3	43.8	37.3	32.5	25.1	20.0
1920-------	1947	101.4	94.7	86.9	71.3	66.0	57.5	50.9	42.4	38.8	30.2	24.7	20.5
1921-------	1948	110.6	103.3	88.5	79.0	71.9	60.5	53.0	47.1	39.0	31.4	26.2	18.1
1922-------	1949	121.9	107.0	96.8	85.8	75.3	65.5	57.7	49.8	41.0	34.0	23.7	19.9
1923-------	1950	127.6	112.2	102.3	90.4	82.4	68.5	63.1	52.2	42.8	31.0	25.9	21.9
1924-------	1951	131.7	118.9	109.5	99.0	84.5	72.6	63.0	53.4	41.2	33.6	28.4	21.7
1925-------	1952	140.4	128.3	116.0	100.2	86.4	75.0	64.0	51.8	43.2	35.4	28.6	22.3
1926-------	1953	153.1	137.9	124.0	103.2	94.9	76.9	67.3	57.5	44.8	38.4	28.8	22.4
1927-------	1954	157.1	143.6	127.8	113.8	94.6	80.7	71.8	56.8	50.4	39.7	29.1	23.7
1928-------	1955	166.5	149.3	136.5	111.2	99.4	86.7	71.9	61.9	49.3	38.2	31.7	22.3
1929-------	1956	177.1	157.8	134.2	117.5	105.9	88.0	76.1	63.8	50.2	42.0	31.4	26.0
1930-------	1957	185.5	156.5	142.0	125.6	109.9	91.6	80.0	61.1	52.9	41.1	33.5	25.8
1931-------	1958	183.6	164.7	150.0	128.9	108.8	96.6	75.8	66.2	52.7	45.3	35.5	28.3
1932-------	1959	186.7	164.0	149.1	122.8	110.8	86.7	78.3	61.1	54.2	42.0	36.2	27.0
1933-------	1960	181.7	162.9	139.3	120.7	104.4	88.4	72.0	62.4	52.2	45.0	34.4	26.4
1934-------	1961	179.6	156.9	136.4	115.2	101.6	82.2	69.5	61.3	51.2	42.3	32.0	25.3
1935-------	1962	172.1	148.2	130.7	111.6	95.0	78.4	71.6	59.2	49.6	38.5	34.3	22.3
1936-------	1963	162.9	141.9	126.4	107.1	91.4	80.4	70.3	59.2	47.3	40.0	28.7	
1937-------	1964	159.1	140.0	123.2	103.2	91.7	81.3	71.5	57.6	48.7	36.4		
1938-------	1965	153.5	137.9	120.6	104.0	96.4	86.6	72.8	57.5	47.6			
1939-------	1966	152.3	135.6	121.2	112.3	103.6	88.1	72.3	59.7				
1940-------	1967	149.9	133.2	125.1	116.0	104.5	85.6	71.9					
1941-------	1968	143.2	134.3	127.9	115.9	98.6	83.8						
1942-------	1969	141.6	136.1	122.6	107.5	92.8							
1943-------	1970	146.8	130.7	117.1	102.8								
1944-------	1971	141.2	123.9	111.9									
1945-------	1972	128.4	116.0										
1946-------	1973	120.3											

TABLE 10C. BIRTH PROBABILITIES FOR ALL OTHER WOMEN FOR EACH YEAR 1917-73 BY AGE AND PARITY FOR EACH COHORT FROM 1868 TO 1958--CON.

(PROBABILITIES ARE THE NUMBER OF BIRTHS PER 1,000 WOMEN IN SPECIFIED PARITY AND EXACT AGE GROUP. FIGURES FOR "0 PARITY" SHOW THE PROBABILITY OF FIRST BIRTHS TO "C PARITY" WOMEN, THOSE FOR "1 PARITY" SHOW THE PROBABILITY OF SECOND BIRTHS TO "1 PARITY" WOMEN, ETC. BASED ON CENTRAL BIRTH RATES AND PARITY DISTRIBUTIONS)

PARITY AND COHORT	DIAGONAL LINE FOR JANUARY 1	EXACT AGE										
		39	40	41	42	43	44	45	46	47	48	49
1 PARITY--CON.												
1868----------------												1.9
1869----------------											2.8	0.9
1870----------------										2.7	0.9	0.9
1871----------------									5.4	0.9	0.9	1.8
1872----------------								5.2	1.7	0.9	2.6	0.9
1873----------------							5.9	2.6	2.5	2.5	0.8	0.8
1874----------------						4.1	4.1	3.3	5.0	0.8	0.8	0.8
1875----------------					5.6	5.6	4.0	5.7	1.6	0.8	0.8	0.8
1876----------------				7.8	7.8	5.5	6.3	1.6	0.8	0.8	0.8	0.8
1877----------------			12.1	9.9	7.6	5.4	3.8	1.5	2.3	0.8	1.5	0.8
1878----------------	1917	20.6	14.1	10.4	7.4	6.0	3.0	3.0	2.2	1.5	1.5	0.7
1879----------------	1918	22.3	13.7	9.4	8.7	5.1	3.6	2.2	2.9	0.7	1.5	0.0
1880----------------	1919	21.7	14.1	11.3	7.1	4.3	2.8	2.8	2.1	1.4	0.7	0.7
1881----------------	1920	24.0	14.5	9.7	6.9	3.5	3.5	1.4	2.1	1.4	0.7	0.0
1882----------------	1921	22.1	13.5	8.8	4.7	4.1	2.7	2.0	2.0	1.4	0.7	0.7
1883----------------	1922	21.0	11.9	6.6	4.6	2.0	2.0	2.0	2.0	0.7	0.7	0.0
1884----------------	1923	18.6	9.7	6.5	3.2	2.6	1.9	1.9	1.3	0.6	0.6	0.0
1885----------------	1924	15.0	8.8	6.3	2.5	2.5	1.3	1.3	0.6	0.6	0.6	0.0
1886----------------	1925	12.7	8.5	4.9	3.0	1.2	1.2	0.6	0.6	0.6	0.0	0.6
1887----------------	1926	12.3	6.4	4.7	2.3	1.2	1.2	1.2	1.2	0.0	0.6	0.6
1888----------------	1927	10.3	6.3	4.0	1.7	1.7	1.1	1.1	0.6	0.6	1.1	0.6
1889----------------	1928	9.3	5.5	3.3	1.7	1.7	1.1	1.1	0.6	0.6	0.6	0.6
1890----------------	1929	8.5	5.4	2.7	2.1	1.6	1.1	0.5	0.5	0.5	0.5	0.5
1891----------------	1930	7.8	4.7	3.1	1.6	1.0	1.0	0.5	0.5	0.5	0.5	0.0
1892----------------	1931	8.2	4.6	2.6	1.5	1.5	1.0	1.0	0.5	0.5	0.0	0.0
1893----------------	1932	6.9	4.0	3.0	2.0	1.0	1.0	0.5	0.5	0.0	0.5	0.0
1894----------------	1933	6.0	3.7	2.8	1.4	0.9	0.5	0.5	0.0	0.0	0.0	0.0
1895----------------	1934	5.3	3.1	2.2	1.3	0.9	0.4	0.0	0.4	0.4	0.0	0.0
1896----------------	1935	4.1	3.3	2.1	1.2	0.8	0.4	0.4	0.4	0.4	0.0	0.0
1897----------------	1936	4.3	3.5	2.0	1.2	0.8	0.4	0.8	0.4	0.0	0.0	0.0
1898----------------	1937	5.3	3.2	2.0	1.2	0.8	0.8	0.8	0.4	0.0	0.0	0.0
1899----------------	1938	5.4	2.7	2.3	1.1	1.1	0.8	0.4	0.4	0.0	0.0	0.4
1900----------------	1939	5.2	3.0	2.2	1.5	1.1	0.7	0.4	0.4	0.0	0.4	0.0
1901----------------	1940	5.1	3.3	2.6	1.5	1.1	0.7	0.7	0.0	0.4	0.4	0.0
1902----------------	1941	5.4	4.0	2.5	1.4	1.4	1.1	0.4	0.4	0.4	0.4	0.0
1903----------------	1942	5.8	4.0	2.5	1.8	1.5	0.7	0.4	0.4	0.0	0.4	0.0
1904----------------	1943	6.5	4.3	2.9	1.8	1.4	0.7	0.7	0.4	0.4	0.0	0.0
1905----------------	1944	6.8	4.3	3.2	2.2	1.4	1.1	0.4	0.4	0.0	0.0	0.0
1906----------------	1945	6.5	5.0	3.6	2.2	1.8	0.7	0.4	0.4	0.0	0.4	0.0
1907----------------	1946	8.4	5.5	3.6	2.6	1.8	0.7	0.4	0.4	0.0	0.0	0.0
1908----------------	1947	8.6	5.6	4.1	2.6	1.5	1.1	0.7	0.4	0.0	0.0	0.0
1909----------------	1948	9.1	6.5	5.0	3.4	2.3	1.1	0.8	0.0	0.0	0.0	0.0
1910----------------	1949	10.7	7.5	5.9	3.6	2.0	1.2	0.4	0.4	0.0	0.4	0.0
1911----------------	1950	11.2	9.3	5.6	3.6	2.4	1.2	0.8	0.4	0.4	0.0	0.0
1912----------------	1951	13.3	8.7	6.3	3.8	2.9	1.3	0.8	0.4	0.0	0.0	0.0
1913----------------	1952	12.7	9.4	6.4	4.3	2.6	1.7	0.9	0.4	0.0	0.0	0.0
1914----------------	1953	14.1	9.7	7.1	4.0	2.7	1.3	0.4	0.4	0.0	0.0	0.0
1915----------------	1954	14.5	10.0	6.4	4.1	2.7	1.4	0.5	0.5	0.0	0.0	0.0
1916----------------	1955	14.7	10.0	6.7	4.8	2.9	1.4	0.5	0.5	0.0	0.0	0.0
1917----------------	1956	15.2	10.3	6.9	4.9	2.5	1.5	0.5	0.5	0.0	0.0	0.0
1918----------------	1957	15.4	10.0	6.5	4.0	2.5	1.0	1.0	0.0	0.0	0.0	0.0
1919----------------	1958	14.7	9.9	5.9	4.0	2.5	1.5	0.5	0.0	0.0	0.0	0.0
1920----------------	1959	13.8	8.4	6.0	4.0	2.5	1.5	0.5	0.5	0.0	0.0	0.0
1921----------------	1960	13.6	9.4	6.8	4.2	2.6	1.6	0.5	0.5	0.0	0.0	0.0
1922----------------	1961	15.5	11.0	7.0	4.1	2.9	1.2	0.6	0.6	0.0	0.0	0.0
1923----------------	1962	16.6	10.5	6.8	4.4	3.1	1.3	0.6	0.0	0.0	0.0	0.0
1924----------------	1963	15.5	11.0	7.2	4.6	2.0	2.0	0.7	0.0	0.0	0.0	0.0
1925----------------	1964	15.6	10.9	7.5	4.8	3.4	2.1	0.7	0.0	0.0	0.0	
1926----------------	1965	18.0	11.3	8.4	5.3	3.8	1.5	0.8	0.0	0.0		
1927----------------	1966	17.3	14.1	7.5	6.7	3.4	1.7	0.8	0.0			
1928----------------	1967	18.0	11.8	10.0	5.5	3.7	1.8	0.9				
1929----------------	1968	18.4	13.7	8.8	6.9	3.9	2.0					
1930----------------	1969	18.7	13.6	9.4	6.3	3.2						
1931----------------	1970	20.9	14.4	11.2	5.6							
1932----------------	1971	19.6	14.3	8.8								
1933----------------	1972	19.2	12.9									
1934----------------	1973	17.4										

TABLE 10C. BIRTH PROBABILITIES FOR ALL OTHER WOMEN FOR EACH YEAR 1917-73 BY AGE AND PARITY FOR EACH COHORT FROM 1868 TO 1958--CON.

(PROBABILITIES ARE THE NUMBER OF BIRTHS PER 1,000 WOMEN IN SPECIFIED PARITY AND EXACT AGE GROUP. FIGURES FOR "0 PARITY" SHOW THE PROBABILITY OF FIRST BIRTHS TO "0 PARITY" WOMEN, THOSE FOR "1 PARITY" SHOW THE PROBABILITY OF SECOND BIRTHS TO "1 PARITY" WOMEN, ETC. BASED ON CENTRAL BIRTH RATES AND PARITY DISTRIBUTIONS)

PARITY AND COHORT	DIAGONAL LINE FOR JANUARY 1	EXACT AGE											
		15	16	17	18	19	20	21	22	23	24	25	26
2 PARITY													
1891-------													198.2
1892-------												224.2	191.6
1893-------											283.4	259.2	218.4
1894-------										299.3	279.7	243.6	225.7
1895-------									290.3	303.5	263.4	250.8	227.7
1896-------								297.8	296.9	283.6	269.4	260.0	202.4
1897-------							286.1	307.5	281.8	288.4	285.0	238.2	200.0
1898-------						290.3	291.6	290.8	286.4	308.7	266.2	242.4	217.8
1899-------					267.2	308.0	286.4	305.0	312.4	294.6	275.3	263.3	210.8
1900-------				*	278.8	306.7	303.5	333.9	299.4	311.8	305.1	250.7	201.6
1901-------			*	*	279.6	327.1	332.9	307.8	304.7	333.6	279.8	226.0	185.2
1902-------	1917	*	*	*	308.5	367.4	300.9	313.5	329.3	299.0	251.0	205.1	161.9
1903-------	1918	*	*	*	341.7	308.2	302.4	331.4	294.5	272.7	235.8	188.3	147.9
1904-------	1919	*	*	*	287.6	328.1	325.9	305.8	284.6	265.5	222.6	179.8	149.1
1905-------	1920	*	*	*	334.7	351.3	301.4	296.6	280.9	249.3	213.6	183.1	151.4
1906-------	1921	*	*	*	346.2	330.1	306.2	293.8	266.5	245.1	218.4	180.5	153.8
1907-------	1922	*	*	*	320.8	334.0	295.1	281.0	258.9	248.2	212.2	185.1	150.4
1908-------	1923	*	*	*	340.0	321.4	288.7	280.3	264.6	241.8	217.7	182.0	152.1
1909-------	1924	*	*	*	314.6	311.7	281.4	286.6	260.0	252.9	219.4	187.8	149.4
1910-------	1925	*	*	*	303.7	305.9	288.8	278.7	271.1	251.6	229.3	182.7	145.2
1911-------	1926	*	*	317.8	288.4	304.2	281.0	292.1	263.7	263.3	222.1	179.0	152.6
1912-------	1927	*	*	*	279.7	303.8	294.6	274.4	275.6	253.9	215.0	185.3	157.0
1913-------	1928	*	*	*	288.5	317.6	275.1	288.5	271.9	249.6	227.8	191.5	155.8
1914-------	1929	*	*	*	298.4	299.0	291.2	292.1	270.3	262.0	234.3	191.8	156.5
1915-------	1930	*	*	*	289.2	319.8	302.4	291.2	286.7	272.4	237.4	197.3	163.7
1916-------	1931	*	*	*	316.7	336.1	304.0	306.9	294.1	273.7	244.7	204.5	165.1
1917-------	1932	*	*	*	325.0	326.1	313.5	305.9	287.2	280.7	250.9	203.3	169.5
1918-------	1933	*	*	*	328.1	334.6	307.6	290.7	291.4	282.6	243.6	204.4	170.4
1919-------	1934	*	*	*	321.2	323.3	296.9	295.4	290.5	272.9	238.3	196.9	156.7
1920-------	1935	*	*	333.3	311.6	322.0	317.6	290.6	281.4	267.9	227.5	180.1	171.4
1921-------	1936	*	*	327.6	339.9	364.7	316.7	291.9	278.5	255.2	207.7	194.9	180.2
1922-------	1937	*	*	362.1	421.7	364.2	315.1	300.2	274.2	234.7	226.9	204.8	188.2
1923-------	1938	*	*	449.2	429.9	359.8	324.5	294.8	255.6	256.3	234.1	220.9	194.0
1924-------	1939	*	*	429.7	407.5	365.7	314.4	274.4	280.6	264.0	255.6	223.8	203.1
1925-------	1940	*	*	471.8	378.9	335.2	283.3	293.5	284.6	284.4	254.3	229.2	209.5
1926-------	1941	*	*	405.9	334.9	301.2	305.8	307.1	308.2	287.4	264.7	236.5	207.5
1927-------	1942	*	*	336.6	302.5	317.4	323.9	331.4	315.6	298.1	272.7	235.0	209.6
1928-------	1943	*	*	331.6	325.4	348.9	353.6	341.4	327.8	306.4	268.9	241.0	211.4
1929-------	1944	*	*	351.1	359.7	369.6	360.6	350.9	333.0	304.0	272.0	241.9	216.7
1930-------	1945	*	*	388.3	371.9	379.5	367.4	355.8	328.8	300.0	278.4	245.4	220.9
1931-------	1946	*	*	379.6	384.3	378.4	366.6	345.8	319.7	305.3	277.4	249.6	223.9
1932-------	1947	*	*	390.2	372.6	378.0	358.8	339.2	330.7	309.9	284.7	252.1	214.2
1933-------	1948	*	*	369.6	364.8	370.4	356.0	349.8	334.1	314.7	284.1	245.4	213.7
1934-------	1949	*	*	390.7	382.6	379.6	376.5	363.5	350.5	320.1	285.1	248.3	208.5
1935-------	1950	*	*	397.1	389.0	395.6	384.1	375.4	355.5	325.0	287.5	242.3	205.1
1936-------	1951	*	*	409.8	406.0	404.2	393.5	381.4	351.9	317.7	278.7	237.9	200.4
1937-------	1952	*	*	423.7	411.3	411.2	401.8	376.3	347.1	314.0	276.6	230.0	193.8
1938-------	1953	*	*	425.3	419.4	415.4	395.4	370.5	343.4	310.3	268.2	222.8	188.5
1939-------	1954	*	*	434.9	416.5	413.7	395.1	369.8	338.6	301.0	259.6	215.6	175.4
1940-------	1955	*	*	426.0	422.0	412.2	391.8	362.8	334.4	287.5	244.6	193.6	156.0
1941-------	1956	*	*	426.5	420.9	408.2	384.6	359.2	319.6	275.5	221.8	177.6	144.8
1942-------	1957	*	*	439.6	417.9	409.3	385.6	348.9	307.9	249.3	200.0	161.4	128.5
1943-------	1958	*	*	433.0	425.6	409.1	381.8	340.3	284.7	228.2	181.8	146.3	129.7
1944-------	1959	*	*	448.7	424.7	400.0	367.0	312.7	257.5	202.9	166.8	146.4	134.2
1945-------	1960	*	*	456.3	415.4	392.5	343.0	285.4	228.5	189.8	166.4	151.1	130.2
1946-------	1961	*	*	428.6	413.3	367.5	312.2	255.0	210.0	186.1	168.8	144.1	108.8
1947-------	1962	*	*	438.5	388.4	332.2	284.8	233.3	205.3	186.2	161.9	122.2	101.0
1948-------	1963	*	*	413.2	355.3	308.9	253.1	221.6	206.3	175.4	133.9	111.8	
1949-------	1964	*	*	375.0	328.1	277.3	243.9	226.3	193.6	148.1	124.4		
1950-------	1965	*	*	348.0	289.5	263.3	246.4	205.3	162.4	138.6			
1951-------	1966	*	*	312.5	284.8	264.3	223.7	180.2	154.1				
1952-------	1967	*	*	298.6	281.9	240.6	199.0	172.4					
1953-------	1968	*	*	309.6	262.2	215.8	189.8						
1954-------	1969	*	*	286.4	231.3	207.4							
1955-------	1970	*	*	248.7	222.2								
1956-------	1971	*	*	243.2									
1957-------	1972	*	*										
1958-------	1973	*											

TABLE 10C. BIRTH PROBABILITIES FOR ALL OTHER WOMEN FOR EACH YEAR 1917-73 BY AGE AND PARITY FOR EACH COHORT FROM 1868 TO 1958--CON.

(PROBABILITIES ARE THE NUMBER OF BIRTHS PER 1,000 WOMEN IN SPECIFIED PARITY AND EXACT AGE GROUP. FIGURES FOR "0 PARITY" SHOW THE PROBABILITY OF FIRST BIRTHS TO "0 PARITY" WOMEN, THOSE FOR "1 PARITY" SHOW THE PROBABILITY OF SECOND BIRTHS TO "1 PARITY" WOMEN, ETC. BASED ON CENTRAL BIRTH RATES AND PARITY DISTRIBUTIONS)

PARITY AND COHORT	DIAGONAL LINE FOR JANUARY 1	EXACT AGE 27	28	29	30	31	32	33	34	35	36	37	38
2 PARITY--CON.													
1879-------													43.6
1880-------												55.3	51.3
1881-------											68.2	64.8	49.5
1882-------										70.3	76.9	61.7	58.0
1883-------									71.7	76.2	70.4	71.0	49.7
1884-------								75.8	76.9	71.9	81.4	60.2	48.9
1885-------							80.9	76.9	71.9	79.1	68.2	57.7	43.5
1886-------						104.0	82.1	75.0	76.1	67.8	64.6	52.1	42.7
1887-------					113.5	105.4	79.4	76.5	68.6	63.6	58.4	50.6	38.9
1888-------				145.6	117.8	106.6	83.8	75.4	66.2	60.1	59.4	44.7	34.6
1889-------			161.7	150.7	120.3	115.0	84.4	73.7	65.2	63.6	53.5	42.7	31.4
1890-------	1917	185.3	161.5	149.7	127.0	112.1	80.6	71.0	68.0	60.9	50.7	37.4	24.4
1891-------	1918	182.2	156.1	155.6	123.8	104.7	75.9	74.2	63.8	56.9	42.9	29.0	23.3
1892-------	1919	173.4	161.7	151.1	110.5	96.7	78.1	66.6	60.3	44.4	34.0	25.6	20.9
1893-------	1920	214.8	191.5	160.3	124.8	121.7	83.2	77.3	57.6	46.7	40.1	30.1	22.8
1894-------	1921	212.4	164.4	150.3	128.0	102.4	75.2	61.7	48.4	42.3	34.9	28.2	22.2
1895-------	1922	185.6	158.7	157.1	114.0	89.1	66.1	52.1	46.3	37.8	31.4	26.5	19.0
1896-------	1923	181.7	166.8	141.2	99.7	82.5	54.6	48.3	42.4	35.6	30.1	23.6	18.7
1897-------	1924	194.0	153.4	129.9	91.9	69.5	50.2	45.2	39.2	33.0	27.5	22.7	17.8
1898-------	1925	178.9	146.1	116.7	79.8	65.9	50.3	46.1	38.6	31.6	27.6	21.9	18.7
1899-------	1926	178.4	138.0	110.6	82.5	69.9	52.2	49.6	40.3	37.3	30.8	25.1	20.9
1900-------	1927	166.5	123.8	109.7	85.5	69.2	55.4	49.6	44.3	37.1	30.5	27.2	21.3
1901-------	1928	145.3	116.9	107.6	77.0	67.1	51.9	50.2	40.0	32.8	30.5	23.9	19.7
1902-------	1929	129.9	110.5	95.6	70.7	62.4	49.2	41.0	35.7	32.7	28.1	22.5	18.4
1903-------	1930	126.8	104.6	91.4	70.5	60.2	43.9	38.7	35.1	32.2	26.0	21.2	18.9
1904-------	1931	129.2	105.0	95.2	69.6	60.3	44.6	41.9	36.7	32.1	26.5	23.4	20.1
1905-------	1932	130.7	106.6	93.1	71.3	56.6	44.4	42.4	37.1	32.4	28.5	25.3	23.7
1906-------	1933	128.5	107.2	93.1	68.8	59.3	47.6	44.0	37.7	35.5	28.9	29.0	25.8
1907-------	1934	130.3	103.2	89.5	69.3	61.2	48.8	44.3	41.3	36.5	33.3	31.7	25.9
1908-------	1935	123.9	101.1	91.7	72.1	61.7	49.2	47.9	44.0	41.6	35.9	32.7	27.7
1909-------	1936	122.5	105.2	96.0	72.0	62.3	53.9	52.6	48.7	44.0	39.1	37.7	31.9
1910-------	1937	127.4	111.3	95.2	72.8	68.0	57.9	58.3	51.1	46.3	43.2	40.0	32.5
1911-------	1938	135.0	110.2	94.7	77.7	70.4	63.5	61.4	54.3	52.1	47.4	40.8	34.9
1912-------	1939	132.7	109.4	99.3	82.3	77.2	66.4	64.2	57.2	54.1	48.4	41.9	37.0
1913-------	1940	133.7	113.8	104.3	88.5	81.8	69.3	69.0	61.9	57.9	50.6	45.0	38.6
1914-------	1941	138.5	119.8	110.1	92.6	81.1	76.7	72.2	67.4	61.1	52.4	49.5	40.8
1915-------	1942	142.6	126.6	116.2	91.6	92.7	81.0	79.4	73.2	63.0	60.3	49.4	43.0
1916-------	1943	150.6	132.9	112.0	104.7	97.7	87.2	84.2	74.0	71.5	54.1	53.5	43.1
1917-------	1944	153.4	122.9	124.5	109.9	102.0	90.9	85.2	78.1	66.9	60.9	53.3	42.2
1918-------	1945	139.3	137.1	129.1	113.6	106.9	94.8	88.1	79.9	70.5	64.1	51.3	42.9
1919-------	1946	156.9	142.7	135.6	120.7	110.6	96.8	94.8	81.4	72.7	61.5	51.4	41.1
1920-------	1947	161.3	150.2	141.1	123.0	112.6	100.6	95.4	82.9	72.0	58.9	50.7	40.8
1921-------	1948	169.8	155.2	141.6	125.8	113.1	103.4	90.9	80.6	69.0	60.0	47.2	38.9
1922-------	1949	172.9	157.3	146.8	125.4	119.4	100.9	92.9	80.0	69.9	57.5	47.3	37.0
1923-------	1950	179.6	165.8	147.3	129.5	116.4	102.0	93.7	81.5	67.6	55.1	45.2	36.9
1924-------	1951	189.9	166.3	153.2	133.3	118.6	105.1	94.0	80.2	66.4	54.2	44.9	36.0
1925-------	1952	187.0	166.1	151.5	128.9	118.8	102.6	89.8	74.3	62.2	52.8	43.7	32.9
1926-------	1953	188.8	168.0	151.3	130.9	118.8	97.4	87.8	71.7	62.6	51.4	38.8	32.1
1927-------	1954	188.5	171.3	155.0	136.4	113.8	97.5	84.9	72.8	62.5	46.4	39.0	30.7
1928-------	1955	194.9	172.3	160.1	127.7	116.4	97.7	85.1	72.8	58.2	48.0	38.3	28.9
1929-------	1956	197.0	178.5	150.8	130.6	115.4	100.3	83.8	69.6	59.0	46.6	36.6	30.8
1930-------	1957	200.6	168.8	151.1	131.2	117.1	93.8	82.3	68.6	55.2	44.7	36.9	26.4
1931-------	1958	191.0	167.9	146.0	130.4	107.0	91.2	79.1	63.8	53.2	40.0	32.1	24.8
1932-------	1959	189.8	162.5	146.4	120.3	103.4	86.3	72.7	61.4	46.9	39.5	31.2	24.8
1933-------	1960	179.6	159.0	135.8	116.0	98.9	80.0	68.9	52.9	46.7	36.9	31.0	22.9
1934-------	1961	180.9	155.6	134.2	109.6	94.6	76.9	62.1	53.7	46.4	37.5	28.4	21.1
1935-------	1962	176.0	152.0	129.6	105.1	87.3	71.8	61.4	53.1	45.2	35.3	27.0	19.2
1936-------	1963	168.9	144.5	121.9	97.3	83.4	68.0	62.4	53.7	42.3	33.1	24.3	
1937-------	1964	165.7	137.9	112.5	94.2	78.7	70.3	62.4	51.4	38.9	31.0		
1938-------	1965	156.3	124.1	106.3	88.5	81.5	72.8	60.4	44.7	37.1			
1939-------	1966	141.0	117.5	98.8	90.6	83.0	70.0	53.0	43.5				
1940-------	1967	131.3	106.3	99.9	91.9	78.4	60.6	47.9					
1941-------	1968	115.5	107.1	102.8	89.1	68.5	54.3						
1942-------	1969	117.0	110.7	97.9	74.7	61.6							
1943-------	1970	122.7	107.0	82.1	68.6								
1944-------	1971	116.5	90.0	76.5									
1945-------	1972	99.4	83.9										
1946-------	1973	92.5											

TABLE 10C. BIRTH PROBABILITIES FOR ALL OTHER WOMEN FOR EACH YEAR 1917-73 BY AGE AND PARITY FOR EACH COHORT FROM 1868 TO 1958--CON.

(PROBABILITIES ARE THE NUMBER OF BIRTHS PER 1,000 WOMEN IN SPECIFIED PARITY AND EXACT AGE GROUP. FIGURES FOR "0 PARITY" SHOW THE PROBABILITY OF FIRST BIRTHS TO "0 PARITY" WOMEN, THOSE FOR "1 PARITY" SHOW THE PROBABILITY OF SECOND BIRTHS TO "1 PARITY" WOMEN, ETC. BASED ON CENTRAL BIRTH RATES AND PARITY DISTRIBUTIONS)

PARITY AND COHORT	DIAGONAL LINE FOR JANUARY 1	EXACT AGE										
		39	40	41	42	43	44	45	46	47	48	49
2 PARITY--CON.												
1868----------------												1.2
1869----------------											2.3	2.3
1870----------------										4.5	4.5	1.1
1871----------------									7.7	7.7	2.2	1.1
1872----------------								7.6	14.0	3.3	3.3	1.1
1873----------------							6.3	13.7	5.3	5.3	1.1	1.1
1874----------------						5.2	10.4	6.2	8.3	3.1	1.0	1.0
1875----------------					7.1	8.1	5.1	9.2	5.1	3.1	1.0	1.0
1876----------------				12.0	11.1	6.0	8.0	6.0	5.0	2.0	2.0	1.0
1877----------------			17.9	18.9	7.0	8.0	6.0	6.0	4.0	3.0	2.0	2.0
1878----------------	1917	31.4	25.6	12.9	9.9	7.9	6.0	5.0	6.0	2.0	3.0	0.0
1879----------------	1918	39.1	20.7	18.8	10.9	7.0	5.0	7.0	5.0	4.0	1.0	1.0
1880----------------	1919	35.3	27.6	20.9	10.0	8.0	6.0	6.0	5.0	1.0	1.0	1.0
1881----------------	1920	44.2	27.8	19.0	11.0	7.0	7.0	6.1	4.1	2.0	1.0	0.0
1882----------------	1921	41.2	26.7	19.9	10.0	7.0	6.0	4.0	2.0	1.0	0.0	1.0
1883----------------	1922	38.7	25.4	16.7	9.9	6.0	5.0	2.0	3.0	1.0	2.0	1.0
1884----------------	1923	36.9	23.5	14.8	7.9	6.0	3.0	3.0	3.0	2.0	2.0	1.0
1885----------------	1924	34.4	24.2	12.7	7.8	3.9	3.0	3.9	3.0	1.0	1.0	1.0
1886----------------	1925	33.9	19.1	11.5	4.8	3.9	2.9	1.9	1.9	1.0	1.9	1.0
1887----------------	1926	27.6	15.8	8.4	5.6	2.8	2.8	1.9	1.9	1.9	0.9	0.9
1888----------------	1927	24.0	13.0	9.3	4.7	2.8	2.8	1.9	1.9	0.9	0.9	0.0
1889----------------	1928	21.5	14.1	9.4	3.8	3.8	2.8	1.9	0.9	0.9	0.9	0.9
1890----------------	1929	20.0	13.7	6.4	4.6	3.7	2.8	1.8	1.8	0.9	0.9	0.9
1891----------------	1930	19.1	9.6	7.9	4.4	3.5	1.8	1.8	0.9	0.9	0.9	0.9
1892----------------	1931	15.4	10.5	7.3	4.1	3.3	2.5	1.6	0.8	0.8	0.8	0.8
1893----------------	1932	19.1	11.5	7.7	4.8	2.9	1.9	1.0	1.0	1.0	1.0	0.0
1894----------------	1933	17.0	10.8	7.2	3.6	3.6	1.8	0.9	0.9	0.9	0.9	0.0
1895----------------	1934	15.6	10.5	6.1	3.5	1.8	1.8	0.9	0.9	0.9	0.0	0.0
1896----------------	1935	15.4	9.5	6.0	3.5	1.7	1.7	0.9	0.9	0.0	0.9	0.0
1897----------------	1936	15.3	8.6	6.0	3.4	1.7	1.7	1.7	0.9	0.9	0.9	0.0
1898----------------	1937	14.5	10.3	6.0	3.5	1.7	2.6	1.7	0.9	0.9	0.9	0.9
1899----------------	1938	16.7	10.6	6.2	3.5	2.7	1.8	1.8	0.9	0.9	0.9	0.9
1900----------------	1939	16.9	10.7	7.2	3.6	2.7	2.7	1.8	1.8	0.9	0.9	0.9
1901----------------	1940	15.5	10.4	6.9	3.5	3.5	2.6	1.7	0.9	0.9	0.9	0.0
1902----------------	1941	15.1	10.1	6.7	4.2	3.4	1.7	0.8	0.8	0.8	0.0	0.8
1903----------------	1942	16.4	10.7	7.4	5.0	3.3	2.5	1.7	0.8	0.0	0.8	0.0
1904----------------	1943	18.4	11.8	8.4	5.1	4.2	2.5	1.7	0.8	0.8	0.0	0.0
1905----------------	1944	20.4	13.6	7.7	6.8	4.3	2.6	1.7	0.9	0.0	0.9	0.0
1906----------------	1945	20.7	12.1	10.4	7.0	4.4	2.6	1.7	0.9	0.9	0.0	0.0
1907----------------	1946	20.8	15.6	10.4	7.0	4.4	2.6	1.7	1.7	0.0	0.9	0.0
1908----------------	1947	23.4	15.7	10.5	6.1	5.2	2.6	1.7	0.9	0.9	0.9	0.0
1909----------------	1948	25.1	16.5	11.3	8.7	6.1	3.5	0.9	0.9	0.9	0.0	0.0
1910----------------	1949	25.8	18.1	13.8	9.5	6.1	2.6	2.6	0.9	0.9	0.9	0.0
1911----------------	1950	29.1	19.8	14.6	9.5	6.0	4.3	1.7	0.9	0.9	0.0	0.0
1912----------------	1951	28.8	20.4	14.5	10.2	6.8	2.6	1.7	0.9	0.0	0.0	0.0
1913----------------	1952	32.9	21.3	16.2	9.4	6.0	3.4	1.7	0.9	0.0	0.0	0.0
1914----------------	1953	31.9	22.8	15.2	10.2	7.7	3.4	1.7	1.7	0.0	0.0	0.0
1915----------------	1954	31.5	23.1	16.3	10.3	5.2	3.5	2.6	0.9	0.0	0.0	0.0
1916----------------	1955	33.2	24.0	15.5	8.6	6.1	4.3	1.7	0.9	0.0	0.0	0.0
1917----------------	1956	34.3	21.9	13.5	11.0	5.9	3.4	1.7	0.9	0.0	0.0	0.0
1918----------------	1957	31.0	20.5	15.7	9.1	6.7	2.5	1.7	0.8	0.0	0.0	0.0
1919----------------	1958	29.8	22.9	14.3	10.4	4.8	3.2	1.6	0.8	0.8	0.0	0.0
1920----------------	1959	30.5	20.8	15.5	7.8	5.5	3.1	1.6	0.8	0.0	0.0	0.0
1921----------------	1960	29.0	21.8	13.6	8.4	6.1	3.1	1.5	0.8	0.0	0.0	0.0
1922----------------	1961	29.2	19.7	12.2	9.1	4.6	3.1	2.3	0.8	0.8	0.0	0.0
1923----------------	1962	28.4	18.1	12.9	7.6	5.3	3.8	1.5	0.8	0.0	0.0	0.0
1924----------------	1963	25.2	19.4	11.3	7.5	5.3	2.3	1.5	0.8	0.8	0.0	0.0
1925----------------	1964	26.0	16.8	11.7	7.3	4.4	2.9	1.5	0.7	0.0	0.0	
1926----------------	1965	23.8	16.7	11.7	6.6	4.4	2.2	1.5	0.7	0.0		
1927----------------	1966	22.1	17.1	9.0	6.0	3.7	1.5	0.7	0.7			
1928----------------	1967	25.3	13.9	10.1	6.2	3.1	2.3	0.8				
1929----------------	1968	19.5	14.9	9.4	4.7	3.1	1.6					
1930----------------	1969	20.3	12.6	8.7	5.5	2.4						
1931----------------	1970	18.9	13.7	8.4	5.3							
1932----------------	1971	18.4	12.6	7.4								
1933----------------	1972	16.1	10.5									
1934----------------	1973	14.4										

TABLE 10C. BIRTH PROBABILITIES FOR ALL OTHER WOMEN FOR EACH YEAR 1917-73 BY AGE AND PARITY FOR EACH COHORT FROM 1868 TO 1958--CON.

(PROBABILITIES ARE THE NUMBER OF BIRTHS PER 1,000 WOMEN IN SPECIFIED PARITY AND EXACT AGE GROUP. FIGURES FOR "0 PARITY" SHOW THE PROBABILITY OF FIRST BIRTHS TO "0 PARITY" WOMEN, THOSE FOR "1 PARITY" SHOW THE PROBABILITY OF SECOND BIRTHS TO "1 PARITY" WOMEN, ETC. BASED ON CENTRAL BIRTH RATES AND PARITY DISTRIBUTIONS)

PARITY AND COHORT	DIAGONAL LINE FOR JANUARY 1	EXACT AGE 15	16	17	18	19	20	21	22	23	24	25	26
3 PARITY													
1891-------													228.6
1892-------												268.4	216.4
1893-------											266.9	240.7	202.0
1894-------										289.7	273.7	242.5	227.7
1895-------									280.1	308.9	271.1	266.3	240.3
1896-------								296.0	304.7	299.0	291.8	290.7	225.8
1897-------							289.5	325.8	294.9	312.8	326.4	275.5	227.5
1898-------						*	322.0	318.7	313.8	361.0	313.5	286.5	254.3
1899-------					*	*	315.3	333.3	355.1	342.0	320.6	304.4	265.6
1900-------				*	*	*	326.4	376.4	332.2	356.8	339.4	306.5	269.5
1901-------			*	*	*	*	365.1	342.3	340.8	366.6	337.0	304.1	247.9
1902-------	1917	*	*	*	*	*	338.2	359.0	355.4	355.4	328.3	276.2	229.7
1903-------	1918	*	*	*	*	*	363.2	367.6	353.2	355.3	310.6	261.4	223.3
1904-------	1919	*	*	*	*	*	359.8	373.5	367.5	341.4	299.8	261.0	222.9
1905-------	1920	*	*	*	*	*	373.9	386.0	357.8	326.4	295.6	264.7	231.7
1906-------	1921	*	*	*	*	*	391.9	368.3	336.2	315.1	303.1	266.2	245.4
1907-------	1922	*	*	*	*	*	368.2	347.7	319.5	332.4	297.8	277.3	235.3
1908-------	1923	*	*	*	*	415.8	352.2	331.6	329.3	314.9	303.9	270.5	244.7
1909-------	1924	*	*	*	*	432.7	339.2	337.7	321.1	322.7	303.4	281.2	238.3
1910-------	1925	*	*	*	*	394.2	327.4	328.2	325.7	319.2	308.1	272.4	234.0
1911-------	1926	*	*	*	*	405.9	340.9	346.5	321.1	337.9	312.0	271.7	239.3
1912-------	1927	*	*	*	*	*	347.4	323.7	340.5	340.3	302.8	280.3	242.6
1913-------	1928	*	*	*	*	*	333.3	359.7	357.7	335.7	321.3	284.4	243.2
1914-------	1929	*	*	*	*	*	361.0	374.3	351.7	356.9	326.3	284.7	245.7
1915-------	1930	*	*	*	*	*	371.4	364.6	363.1	350.7	317.2	289.9	239.7
1916-------	1931	*	*	*	*	*	368.7	366.8	351.5	341.4	334.5	287.1	239.6
1917-------	1932	*	*	*	*	*	360.4	352.5	338.4	371.7	334.5	280.3	249.2
1918-------	1933	*	*	*	*	403.8	350.2	338.1	374.6	373.5	324.5	291.3	249.2
1919-------	1934	*	*	*	*	409.1	336.0	372.1	367.7	356.3	326.2	286.2	237.4
1920-------	1935	*	*	*	*	394.7	387.6	348.0	364.8	355.4	323.0	270.0	249.5
1921-------	1936	*	*	*	*	460.9	343.5	356.1	349.9	344.5	294.6	275.6	243.2
1922-------	1937	*	*	*	*	388.2	355.1	349.4	345.6	309.8	299.9	268.1	238.6
1923-------	1938	*	*	*	*	397.6	354.2	348.3	316.1	321.0	294.6	272.2	247.2
1924-------	1939	*	*	*	*	401.2	357.6	326.5	333.3	320.4	309.7	283.1	263.1
1925-------	1940	*	*	*	*	389.2	331.4	339.0	331.0	337.1	317.8	291.9	272.0
1926-------	1941	*	*	*	*	369.8	347.1	346.4	349.3	343.7	321.9	299.4	271.3
1927-------	1942	*	*	*	*	371.6	360.2	366.4	362.3	342.2	332.3	301.7	270.1
1928-------	1943	*	*	*	*	395.7	381.5	376.0	355.7	356.8	329.2	299.6	273.5
1929-------	1944	*	*	*	*	412.1	390.5	368.8	369.6	356.6	335.3	305.1	271.8
1930-------	1945	*	*	*	*	401.8	373.9	373.9	368.1	352.1	332.1	298.1	269.8
1931-------	1946	*	*	*	*	396.2	374.3	380.6	366.6	353.7	330.2	304.1	266.0
1932-------	1947	*	*	*	393.2	395.1	388.1	372.2	368.9	354.2	335.0	295.2	259.9
1933-------	1948	*	*	*	398.4	419.5	397.5	384.7	378.1	367.4	333.6	294.5	260.8
1934-------	1949	*	*	*	417.9	414.8	403.5	390.5	390.0	359.1	327.1	296.5	251.0
1935-------	1950	*	*	*	428.6	427.2	409.0	408.7	387.8	356.5	327.5	283.2	247.5
1936-------	1951	*	*	*	439.4	427.2	424.9	408.0	385.9	363.6	321.2	279.5	240.4
1937-------	1952	*	*	*	439.4	441.3	433.4	408.3	390.1	352.7	319.0	276.0	232.8
1938-------	1953	*	*	*	469.7	447.9	433.6	417.8	381.8	351.6	312.5	261.1	216.9
1939-------	1954	*	*	*	455.9	454.0	436.6	400.4	385.5	342.3	297.0	249.0	202.2
1940-------	1955	*	*	*	467.6	453.2	422.4	405.0	368.2	323.3	282.2	223.0	175.0
1941-------	1956	*	*	*	464.3	444.4	434.3	394.3	359.1	313.9	256.6	203.7	160.6
1942-------	1957	*	*	*	461.0	448.9	421.0	385.8	344.6	283.9	229.5	181.0	147.3
1943-------	1958	*	*	*	474.1	436.3	412.8	368.9	317.6	254.7	202.2	166.3	144.3
1944-------	1959	*	*	*	449.3	431.3	399.6	342.9	278.9	220.4	185.5	161.9	148.7
1945-------	1960	*	*	*	420.3	405.2	366.7	301.7	246.0	207.3	182.7	165.5	138.9
1946-------	1961	*	*	*	423.1	394.6	326.8	271.6	230.5	206.0	184.4	155.3	118.2
1947-------	1962	*	*	*	415.4	349.8	309.6	255.8	226.8	206.3	174.0	130.3	105.7
1948-------	1963	*	*	*	363.6	323.1	271.5	246.0	228.9	190.7	145.4	116.5	
1949-------	1964	*	*	*	357.8	292.4	266.8	250.9	208.4	165.5	133.2		
1950-------	1965	*	*	*	306.9	291.1	276.4	228.2	187.7	151.2			
1951-------	1966	*	*	*	*	286.4	247.9	204.5	170.5				
1952-------	1967	*	*	*	*	273.2	221.5	193.0					
1953-------	1968	*	*	*	*	231.2	211.9						
1954-------	1969	*	*	*	*	234.2							
1955-------	1970	*	*	*	*								
1956-------	1971	*	*	*									
1957-------	1972	*	*										
1958-------	1973	*											

TABLE 10C. BIRTH PROBABILITIES FOR ALL OTHER WOMEN FOR EACH YEAR 1917-73 BY AGE AND PARITY FOR EACH COHORT FROM 1868 TO 1958--CON.

(PROBABILITIES ARE THE NUMBER OF BIRTHS PER 1,000 WOMEN IN SPECIFIED PARITY AND EXACT AGE GROUP. FIGURES FOR "0 PARITY" SHOW THE PROBABILITY OF FIRST BIRTHS TO "0 PARITY" WOMEN, THOSE FOR "1 PARITY" SHOW THE PROBABILITY OF SECOND BIRTHS TO "1 PARITY" WOMEN, ETC. BASED ON CENTRAL BIRTH RATES AND PARITY DISTRIBUTIONS)

PARITY AND COHORT	DIAGONAL LINE FOR JANUARY 1	EXACT AGE											
		27	28	29	30	31	32	33	34	35	36	37	38
3 PARITY--CON.													
1879-------													60.5
1880-------												71.7	62.8
1881-------											89.9	74.7	65.6
1882-------										99.7	93.0	77.6	71.2
1883-------									96.7	97.0	92.0	79.0	62.7
1884-------								92.3	94.6	95.4	92.0	69.4	54.9
1885-------							92.3	90.6	94.4	97.4	83.3	62.9	50.0
1886-------						126.0	95.3	95.9	100.1	95.2	78.9	59.9	51.3
1887-------					152.0	133.7	102.3	102.2	102.4	92.5	77.6	63.6	53.4
1888-------				195.8	150.4	136.6	104.5	103.0	95.6	88.2	77.4	65.5	53.7
1889-------			193.6	178.7	144.5	130.5	99.3	91.9	87.6	83.5	70.5	58.9	42.1
1890-------	1917	213.4	178.7	175.3	145.6	127.9	91.1	88.2	85.9	73.0	65.6	48.3	35.9
1891-------	1918	199.3	178.3	184.6	146.5	119.8	88.9	89.6	75.4	74.3	56.4	43.0	32.0
1892-------	1919	201.0	193.3	187.2	135.5	118.1	91.4	84.4	79.5	62.2	46.9	38.8	32.2
1893-------	1920	204.0	183.6	159.7	123.3	112.6	84.7	81.3	63.4	48.8	41.5	33.9	28.6
1894-------	1921	213.8	170.2	159.8	132.2	114.3	87.2	72.4	56.9	52.0	40.5	34.3	28.8
1895-------	1922	199.5	170.7	174.2	132.3	114.3	79.0	65.5	59.8	49.0	42.1	33.2	27.4
1896-------	1923	202.1	190.0	177.8	134.2	106.7	71.6	67.5	55.6	50.9	40.0	34.9	27.1
1897-------	1924	222.8	199.0	175.5	124.9	97.3	70.9	63.0	58.3	49.0	40.3	35.0	27.7
1898-------	1925	235.4	198.5	169.4	119.0	98.3	73.2	68.5	59.8	50.0	43.7	35.1	28.3
1899-------	1926	240.4	192.3	162.6	118.5	103.8	78.8	75.2	62.3	57.1	45.4	39.5	30.5
1900-------	1927	226.6	180.7	157.3	127.4	106.8	86.0	76.3	69.1	57.4	50.5	41.4	37.3
1901-------	1928	207.9	170.1	160.5	124.0	110.1	82.5	78.6	66.7	60.1	48.9	43.8	36.4
1902-------	1929	194.5	171.5	160.0	124.1	105.4	81.5	76.1	64.1	53.7	48.3	43.0	35.3
1903-------	1930	195.1	174.7	160.5	122.1	103.0	82.5	69.4	60.0	54.7	48.1	41.5	34.8
1904-------	1931	205.1	181.4	164.0	126.5	109.5	76.9	70.8	63.1	56.5	48.5	41.7	37.0
1905-------	1932	212.5	179.7	167.8	126.4	102.2	79.0	75.2	66.3	55.9	48.8	45.3	40.6
1906-------	1933	210.8	190.6	165.9	126.5	108.8	86.0	80.9	66.7	58.2	54.5	49.9	44.9
1907-------	1934	221.2	181.6	163.3	128.0	112.4	90.3	80.1	70.6	68.4	58.6	55.0	47.2
1908-------	1935	210.0	178.3	164.3	130.5	114.5	88.6	84.5	81.5	73.2	63.1	58.1	47.6
1909-------	1936	210.4	180.7	170.6	133.6	113.1	93.4	93.0	87.6	78.0	69.4	61.9	49.9
1910-------	1937	210.6	188.9	168.8	131.1	117.9	97.0	100.4	91.3	80.7	71.0	62.0	52.8
1911-------	1938	218.8	189.4	169.6	135.5	114.4	105.3	104.9	90.8	83.8	76.3	63.6	54.6
1912-------	1939	219.2	192.3	172.9	138.8	124.5	111.5	103.8	95.4	89.7	73.5	65.7	58.1
1913-------	1940	222.7	193.9	168.5	147.2	130.7	111.7	113.6	100.8	88.7	76.0	70.9	62.2
1914-------	1941	222.7	191.4	177.3	150.9	134.5	123.9	112.5	100.4	89.0	83.7	76.7	63.3
1915-------	1942	212.1	194.6	174.7	145.0	137.7	114.8	109.8	97.7	93.5	81.2	71.7	61.5
1916-------	1943	221.1	194.4	171.3	150.0	134.4	114.6	110.4	104.0	94.2	83.8	73.4	65.6
1917-------	1944	220.2	183.9	175.1	150.9	136.1	118.9	115.8	103.8	92.8	82.3	74.8	63.1
1918-------	1945	210.8	194.6	183.3	157.1	143.3	127.0	123.0	109.3	97.7	87.2	75.6	60.1
1919-------	1946	224.1	203.8	194.6	162.5	148.9	135.2	129.9	113.5	103.6	89.8	74.0	65.1
1920-------	1947	228.5	210.8	193.7	166.8	159.8	143.0	129.4	117.2	102.0	86.7	79.4	59.3
1921-------	1948	226.9	203.8	190.8	172.8	156.5	136.3	129.1	114.4	99.4	86.2	68.0	54.2
1922-------	1949	224.1	208.2	197.9	170.8	154.8	137.9	126.2	109.9	96.3	76.2	62.8	53.9
1923-------	1950	234.5	218.9	199.3	175.4	162.2	139.4	128.0	110.3	90.6	74.1	66.4	53.5
1924-------	1951	246.4	222.4	207.2	182.6	161.0	138.7	126.6	102.1	87.0	74.7	65.0	50.0
1925-------	1952	248.2	227.6	211.9	180.1	160.5	138.7	118.4	99.3	87.5	75.9	60.6	45.6
1926-------	1953	249.4	229.3	206.9	175.6	155.3	129.7	110.4	96.5	85.5	66.1	50.9	41.3
1927-------	1954	254.4	225.4	205.7	171.9	151.3	123.2	110.1	97.8	77.4	60.0	53.1	38.7
1928-------	1955	247.8	221.8	194.3	165.0	143.5	120.3	109.8	90.1	70.2	59.4	45.3	34.9
1929-------	1956	250.4	217.6	190.0	166.8	142.4	126.4	107.2	84.2	72.9	56.5	44.7	34.3
1930-------	1957	239.5	205.4	189.2	154.6	139.7	114.3	97.6	78.5	65.1	50.0	40.8	28.3
1931-------	1958	233.6	206.8	173.9	157.0	127.8	109.5	92.9	74.3	56.7	46.2	33.5	28.9
1932-------	1959	232.1	191.1	175.1	139.8	124.1	98.8	84.5	62.8	51.9	39.9	34.1	27.6
1933-------	1960	222.7	200.3	166.6	139.8	117.0	95.0	74.6	62.0	48.9	40.4	34.8	24.2
1934-------	1961	221.7	186.8	157.0	129.3	107.3	83.8	71.3	54.8	47.4	39.9	29.8	23.1
1935-------	1962	213.1	177.0	151.0	118.9	98.2	82.5	63.3	54.7	47.4	36.9	28.4	19.2
1936-------	1963	201.3	169.8	139.5	110.8	89.4	70.6	62.7	54.8	44.5	32.9	23.9	
1937-------	1964	193.3	159.6	124.0	98.9	80.6	70.7	62.9	51.3	36.7	29.0		
1938-------	1965	179.7	134.1	110.6	89.0	82.1	72.3	57.0	41.9	35.0			
1939-------	1966	153.0	125.2	102.9	91.6	82.2	66.2	48.1	40.0				
1940-------	1967	142.3	114.9	104.6	93.0	77.9	56.3	45.7					
1941-------	1968	132.9	116.4	105.8	90.9	64.9	51.6						
1942-------	1969	130.4	119.8	102.9	76.0	59.4							
1943-------	1970	135.4	113.0	86.6	67.5								
1944-------	1971	124.3	96.7	76.8									
1945-------	1972	106.8	85.2										
1946-------	1973	95.1											

TABLE 10C. BIRTH PROBABILITIES FOR ALL OTHER WOMEN FOR EACH YEAR 1917-73 BY AGE AND PARITY FOR EACH COHORT FROM 1868 TO 1958--CON.

(PROBABILITIES ARE THE NUMBER OF BIRTHS PER 1,000 WOMEN IN SPECIFIED PARITY AND EXACT AGE GROUP. FIGURES FOR "0 PARITY" SHOW THE PROBABILITY OF FIRST BIRTHS TO "0 PARITY" WOMEN, THOSE FOR "1 PARITY" SHOW THE PROBABILITY OF SECOND BIRTHS TO "1 PARITY" WOMEN, ETC. BASED ON CENTRAL BIRTH RATES AND PARITY DISTRIBUTIONS)

PARITY AND COHORT	DIAGONAL LINE FOR JANUARY 1	EXACT AGE										
		39	40	41	42	43	44	45	46	47	48	49
3 PARITY--CON.												
1868												2.6
1869											5.1	6.4
1870										5.1	11.4	1.3
1871									8.7	12.5	3.8	2.5
1872								8.6	22.1	3.7	4.9	2.5
1873							10.9	19.4	7.3	4.9	3.6	1.2
1874						11.9	19.1	7.2	9.6	3.6	2.4	1.2
1875					14.0	10.6	9.4	10.6	8.3	2.4	2.4	1.2
1876				24.1	12.7	9.3	11.6	9.3	5.8	2.3	3.5	1.2
1877			34.8	22.8	12.6	11.5	10.3	6.9	5.8	3.5	2.3	2.3
1878	1917	52.9	34.8	22.5	14.8	12.5	8.0	6.9	6.9	3.4	3.4	0.0
1879	1918	53.6	35.3	27.9	15.7	9.0	7.9	7.9	5.7	4.5	1.1	1.1
1880	1919	55.7	41.4	28.7	11.1	10.0	10.0	6.7	7.8	2.2	1.1	1.1
1881	1920	62.2	40.7	21.6	11.9	11.9	6.5	9.8	5.5	2.2	2.2	1.1
1882	1921	59.4	33.9	22.3	14.9	8.6	10.7	7.5	5.4	2.2	2.2	0.0
1883	1922	49.6	32.1	26.2	14.2	10.2	8.2	6.2	4.1	2.1	1.0	2.1
1884	1923	45.8	33.7	23.3	9.8	9.8	6.9	4.0	4.0	1.0	3.0	2.0
1885	1924	46.5	30.7	17.4	10.7	6.8	4.9	4.9	3.9	2.0	2.0	1.0
1886	1925	43.7	27.0	16.1	9.1	6.1	5.1	4.1	3.1	2.0	1.0	1.0
1887	1926	45.4	23.6	15.1	7.6	6.5	5.4	3.3	3.3	2.2	1.1	2.2
1888	1927	36.3	19.4	14.1	7.6	5.4	5.5	4.4	3.3	1.1	2.2	0.0
1889	1928	32.6	18.9	14.0	7.0	6.0	5.1	4.0	3.0	2.0	1.0	1.0
1890	1929	29.8	19.7	12.3	6.6	4.8	4.8	2.9	1.9	1.0	1.0	1.0
1891	1930	29.6	17.2	10.0	6.4	5.5	3.7	2.8	1.8	0.9	0.9	0.9
1892	1931	27.3	16.9	11.6	7.2	4.5	3.6	2.7	1.8	0.9	0.9	0.9
1893	1932	24.1	15.4	9.8	5.7	4.1	3.3	1.6	1.6	0.8	0.8	0.8
1894	1933	24.1	14.2	10.1	5.9	4.2	2.5	1.7	1.7	0.8	0.8	0.0
1895	1934	22.5	13.9	8.7	6.1	3.5	1.8	1.8	0.9	0.9	0.0	0.0
1896	1935	21.9	12.8	10.1	5.5	3.7	2.8	1.9	1.9	0.0	0.0	0.9
1897	1936	22.1	14.5	8.7	4.9	3.9	2.9	2.9	1.0	0.0	1.0	1.0
1898	1937	23.4	15.4	9.2	6.2	4.1	4.1	3.1	1.0	1.0	1.0	0.0
1899	1938	27.5	14.9	10.7	6.4	6.4	4.3	2.2	2.2	1.1	1.1	0.0
1900	1939	27.7	16.8	12.3	7.9	7.9	4.5	3.4	2.3	1.1	0.0	1.1
1901	1940	27.6	17.3	11.6	9.3	8.2	4.7	3.5	1.2	1.2	1.2	0.0
1902	1941	28.5	17.9	14.4	9.6	6.0	4.8	2.4	1.2	1.2	0.0	0.0
1903	1942	29.0	19.4	14.6	9.8	7.4	4.9	2.5	1.2	1.2	0.0	0.0
1904	1943	31.1	21.2	16.3	11.3	7.6	3.8	2.5	2.5	0.0	1.3	0.0
1905	1944	33.2	24.3	16.7	11.6	7.8	5.2	3.9	1.3	0.0	0.0	1.3
1906	1945	38.5	26.7	18.8	12.1	9.5	6.8	4.1	1.4	1.4	1.4	0.0
1907	1946	39.3	27.3	20.5	12.4	9.6	6.9	2.8	1.4	1.4	1.4	0.0
1908	1947	38.3	27.4	19.2	12.4	11.0	4.1	2.8	2.8	1.4	0.0	0.0
1909	1948	43.2	29.8	19.0	15.0	9.5	6.8	4.1	2.7	0.0	0.0	1.4
1910	1949	43.7	29.2	23.9	13.3	10.7	6.7	4.0	1.3	0.0	1.3	0.0
1911	1950	44.3	32.6	24.8	15.7	13.1	7.9	2.6	1.3	1.3	0.0	0.0
1912	1951	49.1	37.7	24.8	19.7	11.8	6.6	4.0	1.3	1.3	0.0	0.0
1913	1952	49.7	35.7	29.4	18.0	10.3	5.2	2.6	2.6	0.0	0.0	0.0
1914	1953	52.2	41.3	26.4	16.4	11.4	5.1	5.1	1.3	0.0	0.0	0.0
1915	1954	54.7	37.6	23.7	16.6	9.5	7.1	3.6	1.2	1.2	0.0	0.0
1916	1955	51.3	34.4	24.2	16.2	10.4	5.8	3.5	1.2	0.0	0.0	0.0
1917	1956	47.1	33.0	25.4	14.5	8.9	6.7	3.3	1.1	1.1	0.0	0.0
1918	1957	48.4	34.7	23.0	16.4	11.0	4.4	2.2	1.1	0.0	0.0	0.0
1919	1958	49.1	34.8	24.3	17.0	9.6	5.4	2.1	1.1	0.0	1.1	0.0
1920	1959	47.5	33.6	23.5	14.4	9.3	4.1	3.1	1.0	1.0	0.0	0.0
1921	1960	43.9	30.7	22.2	14.5	7.8	4.9	2.9	1.0	0.0	0.0	0.0
1922	1961	41.4	28.7	20.5	12.2	8.4	4.7	1.9	0.9	0.9	0.0	0.0
1923	1962	40.3	30.4	20.4	13.0	7.5	3.7	2.8	0.9	0.0	0.0	0.0
1924	1963	38.0	26.7	18.8	11.7	6.3	3.6	1.8	0.9	0.0	0.0	0.0
1925	1964	36.3	25.2	17.5	10.5	6.2	3.5	1.8	0.9	0.0	0.0	
1926	1965	32.3	21.6	13.4	9.2	5.9	3.3	1.7	0.8	0.0		
1927	1966	28.9	19.1	14.1	9.2	5.9	3.4	1.7	0.8			
1928	1967	26.1	18.7	13.9	9.0	4.1	2.5	0.8				
1929	1968	24.6	19.7	14.0	8.3	4.2	1.7					
1930	1969	26.0	17.4	11.1	6.4	3.2						
1931	1970	23.7	16.1	9.2	5.4							
1932	1971	19.7	13.1	8.0								
1933	1972	17.8	11.4									
1934	1973	15.0										

TABLE 10C. BIRTH PROBABILITIES FOR ALL OTHER WOMEN FOR EACH YEAR 1917-73 BY AGE AND PARITY FOR EACH COHORT FROM 1868 TO 1958--CON.

(PROBABILITIES ARE THE NUMBER OF BIRTHS PER 1,000 WOMEN IN SPECIFIED PARITY AND EXACT AGE GROUP. FIGURES FOR "0 PARITY" SHOW THE PROBABILITY OF FIRST BIRTHS TO "C PARITY" WOMEN, THOSE FOR "1 PARITY" SHOW THE PROBABILITY OF SECOND BIRTHS TO "1 PARITY" WOMEN, ETC. BASED ON CENTRAL BIRTH RATES AND PARITY DISTRIBUTIONS)

PARITY AND COHORT	DIAGONAL LINE FOR JANUARY 1	EXACT AGE											
		15	16	17	18	19	20	21	22	23	24	25	26
4 PARITY													
1891-------													234.0
1892-------												268.8	224.9
1893-------											268.5	243.3	238.1
1894-------										285.4	272.7	276.8	259.3
1895-------									276.4	300.8	306.4	299.5	285.5
1896-------								291.3	299.5	331.4	332.7	337.0	272.2
1897-------							*	315.3	326.8	347.8	375.3	322.1	282.8
1898-------						*	*	355.8	347.4	398.7	361.9	337.7	314.9
1899-------					*	*	*	*	395.6	394.3	381.2	366.7	304.3
1900-------				*	*	*	*	*	386.2	421.7	408.6	350.3	308.0
1901-------			*	*	*	*	*	*	404.4	443.0	384.9	345.6	304.5
1902-------	1917	*	*	*	*	*	*	*	429.3	398.1	362.9	334.4	277.7
1903-------	1918	*	*	*	*	*	*	432.7	376.2	370.4	349.6	299.7	278.2
1904-------	1919	*	*	*	*	*	*	407.1	382.9	366.4	334.0	312.4	272.7
1905-------	1920	*	*	*	*	*	*	414.6	362.8	355.9	343.1	309.6	277.5
1906-------	1921	*	*	*	*	*	*	398.4	371.0	366.1	351.9	309.8	288.5
1907-------	1922	*	*	*	*	*	*	416.0	361.9	366.8	331.8	310.8	279.3
1908-------	1923	*	*	*	*	*	*	377.0	367.1	343.8	328.8	302.8	286.4
1909-------	1924	*	*	*	*	*	*	374.0	343.0	332.3	319.1	312.9	273.7
1910-------	1925	*	*	*	*	*	*	373.9	350.0	339.7	337.9	308.0	280.3
1911-------	1926	*	*	*	*	*	*	370.7	341.5	355.3	334.8	300.2	283.5
1912-------	1927	*	*	*	*	*	*	380.5	367.9	365.4	325.1	314.4	288.0
1913-------	1928	*	*	*	*	*	*	378.4	373.1	338.5	335.6	319.5	288.2
1914-------	1929	*	*	*	*	*	*	415.9	374.4	367.9	343.8	324.3	289.9
1915-------	1930	*	*	*	*	*	*	421.1	386.1	371.5	354.0	338.7	294.4
1916-------	1931	*	*	*	*	*	*	418.8	372.0	381.8	376.4	341.5	292.9
1917-------	1932	*	*	*	*	*	*	393.2	382.1	429.4	384.0	332.2	300.8
1918-------	1933	*	*	*	*	*	*	395.2	421.3	434.7	371.9	343.6	299.1
1919-------	1934	*	*	*	*	*	*	448.8	426.1	408.3	378.0	340.6	300.6
1920-------	1935	*	*	*	*	*	*	425.5	422.6	406.4	373.5	321.8	301.9
1921-------	1936	*	*	*	*	*	*	424.1	388.1	386.1	337.1	320.6	286.7
1922-------	1937	*	*	*	*	*	*	398.8	375.4	345.2	333.3	307.2	290.8
1923-------	1938	*	*	*	*	*	346.2	385.0	348.8	350.7	329.0	318.3	295.9
1924-------	1939	*	*	*	*	*	348.6	360.8	347.8	348.1	339.4	324.8	307.3
1925-------	1940	*	*	*	*	*	310.3	360.4	352.0	358.0	349.5	331.0	306.3
1926-------	1941	*	*	*	*	*	316.2	378.8	359.2	370.9	354.7	337.2	315.3
1927-------	1942	*	*	*	*	*	354.0	399.0	383.4	368.2	361.1	336.9	319.4
1928-------	1943	*	*	*	*	*	359.0	418.6	378.2	374.1	351.6	336.3	318.5
1929-------	1944	*	*	*	*	*	378.0	406.8	384.2	371.1	360.6	340.2	310.2
1930-------	1945	*	*	*	*	*	369.6	417.0	386.4	386.7	367.5	344.5	317.4
1931-------	1946	*	*	*	*	*	368.8	408.8	404.5	391.1	375.6	352.4	316.0
1932-------	1947	*	*	*	*	*	367.2	391.4	390.6	388.5	369.0	342.7	307.8
1933-------	1948	*	*	*	*	*	311.2	396.1	389.2	381.2	367.4	338.3	304.3
1934-------	1949	*	*	*	*	*	351.0	405.0	396.0	388.7	368.1	337.3	290.2
1935-------	1950	*	*	*	*	*	366.2	409.7	402.1	389.4	368.9	322.7	291.0
1936-------	1951	*	*	*	*	*	371.6	427.5	403.7	389.0	352.7	320.3	285.4
1937-------	1952	*	*	*	*	*	393.7	434.8	405.4	374.8	352.1	318.2	275.4
1938-------	1953	*	*	*	*	*	386.0	411.5	380.9	368.2	344.9	296.6	253.7
1939-------	1954	*	*	*	*	*	368.6	396.1	386.0	361.7	327.3	284.1	228.0
1940-------	1955	*	*	*	*	*	361.0	407.3	374.2	349.8	316.5	257.2	200.7
1941-------	1956	*	*	*	*	*	369.3	401.9	370.4	335.9	281.6	225.2	174.8
1942-------	1957	*	*	*	*	*	367.1	392.4	343.3	300.5	250.0	193.9	153.9
1943-------	1958	*	*	*	*	*	364.0	371.4	319.8	265.6	220.5	172.8	152.0
1944-------	1959	*	*	*	*	*	337.8	345.1	275.2	236.7	198.2	174.2	159.4
1945-------	1960	*	*	*	*	*	326.9	307.7	264.4	222.4	200.6	183.9	155.7
1946-------	1961	*	*	*	*	*	292.9	282.5	237.0	217.5	197.5	168.0	127.7
1947-------	1962	*	*	*	*	*	269.7	251.8	224.5	206.1	180.6	138.2	109.3
1948-------	1963	*	*	*	*	*	243.4	255.3	215.2	195.1	156.1	125.8	
1949-------	1964	*	*	*	*	*	250.0	251.2	210.7	170.0	139.7		
1950-------	1965	*	*	*	*	*	247.7	239.1	190.3	153.6			
1951-------	1966	*	*	*	*	*	*	207.3	167.4				
1952-------	1967	*	*	*	*	*	*	190.1					
1953-------	1968	*	*	*	*	*	*						
1954-------	1969	*	*	*	*	*							
1955-------	1970	*	*	*	*								
1956-------	1971	*	*	*									
1957-------	1972	*	*										
1958-------	1973	*											

TABLE 10C. BIRTH PROBABILITIES FOR ALL OTHER WOMEN FOR EACH YEAR 1917-73 BY AGE AND PARITY FOR EACH COHORT FROM 1868 TO 1958--CON.

(PROBABILITIES ARE THE NUMBER OF BIRTHS PER 1,000 WOMEN IN SPECIFIED PARITY AND EXACT AGE GROUP. FIGURES FOR "0 PARITY" SHOW THE PROBABILITY OF FIRST BIRTHS TO "0 PARITY" WOMEN, THOSE FOR "1 PARITY" SHOW THE PROBABILITY OF SECOND BIRTHS TO "1 PARITY" WOMEN, ETC. BASED ON CENTRAL BIRTH RATES AND PARITY DISTRIBUTIONS)

PARITY AND COHORT	DIAGONAL LINE FOR JANUARY 1	EXACT AGE											
		27	28	29	30	31	32	33	34	35	36	37	38
4 PARITY--CON.													
1879-------													78.7
1880-------												92.9	75.7
1881-------											116.2	88.7	81.3
1882-------										126.2	110.6	93.8	83.3
1883-------									135.4	124.0	117.4	97.2	81.8
1884-------								126.5	131.5	126.0	116.1	92.0	77.0
1885-------							126.2	123.8	131.0	121.0	109.3	85.8	66.5
1886-------						147.2	121.3	117.8	120.0	114.5	99.5	72.6	67.6
1887-------					151.5	141.6	116.4	105.7	117.9	104.3	84.8	74.0	63.2
1888-------				183.1	145.1	139.3	105.7	110.8	108.8	93.5	87.2	71.0	55.2
1889-------			186.5	173.2	149.9	129.9	113.6	104.2	102.1	96.4	83.6	66.6	55.0
1890-------	1917	213.4	175.7	186.6	147.5	142.0	108.9	105.1	105.9	93.5	84.9	65.0	48.6
1891-------	1918	203.3	197.1	192.4	161.5	138.6	111.9	107.1	103.7	94.7	74.6	59.3	47.7
1892-------	1919	229.1	208.9	209.1	156.0	142.9	114.8	111.5	102.9	86.7	71.7	59.5	54.1
1893-------	1920	230.8	213.6	188.3	151.5	138.2	111.3	100.6	90.1	77.9	66.8	58.0	46.0
1894-------	1921	252.2	202.9	196.4	162.7	142.3	115.3	100.3	87.5	78.0	69.9	54.8	42.8
1895-------	1922	241.3	214.2	217.2	168.2	153.2	112.7	101.6	88.6	84.3	68.7	55.3	45.9
1896-------	1923	254.2	241.1	219.0	177.9	148.8	109.3	98.0	96.9	77.7	71.7	56.6	46.5
1897-------	1924	282.7	239.1	220.0	172.9	144.8	106.8	107.4	91.3	83.1	70.0	60.0	46.9
1898-------	1925	273.0	231.5	221.1	163.9	143.8	114.7	98.6	93.9	81.0	71.3	55.9	45.0
1899-------	1926	275.1	243.6	216.2	174.6	154.6	114.6	115.2	101.3	92.0	74.0	61.7	54.3
1900-------	1927	282.4	234.2	225.7	179.5	150.5	127.7	120.0	107.1	91.8	75.7	66.8	56.4
1901-------	1928	259.3	237.3	225.4	175.4	158.6	125.8	124.5	104.0	90.4	77.3	66.8	51.3
1902-------	1929	261.2	233.0	216.5	178.3	153.6	126.5	111.3	97.1	85.6	75.3	61.4	54.2
1903-------	1930	250.0	224.0	218.3	167.6	153.7	114.5	107.3	96.7	85.5	69.0	66.5	58.2
1904-------	1931	252.8	232.9	222.1	178.4	148.3	113.0	112.2	100.1	84.0	75.7	72.1	59.1
1905-------	1932	260.6	237.0	229.1	178.2	149.6	122.9	119.8	100.8	92.8	83.3	75.0	66.0
1906-------	1933	266.8	247.1	223.4	171.9	153.4	124.2	117.2	106.5	96.1	83.3	77.7	65.1
1907-------	1934	272.3	235.6	215.7	176.4	150.9	122.1	123.6	109.3	97.0	84.9	77.4	67.9
1908-------	1935	254.5	227.5	217.5	169.7	144.2	126.7	121.7	108.3	99.7	82.9	76.9	64.3
1909-------	1936	255.6	232.9	212.6	163.2	150.4	124.6	120.4	110.9	97.8	89.1	77.2	66.5
1910-------	1937	265.1	232.6	209.7	168.6	149.6	128.6	127.3	111.5	105.7	88.2	79.3	67.3
1911-------	1938	263.5	230.7	209.8	168.4	150.6	135.2	129.1	120.7	104.0	92.2	83.1	68.2
1912-------	1939	268.0	234.3	216.8	179.3	163.4	142.9	139.4	118.0	107.3	97.8	84.6	70.9
1913-------	1940	267.2	240.4	217.1	191.0	170.4	147.9	137.1	122.9	113.7	97.4	88.5	76.2
1914-------	1941	275.5	241.8	230.7	196.4	176.7	143.3	138.8	125.4	113.6	102.0	94.2	77.5
1915-------	1942	271.3	254.5	237.0	197.0	172.7	150.6	143.5	128.6	118.2	105.6	92.0	84.3
1916-------	1943	279.9	253.7	229.5	192.6	170.3	149.3	142.2	130.3	122.3	103.3	97.0	85.6
1917-------	1944	276.7	245.3	227.3	188.2	170.9	148.7	147.9	130.6	118.9	107.5	100.7	81.5
1918-------	1945	274.3	248.6	223.6	191.9	174.5	156.4	147.1	136.1	119.6	109.8	96.4	81.8
1919-------	1946	283.0	249.3	233.4	201.1	185.8	163.1	161.0	139.1	133.1	112.5	98.2	83.1
1920-------	1947	275.2	257.2	237.7	204.5	191.0	174.7	161.7	153.6	131.6	115.4	103.4	83.4
1921-------	1948	276.2	251.6	234.7	213.9	197.8	175.3	174.7	148.9	130.6	113.8	97.1	78.4
1922-------	1949	273.8	252.2	242.3	212.7	198.6	178.7	164.1	144.2	125.7	106.1	92.8	70.2
1923-------	1950	281.8	257.0	241.0	213.8	194.7	168.9	158.0	138.2	116.7	97.6	79.5	69.4
1924-------	1951	280.0	262.7	245.7	213.9	192.3	169.4	155.0	129.5	114.8	88.7	80.2	61.6
1925-------	1952	294.0	269.0	251.3	214.1	199.2	172.3	147.1	129.7	105.8	91.7	74.7	57.7
1926-------	1953	298.3	279.3	248.8	217.4	194.4	158.7	148.1	122.9	103.9	86.3	70.1	54.8
1927-------	1954	303.5	267.3	246.5	212.4	179.0	159.0	136.7	113.9	95.9	80.3	63.0	49.7
1928-------	1955	290.0	255.9	235.2	192.8	176.8	145.9	129.5	108.9	87.6	69.9	57.1	45.4
1929-------	1956	288.9	256.2	222.4	196.3	167.0	140.4	125.0	99.3	81.3	67.3	51.6	37.5
1930-------	1957	287.9	247.8	227.3	190.5	167.0	140.6	116.5	96.3	78.0	61.2	47.8	35.2
1931-------	1958	280.1	250.7	220.1	186.9	158.3	131.1	113.7	89.6	69.6	54.8	44.2	34.7
1932-------	1959	279.0	238.9	217.0	175.3	153.0	122.4	102.2	79.1	63.9	51.0	43.4	33.1
1933-------	1960	263.8	235.9	197.7	168.3	139.6	110.7	88.7	70.1	58.6	47.3	37.6	30.2
1934-------	1961	262.9	224.2	192.4	156.6	127.6	99.0	80.0	63.1	55.2	45.0	35.4	24.4
1935-------	1962	252.0	217.4	182.6	142.1	113.3	90.4	70.6	62.0	53.5	40.4	29.7	22.0
1936-------	1963	246.4	204.7	164.6	124.9	103.1	77.5	70.1	61.5	46.9	36.9	27.1	
1937-------	1964	227.5	181.6	141.8	112.2	88.6	78.1	70.1	54.0	42.5	32.0		
1938-------	1965	203.9	154.8	124.2	98.1	87.9	78.5	62.8	49.8	37.1			
1939-------	1966	175.5	136.9	109.1	97.9	87.3	71.3	55.2	43.3				
1940-------	1967	157.1	122.9	111.6	99.8	84.3	62.9	49.8					
1941-------	1968	136.7	122.8	112.1	95.3	69.6	54.3						
1942-------	1969	135.7	126.4	106.3	78.2	61.6							
1943-------	1970	142.9	120.3	89.0	67.1								
1944-------	1971	135.1	99.8	78.4									
1945-------	1972	114.6	87.0										
1946-------	1973	99.2											

TABLE 10C. BIRTH PROBABILITIES FOR ALL OTHER WOMEN FOR EACH YEAR 1917-73 BY AGE AND PARITY FOR EACH COHORT FROM 1868 TO 1958--CON.

(PROBABILITIES ARE THE NUMBER OF BIRTHS PER 1,000 WOMEN IN SPECIFIED PARITY AND EXACT AGE GROUP. FIGURES FOR "0 PARITY" SHOW THE PROBABILITY OF FIRST BIRTHS TO "0 PARITY" WOMEN, THOSE FOR "1 PARITY" SHOW THE PROBABILITY OF SECOND BIRTHS TO "1 PARITY" WOMEN, ETC. BASED ON CENTRAL BIRTH RATES AND PARITY DISTRIBUTIONS)

PARITY AND COHORT	DIAGONAL LINE FOR JANUARY 1	EXACT AGE										
		39	40	41	42	43	44	45	46	47	48	49
4 PARITY--CON.												
1868----------------												2.7
1869----------------											5.3	2.6
1870----------------										6.6	6.6	2.6
1871----------------									11.8	9.2	3.9	2.6
1872----------------								13.1	15.7	5.2	5.2	1.3
1873----------------							14.3	14.4	10.4	7.8	3.9	1.3
1874----------------						15.6	15.7	11.7	13.1	5.2	3.9	2.6
1875----------------					19.4	15.6	13.0	13.1	7.9	5.2	5.2	2.6
1876----------------				31.7	20.4	14.1	14.2	9.0	7.7	6.5	3.9	2.6
1877----------------			44.4	34.7	17.5	15.1	10.1	8.8	11.3	6.3	2.5	1.3
1878----------------	1917	69.7	46.2	31.9	19.8	13.6	9.9	11.2	11.2	2.5	3.8	1.3
1879----------------	1918	69.0	45.7	36.4	18.3	12.2	12.2	11.1	8.6	4.9	2.5	2.5
1880----------------	1919	71.5	49.8	33.3	15.5	13.2	13.2	9.6	7.2	4.8	2.4	2.4
1881----------------	1920	76.3	46.6	29.2	16.5	14.2	13.0	7.1	7.1	4.7	3.6	2.4
1882----------------	1921	72.5	43.4	28.7	17.3	15.0	9.3	8.1	5.8	4.6	2.3	1.2
1883----------------	1922	68.8	41.8	31.5	21.0	12.9	9.4	7.0	5.9	3.5	3.5	2.4
1884----------------	1923	61.9	43.8	25.5	16.2	11.6	8.1	7.0	5.8	3.5	2.3	1.2
1885----------------	1924	64.7	34.4	26.3	14.9	10.4	8.1	6.9	8.1	2.3	1.2	1.2
1886----------------	1925	50.7	34.3	21.1	12.2	7.8	8.9	7.8	4.5	2.3	2.3	2.3
1887----------------	1926	49.9	29.9	20.4	9.7	9.7	7.6	5.4	3.3	2.2	2.2	1.1
1888----------------	1927	46.1	28.0	16.7	11.5	7.4	6.3	4.2	3.2	2.1	1.1	2.1
1889----------------	1928	42.5	24.5	19.5	9.3	8.3	5.2	4.1	3.1	2.1	2.1	1.0
1890----------------	1929	39.8	28.8	17.6	11.4	7.3	6.3	4.2	3.1	1.1	1.1	1.1
1891----------------	1930	47.2	27.1	18.9	9.5	7.4	6.4	4.2	3.2	1.1	2.1	1.1
1892----------------	1931	41.2	25.6	17.1	9.7	7.5	5.4	3.2	1.1	2.2	2.2	1.1
1893----------------	1932	34.3	23.3	15.3	10.2	7.2	5.1	2.1	2.1	2.1	1.0	1.0
1894----------------	1933	36.8	23.3	17.0	9.6	6.4	3.2	3.2	2.1	2.1	1.1	0.0
1895----------------	1934	38.5	26.3	16.1	8.1	4.6	3.5	3.5	2.3	1.2	0.0	1.2
1896----------------	1935	39.8	24.4	13.5	8.6	4.9	3.7	2.5	2.5	1.2	1.2	0.0
1897----------------	1936	38.4	23.3	15.6	9.1	6.5	3.9	3.9	2.6	1.3	1.3	1.3
1898----------------	1937	38.9	27.5	17.2	10.6	6.6	6.7	4.0	2.7	2.7	1.3	0.0
1899----------------	1938	44.1	27.8	19.6	11.3	9.9	7.1	5.7	2.8	1.4	1.4	0.0
1900----------------	1939	42.7	30.1	20.2	11.6	8.7	7.3	4.4	2.9	1.5	1.5	0.0
1901----------------	1940	45.7	31.3	18.0	10.5	10.5	6.0	4.5	3.0	1.5	1.5	1.5
1902----------------	1941	47.1	29.2	18.5	12.4	10.8	7.8	3.1	1.6	1.6	1.6	0.0
1903----------------	1942	46.6	29.8	20.5	15.8	11.1	4.8	3.2	3.2	1.6	1.6	0.0
1904----------------	1943	48.5	32.6	24.5	14.8	9.9	6.6	3.3	1.6	1.6	1.6	0.0
1905----------------	1944	53.1	39.7	24.3	17.4	10.5	7.0	3.5	1.7	1.7	0.0	0.0
1906----------------	1945	56.9	33.0	26.0	15.6	10.4	6.9	3.5	1.7	1.7	0.0	1.7
1907----------------	1946	53.1	37.8	24.1	15.5	12.0	6.9	3.4	1.7	0.0	1.7	0.0
1908----------------	1947	53.1	35.1	26.8	16.8	11.8	5.0	3.4	1.7	1.7	0.0	0.0
1909----------------	1948	54.2	38.4	27.3	17.7	11.3	9.7	3.2	3.2	1.6	0.0	0.0
1910----------------	1949	56.6	37.9	30.1	17.5	15.9	8.0	4.8	3.2	1.6	0.0	0.0
1911----------------	1950	54.4	43.6	28.2	23.4	14.1	7.8	4.7	3.1	0.0	0.0	1.6
1912----------------	1951	63.0	42.7	33.1	22.1	14.2	7.9	6.3	1.6	1.6	1.6	0.0
1913----------------	1952	63.8	46.8	31.3	21.8	17.1	9.4	4.7	3.1	1.6	0.0	0.0
1914----------------	1953	66.9	47.3	33.4	22.8	16.8	7.7	4.6	3.1	0.0	1.5	0.0
1915----------------	1954	68.1	48.3	37.7	24.3	13.7	9.2	4.6	1.5	1.5	1.5	0.0
1916----------------	1955	66.9	50.9	35.2	20.6	16.2	7.4	4.4	3.0	1.5	1.5	0.0
1917----------------	1956	68.8	46.7	32.7	24.2	14.3	7.2	4.3	1.4	1.4	0.0	0.0
1918----------------	1957	64.8	46.1	32.6	23.2	13.7	6.8	4.1	2.7	1.4	0.0	0.0
1919----------------	1958	66.3	45.8	34.1	19.7	14.5	7.9	4.0	2.6	1.3	0.0	0.0
1920----------------	1959	65.1	44.9	28.3	23.1	14.2	7.8	3.9	2.6	1.3	0.0	0.0
1921----------------	1960	59.3	42.1	31.1	19.9	11.2	7.5	3.8	1.3	0.0	1.3	0.0
1922----------------	1961	55.9	38.1	29.8	18.0	12.0	6.0	3.6	1.2	1.2	0.0	0.0
1923----------------	1962	49.8	36.5	26.6	16.6	8.9	4.4	3.3	1.1	1.1	0.0	0.0
1924----------------	1963	46.0	34.6	24.2	14.7	8.4	5.3	2.1	1.1	0.0	0.0	0.0
1925----------------	1964	44.7	31.6	21.4	12.3	7.2	5.1	2.0	1.0	1.0	0.0	
1926----------------	1965	41.0	31.1	17.1	12.1	9.1	4.0	3.0	1.0	0.0		
1927----------------	1966	38.4	23.2	15.5	11.6	6.8	4.8	1.9	1.0			
1928----------------	1967	31.7	20.5	15.8	10.3	5.6	3.7	1.9				
1929----------------	1968	26.8	19.6	15.1	8.0	5.3	2.7					
1930----------------	1969	29.0	21.7	11.8	8.2	4.5						
1931----------------	1970	26.7	16.9	10.7	7.1							
1932----------------	1971	24.4	15.7	10.5								
1933----------------	1972	19.6	13.9									
1934----------------	1973	18.1										

TABLE 10C. BIRTH PROBABILITIES FOR ALL OTHER WOMEN FOR EACH YEAR 1917-73 BY AGE AND PARITY FOR EACH COHORT FROM 1868 TO 1958--CON.

(PROBABILITIES ARE THE NUMBER OF BIRTHS PER 1,000 WOMEN IN SPECIFIED PARITY AND EXACT AGE GROUP. FIGURES FOR "0 PARITY" SHOW THE PROBABILITY OF FIRST BIRTHS TO "0 PARITY" WOMEN, THOSE FOR "1 PARITY" SHOW THE PROBABILITY OF SECOND BIRTHS TO "1 PARITY" WOMEN, ETC. BASED ON CENTRAL BIRTH RATES AND PARITY DISTRIBUTIONS)

PARITY AND COHORT	DIAGONAL LINE FOR JANUARY 1	EXACT AGE											
		15	16	17	18	19	20	21	22	23	24	25	26
5 PARITY													
1891-------													317.0
1892-------												371.0	335.1
1893-------											352.9	350.2	341.1
1894-------										412.7	429.3	419.8	399.4
1895-------									*	*	503.2	473.0	455.4
1896-------								*	*	*	547.3	539.1	440.3
1897-------							*	*	*	*	642.9	526.5	443.0
1898-------						*	*	*	*	*	609.6	521.7	487.4
1899-------					*	*	*	*	*	*	597.3	550.4	461.8
1900-------				*	*	*	*	*	*	*	628.2	520.2	478.9
1901-------			*	*	*	*	*	*	*	*	581.3	544.7	429.9
1902-------	1917	*	*	*	*	*	*	*	*	*	594.9	467.2	369.2
1903-------	1918	*	*	*	*	*	*	*	*	*	503.2	408.6	359.9
1904-------	1919	*	*	*	*	*	*	*	*	*	462.4	405.4	344.0
1905-------	1920	*	*	*	*	*	*	*	*	*	444.4	386.1	356.1
1906-------	1921	*	*	*	*	*	*	*	*	*	431.0	381.3	333.3
1907-------	1922	*	*	*	*	*	*	*	*	460.0	415.2	350.8	326.3
1908-------	1923	*	*	*	*	*	*	*	*	*	386.5	360.7	345.8
1909-------	1924	*	*	*	*	*	*	*	*	*	401.3	385.6	332.3
1910-------	1925	*	*	*	*	*	*	*	*	*	412.9	370.8	339.6
1911-------	1926	*	*	*	*	*	*	*	*	*	427.7	376.0	346.9
1912-------	1927	*	*	*	*	*	*	*	*	*	416.1	395.0	357.6
1913-------	1928	*	*	*	*	*	*	*	*	*	436.7	389.1	352.9
1914-------	1929	*	*	*	*	*	*	*	*	*	417.6	375.5	349.1
1915-------	1930	*	*	*	*	*	*	*	*	465.3	413.8	381.7	340.0
1916-------	1931	*	*	*	*	*	*	*	*	480.0	443.8	380.1	341.6
1917-------	1932	*	*	*	*	*	*	*	*	550.0	441.5	379.8	339.6
1918-------	1933	*	*	*	*	*	*	*	*	566.0	432.2	385.7	346.5
1919-------	1934	*	*	*	*	*	*	*	*	517.2	448.3	392.6	346.4
1920-------	1935	*	*	*	*	*	*	*	*	523.8	438.7	376.6	350.5
1921-------	1936	*	*	*	*	*	*	*	*	492.5	401.8	374.6	338.3
1922-------	1937	*	*	*	*	*	*	*	*	426.6	394.7	364.8	339.2
1923-------	1938	*	*	*	*	*	*	*	*	434.5	404.3	370.3	352.4
1924-------	1939	*	*	*	*	*	*	*	*	451.4	416.7	400.0	365.2
1925-------	1940	*	*	*	*	*	*	*	*	458.3	442.1	397.6	379.3
1926-------	1941	*	*	*	*	*	*	*	*	489.9	433.2	401.7	374.7
1927-------	1942	*	*	*	*	*	*	*	*	448.5	419.7	390.5	369.3
1928-------	1943	*	*	*	*	*	*	*	*	433.2	412.3	391.9	365.7
1929-------	1944	*	*	*	*	*	*	*	463.0	449.8	413.5	383.8	353.8
1930-------	1945	*	*	*	*	*	*	*	491.7	441.6	410.4	380.3	360.5
1931-------	1946	*	*	*	*	*	*	*	488.9	444.0	407.1	398.3	355.8
1932-------	1947	*	*	*	*	*	*	*	531.5	460.7	444.2	400.4	360.9
1933-------	1948	*	*	*	*	*	*	*	541.1	478.3	441.6	392.1	348.7
1934-------	1949	*	*	*	*	*	*	*	506.3	474.7	427.9	383.7	344.9
1935-------	1950	*	*	*	*	*	*	*	541.7	466.0	427.4	385.8	358.1
1936-------	1951	*	*	*	*	*	*	*	511.2	472.2	420.1	385.3	347.3
1937-------	1952	*	*	*	*	*	*	*	500.0	452.4	421.1	382.6	325.5
1938-------	1953	*	*	*	*	*	*	*	516.5	467.5	428.9	361.7	315.1
1939-------	1954	*	*	*	*	*	*	*	539.3	460.8	394.5	346.3	280.9
1940-------	1955	*	*	*	*	*	*	*	522.2	438.1	388.3	310.7	239.8
1941-------	1956	*	*	*	*	*	*	*	483.5	417.2	334.1	266.1	212.4
1942-------	1957	*	*	*	*	*	*	*	473.7	370.6	307.9	250.5	193.7
1943-------	1958	*	*	*	*	*	*	*	412.5	340.8	278.2	218.0	191.3
1944-------	1959	*	*	*	*	*	*	*	400.0	327.5	251.6	218.8	197.8
1945-------	1960	*	*	*	*	*	*	*	365.9	282.2	242.8	217.8	174.2
1946-------	1961	*	*	*	*	*	*	*	324.1	283.2	249.0	200.6	155.5
1947-------	1962	*	*	*	*	*	*	*	*	289.7	234.1	172.3	137.9
1948-------	1963	*	*	*	*	*	*	*	*	275.0	195.4	154.9	
1949-------	1964	*	*	*	*	*	*	*	*	219.0	173.3		
1950-------	1965	*	*	*	*	*	*	*	*	*			
1951-------	1966	*	*	*	*	*	*	*	*				
1952-------	1967	*	*	*	*	*	*	*					
1953-------	1968	*	*	*	*	*	*						
1954-------	1969	*	*	*	*	*							
1955-------	1970	*	*	*	*								
1956-------	1971	*	*	*									
1957-------	1972	*	*										
1958-------	1973	*											

TABLE 10C. BIRTH PROBABILITIES FOR ALL OTHER WOMEN FOR EACH YEAR 1917-73 BY AGE AND PARITY FOR EACH COHORT FROM 1868 TO 1958--CON.

(PROBABILITIES ARE THE NUMBER OF BIRTHS PER 1,000 WOMEN IN SPECIFIED PARITY AND EXACT AGE GROUP. FIGURES FOR "0 PARITY" SHOW THE PROBABILITY OF FIRST BIRTHS TO "0 PARITY" WOMEN, THOSE FOR "1 PARITY" SHOW THE PROBABILITY OF SECOND BIRTHS TO "1 PARITY" WOMEN, ETC. BASED ON CENTRAL BIRTH RATES AND PARITY DISTRIBUTIONS)

PARITY AND COHORT	DIAGONAL LINE FOR JANUARY 1	EXACT AGE											
		27	28	29	30	31	32	33	34	35	36	37	38
5 PARITY--CON.													
1879-------													136.8
1880-------												162.2	166.7
1881-------											205.7	203.0	176.5
1882-------										236.2	256.8	217.9	192.5
1883-------									258.9	287.5	274.0	235.3	208.9
1884-------								248.7	281.1	278.1	265.7	227.5	187.8
1885-------							232.0	244.1	250.9	250.9	238.4	189.0	168.1
1886-------						238.4	205.7	196.6	207.5	215.2	182.1	155.7	131.5
1887-------					210.0	217.3	169.9	166.0	192.1	172.7	156.3	127.9	117.7
1888-------				259.7	223.8	214.5	172.0	196.5	186.9	182.7	157.6	137.5	115.6
1889-------			256.8	270.9	227.2	218.0	203.4	194.7	201.0	190.7	170.4	153.8	118.0
1890-------	1917	294.2	265.2	288.6	241.0	260.1	202.3	213.3	218.2	203.5	196.0	150.5	115.5
1891-------	1918	309.6	299.0	316.6	285.7	260.0	223.8	240.6	238.4	232.6	185.0	151.3	118.8
1892-------	1919	349.1	335.4	366.9	285.2	286.2	250.0	255.8	245.5	209.5	179.5	147.3	134.5
1893-------	1920	356.5	351.7	336.4	282.1	292.6	242.1	238.2	209.8	188.4	164.3	151.3	123.1
1894-------	1921	417.7	357.4	364.9	327.5	307.1	253.0	238.3	209.6	197.4	172.6	146.7	143.9
1895-------	1922	412.5	370.2	414.7	333.3	303.1	248.0	222.2	211.1	196.0	173.4	167.4	120.1
1896-------	1923	420.4	425.9	399.6	334.0	291.1	227.1	218.2	205.2	186.3	181.6	141.1	120.4
1897-------	1924	476.2	397.2	400.4	308.5	278.0	211.3	220.8	197.8	195.1	156.5	138.8	107.8
1898-------	1925	427.1	403.6	375.8	288.9	259.1	219.1	204.5	205.1	175.6	157.9	129.4	106.3
1899-------	1926	455.5	394.5	353.7	276.2	266.7	214.3	226.5	197.0	187.4	153.2	129.6	106.6
1900-------	1927	427.5	341.3	336.0	277.8	257.6	225.5	215.7	201.2	171.7	145.4	126.4	112.6
1901-------	1928	366.5	321.1	324.1	268.7	254.8	210.6	211.7	178.1	154.7	136.1	123.3	101.4
1902-------	1929	347.0	309.2	306.8	257.3	236.4	196.9	182.0	161.9	144.7	128.5	115.7	94.2
1903-------	1930	325.2	307.4	311.5	245.5	228.6	179.6	172.4	150.8	138.1	121.3	111.1	92.9
1904-------	1931	333.3	314.9	306.9	246.5	219.1	177.1	170.1	151.5	136.6	118.0	110.9	92.3
1905-------	1932	338.4	308.4	304.4	242.4	211.7	180.5	172.8	147.9	133.2	119.7	103.7	95.7
1906-------	1933	327.5	305.8	285.4	229.8	212.9	180.2	170.8	146.4	132.6	112.5	104.7	96.8
1907-------	1934	335.0	286.0	276.7	236.3	215.0	181.1	171.9	149.8	135.9	118.0	108.2	98.3
1908-------	1935	310.1	287.4	288.8	232.7	217.1	185.1	178.1	160.5	149.5	124.7	117.1	93.4
1909-------	1936	316.1	298.2	287.6	234.8	218.5	187.8	181.6	171.0	153.8	136.2	114.9	99.5
1910-------	1937	324.7	303.7	290.0	237.8	223.6	194.0	194.0	179.0	160.4	136.8	122.2	102.5
1911-------	1938	341.9	312.5	298.9	245.7	225.3	209.1	205.2	180.0	160.4	141.6	124.4	108.8
1912-------	1939	351.7	327.0	312.9	260.0	248.9	224.4	205.4	182.8	168.9	145.5	133.9	114.2
1913-------	1940	355.7	329.4	297.5	266.8	251.1	210.0	199.1	178.6	157.5	141.6	126.9	109.6
1914-------	1941	350.0	308.4	295.5	266.5	238.7	201.2	196.7	168.8	155.6	132.8	127.8	105.2
1915-------	1942	325.3	303.5	296.5	250.5	220.5	192.2	185.5	166.0	144.5	135.7	120.2	101.0
1916-------	1943	324.7	310.1	288.0	235.9	216.1	195.8	184.8	158.1	150.7	132.7	121.5	104.3
1917-------	1944	330.3	294.0	269.5	227.4	219.6	189.7	179.8	164.9	151.6	135.1	123.9	108.9
1918-------	1945	324.3	290.4	269.2	236.5	217.6	191.3	188.6	173.8	160.5	143.4	125.4	109.3
1919-------	1946	326.7	291.2	281.7	247.7	229.5	209.8	203.5	179.0	166.1	144.1	130.1	108.3
1920-------	1947	321.6	304.8	286.8	254.9	243.9	213.1	198.0	186.2	163.7	141.7	128.0	98.9
1921-------	1948	328.3	303.5	296.4	264.4	239.9	207.5	206.3	179.8	159.5	141.8	114.2	102.7
1922-------	1949	326.9	312.1	305.1	261.2	241.8	222.2	200.6	178.6	161.6	129.7	119.8	96.0
1923-------	1950	339.0	325.1	301.6	273.6	248.8	218.3	207.9	182.9	151.8	134.4	112.6	92.4
1924-------	1951	358.5	329.7	317.2	275.2	253.0	225.8	207.8	170.0	158.4	124.6	105.3	83.6
1925-------	1952	360.3	332.2	310.9	272.6	253.5	218.6	189.9	168.9	139.5	115.9	97.1	76.1
1926-------	1953	355.9	334.3	308.8	273.6	242.9	205.3	189.4	152.0	132.3	108.6	84.8	68.3
1927-------	1954	352.1	316.7	301.5	259.0	229.5	194.9	165.3	146.2	124.3	95.0	77.9	61.4
1928-------	1955	342.5	313.2	295.7	251.8	223.7	180.6	164.7	137.5	107.0	90.3	74.2	54.7
1929-------	1956	336.0	310.0	280.5	242.2	206.3	178.5	157.0	121.8	105.7	83.7	63.5	49.0
1930-------	1957	336.8	304.0	279.2	236.6	206.8	175.1	140.9	124.6	96.1	72.5	57.8	47.8
1931-------	1958	329.1	299.8	267.7	230.8	200.2	159.1	146.0	105.7	82.1	66.4	54.4	37.0
1932-------	1959	327.4	290.1	268.4	220.9	186.1	156.9	122.1	92.0	76.3	61.0	42.7	38.1
1933-------	1960	315.8	294.9	245.3	205.0	175.7	133.5	105.2	83.7	66.8	50.0	42.5	34.2
1934-------	1961	326.9	273.6	232.8	194.6	158.1	120.9	95.6	75.8	62.3	49.9	41.6	30.6
1935-------	1962	311.1	262.0	229.3	177.9	140.8	106.9	86.5	72.0	59.5	50.0	36.2	24.4
1936-------	1963	294.5	256.9	204.7	158.8	124.2	93.9	82.9	69.1	58.4	42.4	31.4	
1937-------	1964	281.2	223.2	175.8	138.3	106.0	88.1	77.5	67.4	47.4	37.2		
1938-------	1965	254.0	195.6	157.4	121.8	104.3	90.5	77.2	54.8	42.8			
1939-------	1966	212.2	169.9	140.9	113.1	106.4	87.0	64.5	50.0				
1940-------	1967	194.7	158.0	134.6	120.3	99.4	74.5	56.8					
1941-------	1968	173.8	148.8	135.0	109.5	83.9	64.7						
1942-------	1969	173.9	151.9	129.2	96.1	73.5							
1943-------	1970	172.6	141.0	108.3	80.3								
1944-------	1971	162.4	125.7	94.8									
1945-------	1972	138.7	104.8										
1946-------	1973	123.2											

TABLE 10C. BIRTH PROBABILITIES FOR ALL OTHER WOMEN FOR EACH YEAR 1917-73 BY AGE AND PARITY FOR EACH COHORT FROM 1868 TO 1958--CON.

(PROBABILITIES ARE THE NUMBER OF BIRTHS PER 1,000 WOMEN IN SPECIFIED PARITY AND EXACT AGE GROUP. FIGURES FOR "0 PARITY" SHOW THE PROBABILITY OF FIRST BIRTHS TO "C PARITY" WOMEN, THOSE FOR "1 PARITY" SHOW THE PROBABILITY OF SECOND BIRTHS TO "1 PARITY" WOMEN, ETC. BASED ON CENTRAL BIRTH RATES AND PARITY DISTRIBUTIONS)

PARITY AND COHORT	DIAGONAL LINE FOR JANUARY 1	EXACT AGE										
		39	40	41	42	43	44	45	46	47	48	49
5 PARITY--CON.												
1868----------------												6.6
1869----------------											8.3	20.1
1870----------------										10.1	23.6	5.1
1871----------------									16.9	30.6	6.9	6.9
1872----------------								20.4	53.0	8.8	8.8	3.5
1873----------------							27.4	55.3	16.1	10.8	5.4	5.4
1874----------------						29.3	57.4	19.9	19.9	5.4	5.4	5.4
1875----------------					37.9	34.8	24.7	23.1	10.7	7.2	7.2	5.4
1876----------------				59.5	45.0	26.4	28.4	14.3	10.8	9.0	7.2	3.6
1877----------------			83.6	71.9	33.3	26.5	23.1	14.4	16.2	9.0	5.4	3.6
1878----------------	1917	122.8	98.2	55.2	34.8	28.1	21.2	19.6	16.1	5.4	5.4	1.8
1879----------------	1918	146.1	87.3	57.8	38.7	26.7	25.2	19.9	12.7	9.1	5.5	3.6
1880----------------	1919	141.4	93.0	67.4	37.0	26.3	26.4	17.1	19.0	11.5	5.8	5.8
1881----------------	1920	155.7	104.7	69.7	38.6	30.8	22.7	22.7	16.7	8.4	8.4	4.2
1882----------------	1921	172.6	108.2	68.9	42.8	34.1	29.7	20.8	16.2	11.7	4.7	4.7
1883----------------	1922	175.2	113.8	77.1	50.3	40.4	23.0	23.1	23.3	7.8	7.8	2.6
1884----------------	1923	166.3	109.8	81.9	48.5	31.0	28.6	26.2	18.6	10.7	8.0	2.7
1885----------------	1924	145.1	100.9	67.3	35.3	26.0	26.1	19.2	14.5	9.6	4.8	4.8
1886----------------	1925	123.2	74.6	48.5	25.5	19.7	19.8	12.0	15.9	4.0	6.0	6.0
1887----------------	1926	91.6	58.8	34.8	21.6	16.7	11.7	15.1	8.4	5.1	5.1	3.4
1888----------------	1927	94.5	54.2	35.2	21.3	16.0	17.8	10.8	10.8	3.6	3.6	3.6
1889----------------	1928	94.3	56.4	39.9	24.8	17.3	13.5	11.6	7.8	3.9	5.8	3.9
1890----------------	1929	96.0	61.1	47.0	26.9	16.6	14.6	10.4	6.3	6.3	4.2	4.2
1891----------------	1930	112.1	71.1	51.8	25.1	18.3	13.8	9.2	9.2	4.6	4.6	2.3
1892----------------	1931	111.9	81.8	48.0	26.6	19.5	12.2	9.8	7.3	4.9	4.9	2.5
1893----------------	1932	117.3	67.0	46.8	26.1	19.0	11.9	7.1	7.2	4.8	2.4	2.4
1894----------------	1933	107.3	72.3	48.2	28.1	18.0	12.9	7.8	7.8	2.6	2.6	0.0
1895----------------	1934	107.5	69.1	43.9	26.0	18.4	13.2	8.0	5.3	5.3	2.7	0.0
1896----------------	1935	95.7	61.2	41.2	23.5	18.4	13.2	5.3	8.0	2.7	2.7	2.7
1897----------------	1936	89.8	63.3	38.7	26.0	18.3	10.5	13.2	5.3	2.7	2.7	2.7
1898----------------	1937	88.9	60.2	40.4	25.4	17.9	15.4	10.3	7.8	5.2	2.6	2.6
1899----------------	1938	93.5	56.1	39.3	24.7	17.4	14.9	10.0	7.5	5.0	2.5	0.0
1900----------------	1939	89.2	55.0	38.5	21.7	19.4	14.6	9.8	7.3	2.5	2.5	2.5
1901----------------	1940	80.6	53.5	30.4	23.4	18.9	11.8	9.5	4.8	2.4	2.4	0.0
1902----------------	1941	79.5	50.5	34.6	23.3	16.4	11.7	7.0	4.7	2.3	2.3	0.0
1903----------------	1942	78.1	51.9	34.2	25.2	18.3	11.5	6.9	4.6	2.3	2.3	0.0
1904----------------	1943	80.0	54.1	40.9	25.2	18.4	9.2	6.9	4.6	2.3	0.0	2.3
1905----------------	1944	81.3	57.9	38.1	24.8	13.6	11.3	6.8	4.5	0.0	2.3	2.3
1906----------------	1945	80.8	55.1	35.7	20.1	15.7	11.2	6.7	2.3	2.3	2.3	0.0
1907----------------	1946	75.1	55.6	33.6	24.7	18.0	9.0	4.5	4.5	2.3	2.3	0.0
1908----------------	1947	80.1	53.0	37.0	25.5	13.9	11.6	4.7	2.3	2.3	0.0	2.3
1909----------------	1948	79.5	56.9	41.1	25.2	20.6	11.5	6.9	4.6	2.3	2.3	2.3
1910----------------	1949	84.7	61.9	43.9	30.0	20.9	11.6	6.9	4.6	2.3	2.3	0.0
1911----------------	1950	91.5	64.8	46.3	32.6	20.9	13.9	7.0	2.3	2.3	2.3	0.0
1912----------------	1951	94.1	65.9	51.9	30.7	23.6	16.5	7.1	4.7	2.4	0.0	2.4
1913----------------	1952	85.7	67.8	48.2	33.0	24.3	11.0	6.6	4.4	2.2	2.2	0.0
1914----------------	1953	88.7	65.8	45.4	33.0	22.7	12.4	8.3	2.1	2.1	2.1	0.0
1915----------------	1954	88.6	65.6	46.5	32.9	19.4	11.7	5.8	3.9	1.9	0.0	0.0
1916----------------	1955	88.9	65.1	42.8	27.8	18.6	13.0	5.6	3.7	1.9	0.0	0.0
1917----------------	1956	88.0	59.2	39.5	25.1	19.6	10.7	5.4	3.6	1.8	0.0	0.0
1918----------------	1957	83.0	52.9	38.5	27.9	17.4	10.5	5.2	3.5	1.7	0.0	0.0
1919----------------	1958	79.5	58.8	40.3	28.5	16.8	8.4	6.7	3.4	0.0	0.0	0.0
1920----------------	1959	85.6	57.3	43.1	25.7	16.0	12.8	6.4	1.6	0.0	0.0	0.0
1921----------------	1960	77.5	59.5	35.4	23.0	16.8	9.2	4.6	1.5	1.5	0.0	0.0
1922----------------	1961	78.5	50.2	36.6	24.4	16.8	9.2	4.6	1.5	0.0	0.0	0.0
1923----------------	1962	68.5	49.2	32.8	23.8	14.9	7.5	3.0	1.5	1.5	0.0	0.0
1924----------------	1963	66.6	45.5	34.1	21.3	12.8	7.1	2.9	2.9	0.0	0.0	0.0
1925----------------	1964	57.8	40.7	28.9	17.1	10.5	6.6	4.0	1.3	0.0	0.0	
1926----------------	1965	52.2	37.3	26.1	15.0	10.0	6.2	2.5	1.2	0.0		
1927----------------	1966	48.4	34.3	21.4	14.3	8.3	4.8	2.4	1.2			
1928----------------	1967	42.9	27.9	19.8	12.8	8.2	3.5	1.2				
1929----------------	1968	37.9	25.8	18.0	11.2	5.6	3.4					
1930----------------	1969	32.4	25.6	16.7	10.0	6.7						
1931----------------	1970	32.5	22.7	14.1	8.7							
1932----------------	1971	28.5	19.0	12.6								
1933----------------	1972	23.1	15.0									
1934----------------	1973	19.7										

TABLE 10C. BIRTH PROBABILITIES FOR ALL OTHER WOMEN FOR EACH YEAR 1917-73 BY AGE AND PARITY FOR EACH COHORT FROM 1868 TO 1958--CON.

(PROBABILITIES ARE THE NUMBER OF BIRTHS PER 1,000 WOMEN IN SPECIFIED PARITY AND EXACT AGE GROUP. FIGURES FOR "0 PARITY" SHOW THE PROBABILITY OF FIRST BIRTHS TO "0 PARITY" WOMEN, THOSE FOR "1 PARITY" SHOW THE PROBABILITY OF SECOND BIRTHS TO "1 PARITY" WOMEN, ETC. BASED ON CENTRAL BIRTH RATES AND PARITY DISTRIBUTIONS)

PARITY AND COHORT	DIAGONAL LINE FOR JANUARY 1	EXACT AGE											
		15	16	17	18	19	20	21	22	23	24	25	26
6 PARITY													
1891-------													296.6
1892-------												340.0	289.7
1893-------											330.2	283.9	319.8
1894-------										*	*	389.3	352.6
1895-------									*	*	*	400.0	464.5
1896-------								*	*	*	*	513.5	415.7
1897-------							*	*	*	*	*	443.5	409.8
1898-------						*	*	*	*	*	*	446.3	443.9
1899-------					*	*	*	*	*	*	*	479.3	417.5
1900-------				*	*	*	*	*	*	*	*	488.4	415.4
1901-------			*	*	*	*	*	*	*	*	*	475.4	378.8
1902-------	1917	*	*	*	*	*	*	*	*	*	*	414.1	354.5
1903-------	1918	*	*	*	*	*	*	*	*	*	*	418.8	352.6
1904-------	1919	*	*	*	*	*	*	*	*	*	*	386.0	360.0
1905-------	1920	*	*	*	*	*	*	*	*	*	*	369.7	342.9
1906-------	1921	*	*	*	*	*	*	*	*	*	*	368.4	329.4
1907-------	1922	*	*	*	*	*	*	*	*	*	*	364.5	329.0
1908-------	1923	*	*	*	*	*	*	*	*	*	*	*	342.1
1909-------	1924	*	*	*	*	*	*	*	*	*	*	*	348.7
1910-------	1925	*	*	*	*	*	*	*	*	*	*	*	349.0
1911-------	1926	*	*	*	*	*	*	*	*	*	*	388.3	370.1
1912-------	1927	*	*	*	*	*	*	*	*	*	*	398.1	346.2
1913-------	1928	*	*	*	*	*	*	*	*	*	*	382.4	352.6
1914-------	1929	*	*	*	*	*	*	*	*	*	*	388.3	367.1
1915-------	1930	*	*	*	*	*	*	*	*	*	*	411.2	362.0
1916-------	1931	*	*	*	*	*	*	*	*	*	*	396.4	376.5
1917-------	1932	*	*	*	*	*	*	*	*	*	*	411.8	374.3
1918-------	1933	*	*	*	*	*	*	*	*	*	*	414.1	367.0
1919-------	1934	*	*	*	*	*	*	*	*	*	*	382.4	358.2
1920-------	1935	*	*	*	*	*	*	*	*	*	*	381.9	346.3
1921-------	1936	*	*	*	*	*	*	*	*	*	*	377.6	343.0
1922-------	1937	*	*	*	*	*	*	*	*	*	*	390.1	366.3
1923-------	1938	*	*	*	*	*	*	*	*	*	*	395.8	367.6
1924-------	1939	*	*	*	*	*	*	*	*	*	*	398.6	369.2
1925-------	1940	*	*	*	*	*	*	*	*	*	*	392.2	360.0
1926-------	1941	*	*	*	*	*	*	*	*	*	*	382.7	375.5
1927-------	1942	*	*	*	*	*	*	*	*	*	392.2	401.1	391.6
1928-------	1943	*	*	*	*	*	*	*	*	*	432.4	400.0	385.4
1929-------	1944	*	*	*	*	*	*	*	*	*	440.0	412.3	385.4
1930-------	1945	*	*	*	*	*	*	*	*	*	456.5	416.3	395.9
1931-------	1946	*	*	*	*	*	*	*	*	*	448.7	431.9	381.3
1932-------	1947	*	*	*	*	*	*	*	*	*	467.8	410.1	375.3
1933-------	1948	*	*	*	*	*	*	*	*	*	446.9	395.8	379.7
1934-------	1949	*	*	*	*	*	*	*	*	*	429.3	409.8	377.4
1935-------	1950	*	*	*	*	*	*	*	*	441.4	436.9	401.3	364.7
1936-------	1951	*	*	*	*	*	*	*	*	478.6	429.9	394.5	357.3
1937-------	1952	*	*	*	*	*	*	*	*	470.6	437.2	386.0	346.0
1938-------	1953	*	*	*	*	*	*	*	*	483.1	415.1	373.9	334.1
1939-------	1954	*	*	*	*	*	*	*	*	458.3	410.4	371.8	300.7
1940-------	1955	*	*	*	*	*	*	*	*	438.0	388.3	321.3	259.0
1941-------	1956	*	*	*	*	*	*	*	*	434.8	357.1	283.6	237.0
1942-------	1957	*	*	*	*	*	*	*	*	381.8	310.3	257.1	204.5
1943-------	1958	*	*	*	*	*	*	*	*	*	289.5	224.9	193.1
1944-------	1959	*	*	*	*	*	*	*	*	*	248.1	219.1	206.3
1945-------	1960	*	*	*	*	*	*	*	*	*	252.3	244.9	192.5
1946-------	1961	*	*	*	*	*	*	*	*	*	*	203.3	162.5
1947-------	1962	*	*	*	*	*	*	*	*	*	*	188.1	156.3
1948-------	1963	*	*	*	*	*	*	*	*	*	*	*	
1949-------	1964	*	*	*	*	*	*	*	*	*	*		
1950-------	1965	*	*	*	*	*	*	*	*	*			
1951-------	1966	*	*	*	*	*	*	*	*				
1952-------	1967	*	*	*	*	*	*	*					
1953-------	1968	*	*	*	*	*	*						
1954-------	1969	*	*	*	*	*							
1955-------	1970	*	*	*	*								
1956-------	1971	*	*	*									
1957-------	1972	*	*										
1958-------	1973	*											

TABLE 10C. BIRTH PROBABILITIES FOR ALL OTHER WOMEN FOR EACH YEAR 1917-73 BY AGE AND PARITY FOR EACH COHORT FROM 1868 TO 1958--CON.

(PROBABILITIES ARE THE NUMBER OF BIRTHS PER 1,000 WOMEN IN SPECIFIED PARITY AND EXACT AGE GROUP. FIGURES FOR "0 PARITY" SHOW THE PROBABILITY OF FIRST BIRTHS TO "C PARITY" WOMEN, THOSE FOR "1 PARITY" SHOW THE PROBABILITY OF SECOND BIRTHS TO "1 PARITY" WOMEN, ETC. BASED ON CENTRAL BIRTH RATES AND PARITY DISTRIBUTIONS)

PARITY AND COHORT	DIAGONAL LINE FOR JANUARY 1	EXACT AGE											
		27	28	29	30	31	32	33	34	35	36	37	38
6 PARITY--CON.													
1879-------													154.4
1880-------												186.2	151.7
1881-------											216.2	182.5	163.9
1882-------										223.7	206.0	190.3	149.3
1883-------									223.7	210.8	209.0	170.8	135.3
1884-------								211.7	208.8	208.5	186.9	154.1	136.6
1885-------							207.6	199.4	203.6	188.0	168.6	156.2	132.6
1886-------						243.3	198.1	189.9	185.9	179.2	171.9	152.6	135.2
1887-------					233.6	234.9	189.8	177.2	190.1	180.4	170.3	157.6	138.0
1888-------				253.9	210.6	217.6	171.2	187.0	181.1	174.8	169.2	158.6	129.6
1889-------			237.1	247.4	222.2	213.4	195.2	188.1	189.9	184.3	182.7	162.3	121.9
1890-------	1917	278.3	228.4	280.1	225.5	248.1	198.6	203.5	203.1	202.0	186.8	153.6	111.3
1891-------	1918	268.2	278.8	281.7	269.2	249.5	213.8	216.0	216.9	209.8	181.8	141.3	114.1
1892-------	1919	329.8	284.9	349.5	264.6	269.8	228.7	231.2	226.9	199.3	166.4	139.6	122.4
1893-------	1920	311.0	348.2	317.2	267.2	272.2	227.1	231.3	211.9	180.8	158.8	135.2	116.0
1894-------	1921	423.7	331.3	344.6	297.2	281.8	244.4	236.0	194.4	181.3	161.0	144.0	127.8
1895-------	1922	390.2	349.2	382.1	303.5	299.8	257.0	213.7	202.5	188.7	168.1	156.4	121.0
1896-------	1923	401.6	390.9	374.7	325.3	299.1	219.2	209.6	204.3	191.8	183.0	147.6	134.5
1897-------	1924	438.5	362.8	373.0	306.0	267.9	206.2	213.5	204.3	193.1	163.4	150.8	124.7
1898-------	1925	397.7	352.9	356.6	274.2	243.3	212.0	214.3	203.0	186.0	165.9	146.9	114.9
1899-------	1926	378.8	346.9	323.2	252.3	250.5	219.5	218.6	204.1	188.4	163.2	141.0	115.7
1900-------	1927	377.3	313.8	309.5	260.3	258.0	221.5	222.0	202.5	178.6	154.2	137.7	123.1
1901-------	1928	344.7	296.3	310.3	268.9	253.3	220.1	218.2	185.7	171.6	157.3	143.2	119.1
1902-------	1929	329.3	315.1	321.2	269.5	251.2	216.9	198.6	179.4	173.0	155.6	142.2	116.4
1903-------	1930	350.4	325.2	334.3	266.7	263.8	203.4	195.2	193.3	175.2	158.0	140.7	127.2
1904-------	1931	347.8	325.2	322.4	275.4	244.3	201.5	203.4	191.7	170.0	149.3	148.6	115.7
1905-------	1932	331.9	309.3	323.4	255.4	227.3	199.5	210.5	183.6	163.8	153.1	135.3	117.0
1906-------	1933	330.4	313.2	300.0	244.6	234.7	214.3	203.4	183.8	168.7	145.7	142.5	124.4
1907-------	1934	334.9	299.3	291.5	262.6	250.0	212.3	217.2	196.4	176.2	157.1	153.8	127.4
1908-------	1935	327.0	297.7	313.9	271.7	247.9	228.1	227.5	200.0	189.8	169.8	148.4	124.3
1909-------	1936	336.6	333.3	337.7	275.4	265.5	239.0	235.0	211.0	201.6	173.6	157.9	132.4
1910-------	1937	354.4	335.9	331.1	284.0	265.5	235.0	237.2	214.5	197.3	176.9	154.9	128.8
1911-------	1938	355.8	337.1	336.5	282.8	269.4	239.1	241.4	221.1	198.9	176.5	153.6	135.5
1912-------	1939	344.2	341.8	332.3	279.2	270.3	240.2	234.7	207.2	186.7	163.3	148.3	127.9
1913-------	1940	362.8	349.1	316.6	290.6	279.6	246.8	232.6	208.2	189.7	167.5	157.2	129.9
1914-------	1941	367.0	320.1	323.1	293.3	272.3	238.6	231.2	207.0	188.0	170.4	151.9	123.4
1915-------	1942	349.8	332.1	334.4	284.5	267.5	241.1	231.7	207.5	189.1	172.5	149.6	134.0
1916-------	1943	356.5	335.7	323.4	279.6	269.9	241.8	227.7	205.4	191.2	165.9	157.4	135.6
1917-------	1944	352.9	324.4	314.0	283.4	269.9	235.7	228.7	209.6	188.5	172.2	157.3	142.5
1918-------	1945	354.6	323.5	318.1	283.1	268.8	241.5	242.2	213.3	190.7	168.6	161.4	139.3
1919-------	1946	339.7	315.6	315.9	286.4	266.7	254.0	235.4	205.2	185.9	167.4	161.5	128.6
1920-------	1947	337.0	323.1	321.7	285.0	276.5	237.9	227.7	210.0	180.5	176.2	154.8	126.5
1921-------	1948	346.9	331.3	321.8	296.7	267.4	239.3	236.0	200.4	198.1	170.2	143.7	122.6
1922-------	1949	357.4	338.5	333.3	286.4	274.9	257.4	227.6	216.1	195.7	157.1	144.5	117.0
1923-------	1950	354.2	346.3	332.5	296.3	281.4	245.4	237.8	214.0	178.8	158.4	135.0	109.1
1924-------	1951	362.7	341.7	337.3	303.2	276.6	249.5	237.7	196.8	183.6	148.5	129.1	100.0
1925-------	1952	365.7	352.5	338.6	297.2	283.3	249.1	220.3	200.7	163.9	141.2	115.1	90.3
1926-------	1953	374.6	361.7	331.3	302.8	276.5	233.7	225.0	183.1	161.7	124.0	104.3	87.4
1927-------	1954	383.1	344.6	346.2	304.9	273.0	240.5	210.3	185.8	147.7	121.4	101.7	80.5
1928-------	1955	366.0	350.6	327.9	292.3	265.6	222.2	204.8	159.9	132.4	111.4	87.7	65.4
1929-------	1956	380.4	340.6	325.4	285.0	254.5	221.6	185.1	148.8	130.7	97.6	77.1	62.9
1930-------	1957	354.1	335.2	311.2	271.1	234.4	196.6	164.8	147.1	109.8	86.1	68.5	53.7
1931-------	1958	358.3	331.0	304.9	262.2	225.5	187.1	167.3	124.8	97.6	76.0	58.4	47.4
1932-------	1959	355.7	321.1	294.5	248.2	214.3	180.8	146.9	111.4	85.7	66.3	55.2	46.1
1933-------	1960	350.0	324.2	277.6	235.2	206.9	161.5	123.5	98.1	76.2	63.8	52.1	44.2
1934-------	1961	344.3	299.0	270.8	223.8	186.6	132.0	111.8	84.9	73.8	59.5	51.7	32.7
1935-------	1962	327.2	294.1	251.8	200.3	146.7	122.3	94.0	78.8	65.6	57.7	40.3	29.2
1936-------	1963	326.7	272.1	227.4	163.4	133.6	100.6	87.5	73.6	65.3	45.2	32.8	
1937-------	1964	306.8	249.2	193.6	150.9	116.3	98.6	86.3	73.2	52.8	40.8		
1938-------	1965	274.1	213.4	168.3	127.7	114.0	95.4	83.3	57.2	48.3			
1939-------	1966	239.8	195.2	151.3	123.0	111.8	95.3	69.2	56.3				
1940-------	1967	211.9	167.0	136.0	117.2	107.5	74.0	61.1					
1941-------	1968	189.5	147.7	138.5	119.3	86.6	69.3						
1942-------	1969	169.0	151.4	135.4	96.8	77.8							
1943-------	1970	186.3	156.1	116.1	90.9								
1944-------	1971	169.2	125.0	97.9									
1945-------	1972	147.3	112.4										
1946-------	1973	125.0											

TABLE 10C. BIRTH PROBABILITIES FOR ALL OTHER WOMEN FOR EACH YEAR 1917-73 BY AGE AND PARITY FOR EACH COHORT FROM 1868 TO 1958--CON.

(PROBABILITIES ARE THE NUMBER OF BIRTHS PER 1,000 WOMEN IN SPECIFIED PARITY AND EXACT AGE GROUP. FIGURES FOR "0 PARITY" SHOW THE PROBABILITY OF FIRST BIRTHS TO "C PARITY" WOMEN, THOSE FOR "1 PARITY" SHOW THE PROBABILITY OF SECOND BIRTHS TO "1 PARITY" WOMEN, ETC. BASED ON CENTRAL BIRTH RATES AND PARITY DISTRIBUTIONS)

PARITY AND COHORT	DIAGONAL LINE FOR JANUARY 1	EXACT AGE										
		39	40	41	42	43	44	45	46	47	48	49
6 PARITY--CON.												
1868----------------												7.7
1869----------------											9.2	13.8
1870----------------										13.7	13.8	7.6
1871----------------									21.3	23.0	9.1	7.6
1872----------------								25.8	36.8	13.6	9.1	4.6
1873----------------							25.8	41.1	21.1	13.7	4.6	6.1
1874----------------						22.8	36.3	25.4	21.1	7.6	6.1	6.1
1875----------------					30.3	27.1	25.6	25.7	12.2	10.7	7.7	4.6
1876----------------				52.5	34.5	23.9	25.4	16.5	16.5	12.1	6.1	1.5
1877----------------			78.5	61.0	32.7	22.4	20.9	19.4	18.1	9.1	3.0	4.5
1878----------------	1917	128.3	85.5	58.3	30.2	27.2	22.7	22.8	16.8	6.1	7.7	1.5
1879----------------	1918	132.9	87.3	54.8	36.7	24.5	24.6	20.0	17.0	10.9	4.7	1.6
1880----------------	1919	140.5	82.9	69.3	34.3	25.0	23.5	20.4	17.4	4.8	4.7	4.7
1881----------------	1920	131.3	92.0	61.9	34.3	25.1	26.7	20.6	12.7	7.9	6.4	3.2
1882----------------	1921	130.4	86.0	61.0	34.0	28.0	20.3	15.6	15.6	7.8	3.1	3.1
1883----------------	1922	126.1	82.0	58.8	32.1	26.0	19.9	16.9	10.8	7.7	4.6	3.1
1884----------------	1923	121.1	81.1	47.2	30.3	22.8	18.3	12.2	10.7	4.6	4.6	1.5
1885----------------	1924	120.8	67.9	52.4	28.0	21.8	14.1	14.1	11.0	4.7	4.7	3.1
1886----------------	1925	110.1	74.2	49.6	24.2	17.8	17.9	14.6	11.4	4.9	4.9	1.6
1887----------------	1926	116.0	68.6	40.5	25.4	23.8	18.8	13.8	12.0	5.2	3.5	3.4
1888----------------	1927	102.8	51.2	39.7	28.3	20.1	16.9	13.5	8.5	5.1	5.1	1.7
1889----------------	1928	88.0	59.3	47.9	27.7	19.1	15.7	10.5	8.8	5.3	3.5	3.5
1890----------------	1929	93.0	69.0	45.0	27.1	21.7	14.6	11.0	9.2	5.5	5.5	3.7
1891----------------	1930	104.8	65.1	46.7	30.0	20.8	15.2	11.5	9.6	5.8	5.8	1.9
1892----------------	1931	102.1	69.9	46.7	27.5	21.7	13.9	12.0	10.0	6.0	4.0	2.0
1893----------------	1932	1C3.4	63.3	44.5	25.3	19.5	13.7	9.8	7.9	4.0	4.0	2.0
1894----------------	1933	101.6	70.0	45.7	27.2	21.0	14.8	8.5	8.5	4.3	2.1	2.1
1895----------------	1934	112.3	66.1	48.8	29.1	20.3	13.6	11.4	6.8	4.6	2.3	2.3
1896----------------	1935	105.7	67.9	47.4	28.7	16.9	16.9	7.3	7.3	4.9	2.4	2.4
1897----------------	1936	102.3	61.6	42.8	23.9	21.5	12.0	9.6	7.2	4.8	2.4	2.4
1898----------------	1937	91.5	64.7	37.3	28.0	18.7	14.1	9.4	7.0	4.7	2.3	2.3
1899----------------	1938	100.0	58.6	40.8	27.3	18.3	13.8	9.2	6.9	4.6	2.3	2.3
1900----------------	1939	94.5	60.0	40.4	24.8	20.4	13.6	9.1	6.8	2.3	2.3	2.3
1901----------------	1940	91.5	60.2	39.6	25.9	18.9	14.2	7.1	4.7	2.4	2.4	0.0
1902----------------	1941	S6.6	61.1	46.8	27.4	22.4	12.5	7.5	5.0	2.5	2.5	0.0
1903----------------	1942	96.1	67.9	47.4	34.5	21.3	13.3	8.0	5.3	2.7	2.7	0.0
1904----------------	1943	101.0	67.9	49.9	34.2	23.8	13.3	8.0	5.3	2.7	2.7	0.0
1905----------------	1944	102.3	69.6	51.7	31.3	20.9	13.1	7.9	5.2	2.6	0.0	2.6
1906----------------	1945	101.8	73.5	50.3	29.3	24.1	13.5	8.1	5.4	0.0	2.7	0.0
1907----------------	1946	103.5	68.9	46.8	30.5	24.9	13.9	11.1	2.8	2.8	2.8	0.0
1908----------------	1947	100.6	70.0	50.7	34.0	22.7	14.3	8.6	2.9	2.9	0.0	0.0
1909----------------	1948	1C8.0	77.4	54.8	37.6	23.3	17.4	8.7	5.8	0.0	2.9	0.0
1910----------------	1949	112.9	78.0	58.7	36.5	28.1	14.1	11.3	2.8	2.8	0.0	2.8
1911----------------	1950	111.7	82.0	54.9	38.5	27.5	16.5	8.3	5.5	2.8	2.8	0.0
1912----------------	1951	105.1	69.4	56.4	38.5	25.8	15.5	7.7	2.6	2.6	2.6	0.0
1913----------------	1952	101.3	77.9	57.0	36.3	28.4	12.9	7.8	5.2	2.6	0.0	0.0
1914----------------	1953	110.3	77.9	52.6	40.0	25.0	12.5	10.0	5.0	2.5	0.0	0.0
1915----------------	1954	109.7	76.9	61.6	34.6	24.5	14.7	9.8	4.9	2.5	0.0	0.0
1916----------------	1955	113.8	82.1	57.8	33.8	26.5	16.9	7.2	4.8	2.4	0.0	0.0
1917----------------	1956	119.2	79.8	58.8	40.3	26.3	16.7	7.2	7.2	0.0	0.0	0.0
1918----------------	1957	112.4	79.2	57.2	39.2	25.4	16.2	9.3	2.3	2.3	2.3	0.0
1919----------------	1958	107.4	75.2	54.4	35.7	25.2	10.5	6.3	2.1	2.1	0.0	0.0
1920----------------	1959	103.2	73.1	51.5	33.6	19.8	11.9	5.9	2.0	0.0	0.0	0.0
1921----------------	1960	93.2	66.3	45.1	32.0	20.8	11.3	3.8	1.9	1.9	0.0	0.0
1922----------------	1961	S2.1	61.7	46.7	30.0	18.7	9.3	3.7	3.7	1.9	0.0	0.0
1923----------------	1962	85.1	61.7	43.6	27.4	14.6	9.1	5.4	1.8	1.8	1.8	0.0
1924----------------	1963	75.7	56.5	37.7	23.9	15.4	10.2	5.1	1.7	0.0	0.0	0.0
1925----------------	1964	72.3	51.5	33.9	22.5	14.5	8.1	4.8	1.6	0.0	0.0	
1926----------------	1965	66.2	43.1	30.7	19.9	12.3	6.1	3.1	1.5	0.0		
1927----------------	1966	56.3	42.4	28.7	16.6	10.6	6.0	4.5	1.5			
1928----------------	1967	52.2	37.6	23.2	14.5	8.7	5.8	1.4				
1929----------------	1968	47.6	32.2	21.0	14.0	9.8	4.2					
1930----------------	1969	40.1	28.1	20.0	12.0	5.3						
1931----------------	1970	36.9	26.3	17.1	9.2							
1932----------------	1971	35.5	21.1	13.1								
1933----------------	1972	27.3	19.4									
1934----------------	1973	23.8										

TABLE 10C. BIRTH PROBABILITIES FOR ALL OTHER WOMEN FOR EACH YEAR 1917-73 BY AGE AND PARITY FOR EACH COHORT FROM 1868 TO 1958--CON.

(PROBABILITIES ARE THE NUMBER OF BIRTHS PER 1,000 WOMEN IN SPECIFIED PARITY AND EXACT AGE GROUP. FIGURES FOR "0 PARITY" SHOW THE PROBABILITY OF FIRST BIRTHS TO "C PARITY" WOMEN, THOSE FOR "1 PARITY" SHOW THE PROBABILITY OF SECOND BIRTHS TO "1 PARITY" WOMEN, ETC. BASED ON CENTRAL BIRTH RATES AND PARITY DISTRIBUTIONS)

PARITY AND COHORT	DIAGONAL LINE FOR JANUARY 1	EXACT AGE											
		15	16	17	18	19	20	21	22	23	24	25	26
7 AND HIGHER PARITY													
1891-------													323.0
1892-------												*	319.1
1893-------											*	*	403.1
1894-------										*	*	*	409.8
1895-------									*	*	*	*	543.9
1896-------								*	*	*	*	*	462.2
1897-------							*	*	*	*	*	*	504.3
1898-------						*	*	*	*	*	*	*	521.4
1899-------					*	*	*	*	*	*	*	*	544.0
1900-------				*	*	*	*	*	*	*	*	*	507.4
1901-------			*	*	*	*	*	*	*	*	*	*	477.6
1902-------	1917	*	*	*	*	*	*	*	*	*	*	*	450.4
1903-------	1918	*	*	*	*	*	*	*	*	*	*	*	398.4
1904-------	1919	*	*	*	*	*	*	*	*	*	*	*	386.6
1905-------	1920	*	*	*	*	*	*	*	*	*	*	*	392.9
1906-------	1921	*	*	*	*	*	*	*	*	*	*	*	385.3
1907-------	1922	*	*	*	*	*	*	*	*	*	*	*	376.2
1908-------	1923	*	*	*	*	*	*	*	*	*	*	*	*
1909-------	1924	*	*	*	*	*	*	*	*	*	*	*	*
1910-------	1925	*	*	*	*	*	*	*	*	*	*	*	*
1911-------	1926	*	*	*	*	*	*	*	*	*	*	*	*
1912-------	1927	*	*	*	*	*	*	*	*	*	*	*	*
1913-------	1928	*	*	*	*	*	*	*	*	*	*	*	*
1914-------	1929	*	*	*	*	*	*	*	*	*	*	*	*
1915-------	1930	*	*	*	*	*	*	*	*	*	*	*	446.6
1916-------	1931	*	*	*	*	*	*	*	*	*	*	*	431.2
1917-------	1932	*	*	*	*	*	*	*	*	*	*	*	423.7
1918-------	1933	*	*	*	*	*	*	*	*	*	*	*	404.8
1919-------	1934	*	*	*	*	*	*	*	*	*	*	*	375.0
1920-------	1935	*	*	*	*	*	*	*	*	*	*	*	393.9
1921-------	1936	*	*	*	*	*	*	*	*	*	*	*	416.7
1922-------	1937	*	*	*	*	*	*	*	*	*	*	*	424.2
1923-------	1938	*	*	*	*	*	*	*	*	*	*	*	423.4
1924-------	1939	*	*	*	*	*	*	*	*	*	*	*	401.4
1925-------	1940	*	*	*	*	*	*	*	*	*	*	*	404.1
1926-------	1941	*	*	*	*	*	*	*	*	*	*	*	409.1
1927-------	1942	*	*	*	*	*	*	*	*	*	*	*	432.1
1928-------	1943	*	*	*	*	*	*	*	*	*	*	*	431.0
1929-------	1944	*	*	*	*	*	*	*	*	*	*	454.5	426.4
1930-------	1945	*	*	*	*	*	*	*	*	*	*	456.0	423.4
1931-------	1946	*	*	*	*	*	*	*	*	*	*	437.5	419.6
1932-------	1947	*	*	*	*	*	*	*	*	*	*	436.7	426.5
1933-------	1948	*	*	*	*	*	*	*	*	*	*	458.3	425.5
1934-------	1949	*	*	*	*	*	*	*	*	*	*	454.0	408.0
1935-------	1950	*	*	*	*	*	*	*	*	*	*	436.5	420.7
1936-------	1951	*	*	*	*	*	*	*	*	*	*	436.8	404.4
1937-------	1952	*	*	*	*	*	*	*	*	*	470.0	438.1	395.6
1938-------	1953	*	*	*	*	*	*	*	*	*	461.5	437.5	368.3
1939-------	1954	*	*	*	*	*	*	*	*	*	461.5	397.9	316.0
1940-------	1955	*	*	*	*	*	*	*	*	*	450.0	322.2	277.0
1941-------	1956	*	*	*	*	*	*	*	*	*	*	289.2	245.9
1942-------	1957	*	*	*	*	*	*	*	*	*	*	268.1	238.8
1943-------	1958	*	*	*	*	*	*	*	*	*	*	267.9	220.1
1944-------	1959	*	*	*	*	*	*	*	*	*	*	*	246.2
1945-------	1960	*	*	*	*	*	*	*	*	*	*	*	224.3
1946-------	1961	*	*	*	*	*	*	*	*	*	*	*	*
1947-------	1962	*	*	*	*	*	*	*	*	*	*	*	*
1948-------	1963	*	*	*	*	*	*	*	*	*	*	*	
1949-------	1964	*	*	*	*	*	*	*	*	*	*		
1950-------	1965	*	*	*	*	*	*	*	*	*			
1951-------	1966	*	*	*	*	*	*	*	*				
1952-------	1967	*	*	*	*	*	*	*					
1953-------	1968	*	*	*	*	*	*						
1954-------	1969	*	*	*	*	*							
1955-------	1970	*	*	*	*								
1956-------	1971	*	*	*									
1957-------	1972	*	*										
1958-------	1973	*											

TABLE 10C. BIRTH PROBABILITIES FOR ALL OTHER WOMEN FOR EACH YEAR 1917-73 BY AGE AND PARITY FOR EACH COHORT FROM 1868 TO 1958--CON.

(PROBABILITIES ARE THE NUMBER OF BIRTHS PER 1,000 WOMEN IN SPECIFIED PARITY AND EXACT AGE GROUP. FIGURES FOR "0 PARITY" SHOW THE PROBABILITY OF FIRST BIRTHS TO "0 PARITY" WOMEN, THOSE FOR "1 PARITY" SHOW THE PROBABILITY OF SECOND BIRTHS TO "1 PARITY" WOMEN, ETC. BASED ON CENTRAL BIRTH RATES AND PARITY DISTRIBUTIONS)

PARITY AND COHORT	DIAGONAL LINE FOR JANUARY 1	EXACT AGE											
		27	28	29	30	31	32	33	34	35	36	37	38
7 AND HIGHER PARITY--CON.													
1879-------													206.9
1880-------												238.8	204.5
1881-------											258.9	233.5	234.3
1882-------										269.9	250.8	265.4	244.6
1883-------									261.3	259.0	283.0	276.4	243.5
1884-------								226.2	250.3	291.9	295.1	277.4	234.6
1885-------							211.0	209.6	276.2	299.7	293.2	266.4	236.6
1886-------						247.5	196.1	225.7	282.2	308.4	281.8	268.0	246.5
1887-------					246.8	232.8	212.4	228.7	302.8	298.2	285.1	280.3	272.8
1888-------				283.7	220.9	246.6	210.0	257.7	286.6	295.5	292.2	296.5	262.1
1889-------			248.7	278.6	261.7	262.5	253.5	262.6	302.1	321.7	335.4	301.0	269.2
1890-------	1917	285.2	242.9	342.3	278.0	315.3	254.3	276.3	329.5	355.9	322.7	303.7	243.6
1891-------	1918	281.4	314.1	355.8	341.4	310.8	262.9	304.4	363.5	342.9	321.5	272.5	237.8
1892-------	1919	364.5	320.9	444.2	317.8	315.2	283.7	335.9	346.2	329.3	282.2	253.3	244.4
1893-------	1920	360.0	413.2	389.8	321.7	332.3	321.3	318.9	325.0	287.9	265.1	259.0	233.9
1894-------	1921	476.2	350.0	409.3	340.1	365.7	303.9	309.5	288.9	276.6	270.7	253.2	246.6
1895-------	1922	397.0	383.1	429.6	364.5	351.1	288.2	272.5	274.2	281.0	255.3	261.2	233.2
1896-------	1923	435.2	395.2	462.3	367.3	327.0	265.9	262.6	284.2	267.0	261.3	246.5	239.4
1897-------	1924	452.6	437.7	466.0	340.0	316.1	254.7	272.0	274.4	272.5	250.0	260.7	223.5
1898-------	1925	515.0	442.2	431.7	326.1	301.0	264.1	273.0	278.3	262.8	263.5	239.9	212.4
1899-------	1926	500.0	408.5	411.8	311.0	313.7	274.7	283.6	277.5	286.9	249.6	234.1	226.2
1900-------	1927	447.0	378.1	388.8	319.3	317.2	275.9	279.8	294.3	265.9	243.9	248.6	227.3
1901-------	1928	435.4	370.0	399.0	335.3	315.8	269.9	302.1	271.4	260.9	257.2	248.9	222.5
1902-------	1929	399.0	364.3	394.2	312.4	288.3	279.0	268.4	264.3	268.3	254.3	253.1	228.9
1903-------	1930	385.9	360.9	381.6	288.7	311.7	253.0	266.1	272.6	266.0	252.8	256.4	234.5
1904-------	1931	379.1	355.0	357.7	315.3	293.3	259.8	278.2	265.7	264.6	255.1	258.7	234.7
1905-------	1932	372.1	340.0	397.1	305.1	297.8	268.1	277.9	269.9	272.7	256.6	252.7	247.4
1906-------	1933	363.6	380.8	385.3	312.2	308.1	273.0	286.3	285.3	277.8	254.1	267.6	250.2
1907-------	1934	421.1	376.7	383.6	324.1	317.1	282.8	310.4	295.0	279.7	267.5	268.5	251.2
1908-------	1935	402.8	361.5	408.9	329.9	321.6	305.9	322.2	301.1	294.3	268.5	277.0	235.4
1909-------	1936	394.4	393.4	397.3	325.8	336.0	307.7	315.5	308.7	291.0	286.0	264.4	239.1
1910-------	1937	426.6	379.6	396.0	344.1	336.0	306.4	327.9	311.2	312.5	276.6	263.2	234.4
1911-------	1938	402.7	390.1	415.3	339.7	324.3	312.1	328.6	319.8	293.7	270.5	259.8	236.7
1912-------	1939	421.8	429.9	419.0	334.9	339.1	318.3	323.5	298.9	289.6	261.2	255.6	229.8
1913-------	1940	463.1	427.3	390.1	349.1	344.1	314.3	310.3	293.3	282.4	259.8	251.2	233.6
1914-------	1941	448.7	394.1	409.2	355.8	338.3	306.7	309.7	290.9	275.3	260.4	260.7	229.5
1915-------	1942	432.1	408.3	411.4	352.9	335.8	305.6	309.6	286.2	281.0	265.6	250.2	219.1
1916-------	1943	427.7	396.1	398.9	343.5	328.0	297.5	296.7	285.9	279.5	253.2	238.3	225.7
1917-------	1944	410.8	379.2	388.0	327.0	320.7	299.3	302.6	280.3	267.4	244.2	243.5	215.3
1918-------	1945	379.5	369.7	362.9	327.9	326.1	299.4	299.9	277.5	265.5	248.1	236.6	219.4
1919-------	1946	385.0	359.9	382.1	342.6	329.6	301.0	301.7	285.1	270.9	250.0	246.7	213.1
1920-------	1947	399.0	387.8	386.0	341.0	327.6	306.0	307.1	290.7	270.8	255.2	233.8	202.7
1921-------	1948	413.8	390.6	381.8	341.6	330.3	307.8	311.8	286.1	274.6	244.6	219.3	200.6
1922-------	1949	407.8	380.0	381.4	335.2	324.2	311.1	308.9	285.6	264.7	231.4	219.2	193.3
1923-------	1950	396.2	389.6	379.7	330.3	335.8	317.0	309.1	285.7	252.1	235.4	213.8	186.5
1924-------	1951	398.2	385.8	372.2	351.5	343.9	314.5	307.9	275.7	259.9	226.9	207.7	172.1
1925-------	1952	414.1	385.3	397.9	354.6	342.4	313.9	297.5	281.1	246.2	224.6	192.4	166.0
1926-------	1953	414.6	402.7	387.3	357.9	338.9	309.1	297.7	263.4	241.5	204.4	180.3	159.0
1927-------	1954	418.9	391.5	404.3	356.9	334.4	306.0	280.4	257.0	225.4	189.5	170.7	139.1
1928-------	1955	424.6	419.2	399.3	350.1	331.9	296.0	279.3	244.5	208.7	185.8	153.6	118.4
1929-------	1956	434.0	402.5	387.7	343.6	320.9	293.9	268.5	229.6	204.8	163.5	130.4	102.9
1930-------	1957	417.4	393.4	372.9	330.7	315.3	281.2	251.1	220.9	178.5	140.8	113.3	88.4
1931-------	1958	414.6	375.4	348.3	324.9	294.3	259.5	236.8	192.1	155.0	119.2	96.7	79.4
1932-------	1959	401.9	354.1	355.2	308.1	281.3	247.1	210.7	166.9	132.8	105.1	89.3	76.4
1933-------	1960	388.5	375.4	341.7	301.0	275.6	222.1	180.7	145.7	116.7	99.1	86.1	69.6
1934-------	1961	396.9	362.8	334.1	292.3	239.4	189.3	159.4	125.8	110.0	96.1	77.0	59.1
1935-------	1962	388.9	349.3	322.1	253.2	205.6	165.3	139.0	118.4	102.7	84.9	66.7	53.6
1936-------	1963	374.5	331.3	280.5	216.7	180.7	148.1	128.1	109.7	97.3	71.9	57.4	
1937-------	1964	348.7	296.0	235.2	193.9	162.5	135.8	119.0	108.8	79.6	62.4		
1938-------	1965	307.2	246.3	211.0	168.7	146.6	132.1	119.0	86.7	65.5			
1939-------	1966	262.8	217.6	184.0	154.3	147.4	129.9	98.1	75.4				
1940-------	1967	226.9	195.8	175.3	154.8	142.7	106.9	88.5					
1941-------	1968	217.8	189.1	173.1	156.7	118.5	95.8						
1942-------	1969	208.3	188.3	174.0	128.1	112.0							
1943-------	1970	220.1	188.0	143.8	120.9								
1944-------	1971	204.5	153.8	139.0									
1945-------	1972	174.8	136.4										
1946-------	1973	146.8											

TABLE 10C. BIRTH PROBABILITIES FOR ALL OTHER WOMEN FOR EACH YEAR 1917-73 BY AGE AND PARITY FOR EACH COHORT FROM 1868 TO 1958--CON.

(PROBABILITIES ARE THE NUMBER OF BIRTHS PER 1,000 WOMEN IN SPECIFIED PARITY AND EXACT AGE GROUP. FIGURES FOR "0 PARITY" SHOW THE PROBABILITY OF FIRST BIRTHS TO "C PARITY" WOMEN, THOSE FOR "1 PARITY" SHOW THE PROBABILITY OF SECOND BIRTHS TO "1 PARITY" WOMEN, ETC. BASED ON CENTRAL BIRTH RATES AND PARITY DISTRIBUTIONS)

PARITY AND COHORT	DIAGONAL LINE FOR JANUARY 1	EXACT AGE										
		39	40	41	42	43	44	45	46	47	48	49
7 AND HIGHER PARITY--CON.												
1868----------------												8.8
1869----------------											15.4	16.2
1870----------------										23.9	29.0	8.9
1871----------------									36.7	45.1	15.6	10.6
1872----------------								44.6	69.6	24.1	19.0	8.1
1873----------------							53.7	73.9	37.4	29.8	14.5	7.4
1874----------------						63.0	75.4	44.7	46.7	23.1	13.1	8.0
1875----------------					74.3	70.1	53.1	53.1	36.8	21.3	14.6	7.3
1876----------------				107.5	83.0	61.1	59.0	45.4	33.8	23.6	13.5	6.2
1877----------------			132.2	121.7	73.3	63.1	56.2	41.8	37.9	22.0	11.5	6.1
1878----------------	1917	192.4	142.5	109.5	76.5	68.7	52.4	46.1	36.2	18.6	11.5	7.4
1879----------------	1918	159.8	142.3	115.9	83.9	65.2	56.2	44.7	34.9	20.2	12.2	8.7
1880----------------	1919	215.2	151.3	127.5	79.5	67.6	56.1	44.0	37.5	17.5	13.6	7.4
1881----------------	1920	226.2	159.5	119.7	81.6	68.0	57.6	46.5	32.4	19.3	13.0	7.8
1882----------------	1921	230.6	150.3	121.5	81.6	71.5	58.8	43.6	32.9	20.8	13.2	7.6
1883----------------	1922	218.8	151.4	120.5	88.2	73.9	57.0	41.3	32.8	19.5	11.6	7.0
1884----------------	1923	221.9	153.7	130.2	91.7	67.6	53.4	40.7	34.4	17.6	12.3	7.9
1885----------------	1924	227.8	170.2	133.4	81.7	63.4	50.6	42.4	31.0	18.7	12.1	9.3
1886----------------	1925	245.0	166.3	127.0	76.0	62.3	52.4	41.1	34.9	15.9	14.4	8.4
1887----------------	1926	243.5	168.0	115.1	77.0	62.5	52.5	45.9	29.9	17.8	13.6	8.3
1888----------------	1927	237.1	146.3	114.0	77.0	62.0	58.3	39.0	29.2	16.7	12.9	7.0
1889----------------	1928	220.3	155.5	122.2	77.8	70.8	53.2	39.8	30.6	17.5	12.4	7.9
1890----------------	1929	220.0	160.9	118.1	85.8	66.6	57.3	40.5	29.9	16.9	13.4	7.0
1891----------------	1930	229.2	154.3	128.0	83.8	74.5	54.2	39.5	29.8	16.7	11.9	7.1
1892----------------	1931	219.2	165.0	122.7	88.5	71.0	52.1	40.3	28.6	15.2	12.1	5.4
1893----------------	1932	231.7	156.6	125.1	84.7	68.3	51.7	37.8	26.0	14.8	9.9	4.9
1894----------------	1933	218.5	158.4	124.2	81.2	67.7	50.2	34.8	27.1	13.2	7.5	5.0
1895----------------	1934	223.9	154.0	115.8	82.2	64.7	45.7	35.9	23.0	12.1	7.6	4.5
1896----------------	1935	210.7	144.0	118.9	80.0	59.5	48.1	32.1	20.9	12.4	6.5	5.2
1897----------------	1936	196.2	148.9	118.4	74.3	63.5	44.8	34.5	20.9	10.1	8.1	4.7
1898----------------	1937	204.4	155.0	111.3	81.7	63.2	51.2	36.7	19.0	13.5	7.4	3.4
1899----------------	1938	208.8	141.2	115.2	79.0	66.2	48.4	30.1	20.0	10.7	6.7	4.0
1900----------------	1939	198.4	145.4	117.2	79.6	68.2	45.7	32.1	18.0	10.7	6.0	2.7
1901----------------	1940	200.5	149.2	109.2	84.2	68.5	48.3	29.0	19.0	9.2	5.6	3.5
1902----------------	1941	211.6	151.1	121.8	89.4	73.5	46.7	30.0	16.5	8.2	6.0	3.0
1903----------------	1942	211.5	163.3	124.8	91.6	71.6	45.1	25.2	14.1	8.6	5.5	3.1
1904----------------	1943	221.1	161.2	127.0	92.3	67.9	42.5	25.6	15.2	8.8	5.6	3.2
1905----------------	1944	221.8	164.5	127.6	88.6	64.6	42.8	25.4	14.7	8.2	4.9	2.4
1906----------------	1945	229.9	160.4	124.3	85.5	67.8	40.4	24.3	14.2	7.5	5.0	2.5
1907----------------	1946	212.0	160.3	116.9	86.4	63.1	38.6	23.1	13.6	6.8	4.2	2.5
1908----------------	1947	212.9	150.7	119.5	80.5	63.9	37.4	24.2	12.9	6.0	3.4	2.6
1909----------------	1948	206.3	156.2	117.4	87.1	63.9	42.3	24.4	11.8	6.7	5.0	1.7
1910----------------	1949	211.5	154.5	125.8	84.6	66.1	42.3	23.1	12.4	8.2	4.1	2.5
1911----------------	1950	205.7	159.8	117.3	84.8	65.1	39.6	23.3	14.4	5.6	4.0	2.4
1912----------------	1951	209.9	151.3	119.5	85.3	64.0	41.8	24.8	12.8	6.4	4.0	2.4
1913----------------	1952	200.7	151.1	114.4	82.5	67.1	42.0	24.5	11.8	6.3	3.9	1.6
1914----------------	1953	199.1	150.3	111.7	86.8	66.8	41.3	21.0	11.6	5.4	3.1	1.5
1915----------------	1954	198.8	143.3	115.8	85.4	62.0	36.1	19.9	9.9	5.3	3.0	0.8
1916----------------	1955	187.9	146.6	113.3	80.0	55.0	34.4	18.6	10.4	5.2	3.0	0.7
1917----------------	1956	192.6	142.4	108.6	74.8	53.4	33.4	18.8	9.4	5.7	2.2	1.4
1918----------------	1957	185.6	139.0	104.2	74.4	53.7	32.3	18.1	9.7	4.2	2.1	0.7
1919----------------	1958	181.8	139.3	103.8	75.2	53.4	33.5	18.0	9.3	4.7	1.3	1.3
1920----------------	1959	179.0	133.7	102.0	71.0	52.5	32.6	16.9	8.4	3.9	1.9	0.6
1921----------------	1960	170.5	130.9	96.1	69.1	49.0	27.5	14.7	7.0	3.2	1.3	0.6
1922----------------	1961	164.2	121.3	88.5	65.2	42.1	26.0	13.9	6.3	2.5	1.3	0.6
1923----------------	1962	153.4	110.9	86.2	55.9	39.9	22.9	10.5	5.5	2.5	1.2	0.6
1924----------------	1963	142.7	113.3	76.8	52.9	35.2	19.0	9.5	5.3	2.4	1.2	0.0
1925----------------	1964	141.4	98.9	70.7	47.3	29.2	16.5	9.7	5.1	2.3	0.6	
1926----------------	1965	125.2	86.9	61.5	39.3	26.4	15.9	8.7	3.8	1.6		
1927----------------	1966	106.9	74.9	51.5	34.9	24.0	14.4	6.4	3.2			
1928----------------	1967	92.4	64.3	45.5	32.7	23.5	10.1	5.8				
1929----------------	1968	79.7	56.8	41.3	31.0	16.2	9.4					
1930----------------	1969	70.2	52.5	39.7	22.6	14.6						
1931----------------	1970	64.4	48.5	32.2	20.4							
1932----------------	1971	61.6	41.6	27.1								
1933----------------	1972	51.8	34.3									
1934----------------	1973	42.5										

APPENDIX I

METHOD OF ESTIMATING NUMBERS OF WOMEN

Estimates of the female population for single years of age 14 through 49 by color (white and all other) for 1917-73 were prepared for this report by the U.S. Bureau of the Census. The estimates have been corrected for net census undercount and are consistent within cohorts from year to year. The methods of estimation are summarized in the first three sections. The last section describes the adjustment to obtain appropriate denominators for central birth rates of cohorts.

1950

The corrected estimates begin with a 1950 female population corrected for net census undercount and misstatement of age. The white population benchmark was developed from estimates for native U.S. white females prepared by Coale and Zelnik and presented in *New Estimates of Fertility and Population in the United States.*[5] These estimates were converted to figures for total white females by assuming that the percent of net census undercount was the same for foreign-born females as for native females by 5-year age groups. Single year of age data for foreign-born females were estimated by osculatory interpolation. Comparable data for the population of all other races were not available from this source. The 1950 benchmark for this segment of the population was developed from estimates prepared by Coale and presented in "The Population of the United States in 1950 Classified by Age, Sex and Color—A Revision of Census Figures;"[6] single year of age data were estimated by osculatory interpolation.

1951-73

In carrying the female population forward from 1950, white and all other women were treated in a similar manner. Components of change (births, deaths, and immigration) consistent with *Current Population Reports,* Series P-25, No. 310, were used to carry the population forward to 1960. The 1960 census count of females was corrected for undercount using data presented by Siegel and Zelnik in "An Evaluation of Coverage in the 1960 Census of Population by Techniques of Demographic Analysis and by Composite Methods"[7] and carried forward to July 1. Since the two sets of estimates for 1960 were very close, the corrected census estimates were used with no adjustment of earlier years for error of closure. The 1960 estimates were carried forward to 1973 using unpublished data on components of change. Estimates for 1970 are consistent with data from the 1970 census.

1917-49

In carrying the 1950 population backward through time, the two color groups were treated differently due to the basic character of the available data. However, the estimates appear to be mutually consistent, since a review of the ratios of the native white population to the population of all other races by age showed them to be reasonable.

For the white population, benchmarks similar to that for 1950 were available for 1940, 1930, 1920, and 1910. Estimates for each year from 1950 back to 1940 were obtained by reviving the population using data on components of change consistent with those in *Current Population Reports,* Series P-25, No. 98. The estimates for 1940 to 1950 were adjusted pro rata by cohort for the error of closure. Unpublished data were used to revive the population from 1940 to 1930 and then from 1930 to 1920 and on to 1917. The data developed in this way for intervening years were adjusted for the error of closure as described for 1940 to 1950.

For the population of all races other than white there were no benchmarks similar to that for 1950 available for 1940, 1930, and 1920. Therefore the revived estimates of the population were not adjusted for errors of closure for the census years. The 1950 corrected population was revived to 1940 using components of change consistent with P-25, No. 98. Before 1940, estimates of the components of change were not available for the population of all other races and survival rates developed from appropriate life tables were used. No adjustment was made for immigration for 1917 to 1940. For the last 15 years of this period there was virtually no immigration of all other females. The relatively small number of immigrants in the years from 1917 to 1924 was not taken into account in the absence of appropriate age data.

Adjustment for Denominators of Central Birth Rates of Cohorts

These estimates of the numbers of women in single-year cohorts were further adjusted to represent more adequately the denominators of central birth rates of cohorts in calendar years.

Essentially, what is wanted for the denominator of a central birth rate for age x in calendar year y is the average number of women who are between exact ages x and

---

[5] Coale, A.J. and Zelnik, M.: *New Estimates of Fertility and Population in the United States.* Princeton. Princeton University Press, 1963.

[6] Coale, A.J.: The population of the United States in 1950 classified by age, sex and color - A revision of census figures. *J.Am.Stat.A.* 50 (269), Mar. 1955.

[7] Siegel, J.S. and Zelnik, M.: An Evaluation of Coverage in the 1960 Census of Population by Techniques of Demographic Analysis and by Composite Methods, prepared for the American Statistical Association, Aug. 1966.

$x+1$ (that is, current age x or age x last birthday) during year y. Ideally, to obtain such a denominator an estimate is made for the population age x on every day of the year and is averaged for the result. Figure I shows how to approximate this ideal. It shows the date of birth of three cohorts (1919, 1920, and 1921) plotted against the date at which age 20 or 21 is attained during the year 1940. The horizontal distance between the lines for the 20th and 21st birthdays and the beginning or end of 1940 (shaded portion of the figure is the length of time in 1940 that women born on a particular date (vertical axis) are in current age 20. Assuming that the survivors of the 1920 cohort were distributed evenly with respect to the date that age 20 was attained, they spent an average of 75 percent of 1940 in this year of age. In addition, half of the women in the cohorts of 1919 and 1921 were 20 years old during one or more days in 1940 (again assuming an even distribution of birthdays). They spent an average of 25 percent of 1940 at current age 20. Since only half of the women in the cohorts of 1919 and 1921 were 20 years old in 1940, the weight applied to them is half of 25 percent, or 12.5 percent. Therefore, the denominator for a central birth rate at age x in year y is $.125\ P_{y-x-1} + .75\ P_{y-x} + .125\ P_{y-x+1}$. where P represents the female population of the designated cohort on July 1, of year y.

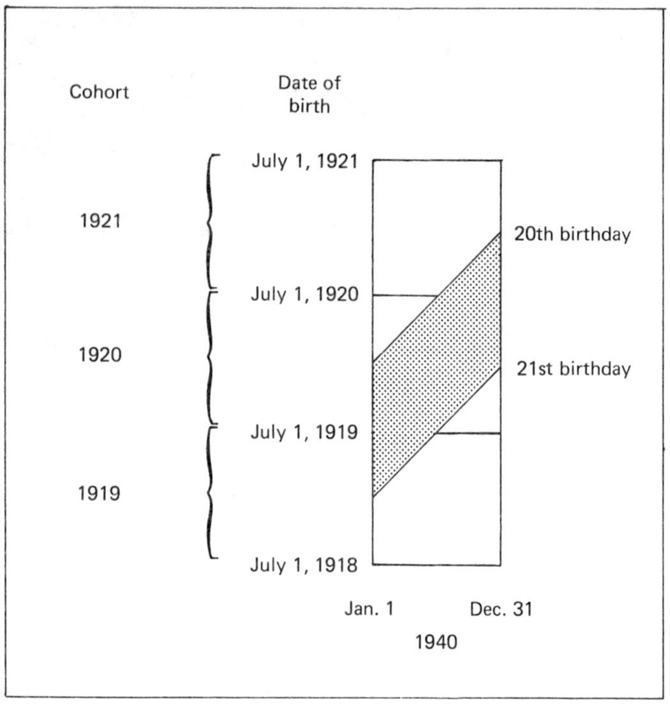

Figure 1. Date in 1940 on which age 20 or 21 is attained by women in the cohorts of 1919, 1920, and 1921.

APPENDIX II

METHOD OF ESTIMATING NUMBERS OF BIRTHS

In order to compute the central birth rates it was necessary to have the number of births in each year from 1917 through 1973, corrected for underregistration, classified by age of mother (single years of age from 14 through 49), live-birth order (each order through the seventh, and eighth and higher orders combined), and color (white and all other). The numbers of registered births tabulated by age, birth order, and color were adjusted to

- Distribute births of unknown age of mother and live-birth order.
- Distribute births of each order by single years of age of mother for years when births were tabulated only for 5-year age groups.
- Estimate "registered" births before 1933 for States not in the birth-registration area.
- Adjust for underregistration of births.

These adjustments were made separately for white and all other births, which were added to obtain total births.

The methods of making these adjustments are described below.

Distributing Births With Unknown Characteristics

Age.—Births to women of unknown age were distributed within each birth-order group like births to women of known age.

Birth order.—Among States for which tabulations of births by age and order were available, births of unknown order were distributed within each age group (single years of age where available or 5-year age groups) like births of known order. From 1939 through 1962, births to residents of Massachusetts, the only State not classifying births by order, were assumed to have the same distribution by order within each age group as births to residents of Connecticut. For 1930-38, births in Massachusetts and other States not classifying births by order were added to other births of unknown order in the United States and distributed, within each age, like births of known order.

Distributing Births by Single Year of Age of Mother When Births Were Tabulated Only for 5-Year Age Groups

Births of each order were distributed among single years of age within 5-year age groups like births in as nearly adjacent a year for which single year of age data were available. The years distributed and the year providing the single year of age pattern are:

Years distributed	*Pattern year*
1942-43	1944
1939-41	1938
1917-23	1924

Estimated births in States not in the birth-registration area in 1924-32 were distributed among single years of age like births in registration-area States.

Estimating "Registered" Births in 1917-32 for States Not in the Birth-Registration Area

Data by age and by birth order for States in the birth-registration area (BRA) were used to estimate numbers of births for States not in the birth-registration area (non-BRA). Estimates of white births were made for all non-BRA States. However, estimates of all other births were not made for eight States with small numbers of all other women (less than 2,500 women 15-44 years of age in the 1920 census). The procedures used are summarized as follows:

a. Calculate rates by age and by order for each BRA State for each year 1917-33.
b. Using rates for 1933, select a guide State for the non-BRA State in 1932. The guide State is the BRA State where rates are most like those of the non-BRA State.
c. Estimate rates by age and by order for 1932 for the non-BRA State, assuming the same relationship between the guide and the estimated State as was observed in 1933. There are now rates for all States in 1932.
d. Estimate "registered" births for non-BRA States.
e. Distribute the age and order marginals obtained in step d to get numbers of births by single year of age by birth order.
f. Repeat steps b-e using rates for 1932 to estimate data for 1931, 1931 to estimate 1930, and so on until numbers of registered births by single year of age of mother, live-birth order, and color have been estimated for each year back to 1917.

These procedures are described in detail below.

a. *Rates by age and by order for BRA States 1917-33.*—For each State registered births with unknown age of mother were distributed within 5-year age groups like births to women of known age. Births of unknown order were similarly distributed. Births to Mexicans were classified as white for all years except 1930-34. Since the number of births identified as Mexican was large enough in some States to significantly affect the proportions of births tabulated as other than white, an adjustment was made. An expected proportion of births of "other races" (races other than white and Negro), excluding Mexicans, for each year from 1930 through 1934 was obtained by straight-line interpolation between proportions for 1928-29 and 1935-36. This was done for each of 11 States with large Mexican populations. The difference between the actual and the expected number of births of "other races" was assumed to be

Mexican births. It was further assumed that the distribution of these births by age and by order was the same as for all births other than white. The estimated numbers of Mexican births were subtracted from all other births and added to white births.

Numbers of females by 5-year age groups for each State were estimated by linear interpolation between censuses of 1910, 1920, 1930, and 1940. Estimates for 1915, 1925, and 1935 were obtained by interpolating cohortwise between censuses. For example, age 25-29 in 1925 is the average of age 20-24 in 1920 and 30-34 in 1930. Estimates for 1917-19, 1921-24, 1926-29, and 1931-33 were the results of linear interpolation within 5-year age groups between data for 1915, 1920, 1925, 1930, and 1935.

Birth rates by age are the number of births to women in a given 5-year age group per 1,000 women of those ages. Rates were computed for the age groups 15-19 through 45-49 years. The rate for ages 15-19 is the number of births to women under 20 per 1,000 women 15-19 years of age. Rates by order are the number of births in each order per 1,000 women 15-44 years of age.

b. *Selecting guide States.*—The birth rates by age and by order for a non-BRA State were compared with the rates for each BRA State using the measure

$$S = \sum_{\text{all } i} \left[\frac{\left(\text{Rate}_{\text{BRA State}} - \text{Rate}_{\text{non-BRA State}} \right)^2}{\text{Rate}_{\text{non-BRA State}}} \right]_i$$

where i is each age and order group. The BRA State for which S was the smallest was chosen as the guide State to estimate rates for the non-BRA State in the previous year. The guide States are shown in tables I and II.

c. *Estimate rates for non-BRA States.*—Assume the ratios of rates for the non-BRA State to the rates for its guide were the same in the year being estimated as they were for the next year, when rates for all States (actual or estimated) were available. This is done for each age and order group. The rate for each group, i, is computed as follows:

$$\text{Rate}_{\text{non-BRA State}, i, Y_e} = \left(\frac{\text{Rate}_{\text{non-BRA State}}}{\text{Rate}_{\text{guide State}}} \right)_{i, Y_{e+1}} X \ \text{Rate}_{\text{guide State}, i, Y_e}$$

where Y_e is the year being estimated. The implied assumption in this procedure is that the rates for the non-BRA State changed by the same percent as for the guide State between Y_e and Y_{e+1}.

d. *Estimate "registered" births for non-BRA States.*—"Registered" births by age and by order are estimated by multiplying the rates obtained in step c by the populations obtained in step a. "Registered" births by age and by order for the United States are the sum of the estimates for non-BRA States and the registered births for the BRA States.

e. *Distribute age and order marginals into age-order cells.*—A first estimate of the age-order distribution of the estimated number of "registered" births in the United States was obtained by using a percent distribution of births in the BRA. This estimate was adjusted first to the control totals for each birth order and then to the control totals for each age group. (The control totals were the numbers estimated in step d.) After each pair of "rakings," first to birth order and then to age controls, the difference between the birth-order controls and the sum of the estimates over all age groups was computed for each birth order. The raking procedure was continued until the absolute difference between the control and the estimate was less than 100 for each birth order.

The numbers that have been obtained for the 15-19 year age group are really for all ages under 20 (see step a). To estimate the under 15 age group (assumed to be age 14) the ratio $\frac{\text{Under 15}}{\text{Under 20}}$ was calculated for the BRA and applied to the estimated births under 20 years of age in the United States. This was done for each birth order.

All 5-year age groups 15-19 through 45-49 were distributed by single years of age as described in the previous section.

Table I. Guide States for estimating birth rates for white women in non-BRA States, 1917-32

State being estimated	Year of estimate															
	1932	1931	1930	1929	1928	1927	1926	1925	1924	1923	1922	1921	1920	1919	1918	1917
	Guide State															
Alabama							Miss.	Miss.	Miss.	Miss.	Miss.	Conn.	Conn.	Conn.	Conn.	Conn.
Arizona								Wis.	Wis.	Minn.	Miss.	Wis.	Wis.	Va.	Va.	Va.
Arkansas							Ky.	Ky.	Ky.	Ky.	Ky.	Ky.	Ky.	Ky.	Ky.	Ky.
California															Wash.	Wash.
Colorado						La.	Nebr.	N.Y.	N.Y.	N.Y.	N.Y.	N.Y.	N.Y.	N.Y.	N.Y.	N.Y.
Delaware													Ohio	Pa.	Pa.	Kans.
Florida										Ind.	Ind.	Ind.	Kans.	Kans.	Kans.	Kans.
Georgia						La.	Ky.	Fla.	Ky.	Ky.	Ky.	Ky.	Ky.	Ky.	Ky.	Ky.
Illinois												N.Y.	D.C.	D.C.	D.C.	D.C.
Iowa										Ill.	Ill.	Ky.	D.C.	D.C.	D.C.	D.C.
Louisiana							Miss.	Miss.	Ky.	Ky.	Ky.	Ky.	Ky.	Kans.	Kans.	Kans.
Mississippi													Md.	Md.	Md.	Md.
Missouri							Ill.	Ill.	Ill.	D.C.	Ill.	D.C.	D.C.	D.C.	D.C.	D.C.
Montana												Wash.	Wash.	Wash.	Wash.	Wash.
Nebraska														Pa.	Ohio	Ohio
New Jersey													Nebr.	Kans.	Kans.	Kans.
New Mexico					Ariz.	Ariz.	Ariz.	Kans.	N.Y.	Minn.	Miss.	Wis.	Wis.	N.C.	N.C.	N.C.
Oklahoma						Iowa	Kans.	Kans.	Iowa	Kans.	Ky.	Ky.	Kans.	Ky.	Ky.	Ky.
Oregon															Minn.	Minn.
South Carolina						Va.	Va.	Va.							Va.	Va.
South Dakota		Minn.	Wash.	Wash.	Wash.	Mont.	Mont.	Mont.	Mont.	Mont.	Mont.	Wash.	Wash.	Calif.	Wash.	Wash.
Tennessee							Ky.	Ky.	Kans.	Kans.	Kans.	Kans.	Kans.	Kans.	Kans.	Kans.
Texas	Okla.	Okla.	Okla.	Okla.	Okla.	Iowa	Kans.	Kans.	Iowa	Kans.	Ky.	Ky.	Ky.	Ky.	Ky.	Ky.
West Virginia									Md.	Md.	Md.	Md.	Md.	Md.	Md.	Md.

Table II. Guide States for estimating birth rates for all other women in non-BRA States, 1917-32

State being estimated	Year of estimate															
	1932	1931	1930	1929	1928	1927	1926	1925	1924	1923	1922	1921	1920	1919	1918	1917
	Guide State															
Alabama----------							Ky.	Miss.	Miss.	Miss.	Miss.	Pa.	Pa.	Pa.	Pa.	Pa.
Arizona----------								Ind.	Fla.	Md.	Ind.	Ind.	Ind.	Ind.	Ind.	Ind.
Arkansas---------							Miss.	Ky.	Ky.	Ky.	Ky.	Ky.	Ky.	Ky.	Ky.	Ky.
California-------															D.C.	D.C.
Colorado---------						Ohio	Ind.	Ind.	Ind.	Ind.	Ind.	Ind.	Ind.	Ind.	Ohio	Ohio
Delaware---------													Ohio	Kans.	Kans.	Kans.
Florida----------										Ind.	Ind.	Ind.	Ind.	Ind.	Ind.	Ind.
Georgia----------						Tenn.	Pa.	Vt.	Vt.	Vt.	Vt.	Vt.	Vt.	Vt.	Vt.	Md.
Idaho------------								Pa.	Pa.	Pa.	Pa.	Pa.	Pa.	Pa.	Pa.	Pa.
Illinois---------												N.Y.	N.Y.	N.Y.	Ohio	Ohio
Iowa-------------										Kans.	Ohio	Ohio	Ohio	Ohio	Ohio	Ohio
Louisiana--------							Pa.	Vt.	Vt.	Vt.	Md.	Md.	Md.	Md.	Md.	Md.
Mississippi------													Pa.	Pa.	Pa.	Pa.
Missouri---------							Ohio	Ohio	Ohio	Md.	Ohio	Ohio	Ohio	Ohio	Ohio	Ohio
Montana----------												Ohio	Ohio	Ohio	Ohio	Kans.
Nebraska---------														N.H.	N.H.	N.H.
Nevada-----------					Wash.	Wash.	Oreg.	Wash.	Oreg.	Oreg.	Oreg.	Oreg.	Oreg.	Oreg.	Wash.	Wash.
New Jersey-------													N.H.	N.H.	N.H.	N.H.
New Mexico-------					W.Va.	W.Va.	W.Va.	W.Va.	N.C.	N.C.	N.C.	N.C.	N.C.	N.C.	N.C.	Utah
North Dakota-----										Minn.	Minn.	Minn.	Minn.	Minn.	Minn.	Minn.
Oklahoma---------						Md.	Md.	Md.	Md.	Md.	Ind.	Ind.	Ind.	Ind.	Ind.	Ind.
Oregon-----------															Wash.	Wash.
Rhode Island-----													Wis.	Wis.		
South Carolina---						Va.	Va.	Va.							Va.	Va.
South Dakota-----		Minn.	Minn.	Minn.	Minn.	N.D.	Minn.	Minn.	Minn.	Minn.	Minn.	Minn.	Minn.	Minn.	Minn.	Minn.
Tennessee--------							Pa.	Vt.	Pa.	Miss.	Miss.	Pa.	Pa.	Pa.	Pa.	Pa.
Texas------------	Ariz.	La.	La.	La.	La.	La.	Ariz.	Mich.	Pa.	Mich.	Mich.	Pa.	Mich.	Mich.	Pa.	Pa.
West Virginia----									Ky.	Ky.	Ky.	Ky.	S.C.	S.C.	Va.	Ky.
Wyoming----------												Mich.	Mich.	Mich.	Mich.	Mich.

Adjusting for Underregistration of Births

There have been three nationwide tests of birth registration completeness (BRT), in 1940, 1950, and 1964-68. These three tests are the basis for estimating the completeness of registration in other years.

The 1950 BRT provided the most detailed results. Data are available for each State by place of delivery (in or out of hospital) and for the United States by age of mother [8] and birth order. The 1940 BRT provided the same information for States, but for the United States no figures were available by birth order. Estimates were made by assuming that for each 5-year age group the relationship by birth order was the same in 1940 as in 1950. Results from these two tests, made in connection with the censuses, may be found in *Vital Statistics of the United States, 1950,* Volume I, Chapter 6.

The 1964-68 BRT was conducted on a sample basis primarily to obtain current national estimates of registration completeness by race. This test is described and the results are shown in "Test of Birth Registration Completeness 1964 to 1968," *Census of Population and Housing, 1970,* Evaluation and Research Program, PHC(E)-2. The test produced estimates for births occurring in and out of hospitals for the United States but not for States. Data by age of mother and birth order are not available.

The methods of estimating registration completeness and numbers of births adjusted for underregistration for nontest years are described below.

1951-73.—Control totals for these years were obtained using national estimates of registration completeness for births in and out of hospital from the 1950 and 1964-68 BRT's. Percents of registration completeness for 1951-65 were obtained by linear interpolation between the test results. The 1964-68 test results were assumed to apply for 1966, the midpoint of the test period, and for later years.

Since age of mother and birth-order data were not available for the 1964-68 BRT, it was assumed that the relationships by these characteristics were the same for all years as in 1950. The first estimates of the number of births adjusted for underregistration obtained using the 1950 percents by age and order were adjusted to the control totals.

1941-49.—For each State the number of births adjusted for underregistration in each of the years between 1940 and 1950 was estimated by assuming a linear trend between the 1940 and 1950 percents of births registered for births in and out of hospital. The national control was the sum of the State estimates. (These are the same totals used by Whelpton and Campbell and are shown in *Vital Statistics of the United States, 1949,* Part I, and elsewhere.)

The numbers of registered births in each year were adjusted using the 1950 percents by age and order. These first estimates were then adjusted to the control totals. This, in effect, assumed a linear change in the registration completeness by age and order.

1917-39.—The total number of births adjusted for underregistration used as control totals for these years are the estimates prepared by P.K. Whelpton and shown in table 1 of "Births and Birth Rates in the Entire United States, 1909-48," *Vital Statistics—Special Reports,* Vol. 33, No. 8. [9] For each of these years it was assumed that the relationships in registration completeness by age and order were the same as in 1940. After the estimates of underregistration for 1940 were applied to the number of "registered" births in 1917-39, the results were adjusted to meet the control totals.

[8] Registration completeness figures from the BRT for 5-year age of mother groups were used for each single year of age within the age group.

[9] National Office of Vital Statistics: Births and birth rates in the entire United States, 1909-48, by P.K. Whelpton. *Vital Statistics—Special Reports,* Vol. 33, No. 8. Public Health Service. Washington, D.C., Sept. 29, 1950.

APPENDIX III

METHOD OF COMPUTING COHORT FERTILITY MEASURES

Central Birth Rates

Central birth rates represent the number of births occurring to women at age *x* (described in appendix II) divided by the number of women of age *x* (described in appendix I). Such rates were computed for all color groups (total, white, and all other) by single year of age 14 through 49 by live-birth order,[10] first through seventh and eighth and higher combined, for each calendar year 1917 through 1973. After the central birth rates were computed, two adjustments were made as described below.

Adjustment to central birth rates of 1899 and 1900 cohorts.—The rates computed for the 1899 and 1900 cohorts appeared to be inconsistent with the rates for preceding and succeeding cohorts, those for the 1899 cohort being too low and those for the 1900 cohort being too high. This probably represented the tendency for some women in the cohort of 1899 to report age as the two right-hand digits of the calendar year when giving information for the birth certificate. Such misreporting was not important for women in the 1901 cohort, perhaps because it raised their age rather than lowering it.

It was assumed that the sum of the births assigned to the 1899 and 1900 cohorts in any calendar year was correct. That is, it was necessary only to redistribute the births already assigned to the two cohorts, subtracting some from the 1900 cohort and adding the same number to the 1899 cohort. This redistribution was done separately for the births of each order because it was found that the misreporting of age was much greater for the higher order births than for those of lower order.

The corrections for each order were calculated on the basis of the sums of central birth rates for the 1898 cohort, the 1899 and 1900 cohorts combined, and the 1901 cohort for 1917 and later years. It was assumed that these sums formed a regular progression, described by a second-degree polynomial that passed through the sums of the rates for the cohorts of 1898 and 1901 and the average of the sums for the 1899 and 1900 cohorts. This procedure yielded a larger sum for the 1899 cohort and a smaller sum for the 1900 cohort. Table III shows the original and corrected sums

[10]No central birth rates are computed for second and higher orders at age 14 or at fifth and higher orders at ages 15-19; an asterisk is shown in the tables for these age-order cells. Before computation of central rates, the few births reported at these ages and orders are added to the youngest age permitted for each order (age 15 for second through fourth orders and age 20 for fifth and higher orders). In addition, the few births reported to women aged 50 and over were added to the number for age 49.

Table III. Sums of central birth rates in 1917 and later years by color and live-birth order, as originally computed for the cohorts of 1898 to 1901 and as revised for the cohorts of 1899 and 1900

Color and live-birth order	Sum of original rates				Sum of revised rates		Percent deviation of revised from original	
	1898	1899	1900	1901	1899	1900	1899	1900
White	2,487.7	2,445.1	2,594.1	2,448.5	2,526.1	2,513.1	3.3	-3.1
First	689.3	734.4	785.1	784.6	743.9	775.6	1.3	-1.2
Second	599.5	593.1	612.0	583.3	605.3	599.8	2.1	-2.0
Third	406.2	386.8	405.2	376.6	400.9	391.1	3.6	-3.5
Fourth	265.9	248.7	264.6	240.8	260.8	252.5	4.9	-4.6
Fifth	176.7	164.0	176.4	157.8	173.4	167.0	5.7	-5.3
Sixth	121.9	111.6	122.3	107.0	119.4	114.5	7.0	-6.4
Seventh	81.1	73.7	81.2	69.9	79.3	75.6	7.6	-6.9
Eighth and higher	147.1	132.8	147.3	128.5	143.2	136.9	7.8	-7.1
All other	2,585.1	2,661.4	3,035.0	2,838.3	2,806.0	2,890.4	5.4	-4.8
First	510.7	610.6	702.0	735.5	618.8	693.8	1.3	-1.2
Second	455.9	479.4	513.9	488.9	491.1	502.2	2.4	-2.3
Third	386.2	383.0	411.2	378.4	398.4	395.8	4.0	-3.7
Fourth	296.5	289.5	326.1	295.3	308.0	307.6	6.4	-5.7
Fifth	226.0	219.6	258.5	230.2	238.3	239.8	8.5	-7.2
Sixth	187.0	179.9	215.6	188.6	197.5	198.0	9.8	-8.2
Seventh	144.1	140.4	166.9	143.7	153.7	153.6	9.5	-8.0
Eighth and higher	378.7	359.0	440.8	377.7	400.1	399.7	11.4	-9.3

of central birth rates for the 1899 and 1900 cohorts with the rates for the 1898 and 1901 cohorts by order of birth for white and all other women.

The number of births to be subtracted from the 1900 cohort and added to the 1899 cohort in each year was found by multiplying the original number of births of each order by the ratio

$$\frac{\text{revised sum of central rates after January 1, 1917}}{\text{original sum of central rates after January 1, 1917}}$$

computed from rates for the 1900 cohort.

This adjustment was applied to white and all other births separately. The revised total number of births for these cohorts is the sum of the revised numbers for the two color groups. After adjustment of the number of births, central birth rates for total women were recomputed for all years.

Adjustment for erratic age pattern of central birth rates.—The central birth rates computed and adjusted as described above were graphed for selected calendar years. These graphs revealed a sawtooth pattern by age, with the peaks at ages ending with 0, 5, 2, and 8. This age preference was more pronounced for women of all other races than for white women and was stronger for the higher order births. The problem had largely disappeared by the early 1930's for the rates for white women and by the late 1940's for the rates for all other women.

To smooth the rates, a three-term average of the central rates was computed for each of the color groups and for the total. The averages were computed within each calendar year using the single year of age rates. For example, the final rate for age 23 was the average of the rates for ages 22, 23, and 24. (The rates for ages 13 and 50 are considered to be zero.) Although the age preference had disappeared by about 1950, the averaging was continued for later years to give a consistent series; it has little effect on the rates for recent years.

Cumulative Birth Rates

Cumulative birth rates by a given exact age represent the total childbearing experience of women in a cohort up to that age. The cumulative birth rate at age 50, assumed to be the end of childbearing, is considered to be the completed fertility rate of a cohort.

Cohorts of 1903-59.—For the cohorts of 1903 through 1959 central birth rates are available from age 14 through the age attained in 1973 (the latest year for which data are included in this report). For these cohorts the cumulative birth rates up to specified ages are the sums of central birth rates for ages 14 forward. That is, the sum of the central birth rates of a cohort during current ages x and younger is referred to as the cumulative birth rate by exact ages $x+1$ and is said to relate to January 1 of a given year. For example, the cumulative birth rate by exact age 30 for the 1910 cohort is the sum of the central birth rates for the 1910 cohort for the years 1924 (when its members were age 14) through 1939 (when they were age 29). This is the cumulative birth rate for exact age 30 on January 1, 1940.

Cohorts of 1863-1902.—Since the cohorts of 1902 and earlier reached age 14 before 1917, the first year for which central birth rates are available, it was not possible to obtain cumulative birth rates for them simply by summing central birth rates. Instead, the cumulative birth rates for these cohorts for ages attained by January 1, 1917, were estimated by other means, and cumulative rates for subsequent years were then obtained by adding central birth rates for 1917 and later years.

Cumulative birth rates up to January 1, 1917, were estimated using 1910 census data on children ever born for women classified in 5-year age groups from 15-19 through 50-54. The census data may be considered as relating to 5-year cohort groups, for current ages rather than exact ages.

Before the census data on children ever born could be used, it was necessary to make certain adjustments. The procedures followed are outlined below in subsections 1-3. The estimation of cumulative birth rates for January 1, 1917, is outlined in subsections 4 and 5.

1. *Estimating numbers of children ever born, by order of birth, from parity distributions for each age group.*—Published tables for the 1910 census do not give numbers of children ever born by order of birth; these numbers must be derived from distributions of women by parity (number of children ever born). The number of births of each order to women reporting number of children ever born was found by cumulating the number of women of each successive parity from the highest parity down to the parity for the order of birth desired. For example, the number of first births was obtained by adding the numbers of women who had borne one or more children. Similarly, the number of fifth births was determined by adding women of fifth and higher parities. The numbers of births of eighth and higher orders were determined by subtracting the calculated numbers for the first seven orders from the published total number of children for all birth orders combined. This was done for the two color groups separately and the results were added to get the total births.

2. *Allowing for births to ever-married women for whom number of children ever born was not reported in 1910 and 1940.*—Reports on the number of children born were not obtained for significant proportions of ever-married women in the 1910 and 1940 censuses (table IV). For native white women and all Negro women in 1940 the U.S. Bureau of the Census estimated the ratio of the fertility of these nonreporters to that of reporters, by age, on the basis of tabulations of number of children under 5 years of age living with mother. Using a similar procedure, these ratios, called "fertility indexes," were computed for white and all other women for 1940; they are shown in table V. The fertility indexes for 1940 were used to estimate the total number of

Table IV. Percent of ever-married women not reporting number of children ever born, by age and race, 1910 and 1940

Age	Native white		Negro	
	1910	1940	1910	1940
15-19 years-------	23.3	22.0	24.4	20.8
20-24 years-------	12.1	15.5	14.0	17.0
25-29 years-------	7.5	12.9	10.4	15.4
30-34 years-------	6.1	11.6	9.6	14.2
35-39 years-------	5.5	11.4	7.8	14.5
40-44 years-------	5.4	11.1	8.6	14.4
45-49 years-------	5.5	11.3	8.1	14.2
50-54 years-------	6.0	11.6	9.5	14.3

Table V. Fertility indexes by age and color, 1940

[Index is the number of children under 5 years living with mother per 1,000 ever-married women for nonreporters divided by the number for reporters]

Age	White	All other
15-19 years	.490	.581
20-24 years	.649	.695
25-29 years	.746	.712
30-34 years	.817	.804
35-39 years	.810	.821
40-44 years	.840	.829
45-49 years	(1)	(1)
50-54 years	(1)	(1)

[1] Not available; assumed to be the same as for 40-44 years.

Table VI. Ratio of cumulative birth rates for exact ages to cumulative birth rates for current ages used to convert 1910 census-based birth rates for all women, by age of mother and live-birth order

Age	Live-birth order		
	1	2	3
15-19 years	.7312	.6180	.5206
20-24 years	.9188	.8663	.8114
25-29 years	.9742	.9473	.9251
30-34 years	.9908	.9774	.9642
35-39 years	.9965	.9916	.9847
40-44 years	.9992	.9985	.9969
45-49 years	1.0000	.9998	.9997
50-54 years	1.0000	1.0000	1.0000

children ever born to the nonreporters in 1910 and hence to reporters and nonreporters combined.

To estimate the number of births of each order to nonreporters, it was assumed that the fertility indexes were constant by order of birth within each age group. This assumption implies that for each age group the parity distribution among women who have given birth was the same for reporters as for nonreporters of children ever born and, therefore, that the difference in the fertility of the two groups was the result of differences in the proportion of ever-married women with no children. Since the fertility of nonreporters was lower than that of reporters, this assumption implies that there were relatively more women with no children among the nonreporters than among the reporters.

The estimates of number of children ever born for white and all other women were added to obtain estimates for all women.

3. *Converting census-based rates from current ages to exact ages.*—The parity distributions published by the Bureau of the Census are by current age of woman, i.e., age at last birthday. In order to use the census-based cumulative fertility rates to supplement the rates based on vital statistics, it was necessary to convert the census rates to an exact age basis. This was done by multiplying the 1910 census-based rates for ages 45-49 and younger by the following ratios, which were derived from vital statistics rates:

$$\frac{\text{cumulative rate for order } N \text{ by exact ages } x \text{ to } x{+}4}{\text{cumulative rate for order } N \text{ by current ages } x \text{ to } x{+}4}$$

Ratios were computed for each 5-year age group 15-19 through 45-49 in each fifth year from 1925 through 1955. The ratios used for the adjustment were the averages of the available ratios for these years.

Adjustment ratios applied to the rates for first, second, and third births to all women are shown in table VI. At the younger ages a difference of 6 months makes a substantial difference in the number of children ever born. The cumulative first birth rates by exact ages 15-19, for example, are 25 to 28 percent below the cumulative rates by current ages 15-19 (or, what is assumed to be the same concept, by exact ages 15½-19½). The census-based cumulative rates estimated for exact ages should be regarded as relating to a date 6 months before the census was taken. The 1910 census date was April 15, 1910, so the cumulative rates by exact age relate to October 15, 1909.

These adjustments were done for each color group and for the total.

4. *Estimation of cumulative birth rates for 5-year cohort groups as of January 1, 1917.*[11] —The method used for births of each order from first through seventh and for eighth and higher orders combined is summarized below:

(a). The cumulative rate by exact age attained on October 15, 1909, was estimated for each 5-year age group from 15-19 through 50-54, as just described.

(b). The cumulative rate by exact ages 15-19 was obtained for the cohorts of 1903-07 as of January 1, 1922, by adding central birth rates for these cohorts for the period 1917-21 and averaging them.

(c). The cumulative rate by exact ages 15-19 was estimated for the cohorts of 1898-1902 as of January 1, 1917, by straight-line interpolation between the rate for 15-19 as of October 15, 1909, mentioned in step (a), and the rate for 15-19 as of January 1, 1922, obtained in step (b).

(d). The cumulative rate by exact ages 20-24 was obtained for the cohorts of 1898-1902 as of January 1, 1922, by adding the cumulative rate by ages 15-19 as of January 1, 1917, obtained in step (c), and their central birth rates for 1917-21.

[11] The cumulative rates for 5-year cohort groups are defined as the average of the rates of each cohort in the group by the ages reached on a specified date. For example, the cumulative rate for the cohorts of 1898-1902 by exact ages 15-19, reached on January 1, 1917, is the average of the following cumulative rates for single cohorts:

Cumulative rate by exact age—	*For the cohort of—*
19	1898
18	1899
17	1900
16	1901
15	1902

Such rates are referred to as cumulative rates for the cohorts of 1898-1902 by ages 15-19 or by January 1, 1917.

Table VII. Estimated cumulative first birth rates for all women by exact ages attained on January 1, 1917, for the cohorts of 1863-1902, and figures on which estimates are based

Age	Cumulative birth rate by exact age on			Sum of central birth rates 1917-21	Cohorts to which the 1917 rates relate
	October 15, 1909[1]	January 1, 1922[2]	January 1, 1917[3]		
15-19 years---	44.9	63.2	55.7	330.0	1898-1902
20-24 years---	344.4	385.7	368.8	279.5	1893-1897
25-29 years---	592.8	648.3	625.5	118.0	1888-1892
30-34 years---	706.7	743.5	728.4	40.2	1883-1887
35-39 years---	762.8	768.6	766.2	13.3	1878-1882
40-44 years---	795.2	779.5	785.9	2.3	1873-1877
45-49 years---	816.5	788.2	799.8	0.2	1868-1872
50-54 years---	826.0	800.0	810.7	...	1863-1867

[1]Estimated by correcting the 1910 census data on number of children ever born for nonreporting and for underreporting and converting the results from a current to an exact age basis. The latter adjustment of 1/2 year of age causes the rates to relate to a date 1/2 year earlier than the census of April 15, 1910.

[2]The rate for ages 15-19 relates to the cohorts of 1903-07 and is based entirely on vital statistics for 1917-21. Rates for other ages are obtained by adding central birth rates for the appropriate cohort group in 1917-21 to the cumulative rate estimated for January 1, 1917.

[3]Estimated by straight-line interpolation between October 15, 1909, and January 1, 1922.

(e). The cumulative rate by exact ages 20-24 was estimated for the cohorts of 1893-97 as of January 1, 1917, by straight-line interpolation between the rate for 20-24 as of October 15, 1909, mentioned in step (a), and the rate for 20-24 as of January 1, 1922, obtained in step (d).

The process described in steps(c)-(e) was repeated for each earlier group of cohorts. The cumulative rate on January 1, 1922, was always estimated by adding central birth rates in 1917-21 to the cumulative rate by the ages reached on January 1, 1917. The cumulative rate on January 1, 1917, was always estimated by straight-line interpolation between cumulative rates by the same exact ages for preceding cohorts on October 15, 1909, and following cohorts on January 1, 1922. The cumulative rates by 1917 and 1922 for first births to all women obtained by this method are shown in table VII. The cumulative rates for all orders combined is the sum of the rates for the first through the seventh and the eighth and higher orders. These procedures were applied to rates for each color group and for the total.

5. *Estimation of cumulative birth rates for single-year cohorts, 1863-1902.*—After estimates had been obtained for cumulative birth rates by January 1, 1917, for 5-year cohort groups (1863-67 through 1898-1902), estimates were derived for single cohorts. Two requirements were imposed on these estimates: they must be consistent with the estimates already derived for 5-year cohort groups, and they must be at approximately the same level as comparable rates for nearby cohorts.

To meet the above requirements, two interpolation procedures were applied. One was applied to the cumulative rates on January 1, 1917, for the more recent groups at the young childbearing ages whose cumulative rates should differ substantially from cohort to cohort. For example, the cohorts of 1903-07 had a cumulative first birth rate of 63.2 by January 1, 1922. This number is an average of five quite different rates for five different cohorts at five different ages. The extent to which these rates for single cohorts would be expected to differ from each other can be seen from the following first birth rates for all women derived from vital statistics for the cohorts of 1903 through 1907:

Cohort	Exact age on January 1, 1922	Cumulative first birth rate on January 1, 1922
1907---------	15	3.8
1906---------	16	15.7
1905---------	17	42.3
1904---------	18	92.0
1903---------	19	162.0
1903-07------	15-19	63.2

To derive such rates for single cohorts in earlier groups, it was assumed that the rate for any single cohort at a given age and birth order is a constant multiplied by the average rate for the next five cohorts at the same age and birth order and that the constant is the same for all cohorts in a given 5-year cohort group. For example, the first birth rate of 3.4 for the 1902 cohort at age 15 is equal to .9655 times the average of the cumulative rate at age 15 for the cohorts of 1903-07. Similarly, the rate of 143.1 for the 1898 cohort at age 19 is equal to the same factor (.9655) times the average of the cumulative rate at age 19 for the cohorts of 1899-1903. Such constants were found for each 5-year cohort group by means of a series of approximations which will not be described. Basically, the algebra is fairly simple, but the derivation of the formulas is too long to warrant a detailed description. The above method was used to derive estimates of cumulative rates on January 1, 1917, for the following cohorts and birth orders:

Cohort	*Birth orders*
1898-1902-----------------	1-4
1893-1897-----------------	1-8 and higher
1888-1892-----------------	3-8 and higher
1883-1887-----------------	6-8 and higher
1878-1882-----------------	8 and higher

Among earlier cohorts than those shown above, the cumulative rates for single cohorts on January 1, 1917, did not differ sufficiently from each other to warrant the use of the rather elabnrate interpolation procedure described. For these earlier groups, cumulative rates for single cohorts on January 1, 1917, were found by osculatory interpolation between values for 5-year cohort groups.

These interpolation procedures were applied to the cumulative birth rates of each order for both color groups and for the total. The cumulative rates for all orders combined for each single year of age is the sum of rates for each of the orders.

Parity Distribution

A parity distribution is a distribution of all the women in a cohort on a per 1,000 basis by the number of children they have ever borne up to a specified exact age. The proportions are computed by subtracting the cumulative birth rates for adjacent orders of birth. The cumulative birth rate for birth order N may be interpreted as the proportion of women who have had at least N children (or who have had N or more children). By subtracting the proportion of women who have had $N+1$ or more children from the proportion who have had N or more children, one finds the proportion of women who have *exactly* N children.

The proportion of zero-parity women is found by subtracting the cumulative first birth rate from 1,000. The proportions of women at parities 1-6 are found from the following formula:

Proportion at N parity =

(cumulative rate, order N) - (cumulative rate, order N+1).

The proportion of women at seventh and higher parities is the cumulative birth rate for seventh order births.

Since no central birth rates are computed for second and higher orders at age 14 or for fifth and higher orders at ages 15-19, there are no cumulative birth rates for second and higher orders at age 15 or for fifth and higher orders at ages 16-20. Consequently, there can be no figures shown in the parity distributions for second and higher parities at age 15 or for fifth and higher parities at ages 16-20.

Birth Probabilities

The age-parity -specific birth probability shows the probability that a woman who has attained N parity by exact age x will have an $(N+1)$th birth during age x. The probabilities are computed using the central birth rates and the parity distributions. The general formula for the probability for age x, parity N is

$$\frac{\text{Central rate, order } N+1}{\text{Proportion of women, parity } N} \quad 1{,}000$$

Since there are no figures for the proportion of women at second and higher parities at age 15 and at fifth and higher parities at ages 16-20, there are no birth probabilities for these groups. In addition, no probability is computed if the proportion of women in an age-parity group is less than 10.0 per 1,000, and an asterisk is shown in the tables.

APPENDIX IV

COMPARISON OF METHODS WITH THOSE OF WHELPTON AND CAMPBELL

With only a few exceptions the methods used by Whelpton and Campbell[12] for the estimation of the numbers of births and for the computation of central and cumulative birth rates have been used in the preparation of estimates for this report. The differences are described in this appendix.

Numbers of Births

The only methodological difference in the estimation of the numbers of births involves the estimates for States not in the birth-registration area (BRA) for 1917-32. Both procedures utilized guide States which were in the BRA in estimating births for States not in the BRA. Whelpton and Campbell selected one set of guide States for the whole period 1917-32. The guide States used in this report were allowed to change in each year. The new method gives, in effect, only different distributions of births by age and by order. Although the estimates were generally lower than Whelpton and Campbell's, this is not a factor in the final estimates since the new figures for the United States were adjusted to the totals prepared by Whelpton and Cambell.

Since Whelpton and Campbell did not prepare estimates by age and by order for white and all other births separately, no comparison between the two methods can be made by color. For the total, however, the numbers are very close. By age group the new estimates are all within 2 percent of the Whelpton and Campbell estimates except for ages 45-49, the least important age group. For the 45-49 age group the difference was 2 percent or less for 1929-32, 3 percent for 1920, 1923-24, and 1928, 4 to 5 percent for 1925-27, 6 to 7 percent for 1921-22, and 8 to 9 percent for 1917-19. For all the years where the difference was 3 percent or greater except one (1918), the new estimates were lower than those of Whelpton and Campbell. By birth order the new estimates are within 3 percent of the Whelpton and Campbell estimates for all orders in all years.

Central Birth Rates

The central birth rates were computed in the same manner as had been done by Whelpton and Campbell, including the adjustment to the cohorts of 1899 and 1900. One additional step was taken in the computation of central birth rates for this report—the 3-year average of central birth rates to remove the sawtooth pattern as described in appendix III, "Central Birth Rates," "Adjustment for erratic age pattern" (page 456).

Cumulative Birth Rates

The estimation of cumulative birth rates for January 1, 1917, involved many steps. Each of the steps, as described by Whelpton and Campbell, was applied to the data for the white population and for the population of all other races. However, the resultant parity distributions for the "all other" women did not appear reasonable—for all ages over 30 nearly 25 percent of the women were at one parity. An examination of the steps used to derive the cumulative birth rates showed the problem to be in a "consistency ratio" relating vital statistics and census cumulative rates. This ratio was used to adjust the census data on children ever born for the omission of births to single women and for the understating of births to ever-married women.

These two factors were posited as accounting for the observed excess of the vital statistics over the census cumulative rates. Whelpton and Campbell used the average of the ratios for 1940 and 1950 to adjust the 1910 census-based cumulative birth rates. However, when ratios were computed for white and all other women separately, those for all other women were not consistent with the logical bias in the census. That is, for all other women for orders 2 and 3, ages 30 and over, and orders 4 and 5, ages 35 and over, the census-based cumulative birth rates were higher than the vital statistics cumulative rates. When the "consistency ratios" (average of 1940 and 1950 ratios) were applied to the 1910 census-based cumulative rates, the result was to increase the rate for first births and to decrease the rate for second births. This yielded an unreasonably high proportion of one-parity women. Since the census rates were higher than vital statistics rates for both 1940 and 1950 for these groups, it was decided not to use any "consistency ratios" on the 1910 census cumulative rates. This resulted in more reasonable parity distributions for January 1, 1917.

A comparison of the new cumulative birth rates for all women with those computed by Whelpton and Campbell for 1940, 1950, and 1960 shows very close agreement. The 1940 rates reflect, in part, the estimated cumulative birth rates for January 1, 1917. For all three years the new rates are within 3 percent of the Whelpton and Campbell rates with two exceptions. At ages 15-19 the new rates were an average of 10 percent higher. The higher orders for younger women (ages 20-24, orders 3 and higher, and ages 25-29, orders 7 and higher) had differences in the same direction ranging up to 10 percent.

12 National Office of Vital Statistics: Fertility tables for birth cohorts of American women, by P.K. Whelpton and A.A. Campbell. *Vital Statistics—Special Reports,* Vol. 51, No. 1. Public Health Service. Washington, D.C., Jan. 29, 1960.

☆ U. S. GOVERNMENT PRINTING OFFICE : 1976 O - 205-071